PRESENT KNOWLEDGE IN NUTRITION

PRESENT KNOWLEDGE IN NUTRITION

CLINICAL AND APPLIED TOPICS IN NUTRITION

VOLUME 2

ELEVENTH EDITION

Edited by

BERNADETTE P. MARRIOTT, PHD
DIANE F. BIRT, PHD
VIRGINIA A. STALLINGS, MD, MS
ALLISON A. YATES, PHD, MSPH, RD

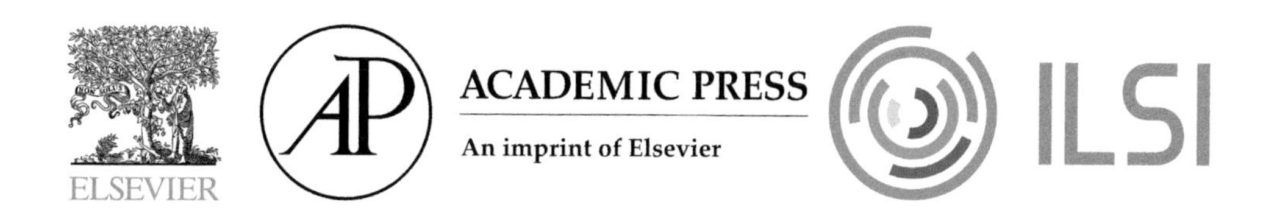

Academic Press is an imprint of Elsevier
125 London Wall, London EC2Y 5AS, United Kingdom
525 B Street, Suite 1650, San Diego, CA 92101, United States
50 Hampshire Street, 5th Floor, Cambridge, MA 02139, United States
The Boulevard, Langford Lane, Kidlington, Oxford OX5 1GB, United Kingdom

Notices
Knowledge and best practice in this field are constantly changing. As new research and experience broaden our understanding, changes in research methods, professional practices, or medical treatment may become necessary.

Practitioners and researchers must always rely on their own experience and knowledge in evaluating and using any information, methods, compounds, or experiments described herein. In using such information or methods they should be mindful of their own safety and the safety of others, including parties for whom they have a professional responsibility.

To the fullest extent of the law, neither the Publisher nor the authors, contributors, or editors, assume any liability for any injury and/or damage to persons or property as a matter of products liability, negligence or otherwise, or from any use or operation of any methods, products, instructions, or ideas contained in the material herein.

Library of Congress Cataloging-in-Publication Data
A catalog record for this book is available from the Library of Congress

British Library Cataloguing-in-Publication Data
A catalogue record for this book is available from the British Library

ISBN: 978-0-12-818460-8

For information on all Academic Press publications visit our website at https://www.elsevier.com/books-and-journals

Publisher: Charlotte Cockle
Acquisitions Editor: Megan R. Bell
Editorial Project Manager: Aleksandra Packowska
Production Project Manager: Omer Mukthar
Cover Designer: Greg Harris

Typeset by TNQ Technologies

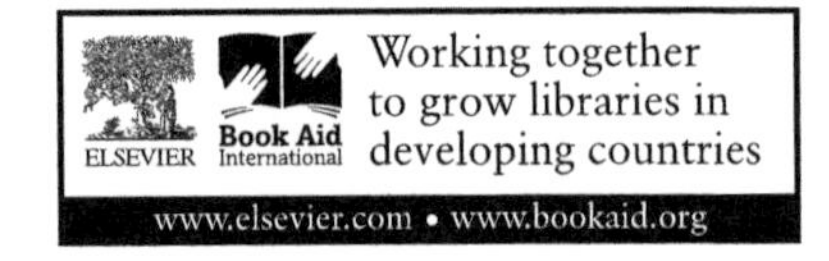

We dedicate this 11th edition of Present Knowledge in Nutrition to members of the global nutrition community who continue to seek the best science, interpret that science for the better good of people worldwide, and persist in countering nonscientifically based nutrition information with evidence-based approaches to better human health. We also dedicate this edition to our own scientific mentors and colleagues who have persuaded and occasionally pushed us in the direction of the highest quality nutrition science—no matter the cost.

Contents of Volume 2

Section C

Clinical Nutrition

Editor Biographies

BERNADETTE P. MARRIOTT, PHD

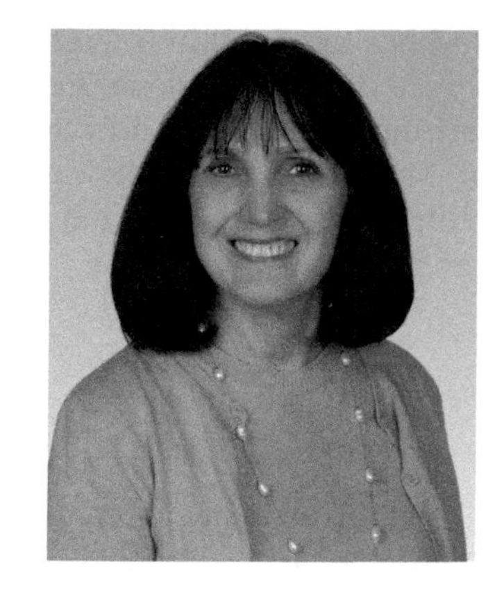

Bernadette P. Marriott holds the position of Professor Emerita and Nutrition Section Director Emerita, Departments of Medicine and Psychiatry, Medical University of South Carolina. Bernadette has over 35 years of experience in the fields of nutrition, psychology, and comparative medicine with expertise in diet, nutrition, and chronic disease. Dr. Marriott has worked in scientific and administration positions in the federal government, the National Academies, universities, and foundations. She was founding director of the Office of Dietary Supplements, NIH and Deputy Director, Food and Nutrition Board, NAS. Her research has focused on both human and animal nutrition and related behavioral studies (in humans: diet and health research and food labeling; in animals: nonhuman primate nutrition and behavioral ecology). She is currently leading or has recently led research projects funded by the Army, DoD, NSF, NIH, USDA, industry, and foundations. Bernadette Marriott has a BSc in biology/immunology from Bucknell University (1970), a PhD in psychology from the University of Aberdeen, Scotland (1976), and postgraduate training in trace mineral nutrition, comparative medicine, and advanced statistics. She has published extensively, is on a number of national committees and university scientific advisory boards, and is a frequent speaker on diet, dietary supplements, and health. She is currently a member of the Food and Nutrition Board, US National Academy of Sciences, and the American Society for Nutrition Committee on Advocacy and Science Policy. In 2016, Dr. Marriott was inducted as a Fellow of the American Society for Nutrition.

DIANE F. BIRT, PHD

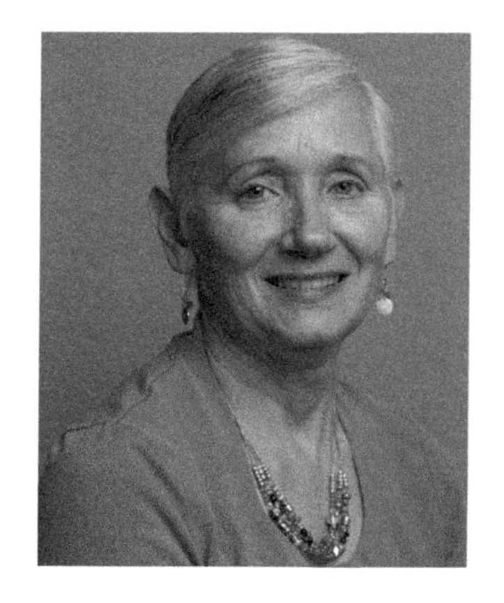

Diane F. Birt is a Distinguished Professor in Food Science and Human Nutrition at Iowa State University. She has BS degrees in Home Economics and Chemistry from Whittier College (1971) and a PhD in Nutrition from Purdue University (1975). Her expertise is in diet and cancer prevention and plant components and health promotion. She was at the University of Nebraska Medical Center (1976–97) before becoming Chair of the Department of Food Science and Human Nutrition (1997–2004) at Iowa State University. Dietary prevention of cancer has been a long-standing interest in the Birt laboratory. More recent research has focused on the prevention of colon cancer by slowly digested maize starches using cell culture and animal models that reflect particular genetic changes that are important in human colon cancer development. She was on the Board of Scientific Counselors for the National Toxicology Program (US Department of Health) and the Food and Nutrition Board of the Institute of Medicine, US National Academy of Sciences. In 2015, Dr. Birt was inducted as a Fellow of the American Society for Nutrition, and in 2016, she was inducted as a member of the National Academy of Medicine.

VIRGINIA A. STALLINGS, MD, MS

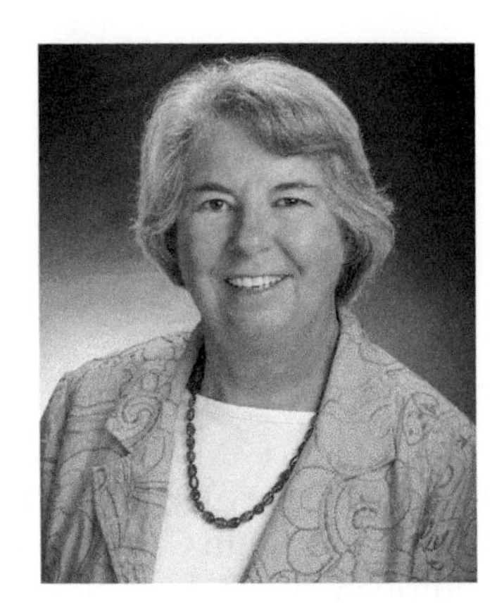

Virginia Stallings is a Professor of Pediatrics at the Children's Hospital of Philadelphia and the Perelman School of Medicine at the University of Pennsylvania and is the recipient of the Jean A. Cortner Endowed Chair in Pediatric Gastroenterology and Nutrition. She holds a BS in Nutrition and Food from Auburn University, MS in Nutrition and Biochemistry from Cornell University, and MD from the University of Alabama Birmingham. Her general pediatric residency was completed at the University of Virginia followed by a subspecialty fellowship in nutrition at the Hospital for Sick Children. Over her career at the Children's Hospital of Philadelphia, she contributed to clinical care, fellow and faculty training, and clinical and translational research in the abnormalities of growth, nutritional status, and health of children with chronic diseases and in those in good health. She has served on many National Academy of Sciences committees to advise on child health, nutrition, and federal nutrition programs and is a member of the National Academy of Medicine. The American Academy of Pediatrics and American Society for Nutrition have recognized her efforts with awards for science, mentoring, and service.

ALLISON A. YATES, PHD, MSPH, RD

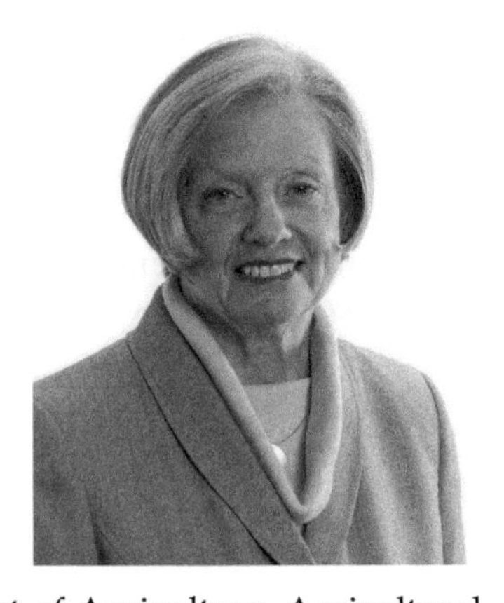

Allison A. Yates holds Bachelor's and Master's degrees from the University of California at Los Angeles in public health and dietetics and a PhD from the University of California at Berkeley in nutrition, and is a registered dietitian having completed a dietetic internship at the VA Center in Los Angeles. She served on the faculties of the University of Texas Health Science Center in Houston, Emory University School of Medicine, and was the founding Dean of the College of Health and Human Sciences at the University of Southern Mississippi, where she led the development of the first accredited public health program in the state. Her research focused on human protein and energy requirements. In 1994, she was named Director of the Food and Nutrition Board of the Institute of Medicine of the US National Academy of Sciences, where, over a 10-year period, she led the expanded approach to establishing human requirements and recommendations for nutrients, termed Dietary Reference Intakes, for the United States and Canada. She then served as Director of the Beltsville Human Nutrition Research Center of the US Department of Agriculture, Agricultural Research Service (ARS), and served as Associate Director for the ARS Beltsville Area region, retiring from USDA in 2014, when she was also inducted as a fellow of the American Society for Nutrition. Since that time, she has led a volunteer effort to establish a framework for establishing reference values for bioactive components in foods.

Contributors to Volume 2

Ajibola Ibraheem Abioye, MD
Harvard University
Cambridge, MA
United States

Katherine Alaimo, PhD
Michigan State University
East Lansing, MI
United States

Stephen Anton, PhD
University of Florida College of Medicine
Gainesville, FL
United States

E. Wayne Askew, PhD
Department of Nutrition and Integrative Physiology
College of Health
University of Utah
Salt Lake City, UT
United States

Joseph L. Baumert, MS, PhD
University of Nebraska, Lincoln
Lincoln, NE
United States

Kirstine J. Bell, APD, CDE, PhD
University of Sydney
Sydney, NSW
Australia

Jennie Brand-Miller, PhD, FAA, FAIFST, FNSA
University of Sydney
Sydney, NSW
Australia

Louise M. Burke, OAM, PhD, APD, FACSM
Australian Sports Commission
Canberra, ACT
Australia

Asta Bye, RD, PhD
Oslo Metropolitan University
Oslo
Norway

Elizabeth J. Campbell, BSc
EAS Consulting Group
Alexandria, VA
United States

Mariana Chilton, PhD, MPH
Drexel University
Philadelphia, PA
United States

Stephen Colagiuri, MBBS, FRACP
University of Sydney
Sydney, NSW
Australia

Charlene Compher, PhD, RD, CNSC, LDN, FADA, FASPEN
University of Pennsylvania
Philadelphia, PA
United States

Jeanne H.M. de Vries, PhD
Wageningen University
Wageningen
Netherlands

Adam Drewnowski, PhD
University of Washington Center for Public Health Nutrition
Seattle, WA
United States

Johanna T. Dwyer, DSc, RD
National Institutes of Health, Office of the Dietary Supplements
Bethesda, MD
United States

Rebecca Egdorf, BS, MS, RD, LD
University of Texas at Tyler
Tyler, TX
United States

Ibrahim Elmadfa, PhD
University of Vienna
Vienna
Austria

Wafaie W. Fawzi, MBBS, MPH, MS, DrPH
Harvard University
Cambridge, MA
United States

Hilda E. Fernandez, MD, MS
New York Presbeterian Hospital
New York, NY
United States

Jimi Francis, BS, MS, PhD, IBCLC, RLC, RDN, LD
University of Texas at Tyler
Tyler, TX
United States

Karl E. Friedl, PhD
US Army Research Institute of Environmental Medicine
Natick, MA
United States

Stephanie P. Gilley, MD, PhD
University of Colorado School of Medicine
Denver, CO
United States

Vi Goh, MD, MS
Children's Hospital of Philadelphia
Philadelphia, PA
United States

Weimin Guo, PhD
Jean Mayer USDA Human Nutrition Research Center on Aging at Tufts University
Boston, MA
United States

David B. Haytowitz, MSc
USDA Agriculture Research Service (Retired)
Silver Spring, MD
United States

Sung Nim Han, PhD, RD
Seoul National University
Seoul
South Korea

Kirsten A. Herrick, PhD, MSc
National Institutes of Health, National Cancer Institute
Bethesda, MD
United States

James E. Hoadley, PhD
EAS Consulting Group
Alexandria, VA
United States

Paul J.M. Hulshof, MSc
Wageningen University
Wageningen
Netherlands

Sharon Y. Irving, PhD, CRNP, FCCM, FAAN
University of Pennsylvania
Philadelphia, PA
United States

Ellisiv Jacobsen, PhD, MPH
Akershus University College
Oslo
Norway

Namrata G. Jain, MD
Columbia University
New York, NY
United States

Marie Johnson, MS, RD
Kaiser Permanente Northwest
Portland, OR
United States

Emily A. Johnston, MPH, RDN, CDE
Pennsylvania State University
University Park, PA
United States

Alexandra M. Johnstone, PhD
The Rowett Institute, University of Aberdeen
Aberdeen
Scotland

Sonya J. Jones, PhD
University of South Carolina
Columbia, SC
United States

Irina Kirpich, PhD
Alcohol Research Center
University of Louisville
Louisville, KY
United States

Nancy F. Krebs, MD, MS
University of Colorado School of Medicine
Denver, CO
United States

Penny M. Kris-Etherton, PhD, RDN
College of Health and Human Development at Pennsylvania State University
University Park, PA
United States

Ellisiv Lærum-Onsager, RN, PhD
Lovisenberg Diaconal University College
Oslo
Norway

Janine L. Lewis, BSc, Grad Dip Nut & Diet, Grad Dip Public Health
Food Standards Australia New Zealand
Majura Park, ACT
Australia

Karen Lindsay, PhD, RD
University of California Irvine School of Medicine
Orange, CA
United States

Asim Maqbool, MD
Children's Hospital of Philadelphia
Philadelphia, PA
United States

Melinda M. Manore, PhD, RD, CSSD, FACSM
Oregon State University
Corvallis, OR
United States

Maria R. Mascarenhas, MBBS
Children's Hospital of Philadelphia
Philadelphia, PA
United States

Craig James McClain, MD
University of Louisville
Louisville, KY
United States

Liam McKeever, PhD, RDN, LDN
University of Pennsylvania
Philadelphia, PA
United States

Sarah A. McNaughton, PhD, APA, FDAA
Deakin University
Melbourne, VIC
Australia

Simin Nikbin Meydani, DVM, PhD
Nutritional Immunology Laboratory,
Jean Mayer USDA Human Nutrition Research Center on Aging at Tufts University
Boston, MA
United States

Alexa L. Meyer, PhD
Nutritional Sciences, University of Vienna
Vienna
Austria

Pablo Monsivais, PhD, MPH
Washington State University
Pullman, WA
United States

Laura M. Nance, MA, RDN
Medical University of South Carolina Friedman Center for Eating Disorders
Charleston, SC
United States

Carolyn Newberry, MD
Cornell University
New York, NY
United States

Thomas L. Nickolas, MD, MS
Columbia University Irving Medical Center
New York, NY
United States

Marga C. Ocké, PhD
National Institute for Public Health and the Environment
Bilthoven
Netherlands

Cynthia L. Ogden, PhD
Centers for Disease Control National Center for Health Statistics
Hyattsville, MD
United States

Elizabeth Prout Parks, MD, MSCE
Children's Hospital of Philadelphia
Philadelphia, PA
United States

Pamela R. Pehrsson, PhD
USDA, ARS Beltsville Human Nutrition Research Center,
Beltsville, MD
United States

Kristina S. Petersen, PhD, BNutDiet(Hons)
Pennsylvania State University
University Park, PA
United States

Robert C. Post, PhD, MEd, MSc
FoodTrition Solutions, LLC
Hackettstown, New Jersey
United States

Renee D. Rienecke, PhD, FAED
Eating Recovery Center/Insight Behavioral Health Centers, Northwestern University
Chicago, IL 60601
United States

Terrence M. Riley, BSc
Pennsylvania State University
University Park, PA
United States

René Rizzoli, MD
Geneva University Hospitals and Faculty of Medicine
Geneva
Switzerland

Donna H. Ryan, MD
Pennington Biomedical Research Center
Baton Rouge, LA
United States

Sarah Safadi, MD
University of Louisville
Louisville, KY
United States

Thomas A.B. Sanders, PhD, DSc
King's College London
London
United Kingdom

Philip A. Sapp, MS
Pennsylvania State University
University Park, PA
United States

David D. Schnakenberg, PhD
Historian of Military Nutrition Science
Vienna, VA
United States

Laura Smart, MD
University of Louisville
Louisville, KY
United States

Juquan Song, MD
University of Texas Medical Branch Dallas
Dallas, TX
United States

Vijay Srinivasan, MBBS, MD, FAAP, FCCM
University of Pennsylvania
Philadelphia, PA
United States

Sylvia Stephen, MSc
The Rowett Institute, University of Aberdeen
Aberdeen
Scotland

Valerie K. Sullivan, RDN
Penn State University
University Park, PA
United States

Paolo M. Suter, MD, MS
University Hospital Zurich, Clinic and Policlinic of Internal Medicine
Zurich
Switzerland

Steve L. Taylor, PhD
University of Nebraska Lincoln
Lincoln, NE
United States

Alyssa M. Tindall, PhD, RDN
College of Health and Human Development, Pennsylvania State University
University Park, PA
United States

Katherine L. Tucker, PhD
University of Massachusetts Lowell
Lowell, MA
United States

Kimberly K. Vesco, MD, MPH
Kaiser Permanente Northwest
Portland, OR
United States

Charles E. Wade, PhD
McGovern School of Medicine, The University of Texas, Houston
Houston, TX
United States

Elizabeth M. Wallis, MD, MS
Medical University of South Carolina
Charleston, SC
United States

Steven E. Wolf, MD
University of Texas Medical Branch
Galveston, TX
United States

Dayong Wu, MD, PhD
Jean Mayer USDA Human Nutrition Research Center on Aging at Tufts University
Boston, MA
United States

Vivian M. Zhao, PharmD
Emory University Hospital
Atlanta, GA
United States

Thomas R. Ziegler, MD
Emory University School of Medicine
Atlanta, GA
United States

Foreword

Timely information regarding nutrition is critical to improving human health and well-being and safeguarding the environment. The mission of the International Life Sciences Institute (ILSI) is in part to provide such information, and we are pleased to present the 11th edition of *Present Knowledge in Nutrition.*

First published in 1953, *Present Knowledge in Nutrition* was launched with the goal of providing readers with the most comprehensive and current information covering the broad fields within the nutrition discipline. Reflecting the global relevance of nutrition, this edition's authors are from a variety of countries and reflect a "who's who" of nutritional science.

ILSI is a worldwide nonprofit organization that seeks to foster science for the public good and collaboration among scientists, all governed by ILSI's core principles of scientific integrity. With 16 entities worldwide, ILSI published 70 scientific articles globally in 2019 and hosted 152 workshops addressing nutrition, food safety, and sustainability. ILSI is a world leader in creating public–private partnerships that advance science for the betterment of public health and achieve positive, real-world impact.

We trust the two volumes of *Present Knowledge in Nutrition* will be valuable resources for researchers, health professionals, clinicians, educators, and advanced nutrition students. ILSI is proud of the contributions made by the authors and editors of this key reference, and we are excited to advance the discipline of nutrition with this publication.

Kerr Dow, ILSI Board of Trustees Co-Chair

Michael Doyle, ILSI Board of Trustees Co-Chair

Preface

As editors, we feel privileged to have been asked to edit the 11th edition of *Present Knowledge in Nutrition*. The 11th edition moves this major nutrition reference source beyond its 65-year history and into an explosion of exciting new methodologies and understandings of the role of diet and nutrition in human health and well-being. In a global survey conducted in 2017, *Present Knowledge in Nutrition* was identified as a key resource for the latest information in the nutrition field for nutrition and dietetic professionals and clinicians. Specifically, survey participants stated that *Present Knowledge in Nutrition* was the source to which they turned when seeking the latest information in an area of nutrition that was outside their main expertise. Further, *Present Knowledge in Nutrition* is valued as an academic text in advanced nutrition courses. Recognizing the important role of the periodic updates of *Present Knowledge in Nutrition* among scientists and practitioners, as editors we have sought to maintain the long-standing tradition of identifying content-thought leaders to provide the most comprehensive and latest information in their fields in the chapters represented in this edition.

The 11th edition of *Present Knowledge in Nutrition* is presented in two companion volumes: *Volume 1: Basic Nutrition and Metabolism* and *Volume 2: Clinical and Applied Topics in Nutrition*. Provision of two volumes enables the reader to more quickly identify the location of relevant materials and makes the printed copies of this 74-chapter edition more physically portable. This 11th edition includes full color illustrations and other color-enhanced features. At the end of each chapter, the authors clearly have identified important research gaps and needs for future research. Volume 1 includes chapters that provide the latest scientific knowledge on requirements for specific nutrients and genomics and chapters that discuss important cross-disciplinary topics including systems biology, the microbiome, and the role of nutrition in regulation of immune function. Volume 2 provides the most recent information on life-stage nutrition, obesity, physical activity, and eating behavior; dietary guidance; and nutrition surveillance, as well as major topics in nutrition and disease processes and medical nutrition therapy.

In addition to print volumes, the 11th edition of *Present Knowledge in Nutrition* is available in electronic format through the website: https://pkn11.org/where-to-buy/. The electronic format provides broader access not only globally but also for educational use.

We believe the authors have done an outstanding job in presenting the latest information in their respective fields and hope this edition will continue the long tradition of being an essential resource broadly in the nutrition field.

Bernadette P. Marriott
Charleston, South Carolina

Diane F. Birt
Ames, Iowa

Virginia A. Stallings
Philadelphia, Pennsylvania

Allison A. Yates
Johnson City, Tennessee

Acknowledgments

Development of a book of this in-depth and highly scientifically current content represents a large commitment of time and effort by many people. First, we would like to thank the authors of the 72 chapters for their commitment to this two-volume reference work and most importantly their dedication to presenting the best information of the current status of the science in their respective fields. Second, this edition would not have come to fruition without the untiring work and guidance of Allison Worden and James Cameron of the International Life Sciences Institute. We appreciated very much the early guidance of two of the editors of the 10th edition, John Erdman and Steven Zeisel, as we were forming the 11th edition concept. Key to any endeavor of this size is the support of family, colleagues, and friends to whom we owe our gratitude for their forbearance during the many hours devoted to this work's development and production.

SECTION A

Lifestage Nutrition and Maintaining Health

CHAPTER

1

INFANT NUTRITION

Stephanie P. Gilley, MD, PhD
Nancy F. Krebs, MD, MS
Department of Pediatrics, Section of Nutrition, University of Colorado Denver School of Medicine, Aurora, CO, United States

SUMMARY

Infancy is a time of rapid growth and development with nutritional needs unique from any other stage of life. Additionally, babies must change from an entirely liquid intake to a diet mostly comprised of solids. Numerous health organizations endorse breastfeeding as the ideal nutrition source for infants during the first year of life. In this chapter, a discussion of common breastfeeding issues and how to support mothers to promote breastfeeding is included. The chapter also addresses formula feeding, the nutritional requirements of premature and hospitalized infants, the transition to complementary foods and how the primary feeding choice influences guidance, common nutritional issues that arise during the first 12 months of life including under- and overnutrition, and a brief comment on the transition to a toddler diet after 1 year.

Keywords: Breastfeeding; Complementary foods; Growth faltering; Inborn errors of metabolism; Infancy; Infant formula; Micronutrient deficiencies; Prematurity.

I. INTRODUCTION

A. Background

The time from conception to 2 years of age, often termed the first 1000 days, represents a uniquely vulnerable window of growth and development with implications for the entire life span. Interventions targeting better nutrition during the first 1000 days may improve health well into adolescence and adulthood. Increasing rates of breastfeeding is a goal of the CDC, the WHO, and the American Academy of Pediatrics and is predicted to promote infant and maternal health in both the long- and short-term, reduce health disparities, and have economic benefits.[1] Although breastfeeding rates have been increasing over the last decade, less than 30% of American children are still receiving any breast milk at 1 year.[1,2]

Since the last edition was published, there have been significant knowledge advances regarding infant nutrition, in particular the adverse effects of early rapid weight gain, the developing microbiome, and ideal timing of introduction of highly allergenic foods. In addition, basic nutrient requirements are fairly well understood. What is less clear is the optimal nutritional composition that is best to assure brain growth, overall development, and long-term health. This chapter presents evidence-based practices, consensus recommendations, and other guidelines for feeding during the first year of life, while highlighting current research gaps that await future investigations.

Present Knowledge in Nutrition, Volume 2
https://doi.org/10.1016/B978-0-12-818460-8.00001-0

B. Key Issues

- Development of gastrointestinal function
- Normal expected growth during infancy
- Human milk feeding
- Formula feeding
- Unique needs of premature infants
- Inborn errors of metabolism
- Introduction of complementary foods
- Issues of concern: breastfeeding contraindications and problems, growth faltering, milk protein intolerance, and micronutrient deficiencies
- Transition to the toddler diet
- Nutritional support of the hospitalized infant

II. PHYSIOLOGICAL DEMANDS OF LIFE STAGES

A. Development of Gastrointestinal Function

At birth, the infant gastrointestinal tract rapidly takes over nutrient absorption functions from the placenta. The gut digestive and absorptive capabilities are immature at birth.[3] The infant diet must therefore match the intestines' level of function. Fats make up 40%–50% of a newborn diet and provide building blocks for neuronal development.[4] Before about 3–6 months of age, however, infants have lower concentrations of pancreatic enzymes including lipases,[5] resulting in only 70%–90% of ingested lipids being absorbed, with lower absorption being noted in premature and formula-fed full-term infants.[6,7] Immature pancreatic function also influences absorption of carbohydrates, since production of amylase does not appear until approximately 1 month and takes up to 2 years to reach maturity.[5] Most carbohydrate digestion occurs via lactase in the intestines.[3]

In addition to digestive functions, the intestines are home to the developing enteric microbiome, which is increasingly recognized for its important role in growth and development.[8] Gestational age, mode of delivery, and primary feeding type, along with other environmental factors, are known to have substantial impact on the microbiome,[9,10] which helps shape developing innate immunity.[11] These differences may have long-term health impacts, as there are numerous studies showing associations between early life microbiome and several diseases including obesity, atopy, inflammatory bowel disease, and neurologic disorders.[10–12]

B. Normal Expected Growth

Weight loss after birth

Immediately following birth, all infants lose weight, evaluated as a percentage of birth weight. The degree of weight loss varies based on numerous factors including maternal intravenous fluid administration during labor and delivery, infant sex, mode of delivery, and method of feeding.[2,13] In general, weight loss of more than 8%–10% of birth weight is considered excessive.[1] Exclusively breastfed infants should have close outpatient follow-up within 1–2 days after hospital discharge. Birth weight is typically regained by 7–10 days of life, although it can take up to 14 days.[1,2] Weight loss of more than 8% of birth weight or failure to return to birth weight by 10 days in an exclusively breastfed infant should trigger an evaluation of feeding effectiveness.

Growth monitoring

Following the initial weight loss, reference growth curves are used to determine whether a child's growth is occurring at an expected rate. For infants up to 24 months, these growth curves examine weight, length, head circumference, and weight-for-length. In 2006, the WHO released standard curves using longitudinal measurements of primarily breastfed infants in six different countries.[14,15] Exclusive use of the WHO curves has been recommended by the CDC and the American Academy of Pediatrics.[1,15,16] In general, infants gain approximately 20–30 g/day for the first 3 months, ~15 g/ day from 3 to 6 months, and 10–12 g/day from 6 to 12 months.[3,16] Birth weight typically doubles by 4–5 months, occurring later in breastfed and female infants.[16,17] Premature infant growth trajectory should be plotted at corrected gestational age until the age of 2–3 years, especially for length.[3] Although not as often used clinically, there are notable changes in body composition, which naturally occur across infancy. Body fat percentage increases steadily until a peak around 6 months of age. After this point, growth of fat-free/lean body mass begins to accelerate and accumulation of fat mass slows.[18]

Growth assessment

Infants who are trending downward across percentiles concern health professionals and parents alike. Some of this fluctuation is expected as infants settle on a growth trajectory based on genetic potential. However, it is important to identify children who are not growing well due to nutritional inadequacy or an underlying medical or genetic condition. Using the weight-for-length chart is useful to help distinguish between normal and unexpected weight gain and to assess degree of thinness. Ideal body weight (IBW) is equal to the weight that corresponds to the 50th percentile for the infant's current length. Percent IBW ([current weight ÷ IBW] × 100%) below 90% is indicative of malnutrition.[3] A weight-for-length z-score below −2 is defined as wasting. Infants who have low weight but normal length typically need an increase in calories. For those 6 months and older, a focus on increasing the protein and fat content of complementary foods may be helpful. If a baby also has diminished length (z-score below −2 is defined as stunting), the differential needs to be expanded, as it could be related to insufficient calories, micronutrient deficiency, or a medical or genetic condition. These cases are concerning and require prompt attention and evaluation. Growth faltering (also called failure to thrive [FTT]) is discussed later in this chapter.

Another adverse growth pattern is early rapid weight gain, which is associated with increased risk of future obesity.[19] This pattern is more common in formula-fed infants compared to those who are exclusively breastfed. Before the age of 2 years, a child with a weight-for-length above the 95th percentile is overweight. The term "obese," defined as excess body fat, is not used in this age group because excessive body fat is not well characterized.[20,21] It is also unknown whether distribution of fat mass (e.g., subcutaneous vs. visceral) influences future disease risk. Parents may be unwilling to accept that their infant is overweight, as in many cultures fatter babies are viewed to be healthier. However, an assessment of energy intake and feeding behaviors should be undertaken, including early introduction of complementary foods, overfeeding by bottle, and consumption of sugar-sweetened beverages or highly processed foods.[21]

C. Term Infants

Recommendations for 0–6 month old infants are based on observed intake by exclusively breastfed infants, and those for 6–12 month olds are based on decreasing consumption of human milk or formula while increasing complementary foods (Table 1.1).[22,23]

Human milk

Innumerable benefits of breastfeeding have been identified for both infant and mother. For the infant, these include reduced risk of ear infection, sudden infant death syndrome, obesity, and hospitalization during the first year of life. Mothers who breastfeed tend to return to prepregnancy weight more quickly and have decreased incidence of stroke, breast and ovarian cancer, type 2 diabetes, and hypertension.[1,2,16,24] The "average" composition of mature human milk is shown in Table 1.2.[3,21] The CDC and WHO have identified increasing breastfeeding rates as an important goal to improve overall population health with resultant economic benefits.[1,3]

Breastfeeding Support; Many women assume that because breastfeeding is natural, it will be easy. However, breastfeeding is a learned skill for both mother and infant, and support from providers knowledgeable in breastfeeding is critical, especially in the first month as milk production is established.[1] A large retrospective study found higher rates of hospitalization in the first month of life for breastfed versus formula-fed babies, primarily due to dehydration or hyperbilirubinemia.[25] This highlights the importance of lactation support, both one-on-one and in a group setting, as well as close monitoring of weight. Women with obesity and/or insulin resistance often experience delayed onset of milk production and may benefit from early lactation support. Additionally, there can be social pressures and strong maternal and family emotional reactions to having difficulty with exclusive breastfeeding. If eligible, encourage women to enroll in the Special Supplemental Nutrition Program for Women, Infants, and Children (WIC), which offers food and nutritional counseling to women and children under 5 years old. Breast pumps can be borrowed from WIC, the infants' growth is followed, and breastfeeding women are provided with additional food to support lactation. Mothers can also be referred to a certified lactation consultant or to the La Leche League website to find local support groups.[1,2] Support from both professionals and lay individuals has a positive impact on breastfeeding continuation, and its importance cannot be overstated.[26]

Expression and storage of human milk; Women who are separated from their infants can express milk either by hand or by using a manual or electric breast pump.[1] For brief separations, manual pumps are easily portable and can be used in the absence of a power source. However, women who will be returning to work or will be otherwise separated from their infant for longer durations should have an electric pump. Since the passage of the Affordable Care Act, US health insurance providers must have some coverage for breast pumps, and employers are required to provide reasonable time and space for milk expression and storage.[1,24] Gentle mixing or shaking can be used to reintegrate the milk and fat layer after natural separation. For milk storage, guidelines

TABLE 1.1 Recommended intakes for term infants by age in both the United States and Europe.

		United States RDA		European union RNI			
Ages included in recommendations:		0–6 months	6–12 months	0–3 months	4–6 months	7–9 months	10–12 months
Nutrient	**Units**						
Vitamin A	mcg	400*	500*	350	350	350	350
Vitamin C/ascorbate	mg	40*	50*	25	25	25	25
Vitamin D	mcg	10*^	10*	8.5–10	8.5–10	8.5–10	8.5–10
Vitamin E	mg	4*	5*				
Vitamin K	mcg	2*	2.5*				
Folate	mcg	65*	80*	50	50	50	50
Vitamin B12	mcg	0.4*	0.5*	0.3	0.3	0.4	0.4
Iron	mg	0.27*	11	1.7	4.3	7.8	7.8
Calcium	mg	200*	260*	525	525	525	525
Phosphorus	mg	100*	275*	400	400	400	400
Sodium	mg	120*	370*	210	280	320	350
Magnesium	mg	30*	75*	55	60	75	80
Zinc	mg	2*	3	4	4	5	5

*, denotes AI; ^, 10mcg vitamin D in the form of cholecalciferol is equivalent to 400 IU.
Values reflect enteral intake. United States RDA and AI values from the national academy of sciences' dietary reference intakes.[1] *European union RNI values from the European food safety authority dietary reference Values.*[2]
AI, *adequate intake; the observed or approximated daily intake of a nutrient by a group of healthy individuals;* IU = *international units;* RDA, *Recommended dietary allowance; intake required to meet the needs of nearly all (97%–98%) healthy individuals in a population;* RNI, *Reference nutrient intake; similar to RDA.*

vary slightly depending on source. Freshly expressed breast milk can be stored for up to 4 h at room temperature, for 4–6 days in the refrigerator, and for 6–12 months in the freezer depending on the temperature.[1,16,27] Previously frozen milk should be used within 24 h of thawing.[16] Breast milk should never be warmed by micro-wave.

Donor milk; Donor milk banks collect, screen, pasteurize, and pool breast milk from multiple women for subsequent distribution. The Human Milk Banking Association of North America helps establish milk banks as well as sets standards for milk processing, pasteurization, and safety. The composition of pasteurized human milk differs from fresh milk, most notably the bioactive components of human milk. For example, the pasteurization process used for donor human milk (DHM) impairs its immunologic properties, including cells, bacteria, enzymes, and immunoglobulins[28,29]; diminishes the activity of digestive enzymes such as amylase and lipase[30]; and eliminates the microbiome.[29,30] Although many studies show benefits in premature infants (discussed below), very few report specifically on DHM use by healthy term infants. Additionally, donor milk is frequently prohibitively expensive for prolonged use.[28] Due to high costs, women sometimes purchase human milk via the Internet or from friends (referred to as direct milk sharing). One study found cow milk contamination of 10% of Internet-purchased human milk[31] and 74% had contamination with potentially pathogenic bacteria.[32] Using milk from a certified bank decreases exposure to medications or narcotics due to pooling of milk from multiple women.[16,28] For these reasons, direct milk sharing is discouraged.

Formula

Despite efforts to promote and support breastfeeding, many women will be either unable or unwilling to breastfeed. Most of these women will choose to formula feed their babies (vs. donor milk). There are different types of formula, as detailed in Table 1.3. Martinez and Ballew have an excellent review covering infant formula composition and different types.[33] In general, a cow milk–based formula is appropriate for most term infants. Consumption of approximately 32oz (1L) of formula per day will meet the recommended daily intake for vitamin D.[3,16,34]

Nutritional composition; Highlighted differences between human milk and cow milk–based formula composition are summarized in Table 1.2 and Fig. 1.1. Standard formulas contain 10–35× higher iron as well as higher protein, zinc, calcium, and sodium compared to human

TABLE 1.2 Composition (amount per 100 kcal) of select nutrients in mature breast milk (after 2–4 weeks), cow milk–based formula, whole cow milk, and almond "milk."

Amount per 100 kcal	Mature breast milk	Cow milk–based formula	Whole cow milk	Almond "milk"
Volume (mL)	150	150–160	167	400–800
Protein (g)	1.3–1.6	2–2.3	5.1–5.7	1.5–2.5
Fat (g)	5	5.1–5.6	5–5.7	4.2–7.5
Carbohydrate (g)	10.3	10.7–11.6	7.3–8	5–13.4
Folic acid (mcg)	12–21	15–16	8*	N/A
Vitamin B12 (mcg)	0.15	0.26–0.33	0.56–1.2	0
Iron (mg)	0.05–0.14	1.5–1.9	0.08	0–0.36
Zinc (mg)	0.1–0.5	0.65–0.8	0.6	N/A
Sodium (mg)	18–38	25–27	83–192	170–450
Vitamin D (IU)	3	60–75	100^	40–100^
Reference(s):	*AAP Pediatric Nutrition*, 7th Edition, *Current Diagnosis and Treatment Pediatrics*, 24th Edition	enfamil.com, gerber.com, abbottnutrition.com	horizon.com, *Current Diagnosis and Treatment Pediatrics*, 24th Edition	silk.com, pacificfoods.com, bluediamond.com

N/A, not available.
* *Goat milk contains only 3.3 mcg folate per 100 kcal.*
^*Reflects fortification.*

TABLE 1.3 Different types of infant formulas, clinical indications for use, and composition.

Formula type	Clinical uses	Composition	Examples
Premature 24+ kcal/oz	Premature hospitalized infants	Higher % of MCT, higher protein, calcium, phosphate, vitamins A and D, zinc, folate, iron; reduced lactose	Similac Special Care Enfamil Premature Gerber Good Start Premature
Transitional (preterm after discharge) 22 kcal/oz	Preterm infants after discharge until 1 year corrected gestational age. Not to be used as a higher calorie alternative for term infants.	Higher % of MCT; higher protein; higher calcium, phosphorus, vitamins A and D, zinc, iron, and folate	EnfaCare NeoSure
Standard 19–20 kcal/oz	Appropriate for most term infants.	Cow milk–based, intact protein	Enfamil Infant, Premium, NeuroPro Similac Advance Earth's Best Organic Dairy Formula
Low lactose	Fussiness, colic, gassiness	Reduced lactose content	Similac Sensitive Gerber Good Start Gentle Earth's Best Sensitivity
Partially hydrolyzed	Term infants with reflux, breastfed infants who require some supplementation (use 100% whey formula), consider for infants with strong family or personal history of atopic disease	Partially hydrolyzed protein; reduced lactose; whey:casein ratio varies, but some are 100% whey	Gerber Good Start, Gentle (*100% whey*) Similac Total Comfort (*100% whey*) Enfamil Gentlease, Reguline
Reflux	Infants with spit up who do not require acid suppression medications	Intact protein; added rice starch; reduced lactose	Similac for Spit Up Enfamil AR
Soy	Infants with galactosemia, lactase deficiency, temporary lactose intolerance following diarrheal illness, or per family preference (vegan/vegetarianism). Not appropriate for premature infants.	Intact soy protein; all are lactose free	Enfamil ProSobee Similac Isomil Gerber Good Start Soy
Extensively hydrolyzed (semielemental)	For infants with malabsorption, short gut syndrome, milk protein intolerance	Extensively hydrolyzed protein. Some have high MCT.	Nutramigen (*not high MCT*) Alimentum Pregestimil
Amino acid–based (elemental)	For infants with malabsorption, short gut syndrome, and milk protein intolerance in which hydrolyzed formulas are not tolerated.	100% free amino acids; lactose free, contains MCT	Elecare Infant Neocate Infant PurAmino Nestle Alfamino

Examples of each type are given, although it is not meant to be an exhaustive list especially as products change frequently.
Note that mention of trade names does not imply endorsement. MCT, medium-chain triglycerides. Table complied with assistance from Bridget Young, PhD; Jill Nyman, RD; Kelly Klaczkiewicz, RD; Alexandra King, MD; Jaime Moore, MD; and Liliane Diab, MD.

milk, which may account for differences in bioavailability. The effects of these differences on long-term health are unknown, including how they may contribute to the variability in outcomes between formula and breastfed infants. For example, there is a known association between high protein intake early in life with higher fat mass, which may lead to increased risk for later obesity.[19,35] Although parents may ask for specific brand recommendations, most standard formulas are nutritionally equivalent. The Infant Formula Act, passed in 1980, regulates the acceptable ranges of nutrient content of any product labeled as an infant formula.

Preparation; Most powdered formulas in the United States use 2 ounces of water for every 1 scoop of powder to yield 19–20 kcal/oz. Some amino acid–based formulas are prepared with 1 ounce of water for every 1 scoop of powder or require packed scoops. Formulas imported from other countries may also be prepared in

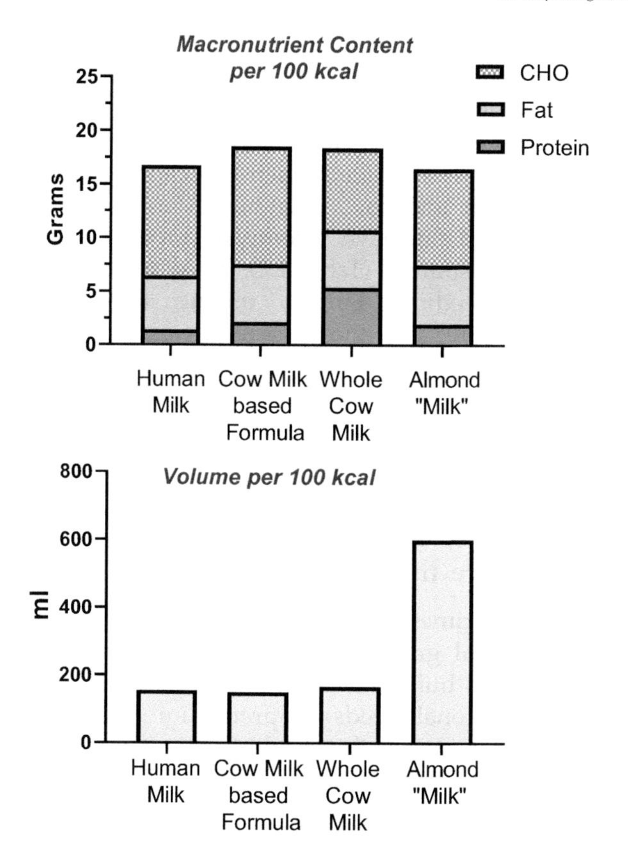

FIGURE 1.1 Comparison of relative composition of mature human milk, infant formula, cow milk, and almond "milk". *CHO*, Carbohydrates.

a different manner, so the container should be examined for instructions. The water should always be measured first, with the powder added second.[16] Once prepared, formula can be refrigerated for up to 24 h and then discarded. If the baby only partially consumes a bottle, the remaining formula should be thrown away after approximately 1 h.[3,16] Formula should never be warmed in the microwave.

Soy formula; Soy formula is an acceptable option for families that prefer to avoid cow milk for personal or religious reasons, such as following a vegan diet, as well as for infants with the rare conditions galactosemia or lactase deficiency.[16,36] Soy formula may also be an option for infants with milk protein allergy, although since there is a 30%–50% chance of soy intolerance in these infants, an extensively hydrolyzed formula is a more appropriate alternative in most cases (see text on MPI given below).[33,36] Soy formula is not recommended for premature infants as their kidneys are unable to handle the higher levels of aluminum that soy formula contains.[16] Soy formula supports infant growth similarly to cow milk–based formulas.[36–38] Although animal studies showed an association between ingestion of soy-based phytoestrogens and infertility, studies in humans have not shown evidence of short- or long-term effects on growth, bone mineralization, reproduction, or neurodevelopment.[33,36,39]

Hydrolyzed and amino acid–based formula; Hydrolyzed formulas are heat and enzymatically treated to break down proteins, specifically casein, into oligopeptides. Formulas may be either partially hydrolyzed (PHF) or extensively hydrolyzed (EHF). Elemental/amino acid–based formulas contain only individual free amino acids.[33] PHFs are generally similar in price to cow milk formulas, while EHF and amino acid–based formulas may be 2–3 times the cost.[40] These formulas also support normal infant growth and may more closely mimic the slower weight gain patterns seen in breastfed infants.[41,42] This is of particular interest in the setting of increased prevalence of childhood obesity, since early rapid weight gain in infancy is a known risk factor.[19] One study of about 80 infants found that those fed a cow milk–based formula demonstrated rapid weight gain, while those fed EHF did not.[42,43] This same group also investigated neurodevelopment differences between these two feeding groups. Infants fed EHF for at least 1 month showed slightly improved gross motor and visual reception scores compared to exclusive cow milk formula feeding.[44] The differences were small and unlikely to be clinically significant, but additional studies may help clarify the ideal formula composition (see Research Gaps at the end of this chapter).

There are several indications for use of hydrolyzed and elemental formulas. EHF and elemental formulas (but not PHF) are useful for cow milk protein intolerance (MPI) as discussed in more detail below.[33] Multiple randomized control trials and meta-analyses have also demonstrated benefit of PHF (but not EHF) formulas in reducing atopic dermatitis in high-risk infants (those with severe eczema or a first-degree relative with anaphylactic food allergy),[41,45,46] although recent analyses and long-term follow-up studies have called these conclusions into question.[47] Other atopic diseases such as asthma have not been as well studied. The American Academy of Pediatrics has concluded that there is not enough evidence to support recommendation for infants at high risk of atopic disease.[47] However, others have argued that PHFs are not significantly more expensive than cow milk formula and there does not appear to be evidence of harm and therefore recommend their use.[45,46]

Prebiotic and probiotic additives; Human milk contains a wide variety of bacteria as well as bioactive components, such as lactoferrin, that support growth of healthy bacteria. The infant intestinal microbiome varies based on feeding type, and its importance for development of innate immunity and long-term health is being increasingly recognized.[48] To help promote growth of commensal bacteria in formula-fed infants to more closely reflect those of breastfed infants, pre- and probiotics are often added to formulas.[33,49] Overall, the data are mixed as to whether there is a benefit to the use of probiotics. Meta-analyses are difficult due to relatively small sample sizes, the wide variety of strains used, and differing outcome measures.[48–51] There is some evidence that giving *Lactobacillus* to breastfed infants may reduce colic, but these results have not been replicated in formula-fed infants.[52] Preterm infants may benefit from probiotic administration. Limited evidence from meta-analyses supports a reduced incidence of necrotizing enterocolitis, late-onset sepsis, and mortality, particularly in infants weighing less than 1500 g at birth, but efficacy varies among strains and more work is needed to precisely develop treatment regimens.[50,51,53] Less is known about prebiotics, but they may be a safer option for premature infants. There have been reports of probiotic-related sepsis in this relatively immunocompromised population[51] and concerns about transference of antibiotic resistance.[48,54] For these reasons, prebiotics warrant further investigation.

Other bioactive compounds; There are numerous non-nutritive components within breast milk that are absent from formula and which are thought to influence development and immunity. It is possible that these factors may be responsible for some of the differences noted between breast- and formula-fed infants. These components include cells, immunoglobulins, cytokines, growth factors, hormones, human milk oligosaccharides, and many others.[55] Formula manufacturers have interest in adding some of these components to their products. For example, milk fat globule membranes (MFGM) are bioactive lipid membranes present in breast milk, which have recently been isolated from bovine milk and added to some formulas.[56] There is some evidence that addition of MFGM to formula reduces incidence of acute otitis media[57] and improves cognitive outcomes.[58] However, the vast majority of clinical research findings on MFGM stems from one randomized controlled trial, which also adjusted macronutrient composition of the experimental formula,[58] making the conclusions and associations difficult to interpret.

Homemade formula; There is recent interest in homemade formulas, which typically involve a combination of raw cow, goat, or plant-based "milk," cod liver oil, molasses, and other ingredients. Multiple recipes are available online. There are significant risks from using a homemade formula. Raw animal milk can contain bacteria such as *Listeria* or *Salmonella*, which can cause devastating infections, including meningitis, in infants. Unmodified cow and goat milk contain high concentrations of protein, sodium, and other minerals (Table 1.2), which increase the renal solute load and can cause electrolyte imbalances.[3] Goat milk is particularly low in folate, which can cause deficiency and macrocytic anemia.[34] Plant-based "milks" are low in calories and fat, have incomplete protein, and are often high in sodium (Table 1.2). They are unsuitable for infant feeding. Finally, mixing the formula incorrectly can put unnecessary stress on infant kidneys and intestines and may not provide sufficient calories.[3] Use of all of these formulas should be discouraged in all situations, especially when used as the sole food for the young infant.

D. Premature Infants

The third trimester of gestation is characterized by significant fetal growth, bone mineralization, transfer of nutrients to build stores, and lung maturation. The unique nutritional needs of premature infants stem from needing to mimic this third trimester to adequately support growth.[59] About half of premature infants have growth restriction at the time of hospital discharge, although the prevalence is decreasing.[60] Much of this growth failure results from inadequate nutrition and is, therefore, preventable.[61,62] There are relatively high protein and caloric requirements to support appropriate growth.[59,61,63] These amounts may be further increased in times of significant illness and stress.[64] Table 1.4[3] lists consensus recommended intakes for premature infants based on weight.

Parenteral nutrition

Infants born before 33–34 weeks gestation are unlikely to tolerate full enteral feeds at birth, and early initiation of parenteral nutrition (PN) is an important aspect of their care.[65] Calorie intake from PN should be 90–105 kcal/kg/day for infants weighing 1000–1500 g, and 105–115 kcal/kg/day for infants with a weight below 1000 g.[3,65] Calorie composition is similar in premature and term infants. About 30%–40% of total calories should be from lipids, 10%–20% from protein, and the remaining calories derived from dextrose. Better tolerance is achieved with a 20% lipid preparation, which can be initiated at 1–2 g/kg/day and increased to goal intake.[3,65] Protein administration can be started directly at goal intake, with higher needs in more premature, smaller infants.[3,59,65] Sodium administration is initially restricted until the initial diuresis has begun as measured by increased urine output and weight loss.[3] See Table 1.4 for micronutrient and vitamin recommendations specific to PN.

TABLE 1.4 Consensus recommendations for enteral and parenteral nutrition in premature infants are based on current body weight.

		Enteral		Parenteral	
Macronutrients	Units	Weight <1000 g	Weight 1000–1500 g	Weight <1000 g	Weight 1000–1500 g
Energy	kcal/kg/day	130–150	110–130	105–115	90–100
Carbohydrate	g/kg/day	9–20	7–17	13–17	9.7–15
Fat	g/kg/day	6.2–8.4	5.3–7.2	3–4	3–4
Protein	g/kg/day	3.8–4.4	3.4–4.2	3.5–4.0	3.2–3.8
Micronutrients					
Vitamin A	IU/kg/day	700–1500		700–1500	
Vitamin C/ascorbate	mg/kg/day	18–24		15–25	
Vitamin D	IU/kg/day	150–400		40–160	
Vitamin E	IU/kg/day	6–12		2.8–3.5	
Vitamin K	mcg/kg/day	8–10		10	
Folate	mcg/kg/day	25–50		56	
Iron	mg/kg/day	2–4		0.1–0.2	
Calcium	mg/kg/day	100–220		60–80	
Phosphorus	mg/kg/day	60–140		45–60	
Sodium	mg/kg/day	69–115		69–115	
Potassium	mg/kg/day	78–117		78–117	
Magnesium	mg/kg/day	7.9–15		4.3–7.2	
Zinc	mg/kg/day	1–3		0.4	
Choline	mg/kg/day	14.4–28		14.4–28	
Carnitine	mg/kg/day	2.9		2.9	
Taurine	mg/kg/day	4.5–9.0		1.88–3.75	

Adapted from Pediatric Nutrition 7th Edition from the American Academy of Pediatrics.[3]

Enteral nutrition

Introduction of feeds; Early and progressive initiation of enteral feeds in premature infants, particularly mother's own milk, has multiple benefits including decreased risk of necrotizing enterocolitis, decreased total central line days, and improved growth.[3,62,66] It is important to introduce enteral feeds within the first few days of life, ideally within the first day,[61] as infants with delayed enteral feeding take longer to establish full feeding.[67] Neonatal intensive care units should develop and follow a feeding protocol that addresses progression of volumes, timing of feeds, and introduction of fortification. Careful attention should be paid to the infant's total fluid volume, caloric, and protein intake as PN is decreased and enteral intake increased.[3,61]

Maternal milk; Whenever available, mother's own milk is preferred for all feeds as it has numerous benefits in premature infants including protection against necrotizing enterocolitis, late-onset sepsis, and possibly improved neurodevelopment.[24,63,66,68,69] In addition, the breast milk of mothers who have premature infants differs from those who gave birth at term. Breast milk produced in the first month after premature birth contains higher immunologically active proteins (including immunoglobulin A), growth factors, total protein, and oligosaccharides compared to mature milk.[3,30] Colostrum should be administered in the mouth as soon as it is available to provide important immune system benefits.[62] Although infants may show slightly better growth with formula feeding during hospitalization,[70] the other risks of formula feeding outweigh these growth benefits, and breast milk should be used when possible. To meet the higher nutrient requirements of the preterm infant, human milk requires fortification,[1,24,71] discussed in detail below. Despite the known importance of receiving maternal milk, rates of breastfeeding in premature infants remains low.[72]

Access to breastfeeding education, lactation consultants, electric double breast pumps, and private spaces to express milk are extremely important to adequately support mothers while their child is hospitalized.[1,72,73] Early and continuous skin-to-skin contact between mother and infant (kangaroo care) has also been shown to improve breastfeeding rates in multiple studies.[74]

Donor milk; The use of banked DHM for premature infants has grown in popularity over the last decade[3,30] due to small but consistent clinical benefits.[68,69] DHM typically performs better than formula, but slightly less well than mother's own milk, at reducing morbidity and mortality.[29,62,68,69] Meta-analyses show that, compared to formula, exclusive human milk (whether fresh or pasteurized) reduces bronchopulmonary dysplasia,[75] necrotizing enterocolitis,[68] and late-onset sepsis.[69] Because of these findings, DHM has become standard of care when maternal milk is unavailable, especially for infants born weighing less than 1500 g.[1,30] DHM is known to have altered composition compared to fresh preterm human milk including lower fat, protein, and calories,[29,30] which may account for the faster weight gain in neonates receiving mother's own milk compared to DHM.[29] The pasteurization process used for DHM also impairs its bioactive properties[28–30] and slightly influences micronutrient composition.[76,77] However, knowledge gaps remain regarding which clinical variations are attributable to pasteurization versus other differences such as freeze-thaw cycles, container transfers, or composition differences between the infant's own mother's milk versus that from mothers of older term infants.[29,30]

Fortification; Although human milk is the preferred food for the preterm infant, it requires fortification, specifically calories, protein, zinc, calcium, and phosphorous.[1,33,71,78] Options for fortification include human milk fortifiers and cow milk–based fortifiers, usually either in a powdered or concentrated liquid form. Due to challenges with sterilization of powdered products, liquid fortifiers are generally preferred.[61,71] An additional benefit of liquid protein fortifiers is the increased protein provided: 1.7 g of protein per 100 mL of milk, compared to powdered products which supply about 1 g per 100 mL.[61] Fortifier is typically added to human milk once the infant is tolerating 80–100 mL/kg/day of enteral feeds.[1] Human milk fortifiers vary in their iron content. Because premature infants have higher iron needs (approximately 2–4 mg/kg/day),[3] their iron status needs to be followed with measurement of hemoglobin, ferritin, and a marker of inflammation. Iron supplements can be given separately from enteral feeds if a noniron-containing fortifier is used.

Assessing growth

During hospitalization, premature infants should have their growth followed closely with daily weights and weekly length and head circumference measurements. These points are plotted on premature infant-specific curves by gestational age.[79] Various options exist including the Fenton curves,[80] Olsen,[81] INTERGROWTH-21st,[82] and others. Although these curves have differences, a commonality is approximate goal growth of 15–20 g/kg/day.[1]

After discharge

Outpatient providers should continue to correct growth for prematurity until 2–3 years of life. Premature infants continue to need more calories, protein, iron, calcium, zinc, and phosphorous compared to infants born at term. Special formulas (Table 1.3) contain the appropriate balance of macro- and micronutrients to support growth of these babies. Premature formulas contain 22 kcal/oz, compared to 19–20 kcal/oz for standard formulas as well as more protein, calcium, and phosphorous.[33,63] Breastfed premature infants can continue to do so by giving expressed breast milk fortified to 22 or 24 kcal/oz with a premature formula or by substituting 2–3 feeds per day with a premature infant formula.[1] They should also receive an iron supplement (2 mg/kg/day) as even late preterm infants are at risk for early iron deficiency,[1,16,62] as well as a vitamin D supplement similar to term breastfed infants.[83]

E. Inborn Errors of Metabolism

There are multiple inborn errors of metabolism that require dietary modification early in infancy. Discussion of the specific symptoms and diagnosis of these disorders is beyond the scope of this text. Generally, however, infants may present with feeding difficulties, lethargy, vomiting, rapid breathing, and in some cases seizures.[84]

The first error of metabolism which was approved for newborn screening was phenylketonuria (PKU), a congenital absence of the enzyme phenylalanine hydroxylase which is required for conversion of the amino acid phenylalanine to tyrosine. Toxic levels of phenylalanine will begin to accumulate if PKU is not diagnosed early, and children can suffer irreversible brain damage.[85,86] Fortunately, long-term adherence to a diet low in phenylalanine can lead to normal or nearly normal growth and development.[85,87] Previously, infants were placed on low-phenylalanine formulas and counseled against breastfeeding, partially due to the increased difficulty in controlling phenylalanine intake. However, regimens have been developed to augment breastfeeding with phenylalanine-free formula and an amino acid–based protein supplement.[24,88] A small study showed that breastfeeding resulted in slightly better serum phenylalanine control.[87] More research with a larger sample size is needed, and a consensus should be established as feeding practices are widely variable.[89] No matter which feeding method is utilized, infants diagnosed with PKU will need to have phenylalanine levels and long-term growth closely followed by a pediatric metabolic disease specialist. Multiple applications for electronic devices are available, which allow families to track phenylalanine intake and help with dietary planning.

Breastfeeding is not well studied in other metabolic disorders. Most inborn errors of metabolism can include some breastfeeding and close monitoring,[88] but consultation with a metabolic specialist is recommended. Two notable exceptions are galactosemia and congenital lactase deficiency. Galactosemia is a congenital inability to properly metabolize the sugar galactose due a complete absence of galactose-1-phosphate uridylyltransferase (GALT) enzymatic activity. Because the primary sugar in breast milk is lactose (glucose + galactose), galactosemia is a true contraindication to breastfeeding.[16,24,88] Congenital lactase deficiency is also a contraindication since these children are unable to break down lactose and present with severe watery diarrhea.[90] Both of these conditions are extremely rare. There is recent evidence that children with Duarte galactosemia (characterized by partial impairment GALT activity) may not have adverse developmental outcomes when exposed to galactose in formula or breast milk.[91]

III. NUTRITIONAL REQUIREMENTS

A. Basis for Key Nutrient Recommendations

Global differences

There are differences among international expert committees regarding recommended intakes for infants, which also vary by age. See Table 1.1 for additional information.

Supplementation

Vitamin D supplementation; Breast milk is low in vitamin D, particularly since many women have marginal vitamin D status themselves. The American Academy of Pediatrics recommends that all infants who are exclusively breastfed receive vitamin D supplementation of 400 IU daily.[1–3,34,92] One randomized clinical trial showed noninferiority of maternal supplementation with 6400 IU/day of vitamin D3.[93] This has the added benefit of addressing maternal vitamin D deficiency, but evidence is currently too limited to support this as a sufficient and reliable alternate vitamin D source.[16]

Iron supplementation; The iron stores conferred during the third trimester and through delayed cord clamping begin to be depleted by 4–6 months of age in healthy, term, breastfed infants.[94,95] Human milk contains a small amount of iron (<0.5 mg/L). Although the iron has favorable bioavailability, human milk becomes inadequate after the third trimester endowment is exhausted. Iron-containing complementary foods, such as red meat, lentils, soybeans, dark leafy greens, and fortified foods like infant cereals, are therefore critical sources of iron in breastfed infants and should be prioritized.[95] An iron supplement can be initiated with a liquid vitamin, but there are few data to show benefit of universal iron supplementation in high-resource settings. There is evidence in low-resource settings that excess iron in nonanemic older infants and young children may cause harm.[96,97] Iron deficiency is specifically addressed later in this chapter. It is worth noting that many infant multivitamins with iron also contain vitamin D, so any separate vitamin D supplements can be discontinued. Healthy term infants consuming iron-fortified formulas do not need additional supplementation but should also be provided iron-containing foods. Premature infants have higher iron needs as discussed earlier.

Risk of micronutrient deficiencies

Iron; Iron deficiency without anemia has been shown to alter neurodevelopment and to result in deficits which persist beyond successful treatment.[98–100] It is therefore important to detect and treat promptly. Risk factors for iron deficiency include exclusive breastfeeding, maternal iron deficiency, premature birth, small-for-gestational age or birth weight below 2500 g, low intake of high iron complementary foods, rapid rate of growth, and elevated BMI z-score.[94,100,101] Although it is common in the United States to test hemoglobin concentration around 1 year of life, this alone is not sufficient screening for iron deficiency, as many other conditions can cause anemia and iron deficiency can be present without anemia.[102] One study looked at using serum ferritin in a primary care setting and found that screening around 15–18 months of age had greater sensitivity and specificity to detect iron deficiency compared to hemoglobin.[102] However, breastfed infants are at risk as early as 6–8 months, so this timeline would be too late for universal screening. A more appropriate scenario would be development of different screening guidelines for breast versus formula-fed infants. The overall risk of iron deficiency for formula-fed infants in the first year of life is minimal due to the high iron content of US formulas. However, formula-fed infants can develop deficiency after stopping formula if there is insufficient iron intake from food. Prevention of iron deficiency starts prior to birth, with supplementation of iron-deficient mothers during pregnancy. Delayed cord clamping also reduces risk for iron deficiency, especially in breastfed infants.[100,103] For repletion of iron, start 3–6 mg/kg/day divided into twice daily dosing after resolution of acute inflammatory processes.[21]

Zinc; Zinc is a micronutrient critical for proper growth, taste, and function of the gastrointestinal tract and the immune system.[78,95] Clinical presentation of mild to moderate zinc deficiency is most common and typically includes such nonspecific signs as growth impairment (both weight and linear), loss of appetite, and immune impairment. Severe deficiency is characterized by an erythematous eczematous skin rash on the extremities and around the mouth and perineum, weakened immunity, and diarrhea.[21,78] The best dietary sources of zinc for complementary foods include meats and some brands of fortified infant cereals. Fruits and vegetables are low in zinc content. Although zinc is moderately high in whole grains and legumes, bioavailability from these sources is low. Children raised on a vegan/vegetarian diet are at risk for deficiency, especially if exclusively breastfed from 0 to 6 months and with continued predominant breastfeeding thereafter.[78] Parents should be counseled on ways to increase zinc intake from foods such as fortified cereals, lentils, nut butters, and, if not restricting these foods, meats and eggs. Providers should have a low threshold for starting zinc supplementation particularly for children with growth concerns (starting dose: 1 mg elemental Zn/kg/day).[21] Most, if not all, liquid infant multivitamins do not contain zinc. Liquid zinc supplements (e.g., 15 mg elemental zinc per 10 drops) are available online and are less expensive than prescription formulations.

Vitamin B12; Deficiency in vitamin B12 is primarily an issue in children who are exclusively breastfed and who then receive complementary foods absent of all animal products.[21,34] Deficiency occurs more readily in infants compared to adults.[34] There are several products currently available for vitamin B12 supplementation. Zarbee's Naturals Baby Multivitamin with Iron Supplement and NovaFerrum Multivitamin with Iron Pediatric drops contain vitamin B12. Of note, Enfamil's Poly-Vi-Sol without iron includes vitamin B12; the version with iron does not.

Other micronutrients; Deficiencies of other micronutrients and vitamins are less common, although specific situations that may increase an infant's risk exist. The following list is not exhaustive but illustrates some important clinical scenarios that should heighten concern for deficiencies. Exclusively breastfed infants who do not receive intramuscular vitamin K prophylaxis at birth can present with bruising or bleeding due to deficiency; the most devastating sequela is intracranial hemorrhage.[21,34] Vitamin A, copper, and selenium deficiency can develop in premature infants in association with inadequately supplemented PN. Premature infants are also at risk for calcium and phosphorus deficiency if fed unfortified breast milk. Renal disease predisposes to magnesium and selenium deficiencies. Lastly, maternal insufficiency or deficiency can predispose breastfed infants to many micronutrient deficiencies including vitamin B12, thiamin, and iodine.[21]

B. Dietary Guidance

Practices

Expected calories/volumes; A common question parents ask is how much their baby should be consuming. Parents should be encouraged to focus on responsive feeding, such as watching for satiety cues, rather than focusing on exact numbers. Clinical providers should use weight and growth trends to assess adequacy of intake. Recommendations based purely on caloric intake can result in overfeeding, which carries its own risks. As a guide, approximate caloric intake and expected volumes by age are shown in Table 1.5.[1,21]

Complementary foods; The introduction of complementary foods is recommended to start by approximately 6 months. Infants are generally ready to trial solid foods if they have good head control while upright, can sit with support, seem interested in food, willingly open their mouth to accept a spoon, and have lost the tongue extrusion reflex (where the tongue protrudes from the mouth to remove nonliquids).[16] Biologically, breast milk becomes an inadequate source of calories, iron and zinc around this 4–6 month window.[78,95] Introducing solid foods earlier than 4 months may be associated with obesity[95] while waiting much beyond 6 months may lead to micronutrient deficiencies, poor growth, and feeding rejection and difficulties.[16]

The foods that should be emphasized differ in formula versus breastfed infants. Exclusively breastfed infants are dependent on complementary foods for adequate intake of zinc and iron.[95] It is therefore important to include foods such as meat, eggs, fortified cereals, and dark green vegetables with early feeding experiences. The variety of foods introduced is less critical to meet nutrient needs in formula-fed infants, but exposure to a diversity of flavors and textures is important. However, emerging data suggest that protein quality may impact long-term growth.[104,105] Whole, unprocessed foods without added sugar should be prioritized for both formula-fed and breastfed infants.[95] Other than honey and choking hazards (highest risk foods are hot dogs, whole nuts/seeds, carrots, popcorn, hard candy/gum, apples, and whole grapes[3]), no specific foods or food groups are off limits for introduction.

TABLE 1.5 Average calorie requirements and estimated volumes for infants by age.

Age	Average calorie requirement (kcal/kg/day)	Approximate volume per day (mL)*	Breastfed		Formula	
			Feeds per day	Estimated volume per feed	Feeds per day	Volume per feed
0–24 h			>6	Drops		5–10 mL
24–48 h			>8	5 mL		10–20 mL
48–72 h			>8	15 mL		20–30 mL
72–96 h			8–12	30 mL		30–40 mL
4–9 days			8–12	30–50 mL		40–50 mL
10–30 days	120	740–800	8–12	2–4 oz	6–8	2–4 oz
1–2 months	115	880–950	8–12	3–5 oz	5–7	3–5 oz
2–3 months	105	910–1010	8–12	4–6 oz	4–6	4–7 oz
3–4 months	95	910–1010	8–12	4–6 oz	4–6	5–8 oz
4–6 months	95	1025–1055	6–10	4–6 oz	4–6	6–8 oz
6–12 months	90 (70 from milk/formula)	575–630	5–8	4–6 oz	3–5	6–8 oz
References	*Current Diagnosis and Treatment Pediatrics*, 24th Edition,[4] *Breastfeeding Handbook for Physicians*, 2nd edition[5]					

Targeting caloric intake alone can result in overfeeding, which can result in detrimental health outcomes. Breast- and formula-fed infants will have different feeding patterns. Note that from 24 to 48 h of life, infants may breastfeed up to every hour before the milk comes in. This is important to stimulate milk production and does not indicate that supplementation is necessary.
* *calculated by taking average kcal/kg/day and multiplying by 50th percentile weight for both males and females to obtain kcal/day.*

The general recommendation is to introduce only one new food every few days to be able to identify the source of an allergic reaction.[3] Older infants can be offered small amounts of water (1–2oz) in a cup with meals but should not be given other liquids including cow or other animal milk, plant-based milks, or sugar-sweetened or carbonated beverages. Fruit juice is also not recommended before the age of one.[3,95,106]

Introduction of highly allergenic foods; Infants with severe, difficult-to-control eczema or with a strong family history of anaphylactic food allergies are at high risk for developing food allergies.[47,107] Although delaying introduction beyond 1 year was previously recommended for highly allergenic foods (particularly peanuts and eggs, but also milk, shellfish, sesame, soy, tree nuts, and wheat), randomized trials have now shown that earlier introduction is likely to be protective against future food allergies in high-risk infants.[47,107–109] High-risk children should be referred to a pediatric allergy specialist around age 4–6 months to guide introduction of allergenic foods.[16,107] Ideally, these infants would have skin or serum testing prior to introduction of peanuts.[47,107] For lower-risk infants, small amounts of highly allergenic foods can be introduced at home in age-appropriate forms with the serving size increased over time if no signs of allergy are seen.[16,47,107]

Vegan/vegetarian diets; The specific foods that are avoided are variable among individuals who use vegan or vegetarian to describe their diets.[3] It is necessary to clarify with parents what foods are eliminated. Iron and zinc are often a concern for vegan/vegetarian infants over 6 months if they have been primarily breastfed. This is because the best sources of these micronutrients are meats (if formula-fed, this not an issue as discussed elsewhere in this chapter). Absorption of plant-based iron is increased by combining iron sources with coingestion of vitamin C and separated from high calcium sources. Vitamin B12 deficiency occurs more readily in infants compared to adults and can occur if there is minimal or no intake of animal products.[34] Supplementation for prevention of micronutrient deficiencies was discussed earlier.

Issues of concern

Contraindications to breastfeeding, infant, and maternal; There are few infant contraindications to receiving breast milk. Galactosemia is the most commonly cited.[1,16,24] Maternal contraindications are more common. There are some infectious diseases that may require temporary or complete avoidance of breastfeeding. Because recommendations change frequently, the CDC and WHO websites can be referenced for the most up-to-date advice. Breastfeeding mothers are often told to "pump and dump" (i.e., express breast milk and then dispose of it) while taking certain medications. This is often unnecessary as most medications are safe for breastfeeding.[1] There are several references and electronic device applications that can provide the most current advice, including LactMed from the NIH[16,24] or the Infant Risk Center from Texas Tech University Health Sciences Center.[2] Generally, amphetamines, chemotherapy agents, ergotamines, and statins are not compatible with breastfeeding.[24]

Recreational drugs; A rising issue in the United States with more states legalizing marijuana (MJ) is its use by pregnant and breastfeeding mothers. MJ and its metabolites are detectable in breast milk up to 6 days after the last use.[110] Many of these compounds are readily absorbed in fat, which makes up 3%–5% of breast milk. Furthermore, although studies regarding infant outcomes are limited,[1] the infant brain contains a large percentage of fat and may concentrate psychoactive compounds. Women should be encouraged not to use MJ in any form while pregnant and breastfeeding.[2,16]

Mothers should also be counseled against tobacco use. However, even if there is no intention for smoking cessation, mothers should be encouraged to continue breastfeeding.[1] Women who smoke are less likely to breastfeed, but human milk may have added benefits in protecting against some of the negative health effects of tobacco smoke exposure.[72] Finally, alcohol consumption should be avoided or minimized. Although there may not be an impact on long-term development,[111] there is evidence that alcohol exposure can impact infants including sleep patterns.[112] It is generally accepted that one to two alcoholic beverage(s) consumed at least 2–3 h prior to a nursing session results in minimal alcohol being transferred in the breast milk and that it is safe to do so on occasion.[1,24]

Breastfeeding problems; Breastfeeding mothers encounter numerous issues. One of the most common concerns is actual or perceived insufficient milk supply especially in the first few weeks of life. It is normal for newborns to feed 8–12 times in a 24 h period (Table 1.5).[1,2] To assess milk intake, follow the infant's weight and output, looking for the appearance of yellow-seedy stools around day 4–5 of life, and at least 7–8 voids in 24 h by 1 week of life.[1] Asking a mother to pump after feeds at least 2–3 times per day in addition to direct breastfeeding can help determine and increase milk supply. This is especially critical in late preterm infants (born at 35–36 weeks gestation) as they may have less stamina and less effective milk transfer than term infants, which can lead to insufficient breast emptying and therefore inadequate stimulation of milk production. Women who are obese, have a history of gestational diabetes, or have type 2 diabetes frequently have delayed onset of lactogenesis and may need support to successfully initiate and sustain breastfeeding. The triple feeds approach is comprised of (1) breastfeeding, (2) bottle feeding of human milk or formula, and (3) pumping milk to maintain supply, and is sometimes indicated.[1] To evaluate milk transfer at the breast, it can be helpful to do a weight before and after a feed (called a test weigh or pre/post weights); this requires a scale accurate to 1–2 g. However, we again caution against focusing on precise numbers and instead evaluating latch, overall growth trend, number of stools and voids, and infant satiety after feeding at the breast. Other common breastfeeding concerns include pain, sleep deprivation, returning to work, and teething.[1,2,24] Providers can anticipate these challenges and counsel mothers accordingly to encourage breastfeeding success. For more information on these and other breastfeeding questions, see recent reviews[2,24] or the American Academy of Pediatrics' Breastfeeding Handbook for Physicians for a comprehensive guide.[1] There should be a low threshold to refer to a lactation professional for evaluation and assistance.

Growth faltering; Growth faltering, commonly called FTT, is defined as growth (whether weight, length, or weight-for-length) below norms for age and sex[3] or which declines across more than two major percentile lines.[21] It is important to ensure that the correct growth chart (WHO curve for term infants to age 24 months) is being used and that premature infants are corrected for gestational age.[16,24] See earlier text on Growth monitoring for further discussion of growth assessment. After the diagnosis is made, the first step is to diagnose the underlying etiology.

Growth faltering has historically been divided into nonorganic and organic causes although this classification is losing popularity. Nonorganic refers to insufficient caloric intake in an otherwise normal infant or child. The vast majority of infants will fall into this category.[21] For breastfed infants, this is most commonly due to insufficient milk intake, whether due to ineffective transfer of milk at the breast or low milk supply. Weighted feedings/test weighs can be helpful to estimate the volume of milk being transferred. Evaluate the latch at the breast and listen for swallowing with every few sucks. Encourage the mother to pump after at least two to three feeds every day to help evaluate and increase supply. Triple feeds as described above can be initiated for a brief time. For formula-fed infants, weight faltering may be due to improper mixing of formula, intentional dilution of formula to try to make it last longer due to food insecurity, or use of alternatives (such as cow, almond, soy, or rice milk) as a substitute for infant formula. To evaluate for these different possibilities, take a 24 h feeding recall, ask how formula is being mixed, and ask about food insecurity in the home. Refer low-income families to the WIC program.[3] The other traditional main category of FTT is due to an "organic" cause that typically results from an underlying condition that results in excessive caloric needs (e,g., congenital heart disease), malabsorption (e.g., cystic fibrosis, chronic diarrhea), or underlying genetic disorder leading to a different growth pattern.

Calorie requirements for catch-up growth are an approximate increase of intake over and above maintenance needs by 5 kcal per gram of catch-up growth needed (i.e., per gram of weight deficit). Alternatively, goal caloric intake can be determined by IBW instead of current body weight. Caloric goals are intended for clinical providers and not meant for parents to initiate calorie counting for their infant. Increased calorie intake can often be achieved by mixing formula or fortifying expressed breast milk to 24–26 kcal/oz. If over 6 months, caloric intake can be increased by emphasis on calorically dense, high fat complementary foods (e.g., meats, eggs, nut butters, and adding oil or butter to fruits and vegetables). Micronutrient deficiencies should be corrected (see above).

MPI; Cow MPI occurs in about 2%–3% of formula-fed infants[33] with lower incidence in breastfed babies.[2,40] The most common manifestation of MPI is blood and sometimes mucus in the stool.[16] Infants may also have poor growth, colic, constipation, feeding refusal, or excessive spitting up or reflux that is difficult to control despite medical therapy.[40] If the infant is being formula-fed, an extensively hydrolyzed formula is likely to be required.[33,40] Although soy formula can be trialed if cost or availability are major concerns, between 30% and 50% of infants with MPI will also have a sensitivity to soy. For the most severe cases, an amino acid–based/elemental formula can be used. A formula trial should last at least 1 week before changing and declaring a treatment failure. Most dairy-sensitive infants will also react to the milk from other animals such as goat or sheep milk, so infant formulas from these sources are not appropriate alternatives. For infants who are breastfed, treatment requires elimination of all milk products (and sometimes soy) from the mother's diet as these proteins are transferred into breast milk.[16] Mothers should be given a list of milk-related ingredients to avoid including casein, lactalbumin, lactoferrin, lactulose, and rennet casein.[40] Consider referral to a pediatric gastroenterologist or pediatric nutrition specialist if there is significant weight loss, failure to gain weight or failure of symptom resolution despite adherence to dietary restrictions, or feeding aversion.[16,40] Since most babies outgrow MPI, it is generally safe to trial reintroduction of milk products around the age of 1 year with monitoring of symptoms.[16,40]

C. Other Guidance

Beyond one year: transition to toddler diet

Breastfeeding can be continued for as long as it is mutually desired by mother and child. There are continued benefits to breastfeeding beyond 1 year and the WHO recommends breastfeeding until 2 years and beyond.[113] Excessive human milk intake at the expense of other foods can impact the total daily intake and lead to poor weight gain and/or micronutrient deficiencies. It is therefore recommended that some structure in feeding schedule be placed after 12 months of age so that the child is offered table foods prior to nursing and that the child is not allowed to frequently consume small volumes of breast milk throughout the day. A cup with water may be given at meals, or cow milk can be introduced while breastfeeding is continued. Formula-fed infants may be switched to whole cow milk after the age of 1 year. Alternative milks such as soy, almond, and coconut "milk" have much lower total and lower quality protein, as well as lower fat content and therefore lower caloric density (Table 1.2 and Fig. 1.1). Mineral content, including sodium, also varies widely among alternative fluids, including several-fold differences relative to caloric intake (Table 1.2 and Fig. 1.1). If one of these nondairy milks is used, parents will need to plan their child's diet carefully to include healthy sources of fat and complete protein to support appropriate growth and brain development.[3] Toddlers on a vegan diet will require supplementation with vitamin B12 and possibly other micronutrients. Many toddlers have intakes of fruits and vegetables below recommendations, and a major goal of early childhood feeding experiences should be to develop acceptance of a broad range of foods and healthy habits that can be continued throughout life.[3] Emphasizing this fact with families is of primary importance. Lastly, all toddlers also have relatively high protein, iron, and zinc requirements compared to adults. Diverse diets including foods from all major food groups is a priority, with minimal intake of highly processed foods, added sugars, salts, and refined carbohydrates. Toddlers should be encouraged to eat the same foods consumed by their family.

Hospitalized infant

Hospitalized infants are at risk for decreased intake and therefore poor nutritional status, which can impair healing and recovery particularly in critically ill infants.[114,115] Please note that nutritional support for infants 30 days or younger typically follow neonatal guidelines[115] as discussed earlier in this chapter.

Nutritional assessment; An evaluation of the infant's nutritional status should first occur at the time of admission.[114,115] It should account not only for the infant's weight/growth status at that time but also for what needs are anticipated based on the illness. Studies have shown that a relatively high portion of children already have some degree of malnutrition at the time of admission.[114–116] Young infants are at high risk for rapid deterioration in nutritional status due to relatively high requirements for normal growth. Nutritional intake, fluid status, and the patient's weight should be assessed daily throughout the entire admission, and length should be measured weekly for prolonged hospitalizations. Early initiation of nutrition support is important to supporting adequate recovery. However, a large portion of patients, especially those who are critically ill, still do not achieve caloric and protein goals.[115,116]

Fluid requirements; A general rule of thumb to estimate fluid requirements in pediatric patients is 100 mL/kg/day for the first 10 kg of body weight; an additional 50 mL/kg/day for each kg above 10 kg; and a final 20 mL/kg/day for each kilogram over 20 kg. As many infants weigh less than 10 kg, weight can be multiplied by 100 mL to determine daily fluid needs.[3]

Calorie and protein needs; Caloric and protein needs typically increase somewhat during illness,[114] with further increased protein needs with extracorporeal membrane oxygenation, renal dialysis, and severe burns, trauma, or wounds. Prolonged fever increases calorie needs by 12%–13% for every degree above 37°C during the time of critical illness. Minimum protein requirements for ill children are 1.5 g/kg/day with intake as high as 3 g/kg/day sometimes needed to balance catabolic losses.[115] While it is important to not underfeed a hospitalized child, it is equally important not to overfeed, which also increases morbidity and mortality.[115,117] Calorie and fluid requirements are reduced with mechanical ventilation or sedation. The importance of daily assessment of fluid and caloric intake cannot be overemphasized to avoid either over- or underestimating nutritional support.

Enteral; When medically possible, enteral nutrition is preferred over parenteral.[115] Breastfed infants can continue to directly breastfeed or, if receiving feeds through a nasogastric or nasojejunal (transpyloric) tube, can receive expressed breast milk. Mothers should receive support from a lactation specialist in order to discuss frequency of breast emptying via pump to maintain milk production.[73] This is especially important if the infant is medically prevented from having oral feeds for a significant duration, such as prior to a procedure. Formula-fed infants can continue to receive the same or equivalent formula to what they are fed at home. Overall caloric recommendations are in Table 1.5 but need to be adjusted on a patient-to-patient basis. Guidelines for preprocedure fasting as supported by the American Society of Anesthesiologists include 2 h for clear liquids, 4 h for breast milk, 6 h for infant formula, and 8 h for everything else.[118]

TABLE 1.6 Important areas for future research.

Research gaps	
Breastfeeding barriers and effect of maternal phenotype	Overweight and obese mothers have lower rate of success. Additionally, milk composition may be influenced, the effect of which on the infant is not yet known.
Long-term outcomes in infants who are breastfed versus formula-fed	Particularly studies into adolescence and adulthood.
Ideal formula composition	What is the impact on offspring growth and obesity risk of the high iron and protein content relative to breast milk?
Ideal complementary feeding based on feeding type	Randomized control trials that investigate complementary foods while also accounting for breast or formula feeding. Should include body composition and long-term outcomes.
Impact of early feeding on later risk of adult-onset medical conditions	Little is known about influence of early nutritional exposures on immune development or propensity for development of cancer, Alzheimer's disease, kidney disease, and other conditions.
Ideal weight gain, especially in premature infants	Both rapid weight gain and poor catch-up growth have risks, but it is still not known whether growth of premature infants should target growth rates of the fetus or another metric.
Screening for iron deficiency anemia	Future studies are needed to determine the ideal time and method for testing while accounting for primary feeding type (human milk vs. iron-fortified formula).
Nutritional influences on disease states	More research is needed to fully understand the impact of nutrigenetics and nutriepigenetics on health and disease over the entire life span.
Nutritional exposures on health	The American Academy of Pediatrics released a statement in 2018 calling for the FDA to update the food chemical safety assessment program and to retest chemicals already labeled as safe taking infant and children into account.

Parenteral; Although directly feeding the gut is ideal, there are instances when PN will be required. Energy requirements are approximately 10% lower with PN due to the lack of thermic effect of food. Many micronutrient requirements are also lower as the incomplete absorption from the gut is not a factor. To determine PN composition, first calculate total fluid and calorie needs. About 30%–40% of total calories should be from lipids, 10%–20% from protein, and the remaining calories derived from dextrose. Amino acids can be started at goal in the absence of hepatic dysfunction. Start lipids at 0.5–1 g/kg/day and increase by 1 g/kg/day to goal. Glucose infusion rate (= [mL/h infusion rate × % dextrose] ÷ [kg × 6]) can be increased by about 2.5%–5% per day to goal.[3] Maximum glucose infusion rate is determined by serum glucose, by the location of intravenous line placement (i.e., central vs. peripheral), the patient's age, other medications, and the patient's metabolic state in relation to illness. Laboratory monitoring should occur at least daily while the PN composition is being adjusted.

RESEARCH GAPS

Although there have been significant research advances in the field of infant nutrition, there remain large knowledge gaps (Table 1.6). Research in these areas has the potential to improve growth, development, and health from infancy and into adulthood.

IV. REFERENCES

1. *Breastfeeding Handbook for Physicians.* 2nd ed. Elk Grove Village, Illinois: American Academy of Pediatrics; 2014.
2. Bunik M. The pediatrician's role in encouraging exclusive breastfeeding. *Pediatr Rev.* 2017;38(8):353–368.
3. American Academy of Pediatrics Committee on Nutrition. *Pediatric Nutrition.* 7th ed. Elk Grove Village, IL: American Academy of Pediatrics; 2014.
4. Manson WG, Weaver LT. Fat digestion in the neonate. *Arch Dis Child Fetal Neonatal Ed.* 1997;76(3):F206–F211.
5. McClean P, Weaver LT. Ontogeny of human pancreatic exocrine function. *Arch Dis Child.* 1993;68(1 Spec No):62–65.

6. Poquet L, Wooster TJ. Infant digestion physiology and the relevance of in vitro biochemical models to test infant formula lipid digestion. *Mol Nutr Food Res*. 2016;60(8):1876–1895.
7. Lindquist S, Hernell O. Lipid digestion and absorption in early life: an update. *Curr Opin Clin Nutr Metab Care*. 2010;13(3): 314–320.
8. Robertson RC, Manges AR, Finlay BB, Prendergast AJ. The human microbiome and child growth – first 1000 days and beyond. *Trends Microbiol*. 2019;27(2):131–147.
9. Hill CJ, Lynch DB, Murphy K, et al. Evolution of gut microbiota composition from birth to 24 weeks in the INFANTMET Cohort. *Microbiome*. 2017;5(1):4.
10. Tamburini S, Shen N, Wu HC, Clemente JC. The microbiome in early life: implications for health outcomes. *Nat Med*. 2016;22(7): 713–722.
11. Pronovost GN, Hsiao EY. Perinatal interactions between the microbiome, immunity, and neurodevelopment. *Immunity*. 2019; 50(1):18–36.
12. Videhult FK, West CE. Nutrition, gut microbiota and child health outcomes. *Curr Opin Clin Nutr Metab Care*. 2016;19(3): 208–213.
13. Thulier D. Weighing the facts: a systematic review of expected patterns of weight loss in full-term, breastfed infants. *J Hum Lactation*. 2016;32(1):28–34.
14. Cole TJ. The development of growth references and growth charts. *Ann Hum Biol*. 2012;39(5):382–394.
15. Grummer-Strawn LM, Reinold C, Krebs NF. Use of world health organization and CDC growth charts for children aged 0–59 months in the United States. *MMWR Recomm Rep*. 2010; 59(RR-9):1–15.
16. DiMaggio DM, Cox A, Porto AF. Updates in infant nutrition. *Pediatr Rev*. 2017;38(10):449–462.
17. Neumann CG, Alpaugh M. Birthweight doubling time: a fresh look. *Pediatrics*. 1976;57(4):469–473.
18. Demerath EW, Fields DA. Body composition assessment in the infant. *Am J Hum Biol*. 2014;26(3):291–304.
19. Singhal A. Long-term adverse effects of early growth acceleration or catch-up growth. *Ann Nutr Metab*. 2017;70(3):236–240.
20. Krebs NF, Himes JH, Jacobson D, Nicklas TA, Guilday P, Styne D. Assessment of child and adolescent overweight and obesity. *Pediatrics*. 2007;120(Suppl 4):S193–S228.
21. Haemer MA, Primak LE, Krebs NF. Normal childhood nutrition and its disorders. In: Hay Jr WW, Levin MJ, Deterding RR, Abzug MJ, eds. *Lange Current Diagnosis and Treatment: Pediatrics*. 24th ed. Chicago, IL, USA: McGraw-Hill Education; 2018.
22. National Academies of Sciences. Dietary Reference Intakes Tables and Application. http://nationalacademies.org/hmd/Activities/Nutrition/SummaryDRIs/DRI-Tables.aspx. Accessed April 1, 2019.
23. European Food Safety Authority. Dietary Reference Values. https://www.efsa.europa.eu/en/topics/topic/dietary-reference-values. Accessed April 1, 2019.
24. American Academy of Pediatrics Section on Breastfeeding. Breastfeeding and the use of human milk. *Pediatrics*. 2012;129(3):e827–841.
25. Flaherman V, Schaefer EW, Kuzniewicz MW, Li SX, Walsh EM, Paul IM. Health care utilization in the first month after birth and its relationship to newborn weight loss and method of feeding. *Acad Pediatr*. 2018;18(6):677–684.
26. McFadden A, Gavine A, Renfrew MJ, et al. Support for healthy breastfeeding mothers with healthy term babies. *Cochrane Database Syst Rev*. 2017;2:Cd001141.
27. Eglash A, Simon L. ABM clinical protocol #8: human milk storage information for home use for full-term infants, revised 2017. *Breastfeed Med*. 2017;12(7):390–395.
28. Committee on Nutrition Section on Breastfeeding Committee on Fetus and Newborn. Donor human milk for the high-risk infant: preparation, safety, and usage options in the United States. *Pediatrics*. 2017;139(1).
29. Hard AL, Nilsson AK, Lund AM, Hansen-Pupp I, Smith LEH, Hellstrom A. Review shows that donor milk does not promote the growth and development of preterm infants as well as maternal milk. *Acta Paediatr*. 2019;108(6):998–1007.
30. Meier P, Patel A, Esquerra-Zwiers A. Donor human milk update: evidence, mechanisms, and priorities for research and practice. *J Pediatr*. 2017;180:15–21.
31. Keim SA, Kulkarni MM, McNamara K, et al. Cow's milk contamination of human milk purchased via the internet. *Pediatrics*. 2015; 135(5):e1157–1162.
32. Keim SA, Hogan JS, McNamara KA, et al. Microbial contamination of human milk purchased via the Internet. *Pediatrics*. 2013; 132(5):e1227–1235.
33. Martinez JA, Ballew MP. Infant formulas. *Pediatr Rev*. 2011;32(5): 179–189. quiz 189.
34. Diab L, Krebs NF. Vitamin excess and deficiency. *Pediatr Rev*. 2018; 39(4):161–179.
35. Rzehak P, Oddy WH, Mearin ML, et al. Infant feeding and growth trajectory patterns in childhood and body composition in young adulthood. *Am J Clin Nutr*. 2017;106(2):568–580.
36. Vandenplas Y, Castrellon PG, Rivas R, et al. Safety of soya-based infant formulas in children. *Br J Nutr*. 2014;111(8):1340–1360.
37. Andres A, Cleves MA, Bellando JB, Pivik RT, Casey PH, Badger TM. Developmental status of 1-year-old infants fed breast milk, cow's milk formula, or soy formula. *Pediatrics*. 2012;129(6): 1134–1140.
38. Mendez MA, Anthony MS, Arab L. Soy-based formulae and infant growth and development: a review. *J Nutr*. 2002;132(8):2127–2130.
39. Testa I, Salvatori C, Di Cara G, et al. Soy-based infant formula: are phyto-oestrogens still in doubt? *Front Nutr*. 2018;5:110.
40. Brill H. Approach to milk protein allergy in infants. *Can Fam Physician*. 2008;54(9):1258–1264.
41. Sauser J, Nutten S, de Groot N, et al. Partially hydrolyzed whey infant formula: literature review on effects on growth and the risk of developing atopic dermatitis in infants from the general population. *Int Arch Allergy Immunol*. 2018;177(2):123–134.
42. Mennella JA, Inamdar L, Pressman N, et al. Type of infant formula increases early weight gain and impacts energy balance: a randomized controlled trial. *Am J Clin Nutr*. 2018;108(5):1015–1025.
43. Mennella JA, Papas MA, Reiter AR, Stallings VA, Trabulsi JC. Early rapid weight gain among formula-fed infants: impact of formula type and maternal feeding styles. *Pediatr Obes*. 2019;14:e12503.
44. Mennella JA, Trabulsi JC, Papas MA. Effects of cow milk versus extensive protein hydrolysate formulas on infant cognitive development. *Amino Acids*. 2016;48(3):697–705.
45. Alexander DD, Schmitt DF, Tran NL, Barraj LM, Cushing CA. Partially hydrolyzed 100% whey protein infant formula and atopic dermatitis risk reduction: a systematic review of the literature. *Nutr Rev*. 2010;68(4):232–245.
46. Vandenplas Y, Latiff AHA, Fleischer DM, et al. Partially hydrolyzed formula in non-exclusively breastfed infants: a systematic review and expert consensus. *Nutrition*. 2019;57:268–274.
47. Greer FR, Sicherer SH, Burks AW. The effects of early nutritional interventions on the development of atopic disease in infants and children: the role of maternal dietary restriction, breastfeeding, hydrolyzed formulas, and timing of introduction of allergenic complementary foods. *Pediatrics*. 2019;143(4). pii: e20190281.
48. Aceti A, Beghetti I, Maggio L, Martini S, Faldella G, Corvaglia L. Filling the gaps: current research directions for a rational use of probiotics in preterm infants. *Nutrients*. 2018;10(10).
49. Braegger C, Chmielewska A, Decsi T, et al. Supplementation of infant formula with probiotics and/or prebiotics: a systematic review and comment by the ESPGHAN committee on nutrition. *J Pediatr Gastroenterol Nutr*. 2011;52(2):238–250.
50. Aceti A, Maggio L, Beghetti I, et al. Probiotics prevent late-onset sepsis in human milk-fed, very low birth weight preterm infants: systematic review and meta-analysis. *Nutrients*. 2017;9(8).

51. van den Akker CHP, van Goudoever JB, Szajewska H, et al. Probiotics for preterm infants: a strain-specific systematic review and network meta-analysis. *J Pediatr Gastroenterol Nutr.* 2018; 67(1):103–122.
52. Sung V, D'Amico F, Cabana MD, et al. Lactobacillus reuteri to treat infant colic: a meta-analysis. *Pediatrics.* 2018;141(1).
53. Thomas JP, Raine T, Reddy S, Belteki G. Probiotics for the prevention of necrotising enterocolitis in very low-birth-weight infants: a meta-analysis and systematic review. *Acta Paediatr.* 2017;106(11): 1729–1741.
54. Kolacek S, Hojsak I, Berni Canani R, et al. Commercial probiotic products: a call for improved quality control. A position paper by the ESPGHAN working group for probiotics and prebiotics. *J Pediatr Gastroenterol Nutr.* 2017;65(1):117–124.
55. Ballard O, Morrow AL. Human milk composition: nutrients and bioactive factors. *Pediatr Clin N Am.* 2013;60(1):49–74.
56. Hernell O, Timby N, Domellof M, Lonnerdal B. Clinical benefits of milk fat globule membranes for infants and children. *J Pediatr.* 2016;173(Suppl):S60–S65.
57. Timby N, Hernell O, Vaarala O, Melin M, Lonnerdal B, Domellof M. Infections in infants fed formula supplemented with bovine milk fat globule membranes. *J Pediatr Gastroenterol Nutr.* 2015;60(3):384–389.
58. Timby N, Domellof E, Hernell O, Lonnerdal B, Domellof M. Neurodevelopment, nutrition, and growth until 12 mo of age in infants fed a low-energy, low-protein formula supplemented with bovine milk fat globule membranes: a randomized controlled trial. *Am J Clin Nutr.* 2014;99(4):860–868.
59. Denne SC. Protein and energy requirements in preterm infants. *Semin Neonatol.* 2001;6(5):377–382.
60. Horbar JD, Ehrenkranz RA, Badger GJ, et al. Weight growth velocity and postnatal growth failure in infants 501 to 1500 grams: 2000–2013. *Pediatrics.* 2015;136(1):e84–92.
61. Hay WW, Ziegler EE. Growth failure among preterm infants due to insufficient protein is not innocuous and must be prevented. *J Perinatol.* 2016;36(7):500–502.
62. Cleminson JS, Zalewski SP, Embleton ND. Nutrition in the preterm infant: what's new? *Curr Opin Clin Nutr Metab Care.* 2016; 19(3):220–225.
63. Hay Jr WW, Hendrickson KC. Preterm formula use in the preterm very low birth weight infant. *Semin Fetal Neonatal Med.* 2017;22(1): 15–22.
64. Ramel SE, Brown LD, Georgieff MK. The impact of neonatal illness on nutritional requirements-one size does not fit all. *Curr Pediatr Rep.* 2014;2(4):248–254.
65. Patel P, Bhatia J. Total parenteral nutrition for the very low birth weight infant. *Semin Fetal Neonatal Med.* 2017;22(1):2–7.
66. Corpeleijn WE, Kouwenhoven SM, Paap MC, et al. Intake of own mother's milk during the first days of life is associated with decreased morbidity and mortality in very low birth weight infants during the first 60 days of life. *Neonatology.* 2012;102(4): 276–281.
67. Morgan J, Young L, McGuire W. Delayed introduction of progressive enteral feeds to prevent necrotising enterocolitis in very low birth weight infants. *Cochrane Database Syst Rev.* 2014;(12): Cd001970.
68. Miller J, Tonkin E, Damarell RA, et al. A systematic review and meta-analysis of human milk feeding and morbidity in very low birth weight infants. *Nutrients.* 2018;10(6).
69. de Halleux V, Pieltain C, Senterre T, Rigo J. Use of donor milk in the neonatal intensive care unit. *Semin Fetal Neonatal Med.* 2017; 22(1):23–29.
70. Quigley M, Embleton ND, McGuire W. Formula versus donor breast milk for feeding preterm or low birth weight infants. *Cochrane Database Syst Rev.* 2018;6:Cd002971.
71. Pillai A, Albersheim S, Matheson J, et al. Evaluation of a concentrated preterm formula as a liquid human milk fortifier in preterm babies at increased risk of feed intolerance. *Nutrients.* 2018;10(10).
72. Gertz B, DeFranco E. Predictors of breastfeeding non-initiation in the NICU. *Matern Child Nutr.* 2019:e12797.
73. Geraghty SR, Riddle SW, Shaikh U. The breastfeeding mother and the pediatrician. *J Hum Lactation.* 2008;24(3):335–339.
74. Boundy EO, Dastjerdi R, Spiegelman D, et al. Kangaroo mother care and neonatal outcomes: a meta-analysis. *Pediatrics.* 2016;137(1).
75. Villamor-Martínez E, Pierro M, Cavallaro G, Mosca F, Kramer BW, Villamor E. Donor human milk protects against bronchopulmonary dysplasia: a systematic review and meta-analysis. *Nutrients.* 2018;10(2).
76. Mohd-Taufek N, Cartwright D, Davies M, et al. The effect of pasteurization on trace elements in donor breast milk. *J Perinatol.* 2016;36(10):897–900.
77. Young BE, Borman LL, Heinrich R, Long J, Pinney S, Westcott J, Krebs NF. Effect of pooling practices and time postpartum of milk donations on the energy, macronutrient, and zinc concentrations of resultant donor human milk pools. *J Pediatr.* 2019;214: 54–59.
78. Krebs NF. Update on zinc deficiency and excess in clinical pediatric practice. *Ann Nutr Metab.* 2013;62(Suppl 1):19–29.
79. Bhatia J. Growth curves: how to best measure growth of the preterm infant. *J Pediatr.* 2013;162(3 Suppl):S2–S6.
80. Fenton TR, Kim JH. A systematic review and meta-analysis to revise the Fenton growth chart for preterm infants. *BMC Pediatr.* 2013;13:59.
81. Olsen IE, Groveman SA, Lawson ML, Clark RH, Zemel BS. New intrauterine growth curves based on United States data. *Pediatrics.* 2010;125(2):e214–224.
82. Villar J, Giuliani F, Fenton TR, Ohuma EO, Ismail LC, Kennedy SH. INTERGROWTH-21st very preterm size at birth reference charts. *Lancet.* 2016;387(10021):844–845.
83. Abrams SA. Calcium and vitamin d requirements of enterally fed preterm infants. *Pediatrics.* 2013;131(5):e1676–1683.
84. Burton BK. Inborn errors of metabolism in infancy: a guide to diagnosis. *Pediatrics.* 1998;102(6):E69.
85. Berry SA, Brown C, Grant M, et al. Newborn screening 50 years later: access issues faced by adults with PKU. *Genet Med.* 2013; 15(8):591–599.
86. Brown CS, Lichter-Konecki U. Phenylketonuria (PKU): a problem solved? *Mol Genet Metab Rep.* 2016;6:8–12.
87. Kose E, Aksoy B, Kuyum P, Tuncer N, Arslan N, Ozturk Y. The effects of breastfeeding in infants with phenylketonuria. *J Pediatr Nurs.* 2018;38:27–32.
88. Lawrence RM. Circumstances when breastfeeding is contraindicated. *Pediatr Clin N Am.* 2013;60(1):295–318.
89. Pinto A, Adams S, Ahring K, et al. Early feeding practices in infants with phenylketonuria across Europe. *Mol Genet Metab Rep.* 2018;16:82–89.
90. Wanes D, Husein DM, Naim HY. Congenital lactase deficiency: mutations, functional and biochemical implications, and future perspectives. *Nutrients.* 2019;11(2).
91. Carlock G, Fischer ST, Lynch ME, et al. Developmental outcomes in Duarte galactosemia. *Pediatrics.* 2019;143(1).
92. Wagner CL, Greer FR. Prevention of rickets and vitamin D deficiency in infants, children, and adolescents. *Pediatrics.* 2008; 122(5):1142–1152.
93. Hollis BW, Wagner CL, Howard CR, et al. Maternal versus infant vitamin D supplementation during lactation: a randomized controlled trial. *Pediatrics.* 2015;136(4):625–634.
94. Krebs NF, Sherlock LG, Westcott J, et al. Effects of different complementary feeding regimens on iron status and enteric microbiota in breastfed infants. *J Pediatr.* 2013;163(2):416–423.

95. Young BE, Krebs NF. Complementary feeding: critical considerations to optimize growth, nutrition, and feeding behavior. *Curr Pediatr Rep*. 2013;1(4):247–256.
96. Sazawal S, Black RE, Ramsan M, et al. Effects of routine prophylactic supplementation with iron and folic acid on admission to hospital and mortality in preschool children in a high malaria transmission setting: community-based, randomised, placebo-controlled trial. *Lancet*. 2006;367(9505):133–143.
97. Tang M, Frank DN, Hendricks AE, et al. Iron in micronutrient powder promotes an unfavorable gut microbiota in Kenyan infants. *Nutrients*. 2017;9(7).
98. Georgieff MK. Long-term brain and behavioral consequences of early iron deficiency. *Nutr Rev*. 2011;69(Suppl 1):S43–S48.
99. Lozoff B, Clark KM, Jing Y, Armony-Sivan R, Angelilli ML, Jacobson SW. Dose-response relationships between iron deficiency with or without anemia and infant social-emotional behavior. *J Pediatr*. 2008;152(5):696–702, 702.631-693.
100. Cusick SE, Georgieff MK, Rao R. Approaches for reducing the risk of early-life iron deficiency-induced brain dysfunction in children. *Nutrients*. 2018;10(2).
101. Sypes EE, Parkin PC, Birken CS, et al. Higher body mass index is associated with iron deficiency in children 1 to 3 years of age. *J Pediatr*. 2019;207:198–204. e1.
102. Oatley H, Borkhoff CM, Chen S, et al. Screening for iron deficiency in early childhood using serum ferritin in the primary care setting. *Pediatrics*. 2018;142(6).
103. Andersson O, Hellstrom-Westas L, Andersson D, Domellof M. Effect of delayed versus early umbilical cord clamping on neonatal outcomes and iron status at 4 months: a randomised controlled trial. *BMJ*. 2011;343:d7157.
104. Tang M, Hendricks AE, Krebs NF. A meat- or dairy-based complementary diet leads to distinct growth patterns in formula-fed infants: a randomized controlled trial. *Am J Clin Nutr*. 2018; 107(5):734–742.
105. Tang M, Andersen V, Hendricks AE, Krebs NF. Different growth patterns persist at 24 months of age in formula-fed infants randomized to consume a meat- or dairy-based complementary diet from 5 to 12 months of age. *J Pediatr*. 2019;206:78–82.
106. Heyman MB, Abrams SA. Fruit juice in infants, children, and adolescents: current recommendations. *Pediatrics*. 2017;139(6).
107. Togias A, Cooper SF, Acebal ML, et al. Addendum guidelines for the prevention of peanut allergy in the United States: report of the National Institute of Allergy and Infectious Diseases-sponsored expert panel. *J Allergy Clin Immunol*. 2017;139(1):29–44.
108. Du Toit G, Roberts G, Sayre PH, et al. Randomized trial of peanut consumption in infants at risk for peanut allergy. *N Engl J Med*. 2015;372(9):803–813.
109. Perkin MR, Logan K, Tseng A, et al. Randomized trial of introduction of allergenic foods in breast-fed infants. *N Engl J Med*. 2016; 374(18):1733–1743.
110. Bertrand KA, Hanan NJ, Honerkamp-Smith G, Best BM, Chambers CD. Marijuana use by breastfeeding mothers and cannabinoid concentrations in breast milk. *Pediatrics*. 2018;142(3).
111. Little RE, Northstone K, Golding J. Alcohol, breastfeeding, and development at 18 months. *Pediatrics*. 2002;109(5):E72.
112. Mennella JA, Gerrish CJ. Effects of exposure to alcohol in mother's milk on infant sleep. *Pediatrics*. 1998;101(5):E2.
113. World Health Organization. *Breastfeeding*; 2019. https://www.who.int/nutrition/topics/exclusive_breastfeeding/en/. Accessed January 14, 2019.
114. Hartman C, Shamir R, Hecht C, Koletzko B. Malnutrition screening tools for hospitalized children. *Curr Opin Clin Nutr Metab Care*. 2012;15(3):303–309.
115. Mehta NM, Skillman HE, Irving SY, et al. Guidelines for the provision and assessment of nutrition support therapy in the pediatric critically ill patient: society of critical care medicine and American society for parenteral and enteral nutrition. *J Parenter Enter Nutr*. 2017;41(5):706–742.
116. Leroue MK, Good RJ, Skillman HE, Czaja AS. Enteral nutrition practices in critically ill children requiring noninvasive positive pressure ventilation. *Pediatr Crit Care Med*. 2017;18(12):1093–1098.
117. Ladd AK, Skillman HE, Haemer MA, Mourani PM. Preventing underfeeding and overfeeding: a clinician's guide to the acquisition and implementation of indirect calorimetry. *Nutr Clin Pract*. 2018;33(2):198–205.
118. American Society of Anesthesiologists. Practice guidelines for preoperative fasting and the use of pharmacologic agents to reduce the risk of pulmonary aspiration: application to healthy patients undergoing elective procedures: an updated report by the American society of anesthesiologists task force on preoperative fasting and the use of pharmacologic agents to reduce the risk of pulmonary aspiration. *Anesthesiology*. 2017;126(3): 376–393.

CHAPTER

2

NUTRIENT NEEDS AND REQUIREMENTS DURING GROWTH

Elizabeth Prout Parks[1,2], *MD, MSCE*
Maria R. Mascarenhas[1,2], *MBBS*
Vi Goh[1,2], *MD, MS*

[1]Perelman School of Medicine, University of Pennsylvania, Philadelphia, PA, United States
[2]Gastroenterology, Hepatology and Nutrition, The Children's Hospital of Philadelphia, Philadelphia, PA, United States

SUMMARY

Childhood and adolescence are important periods during which major biological, social, physiological, and cognitive changes take place and nutrition plays a key role. The nutritional requirements of children change as they grow and develop and depend on growth rate, total body size, and activity levels. In adolescents, these requirements are even higher than those of children because of the growth spurt, sexual maturation, changes in body composition, skeletal mineralization, and changes in physical activity. In this chapter, we will review the nutritional needs for children and adolescents with special emphasis on feeding recommendations for children and obesity and pregnancy in adolescents.

Keywords: Adolescence; Childhood; Feeding; Nutrient needs; Obesity; Pregnancy.

I. INTRODUCTION

Nutrition plays an important role in the growth and development of all children from birth through adolescence. When nutritional needs are not met then, growth and development are affected resulting in malnutrition, stunting, developmental, and cognitive delays. This is true not only for macronutrients but also for micronutrients with strong supportive evidence for iron and zinc. In this chapter, we will review the needs for children and adolescents (infant requirements, Section B, Chapter 1).

II. CHILDHOOD

The nutritional requirements of children change as they grow and develop. Children require adequate intakes of energy, protein, and other essential nutrients for the typical patterns of growth and development. Nutrient needs vary depending on growth rate, total body size, and physical activity levels. Toddlers have slower growth rate compared to infants, and this growth rate continues through childhood until the growth spurt of adolescence. Healthy food patterns will provide children with adequate nutrients for growth and development.

A. Growth Rates

Anthropometric assessment is the best way to determine whether children are well nourished. In healthy children with well-balanced diets, their growth rates are usually predictable. A child's birth weight typically triples by 12 months of age and quadruples by 2 years of age. Average weight gain is 7 g/day by the end of second year and slows to relatively steady rate of 2–3 kg/year until adolescent growth spurt begins.[1]

Linear growth is approximately 9 cm a year at the end of second year and 8 cm a year at the end of third year. A child typically reaches 50% of adult height at 2 years of age and approximately 80% of adult height at 10 years of age. The height gain velocity in both males and females is consistent at 5–8 cm/year from

Present Knowledge in Nutrition, Volume 2
https://doi.org/10.1016/B978-0-12-818460-8.00002-2

3 to 10 years of age.[1] The average head circumference of a newborn in the United States (US) is approximately 34 cm, doubles during first year of life, and increases to 50 cm by 3 years of age. Thereafter, head circumference does not change markedly.[2,3] Weight and height (or length for children < 24 months old) are plotted on growth charts to determine whether they are maintaining their growth trajectory. The current US recommendation is to plot children <24 months of age on the WHO growth charts (Fig. 2.1) and those >24 months of age on the CDC growth charts (Fig. 2.2). For children <24 months old, the relationship between weight and length can be plotted on the WHO weight for length chart and >24 months old, and the body mass index (BMI) can be plotted on the CDC growth chart. Appropriate weights and lengths/heights, according to age and sex, lie between the 5th and 85th percentiles, allowing for individual differences in body build.

B. Nutrient Requirements

Energy

Energy intake recommendations are intended to maintain health, promote optimal growth and maturation, and support a desirable level of physical activity. Energy needs are highly variable in children and depend on basal metabolism, rate of growth, physical activity, body size, and sex. Since the annual weight gain, length/height gain, and growth in head circumferences decrease between years 1 and 3, there is concurrent decrease in energy needs when expressed per kilo body weight.

Between 15 and 24 months of age, most children are eating the same foods as the rest of the family, and approximately 60% of energy comes from table foods.[4] Milk is still the leading source of daily energy (approximately 25%), macronutrients, and many vitamins and minerals, including vitamins A and D, calcium, and zinc.[5] At this time, a diet based on an appropriate number of servings and portion sizes from the various food groups in additional to milk will provide adequate amounts of most nutrients.

As the child gets older and intake of solid foods increases, the intake of milk decreases. It is important at this stage to provide well-balanced, appropriate portion size foods and to model healthy eating patterns for children during mealtime and snacks to promote long-term healthy eating habits. In the preadolescent age (7–9 years old), children are laying down energy reserves in preparation for the adolescent growth spurt and energy intake may increase. However, excessive weight gain in anticipation of this growth spurt may result in childhood weight problems with increased risk of overweight/obesity.

Most children's diets contain adequate amount of energy, carbohydrate, protein, and fat. However, children's intake of "extra" or additional calories from sugars are notably high especially from snacks representing nearly 28%–44% of daily energy intake, 32% of carbohydrate, and 39% of added sugars.[6–8] Sweetened beverages contribute to 25% of all added sugars obtained from snacks. Approximately 50% of 3-year-olds in the US consume sweetened beverages and 75% consume desserts or candies on any given day,[9] and they are top sources of sugar intake in children. This snacking pattern results in high-energy intakes in preschool- and school-aged children.[6,10,11] Increased frequency of snacking has also been associated with greater intake of energy-rich, nutrient-poor foods. Juice intake should be limited to 4oz/day in children 1- to 3-year-olds, to 4–6 oz/day for 4- to 6-year-olds, and 8 oz/day for 7- to 18-year-olds.

Protein

Similar to energy needs, protein needs correlate more closely with a child's growth pattern than with chronological age. The Dietary Reference Intake (DRI) for protein is based on the amount of protein needed for age, sex, and growth and positive nitrogen balance. Average protein intake of US children is well above the Recommended Dietary Allowance (RDA) for all age groups. The RDA of protein for 1 to 3-year-olds is 1.05 g/kg/day and 4- to 8-year-olds is 0.95 g/kg/day.[12] When total energy intake is inadequate, dietary protein may be used to meet energy needs, making it unavailable for synthesis of new tissue or for tissue repair. This may lead to reduction in growth rate and a decrease in lean body mass. Excess protein consumption, whether from food or supplements (as in adolescent athletes), could lead to excessive weight gain and calcium loss and potentially affect renal function.

Fat

In healthy children younger than 2 years of age, the American Academy of Pediatrics (AAP) recommends against fat restriction due to rapid growth and development requiring high energy intake.[13] Therefore, skimmed or low-fat milks are not recommended for use during the first 2 years of life. Fat intake after 2 years of age should subsequently be decreased gradually to provide approximately 30% of total energy[13,14]. Transitioning the diet to provide less energy from fat can be achieved by increasing the intake of naturally low-fat products such as fruits, vegetables, beans, lean meat, fish, and whole grain foods.

There have been concerns that some parents may have overinterpreted the emphasis on supporting lower fat diets. Indeed, 23% of toddlers 12–23 months of age and 47% of preschool-aged children 24–47 months of age consume less total fat than recommended.[7] At the

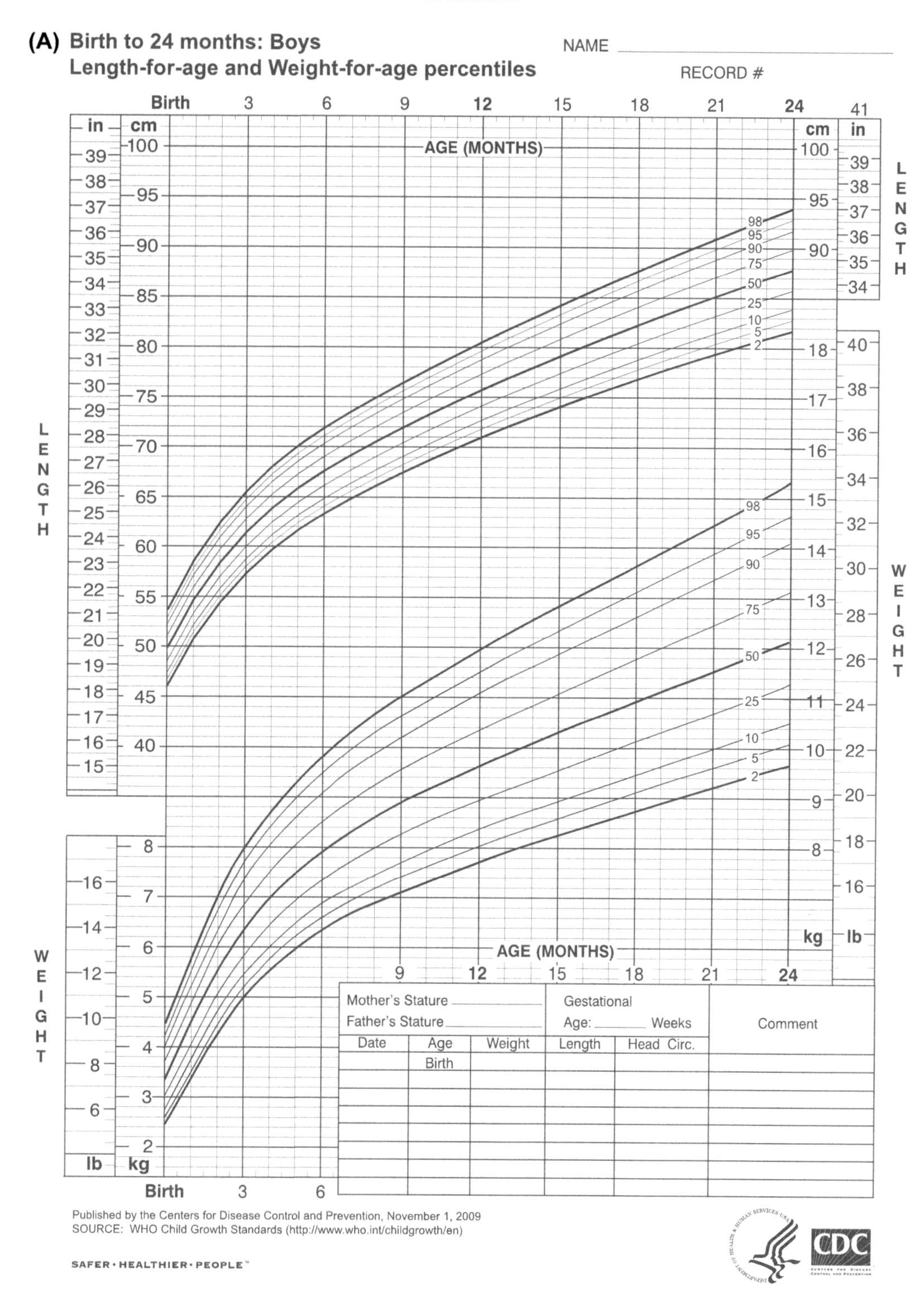

FIGURE 2.1 (A) Birth to 24 months: boys length-for-age percentiles and weight-for-age percentiles, (B) Birth to 24 months: boys weight-for-length percentiles and head circumference-for-age percentiles, (C) Birth to 24 months: girls length-for-age percentiles and weight-for-age percentiles, (D) Birth to 24 months: girls weight-for-length percentiles and head circumference-for-age percentiles

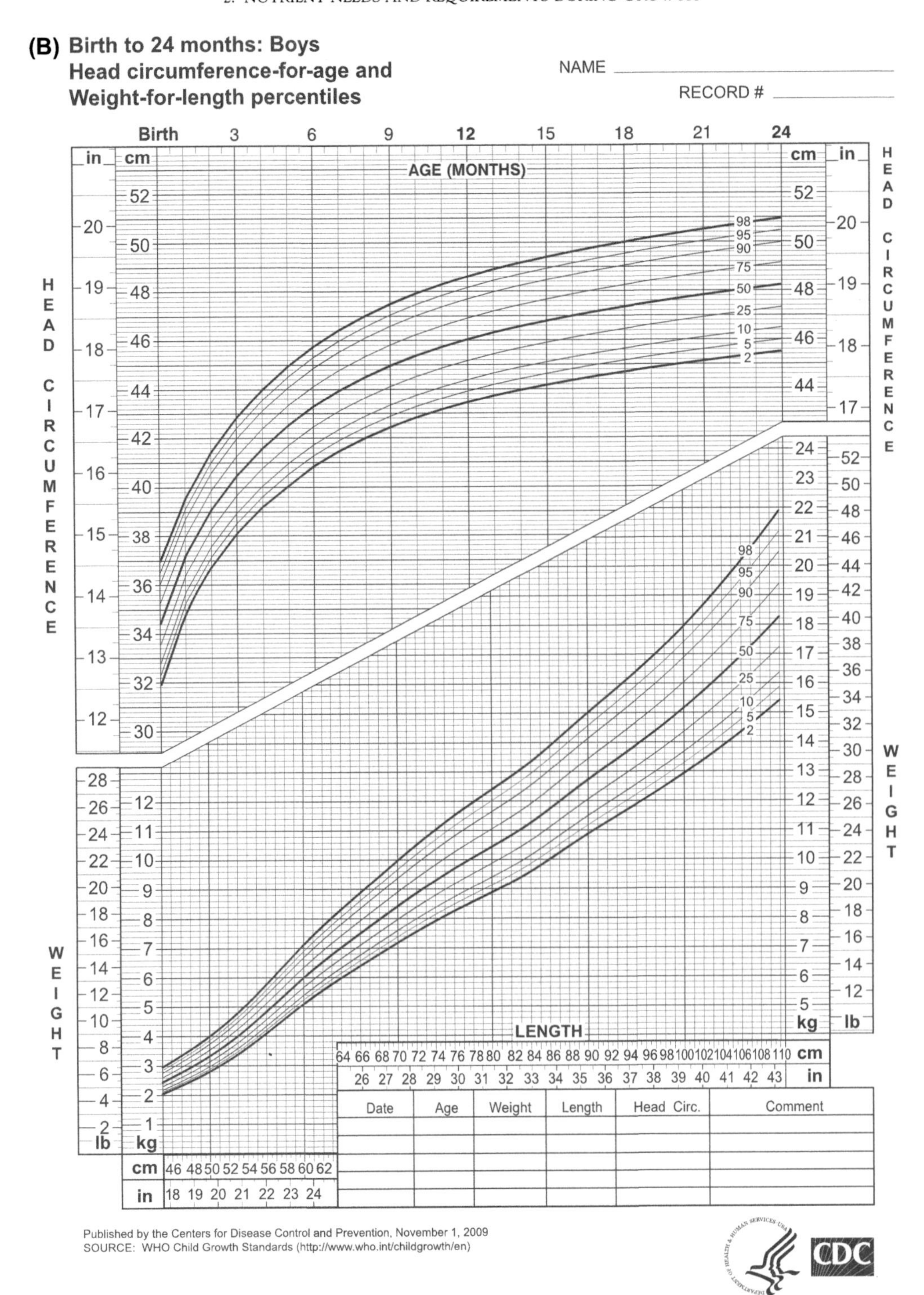

FIGURE 2.1 Cont'd

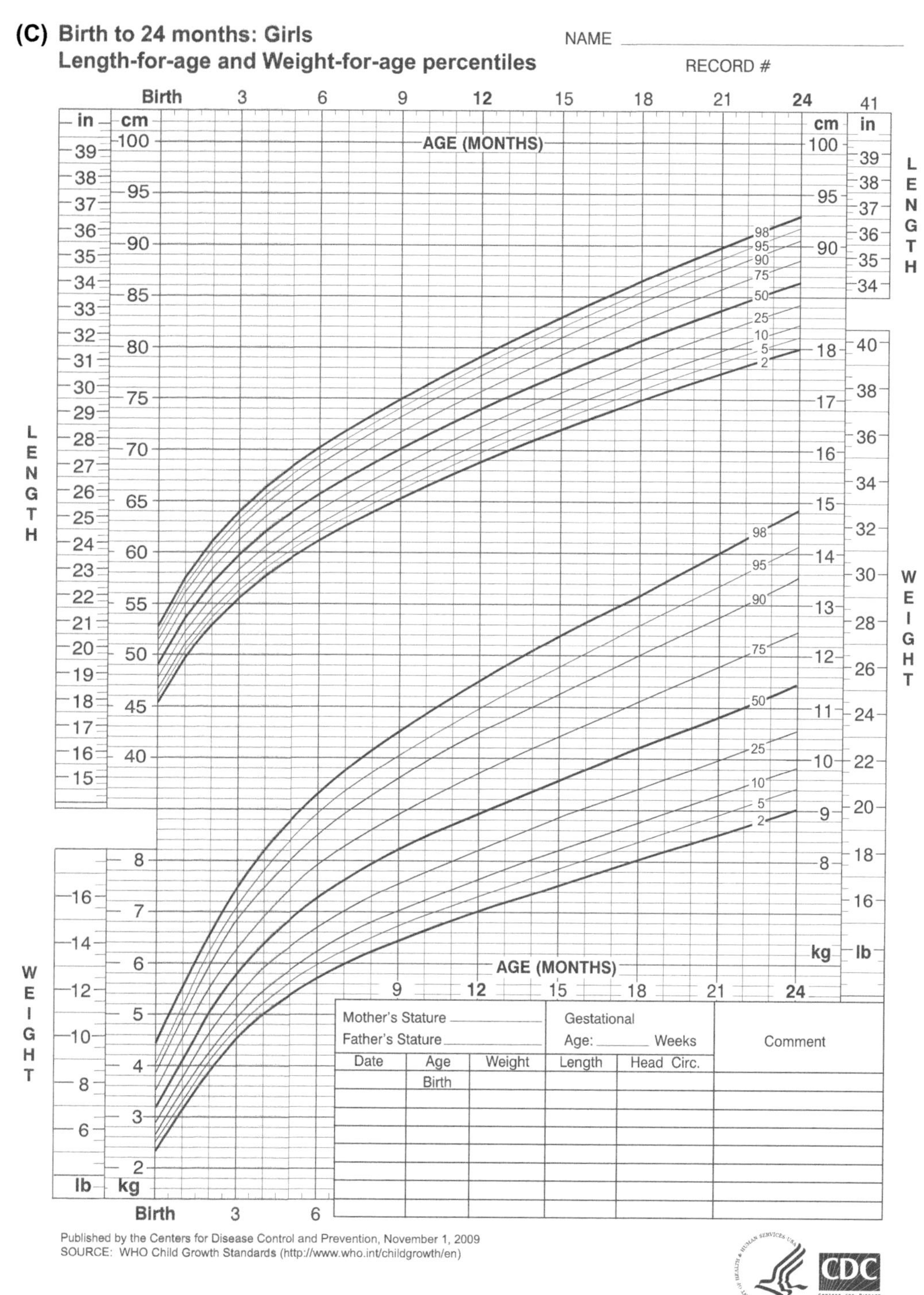

FIGURE 2.1 Cont'd

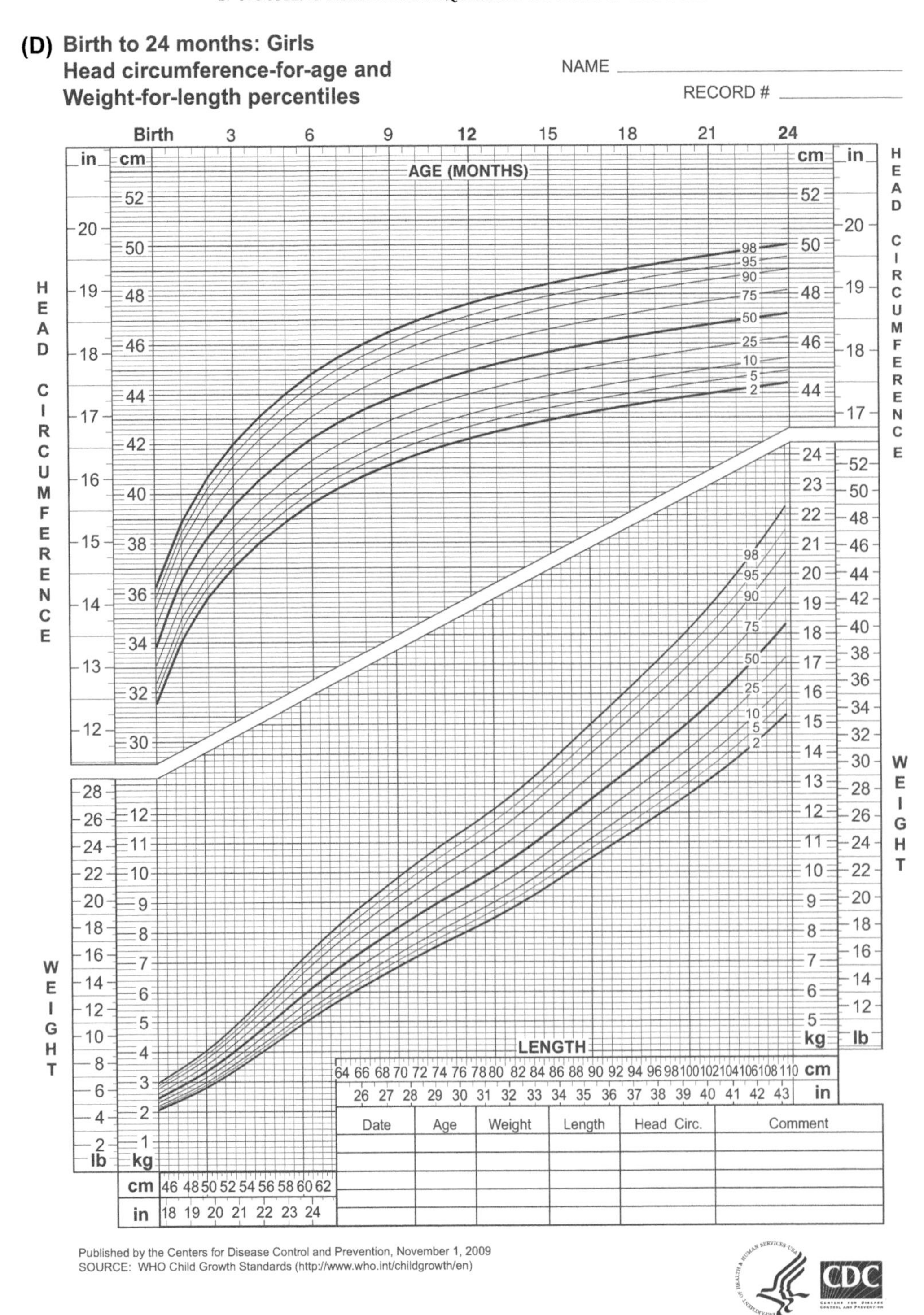

FIGURE 2.1 Cont'd

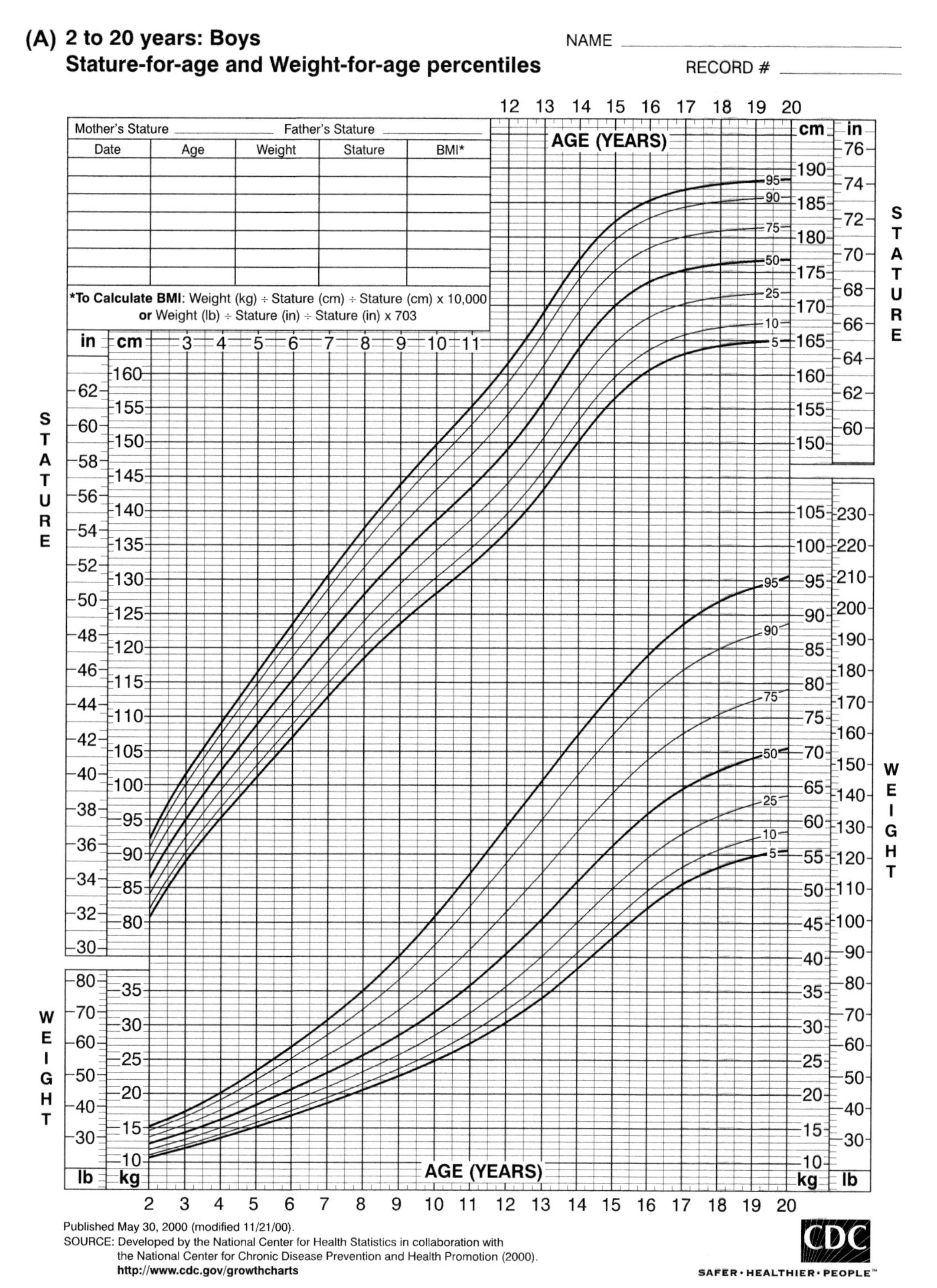

FIGURE 2.2 (A) 2 to 20 years: Boys stature-for-age and weight-for-age, (B) 2 to 20 years: Boys BMI-for-age, (C) 2 to 20 years: Girls stature-for-age and weight-for-age, (D) 2 to 20 years: Girls BMI-for-age

(B) 2 to 20 years: Boys
Body mass index-for-age percentiles

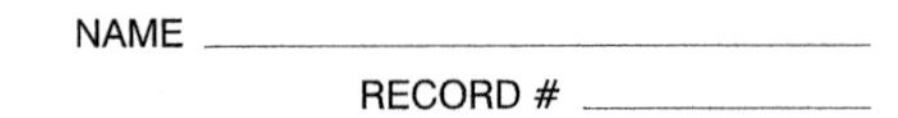

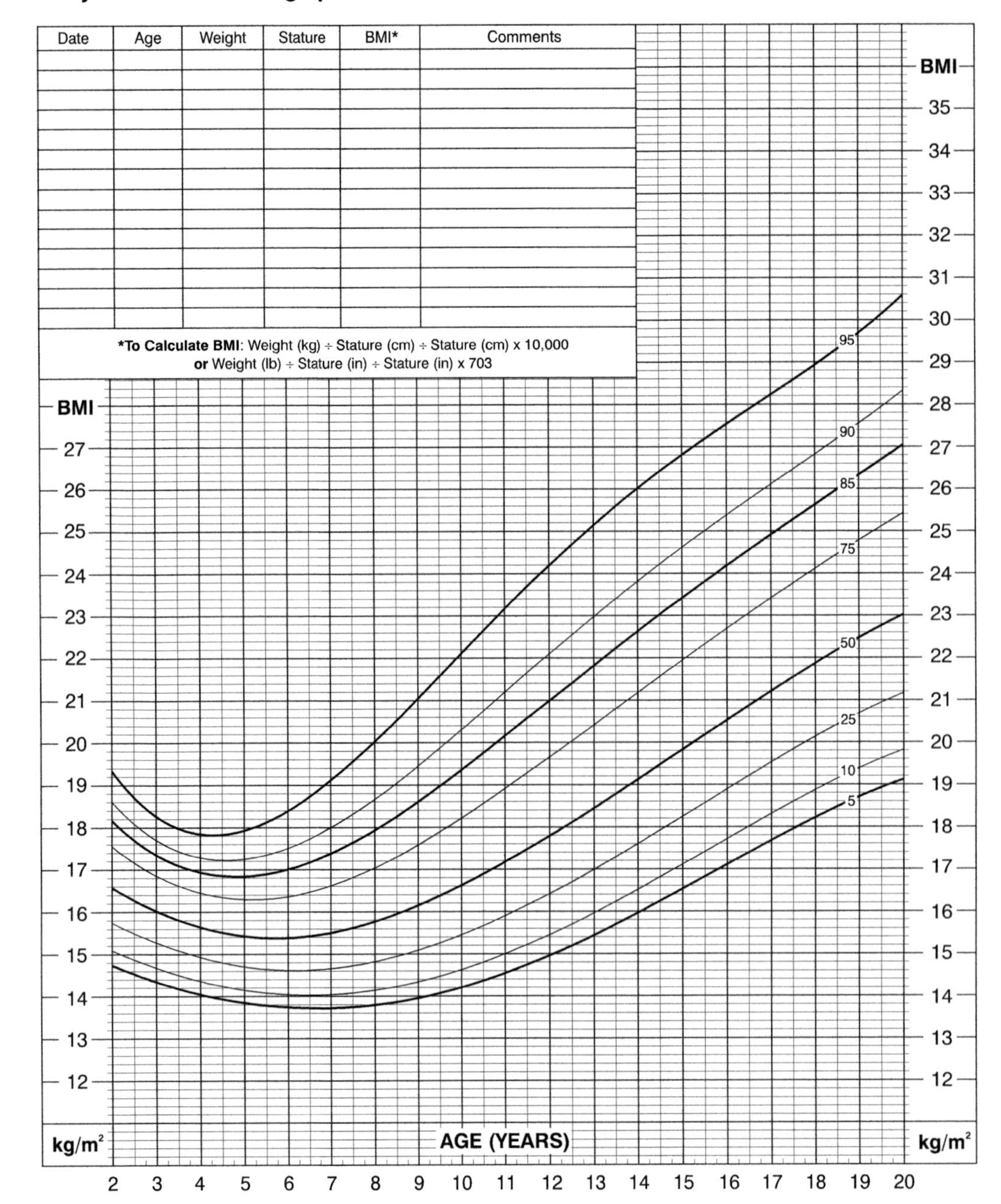

Published May 30, 2000 (modified 10/16/00).
SOURCE: Developed by the National Center for Health Statistics in collaboration with the National Center for Chronic Disease Prevention and Health Promotion (2000).
http://www.cdc.gov/growthcharts

CDC
SAFER • HEALTHIER • PEOPLE™

FIGURE 2.2 Cont'd

(C) 2 to 20 years: Girls
Stature-for-age and Weight-for-age percentiles

NAME ______________________

RECORD # __________

Mother's Stature ______________ Father's Stature ______________

Date	Age	Weight	Stature	BMI*

***To Calculate BMI**: Weight (kg) ÷ Stature (cm) ÷ Stature (cm) x 10,000
or Weight (lb) ÷ Stature (in) ÷ Stature (in) x 703

AGE (YEARS)

12 13 14 15 16 17 18 19 20

STATURE (in): 30 32 34 36 38 40 42 44 46 48 50 52 54 56 58 60 62 64 66 68 70 72 74 76

STATURE (cm): 80 85 90 95 100 105 110 115 120 125 130 135 140 145 150 155 160 165 170 175 180 185 190

Percentiles: 5 10 25 50 75 90 95

WEIGHT (kg): 10 15 20 25 30 35 40 45 50 55 60 65 70 75 80 85 90 95 100 105

WEIGHT (lb): 30 40 50 60 70 80 90 100 110 120 130 140 150 160 170 180 190 200 210 220 230

AGE (YEARS)

2 3 4 5 6 7 8 9 10 11 12 13 14 15 16 17 18 19 20

Published May 30, 2000 (modified 11/21/00).
SOURCE: Developed by the National Center for Health Statistics in collaboration with the National Center for Chronic Disease Prevention and Health Promotion (2000).
http://www.cdc.gov/growthcharts

CDC
SAFER · HEALTHIER · PEOPLE™

FIGURE 2.2 Cont'd

(D) 2 to 20 years: Girls
Body mass index-for-age percentiles

NAME ______________

RECORD # ______________

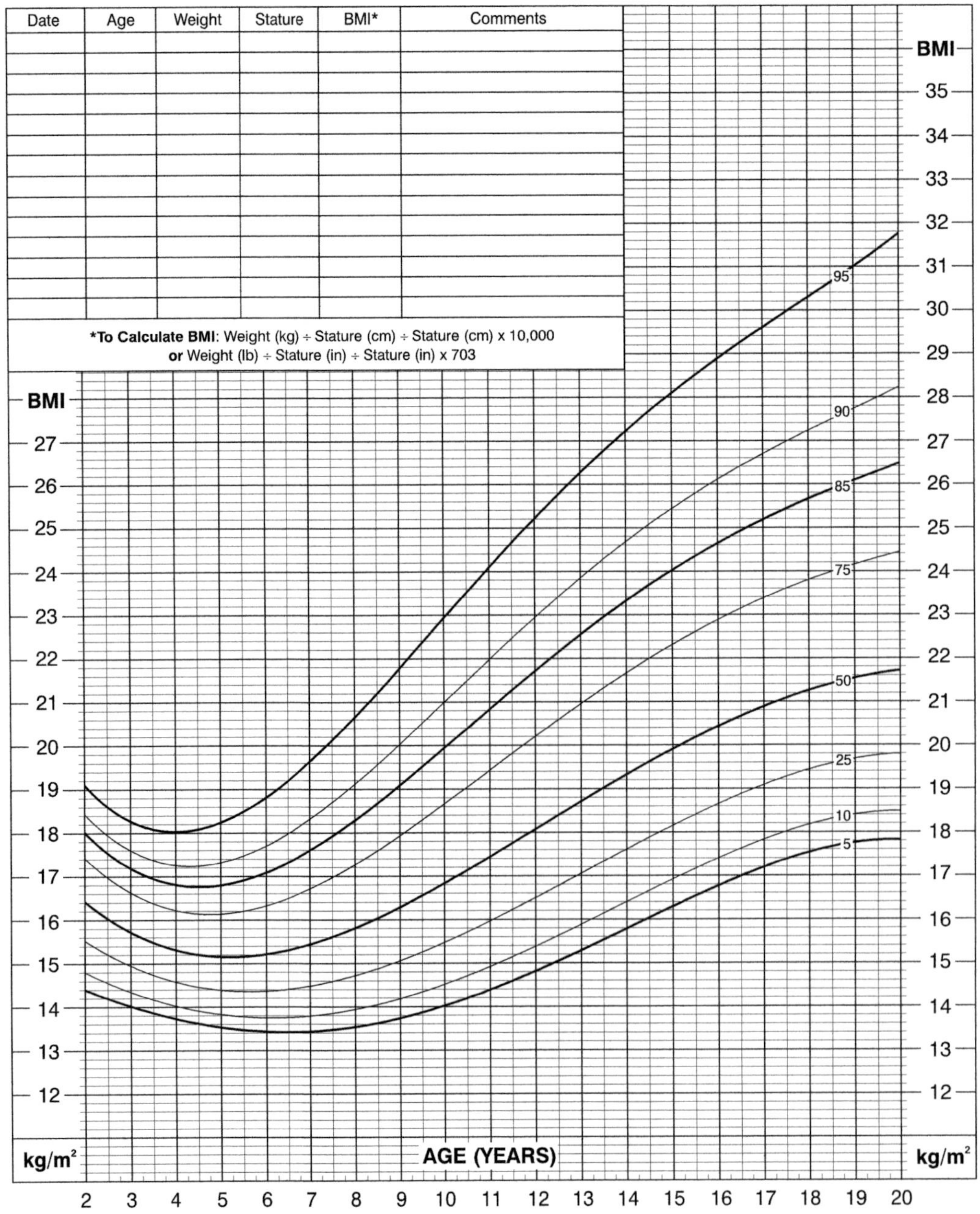

Date	Age	Weight	Stature	BMI*	Comments

***To Calculate BMI**: Weight (kg) ÷ Stature (cm) ÷ Stature (cm) x 10,000
or Weight (lb) ÷ Stature (in) ÷ Stature (in) x 703

BMI
35
34
33
32
31
30
29
28
27
26
25
24
23
22
21
20
19
18
17
16
15
14
13
12
kg/m²

95
90
85
75
50
25
10
5

AGE (YEARS)
2 3 4 5 6 7 8 9 10 11 12 13 14 15 16 17 18 19 20

Published May 30, 2000 (modified 10/16/00).
SOURCE: Developed by the National Center for Health Statistics in collaboration with the National Center for Chronic Disease Prevention and Health Promotion (2000).
http://www.cdc.gov/growthcharts

CDC
SAFER • HEALTHIER • PEOPLE™

FIGURE 2.2 Cont'd

same time, about 6% of preschool-aged children consume higher levels of saturated fats than recommended. Yogurt consumption in children has been associated with lower total fat and saturated intakes and lower body fat composition.[15] Essential fatty acids (linoleic and alpha-linolenic acid) need to be consumed in adequate amount to prevent deficiency that has been shown in infants and children consuming low-fat diet or with severe fat malabsorption with certain diseases.[16,17] Essential fatty acids are required for normal function of tissues. Deficiency can result in wide variety of symptoms including dermatitis, reduced growth rate, hair loss, increased susceptibility to infections, liver dysfunction, depressed adenosine triphosphate synthesis, changes in brain, and retinal development in children.[18]

Micronutrients

Vitamins and minerals play an important role in the health and growth of children. Parent often give vitamins and minerals supplementation to their children, with recent estimation that approximately 21% of toddlers and 40% preschool-aged children are given some types of daily supplement. Children may not need vitamin or mineral supplements if they are healthy children who consume a well-balanced diet. Prior to prescribing a vitamin/mineral supplement, an evaluation of dietary intake should be completed. For children and adolescent who cannot or will not consume adequate amount of micronutrients, the use of mineral supplements should be considered. Vitamin D is the most common dietary supplement with 20% of toddlers and approximately 40% of preschool children taking vitamin D. The AAP recommends that healthy children receiving a well-balanced diet do not need vitamin supplementation over the RDA, which is 600 IU/day of vitamin D for children over 1 year of age. Iron supplements on the other hand were consumed by fewer than 10%.[7,19] Iron deficiency causes anemia, depressed mental and motor development, impaired cognitive performance including depressed school achievement into middle childhood, poor immune function, and decreased work performance.[20–22] The mechanism of the role of iron in cognitive development is not fully understood, but some studies have identified the role of iron in normal myelination and neurotransmitter function[21,23]. For children >2 years of age, short-term treatment of iron deficiency is associated with improvement in cognition but not in school achievement.[21] Due to the evidence of adverse effect of iron deficiency in children, the goal is to prevent iron deficiency by encouraging dietary intake of diverse foods with bioavailable iron, fortification of foods targeted for children, and providing iron supplementation when indicated by high risk of iron deficiency. Approximately 25% of 2-year-olds consume salty snacks daily and nearly 50% consume higher than recommended intake of sodium,[7,9] which could potentially lead to other long-term health risks of hypertension and cardiovascular disease.

Due to the many health benefits of the micronutrient-rich fruits and vegetables, the US Dietary Guidelines recommend 2 cups of fruit and 2 ½ cups of vegetables per day for an older child or a young adult consuming 2000 calories. The daily recommendation for fruit and vegetable intake is 1 cup for 2- to 3-year-olds and 1.5 cups for 4- to 8-year-olds, respectively.[24] Fruit and vegetable intake among young children is below recommendations.[25,75] Approximately one-third of 2-year-olds do not consume any vegetables or fruit on a given day. The most commonly consumed vegetables are French fries and fried potatoes,[9] and the most commonly consumed fruits are applesauce and fruit cocktail, which are low-fiber fruits.[26] As such, a majority of preschool-aged children consume less than the recommended amounts of fiber.[7] Despite low fruit and vegetable intake, most healthy children ingest sufficient amount of vitamins and minerals from fruit, vegetable, and other food groups. Recent comparison of nutrient intakes from the feeding infant and toddlers study in the US showed that toddlers 12–23.9 months old were consuming diets low in vitamin D, vitamin K, iron, potassium, and calcium, whereas toddlers 2–4 years of age were consuming diets low in potassium, vitamin A, vitamin D, dietary fiber, and iron.[27] It has also been shown that children who consume high levels of added sugar (>25% of daily energy) have lower micronutrient intake, particularly calcium, potassium, and vitamins A and E.[28] Increased consumption of vegetables is required to address nutrient shortfalls of potassium, vitamin A, and dietary fiber.

C. Feeding Behavior

Toddlers (1–3 years)

Feeding behavior develops progressively during the toddler years with eventual acquisition of self-feeding skills. Oral and neuromuscular development improves the ability to eat; toddlers achieve gross motor skills required for holding a spoon and then develop fine motor skills needed to scoop food, dip food, and bring food to mouth with limited spilling.[29,30] The appearance of most of the primary teeth also leads toddlers to be able to bite and chew and support self-feeding and participation in family meals. The acquisition of language skills enables the toddler to verbally express eating preferences, hunger, and satiety. Use of finger foods, spoons, and cups should be encouraged to improve the development of manual dexterity and coordination. Supporting the acquisition of self-feeding skills is thought to encourage the maintenance of self-regulation of energy intake, the mastery of feeding skills, and the socialization of eating behaviors. Given earlier opportunities for mastery of self-feeding skills, the older toddler is ready to consume most of the same foods offered to the rest of the family in an age appropriate portion size. The AAP offers guidance on the numbers of meals and snacks in order to provide constant supply of nutrients to fuel children's activities; specifically, children 1–4 years of age should be given three main meals and two to three snacks spread throughout the day.[31] Toddlers should be seated at the high chair or at the dinner table at mealtime. Foods that could cause choking or aspiration such as nuts, hot dogs, uncut grapes, and popcorn should be avoided. Limits should be set so that the child is not eating throughout the day. It is common to have variable food intake at this stage. Most toddlers have decreased food intake relative to body size, compared to infancy, related to the reduction in growth rate with aging. Food preferences may be erratic, with foods readily accepted 1 day or for a period of time and then being rejected the next day. Toddlers may also become more selective with only consuming particular foods, and this is often worrisome to parents. The use of growth charts to demonstrate adequate growth and guidance about typical eating behavior will help reassure parents. New foods should be offered multiple times (up to 10 exposures) to promote acceptance. Although intake may appear erratic from meal to meal, most children have the capacity to adjust food intake such that daily energy intake remains fairly constant.[32] Toddlers should be offered a variety of foods from each of the six food groups, at regular intervals, with limited distractions. A typical pattern is 3 meals a day with two to three snacks. Goals of early childhood nutrition are to establish healthy eating habits and offer foods that are developmentally appropriate. Milk consumption usually gradually decreases as solid food intake increases. Around 12 months of age, children learn to drink from a cup, although some may still breastfeed or desire formula bottle feeding. Bottle weaning should start around 12–15 months, as extended bottle use has been associated with iron deficiency, obesity, and dental caries.[33–36] Bedtime bottles and use of fruit juice or sugar-sweetened beverages in bottles are discouraged because of the association with dental carries.[37] Unless being used at mealtime for milk, sippy cup devices should only contain water to prevent caries.

Early childhood (4–6 years)

Children 4–6 years of age are able to self-feed without assistance and although children's appetites may be variable. At this age, it has been shown that children may increase food portion size and consume more store-bought processed foods as they spend time away from home either at school or daycare.[38–40] With anticipatory guidance for parents regarding basic principles of nutrition and meal planning, nutritional deficiencies or excesses can be prevented. The nutrient quality of foods from all food groups should still be emphasized. Parents and caregivers are responsible for providing variety of nutritious foods, defining the structure and timing of meals. Children are responsible for their choices from food provided and have primary responsibility for determining how much is consumed at each eating occasion. Snacks or desserts high in sweets or of low nutritional value should be offered infrequently to prevent obesity and dental caries. Skim or low-fat milk may be substituted for whole milk, especially if the child is at risk of becoming overweight to decrease total caloric intake per day.[41]

Middle childhood (7–9 years)

Preadolescents' eating habits are often influenced more by peer pressure than by parents. Adaptation to school and peer eating habits may present nutritional problems. Meals may be skipped due to school schedules or preferences and snacks during the day may be unsupervised.[42,43] These adaptations may be less of a problem if sound eating habits were established earlier in life, such as the development of personal food preferences for healthier foods.[44,45] The progression from being dependent on parents providing healthful foods to making their own food choices occurs during this period in life. Children should also be educated on the basic nutrition principles and how to apply to their daily lives.[44,45] This will allow children to accept more responsibilities for their health and optimize dietary habits in adolescence and adulthood.

III. ADOLESCENCE

Adolescence is an important period during which major biological, social, physiological, and cognitive changes take place. Adolescence is divided into two developmental periods: early adolescence (10–14 years of age) and late adolescence (15–19 years of age). Young adulthood is the period between 20 and 24 years of age.[46] Adolescents have special nutritional needs due to rapid growth and maturational changes associated with the onset of puberty. Dietary surveys show that many adolescents do not meet nutrient recommendations for their age group and have inadequate intake of calcium, iron, thiamin, riboflavin, and vitamins A and C.[47] Clinically, however, despite their poor dietary intake patterns, the only biochemical nutrient deficiency commonly seen among adolescents is iron deficiency anemia. Increasingly seen are problems with dietary excesses and obesity.

A. Growth

Adolescents vary considerably as to age at onset of puberty and rate of progression through puberty.[48] The hormonal changes of puberty result in characteristic alterations in body size, body composition (muscle, fat, bone), and skeletal and sexual maturation. Such alterations are the basis for the increased dietary requirements for energy, protein, and most micronutrients. Height and weight growth during adolescence account for 50% of total body weight. Nutrition requirements during puberty are high.[46] The adolescent growth spurt occurs about 2 years later in boys than in girls, and so boys and girls of similar age often differ in nutritional requirements. Undernutrition and many chronic diseases can delay the onset of puberty.[49] Furthermore, growth is not a continuous process, but it proceeds as a series of small growth spurts that vary in amplitude and frequency.[50] All of these factors influence an individual adolescent's nutritional needs, which will vary between and within individuals over time. Above all, it is important to recognize that adequate nutritional intake is necessary to assure normal growth and maturation.

Now, the onset of puberty occurs at an earlier age than previously documented, with variability among ethnic groups. Among a national sample of US boys and girls from the National Health and Nutrition Examination Survey (NHANES) III 1988–94, evaluated at 8–19 years of age,[51] the median ages of onset of pubic hair development were 11.2, 12.0, and 12.3 years for non-Hispanic black, non-Hispanic white, and Hispanic boys, respectively, and 9.4, 10.6, and 10.4 years for non-Hispanic black, non-Hispanic white, and Hispanic girls, respectively. In another large sample of US from 1997, in girls evaluated at ages 3–12, the average age at menarche was 12.2 years for African Americans and 12.9 years for whites.[52] Menarche usually occurs just after the adolescent growth spurt.[48] At the peak of adolescent linear growth, the rate of increase in height is about 10.3 cm/year for boys (range 7.2–13.4) and 9.0 cm/year for girls (range 7.0–11.0).[48] From the onset of the adolescent linear growth to the attainment of adult stature, both boys and girls gain about 17% of final height.[53]

Adolescent growth in height is followed by rapid accrual of bone mass. Peak bone mass, the maximum amount of bone gained during the life cycle, is achieved by the end of adolescence or in early adulthood.[54,55] Epidemiological evidence suggests that a higher peak bone mass is associated with physical activity, greater dietary calcium and vitamin D intake.[56] Higher calcium intake is associated with lower rates of hip fracture later in life.[55] Thus, adequate calcium and vitamin D intake to assure optimal accrual of bone mass during childhood and adolescence may have important lifelong health implications.[56]

Bone mineral density (g/cm^2) increases through puberty.[54] A longitudinal growth study by Bailey et al.[56,57] showed that the peak accrual in whole body bone mineral content (g) occurred after the adolescent growth in height. Accordingly, to accommodate these rapid adolescent gains, calcium requirements are considerably higher for adolescents (1300 mg) than for children or adults (Table 2.1). Although recommended calcium intake is 63% higher for adolescents than children, results from NHANES III national survey show that dietary calcium intake declines as children become adolescents (Table 2.2), and calcium intake is lower in non-Hispanic black compared to non-Hispanic white and Hispanic children and adolescents.[59] In a recently published survey of a mixed ethnic sample from NHANES 1999–2000,[60] girls still showed a decline in dietary calcium intake from childhood to adolescence; however, calcium intake in boys remained stable and well below the 1300 mg/day recommended during adolescence.[61] Net calcium absorption is highest in infancy and adolescence.[62] However, it is unlikely that increased calcium absorption efficiency in the context of inadequate dietary intake is sufficient to optimize peak bone mass. Calcium supplementation can increase-bone mineral density in children,[63] a finding that underscores the importance of adequate calcium intake. Increased calcium intake must be sustained to maintain the effect on accretion of bone mineral density.

Other factors that influence bone mass accrual during growth include vitamin D status and physical activity. Adequate vitamin D concentrations are necessary to facilitate calcium absorption in the gut. Vitamin D is absorbed through the skin and is adversely affected by latitude away form the equator, seasonal fluctuation, sunblock use, darker skin pigmentation, and obesity. A part from these factors, casual daily sunlight exposure to the hands and face is usually sufficient to achieve adequate vitamin D status in healthy children and

TABLE 2.1 Recommended calcium intake (mg/day) levels, from two sources.[a].

Age range (years)	RDA (2010)	NIH
1–3	700	700
4–8	1000	800–1200
9–18	1300	1200–1500[b]
14–18	1300	1200–1500

[a]*RDA, the National Academy's Recommended Dietary Allowance*[12]*; NIH, National Institutes of Health Consensus Development Panel on Optimal Calcium Intake.* [58].
[b]*Changes at age 11.*

TABLE 2.2 Calcium intake (mg/day) for males and females, from the National Health and Nutrition Examination 1999–2014 Surveys.

	Males		Females	
1988–1992*	**6–11 years**	**12–15 years**	**6–11 years**	**12–15 years**
Non-Hispanic white	994	822	822	744
Non-Hispanic black	761	688	688	613
Mexican American	986	890	890	790
1999–2000**	6–11 years	12–19 years	6–11 years	12–19 years
All race/ethnic groups	843	956	812	661

*Source: * Alaimo et al.* [59]*, ** Ervin et al.* [60].

adolescents.[64] The RDA for vitamin D3 is 600 IU/day for adolescents.[61] Also, weight-bearing physical activity is important to strengthen bone and increase muscle mass.[65] Exercise before and during adolescence is also of great importance to bone formation.[66]

B. Nutritional Needs of Adolescents

Nutritional needs of adolescents are higher than those of children because of the growth spurt, sexual maturation, changes in body composition, skeletal mineralization, and changes in physical activity. Physical activity is not necessarily increased, but total energy needs are increased because of larger body size. Unlike children, adolescent males and females differ in their nutritional needs, and these continue into adulthood. Reasons include the earlier maturation of females and the considerable variability of puberty and nutrient requirements.[67] Nutrient needs are increased for protein, energy, calcium, iron, and zinc. Additionally, increased nutritional requirements occur with adolescent pregnancy, many chronic diseases, and rigorous physical conditioning. Some common adolescent illnesses, such as the eating disorders of anorexia nervosa and bulimia, may affect nutritional status and maturation. Recommended dietary intake for adolescents[68] often represent interpolations based on known requirements for children and adults rather than evidence based on adolescent research subjects. Nutrient requirements are usually greater for males than females and for pregnant and lactating females.

Often, adolescents' dietary habits differ from those of children and adults. Changes in adolescent dietary patterns can adversely[69] affect growth during this period. Adolescents tend to skip meals, eat more meals outside their home, and eat snacks, especially sugar-sweetened beverages, candy, and diet or fast foods. Some develop strong food beliefs, adopt food fads, or become vegetarians/vegans. These diet fads may reflect an expression of independence, a busy life style, problems with body image, or a search for self-identity, or they may be secondary to peer and social pressures.[69]

Typically, dietary intake data show insufficient intake of calcium, iron, and vitamins A and C in the diets of US adolescents. The average intake for males was closer to the RDA than that for females. Adolescents often have high intakes of soda, coffee, tea, and alcohol and low intakes of milk and juice than children, a pattern seen more often in white adolescents.[67] In a large survey of 12,500 children aged 11–18 years, Cavadini et al. showed that total energy intake, as well as the proportion of energy from total fat and saturated fat, decreased from 1965 to 1996.[70] Total milk consumption decreased, accompanied by an increase in sugar-sweetened beverages and noncitrus juices. Among US high school students surveyed between 1999 and 2003, only 16%–18% reported drinking more than three glasses of milk daily.[71] Vegetable intake was lower than the recommended five servings per day, and folate, iron, and calcium intakes were lower than recommendations for females.[61,68,70,72] In adolescent females and low-income youth, vitamins B6, A, and E, iron, calcium, and zinc intakes were low.[73] In the typical American adolescent diet, French fried potatoes make up 25% of all the vegetables consumed, intake of simple sugars exceeded the intake of complex carbohydrates, and more than a third of the dietary fat (which accounts for >33% of calories consumed) was saturated fat. Additionally "junk" or processed food with few nutrients and high-fat fast food accounted for >33% of the daily caloric intake.[25,74] Although MyPlate (USDA guide to healthy eating) suggests that an appropriate intake of fruit and vegetables is > 5 servings per day, adolescents have lower intakes. Only 8.5% of high school students surveyed between 2007 and 2010 in the National Youth Risk Behavior Survey ate ≥1.42 cups of fruits and ate ≥2.53 cups of vegetables per day.[71]

Recommendations for adolescent food intake from various sources stress the following: increased intake of calcium-rich and iron-containing foods in adolescent girls; limitation of foods high in simple sugars; decreas ed intake of complex carbohydrate foods that could be retained in the mouth and contribute to dental caries; use of fluoridated water, dentifrices, topical treatments, and rinses to prevent dental caries; limitation of total fat to <30% of energy intake, with saturated fat <10% and dietary cholesterol <300 mg/day; and limitation of salt intake to 2500 mg (girls) and 2.500–3000 mg/day (boys) and daily protein intake <2 times the RDA.[75,76] The AAP recommends a fat intake of about 20%–30% of energy because of the rapid growth that occurs in adolescence.[77]

Energy

Exact energy requirements of the individual growing adolescent are difficult to determine.[78] The DRI provides a method to estimate energy needs as Estimated Energy Requirements (EERs, kcal/d) prediction equations (Table 2.3).[79] Additionally, an activity factor should be used to account for different levels of physical activity (sedentary, low active, moderate active, and high active). Peak energy requirements occur in girls at about 15–16 years of age and in boys at about 18 years and correspond to the increased needs of later pubertal growth and development. Adolescent females at the moderate active level require about 2300 kcal/day, whereas males require 2600–3300 kcal/day. Energy needs increase and vary during the second and third trimester of pregnancy and during the first and second 6 months of lactation.[79] Predictive formulas are also available to calculate the EER-based energy needs for obese adolescent females and males.[79]

Data from NHANES III showed energy intakes were higher for males than for females, and intakes peaked in late adolescence.[80] Although mean dietary intakes in some adolescents were less than the RDAs, there has been an increase in the prevalence of overweight and obese adolescents. Despite a trend toward decreased dietary fat intake, fat intake is still higher than recommended.[67]

TABLE 2.3 Estimated Energy Requirement (EER) for boys and girls 13 through 18 years of age.

Boys age (y)	Reference weight* (kg [lb])	Reference height* (m [in])	Sedentary PAL**	Low active PAL	Active PAL	Very active PAL
13	45.6 (100.4)	1.56 (61.4)	1935	2276	2618	3038
14	51.0 (112.3)	1.64 (64.6)	2090	2459	2829	3283
15	56.3 (124.0)	1.70 (66.9)	2223	2618	3013	3499
16	60.9 (134.1)	1.74 (68.5)	2320	2736	3152	3663
17	64.6 (142.3)	1.75 (68.9)	2366	2796	3226	3754
18	67.2 (148.0)	1.76 (69.3)	2383	2823	3263	3804
Girls age (y)	Reference weight (kg [lb])	Reference height (m [in])	Sedentary PAL	Low active PAL	Active PAL	Very active PAL
13	45.8 (100.4)	1.57 (61.8)	1684	1992	2281	2762
14	49.4 (112.3)	1.60 (63.0)	1718	2036	2334	2831
15	52.0 (124.0)	1.62 (63.8)	1731	2057	2362	2870
16	53.9 (134.1)	1.63 (64.2)	1729	2059	2368	2883
17	55.1 (142.3)	1.63 (64.2)	1710	2042	2353	2871
18	56.2 (148.0)	1.63 (64.2)	1690	2024	2336	2858

**PAL = physical activity level.
* *Table adapted from: Institute of Medicine, Food and Nutrition Board. Dietary Reference Intakes for energy, carbohydrate, fiber, fat, fatty acids, cholesterol, protein and amino acids. Washington DC: National Academy Press, 2002* [79].

Protein

Protein recommendations are shown in Table 2.4. Most adolescents easily achieve these levels in the US, as seen in the NHANES III survey.[80] Experimental data on adolescent protein requirements are not available, and the recommendations are interpolated from results of studies in infants and adults. Peak protein intake coincides with peak energy intake. Protein should account for 12%–14% of energy intake. Adolescents at risk for low protein intake are those with eating disorders, malabsorption, chronic disease, and socioeconomic limitations resulting in food insecurity. In the event of inadequate energy intake, protein is used for energy needs and results in malnutrition.

Minerals

Some adolescents have inadequate intakes of minerals, including calcium, iron, zinc, and magnesium. Calcium and phosphorus are essential for good bone health. Though dietary phosphorus intake is usually adequate, calcium intake is often inadequate in adolescents. As previously discussed in the bone health section, national surveys show that calcium intake is less than recommended and has either declined or not increased over the last 20 years. Among females aged 15–18 years, the average calcium intake dropped from 680 mg/day in 1980 to 600 mg/day in 1990.[81] Among females aged 12–19 years in the NHANES 1999–2000 dietary survey,[60] median calcium intake was 611 mg/day, which is only 51% of the currently recommended amount of 1300 mg/day.[61] The best way to meet nutritional requirements for calcium is through foods rather than through calcium supplements, and calcium is more efficiently absorbed in combination with lactose. Dairy products provide about 55% of the calcium intake in the US diet. Calcium absorption from other dietary sources is important,

TABLE 2.4 Dietary reference intake for protein.

	Males		Females	
	g/kg/day	g/day	g/kg/day	g/day
9 to 13 y	0.95	34	0.95	34
14 to 18 y	0.85	52	0.85	46
Pregnancy*	–	–	1.10	+25

* *For pregnant adolescents, an additional 25 g of protein daily is recommended. For a 14–18 year old pregnant adolescent girl, 71 g of protein daily (46 + 25 g/day) is recommended.*
Table adapted from: Institute of Medicine, Food and Nutrition Board. Dietary Reference Intakes for energy, carbohydrate, fiber, fat, fatty acids, cholesterol, protein and amino acids. Washington DC: National Academy Press, 2002. [79].

however, especially in communities where dairy products are not easily available for adolescents who have lactose intolerance. Despite iron fortification of many cereal grains, iron deficiency remains common. Iron needs are higher during adolescence because of increases in blood volume and muscle mass. Females' needs are further increased by menstrual losses. The adolescent females who are at increased risk for iron deficiency include the older adolescent female, the pregnant adolescent, and female athletes. Median iron intake for 12–19 year old females in the NHANES 1999–2000 survey was 11.7 mg/day, 78% of the 15 mg/day recommended for females aged 14–18 years.[60,72] Iron deficiency during pregnancy results in an increased risk of preterm birth and low birth weight infants. Because of their rapid growth, young pubertal males are also at risk for iron deficiency anemia. Iron needs decrease with slower growth after puberty. Iron deficiency is more common among low-income youth and is seen more often in adolescent females than in adolescent males.[67] The prevalence of iron deficiency anemia among adolescents varies from 2% to 10% and is more frequent in males aged 11–14 years and in females aged 15–19 years.[73] Increased zinc is needed for growth and puberty, and zinc intake is often low in adolescents. Zinc deficiency is associated with growth retardation and hypogonadism, and zinc supplementation results in reversal of these clinical manifestations. Data from the NHANES 1999–2000 survey[60] show that magnesium intake among US adolescents aged 12–19 years did not meet recommendations.[61]

Vitamins

The vitamins that are at risk for insufficient amounts in the diets of adolescents include vitamins A, B6, E, D, and C and folic acid. Because females have lower food intakes than males, vitamin deficiencies are more common among females. Data from NHANES 1999–2000 survey[82] show that median intake of vitamins A, E, and C and folic acid for adolescents aged 12–19 years, in general, does not meet recommendations.[68,72]

Fiber

Adolescents ingest less than recommended amounts of fiber. Average fiber intake is about 12 g/day in comparison to the 25 g/day recommended by the American Heart Association for blood cholesterol reduction and the 35–45 g/day recommended for reduction of colon cancer risk.[83] DRI[79] recommendations are for males 9–13 years of age to consume 31 g/day of total fiber and 14–18 years of age to consume 38 g/day. Female intake is recommended as 26 g/day for 9–18 years of age. Data from the NHANES III survey (1988–94) show that adolescent fiber intake was 11–16 g/day for adolescents 12–19 years of age, much less than the recommended 26–38 g/day.[80,84]

C. Nutritional and Pubertal Assessment

During the adolescent years, anthropometric assessment of nutritional status (weight, height, and body composition) is influenced by puberty. Still, it is an important period for careful monitoring of nutritional status because of the heightened risk of nutritional disorders, such as obesity and anorexia nervosa. In addition to CDC weight, height and BMI growth charts,[85] height velocity growth charts,[86] which include a classification for early and late onset of puberty, are useful to assess height relative to maturity status. For early or late maturing children whose linear growth deviates significantly from their previous growth patterns or from standard growth curves, these charts are useful for the interpretation of growth measurements in individual adolescents. Assessment of sexual maturity status is classified according to the stages described by Tanner[48] for pubic hair growth and genital development in boys and for pubic hair and breast development in girls. A self-assessment pictorial questionnaire can be used to document puberty stage.[87] For assessment of weight-for-height status, the BMI (expressed in kg/m^2) may be used. CDC growth charts for children 2 through 20 years of ages include a BMI chart. Sex and age-specific BMI percentile can be plotted in the same manner as for weight and height. There are no clear guidelines on how to assess BMI relative to early or late sexual maturity.[88] For assessment of overweight, obesity, and severe obesity, BMI should be combined with triceps skinfold measurement.[89] For children and adolescents with a BMI percentile greater than the 95th percentile, extended BMI percentile curves should be utilized.[90]

D. States of Altered Growth Patterns

Obesity

The prevalence of obesity in children and adolescents has tripled over the last several decades. Based upon national surveys, the prevalence of obesity in children 2–19 years of age (BMI at the 95th percentile or higher)[91] has increased from 5% to 6% in the 1980s to 18.5% in 2016. According to the NHANES 2015–16 survey, overweight (BMI $\geq$85th percentile) is present in 34.3% of children between the ages of 2–19 years, obesity (BMI $\geq$95th percentile) in 18.5%, and severe obesity (BMI $\geq$ 120% > 95th percentile or BMI $\geq$ 35 kg/m^2) in 5.6% of children.[92,108] The prevalence increases in adolescents for all obesity-related categories: overweight (20%–24%), obesity (21%), and severe obesity (8%).[92,93] Obesity affects non-Hispanic black males (20%) and females (29%) and Hispanic males (27%%) and females (17%) adolescents disproportionately compared with non-Hispanic white males (17%) and females (15%%)[94] (Table 2.5).

The adolescent period presents with physiologic developmental, familial, and social challenges that lend themselves to increased risk/exacerbation of obesity. The early adolescent pubertal development period is a period of natural body fat deposition, particularly in girls. Additionally, the transition from Tanner stage 1 to Tanner stage 3 is associated with a 32% reduction in insulin sensitivity, which is further exacerbated in adolescents who experience early menarche (<11.9 yrs of age).[95,96] These normal physiologic changes can increase the likelihood for a child who is overweight to cross over into the obese category during adolescence. Additionally, physical activity decreases in adolescent girls, particularly in non-Hispanic black and Hispanic girls, which provides an additional challenge as physical activity improves insulin sensitivity.[97]

Adolescence is a time of increased independence, where peers often times have a strong influence over choices. For example, an adolescent may not wish to take a lunch to school because it is not considered to be socially acceptable. Additionally, adolescents may have their own money to purchase food from fast food restaurants and convenience stores. Physical activity decreases in adolescent girls, particularly in non-Hispanic black and Hispanic girls, which provides an additional challenge as physical activity improves insulin sensitivity and weight maintenance.[97]

The risk of becoming obese as a child, and remaining obese as an adult, is influenced by family history and by the child's age. Data from the Cardiovascular Risk in Young Finns Study, which followed children from age 6–49 years, demonstrated that children with obesity who remain obese as adults had a BMI trajectory that increased linearly until age 25 years. In contrast, children who did not develop obesity as adults transition to a null-growth BMI trajectory at 16 years for girls and 21 years for boys.[98] Children with obesity who did not develop obesity as adults have a lower BMI at age 6 and slower rate of BMI change during adolescence.[98] There is an 80% chance of an obese adolescent becoming an obese adult.[99] Further, children with obesity have increased cardiovascular risk as adults.[98]

TABLE 2.5 Prevalence of obesity in adolescents (ages 2–19 years).

	Non-Hispanic white	Non-Hispanic black	Hispanic
Boys			
1976–1980	3.8	6.1	7.7
1988–1994	11.6	10.7	14.1
1999–2002	14.6	18.7	24.7
2007–2008	16.7	19.8	25.5
2013–2016	15.3	17.9	24.3
Girls			
1976–1980	4.6	10.7	8.8
1988–1994	8.9	16.3	13.4
1999–2002	12.7	23.6	19.6
2007–08	14.5	29.2	17.5
2013–16	14.1	23.0	22.9

Prevalence >95th percentile BMI.
Sources: Ogden CL et al. [94]

Obesity is caused by a positive energy imbalance in which individuals expend less energy than consumed. A chronic, small positive energy imbalance will have a large effect on weight gain over time. Finding the cause of such a small energy surplus makes the prevention and treatment of obesity challenging. In general, the search for the causes for obesity has focused on four areas: genetics, environment, energy expenditure, and dietary factors.

Genetics; Even though some genetic syndromes (e.g., Prader–Willi syndrome, Down syndrome), single-gene mutations (e.g., leptin receptor deficiency, MC4-R), and clinical syndromes of other etiology (e.g., Cushing's syndrome) are associated with obesity, these represent <1% of the cases of obesity in children. Most adolescents with a medical cause of obesity may be identified earlier in life, but acquired clinical syndromes (e.g., hypothyroidism) may present in adolescence. Although genetic influence on obesity is supported by the clustering of obesity within families and by studies of adopted and twin children, genetics is unlikely to explain the current trend of increasing prevalence of obesity in adolescents.[96,100] The relative weight of adults who were adopted as children is positively associated with the relative weight of their biological parents. No such relationship exists between these children and their adoptive parents.[96,100] Similarly, the weights of adoptive twins reared apart in different family environments are similar to that of twins reared together. The discovery of the leptin hormone and the leptin gene in animal models raised the hope that obesity genes would be identified; however, the search has not yet been fruitful in humans.

Environmental and behavioral; As noted above, adolescence is a time of increased independence, where peers have a strong influence over choices and behaviors. Environmental influences such as supermarket availability, the number of fast food restaurants in the neighborhood, neighborhood safety, presence of a television in the bedroom, eating meals as a family, and socioeconomic status play important roles. Childhood and adolescent socioeconomic factors such as parental education, family size, region of the country, and urban versus rural factors are all associated with obesity.[101] An important environmental influence is the amount of time spent watching television and other screen time. A relationship between television watching and obesity has been clearly described in older children, including a dose response.[97] Preadolescents and young adolescents were 5.5 times as likely to be overweight if they watched >5 h/day, as compared to those who watched <2 h/day.

Resting energy expenditure (REE); Altered REE, lower energy of physical activity, and total energy expenditure are potential causes for excessive weight gain. Many obese adolescents and their families believe the cause of the weight gain is/was low metabolic rate, but data do not consistently support this. Although these studies specifically evaluated children and adults, similar findings would be expected in adolescents. A recent finding has been a lower REE among African American children and adults. Decreased total daily energy expenditure through a pattern of decreased physical activity could induce a positive energy balance, resulting in excessive weight gain. Obese children may be less physically active than nonobese children; however, some evidence suggests that obese individuals expend extra energy to carry their excess body mass. Therefore, they expend as much or more total energy completing these activities of daily living as do nonobese children. Despite these mixed findings, the improved clinical outcome with weight management that includes exercise[99,103–105] supports the negative influence of the pattern of sedentary physical activity on the development and treatment of obesity.

Dietary intake; Data on dietary intake and obesity suggest that obese children tend to eat high-fat diets and thus higher energy diets. Humans also have a taste preference for energy-dense foods. In our current environment with easy access to an abundance of high-fat, energy-dense foods, this preference may underlie the increasing prevalence of obesity. Assessing dietary intake and energy needs is difficult. Obese adolescents often underreport energy intake by 40%–60%.[100,106] Standardized prediction equations to calculate energy requirements of obese children are available.[79] Measuring REE is available in some clinical settings and provides an accurate estimate of this component of energy needs.

Evaluation and treatment; True assessment of the degree of adiposity is difficult. One of the most commonly used measures to assess relative weight is BMI. In adults, a BMI ≥25 defines overweight and ≥30 defines obesity. However, BMI normally increases as children grow in height and weight; therefore, a particular BMI cutoff point in kg/m^2 cannot be set to define obesity in adolescents. Generally, for adolescents, BMI percentile for age and sex is used. A BMI ≥85th percentile identifies overweight, and a BMI ≥95th percentile identifies obesity. The 2000 CDC growth charts include age- and sex-specific BMI percentile curves and suggest the clinical use of BMI to assess relative weight.[85] The area between the 85th and 95th percentiles is defined as at risk for overweight, whereas points above the 95th percentile are defined as overweight.[91] However, current CDC BMI curves are unable to accurately determine extreme values of BMI, and an extended BMI curve is available to define severe obesity as 120% of the 95th BMI percentile.[90,103,107] It has also been suggested for children and adolescents with severe obesity to examine a child's sex and age BMI as the 95th percentile.[90]

The assessment of an obese child should include a routine history and physical, which includes a review for signs of obesity-related syndromes or conditions. Screening for associated important clinical conditions (e.g., hyperlipidemia, insulin resistance, and hypertension) or contributing processes (e.g., low metabolic rate) should be considered. Significant family dysfunction or adolescent psychological problems need to be evaluated as part of the weight management evaluation and treatment program.

Several treatment methods, including behavioral modification, diet, exercise, school-based programs, pharmacologic interventions, and surgery, have been devised for obese adolescents. Most pediatric weight management programs have targeted younger age groups. Treatment is more successful when a comprehensive behavioral program, in conjunction with specific diet and exercise prescriptions, is used.[106,109–111] An important component of adolescent treatment is parental and family participation. In addition to attending group sessions, the parent must work with the adolescent to restructure the home and play environments and to monitor progress. Obesity treatment and specific cardiovascular risk factors are reviewed elsewhere.

Adolescent pregnancy

Adolescent females continue to grow in stature and fat-free mass during pregnancy. This growth may occur at the expense of the fetus and result in decreased birth weight despite increased maternal weight gain or in suboptimal maternal nutritional status and growth. Additionally, reduced maternal ferritin, cord ferritin, and folate blood concentrations were noted in the adolescents who gained height during pregnancy.[112,113] The fact that pregnant adolescent females continue to grow implies that nutrient needs for pregnant adolescents are even greater than those for nonadolescent pregnant women.

To accommodate the potential growth, it is recommended that pregnant teens gain weight at the upper end of the recommended range for their prepregnancy weight.[114] Weight gain in the first and second trimesters is related to improved birth weight.[115] Pregnant and lactating females also need additional calories[79] and protein (Table 2.4), calcium, iron, vitamins B6, C, A, and D, and folate. A prenatal supplement that contains vitamins A and D, zinc, calcium, folate, and iron is recommended. Nutritional education and counseling are an important part of prenatal care for adolescents.

There is an increased incidence of medical complications in adolescent pregnancy, especially among adolescents <17 years of age. The maternal mortality rate is twice that of adult pregnant women. Other medical problems include poor maternal weight gain, prematurity, hypertension, anemia, sexually transmitted diseases, low birth weight infants, and increased neonatal death. These latter two complications are more common in adolescent mothers <14 years of age and in the African American population. Factors responsible for all of the above complications include low prepregnancy weight and height, parity, poor pregnancy weight gain, poverty, unmarried status, low educational attainment, drug use, and inadequate prenatal care.[112]

IV. CONCLUSION

Childhood and adolescence are critical periods during which it is important that nutritional needs be met. Certain micronutrient deficiencies are more common in different age groups. Lack of normal feeding patterns can lead to subsequent problems. Obesity and adolescent pregnancy are complicating conditions, which need to be addressed in the growing adolescent.

RESEARCH GAPS

There are several gaps in our knowledge of the nutrient needs for growth in children and adolescents. While we know the impact of micronutrient deficiencies on cognitive function, there are few studies looking at micronutrient needs and mental health in children. There are no long-term prospective studies evaluating the long-term impact of nutrition interventions (nutrient quality, micronutrient intake) in childhood and adolescence on obesity, metabolic diseases, and mental health in adulthood. Given the exploding knowledge of the interactions of specific nutrients and the microbiome, understanding optimal food composition in children for health is important.

Acknowledgments

This chapter is an update of the chapter titled "41. Adolescence" by Asim Maqbool, Kelly A. Dougherty, Elizabeth P. Parks and Virginia A. Stallings, in Present Knowledge in Nutrition, 10th Edition, edited by Erdman JW, Macdonald IA, and Zeisel SH and published by Wiley-Blackwell. © 2012 International Life Sciences Institute. Portions of this update are from the previously published chapter and the contributions of previous authors are acknowledged.

V. REFERENCES

1. World Health Organization, M.G.R.S.G. *Length/Heightfor-Age, Weight-for-Age, Weight-for-Length, Weight-for-Height and Body Mass Index-Forage: Methods and Development*. Geneva, Switzerland: World Health Organization; 2006. July 14, 2019; Available from: https://www.who.int/childgrowth/standards/technical_report/en/.
2. Data Table for Girls Weight-for-Length and Head Circumference-for-Age Charts. July 14, 2019; Available from: https://www.cdc.gov/growthcharts/who/girls_weight_head_circumference.htm.
3. Data Table for Boys Weight-for-Length and Head Circumference-for-age Charts. July 14, 2019; Available from: www.cdc.gov/growthcharts/whocharts.htm.
4. Briefel RR, et al. Toddlers' transition to table foods: impact on nutrient intakes and food patterns. *J Am Diet Assoc*. 2004;104(1 Suppl 1):s38–44.
5. Fox MK, et al. Sources of energy and nutrients in the diets of infants and toddlers. *J Am Diet Assoc*. 2006;106(1 Suppl 1):S28–S42.
6. Shriver LH, et al. Contribution of snacks to dietary intakes of young children in the United States. *Matern Child Nutr*. 2018;14(1).
7. Butte NF, et al. Nutrient intakes of US infants, toddlers, and preschoolers meet or exceed dietary reference intakes. *J Am Diet Assoc*. 2010;110(12 Suppl):S27–S37.
8. Reedy J, et al. Comparing 3 dietary pattern methods—cluster analysis, factor analysis, and index analysis—with colorectal cancer risk: the NIH-AARP diet and health study. *Am J Epidemiol*. 2010; 171(4):479–487.
9. Fox MK, et al. Food consumption patterns of young preschoolers: are they starting off on the right path? *J Am Diet Assoc*. 2010;110(12 Suppl):S52–S59.
10. Leahy KE, et al. Reductions in entree energy density increase children's vegetable intake and reduce energy intake. *Obesity*. 2008; 16(7):1559–1565.
11. Mendoza JA, et al. Dietary energy density is associated with selected predictors of obesity in U.S. Children. *J Nutr*. 2006; 136(5):1318–1322.
12. (US), National Research Council. Protein and amino acids. In: Commission on Life Science National Research Council, Food and Nutrition Board, ed. *Recommended Dietary Allowances*. Washington DC: National Academies Press; 1989.
13. Daniels SR, Greer FR, Committee on Nutrition. Lipid screening and cardiovascular health in childhood. *Pediatrics*. 2008;122(1):198–208.
14. American Academy of Pediatrics, Committee on Nutrition. Statement on cholesterol. *Pediatrics*. 1998;101(1):141–147.

15. Albertson AM, Gugger CK, Hill Gallant KM, Holschuh NM, Keast DR. Associations between yogurt, dairy, calcium, and vitamin D intake and obesity among U.S. children aged 8-18 years: NHANES, 2005–2008. *Nutrients*. 2015;7(3):1577–1593.
16. Wiese HF, Hansen AE, Adam DJ. Essential fatty acids in infant nutrition. I. Linoleic acid requirement in terms of serum di-, tri- and tetraenoic acid levels. *J Nutr.* 1958;66(3):345–360.
17. Christensen MS, Hoy CE, Jeppesen PB, Mortensen PB. Essential fatty acid deficiency in patients with severe fat malabsorption. *Am J Clin Nutr.* 1997;65(3):837–843.
18. Alberda C, Bistrian B, Driscoll D. Essential fatty acid deficiency in 2015: the impact of novel intravenous lipid emulsions. *J Parenter Enter Nutr.* 2015;39(1 suppl), 61S–6S.
19. Bailey RL, et al. Total usual nutrient intakes of US children (under 48 Months): findings from the feeding infants and toddlers study (FITS) 2016. *J Nutr.* 2018;148(9S):1557S–1566S.
20. Scholl TO, Reilly T. Anemia, iron and pregnancy outcome. *J Nutr.* 2000;130(2S Suppl):443S–447S.
21. Grantham-McGregor S, Ani C. A review of studies on the effect of iron deficiency on cognitive development in children. *J Nutr.* 2001; 131(2):649S–668S.
22. Lozoff B, et al. Poorer behavioral and developmental outcome more than 10 years after treatment for iron deficiency in infancy. *Pediatrics*. 2000;105(4):E51.
23. Angulo-Kinzler RM, et al. Spontaneous motor activity in human infants with iron-deficiency anemia. *Early Hum Dev.* 2002;66(2):67–79.
24. United States Department of Agriculture. ChooseMyPlate. July 14, 2019; Available from: https://www.choosemyplate.gov.
25. Alberda C, Clevland L, Cook A, Friday J, Kahle LL, Krebs-Smith SM. Fruit and vegetable intakes of children and adolescents in the United States. *Arch Pediatr Adolesc Med.* 1996;150(1):81–86.
26. Kranz S, et al. Dietary fiber intake by American preschoolers is associated with more nutrient-dense diets. *J Am Diet Assoc.* 2005;105(2):221–225.
27. Eldridge AL, et al. Trends in mean nutrient intakes of US infants, toddlers, and young children from 3 feeding infants and toddlers studies (FITS). *J Nutr.* 2019;149(7):1230–1237.
28. Connor P, Hadden L, Marriott BP, Olsho L. Intake of added sugars and selected nutrients in the United States, National Health and Nutrition Examination Survey (NHANES) 2003–2006. *Crit Rev Food Sci Nutr.* 2010;50(3):228–258.
29. Carruth BR, et al. Developmental milestones and self-feeding behaviors in infants and toddlers. *J Am Diet Assoc.* 2004;104(1 Suppl 1):s51–s56.
30. Carruth BR, Skinner JD. Feeding behaviors and other motor development in healthy children (2–24 months). *J Am Coll Nutr.* 2002;21(2):88–96.
31. American Academy of Pediatrics. Promoting healthy nutrition. In: Hagab S, Duncan, eds. *Bright Futures: Guidelines for Health Supervision of Infants, Children, and Adolescents.* Elk Grove Village, IL USA: AAP; 2008.
32. Birch LL, et al. The variability of young children's energy intake. *N Engl J Med.* 1991;324(4):232–235.
33. Gooze RA, Anderson SE, Whitaker RC. Prolonged bottle use and obesity at 5.5 years of age in US children. *J Pediatr.* 2011;159(3): 431–436.
34. Brotanek JM, et al. Reasons for prolonged bottle-feeding and iron deficiency among Mexican-American toddlers: an ethnographic study. *Acad Pediatr.* 2009;9(1):17–25.
35. Brotanek JM, et al. Iron deficiency, prolonged bottle-feeding, and racial/ethnic disparities in young children. *Arch Pediatr Adolesc Med.* 2005;159(11):1038–1042.
36. Kimbro RT, Brooks-Gunn J, McLanahan S. Racial and ethnic differentials in overweight and obesity among 3-year-old children. *Am J Public Health.* 2007;97(2):298–305.
37. American Academy of Pediatrics, Section on Pediatric Dentistry and Oral Health. Preventive oral health Intervention of pediatricians. *Pediatrics*. 2008;122(6):1387–1394.
38. Poti JM, Popkin BM. Trends in energy intake among US children by eating location and food source, 1977–2006. *J Am Diet Assoc.* 2011;111(8):1156–1164.
39. Jahns L, Siega-Riz AM, Popkin BM. The increasing prevalence of snacking among US children from 1977 to 1996. *J Pediatr.* 2001; 138(4):493–498.
40. Bowman SA, et al. Effects of fast-food consumption on energy intake and diet quality among children in a national household survey. *Pediatrics*. 2004;113(1 Pt 1):112–118.
41. Rehm CD, Drewnowski A, Monsivais P. Potential population-level nutritional impact of replacing whole and reduced-fat milk with low-fat and skim milk among US children aged 2–19 years. *J Nutr Educ Behav.* 2015;47(1), 61-68 e1.
42. Drewnowski A, Rehm CD, Vieux F. Breakfast in the United States: food and nutrient intakes in relation to diet quality in National Health and Examination Survey 2011(–)2014. A study from the International Breakfast Research Initiative. *Nutrients*. 2018;10(9).
43. Bevans KB, et al. Children's eating behavior: the importance of nutrition standards for foods in schools. *J Sch Health.* 2011;81(7): 424–429.
44. Birch LL, Fisher JO. Development of eating behaviors among children and adolescents. *Pediatrics*. 1998;101(3 Pt 2):539–549.
45. Patrick H, Nicklas TA. A review of family and social determinants of children's eating patterns and diet quality. *J Am Coll Nutr.* 2005; 24(2):83–92.
46. Da JK, Salam RA, Thornburg KL, et al. Nutrition in adolescents: physiology, metabolism, and nutritional needs. *Ann N Y Acad Sci.* 2017;1393(1):21–33.
47. Skiba A,LE, Orr DP. Nutritional screening and guidance for adolescents. *Adolesc Health Update.* 1997;9(1–8).
48. James Mourilyan T. *Growth at Adolescence*. Oxford: Blackwell Publications; 1962.
49. Pozo J, Argente J. Delayed puberty in chronic illness. *Best Pract Res Clin Endocrinol Metabol.* 2002;16(1):73–90.
50. Lampl M, Johnson ML. A case study of daily growth during adolescence: a single spurt or changes in the dynamics of saltatory growth? *Ann Hum Biol.* 1993;20(6):595–603.
51. Sun SS, et al. National estimates of the timing of sexual maturation and racial differences among US children. *Pediatrics*. 2002;110(5): 911–919.
52. Herman-Giddens ME, et al. Secondary sexual characteristics and menses in young girls seen in office practice: a study from the pediatric research in office settings network. *Pediatrics*. 1997;99(4): 505–512.
53. Abbassi V. Growth and normal puberty. *Pediatrics*. 1998;102(2 Pt 3):507–511.
54. Theintz G BB, Rizzoli R, Slosman D, Clavien H, Sizonenko PC, Bonjour JP. Longitudinal monitoring of bone mass accumulation in healthy adolescents: evidence for a marked reduction after 16 years of age at the levels of lumbar spine and femoral neck in female subjects. *J Clin Endocrinol Metab.* 1992;75(4):1060–1065.
55. Matkovic V. Calcium and peak bone mass. *J Intern Med.* 1992; 231(2):151–160.
56. Weaver CM PM, Johnston Jr CC. Adolescent nutrition in the prevention of postmenopausal osteoporosis. *J Clin Endocrinol Metab.* 1999;84(6):1839–1843.
57. Bailey DA MH, Mirwald RL, Crocker PR, Faulkner RA. A six-year longitudinal study of the relationship of physical activity to bone mineral accrual in growing children: the University of Saskatchewan Bone Mineral Accrual Study. *J Bone Miner Res.* 1999;14(10): 1672–1679.

58. Bilezikian JP, Elmer PJ, Bailey L, et al. NIH Consensus conference. Optimal calcium intake. NIH Consensus Development Panel On Optimal Calcium Intake. *J Am Med Assoc*. 1994;272(24):1942–1948.
59. Alaimo K, McDowell M, Briefel RR, et al. Dietary intake of vitamins, minerals, and fiber of persons ages 2 months and over in the United States: Third National Health and Nutrition Examination Survey. *Adv Data*. 1994;14(258):1–28.
60. Ervin RB, Wang C, Wright JD, Kennedy-Stephenson J. Dietary intake of selected minerals for the United States population: 1999–2000. *Adv Data*. 2004;(341):1–5.
61. Institute of Medicine (US) Standing Committee on the Scientific Evaluation of Dietary Reference Intake. *Dietary Reference Intakes for Calcium, Phosphorus, Magnesium, Vitamin D, and Fluoride*. 1997.
62. Matkovic V. Calcium metabolism and calcium requirements during skeletal modeling and consolidation of bone mass. *Am J Clin Nutr*. 1991;54(1):245S–260S.
63. Johnston Jr CC, Miller J, Slemenda CW, et al. Calcium supplementation and increases in bone mineral density in children. *N Engl J Med*. 1992;327(2):82–87.
64. Holick MF. *Vitamin D. Photobiology of Vitamin D*. 1997.
65. Specker BL. Evidence for an interaction between calcium intake and physical activity on changes in bone mineral density. *J Bone Miner Res*. 1996;11(10):1539–1544.
66. Marcus R. Exercise: moving in the right direction. *J Bone Miner Res*. 1998;13(12):1793–1796.
67. JT D. Present knowledge in nutrition. In: *Adolescence*. 7th ed. Washington D.C.: ILSI Press; 1996.
68. Institute of Medicine (US), Standing committee on the Scientific Evaluation of Dietary Reference Intakes and its Panel on Folate, Other B Vitamins, and Choline. *Dietary Reference Intakes for Thiamin, Riboflavin, Niacin, Vitamin B_6, Folate, Vitamin B_{12}, Pantothenic Acid, Biotin and Choline*. 1998.
69. Story M, Neumark-Sztainer D, French S. Individual and environmental influences on adolescent eating behaviors. *J Am Diet Assoc*. 2002;102(3 Suppl):S40–S51.
70. Cavadini C, Siega-Riz A, Popkin BM. US adolescent food intake trends from 1965 to 1996. *Arch Dis Child*. 2000;83(1):18–24.
71. Services, D.o.H.a.H.. *Trends in the Prevalence of Dietary Behaviors and Weight Control Practices. National Youth Risk Behavior Survey: 1991–2003. DHHS, Centers for Disease Control and Prevention*. 2005.
72. Institute of Medicine (US) Panel on Micronutrients. *Dietary Reference Intakes for Vitamin A, Vitamin K, Arsenic, Boron, Chromium, Copper, Iodine, Iron, Manganese, Molybdenum, Nickel, Silicon, Vanadium, and Zinc*. 2001.
73. Story M, Alton I. Adolescent nutrition: current trends and critical issues. *Top Clin Nutr*. 1996;11:56–69.
74. Muñoz KA, Krebs-Smith S, Ballard-Barbash R, Cleveland LE. Food intakes of US children and adolescents compared to recommendations. *Pediatrics*. 1997;100(3 Pt 1):323–329.
75. National Academies of Sciences, Engineering, and Medicine. *Dieteary Reference Intakes for Sodium and Potassium. 2019*. Washington, DC: The National Academies; 2019.
76. Dietary Guidelines Advisory Committee. *Scientific Report of the 2015 Dietary Guidelines Advisory Committee:Advisory Report to the Secretary of Health and Human Services and the Secretary of Agriculture*. 2015.
77. Committee on Nutrition, K.R. *Adolescent Nutrition*. American Academy of Pediatrics; 2004:149–154.
78. Gong EJ, Heald F. *Diet, Nutrition and Adolescence*. 1999:857–869.
79. Trumbo P, S.S., Yates AA, Poos M, Food and Nutrition Board of the Institute of Medicine, The National Academies. Dietary reference intakes for energy, carbohydrate, fiber, fat, fatty acids, cholesterol, protein and amino acids. *J Am Diet Assoc*. 2002;102(11): 1621–1630.
80. Bialostosky K, Wright J, Kennedy-Stephenson J, McDowell M, Johnson CL. Dietary intake of macronutrients and other dietary constituents: United States. *Vital Health Stat*. 2002;11(245):1–158.
81. Albertson AM, Tobelmann R, Marquart L. Estimated dietary calcium intake and food sources for adolescent females: 1980–1992. *J Adolesc Health*. 1997;20(1):20–26.
82. Ervin RB, Wang C, Wright JD, Kennedy-Stephenson J. Dietary intake of selected vitamins for the United States population: 1999–2000. *Adv Data*. 2004;(339):1–4.
83. Nicklas TA, Myers L, Berenson GS. Dietary fiber intake of children: the Bogalusa Heart Study. *Pediatrics*. 1995;96(5 Pt 2):988–994.
84. Williams CL, Bollella M, Wynder EL. A new recommendation for dietary fiber in childhood. *Pediatrics*. 1995;96(5 Pt 2):985–988.
85. Kuczmarski RJ, Ogden C, Grummer-Strawn LM, et al. CDC growth charts: United States. *Adv Data*. 2000;8(314):1–27.
86. Tanner JM, Davies P. Clinical longitudinal standards for height and height velocity for North American children. *J Pediatr*. 1985; 107(3):317–329.
87. Morris NM, Udry J. Validation of a self-administered instrument to assess stage of adolescent development. *J Youth Adolesc*. 1980; 9(3):271–280.
88. Himes JH. *Auxology Advances in the Study of Human Growth and Development. Growth Reference Data for Adolescents: Maturation-Related Misclassification and its Accommodation*. London: Smith Gordon; 1999.
89. Must A, Dallal G, Dietz WH. Reference data for obesity: 85th and 95th percentiles of body mass index (wt/ht2) and triceps skinfold thickness. *Am J Clin Nutr*. 1991;53(4):839–846.
90. Kelly AS, Barlow SE, Gaoutham R, et al. Severe obesity in children and adolescents: identification, associated health risks, and treatment approaches: a scientific statement from the American Heart Association. *Circulation*. 2013;128(15):1689–1712.
91. Kuczmarski RJ, Ogden C, Guo SS, et al. 2000 CDC Growth Charts for the United States: methods and development. *Vital Health Stat*. 2002;(246):1–190.
92. Hales CM, Frayar CD, Carroll MD, et al. Trends in obesity and severe obesity prevalence in US youth and adults by sex and age, 2007–2008 to 2015–2016. *J Am Med Assoc*. 2018;319(16):1723–1725.
93. Skinner AC, et al. Prevalence of obesity and severe obesity in US children, 1999–2016. *Pediatrics*. 2018;141(3).
94. Ogden CL, et al. Differences in obesity prevalence by demographics and urbanization in US children and adolescents, 2013–2016. *J Am Med Assoc*. 2018;319(23):2410–2418.
95. Goran MI, et al. Deterioration of insulin sensitivity and beta-cell function in overweight Hispanic children during pubertal transition: a longitudinal assessment. *Int J Pediatr Obes*. 2006;1(3): 139–145.
96. Chumlea WM, Demerath EW, Remsberg KE, Schubert CM, Siervogel RM, Sun SS. Early menarche and the development of cardiovascular disease risk factors in adolescent girls: the Fels Longitudinal Study. *J Clin Endocrinol Metab*. 2005;90(5):2718–2724.
97. Renna F, Grafova I, Thakur N. The effect of friends on adolescent body weight. *Econ Hum Biol*. 2008;6(3):377–387.
98. Buscot MJ, et al. BMI trajectories associated with resolution of elevated youth BMI and incident adult obesity. *Pediatrics*. 2018; 141(1).
99. Whitaker RC, Wright J, Pepe MS, Seidel KD, Dietz WH. Predicting obesity in young adulthood from childhood and parental obesity. *N Engl J Med*. 1997;337(13):869–873.
100. Stunkard AJ, Sørensen T, Hanis C, et al. An adoption study of human obesity. *N Engl J Med*. 1986;314(4):193–198.
101. Kumanyika SK. Environmental influences on childhood obesity: ethnic and cultural influences in context. *Physiol Behav*. 2008; 94(1):61–70.
102. Deleted in review
103. Davis MM, McGonagle K, Schoeni RF, Stafford F. Grandparental and parental obesity influences on childhood overweight: implications for primary care practice. *J Am Board Fam Med*. 2008; 21(6):549–554.

104. Epstein LH, Wing R, Penner BC, Kress MJ. Effect of diet and controlled exercise on weight loss in obese children. *J Pediatr.* 1985;107(3):358–361.
105. Shick SM, Wing R, Klem ML, McGuire MT, Hill JO, Seagle H. Persons successful at long-term weight loss and maintenance continue to consume a low-energy, low-fat diet. *J Am Diet Assoc.* 1998;98(4):408–413.
106. Bandini LG, Schoeller D, Cyr HN, Dietz WH. Validity of reported energy intake in obese and nonobese adolescents. *Am J Clin Nutr.* 1990;52(3):421–425.
107. Gulati AK, Kaplan DW, Daniels SR. Clinical tracking of severely obese children: a new growth chart. *Pediatrics.* 2012;130(6):1136–1140.
108. Freedman DS, Berenson GS. Tracking of BMI z scores for severe obesity. *Pediatrics.* 2017;140(3).
109. Freedman DS, Srinivasan S, Harsha DW, Webber LS, Berenson GS. Relation of body fat patterning to lipid and lipoprotein concentrations in children and adolescents: the Bogalusa Heart Study. *Am J Clin Nutr.* 1989;50(5):930–939.
110. Epstein LH, Myers M, Raynor HA, Saelens BE. Treatment of pediatric obesity. *Pediatrics.* 1998;101(3 pt. 2):554–570.
111. Wilson GT. Behavioral treatment of obesity: thirty years and counting. *Adv Behav Res Ther.* 1993;16(1):31–75.
112. Rafiroiu C, Sargent R, Parra-Medina D, Drane WJ, Valois RF. Covariations of adolescent weight-control, health-risk and health-promoting behaviors. *Am J Health Behav.* 2003;27(1):3–14.
113. Woo T. Pharmacotherapy and surgery treatment for the severely obese adolescent. *J Pediatr Health Care.* 2009;23(4):206–212.
114. Strong JP. Landmark perspective: Coronary atherosclerosis in soldiers: a clue to the natural history of atherosclerosis in the young. *J Am Med Assoc.* 1986;256(20):2863–2866.
115. Strong JP, Malcom G, McMahan CA, et al. Prevalence and extent of atherosclerosis in adolescents and young adults: implications for prevention from the Pathobiological Determinants of Atherosclerosis in Youth Study. *J Am Med Assoc.* 1999;281(8): 727–735.

C H A P T E R

3

MATERNAL NUTRIENT METABOLISM AND REQUIREMENTS IN PREGNANCY

Kimberly K. Vesco[1], *MD, MPH*
Karen Lindsay[2], *PhD, RD*
Marie Johnson[3], *MS, RD*

[1]Department of Obstetrics & Gynecology, Kaiser Permanente Northwest, Science Programs Department, Kaiser Permanent Center for Health Research, Portland, OR, United States
[2]Department of Pediatrics, UCI School of Medicine, Susan and Henry Samueli College of Health Sciences, University of California, Irvine, Orange, CA, United States
[3]Department of Regional Clinical Nutrition, Kaiser Permanente Northwest, Portland, OR, United States

SUMMARY

This chapter describes how the additional nutrient requirements of pregnancy are met by a combination of physiological events that affect maternal nutrient utilization, fetal nutrient transfer, and increased dietary intakes. The physiological changes of pregnancy complicate the interpretation of nutritional status measures. The adverse effects of consuming an inadequate amount of most vitamins and minerals during pregnancy are partially understood, but little is known of the subclinical or long-term effects of deficiencies or their role in specific adverse pregnancy outcomes. With rising rates of maternal obesity on entering pregnancy, excess gestational weight gain, and complications such as gestational diabetes mellitus, there is a need for clearer guidance on optimal macronutrient balance and dietary patterns for pregnant women to reduce the risk of adverse outcomes and long-term health problems for both mother and offspring.

Keywords: Dietary patterns in pregnancy; Gestational diabetes; Gestational weight gain; Maternal nutrition; Maternal obesity; Nutrient metabolism in pregnancy; Nutrient requirements for fetal growth.

I. INTRODUCTION

A. Background

It has long been a worldwide public health priority to enable pregnant women to meet their nutrient needs. This priority is based on evidence that undernutrition prior to and during the period of reproduction can have serious short- and long-term adverse effects on mother and child. There is increasing information about how variability in diet, nutrient metabolism, and individual nutritional needs affects pregnancy weight gain, fetal growth, risk of preterm delivery, birth defects, and other pregnancy outcomes. Well-designed studies on undernourished women in developing countries have revealed the impact that improved maternal nutrition can have on maternal and infant health. However, rates of preterm delivery, low birth weight, birth defects, and other pregnancy complications are still unacceptably high, even in wealthier countries. Furthermore, the increased prevalence of maternal obesity and overnutrition as a result of poor quality diets presents new challenges for the development of pregnancy complications, excess fetal growth, and long-term adverse

https://doi.org/10.1016/B978-0-12-818460-8.00003-4

outcomes for both mother and offspring. There is much to be learned about optimal maternal nutrient requirements and dietary intake patterns during pregnancy.

B. Key Issues

This chapter discusses the physiological changes that occur during pregnancy, maternal macro- and micronutrient requirements to support optimal fetal growth and development and to reduce risk of pregnancy complications, and the nutritional challenges provided by maternal obesity and gestational diabetes mellitus (GDM). New research developments on dietary patterns that may improve pregnancy outcomes are also discussed, as well as concerns regarding food safety and the suitability of following popular diets in the prenatal period. There are many aspects of prenatal nutrition that require further research, as outlined in the section on Research Gaps.

II. PHYSIOLOGICAL DEMANDS OF PREGNANCY

A. Hormonal Changes

In pregnancy, larger amounts of nutrients are required for the growth and metabolism of maternal and fetal tissues and for storage in the fetus. Some of these needs are met by increased maternal food intake, but regardless of dietary intake, there are enormous metabolic adjustments in nutrient utilization that support the development of the fetus. Some of the most important changes are in serum hormone concentrations and in tissue deposition and metabolism and are summarized in Table 3.1.

Human chorionic gonadotropin (hCG) is produced almost exclusively by the placenta (low levels produced by the fetal kidney) and begins to enter the maternal bloodstream after implantation, becoming detectable in the plasma of pregnant women about 8 days after ovulation.[1] The primary function of hCG is to help sustain the corpus luteum, which produces steroid hormones to support the pregnancy until placental steroid production is sufficient. The transition of steroid hormone production from the corpus luteum to the placenta (known as the luteal–placental shift) takes place at 7–10 weeks of gestation. Blood hCG peaks (~100,000 IU/L) at about 8–10 weeks' gestation and then declines to much lower levels (~10,000–20,000 IU/L) by 18–20 weeks, where it remains until term.

Blood progesterone concentrations rise substantially during pregnancy. In early pregnancy, the primary source of progesterone is the corpus luteum. After the luteal–placental shift, the placenta becomes the major source of progesterone synthesis.[1] Progesterone relaxes the smooth muscle cells of the gastrointestinal tract[2] and uterus,[3] stimulates maternal respiration,[4] promotes development of mammary gland lobules, and prevents milk secretion from occurring during pregnancy.[5]

The biosynthesis of estrogens (estrone, estradiol, and estriol) increases substantially during pregnancy, and blood estrogen concentrations continue to rise throughout gestation.[3] Estrogen plays an important role in promoting uterine blood flow and contractility and may play a role in fetal development and organ maturation. Estrogen also influences carbohydrate, lipid, and bone metabolism[6] and, in preparation for lactation, promotes ductal proliferation in the breast and stimulates the synthesis and release of prolactin from the pituitary lactotrophs.[7]

TABLE 3.1 Changes in hormone concentrations and in tissue and nutrient deposition during pregnancy.

Serum hormones, tissues, and metabolic processes	Week of gestation			
	10	20	30	40
Serum placental hormones				
Human chorionic gonadotropin (10^4U/L)	1.3	4.0	3.0	2.5
Human placental lactogen (nmol/L)	23	139	255	394
Estradiol (pmol/L)	5	22	55	66
Products of conception				
Fetus (g)	5	300	1500	3400
Placenta (g)	20	170	430	650
Amniotic fluid (g)	30	250	750	800
Maternal tissue gain				
Uterus (g)	140	320	600	970
Mammary gland (g)	45	180	360	405
Plasma volume (mL)	50	800	1200	1500
Nutrient metabolism and accretion in mother + fetus				
Increase in basal metabolism/day	80[a] 0.19[b]	170 0.41	260 0.62	400 0.95
Fat deposition (g)	328	2064	3594	3825
Protein deposition (g)	36	165	498	925
Iron accretion (mg)				565
Calcium accretion (g)				30
Zinc accretion (mg)				100
Hemoglobin (g/L)	125	117	119	130

[a]*kcal.*
[b]*MJ.*
Data from King (2000a).

Human placental lactogen (hPL) is produced by the placenta. Its blood level correlates with placental and fetal weight, steadily increasing during pregnancy until the last 4 weeks, at the time at which the level reaches a plateau.[1] hPL supports placental and fetal growth by stimulating maternal fat breakdown to increase the circulating levels of free fatty acids, which can be used as an energy source for maternal and fetal nutrition. It also stimulates insulin secretion and production of insulin-like growth factor and induces insulin resistance and carbohydrate intolerance. Additionally, it stimulates mammary gland development in preparation for lactation.[8]

A period of increasing insulin resistance occurs during normal pregnancy. Hormones such as progesterone, placentally derived growth hormone, prolactin, cortisol, and leptin, and cytokines such as tumor necrosis factor all play a role in the insulin resistance of pregnancy. The increase in insulin resistance serves to provide a steady flow of glucose to the fetus.[9]

Although the weight of the fetus increases throughout pregnancy, about 90% of fetal ponderal growth occurs in the last 20 weeks of gestation (Table 3.1). Fetal growth is accompanied by expansion of the placenta, uterus, and mammary glands. The additional tissues cause maternal metabolic rate to increase by 60% during the last half of pregnancy, creating a need for additional dietary energy.[6] The protein, fat, minerals, and vitamins deposited in fetal and maternal tissues come from increased maternal food intake and/or more efficient intestinal absorption or renal reabsorption, depending on the specific nutrient.

B. Changes in Blood and Other Fluids

Plasma volume expansion begins at 6–8 weeks of gestation and increases by approximately 45% (1.2–1.6 L) by late pregnancy, whereas red cell mass increases by only 20%–30% (250–450 mL).[10] The larger proportional increase in plasma volume relative to red cell mass leads to a "hemodilution of pregnancy," especially during the second trimester, when there is the largest rise in plasma volume (Table 3.1). Hemodilution may lead to declines in blood serum concentrations of certain minerals, such as potassium.[9] The hypervolemia of pregnancy is needed to meet the increasing demands of the growing uterus to transport nutrients and elements to the fetus and to protect the mother against parturition-related blood loss.[9]

Albumin serves as a carrier for various minerals, hormones, and fatty acids and helps to maintain oncotic pressure in the capillaries.[11] Concentrations of serum albumin decline during pregnancy; as a result, the concentrations of nutrients that bind to albumin (such as calcium) may decline as well. In contrast, there is a higher level of most globulins, lipids (especially triacylglycerol), and vitamin E. Renal plasma flow increases by 80% and glomerular filtration rate by 50%, accompanied by higher urinary excretion of glucose, amino acids, and water-soluble vitamins, and serum creatinine levels decline.[9]

C. Weight Gain During Pregnancy

Weight gain is a normal aspect of pregnancy that occurs as the mother's body adapts to support fetal growth, parturition, and lactation. The products of conception (amniotic fluid, fetus, and placenta) and maternal structural changes, such as an increase in uterine size and fat stores, expanded blood and extravascular fluid volumes, and accumulation of cellular water and protein, all contribute to gestational weight gain.[9,12]

Guidelines for gestational weight gain were revised by the US Institute of Medicine (IOM) in 2009. They were based on the best available evidence at that time, taking into consideration both the welfare of the mother and her offspring. The recommended weight gains (Table 3.2) are those associated with lowest prevalence of cesarean delivery, postpartum weight retention, preterm birth, small- (<10th percentile) and large-for-gestational-age (>90th percentile) infants, and childhood obesity. The amount of weight gain that optimizes these outcomes varies by maternal body mass index (BMI, kg/m^2) prior to pregnancy. The IOM recommendations for total weight gain and the rate of second- and third-trimester weight gain for women carrying a single fetus are categorized by World Health Organization (WHO) BMI groupings, as shown in Table 3.2.[12]

The IOM guidelines contain provisional weight gain recommendations for women with multifetal pregnancies with normal weight, overweight, and obesity prepregnancy (Table 3.2). The available data sources by which to make these provisional recommendations were limited, and there was insufficient evidence to make recommendations for women with multifetal pregnancies in the underweight BMI category. In addition, the IOM committee concluded that there was insufficient evidence to support modification of the weight gain recommendations based on racial/ethnic group, parity, and for adolescents or women of short stature. Although recent studies have suggested that the IOM weight gain guidelines may not be appropriate for Asian pregnant populations,[13–16] a metaanalysis of the data found that these guidelines are applicable if regional BMI categories are used to classify East Asian women.[16] Although several countries outside of the United States follow the IOM guidelines, there is currently no global consensus on optimal gestational weight gain, and further research to establish ethnicity-specific guidelines is warranted.[17]

TABLE 3.2 Institute of Medicine weight gain recommendations for pregnancy, by prepregnancy BMI.

Body mass index (BMI) category	Total pregnancy weight gain for singleton pregnancies		Rate of weight gain for singleton pregnancies in second and third trimester		Total weight gain for multifetal pregnancies[a]	
	Range in kg	**Range in lbs**	**Mean (range) in kg/week**	**Mean (range) in lbs/week**	**Range in kg**	**Range in lbs**
Underweight (BMI <18.5)	12.5–18	28–40	0.51 (0.44–0.58)	1 (1–1.3)	–	–
Normal (BMI 18.5–24.9)	11.5–16	25–35	0.42 (0.35–0.50)	1 (0.8–1)	17–25	37–54
Overweight (BMI 25.0–29.9)	7–11.5	15–25	0.28 (0.23–0.33)	0.6 (0.5–0.7)	14–23	31–50
Obese (BMI ≥30.0)	5–9	11–20	0.22 (0.17–0.27)	0.5 (0.4–0.6)	11–19	25–42

[a] *Provisional guidelines are available for women with a multifetal pregnancy, but not for those with a prepregnancy BMI in the underweight category. Recommendations on the rate of weight gain for multifetal pregnancies also have not been established.*

Adapted from Institute of Medicine and National Research Council. 2009. Weight Gain During Pregnancy: Reexamining the Guidelines. *Washington, DC: The National Academies Press.*

Women who smoke are at increased risk for delivering a small-for-gestational-age (SGA) infant; however, based on data from gestational weight gain studies of women who smoke, a substantially higher weight gain would be required to reduce the risk of SGA. The IOM committee noted that at least some of the effect of smoking on birth weight was independent of weight gain and concluded that asking women who smoke to gain a higher amount of weight would result in an unfavorable trade-off between significantly increased maternal postpartum weight retention and a small likelihood of reducing SGA.[12]

One controversial topic is the recommendation of limited weight gain or weight maintenance during pregnancy for women with obesity, particularly for women with BMI $\geq$35 kg/m^2 (Class 2 obesity or greater). There are data to suggest weight gain below the current IOM guidelines, or even weight loss, may optimize perinatal outcomes for women with obesity.[12,18,19] However, the IOM guidelines committee concluded that the evidence was insufficient to recommend lower weight gain for women with obesity. Their concern was the potential for risk of fetal growth restriction and harm to the fetus secondary to ketonemia, which might occur with severe dietary restriction, and that women and their health care providers might be inadequately equipped to implement a nutritionally balanced, calorie-restricted diet that would avoid ketonemia.[12]

In contrast, low weight gain is a significant concern for women who are underweight as they have the highest risk of delivering a low birth weight infant and low weight gain further increases the risk of poor fetal growth.

Internationally, both excessive and inadequate gestational weight gain are of concern and are associated with increased risk of adverse maternal and fetal outcomes. Data from a systematic review and metaanalysis of over 1 million pregnancies from diverse international cohorts indicate that globally 47% of women gain too much and 23% of women gain too little weight during pregnancy.[16]

To help women optimize their pregnancy weight gain, the IOM committee recommended that health care providers establish a weight gain goal with each woman at the beginning of her pregnancy, chart her weight gain during pregnancy and review her progress toward her weight gain goal at each prenatal visit, and provide guidance on dietary intake and physical activity.[12]

There are multiple resources for BMI-specific gestational weight gain charts for use by patients and providers.[12,20] Conversely, in the United Kingdom, the National Institute for Health and Clinical Excellence (NICE) recommends against routine weighing of women during pregnancy and states that weight tracking should only be "confined to circumstances in which clinical management is likely to be influenced."[21] While NICE emphasizes the importance of addressing diet and physical activity among women who enter pregnancy with a BMI $\geq$30 kg/m^2, it concludes that there is insufficient experimental evidence that monitoring gestational weight gain will lead to improved birth outcomes.

It is also important for providers to assist women in returning to their prepregnancy weight after delivery. Many studies have demonstrated that interpregnancy weight gain or increase in weight from the onset of one pregnancy to the next is associated with increased risk for adverse pregnancy outcomes, such as preeclampsia, gestational diabetes, large-for-gestational-age infants, and cesarean delivery, in subsequent pregnancies.[22–27]

III. NUTRITIONAL REQUIREMENTS

A. Basis for Key Nutrient Recommendations

The profound physiological changes that cause hemodilution, changes in the ratio of free to bound forms of nutrients, and alterations in nutrient turnover and homeostasis affect our ability to assess nutritional status and requirements during pregnancy. For most nutrients, the recommended intake is calculated using a factorial approach. This involves adding estimates of the amount of the nutrient deposited in the mother and fetus, and a factor to cover the inefficiency of utilization for tissue growth, to the requirements for nonpregnant women. For a few nutrients, including folate, some experimental data exist so recommendations can be based on the amount needed to maintain tissue levels and nutrient-dependent function. A summary of recommended nutrient intakes for pregnancy is provided in Table 3.3.

B. Dietary Guidance

Energy

During pregnancy, energy requirements increase to cover energy deposited in the mother and fetus (~180 kcal/day, for a total of 3.8 kg fat and 925 g protein over pregnancy).[28] In addition, energy expenditure increases by 8 kcal/d/week due to the cost of additional fetal and maternal metabolism. These increased needs start primarily in the second trimester when the estimated energy requirement (EER) = *nonpregnant requirement* + *(8 kcal/d/week* × *20 weeks)* + *180 kcal/day*. In the third trimester, the EER = *nonpregnant requirement* + *(8 kcal/d/week* × *34 weeks)* + *180 kcal/day*. The actual amount of energy required varies greatly among pregnant women

TABLE 3.3 Recommended daily intakes of nutrients for nonpregnant and pregnant adult women.

Nutrient	Adult women	Pregnancy
Energy (kcal)	2000–2200[a]	+340[b], +452[c]
Energy (MJ)	8.37–9.21[a]	+1.42[b], +1.89[c]
Protein (g/kg)	0.8	1.1
Carbohydrate (g)	130	175
Fiber (g)	14	14
Linoleic acid (g)	12	13
α-Linolenic acid (g)	1.1	1.4
Vitamin A (μg retinol equivalents)	700	770
Vitamin D (μg)	15 (600 IU)	15 (600 IU)
Vitamin E (mg α-tocopherol)	15	15
Vitamin K (μg)	90	90
Vitamin C (mg)	75	85
Thiamin (mg)	1.1	1.4
Riboflavin (mg)	1.1	1.4
Vitamin B_6 (mg)	1.3	1.9
Niacin (mg niacin equivalents)	14	18
Folate (μg dietary folate equivalents)	400	600
Vitamin B_{12} (μg)	2.4	2.6
Pantothenic acid (mg)	5	6
Biotin (μg)	30	30
Choline (mg)	425	450
Calcium (mg)	1000	1000
Phosphorus (mg)	700	700
Magnesium (mg)	310[d], 320[e]	350
Iron (mg)	18	27
Zinc (mg)	8	11
Iodine (μg)	150	220
Selenium (μg)	55	60
Fluoride (mg)	3	3

Values represent recommendations of the Institute of Medicine, 2006, except for calcium and vitamin D recommendations, which were updated by the Institute of Medicine in 2011. Values are recommended dietary intakes (RDAs) except for vitamin K, pantothenic acid, biotin, choline, and fluoride, where the value is an Adequate Intake.
[a]*Assuming moderately active woman.*
[b]*Trimester 2.*
[c]*Trimester 3.*
[d]*Nonpregnant women aged 19–30 years.*
[e]*Nonpregnant women aged 31–50 years.*

because of differences in the amount of weight and fat gain and energy expenditure. One study of 10 healthy North American women reported that the cumulative energy costs of tissue metabolism and deposition ranged from 60,000 to 170,000 kcal (252–714 MJ) over the course of gestation.[29] It is unclear how this almost threefold variability in energy deposition can be translated into recommended energy intakes.

Higher energy intakes by underweight pregnant women can improve birth weight and length and reduce stillbirths and perinatal mortality.[30,31] A higher energy intake causes more maternal fat deposition as well as a higher metabolic rate across well- and poorly nourished populations.[32] In Gambia, the midpregnancy resting metabolic rate of undernourished women actually fell below prepregnancy values, presumably to conserve energy for fetal development, but the resting metabolic rate increased significantly when the women received supplemental energy. It is evident that although there are adaptations in energy expenditure and deposition depending on energy availability, they do not necessarily promote optimal fetal development and long-term health.[33] For example, an individual who suffered nutritional restriction in utero has a "thrifty genotype" or "thrifty phenotype," such that their metabolism is programmed to preferentially store fat and reduce energy expenditure. While this may help survival in conditions of nutrient restriction, it may also increase the risk of obesity and type 2 diabetes when the food supply is plentiful. Risk of coronary heart disease, hypercholesterolemia, and hypertension is higher for adults who were born small.[34] In utero undernutrition may also adversely affect later adult immunocompetence.[33] In Gambia, for example, adults born during the hungry season had an 11-fold higher risk of dying prematurely of infectious diseases than those born during the rest of the year.[30] It is becoming increasingly evident that undernutrition in utero has serious long-term consequences for poor health.[35]

At present, the best strategy may be to monitor weight gain closely and counsel women to either consume more dietary energy or consume less as needed. Because the requirement for most nutrients increases substantially more than that for energy, however, recommendations of lower energy intake must be made with caution to avoid compromising nutrient density of the diet. Advice to improve dietary quality and to obtain sufficient exercise is usually appropriate.

Fats and essential fatty acids

Dietary fat is required during pregnancy to provide a maternal source of fuel, for fetal brain and eye development, and to increase maternal fat stores in preparation for lactation. The recommended intake of total fat as a percent of daily energy is the same as for the nonpregnant population, i.e., 20%–35% energy. Pregnant women should emphasize intake of mono- and polyunsaturated fats and minimize saturated fats, particularly those from processed animal foods. A very low-fat diet (≤20% energy from fat) may compromise fetal development through insufficient maternal supply of essential polyunsaturated fatty acids (PUFAs).

Essential PUFAs, which must be consumed in the diet, are linoleic acid (LA, 18:2n-6) and α-linolenic acid (ALA, 18:3n-3), found mainly in vegetable and seed oils, nuts, and seeds. Their long-chain more unsaturated derivatives include arachidonic acid (AA) and dihomo-γ-linolenic acid derived from LA and eicosapentaenoic acid (EPA) and docosahexanoic acid (DHA) derived from ALA. EPA is a precursor of prostanoids, while AA and DHA play critical roles in fetal and infant central nervous system (CNS) development.[36,37] The fetal supply of PUFAs depends on maternal PUFA status, and the developing fetal brain is particularly susceptible to nutritional deficiencies in the third trimester, when fetal long-chain PUFA accumulation is at its peak.[38] Indeed, suboptimal PUFA status of some pregnant women has been found to be inadequate to support optimal neonatal status, especially if there are multiple births.[39] Aberrant long-chain PUFA metabolism has also been associated with pregnancies complicated by GDM[40] and the pathogenesis of preeclampsia.[41]

The Adequate Intake recommendation for LA increases from 12 to 13 g/day for pregnancy, and for ALA from 1.1 to 1.4 g/day, based on usual population intakes. However, since endogenous conversion of ALA to the long-chain omega-3 EPA and DHA is less than 10%,[42] pregnant women are advised to increase their long-chain omega-3 fatty acid consumption through fatty fish, particularly those low in mercury (e.g., salmon, sardines, anchovies), due to the potential for fetal neurotoxicity from excess mercury intake from larger, predatory fish. Consumption of Westernized diets rich in highly processed foods and vegetable oils typically predisposes to an imbalanced ratio of n-6:n-3 fatty acids (>1:1). There are some suggestions that such PUFA imbalances in pregnant women are associated with greater adiposity and emotional and behavioral problems in their offspring,[43,44] although this is an ongoing area of research. Higher intakes of *trans* fatty acids are associated with poorer maternal and neonatal PUFA status; however, this is rarely a concern today as most *trans* fatty acids have been eradicated from the food supply.

Carbohydrate

To support normal fetal growth and brain development, carbohydrates should comprise 45%−65% of daily calories consumed. The Recommended Daily Allowance (RDA) for carbohydrates is a minimum of 175 g daily for women who are pregnant.[45] To promote good glycemic control and provide adequate fiber, the majority of carbohydrate intake should come from whole grains, vegetables, and fruit, with a minimum of simple sugars. Although a low−glycemic index (GI) diet has been popularized for its glycemic moderating effects, there is inconclusive evidence from clinical trials that following a low-GI diet during pregnancy is helpful for preventing GDM, excess fetal growth, or other adverse perinatal outcomes.[46]

The total quantity of carbohydrate in the maternal diet has been a topic of much research in recent years, particularly with increased prevalence of maternal obesity, insulin resistance, and GDM. In addition to recommending a minimal intake of simple sugars, it has long been accepted clinical practice to advise patients with GDM to restrict total carbohydrate intake to improve glycemic control.[47] The Endocrine Society Clinical Practice Guidelines suggest that women with GDM consume 35%−45% of total calories from carbohydrate.[48] However, there is also concern that replacing a proportion of carbohydrates with dietary fat in pregnancies complicated by GDM may increase levels of maternal plasma triglycerides and contribute to excess fetal fat deposition.[49] Further research is required to determine the optimal proportion of dietary carbohydrate for pregnant women with obesity or GDM. Women who are pregnant or plan to become pregnant should use caution when following a very−low-carbohydrate (<30% energy) or ketogenic diet due to a risk of nutrition inadequacy, potentially leading to negative outcomes such as altered fetal neurodevelopment and organ growth (see Section III.C.vi).[50]

Protein

From very early in pregnancy, there are adaptations in maternal nitrogen metabolism that increase nitrogen and protein deposition in the mother and fetus. These include lower urea production and excretion, lower plasma α-amino nitrogen, and a lower rate of branched chain amino acid transamination.[51] The RDAs provide for an additional 925 g of protein deposited in the mother and fetus, of which an additional ~8 g/day is needed during the second trimester and ~17 g/day during the third.[28] Thus, the total RDA is 1.1 g/kg/day or +25 g/day additional protein. Most pregnant women in industrialized countries, and probably the majority in developing countries, consume at least the recommended amount of protein.

Vitamin A

Vitamin A is involved in immune function, vision, reproduction, and cellular communication.[52,53] Vitamin A deficiency during pregnancy and lactation is rare in industrialized countries but of concern worldwide, particularly in Africa and Southeast Asia.[54] It is a significant cause of night blindness among pregnant women.[54] Among children, it is the leading cause of preventable blindness and increases the risk of disease and death from severe infections.[55,56]

The RDAs for vitamin A are given as micrograms (mcg) of retinol activity equivalents (RAEs) to account for the different bioactivities of retinol and provitamin A carotenoids. The RAE for pregnancy is 770 mcg/day, which is just slightly higher than the RAE of 700 mcg/day recommended for nonpregnant women of reproductive age.

Current evidence indicates that vitamin A supplementation during pregnancy does not reduce the risk of illness or death in mothers or their infants.[54] The WHO recommends vitamin A supplementation (to prevent night blindness) only among pregnant women in areas where vitamin A deficiency is a severe public health problem. There is conflicting evidence as to whether vitamin A supplementation among women with HIV decreases maternal–fetal HIV transmission, and further investigation is needed.[57]

Excessive supplementation with retinol or the analog isotretinoin, which is a drug used to treat severe cystic acne, is associated with birth defects, including abnormalities of the CNS and craniofacial and cardiovascular defects.[53,55] The first trimester is the most vulnerable stage because the malformations are derived from cranial neural crest cells.[55]

The upper safe limit of preformed vitamin A has been set at 3000 μg/day RAE (10,000 IU) for women of reproductive age and in pregnancy.[55] Large intakes of β-carotene do not have a teratogenic effect.[58]

Vitamin D

Adequate vitamin D status is important during pregnancy to promote normal skeletal development in the fetus and to prevent neonatal vitamin D deficiency. The conversion of vitamin D3 to 25-hydroxyvitamin D (25(OH)D) during pregnancy is largely unchanged from the nonpregnant state. However, the conversion of 25(OH)D to the active form 1,25-dihydroxyvitamin D ($1,25(OH)_2D$) increases substantially by the end of the first trimester compared to nonpregnant women, driven by increases in renal synthesis plus placenta/decidual tissue production.[59,60] Maternal serum levels of $1,25(OH)_2D$ are more than doubled by late pregnancy, and maternal and neonatal levels are highly correlated at delivery. Thus, depending on maternal 25(OH)D substrate availability, fetal $1,25(OH)_2D$ levels also rise with advancing gestation.[61] This increase in maternal/fetal $1,25(OH)_2D$ across pregnancy does not appear to be driven by calcium homeostatic mechanisms but rather may have important immunomodulatory properties by ensuring maternal tolerance to the fetus.[62,63] Some evidence exists for vitamin D playing a role in prevention of hypertensive disorders of pregnancy, including preeclampsia.[64] Maternal vitamin D insufficiency has also been implicated as a risk factor for GDM, preterm birth and SGA.[65,66]

Currently, there is a lack of adequate evidence to determine the optimal intake of vitamin D levels for pregnancy. As a result, most agencies provide the same dietary recommendation for pregnant adults as they do for nonpregnant adults in order to prevent maternal vitamin D deficiency. In the United States and Canada, the RDA is set at 600 IU/day (15 μg).[67] The WHO recommends a lower intake of 200 IU/day (5 μg), and it does not recommend vitamin D supplementation for pregnant women, unless they already have been diagnosed with vitamin D deficiency.[68] However, it has been argued that higher doses may be required to protect against neonatal deficiency.[61,62,69] This may be particularly important for women at higher risk of inadequate vitamin D status on entering pregnancy, such as those living at northerly latitudes, with darker skin pigmentation, and who have a low intake of vitamin D from fortified foods and supplements.[70,71] Additionally, seasonal variation in maternal serum 25(OH)D levels has been reported,[72–74] which may further exacerbate maternal and infant vitamin D deficiency in the absence of supplementation, increasing the risk of abnormal skeletal development among offspring with winter gestations.

Vitamin B6

The vitamin B6 RDA for women who are pregnant is 1.9 mg/day. Vitamin B6 primarily plays a role as a coenzyme for protein metabolism.[75] Although plasma concentrations of pyridoxal and pyridoxal phosphate decline more than can be accounted for by hemodilution, this is probably caused by hormonal changes rather than by poorer vitamin status.[75] Pyridoxal is transferred via active diffusion to the placenta, which converts it to pyridoxal phosphate.[76]

In the United States, nonpregnant women's intake of vitamin B6 averages about 1.5 mg per day, but there is no evidence of a significant vitamin B6 deficiency problem. In Japan, a maternal B6 supplement of 2 mg per day of the vitamin improved vitamin B6 status and growth of the newborn.[77] Furthermore, vitamin B6 is often prescribed during pregnancy to treat hyperemesis gravidarum.[78]

Folate

There is a marked increase in folate utilization during pregnancy as a result of the acceleration of reactions requiring single-carbon transfer, the rapid rate of cell division in maternal and fetal tissues, and deposition in the fetus. A higher intake of folate from diet plus supplements,[79,80] or higher erythrocyte folate concentrations,[81] is inversely related to neural tube defect (NTD) risk. The metabolic defect that causes NTDs and the mechanisms by which folic acid lowers NTD risk are not fully understood, although disruption of the folate-metabolizing enzyme, serine hydroxymethyltransferase 1, has been implicated.[82]

Randomized controlled trials have proven that taking folic acid supplements before conception and through about the first 4 weeks of pregnancy lowers the risk of genetically predisposed women having a baby with an NTD.[83,84] Unfortunately, most women are unaware that they are pregnant at this early stage. NTDs occur in about 5.5/10,000 births in the United States and up to 40/10,000 in other countries and tend to recur in subsequent pregnancies.

The RDA for folic acid in pregnancy is 600 μg of dietary folic acid equivalents and is based on the amount that maintained erythrocyte folate concentrations in clinical trials. Since 1998, in an effort to ensure folate adequacy on a population level for NTD prevention, the FDA has required fortification of all enriched grain products in the United States to reach a level of 140 μg folic acid/100g of product.[85] Folate found in food has only about half the bioavailability of the synthetic form. Therefore, to reduce the risk of NTD, women are widely recommended to take 400 μg/day of synthetic folic acid from fortified foods and/or supplements during both the preconception and prenatal periods, in addition to consuming food folate from a varied diet.[75,86,87] This amount is expected to maintain normal folate status in pregnancy and prevent elevated plasma homocysteine concentrations. Maternal supplements of 400 μg folic acid/day reduced the occurrence of NTDs in Northern China by up to 80%,[88] and by 70% in New England, 35% in California, and 28% overall in the United States; the percent reduction is higher in populations with a higher initial prevalence of NTDs.[83]

The American College of Obstetricians and Gynecologists (ACOG) recommends that women at increased risk of NTDs should supplement with a higher daily dose of folic acid, 4000 mcg (4 mg) rather than 400 mcg, starting from 3 months prior to conception through 12 weeks gestation. This group of woman at risk includes those with a previous pregnancy affected by an NTD, women who are affected with an NTD themselves, those who have a partner who is affected, or those with a partner with a previous affected child.[87]

Another consideration is that the efficiency of conversion of inactive folic acid to its biologically active form, L-methylfolate, can be compromised by a genetic polymorphism of the methylenetetrahydrofolate reductase (MTHFR) enzyme. Up to 25% of certain populations are homozygous for these genetic variations.[89] Women who may become pregnant may benefit from supplementing directly with L-methylfolate rather than folic acid to improve their folate status,[90,91] although further research is required on the efficacy of preconception and prenatal L-methylfolate supplementation before being widely recommended.

Calcium

Maternal calcium absorption doubles during pregnancy. There is both increased calcium absorption from the intestine and increased maternal excretion of urinary calcium due to increased calcium clearance.[92] Calcium is transferred across the placenta daily to meet fetal needs. The rate of transfer is greatest in the late third trimester, ranging from 300 to 350 mg/day.[93]

The IOM recommends a calcium intake of 1000 mg/day, the same as for nonpregnant women aged 19–50 years.[94] For pregnant women under 18 years of age, the recommended intake is 1300 mg/day. Data are conflicting as to whether calcium supplementation benefits maternal and neonatal bone mineral content for women with low dietary calcium intake.[95,96] Although there is a modest amount of maternal bone resorption during pregnancy, this loss is generally reversible, recovering within 6–12 months of weaning.[92]

Several randomized trials have been conducted to assess the effect of calcium supplements for reducing the risk of pregnancy-related hypertensive disorders. These disorders arise after 20 weeks' gestation and include gestational hypertension, i.e., new-onset hypertension without other signs or symptoms and preeclampsia and eclampsia. Preeclampsia occurs when there is both hypertension and other signs or symptoms, such as proteinuria, thrombocytopenia; impaired liver function, indicated by elevated blood concentrations of liver enzymes and severe persistent right upper quadrant or epigastric pain unresponsive to medication; renal insufficiency; pulmonary edema; new-onset headache unresponsive to medication; and visual disturbances.[97] Eclampsia refers to the occurrence of grand mal seizures in a patient with gestational hypertension or preeclam psia.[97,98] Worldwide, preeclampsia-eclampsia is one of the three leading causes of maternal morbidity and mortality, affecting an estimated 2%–8% of pregnancies[98] and accounting for approximately 14% of all maternal deaths.[99]

Trials have shown conflicting results about the impact of calcium supplementation for reducing the incidence of preeclampsia and its related morbidity and mortality.[100–102] However, a systematic review, which included 27 randomized trials of calcium supplementation for the prevention of preeclampsia, suggests that high-dose calcium supplementation (≥1 g/day) may reduce the risk of preeclampsia and preterm birth, among women with a history of a low-calcium diet (<900 mg/day).[99,103]

Due to the substantial morbidity and mortality attributable to preeclampsia-eclampsia and the existing scientific evidence regarding calcium supplementation during pregnancy, the WHO recommends daily calcium supplementation (1.5–2.0 g oral elemental calcium) for pregnant women with low dietary calcium intake to reduce the risk of preeclampsia.[99] The ACOG does not currently recommend calcium supplementation for preeclampsia prevention.[104]

Iron

During pregnancy, the amount of iron a woman needs to absorb rises substantially, increasing from 1.2 mg/day in the first trimester to 4.7 mg/day and 5.6 mg/day in the second and third trimesters, respectively.[105] The total estimated additional iron requirement of pregnancy is 1130 mg.[106] The greatest proportion of additional iron is used for expansion of maternal red cell mass (450 mg), followed by fetal requirements (270 mg). The fetus preferentially obtains iron from the mother. Maternal iron is carried by transferrin and actively transferred to the fetus via transferrin receptors on the placenta. Iron is also retained in the placenta and umbilical cord (90 mg) and lost through normal maternal excretion routes (170 mg), such as the gastrointestinal tract, and through blood loss at delivery (150 mg).

Iron deficiency is the most common cause of anemia worldwide, affecting nearly one-third of women of reproductive age.[105,107] Internationally, iron deficiency anemia affects 43% of pregnant women, with the highest prevalence in Central and West Africa (56%) and South Asia (52%).[107] The Centers for Disease Control and Prevention (CDC) estimated the prevalence of anemia among pregnant women using NHANES 2003–12 data and found an overall prevalence of 8.8%, although race–ethnicity disparities existed; prevalence of anemia among black pregnant women was 24.2%. From the same study, prevalence of iron deficiency among US pregnant females aged 22–49 years was found to increase as pregnancy progressed, with prevalence estimates of 5.3%, 12.7%, and 27.5%, in the first, second, and third trimester, respectively.[108]

The increase in prevalence of anemia across trimesters of pregnancy parallels the increasing demand for iron during pregnancy. Iron deficiency anemia during pregnancy has been associated with an increased risk of low birth weight, preterm birth, and perinatal mortality.[105,109] There may also be an association of maternal iron deficiency anemia with postpartum depression and poorer results on mental and psychomotor performance testing in the offspring.[109]

Many organizations, including the WHO, recommend screening for anemia at the first prenatal visit.[105,109,110] Hemoglobin concentrations decline during pregnancy, reaching their lowest point in the second trimester.[111] The WHO, CDC, and ACOG recommend a lower cut point for anemia in the second trimester (hemoglobin <105 g/L or hematocrit <32%) compared to the first and third trimesters (hemoglobin <110 g/L or hematocrit <33%).[109,110,112]

All diagnostic thresholds for anemia in pregnancy are lower relative to the cut point for nonpregnant women (hemoglobin of <120 g/L for women age 15 years or older).[111]

The RDA for iron intake in pregnancy is 27 mg/day.[105,113] Recommendations for iron supplementation in pregnancy vary across institutions. The WHO recommends pregnant women take a daily iron supplement with 30–60 mg of elemental iron (equivalent to 300 mg ferrous sulfate) to prevent maternal anemia, puerperal sepsis, low birth weight, and preterm birth.[105] The higher daily dose of 60 mg is recommended when the population prevalence of anemia in pregnancy is 40% or greater.[105] For those who cannot tolerate the side effects of daily supplementation and the population prevalence of anemia is <20%, the WHO suggests a weekly oral iron supplement of 120 mg. The CDC also recommends advising pregnant women at their first prenatal visit to start taking a daily oral iron supplement that contains 30 mg/day, and if diagnosed with anemia, treating them with an oral dose of 60–120 mg/day.[110] The ACOG states that perinatal iron supplementation is important because the typical American diet and endogenous iron stores of women are inadequate to meet the demands of pregnancy. They note that most prenatal vitamins have sufficient iron content to meet the RDA of 27 mg daily and only recommend additional iron supplementation for women diagnosed with iron deficiency anemia.[109]

The advantages of routine maternal iron supplementation, regardless of iron status, are uncertain,[114,115] so supplements are not given routinely in some countries, including many in Europe. A large systematic review found that preventive iron supplementation in pregnancy, in which included studies used doses ranging from 20 to 100 mg of elemental iron daily, reduced both the risk of maternal anemia and iron deficiency anemia at term but not maternal mortality or infection.[115] Women taking iron supplements, compared to controls, had a smaller but nonsignificant difference in the proportion of low birth weight newborns and preterm birth and no difference in neonatal death or congenital anomalies. Overall, the authors of this review found that the general quality of the evidence was low, suggesting a need for additional research.

Iron supplementation during pregnancy increases iron stores of the infant for ~6 months, which is an advantage especially in developing countries where complementary foods are low in available iron.[116] Infants are at greatest risk of iron deficiency anemia if they were low birth weight and their mothers were anemic.[117]

An additional measure to reduce the risk of anemia in offspring is delayed umbilical cord clamping. Delayed cord clamping (30–60 s) after birth allows blood to continue to flow between the placenta and neonate and reduces the risk of anemia in the infant through 6 months of life. The WHO, ACOG, and NICE recommend delayed cord clamping for all births of vigorous term and preterm infants.[105,118,119] The NICE and WHO recommend the cord not be clamped earlier than 1 min after birth, whereas ACOG recommends a 30–60 s delay in cord clamping.

Zinc

The estimated additional zinc required for pregnancy is ~100 mg, equivalent to 5%–7% of the mother's body zinc.[120] About half of this zinc is deposited in the fetus and one-quarter in the uterus. The recommendation is to increase zinc intake by an additional 3 mg/day to a total of 11 mg/day among women 19 years of age and older; 12 mg/d is recommended for those aged 14–18 years.[121] Homeostatic adjustments in circulating zinc, zinc absorption, excretion, and whole-body kinetics enable women to meet pregnancy needs over a wide range of intakes.[122] Zinc deficiency is likely to be more prevalent in populations consuming low amounts of animal source foods and high amounts of foods such as beans, grains, nuts, and seeds, which are rich in phytates and inhibit zinc absorption. Nevertheless, a threshold below which zinc homeostatic adjustments cannot be made to support a healthy pregnancy outcome has not been established. The usual decline in plasma zinc concentrations during pregnancy due to expanded plasma volume obviates it as a biomarker of maternal zinc nutrition.[123]

In addition to the zinc accrued by the fetus, it is also deposited in the placenta, amniotic fluid, and uterine and mammary tissue. Zinc plays critical roles in cell division, hormone metabolism, protein and carbohydrate metabolism, and immunocompetence during pregnancy.[124] A metaanalysis of zinc supplementation trials indicated a 14% reduction in preterm deliveries among the supplemented women.[125] Although most studies have not shown a significant effect of maternal zinc supplementation on infant birth weight, no adverse effects have been observed, and there may be a beneficial effect in underweight or zinc-deficient women. Since supplemental zinc may reduce preterm deliveries and improve infant birth weights without any adverse effects, zinc should be included in prenatal supplements for pregnant women in populations at risk for zinc deficiency.

Iodine

Iodine is a critical component of thyroid hormone synthesis, particularly thyroxine (T4) and triiodothyronine (T3).[126,127] During pregnancy, renal clearance of iodine is enhanced and a significant amount of iodine is diverted to the fetoplacental unit to support fetal thyroid hormone production.[128] Iodine, thyroxine, and triiodothyronine cross the placenta.[126,128] Fetal thyroid hormone production begins in midgestation; prior to that time, the fetus relies on an adequate supply of maternal thyroid hormones.[128]

Lack of iodine in the diet can lead to insufficient production of thyroid hormones, resulting in maternal goiter and hypothyroidism.[126] Iodine deficiency during pregnancy can have permanent adverse effects on the infant as thyroid hormones play a critical role in skeletal and CNS development. Hypothyroidism in the fetus or early childhood leads to congenital hypothyroidism.[126] In the most severe cases of congenital hypothyroidism, children may experience severe intellectual disability, short stature with incomplete skeletal development, coarse facial features, and a protruding tongue.[126] Even mild iodine deficiency in pregnancy may result in long-term cognitive effects in offspring.[129,130]

The WHO, United Nations Children's Fund, and former International Council for the Control of Iodine Deficiency (now part of the Iodine Global Network) recommend an increase in iodine intake from 150 μg/day for a woman of reproductive age (15–49 years) to 250 μg/day for pregnant women.[131] The RDA for pregnant women is slightly lower at 220 μg/day.[55]

Iodine deficiency may be corrected by increasing intake of iodized salt or foods rich in iodine or use of iodine supplements. Dairy products, fish, eggs, and seaweed contain iodine, as do fruit, vegetables, and bread in small amounts.[132] However, dietary sources may not provide sufficient amounts to prevent deficiency, particularly in areas where the soils are iodine deficient or iodized salt intake is low.[126,133,134] Despite having a universal salt iodization process in many countries around the world,[131] there is evidence that iodine deficiency is still a widespread concern.[134–136] Iodine intake is considered insufficient to protect the fetus and young child in countries where the proportion of households consuming iodized salt is <90%.[137]

Iodine supplements may be given daily as potassium iodide or annually as a single annual oral dose of 400 mg of iodine as iodized oil.[137] In addition, some multivitamins contain iodine as potassium or sodium iodide.[132]

C. Other Guidance

Alcohol

The adverse effects of alcohol on the fetus were first described in the 1960s.[138] Ethanol readily crosses the placenta. It acts directly as a teratogen and indirectly as a disrupter of normal physiologic processes, including absorption and metabolism of nutrients.[139]

Birth defects related to alcohol include facial dysmorphologies, growth retardation, and CNS neurodevelopmental abnormalities.[139,140] There is a broad range of disabilities among children exposed prenatally to alcohol, which are now known as fetal alcohol spectrum disorders (FASD).[138] FASD are the leading cause of preventable developmental disabilities in the world,[138] and associated behavioral disorders and impaired intellectual development can lead to challenges with school and employment for exposed individuals.[140] The global prevalence of FASD is 22.8 per 1000 births and varies by country, ranging from 1.1 per 1000 in Australia to 113.2 per 1000 in South Africa.[141]

Alcohol use during pregnancy has also been associated with an increased risk of miscarriage and intrauterine fetal death.[139] A safe threshold for alcohol intake during pregnancy has not been determined, and there are no currently approved therapies to prevent, slow, or reverse the damage of prenatal alcohol exposure.[139] It is therefore recommended that pregnant women and those who plan to become pregnant abstain from alcohol consumption.[142]

Caffeine

Caffeine is a stimulant that crosses the placenta and has been detected in the amniotic fluid, umbilical cord, urine, and plasma of fetuses.[143,144] Caffeine metabolism is slower in pregnant women, with an elimination half-life that is 1.5–3.5 times longer than for nonpregnant women.[145] Caffeine can raise maternal catecholamine levels,[146] and physiologic data suggest that it may decrease uteroplacental blood flow.[147] Several studies have examined caffeine intake during pregnancy and risk of pregnancy loss and low birth weight. One large systematic review found no increased risk of miscarriage, preterm birth, congenital anomalies or stillbirth with caffeine intakes <300 mg/day.[148] Some studies suggest a possible increased risk in SGA infants and intrauterine growth restriction (IUGR) as caffeine intake increases from as low as 50 mg/day,[149] whereas other studies have shown no effect of caffeine intake on these outcomes.[150–152] It is unclear why data regarding the effects of caffeine intake on SGA/IUGR differ, although in some studies, adjustment for smoking and other confounders eliminates observed associations between caffeine intake and low birth weight.[150,152] Whether abstinence from caffeine during pregnancy has an impact on low birth weight or other pregnancy outcomes has not yet been determined.[153]

The WHO recommends that pregnant women limit caffeine consumption to <300 mg/day, which is similar to three 8-ounce cups of coffee, six cups of black tea, or eight cans (~96 ounces) of cola. The ACOG and the United Kingdom's Royal College of Obstetricians and Gynaecologists recommend that caffeine consumption not exceed 200 mg/day (~two cups of coffee).[146,154]

Pregnancy in women with obesity

Dramatic increases in the prevalence of obesity in recent decades have also affected women of childbearing age. In the United States, over 50% of women are now either overweight or obese entering pregnancy,[155] with marked disparities evident by race and ethnicity.[156] There is general agreement that even moderate degrees of overweight increase the risk of pregnancy complications and adverse outcomes for offspring, and these risks may be largely independent of gestational weight gain.[157] Women with a prepregnancy BMI $\geq$25 kg/m^2 have about two to six times (increasing with higher BMI) the risk of gestational diabetes, gestational hypertension and preeclampsia, preterm delivery, and cesarean delivery, compared with those with normal weight.[158–160] With respect to infant outcomes, maternal obesity increases the risk of low Apgar scores, admission to the neonatal intensive care unit, macrosomia, large for gestational age, perinatal mortality, NTDs, and difficulty in initiating breastfeeding.[161–163] Furthermore, the Developmental Origins of Health and Disease hypothesis suggests that maternal weight and nutritional status before and during pregnancy exert lifelong impact on the health of the offspring. Indeed, maternal prepregnancy obesity and associated metabolic dysfunction increase the risk of greater infant adiposity,[164,165] and increased propensity for development of childhood obesity and cardiometabolic, immune, and neurodevelopmental disorders in later years.[166–168] The fetal programming mechanisms for the intergenerational transfer of obesity risk have been largely attributed to higher maternal plasma glucose concentrations, leading to fetal insulin resistance.[169,170] Research also reveals a plausible role of excess circulating maternal lipids in the development of offspring adiposity and downstream cardiometabolic disease risk.[171,172]

There is currently limited or inadequate evidence that prenatal intervention studies of dietary and/or exercise programs for women with prepregnancy obesity improve important clinical outcomes for mother or baby, even if reduced gestational weight gain is achieved.[173,174] As such, there is growing consensus that preconception counseling about healthy diet and lifestyle habits for weight reduction may provide greater benefit than interventions initiated during pregnancy. While achieving normal weight status prior to conception is the ideal, this may be an unrealistic goal for many women. However, even modest weight loss (3%–5% body weight) prior to conception provides metabolic benefits for the mother, improves fertility, and does not harm the offspring.[175] The impact of substantial preconception weight loss, which can be achieved through very low calorie diets or bariatric surgery, is less clear. Although these approaches may reduce the risk of maternal pregnancy complications such as GDM, there is concern about increased risk of adverse infant outcomes.[176]

It is important to acknowledge the many social and psychological barriers to adopting healthy lifestyle behaviors among women with obesity. The ACOG recommends incorporation of motivational interviewing techniques to improve the success of lifestyle interventions initiated before and during pregnancy.[177] Once they become pregnant, women with obesity need monitoring for diabetes and hypertension and should be advised to gain lower amounts of weight (see Table 3.2) and to increase physical activity. Even if dietary and activity behaviors initiated during the prenatal period do not reduce the immediate risk of pregnancy complications or adverse infant outcomes, there is potential for sustained health behavior change into the postnatal period, which may aid postpartum weight loss and benefit maternal preconception health for future pregnancies.[178]

Gestational diabetes mellitus

GDM has traditionally been defined as carbohydrate intolerance that is first recognized during preg nancy.[179–181] Screening for GDM usually occurs at 24–28 weeks' gestation. Screening is done via either the two-step method—a nonfasting, 1-h, 50-g oral glucose challenge test, which, if abnormal, is followed by a fasting 3-h, 100-gram oral glucose tolerance test (OGTT)—or the one-step method, which is a fasting, 2-h, 75-g OGTT. Diagnostic thresholds for these tests vary.[179–181] With the increased prevalence of diabetes and obesity among reproductive-aged women, many organizations recommend screening women for diabetes mellitus at the first prenatal visit if they have risk factors for type 2 diabetes[179,180] and classifying women as having preexisting or pregestational diabetes if they meet the standard diagnostic criteria for diabetes mellitus outside of pregnancy.[180,181]

Maternal risks associated with GDM include preeclampsia and cesarean birth. Risks to the offspring include macrosomia (birth weight >4000 g), neonatal hypoglycemia, hyperbilirubinemia, shoulder dystocia, birth trauma, and stillbirth, as well as childhood obesity and diabetes.[179] The Hyperglycemia and Adverse Pregnancy Outcomes study, an international, multicenter study in which over 25,000 pregnant women underwent 75-g, 2-h OGTTs at 24–32 weeks' gestation, found that an increase in maternal glucose levels (fasting, 1- and 2-h postprandial) was associated with increased risk of adverse outcomes such as cesarean delivery, large for gestational age (birth weight >90th percentile), and neonatal hypoglycemia, and that there was no obvious threshold at which risks increased (i.e., there was a continuum of increased risk).[182] Primary prevention of GDM and optimization of maternal glycemic control through healthy preconception and prenatal lifestyles are the goal. However, there currently is inconclusive evidence from clinical trials that any particular prenatal dietary intervention is effective for GDM prevention.[46]

Two large, randomized clinical trials have shown that treatment of GDM with dietary modification, self-monitoring of blood glucose, and the addition of insulin, if necessary, reduce the risk of adverse maternal and neonatal outcomes.[183,184] All women diagnosed with GDM should be referred to a dietitian for at least three sessions of dietary counseling within the first 3 weeks of GDM diagnosis.[185] Medical nutrition therapy for GDM typically involves adjustment in absolute carbohydrate and caloric intake, particularly for women with obesity, as well as redistribution of carbohydrate intake throughout the day to optimize maternal fasting and postprandial glucose levels, fetal growth, and maternal weight gain.[186,187] Various dietary patterns have been investigated for their impact on glycemic control and infant outcomes in pregnancies affected by GDM, including implementation of a low GI diet, reduced carbohydrate with higher fat, increased complex carbohydrate with lower fat, and Mediterranean-type diets. While most studies report a reduction in maternal glucose measures, need for treatment with medication, infant birth weight, and macrosomia, the ideal dietary pattern for optimally reducing risks associated with GDM has not yet been established.[188,189] Exercise has also been shown to have favorable effects on maternal glucose and is recommended for all women with GDM; the goal is 30 min or more per day of moderate-intensity aerobic activity.[179,187]

Diet quality patterns in pregnancy

There is growing consensus that it is more helpful to counsel pregnant women about foods and dietary patterns that promote good dietary quality rather than focus on individual nutrients.[190–192] Studies have investigated a variety of diet quality indices and their associations with biomarkers of interest and maternal pregnancy or child outcomes. Common elements that contribute to high-quality diets across several indices include increased consumption of vegetables, whole fruit, whole grains, low-fat or fat-free dairy products, and fatty fish and poultry and reduced intake of simple sugars, red and processed meats, and processed/fried foods rich in saturated and *trans* fats.[193] Broadly, this type of dietary pattern is expected to provide a wide range of micronutrients, polyunsaturated fats, fiber and protein required for optimal fetal growth, adequate gestational weight gain, and reduced risk of pregnancy complications.[190]

While no single dietary pattern is currently recognized as optimal for pregnancy, evidence is accumulating regarding beneficial effects of the Mediterranean dietary pattern, particularly for reduced risk of GDM and infant atopy,[194] and potential protection against excess offspring adiposity and cardiometabolic disease risk.[195] This dietary pattern is rich in monounsaturated fats, primarily from olive oil and nuts, as well as vegetables, fruits, fatty fish, pulses, and whole grains. It relies on a modest dairy intake and is low in red and processed meats, refined grains, simple sugars, and highly processed food. One randomized clinical study has been published that systematically tested the maternal and offspring health outcomes associated with following a Mediterranean dietary pattern in the prenatal period. The St. Carlos GDM Prevention study conducted in Spain provided an abundant supply of extra virgin olive oil and pistachio nuts as a supplement to Mediterranean dietary advice in the intervention group. The intervention was found to significantly reduce the risk of developing GDM and was associated with less gestational weight gain, reduced rates of cesarean delivery, and fewer large-for-gestational-age and SGA babies.[196–198] Furthermore, among women diagnosed with GDM, glycemic control was significantly improved in those following the Mediterranean diet, with less requirement for insulin therapy.[198] The beneficial metabolic effects of this diet may be attributed to the higher intake of healthy fats from olive oil, as well as additional fiber and phytochemicals from nuts, which collectively have the potential to enhance satiety and thermogenesis, reduce inflammation, carbohydrate loading at mealtimes, and postprandial glycemia, and displace less healthful foods from the diet.[199,200] However, further clinical trials in other geographical settings (such as the United States) are required to determine whether a maternal Mediterranean dietary pattern can exert the same favorable effects on pregnancy outcomes among populations where the standard diet deviates further from this pattern.

Suitability and inadequacies of popular diets in the prenatal period

There is a growing trend in the nonpregnant population, including women of childbearing age, to follow a range of other alternative dietary patterns, which would not typically be advised in clinical practice unless indicated for disease treatment. Some of these dietary patterns may or may not be suitable for pregnancy.

Vegan diet; Although vegetarian diets have been followed for centuries, the more recent advent of veganism has been understudied with respect to nutritional adequacy, particularly at critical life stages such as pregnancy.[201] A vegan diet excludes all animal foods, including eggs and dairy. It is therefore deficient in vitamin B12 (without supplementation) and may provide inadequate amounts or insufficient absorption of protein, iron, zinc, calcium, fat-soluble vitamins, and omega-3 fatty acids.

Women who choose to follow a vegan diet before and during pregnancy should receive dietary counseling to ensure all nutrient requirements are met for optimal fetal development and to prevent vitamin B12 or iron deficiency anemia or other pregnancy complications.[202,203] Special attention should be given to appropriate micronutrient supplementation in these women.

Ketogenic Diet; The application of the Ketogenic Diet and modified Atkins diet has increased in the recent years to improve seizure control, glycemic control, and obesity. It is characterized by extremely low intake of dietary carbohydrates in order to raise levels of ketone bodies in circulation; consequently, this diet is very high in fat ($\geq$70% total energy). The use of the Ketogenic Diet during the gestational period by individuals with pharmacologic-resistant epilepsy is not widely studied and needs further investigation to determine safety and long-term effects.

A case report was made of a 27-year-old pregnant woman with epilepsy who was placed on a 75 g/day carbohydrate restriction, which was later reduced to 47 g/day. Her blood glucose levels ranged from 72 to 106 mg/dL and blood ketone levels ranged from 0.2 to 1.4 mmol/L. The acceptable range for blood ketones in pregnancy is $\leq$ 0.6 mmol/L. As a result, seizure frequency decreased, and fetal growth and development were normal.[204]

In an animal study that compared the embryonic organ growth in mice whose mothers were fed either a standard diet or a ketogenic diet, the ketogenic diet embryo was volumetrically smaller but had an enlarged cervical spine, thalamus, midbrain, and pons.[50] Adherence to a ketogenic diet in the perinatal period may be linked to organ development dysfunction. Due to the lack of consistent results from human and animal studies, a ketogenic diet should not be followed during pregnancy, particularly during embryogenesis. This diet may also be a concern for women planning to conceive as they may not realize they are pregnant for the first few weeks, thereby potentially impacting fetal CNS development.

Low-carbohydrate diet; This diet involves a moderate restriction of carbohydrate intake to approximately 100 g/day (~20% total energy), usually to achieve or maintain weight loss or reduce insulin resistance. Fat and/or protein content of the diet is increased in compensation. While a consistently low intake of carbohydrate would not typically raise blood ketone levels in the nonpregnant state, it is possible that a state of ketosis may be reached in pregnancy due to increased fetal glucose utilization, which might compromise fetal development.

Although modest carbohydrate restriction is typically incorporated into nutrition therapy for women with a diagnosis of GDM, there is insufficient evidence that a low-carbohydrate diet is effective for improving maternal or infant health outcomes.[205,206] A low carbohydrate dietary pattern with high intake of fat and protein from animal sources has even been associated with increased GDM risk.[207,208] Furthermore, reduced intake of grain-based foods on a low-carbohydrate diet may compromise maternal folate status and may increase the risk of NTDs, particularly in countries where folic acid fortification of flours is common practice.[209] This diet also may not provide sufficient fiber if whole grains are restricted.

Paleolithic (or caveman) diet; This diet is characterized by consumption of unprocessed whole foods with a focus on those foods that were available during Paleolithic times: whole fruit and vegetables, nuts and seeds, meat and fish, and eggs and low GI starchy vegetables (e.g., carrots, squash, sweet potato) as the primary carbohydrate sources. This diet restricts grains and grain products (e.g., bread), dairy, simple sugars, fruit juice, and processed meat and fish products. There is currently insufficient evidence for beneficial metabolic effects of a Paleolithic diet in general populations.[210]

While there have been no studies evaluating the effects of a paleolithic diet in pregnancy, the general focus on a variety of whole foods suggests that it may be maintained as a healthy diet through pregnancy, provided carbohydrate intake is not overly restricted. Sufficient calcium intake should also be sought through nondairy sources such as nuts, fatty fish, green vegetables, and fortified nondairy milk alternatives. Avoidance of breads and other grain-based foods may reduce women's intake of folate,[209] as described above for low carbohydrate diets. Appropriate folate supplementation and intake of green leafy vegetables should be advised to ensure adequate folate status throughout pregnancy.

Gluten-free diet; Avoidance of gluten, a protein found naturally in all forms of wheat, barley, and rye, is the primary and critical treatment for celiac disease. However, there is increasing recognition of the existence of nonceliac gluten intolerance/sensitivity, and following a gluten-free diet may benefit digestive processes and reduce abdominal discomfort among certain individuals without a diagnosis of celiac disease.[211]

A gluten-free diet improves pregnancy outcomes for women with celiac disease,[212] but its effects among pregnant women with nonceliac gluten sensitivity has not been evaluated. A gluten-free diet is associated with inadequate micronutrient status, so adequate fruit and vegetable intake and appropriate supplementation, particularly for folate, should be encouraged in pregnancy when following this diet, as well as adequate carbohydrate intake from gluten-free food sources, e.g., starchy vegetables, rice, quinoa, potatoes, pulses, and fruit.

Intermittent fasting/time-restricted feeding; This is the practice of consuming daily food within a restricted time frame so that the overnight fasting period is extended, e.g., 8-h eating window and 16 h fasting. Although there is increasing evidence for a range of beneficial metabolic and cognitive effects of intermittent fasting in nonpregnant individuals,[213] it is not recommended for pregnancy because the extended fasting window induces a state of temporary ketosis, which may be harmful to the fetus.

Food safety and exposure to food-based toxins in pregnancy

Cell-mediated immune function is decreased in pregnancy due to hormonal shifts. As a result, pregnant women are at an increased risk of contracting food-borne pathogens. *Listeria monocytogenes* and *Salmonella enterica* are of special interest as they can lead to perinatal complications such as stillbirth, spontaneous abortion, and low birth weight.[214]

Pregnancy can increase the risk of contracting *L. monocytogenes* by 10 fold. Unpasteurized milk, soft-ripened cheeses, and refrigerated ready-to-eat meats and seafood are associated with the bacterial pathogen *L. monocytogenes.* Ready-to-eat meats such as hot dogs, luncheon meats, and fermented sausage should be heated to 165°F before consuming. All seafood should reach an internal temperature of 145°F before consuming, and raw seafood such as sushi, ceviche, and oysters should be avoided. Soft, unpasteurized cheeses such as brie, queso blanco, feta and Roquefort should also be avoided.[214]

S. enterica is primarily associated with unpasteurized or undercooked eggs, raw sprouts, and undercooked meat or poultry. Eggs should be cooked to an internal temperature of 160°F and foods containing raw eggs such as Caesar salad dressing, eggnog, and tiramisu should be avoided.[214]

The consumption of mercury beyond recommended levels can negatively impact fetal nervous system development. Pregnant women should avoid commercially available fish with the highest mercury concentrations.[215] These include tilefish from the Gulf of Mexico, swordfish, shark, orange roughy, marlin, and king mackerel. However, health messages to pregnant women should emphasize the overall benefits of consuming low mercury content seafood, including salmon, sardines, and anchovies (minimum 12 ounces per week), due to their beneficial high DHA content.[216]

Other toxic chemical exposures from food sources during pregnancy are receiving increasing attention for their potential adverse effects on fetal development. These include plastics from food packaging (e.g., bisphenol A, di(2-ethylhexyl) phthalate), which are known endocrine-disrupting chemicals,[217,218] and pesticides, herbicides, or fertilizers used in some farming practices, which have been associated with offspring endocrine disruption through increased androgen levels in males and females,[219] poorer child neurodevelopmental outcomes,[220,221] and childhood leukemia.[222] No public health guidelines yet exist to advise reducing exposure to plastic-packaged and/or consumption of inorganic foods during pregnancy.

RESEARCH GAPS

Additional studies are needed to determine the following:

- Whether adherence to a Mediterranean diet throughout pregnancy improves maternal and infant outcomes outside Mediterranean regions.
- The optimal dietary pattern and macronutrient distribution for reducing maternal and neonatal risks associated with GDM.
- The role maternal triglycerides play in the development of excess fetal growth and adiposity, particularly among women with obesity and/or GDM, and the importance of providing specific advice for pregnant women about quality of dietary fat.
- Whether vitamin A supplementation among women with HIV decrease maternal-fetal HIV transmission.
- The effectiveness of iron supplementation for primary or secondary prevention of adverse perinatal outcomes.
- Whether L-methylfolate supplementation before and during pregnancy provides greater benefit for the prevention of NTDs than folic acid supplementation on a population level and among women with MTHFR polymorphisms.
- The requirements and adequate serum concentrations for vitamin D in pregnancy to optimize a broader spectrum of maternal and infant outcomes beyond skeletal development alone.
- The impact of caffeine on fetal growth and risk of growth restriction.
- Whether reducing toxic chemical exposures from food sources during pregnancy reduces risk of adverse outcomes in the offspring.
- The optimal gestational weight gain for women with multifetal pregnancies, particularly those with prepregnancy BMI in underweight category.

Acknowledgments

We would like to acknowledge Dr. Lindsay Allen, author of the chapter on Pregnancy and Lactation of the last edition of *Present Knowledge in Nutrition*, and our consultants on the dietary guidance for nutritional requirements in pregnancy: Dr. Janet King of Children's Hospital Oakland Research Institute (zinc and energy); Dr. Andrea Sharma (vitamins A, D, B6, calcium, and iodine) and Dr. Cria Perrine (iodine) of the Centers for Disease Control and Prevention; and Dr. Anne Williams (folate, calcium, and iron) of Emory University.
This chapter is an update of the chapter titled "39. Maternal Nutrient Metabolism and Requirements in Pregnancy and Lactation" by Lindsay H. Allen, in Present Knowledge in Nutrition, 10th Edition, edited by Erdman JW, Macdonald IA, and Zeisel SH and published by Wiley-Blackwell. © 2012 International Life Sciences Institute. Portions of this update are from the previously published chapter and the contributions of previous authors are acknowledged.

IV. REFERENCES

1. Frtiz MA, Speroff L. The endocrinology of pregnancy. In: Frtiz MA, Speroff L, eds. *Clinical Gynecologic Endocrinology and Infertility.* 8th ed. Philiadelphia, PA: Lippincott Williams & Wilkins; 2011:269–327.
2. Kelly TF, Savides TJ. Gastrointestinal disease in pregnancy. In: Resnik R, Lockwood CJ, Moore TR, Greene MF, Copel JA, Silver RM, eds. *Creasy and Resnik's Maternal-Fetal Medicine: Principles and Practice.* 8th ed. Elsevier, Inc; 2019, 1158–1172.e1154.
3. Liu JH. Endocrinology of pregnancy. In: Resnik R, Lockwood CJ, Moore TR, Greene MF, Copel JA, Silver RM, eds. *Creasy and Resnik's Maternal-Fetal Medicine: Principles and Practice.* 8th ed. Elsevier, Inc; 2019, 148–160.e143.
4. Whitty JE, Dombrowski MP. Respiratory diseases in pregnancy. In: Resnik R, Lockwood CJ, Moore TR, Greene MF, Copel JA, Silver RM, eds. *Creasy and Resnik's Maternal-Fetal Medicine: Principles and Practice.* 8th ed. Elsevier, Inc; 2019, 1043–1066.e1043.
5. Lawrence RM, Lawrence RA. The breast and the physiology of lactation. In: Resnik R, Lockwood CJ, Moore TR, Greene MF, Copel JA, Silver RM, eds. *Creasy and Resnik's Maternal-Fetal Medicine: Principles and Practice.* Elsevier, Inc; 2019, 161–180.e163.
6. King JC. Physiology of pregnancy and nutrient metabolism. *Am J Clin Nutr.* 2000;71(5 Suppl):1218s–1225s.
7. Beesley R, Johnson J. *The Breast during Pregnancy and Lactation.* 2008. https://doi.org/10.3843/GLOWM.10305.
8. Cunningham FG, Leveno KJ, Bloom SL, et al. The puerperium. In: *Williams Obstetrics.* 25th ed. New York, NY: McGraw-Hill Education; 2018.
9. Cunningham FG, Leveno KJ, Bloom SL, et al. Maternal physiology. In: *Williams Obstetrics.* 25th ed. New York, NY: McGraw-Hill Education; 2018.
10. Mastrobattista JM, Monga M. Maternal cardiovascular, respiratory, and renal adaptation to pregnancy. In: Resnik RL, Charles J, Moore TR, Greene MF, Copel JA, Silver RM, eds. *Creasy and Resnik's Maternal-Fetal Medicine: Principles and Practice.* 8th ed. Elsevier, Inc; 2019, 141–147.e143.
11. Doweiko JP, Nompleggi DJ. The role of albumin in human physiology and pathophysiology, Part III: albumin and disease states. *J Parenter Enter Nutr.* 1991;15(4):476–483.

12. Institute of Medicine and National Research Council. *Weight Gain during Pregnancy: Reexamining the Guidelines*. Washington, DC: The National Academies Press; 2009.
13. Arora P, Tamber Aeri B. Gestational weight gain among healthy pregnant women from Asia in comparison with Institute of Medicine (IOM) guidelines-2009: a systematic review. *J Pregnancy*. 2019:10.
14. Jiang X, Liu M, Song Y, et al. The Institute of Medicine recommendation for gestational weight gain is probably not optimal among non-American pregnant women: a retrospective study from China. *J Matern Fetal Neonatal Med*. 2019;32(8):1353–1358.
15. Ota E, Haruna M, Suzuki M, et al. Maternal body mass index and gestational weight gain and their association with perinatal outcomes in Viet Nam. *Bull World Health Organ*. 2011;89(2):127–136.
16. Goldstein RF, Abell SK, Ranasinha S, et al. Gestational weight gain across continents and ethnicity: systematic review and meta-analysis of maternal and infant outcomes in more than one million women. *BMC Med*. 2018;16(1):153.
17. Scott C, Andersen CT, Valdez N, et al. No global consensus: a cross-sectional survey of maternal weight policies. *BMC Pregnancy Childbirth*. 2014;14:167.
18. Oken E, Kleinman KP, Belfort MB, Hammitt JK, Gillman MW. Associations of gestational weight gain with short- and longer-term maternal and child health outcomes. *Am J Epidemiol*. 2009;170(2): 173–180.
19. Kiel DW, Dodson EA, Artal R, Boehmer TK, Leet TL. Gestational weight gain and pregnancy outcomes in obese women: how much is enough? *Obstet Gynecol*. 2007;110(4):752–758.
20. Centers for Disease Control and Prevention. *Pregnancy Weight Gain Trackers for Women Pregnant with One Baby. Weight Gain During Pregnancy*; 2019. https://www.cdc.gov/reproductivehealth/maternalinfanthealth/pregnancy-weight-gain.htm#tracking.
21. National Institute for Health and Care Excellence (NICE). *Weight Management before, during and after Pregnancy*. Public Health Guideline [PH27]; 2010.
22. Glazer NL, Hendrickson AF, Schellenbaum GD, Mueller BA. Weight change and the risk of gestational diabetes in obese women. *Epidemiology*. 2004;15(6):733–737.
23. Ehrlich SF, Hedderson MM, Feng J, Davenport ER, Gunderson EP, Ferrara A. Change in body mass index between pregnancies and the risk of gestational diabetes in a second pregnancy. *Obstet Gynecol*. 2011;117(6):1323–1330.
24. Whiteman VE, Aliyu MH, August EM, et al. Changes in prepregnancy body mass index between pregnancies and risk of gestational and type 2 diabetes. *Arch Gynecol Obstet*. 2011;284(1):235–240.
25. Getahun D, Ananth CV, Peltier MR, Salihu HM, Scorza WE. Changes in prepregnancy body mass index between the first and second pregnancies and risk of large-for-gestational-age birth. *Am J Obstet Gynecol*. 2007;196(6):530–538.
26. Hoff GL, Cai J, Okah FA, Dew PC. Pre-pregnancy overweight status between successive pregnancies and pregnancy outcomes. *J Womens Health (Larchmt)*. 2009;18(9):1413–1417.
27. Paramsothy P, Lin YS, Kernic MA, Foster-Schubert KE. Interpregnancy weight gain and cesarean delivery risk in women with a history of gestational diabetes. *Obstet Gynecol*. 2009;113(4):817–823.
28. Institute of Medicine. *Dietary Reference Intakes for Energy, Carbohydrate, Fiber, Fat, Fatty Acids, Cholesterol, Protein, and Amino Acids*. Washington, DC: The National Academies Press; 2005.
29. Bronstein MN, Mak RP, King JC. Unexpected relationship between fat mass and basal metabolic rate in pregnant women. *Br J Nutr*. 2007;75(5):659–668.
30. Moore SE. Nutrition, immunity and the fetal and infant origins of disease hypothesis in developing countries. *Proc Nutr Soc*. 2007; 57(2):241–247.
31. Ceesay SM, Prentice AM, Cole TJ, et al. Effects on birth weight and perinatal mortality of maternal dietary supplements in rural Gambia: 5 year randomised controlled trial. *BMJ (Clin Res ed)*. 1997;315(7111):786–790.
32. Prentice AM, Goldberg GR. Energy adaptations in human pregnancy: limits and long-term consequences. *Am J Clin Nutr*. 2000; 71(5):1226S–1232S.
33. Moore SE. Early life nutritional programming of health and disease in the Gambia. *J Dev Orig Health Dis*. 2016;7(2):123–131.
34. Godfrey KM, Barker DJ. Fetal nutrition and adult disease. *Am J Clin Nutr*. 2000;71(5 Suppl):1344S–1352S.
35. Langley-Evans SC. *Fetal Programming and Adult Disease. Programming of Chronic Disease through Fetal Exposure to Undernutrition*. Wallingford: CABI Publishing; 2006.
36. Birch EE, Castañeda YS, Wheaton DH, Birch DG, Uauy RD, Hoffman DR. Visual maturation of term infants fed long-chain polyunsaturated fatty acid–supplemented or control formula for 12 mo. *Am J Clin Nutr*. 2005;81(4):871–879.
37. Birch EE, Garfield S, Castañeda Y, Hughbanks-Wheaton D, Uauy R, Hoffman D. Visual acuity and cognitive outcomes at 4 years of age in a double-blind, randomized trial of long-chain polyunsaturated fatty acid-supplemented infant formula. *Early Hum Dev*. 2007;83(5):279–284.
38. Wadhwani N, Patil V, Joshi S. Maternal long chain polyunsaturated fatty acid status and pregnancy complications. *Prostagl Leukot Essent Fat Acids*. 2018;136:143–152.
39. Hornstra G. Essential fatty acids in mothers and their neonates. *Am J Clin Nutr*. 2000;71(5):1262S–1269S.
40. Zhao JP, Levy E, Shatenstein B, et al. Longitudinal circulating concentrations of long-chain polyunsaturated fatty acids in the third trimester of pregnancy in gestational diabetes. *Diabet Med*. 2016; 33(7):939–946.
41. Mackay VA, Huda SS, Stewart FM, et al. Preeclampsia is associated with compromised maternal synthesis of long-chain polyunsaturated fatty acids, leading to offspring deficiency. *Hypertension*. 2012;60(4):1078–1085.
42. Burdge GC, Wootton SA. Conversion of α-linolenic acid to eicosapentaenoic, docosapentaenoic and docosahexaenoic acids in young women. *Br J Nutr*. 2007;88(4):411–420.
43. Donahue SM, Rifas-Shiman SL, Gold DR, Jouni ZE, Gillman MW, Oken E. Prenatal fatty acid status and child adiposity at age 3 y: results from a US pregnancy cohort. *Am J Clin Nutr*. 2011;93(4):780–788.
44. Steenweg-de Graaff JCJ, Tiemeier H, Basten MGJ, et al. Maternal LC-PUFA status during pregnancy and child problem behavior: the Generation R Study. *Pediatr Res*. 2014;77:489.
45. Trumbo P, Schlicker S, Yates AA, Poos M. Dietary reference intakes for energy, carbohydrate, fiber, fat, fatty acids, cholesterol, protein and amino acids. *J Acad Nutr Diet*. 2002;102(11):1621–1630.
46. Tieu J, Shepherd E, Middleton P, Crowther CA. Dietary advice interventions in pregnancy for preventing gestational diabetes mellitus. *Cochrane Database Syst Rev*. 2017;1(1). CD006674.
47. Bao W, Li S, Chavarro JE, et al. Low carbohydrate-diet scores and long-term risk of type 2 diabetes among women with a history of gestational diabetes mellitus: a prospective cohort study. *Diabetes Care*. 2016;39(1):43–49.
48. Blumer I, Hadar E, Hadden DR, et al. Diabetes and pregnancy: an endocrine society clinical practice guideline. *J Clin Endocrinol Metab*. 2013;98(11):4227–4249.
49. Barbour LA, Hernandez TL. Maternal lipids and fetal overgrowth: making fat from fat. *Clin Therapeut*. 2018;40(10):1638–1647.
50. Sussman D, van Eede M, Wong MD, Adamson SL, Henkelman M. Effects of a ketogenic diet during pregnancy on embryonic growth in the mouse. *BMC Pregnancy and Childbirth*. 2013;13:109.
51. Kalhan SC. Protein metabolism in pregnancy. *Am J Clin Nutr*. 2000; 71(5):1249S–1255S.
52. US Department of Health and Human Services. *Vitamin A. Fact Sheet For Health Professionals*; 2018. https://ods.od.nih.gov/factsheets/VitaminA-HealthProfessional/. Accessed October 5, 2018.
53. Ross CA. Vitamin A. In: Coates PMB JM, Blackman MR, Cragg GM, Levine M, Moss J, White JD, eds. *Encyclopedia of Dietary Supplements*. 2nd ed. New York: London: Informa Healthcare; 2010:778–791.

54. World Health Organization. *Vitamin A Supplementation during Pregnancy.* e-Library of Evidence for Nutrition Actions (eLENA); 2019. https://www.who.int/elena/titles/vitamina_pregnancy/en/. Accessed February 11, 2019.
55. Institute of Medicine (US) Panel on Micronutrients, ed. *Dietary Reference Intakes for Vitamin A, Vitamin K, Arsenic, Boron, Chromium, Copper, Iodine, Iron, Manganese, Molybdenum, Nickel, Silicon, Vanadium, and Zinc.* Washington, DC: National Academies Press; 2001. https://www.ncbi.nlm.nih.gov/books/NBK222310/.
56. WHO. Global prevalence of vitamin A deficiency in populations at risk 1995–2005. WHO Global Database on Vitamin A Deficiency. Geneva, World Health Organization, 2009. https://apps.who.int/iris/bitstream/handle/10665/44110/9789241598019_eng.pdf?ua=1. Accessed 23 June 2019.
57. World Health Organization. *Vitamin A Supplementation in HIV-Infected Women during Pregnancy.* e-Library of Evidence for Nutrition Actions (eLENA); 2019. https://www.who.int/elena/titles/vitamina_hiv_pregnancy/en/. Accessed February 11, 2019.
58. Johnson EJ, Russell RM. Beta-carotene. In: Coates PMB JM, Blackman MR, Cragg GM, Levine M, Moss J, White JD, eds. *Encyclopedia of Dietary Supplements.* 2nd ed. New York: London: informa healthcare; 2010:115–120.
59. Brannon PM, Picciano MF. Vitamin D in pregnancy and lactation in humans. *Annu Rev Nutr.* 2011;31(1):89–115.
60. Zehnder D, Evans KN, Kilby MD, et al. The ontogeny of 25-hydroxyvitamin D3 1α-hydroxylase expression in human placenta and decidua. *Am J Pathol.* 2002;161(1):105–114.
61. Kiely M, Hemmingway A, O'Callaghan KM. Vitamin D in pregnancy: current perspectives and future directions. *Ther Adv Musculoskelet Dis.* 2017;9(6):145–154.
62. Hollis BW, Wagner CL. New insights into the vitamin D requirements during pregnancy. *Bone Res.* 2017;5:17030.
63. Tamblyn JA, Hewison M, Wagner CL, Bulmer JN, Kilby MD. Immunological role of vitamin D at the maternal–fetal interface. *J Endocrinol.* 2015;224(3):R107–R121.
64. De-Regil LM, Palacios C, Lombardo LK, Peña-Rosas JP. Vitamin D supplementation for women during pregnancy. *Cochrane Database Syst Rev.* 2016;(1):CD008873.
65. Aghajafari F, Nagulesapillai T, Ronksley PE, Tough SC, O'Beirne M, Rabi DM. Association between maternal serum 25-hydroxyvitamin D level and pregnancy and neonatal outcomes: systematic review and meta-analysis of observational studies. *BMJ Br Med J (Clin Res Ed).* 2013;346:f1169.
66. Qin L-L, Lu F-G, Yang S-H, Xu H-L, Luo B-A. Does maternal vitamin D deficiency increase the risk of preterm birth: a meta-analysis of observational studies. *Nutrients.* 2016;8(5).
67. Institute of Medicine. *Dietary Reference Intakes for Calcium and Vitamin D.* Washington, DC: National Academies Press; 2011, 0309163943.
68. World Health Organization. Vitamin D Supplementation During Pregnancy. eLibrary of Evidence for Nutrition Actions (eLENA). https://www.who.int/elena/titles/vitamind_supp_pregnancy/en/. Updated February 11, 2019. Accessed June 24, 2019.
69. March KM, Chen NN, Karakochuk CD, et al. Maternal vitamin D3 supplementation at 50 μg/d protects against low serum 25-hydroxyvitamin D in infants at 8 wk of age: a randomized controlled trial of 3 doses of vitamin D beginning in gestation and continued in lactation. *Am J Clin Nutr.* 2015;102(2):402–410.
70. Fiscaletti M, Stewart P, Munns CF. The importance of vitamin D in maternal and child health: a global perspective. *Publ Health Rev.* 2017;38:19.
71. Roth DE, Abrams SA, Aloia J, et al. Global prevalence and disease burden of vitamin D deficiency: a roadmap for action in low- and middle-income countries. *Ann N Y Acad Sci.* 2018;1430(1):44–79.
72. Luque-Fernandez MA, Gelaye B, VanderWeele T, et al. Seasonal variation of 25-hydroxyvitamin D among non-Hispanic black and white pregnant women from three US pregnancy cohorts. *Paediatr Perinat Epidemiol.* 2014;28(2):166–176.
73. Sloka S, Stokes J, Randell E, Newhook LA. Seasonal variation of maternal serum vitamin D in Newfoundland and Labrador. *J Obstet Gynaecol Can.* 2009;31(4):313–321.
74. Jain V, Gupta N, Kalaivani M, Jain A, Sinha A, Agarwal R. Vitamin D deficiency in healthy breastfed term infants at 3 months & their mothers in India: seasonal variation & determinants. *Indian J Med Res.* 2011;133(3):267–273.
75. Institute of Medicine Food and Nutrition Board, ed. *Dietary Reference Intakes: Thiamin, Riboflavin, Niacin, Vitamin B6, Folate, Vitamin B12, Pantothenic Acid, Biotin, and Choline.* Washington DC: National Academy Press; 1998.
76. Schenker S, Johnson RF, Mahuren JD, Henderson GI, Coburn SP. Human placental vitamin B6 (pyridoxal) transport: normal characteristics and effects of ethanol. *Am J Physiol Regul Integr Comp Physiol.* 1992;262(6):R966–R974.
77. Chang SJ. Adequacy of maternal pyridoxine supplementation during pregnancy in relation to the vitamin B6 status and growth of neonates at birth. *J Nutr Sci Vitaminol.* 1999;45(4):449–458.
78. Shrim A, Boskovic R, Maltepe C, Navios Y, Garcia–Bournissen F, Koren G. Pregnancy outcome following use of large doses of vitamin B6 in the first trimester. *J Obstet Gynaecol.* 2006;26(8):749–751.
79. Werler MM, Shapiro S, Mitchell AA. Periconceptional folic acid exposure and risk of occurrent neural tube defects. *J Am Med Assoc.* 1993;269(10):1257–1261.
80. Shaw GM, Schaffer D, Velie EM, Morland K, Harris JA. Periconceptional vitamin use, dietary folate, and the occurrence of neural tube defects. *Epidemiology.* 1995;6(3):219–226.
81. Daly LE, Kirke PN, Molloy A, Weir DG, Scott JM. Folate levels and neural tube defects. Implications for prevention. *J Am Med Assoc.* 1995;274(21):1698–1702.
82. Beaudin AE, Abarinov EV, Noden DM, et al. Shmt1 and de novo thymidylate biosynthesis underlie folate-responsive neural tube defects in mice. *Am J Clin Nutr.* 2011;93(4):789–798.
83. Heseker HB, Mason JB, Selhub J, Rosenberg IH, Jacques PF. Not all cases of neural-tube defect can be prevented by increasing the intake of folic acid. *Br J Nutr.* 2009;102(2):173–180.
84. Wolff T, Witkop CT, Miller T, Syed SB. Folic acid supplementation for the prevention of neural tube defects: an update of the evidence for the U.S. Preventive Services Task Force. *Ann Intern Med.* 2009;150(9):632–639.
85. US Food and Drug Administration. *Food Standards: Amendments of Standards of Identity for Enriched Grain Products to Require Addition of Folic Acid.* In: *Office of the Federal Register.* Vol. 61. National Archives and Records Administration; 1996:8781–8797.
86. Centers for Disease Control. Recommendations for the use of folic acid to reduce the number of cases of spina bifida and other neural tube defects. *MMWR.* 1992;41(RR-14). Washington DC.
87. ACOG. Neural tube defects. Practice bulletin No. 187. American College of Obstetricians and Gynecologists. *Obstet Gynecol.* 2017; 130:e279–290.
88. Berry RJ, Li Z, Erickson JD, et al. Prevention of neural-tube defects with folic acid in China. China-U.S. Collaborative project for neural tube defect prevention. *N Engl J Med.* 1999;341(20):1485–1490.
89. Greenberg JA, Bell SJ, Guan Y, Yu Y-H. Folic acid supplementation and pregnancy: more than just neural tube defect prevention. *Rev Obstet Gynecol.* 2011;4(2):52–59.
90. Lamers Y, Prinz-Langenohl R, Brämswig S, Pietrzik K. Red blood cell folate concentrations increase more after supplementation with [6 S]-5-methyltetrahydrofolate than with folic acid in women of childbearing age. *Am J Clin Nutr.* 2006;84(1):156–161.
91. Obeid R, Holzgreve W, Pietrzik K. Is 5-methyltetrahydrofolate an alternative to folic acid for the prevention of neural tube defects? *J Perinat Med.* 2013;41:469.

92. Nader S. Other endocrine disorders of pregnancy. In: Resnik RL, Charles J, Moore TR, Greene MF, Copel JA, Silver RM, eds. *Creasy and Resnik's Maternal-Fetal Medicine: Principles and Practice*. 8th ed. Elsevier, Inc; 2019, 1135–1157.e1134.
93. Kovacs CS. Maternal mineral and bone metabolism during pregnancy, lactation, and post-weaning recovery. *Physiol Rev*. 2016; 96(2):449–547.
94. IOM (Institute of Medicine). *Dietary Reference Intakes for Calcium and Vitamin D*; 2011. https://www.ncbi.nlm.nih.gov/books/NBK56070/.
95. Jarjou LM, Prentice A, Sawo Y, et al. Randomized, placebo-controlled, calcium supplementation study in pregnant Gambian women: effects on breast-milk calcium concentrations and infant birth weight, growth, and bone mineral accretion in the first year of life. *Am J Clin Nutr*. 2006;83(3):657–666.
96. Kovacs CS. Calcium and bone metabolism disorders during pregnancy and lactation. *Endocrinol Metab Clin N Am*. 2011;40(4): 795–826.
97. Hypertension in pregnancy. Report of the American College of Obstetricians and Gynecologists' Task Force on hypertension in pregnancy. *Obstet Gynecol*. 2013;122(5):1122–1131.
98. Ghulmiyyah L, Sibai B. Maternal mortality from preeclampsia/eclampsia. *Semin Perinatol*. 2012;36(1):56–59.
99. WHO recommendation. *Calcium Supplementation during Pregnancy for the Prevention of Pre-eclampsia and its Complications*; 2018. https://www.ncbi.nlm.nih.gov/books/NBK535812/.
100. Bucher HC, Cook RJ, Guyatt GH, et al. Effects of dietary calcium supplementation on blood pressure. A meta-analysis of randomized controlled trials. *Jama*. 1996;275(13):1016–1022.
101. Levine RJ, Hauth JC, Curet LB, et al. Trial of calcium to prevent preeclampsia. *N Engl J Med*. 1997;337(2):69–76.
102. Villar J, Abdel-Aleem H, Merialdi M, et al. World Health Organization randomized trial of calcium supplementation among low calcium intake pregnant women. *Am J Obstet Gynecol*. 2006; 194(3):639–649.
103. Hofmeyr GJ, Lawrie TA, Atallah AN, Torloni MR. Calcium supplementation during pregnancy for preventing hypertensive disorders and related problems. *Cochrane Database Syst Rev*. 2018;10: Cd001059.
104. American College of Obstetricians and Gynecologists (ACOG). ACOG practice bulletin No. 202: gestational hypertension and preeclampsia. *Obstet Gynecol*. 2019;133(1):e1–e25.
105. Nutritional anaemias: tools for effective prevention and control. Geneva: World Health Organization; 2017. https://apps.who.int/iris/bitstream/handle/10665/259425/9789241513067-eng.pdf?sequence=1. Accessed 23 June 2019.
106. Kilpatrick SJ, Kitahara S. Anemia and pregnancy. In: Resnik RL, Charles J, Moore TR, Greene MF, Copel JA, Silver RM, eds. *Creasy and Resnik's Maternal-Fetal Medicine: Principles and Practice*. 8th ed. Elsevier; 2018, 991–1006e.
107. Stevens GA, Finucane MM, De-Regil LM, et al. Global, regional, and national trends in haemoglobin concentration and prevalence of total and severe anaemia in children and pregnant and non-pregnant women for 1995–2011: a systematic analysis of population-representative data. *Lancet Glob Health*. 2013;1(1):e16–e25.
108. Gupta PM, Hamner HC, Suchdev PS, Flores-Ayala R, Mei Z. Iron status of toddlers, nonpregnant females, and pregnant females in the United States. *Am J Clin Nutr*. 2017;106(Suppl 6): 1640s–1646s.
109. The American College of Obstetricians and Gynecologists (ACOG). Anemia in pregnancy. *ACOG Practice Bulletin*. 2008; 112(1).
110. Centers for Disease Control and Prevention. Recommendations to prevent and control iron deficiency in the United States. *MMWR Recomm Rep (Morb Mortal Wkly Rep)*. 1998;47(RR-3):1–36.
111. World Health Organization. *Haemoglobin Concentrations for the Diagnosis of Anaemia and Assessment of Severity*. Vitamin and Mineral Nutrition Information System (VMNIS); 2011. https://www.who.int/vmnis/indicators/haemoglobin/en/.
112. World Health Organization. *WHO Recommendations on Antenatal Care for a Positive Pregnancy Experience*; 2016. https://apps.who.int/iris/bitstream/handle/10665/250796/9789241549912-eng.pdf;jsessionid=FC47BF0E3A4F6469C482E16C7875705A?sequence=1.
113. The National Academies of Sciences Engineering Medicine. Key points for iron. In: Otten JJ, Pitzi Hellwig J, Meyers LD, eds. *Dietary Reference Intakes (DRI): The Essential Guide to Nutrient Requirements*. Washington, DC: Insitute of Medicine of the National Academies; 2006.
114. Ziaei S, Norrozi M, Faghihzadeh S, Jafarbegloo E. A randomised placebo-controlled trial to determine the effect of iron supplementation on pregnancy outcome in pregnant women with haemoglobin > or = 13.2 g/dl. *BJOG*. 2007;114(6):684–688.
115. Pena-Rosas JP, De-Regil LM, Garcia-Casal MN, Dowswell T. Daily oral iron supplementation during pregnancy. *Cochrane Database Syst Rev*. 2015;7:Cd004736.
116. Preziosi P, Prual A, Galan P, Daouda H, Boureima H, Hercberg S. Effect of iron supplementation on the iron status of pregnant women: consequences for newborns. *Am J Clin Nutr*. 1997;66:1178–1182.
117. De Pee S, Bloem MW, Sari M, Kiess L, Yip R, Kosen S. The high prevalence of low hemoglobin concentration among Indonesian infants aged 3-5 months is related to maternal anemia. *J Nutr*. 2002;132(8):2215–2221.
118. The American College of Obstetricians and Gynecologists (ACOG). Delayed umbilical cord clamping after birth. *Committee Opin Committee Obstet Practice*. 2017:684.
119. National Institute for Health and Care Excellence (NICE). *Intrapartum Care: Delayed Cord Clamping*. NICE Guidelines: Quality Standard [QS105]; 2017. Quality Statement 6.
120. Swanson CA, King JC. Zinc and pregnancy outcome. *Am J Clin Nutr*. 1987;46(5):763–771.
121. Institute of Medicine. *Dietary Reference Intakes for Vitamin A, Vitamin K, Arsenic, Boron, Chromium, Copper, Iodine, Iron, Manganese, Molybdenum, Nickel, Silicon, Vanadium, and Zinc*. Washington DC: The National Academies Press; 2001.
122. Donangelo CM, King JC. Maternal zinc intakes and homeostatic adjustments during pregnancy and lactation. *Nutrients*. 2012; 4(7):782–798.
123. Swanson CA, King JC. Reduced serum zinc concentration during pregnancy. *Obstet Gynecol*. 1983;62:313–318.
124. King JC, Brown KH, Gibson RS, et al. Biomarkers of nutrition for development (BOND)-Zinc review. *J Nutr*. 2016;146(4):858S–885S.
125. Hess SY, King JC. Effects of maternal zinc supplementation on pregnancy and lactation performance. *Food Nutr Bull*. 2009;30(1): S60–S78.
126. White B, Harrison JR, Mehlmann L. The thyroid gland. In: *Endocrine and Reproductive Physiology*. 5th ed. Elsevier, Inc; 2019.
127. World Health Organization. In: Andersson MdB B, Darnton-Hill I, Delange F, eds. *Iodine Deficiency in Europe: A Continuing Public Health Problem*. Geneva: World Health Organization; 2007. https://apps.who.int/iris/handle/10665/43398.
128. Nader S. Thyroid disease and pregnancy. In: Resnik RL, Charles J, Moore TR, Greene MF, Copel JA, Silver RM, eds. *Creasy and Resnik's Maternal-Fetal Medicine: Principles and Practice*. 8th ed. Elsevier, Inc; 2019, 1116–1134.e1114.
129. Hynes KL, Otahal P, Hay I, Burgess JR. Mild iodine deficiency during pregnancy is associated with reduced educational outcomes in the offspring: 9-year follow-up of the gestational iodine cohort. *J Clin Endocrinol Metab*. 2013;98(5):1954–1962.
130. Bath SC, Steer CD, Golding J, Emmett P, Rayman MP. Effect of inadequate iodine status in UK pregnant women on cognitive

outcomes in their children: results from the Avon Longitudinal Study of Parents and Children (ALSPAC). *Lancet*. 2013; 382(9889):331–337.

131. World Health Organization, United Nations Children's Fund. International Council for the control of iodine deficiency disorders. In: *Assessment of Iodine Deficiency Disorders and Monitoring Their Elimination: A Guide for Programme Managers*. 3rd ed. Geneva, Switzerland: WHO; 2008.
132. US Department of Health and Human Services. *Iodine. Fact Sheet For Health Professionals*; 2018. https://ods.od.nih.gov/factsheets/Iodine-HealthProfessional/. Accessed on 26, September 2018.
133. Gupta PM, Gahche JJ, Herrick KA, Ershow AG, Potischman N, Perrine CG. Use of iodine-containing dietary supplements remains low among women of reproductive age in the United States: NHANES 2011-2014. *Nutrients*. 2018;10(4):422.
134. Zimmermann MB, Jooste PL, Pandav CS. Iodine-deficiency disorders. *Lancet*. 2008;372(9645):1251–1262.
135. Perrine CG, Herrick K, Serdula MK, Sullivan KM. Some subgroups of reproductive age women in the United States may be at risk for iodine deficiency. *J Nutr*. 2010;140(8):1489–1494.
136. Perrine CG, Herrick KA, Gupta PM, Caldwell KL. Iodine status of pregnant women and women of reproductive age in the United States. *Thyroid*. 2019;29(1):153–154.
137. Andersson M, de Benoist B, Delange F, Zupan J. Prevention and control of iodine deficiency in pregnant and lactating women and in children less than 2-years-old: conclusions and recommendations of the Technical Consultation. *Publ Health Nutr*. 2007; 10(12a):1606–1611.
138. Hoyme HE, Kalberg WO, Elliott AJ, et al. Updated clinical guidelines for diagnosing fetal alcohol spectrum disorders. *Pediatrics*. 2016;138(2).
139. Pruett D, Waterman EH, Caughey AB. Fetal alcohol exposure: consequences, diagnosis, and treatment. *Obstet Gynecol Surv*. 2013;68(1):62–69.
140. Denny CHAC, Naimi TS, Kim SY. Consumption of alcohol beverages and binge drinking among pregnant women aged 18–44 years — United States, 2015–2017. *MMWR Morb Mortal Wkly Rep*. 2019;68:365–368.
141. Roozen S, Black D, Peters GY, et al. Fetal alcohol spectrum disorders (FASD): an approach to effective prevention. *Curr Dev Disord Rep*. 2016;3(4):229–234.
142. Centers for Disease Control and Prevention: National Center on Birth Defects and Developmental Disabilities. *Advisory on Alcohol Use in Pregnancy [Press Release]*. 2005.
143. Soyka LF. Caffeine ingestion during pregnancy: in utero exposure and possible effects. *Semin Perinatol*. 1981;5(4):305–309.
144. Goldstein A, Warren R. Passage of caffeine into human gonadal and fetal tissue. *Biochem Pharmacol*. 1962;11:166–168.
145. Knutti R, Rothweiler H, Schlatter C. The effect of pregnancy on the pharmacokinetics of caffeine. *Arch Toxicol Suppl*. 1982;5: 187–192.
146. The American College of Obstetricians and Gynecologists (ACOG). Moderate caffeine consumption during pregnancy. *Committee Opin Committee Obstet Practice*. 2010;116:467–468.
147. Kirkinen P, Jouppila P, Koivula A, Vuori J, Puukka M. The effect of caffeine on placental and fetal blood flow in human pregnancy. *Am J Obstet Gynecol*. 1983;147(8):939–942.
148. Wikoff D, Welsh BT, Henderson R, et al. Systematic review of the potential adverse effects of caffeine consumption in healthy adults, pregnant women, adolescents, and children. *Food Chem Toxicol*. 2017;109(Pt 1):585–648.
149. Chen LW, Wu Y, Neelakantan N, Chong MF, Pan A, van Dam RM. Maternal caffeine intake during pregnancy is associated with risk of low birth weight: a systematic review and dose-response meta-analysis. *BMC Med*. 2014;12:174.
150. Mills JL, Holmes LB, Aarons JH, et al. Moderate caffeine use and the risk of spontaneous abortion and intrauterine growth retardation. *JAMA*. 1993;269(5):593–597.
151. Grosso LM, Rosenberg KD, Belanger K, Saftlas AF, Leaderer B, Bracken MB. Maternal caffeine intake and intrauterine growth retardation. *Epidemiology*. 2001;12(4):447–455.
152. Linn S, Schoenbaum SC, Monson RR, Rosner B, Stubblefield PG, Ryan KJ. No association between coffee consumption and adverse outcomes of pregnancy. *N Engl J Med*. 1982;306(3):141–145.
153. Jahanfar S, Sharifah H. Effects of restricted caffeine intake by mother on fetal, neonatal and pregnancy outcome. *Cochrane Database Syst Rev*. 2009;(2):Cd006965.
154. Royal College of Obstetricians & Gynaecologists. *Healthy Eating and Vitamin Supplements in Pregnancy*. Information for you; 2014. https://www.rcog.org.uk/en/patients/patient-leaflets/healthy-eating-and-vitamin-supplements-in-pregnancy/.
155. Robbins CL, Zapata LB, Farr SL, et al. Core state preconception health indicators - pregnancy risk assessment monitoring system and behavioral risk factor surveillance system, 2009. *MMWR Surveill Summ*. 2014;63(3):1–62.
156. Singh GK, DiBari JN. Marked disparities in pre-pregnancy obesity and overweight prevalence among US women by race/ethnicity, nativity/immigrant status, and sociodemographic characteristics, 2012–2014. *Journal of Obesity*. 2019;2019:13.
157. Voerman E, Santos S, Inskip H, et al. Association of gestational weight gain with adverse maternal and infant outcomes. *Jama*. 2019;321(17):1702–1715.
158. Abenhaim HA, Kinch RA, Morin L, Benjamin A, Usher R. Effect of prepregnancy body mass index categories on obstetrical and neonatal outcomes. *Arch Gynecol Obstet*. 2007;275(1):39–43.
159. Schuster M, Mackeen AD, Neubert AG, Kirchner HL, Paglia MJ. The impact of pre-pregnancy body mass index and pregnancy weight gain on maternal and neonatal outcomes [24A]. *Obstet Gynecol*. 2016;127.
160. Schummers L, Hutcheon JA, Bodnar LM, Lieberman E, Himes KP. Risk of adverse pregnancy outcomes by prepregnancy body mass index: a population-based study to inform prepregnancy weight loss counseling. *Obstet Gynecol*. 2015;125(1).
161. Avci ME, Sanlikan F, Celik M, Avci A, Kocaer M, Gocmen A. Effects of maternal obesity on antenatal, perinatal and neonatal outcomes. *J Matern Fetal Neonatal Med*. 2015;28(17):2080–2083.
162. Liu P, Xu L, Wang Y, et al. Association between perinatal outcomes and maternal pre-pregnancy body mass index. *Obes Rev*. 2016;17(11):1091–1102.
163. Turcksin R, Bel S, Galjaard S, Devlieger R. Maternal obesity and breastfeeding intention, initiation, intensity and duration: a systematic review. *Matern Child Nutr*. 2014;10(2):166–183.
164. Andersson-Hall UK, Järvinen EAJ, Bosaeus MH, et al. Maternal obesity and gestational diabetes mellitus affect body composition through infancy: the PONCH study. *Pediatr Res*. 2019;85(3):369–377.
165. Logan KM, Gale C, Hyde MJ, Santhakumaran S, Modi N. Diabetes in pregnancy and infant adiposity: systematic review and meta-analysis. *Arch Dis Child Fetal Neonatal Ed*. 2017;102(1):F65.
166. Godfrey KM, Reynolds RM, Prescott SL, et al. Influence of maternal obesity on the long-term health of offspring. *Lancet Diabetes Endocrinol*. 2017;5(1):53–64.
167. Gaillard R, Santos S, Duijts L, Felix JF. Childhood health consequences of maternal obesity during pregnancy: a narrative review. *Ann Nutr Metabol*. 2016;69(3–4):171–180.
168. Catalano PM, Farrell K, Thomas A, et al. Perinatal risk factors for childhood obesity and metabolic dysregulation. *Am J Clin Nutr*. 2009;90(5):1303–1313.
169. Catalano PM, Presley L, Minium J, Hauguel-de Mouzon S. Fetuses of obese mothers develop insulin resistance in utero. *Diabetes Care*. 2009;32(6):1076.

170. Freeman DJ. Effects of maternal obesity on fetal growth and body composition: implications for programming and future health. *Semin Fetal Neonatal Med*. 2010;15(2):113–118.
171. Baker 2nd PR, Patinkin Z, Shapiro AL, et al. Maternal obesity and increased neonatal adiposity correspond with altered infant mesenchymal stem cell metabolism. *JCI Insight*. 2017;2(21): e94200.
172. Heerwagen MJR, Miller MR, Barbour LA, Friedman JE. Maternal obesity and fetal metabolic programming: a fertile epigenetic soil. *Am J Physiol Regul Integr Comp Physiol*. 2010;299(3):R711–R722.
173. Oteng-Ntim E, Tezcan B, Seed P, Poston L, Doyle P. Lifestyle interventions for obese and overweight pregnant women to improve pregnancy outcome: a systematic review and meta-analysis. *Lancet*. 2015;386:S61.
174. Flynn AC, Dalrymple K, Barr S, et al. Dietary interventions in overweight and obese pregnant women: a systematic review of the content, delivery, and outcomes of randomized controlled trials. *Nutr Rev*. 2016;74(5):312–328.
175. Price SA, Sumithran P, Nankervis A, Permezel M, Proietto J. Preconception management of women with obesity: a systematic review. *Obes Rev*. 2019;20(4):510–526.
176. Matusiak K, Barrett HL, Callaway LK, Nitert MD. Periconception weight loss: common sense for mothers, but what about for babies? *J Obes*. 2014;2014:10.
177. Practice bulletin no 156: obesity in pregnancy. *Obstet Gynecol*. 2015;126(6).
178. Dalrymple KV, Flynn AC, Relph SA, O'Keeffe M, Poston L. Lifestyle interventions in overweight and obese pregnant or postpartum women for postpartum weight management: a systematic review of the literature. *Nutrients*. 2018;10(11):1704.
179. The American College of Obstetricians and Gynecologists. Medical nutrition therapy and lifestyle interventions [Interim update]. *Med Nutri Therapy Lifestyle Intervent*. 2018;131(2).
180. American Diabetes Association. 2. Classification and diagnosis of diabetes: standards of medical care in diabetes-2019. *Diabetes Care*. 2019;42(Suppl 1):S13–s28.
181. World Health Organization. *Diagnostic Criteria and Classification of Hyperglycaemia First Detected in Pregnancy*. WHO: Diabetes Programme; 2013.
182. Metzger BE, Lowe LP, Dyer AR, et al. Hyperglycemia and adverse pregnancy outcomes. *N Engl J Med*. 2008;358(19):1991–2002.
183. Landon MB, Spong CY, Thom E, et al. A multicenter, randomized trial of treatment for mild gestational diabetes. *N Engl J Med*. 2009; 361(14):1339–1348.
184. Crowther CA, Hiller JE, Moss JR, et al. Effect of treatment of gestational diabetes mellitus on pregnancy outcomes. *N Engl J Med*. 2005;352(24):2477–2486.
185. Duarte-Gardea MO, Gonzales-Pacheco DM, Reader DM, et al. Academy of nutrition and dietetics gestational diabetes evidence-based nutrition practice guideline. *J Acad Nutr Diet*. 2018;118(9):1719–1742.
186. Reader DM. Medical nutrition therapy and lifestyle interventions. *Diabetes Care*. 2007;30(Suppl 2):S188–S193.
187. Academy of Nutrition and Dietetics. GDM: executive summary of recommendations. *Gestational Diabetes (GDM) Guideline*; 2016. https://www.andeal.org/topic.cfm?menu=5288&cat=5538.
188. Hernandez TL, Brand-Miller JC. Nutrition therapy in gestational diabetes mellitus: time to move forward. *Diabetes Care*. 2018;41(7): 1343–1345.
189. Yamamoto JM, Kellett JE, Balsells M, et al. Gestational diabetes mellitus and diet: a systematic review and meta-analysis of randomized controlled trials examining the impact of modified dietary interventions on maternal glucose control and neonatal birth weight. *Diabetes Care*. 2018;41(7):1346–1361.
190. Chen X, Zhao D, Mao X, Xia Y, Baker PN, Zhang H. Maternal dietary patterns and pregnancy outcome. *Nutrients*. 2016;8(6):351.
191. Tobias DK, Zhang C, Chavarro J, et al. Prepregnancy adherence to dietary patterns and lower risk of gestational diabetes mellitus. *Am J Clin Nutr*. 2012;96(2):289–295.
192. Mijatovic-Vukas J, Capling L, Cheng S, et al. Associations of diet and physical activity with risk for gestational diabetes mellitus: a systematic review and meta-analysis. *Nutrients*. 2018; 10(6).
193. Academy of Nutrition and Dietetics. *Pregnancy Nutrition Therapy*; 2018. https://www.eatright.org/health/pregnancy/what-to-eat-when-expecting/the-best-foods-to-eat-during-pregnancy. Accessed August 29, 2019.
194. Amati F, Hassounah S, Swaka A. The impact of mediterranean dietary patterns during pregnancy on maternal and offspring health. *Nutrients*. 2019;11(5):1098.
195. Biagi C, Di Nunzio M, Bordoni A, Gori D, Lanari M. Effect of adherence to mediterranean diet during pregnancy on Children's health: a systematic review. *Nutrients*. 2019;11(5).
196. Assaf-Balut C, García de la Torre N, Duran A, et al. A mediterranean diet with an enhanced consumption of extra virgin olive oil and pistachios improves pregnancy outcomes in women without gestational diabetes mellitus: a sub-analysis of the St. Carlos gestational diabetes mellitus prevention study. *Ann Nutr Metab*. 2019;74(1):69–79.
197. García de la Torre N, Assaf-Balut C, Jiménez Varas I, et al. Effectiveness of following mediterranean diet recommendations in the real world in the incidence of gestational diabetes mellitus (GDM) and adverse maternal-foetal outcomes: a prospective, universal, interventional study with a single group. The St Carlos study. *Nutrients*. 2019;11(6).
198. Assaf-Balut C, García de la Torre N, Durán A, et al. A Mediterranean diet with additional extra virgin olive oil and pistachios reduces the incidence of gestational diabetes mellitus (GDM): a randomized controlled trial: the St. Carlos GDM prevention study. *PLoS One*. 2017;12(10):e0185873.
199. Schwingshackl L, Christoph M, Hoffmann G. Effects of olive oil on markers of inflammation and endothelial function—a systematic review and meta-analysis. *Nutrients*. 2015;7(9).
200. Hernández-Alonso P, Salas-Salvadó J, Baldrich-Mora M, Juanola-Falgarona M, Bulló M. Beneficial effect of pistachio consumption on glucose metabolism, insulin resistance, inflammation, and related metabolic risk markers: a randomized clinical trial. *Diabetes Care*. 2014;37(11):3098.
201. Piccoli GB, Clari R, Vigotti FN, et al. Vegan–vegetarian diets in pregnancy: danger or panacea? A systematic narrative review. *BJOG*. 2015;122(5):623–633.
202. Baroni L, Goggi S, Battaglino R, et al. Vegan nutrition for mothers and children: practical tools for healthcare providers. *Nutrients*. 2018;11(1).
203. Kaiser LL, Campbell CG. Practice paper of the Academy of Nutrition and Dietetics abstract: nutrition and lifestyle for a healthy pregnancy outcome. *J Acad Nutr Diet*. 2014;114(9):1447.
204. van der Louw EJTM, Williams TJ, Henry-Barron BJ, et al. Ketogenic diet therapy for epilepsy during pregnancy: a case series. *Seizure*. 2017;45:198–201.
205. Viana LV, Gross JL, Azevedo MJ. Dietary intervention in patients with gestational diabetes mellitus: a systematic review and meta-analysis of randomized clinical trials on maternal and newborn outcomes. *Diabetes Care*. 2014;37(12):3345.
206. Han S, Middleton P, Shepherd E, Van Ryswyk E, Crowther CA. Different types of dietary advice for women with gestational diabetes mellitus. *Cochrane Database Syst Rev*. 2017;2(2):CD009275.
207. Bao W, Bowers K, Tobias DK, et al. Prepregnancy low-carbohydrate dietary pattern and risk of gestational diabetes mellitus: a prospective cohort study. *Am J Clin Nutr*. 2014;99(6):1378–1384.
208. Looman M, Schoenaker DAJM, Soedamah-Muthu SS, Geelen A, Feskens EJM, Mishra GD. Pre-pregnancy dietary carbohydrate

quantity and quality, and risk of developing gestational diabetes: the Australian Longitudinal Study on Women's Health. *Br J Nutr.* 2018;120(4):435–444.

209. Desrosiers TA, Siega-Riz AM, Mosley BS, Meyer RE, National Birth Defects Prevention S. Low carbohydrate diets may increase risk of neural tube defects. *Birth Defects Res.* 2018; 110(11):901–909.
210. Pitt C. Cutting through the Paleo hype: the evidence for the Palaeolithic diet. *Aust Fam Physician.* 2016;45:35–38.
211. Khan A, Suarez MG, Murray JA. Nonceliac gluten and wheat sensitivity [Review]. *Clin Gastroenterol Hepatol;* 2019. https://dx.doi.org/10.1016/j.cgh.2019.04.009.
212. Tursi A, Giorgetti G, Brandimarte G, Elisei W. Effect of gluten-free diet on pregnancy outcome in celiac disease patients with recurrent miscarriages. *Dig Dis Sci.* 2008;53(11):2925–2928.
213. Patterson RE, Sears DD. Metabolic effects of intermittent fasting. *Annu Rev Nutr.* 2017;37(1):371–393.
214. Tam C, Erebara A, Einarson A. Food-borne illnesses during pregnancy: prevention and treatment. *Canadian family physician Medecin de famille canadien.* 2010;56(4):341–343.
215. Evans EC. The FDA recommendations on fish intake during pregnancy. *J Obstet Gynecol Neonatal Nurs.* 2002;31(6): 715–720.
216. Lando AM, Fein SB, Choinière CJ. Awareness of methylmercury in fish and fish consumption among pregnant and postpartum women and women of childbearing age in the United States. *Environ Res.* 2012;116:85–92.
217. Martínez MA, Rovira J, Prasad Sharma R, Nadal M, Schuhmacher M, Kumar V. Comparing dietary and non-dietary source contribution of BPA and DEHP to prenatal exposure: a Catalonia (Spain) case study. *Environ Res.* 2018;166:25–34.
218. Martínez MA, Rovira J, Sharma RP, Nadal M, Schuhmacher M, Kumar V. Prenatal exposure estimation of BPA and DEHP using integrated external and internal dosimetry: a case study. *Environ Res.* 2017;158:566–575.
219. Manservisi F, Lesseur C, Panzacchi S, et al. The Ramazzini Institute 13-week pilot study glyphosate-based herbicides administered at human-equivalent dose to Sprague Dawley rats: effects on development and endocrine system. *Environ Health.* 2019;18(1):15.
220. González-Alzaga B, Lacasaña M, Aguilar-Garduño C, et al. A systematic review of neurodevelopmental effects of prenatal and postnatal organophosphate pesticide exposure. *Toxicol Lett.* 2014;230(2):104–121.
221. Schmidt Rebecca J, Kogan V, Shelton Janie F, et al. Combined prenatal pesticide exposure and folic acid intake in relation to autism spectrum disorder. *Environ Health Perspect.* 2017;125(9):097007.
222. Bailey HD, Infante-Rivard C, Metayer C, et al. Home pesticide exposures and risk of childhood leukemia: findings from the childhood leukemia international consortium. *Int J Canc.* 2015;137(11): 2644–2663.

CHAPTER

4

NUTRIENT METABOLISM AND REQUIREMENTS IN LACTATION

Jimi Francis, BS, MS, PhD, IBCLC, RLC, RDN, LD
Rebecca Egdorf, BS, MS, RD, LD
College of Nursing and Health Sciences, Department of Health and Kinesiology, University of Texas at Tyler, Tyler, TX, United States

SUMMARY

Breastfeeding, metabolically akin to a performance sport, has unique dietary and caloric needs. For months leading up to the moment of initiation of breastfeeding, mammary tissue has been developing into a branched network of mass-producing secretory cells as mothers' bodies prepare to burn large amounts of calories to keep this production on track once copious milk production begins. Not only does maternal nutrition become important for the infant, it is crucial for long-term maternal health to maintain replete nutrition status throughout her lactation and beyond. Nutrition is the key to supplying the mother with the right ingredients for the highest quality milk output. Understanding how nutrition impacts both mother and baby is a critical step in being able to properly manage and recommend changes in food routines or supplementation to optimize health status. Lactation nutritional needs differ from other life stages. Those differences will be discussed in this chapter.

Keywords: Breastfeeding; Diet; Food intake; Lactation; Metabolism; Nutrient deficiencies; Nutrition.

I. SUMMARY

Lactation is time of high metabolic activity and depending on the age and number of the infants being fed can effectively double maternal energy requirements. In this regard breastfeeding is similar to a performance sport. Some nutrients have increased requirements during lactation while others remain stable. Appropriate nutrient intake is crucial to ensure maternal needs are met to maintain health while providing optimal nutrition for the growing infant.

II. INTRODUCTION

A. Background

Lactation is a special time for mother and infant, emotionally and biophysically. To redirect popular focus, the American Academy of Pediatrics has reaffirmed its recommendation of "exclusive breastfeeding for about 6 months, followed by continued breastfeeding as complementary foods are introduced, with continuation of breastfeeding for 1 year or longer as mutually desired by mother and infant."[1] Metabolic support, in the form of a balanced food patterns containing a wide variety of foods, will support maternal health and provide an optimal concentration of nutrients in the human milk produced during lactation. Food patterns that are chronically deficient in specific nutrients will compromise the mother's health and deplete nutrient stores, and downstream, this may limit the nutritive content of the milk she produces.[2]

B. Key Issues

With a new baby, a mother's routine tasks,[3] such as preparing food and eating, can become difficult, thereby

Present Knowledge in Nutrition, Volume 2
https://doi.org/10.1016/B978-0-12-818460-8.00004-6

decreasing both the balance and variety of the foods a mother consumes. A focus on maternal nutrition is crucial to maintain maternal health and supporting optimal health of the breastfeeding infant, and the quality of maternal food intake during lactation may decrease obesity risk for infants.[4] During early lactation, attention is focused on producing an adequate amount of milk for her infant and settling in to the routine a new baby brings. Physiologically, almost all mothers can produce sufficient amounts of human milk for their infants.

In the first few days of lactation, colostrum is the "first" milk to appear and is driven by the shift in maternal hormones. After the initial hormone-driven period, approximately 72 h after birth, the determinants of milk volume are regularity of milk removal (number of feedings/24-hour period) and the amount of milk removed at each feeding. In the United States, the common recommendation is between 8 and 12 feeds in 24 h, the reported average is 11 times in 24 h.[5] However, to determine what typical feeding behavior is, it is important to evaluate lactation behaviors in societies unbiased by feeding scheduling constraints such as those in developed countries. When assessing feeding practices in developing countries, infants are often fed 14 to 18 times in 24 h.[6] In the first 2–3 weeks of lactation, there may be a wide variety of acceptable feeding routines; however, a range between 8 and 20 feedings per day is considered normal.[7] As lactation progresses over time, the number of feedings declines and often decreases in the amount of time each feeding takes. However, this can vary particularly during infant growth spurts.

Maternal benefits of breastfeeding

The benefits of consumption of human milk for infants are well known. There are numerous maternal health benefits with lactation as well. One of the first effects of breastfeeding immediately after birth is the decrease in postpartum bleeding and increase in rapid uterine involution.[8] These effects translate into less menstrual blood loss during lactation and increased child spacing due to lactational amenorrhea, as long as breastfeeding continues through the night.[9] Given the increase in calorie expenditure to make milk, breastfeeding women return to prepregnancy weight more readily than those who do not breastfeed.[10] Among lifetime benefits, there is a dose response for the lactating woman based on the cumulative months of breastfeeding for decreased risk of breast,[11] ovarian,[12] and endometrial cancers[13] and some evidence of a decreased risk of hypertension for women who breastfeed exclusively for 6 months.[14,15] Breastfeeding is very convenient and may improve maternal sleep patterns.[16]

In addition to these public health benefits, it is also beneficial to the environment and society.[17] Breastfeeding families have less illness, and the parents miss less work.[18] It is environmentally friendly as it neither requires the use of an outside energy source for manufacturing infant formula nor creates waste or air pollution.

Contraindications

The readily accepted contraindications to breastfeeding in the United States include mothers infected with human immunodeficiency virus or infants with inborn errors of metabolism such as classic galactosemia (galactose-1-phosphate uridyltransferase deficiency).[1] Subjective recommendations against breastfeeding are often made to mothers taking prescription or illicit drugs (some examples of common items are shown in Table 4.1) that can transfer into the milk and thus be fed to the baby at unpredictable and harmful levels. It is important to refer to a reliable source for current recommendations for medication use during lactation.

III. PHYSIOLOGICAL DEMANDS OF LACTATION

Lactation is a distinguishing feature of mammals. It is helpful to have a basic understanding of lactation physiology to better understand maternal nutritional needs during this high-calorie expenditure period of a mother's life.[19] Starting with mammary tissue development

TABLE 4.1 Examples of subjective opinions on medications. Refer to a current reputable source.

Medication	Purpose	Use during lactation	Notes
Sudafed	Decongestant	No	Decreases milk supply
Benadryl	Antihistamine	Yes	Small, occasional doses considered safe
Zoloft	Antidepressant	Yes	Seemingly does not pass into milk
Depo-Provera	Contraceptive	Maybe[a]	Do not use before 6 weeks postpartum as it can decrease milk supply
St. John's Wort	Herbal supplement	Maybe[a]	Can interact with other medications, use with caution
Sage	Herbal supplement	Maybe[a]	Purported to decrease milk supply; can cause nausea, vomiting, and diarrhea

[a] *Refer to health care provider.*

during fetal growth, in female infants, reproductive differentiation builds the foundational tissues into parturition. By birth, there is a rudimentary ductal system present, which provides a scaffolding for elongation and bifurcation of the ducts during puberty in response to the increase in estrogen and progesterone hormones. After adolescence, the mammary tissue enters a quiescent phase until pregnancy. During pregnancy, mammary epithelial cells differentiate into lactocytes with the capacity to synthesize unique milk constituents such as the sugar lactose, and this phase is known as secretory differentiation. This process requires the presence of a "lactogenic hormone complex" comprising adrenocorticotropin, thyrotropin, growth hormones, and estrogen, progesterone, and prolactin.[20] By the end of the third trimester, the maternal mammary tissue is ready for the most visible scene of this biochemical ballet. At birth, the high circulating concentrations of progesterone decrease rapidly signaling secretory activation.[21] Secretory activation has an array of steps, starting with the precipitous decrease of progesterone after which the presence of prolactin, insulin, and glucocorticoids causes the tight junctions of the mammary tissue to become less permeable.[22] As secretory activation progresses toward copious milk production, the blood vessels in the mammary tissue dilate and become visible in all colors of skin. Secretory activation is a progressive process in humans rather than an abrupt event as seen in other mammal as only a small volume (~30 mL/24 h) of colostrum is available during the first 30–40 h after birth.[23] Colostrum then transitions to mature milk over the first 7–10 days of lactation.[24] Overall, the change from secretory differentiation to secretory activation at birth increases the amount of energy needed by the mother by at least 300 calories per day from the diet and from maternal adipose tissue,[25] if available.

IV. NUTRITIONAL REQUIREMENTS

A. Basis for Key Nutrient Recommendations

Infants being breastfed exclusively for the first 6 months of life are dependent upon their mother's milk for all their nutritional needs, and lactating women need to supply adequate nutrients for their own health needs as well. It has long been thought that for most healthy women, the nutrient concentrations in milk were consistent among women. It is now known that some nutrients, including vitamins A, C, D, B1, B2, B3, B6, and B12, fatty acids, and iodine, in human milk are influenced by prepartum stores and postpartum daily maternal diet, which will be the focus in this chapter.

B. Dietary Guidance

Practices

Fluid needs; As mother/infant dyads settle in to their new routine, the mother's need for fluids increases. During lactation, water is needed for milk production, which is 87% water.[26] The fluid Adequate Intake (AI) recommendations for a healthy adult woman, between the ages of 19 and 50, is 2.7 L per day, and this increases to 3.8 L per day during lactation.[27] Women may be advised to consume additional fluid if there is a decline in milk production; however, there is insufficient evidence that fluid consumption above the Recommended Daily Allowance (RDA) improves milk production based on a Cochrane review.[28] The Academy of Nutrition and Dietetics' Evidence Analysis Library found no significant relationships between short periods of increased or decreased fluid intake (+25–50% fluid change compared to baseline) in healthy adult lactating women and human milk volume.[29] Women should be encouraged to drink to thirst and to have pale yellow urine, which reflects diluted urine to ensure optimal hydration.[30,31]

Energy needs; Lactation requires greater energy expenditure than needed during pregnancy. In the third trimester, the increased calorie need for a singleton pregnancy is approximately 500 kcal/day above prepartum needs.[25] During lactation, energy expenditure is increased by approximately 600 kcals/day for an average production of 26 ounces of milk in a 24 h period,[32] with approximately 155 kcals/day coming from maternal

TABLE 4.2 Acceptable macronutrient distribution ranges (AMDR) during lactation as a percentage of total daily calorie intake and in grams per day.

				RDA	RDA
Lactation	**Lipid**	**Carbohydrate**	**Protein**	**Carbohydrate in grams**	**Protein in grams**
≤18 yr	20%–35%	45%–65%	15%–35%	210	
19–50yr 1st 6 months of lactation	20%–35%	45%–65%	15%–35%	210	65 g/1000 kcals
31–50 yr 2nd 6 months of lactation	20%–35%	45%–65%	15%–35%	210	62 g/1000 kcals

energy stores.[33] For those women feeding multiple infant/s, energy needs increase significantly. For twins, maternal energy need during lactation is between 1200 and 1500 kcals/day[34] For breastfeeding additional infants, the maternal energy requirement is 500–600 kcals/per infant/day depending on the age and size of the infants. As an example, a mom of triplets exclusively breastfeeding in the first 6 months of lactation would need an additional 1700–2000 kilocalories per day above her nonlactating need.[34] It is rare for moms of triplets to exclusively breastfeed their infants, and this requires significant family support.

Protein; According to the Acceptable Macronutrient Distribution Ranges (AMDR), an adult person should consume between 10% and 35% of total calories from protein. Typically, women, children, and some elderly consume 13%–15%. The RDA for protein is 0.8 g per kilogram of body weight per day for healthy adults. Lactation increases protein requirement.[35] The AMDR ranges for carbohydrate, protein, and lipid as a percentage of total kcal/day intake and RDA for protein are shown in Table 4.2.

While adequate protein intake is important to support maternal health and prevent malnutrition, excess intake of any nutrient including protein should be avoided during lactation. The general health recommendation to avoid high intakes of processed meats that have been associated with certain cancers and animal-derived food sources high in saturated fat that may contribute to heart disease, obesity, and diabetes risk[36] also apply to the lactating woman. High protein intakes should also be avoided in those with chronic kidney disease as it can accelerate loss of kidney function.[37] Protein supplementation is not needed by those with a balanced food routine.

Vegetarians; Vegetarian and vegan mothers should monitor their intake carefully to ensure adequate and complete protein intake during lactation. Each type of vegetarianism has different nutrition implications for maternal risk of nutritional deficiency risks during lactation if not carefully considered. Protein quality is an important consideration during lactation. The type of vegetarian food routine followed will dictate the nutrient recommendations for a lactating woman.[38] Protein sources for lactating vegetarians should include complementary protein patterns such as legumes, seeds, nuts, eggs, dairy products, soy products, peas, and beans. Minerals that may be deficient in vegetarian diets include iron, calcium, zinc, and vitamin B12. Laboratory testing to determine maternal status for these specific nutrients may be indicated.[35] Lactating women following a vegan food routine should be monitored for B12 status.[39]

Lipids; Fatty acids in human milk reflect current maternal diet,[40] prepregnancy food intake, and body lipid stores.[41] The popularity of high lipid food routines such as the Atkins diet brings up the safety of extreme high-fat diets during lactation.[42] These food routines are not appropriate for women during lactation as they are far outside the AMDR recommendations and may alter lactation outcomes,[43,44] and many consist of 60% or more calories from lipids rather than the recommended amount of 35%(see Table 4.2.), which may not be a safe intake of lipids long-term. While excess lipid intake is not recommended, the fatty acids, linolenic (ALA, 18:3 Ω 3)[45] and linoleic acid (LA, 18:2 Ω 6),[46] are essential nutrients and must be obtained from routine intake. These essential fatty acids can be desaturated and elongated to form long-chain polyunsaturated fatty acids, including arachidonic (AA) and docosahexaenoic (DHA) acids. However, this conversion is a competitive process in that high intakes of LA can decrease the conversion of ALA to DHA.[47]

Omega "6 and 3" fatty acids; A balance of ALA (omega 3) and LA (omega 6) is important during lactation to ensure maternal replete status and ensure adequate amounts of DHA in human milk especially for those who do not eat fatty fish and other sources of DHA. DHA has been shown to lower blood pressure, reduce blood viscosity, increase cell membrane fluidity, and alter many basic properties of cell membranes changing the way nutrients, waste, and toxins move into and out of the cells.[48] Maternal intake and stores of omega-3 fatty acids supports infant neurologic development,[49] and higher intakes are associated with long-term maternal health benefits, including protection against heart disease and possibly stroke.[50] New studies are identifying potential benefits of lipid antiinflammatory agents for a wide range of conditions including cancer, inflammatory bowel disease, and autoimmune diseases such as lupus and rheumatoid arthritis.[51]

During infancy, AA acid and DHA must be obtained through breast milk or formula as infants are unable to produce enzymes in sufficient amounts to produce these long-chain fatty acids from essential ALA and LA making DHA and AA conditionally essential fatty acids.[52] Although, as shown in stable isotope studies, infants after birth can convert some ALA and LA into DHA and AA, respectively, their enzyme activity for this process is low. DHA and AA fatty acids are essential for normal infant growth of the eyes, brain, and nervous system.[53]

DHA intake in most American diets is low at an average of 150 mg/day, which is equivalent to 1 fish meal every 10 days, while in Europe, it is 180 mg/day, which is equivalent to 1 fish meal every 7 days.[54] The American Heart Association recommends that people without coronary heart disease take in 300 mg/day, and for people with coronary heart disease, the intake should be 1000 mg/day. While there is not yet a recommendation for the amount of DHA that should be consumed during lactation, it has been suggested that women of childbearing age consume 200 mg of DHA each day.[55] DHA supplementation of mothers has been reported to augment the IQ at 4 years of age and may improve eye and hand coordination at 2 years of age of their breastfed infants.[56,57]

In a study of DHA supplementation versus food in lactating women, after 2 weeks of supplementation, the milk of those in the Intervention group (supplemented with DHA) contained the higher levels of DHA than the Control group (placebo). The Intervention group took in 250 mg/day as a supplement. The Control group took in 70 mg/day from food. The Intervention group had a 28% higher concentration of DHA in their milk after a 14-day supplement treatment. The increase of DHA in the milk was present between 6 and 8 h after taking the supplement.[57]

Carbohydrates; Increasing complex carbohydrate intake may be helpful during lactation. During lactation and early motherhood, it is common to have periods of erratic meals or food intake, "feast and famine," due to difficulty balancing regular meal preparation and having a new baby. Having readily available healthy snacks that combine carbohydrates with protein and lipids can decrease fluctuations in blood glucose due to insulin response to carbohydrate intake. The AMDR recommendation for carbohydrate is between 45% and 65% of total daily kcals. The level of carbohydrate intake will move within this range depending on the individual's needs and health goals. For example, lower levels of carbohydrate can reduce exercise performance in anaerobic activities[58] and decrease the amount of glycogen replenishment after activity.[59]

Vitamins; Water-soluble vitamins (C and B vitamins) and lipid-soluble vitamins (A, D, E, K) are present in human milk, and concentrations are reflective of maternal nutrient status.[35] Maternal micronutrient needs are elevated during lactation for several vitamins and minerals[27] (see Tables 4.3 and 4.4). Vitamin and mineral content of human milk will usually remain consistent in cases of short-term reduced maternal intakes at the expense of maternal stores in well-nourished women.[25,60–62] However, a number of studies show that after prolonged reduced intake of specific micronutrients, milk micronutrient composition may be compromised but milk volume is not impacted.[27,62–66]

Studying the micronutrient composition of human milk has several limitations including the wide variation of nutrient concentrations between milk produced for preterm versus full-term infants, the sex of the infant, stage of lactation, genetic factors, environmental factors, season, method of collection and storage of milk samples, and time of day and the time during a feed at which the milk sample was collected.[62,67] Also, as Allen et al. points out, most current research studies on the topic have small sample sizes and do not offer longitudinal data.[67]

Fat-soluble vitamins; The present vitamin K recommendation for lactating females 19 years of age and older of 90 μg/day (shown in Table 4.3) is based on the amount needed to prevent bleeding. Overall, vitamin K content is low in human milk, and variations in maternal diet do not appear to significantly alter its concentration.[68,69] Concentrated in early colostrum and then lipid-rich portion of mature milk, vitamin K is transported in the core of the milk-fat globule.[70,71] Due to the risk for neonatal hemorrhage syndrome, it is recommended that infants receive a 0.5–1.0 mg dose of vitamin K1 (phytonadione) intramuscularly at birth after the first breastfeed, but no more than 6 hours postpartum as a preventive measure.[1]

Vitamin D deficiency among women and children is a growing concern domestically and internationally.[72,73] Deficiency and insufficiency are becoming common in women of childbearing age[74,75] Nondietary risk factors include inadequate sunlight exposure and darker

TABLE 4.3 Dietary reference intakes (DRIs) for the United States and Canada: Vitamins intake during lactation.

Age	Vitamin A (μg/day)	Vitamin C (μg/day)	Vitamin D (μg/day)	Vitamin E (μg/day)	Vitamin K (μg/day)	Thiamin (mg/day)	Riboflavin (mg/day)	Niacin (mg/day)	Vitamin B6 (mg/day)	Folate (μg/day)	Vitamin B12 (μg/day)	Pantothenic acid (mg/day)	Biotin (μg/day)	Choline (mg/day)
14–18 yr	1200	115	15	19	75	1.4	1.6	17	2.0	500	2.8	7	35	550
19–30 yr	1300	120	15	19	90	1.4	1.6	17	2.0	500	2.8	7	35	550
31–50 yr	1300	120	15	19	90	1.4	1.6	17	2.0	500	2.8	7	35	550

NOTE: An Estimated Average Requirement (EAR) is the average daily nutrient intake level estimated to meet the requirements of half of the healthy individuals in a group. EARs have not been established for vitamin K, pantothenic acid, biotin, choline, chromium, fluoride, manganese, or other nutrients not yet evaluated via the DRI process.

TABLE 4.4 Dietary Reference Intakes (DRIs) for the USA and Canada: Mineral intake during Lactation

Age	Calcium (mg/ day)	Chromium (μg/ day)	Copper (μg/ day)	Fluoride (mg/ day)	Iodine (μg/ day)	Iron (mg/ day)	Magnesium (mg/ day)	Manganese (mg/ day)	Molybdenum (μg/ day)	Phosphorus (mg/ day)	Selenium (μg/ day)	Zinc (mg/ day)	Potassium (g/day)	Sodium (g/day)	Chloride (g/day)
14-18 yr	**1,300**	44*	**1,300**	3*	**290**	**10**	**360**	2.6*	**50**	**1,250**	**70**	**13**	5.1*	1.5*	2.3*
19-30 yr	**1,000**	45*	**1,300**	3*	**290**	**9**	**310**	2.6*	**50**	**700**	**70**	**12**	5.1*	1.5*	2.3*
31-50 yr	**1,000**	45*	**1,300**	3*	**290**	**9**	**320**	2.6*	**50**	**700**	**70**	**12**	5.1*	1.5*	2.3*

NOTE: This table (taken from the DRI reports, see www.nap.edu) presents Recommended Dietary Allowances (RDAs) in bold type and Adequate Intakes (AIs) in ordinary type followed by an asterisk (*). An RDA is the average daily dietary intake level sufficient to meet the nutrient requirements of nearly all (97–98 percent) healthy individuals in a group. It is calculated from an Estimated Average Requirement (EAR). If sufficient scientific evidence is not available to establish an EAR, and thus calculate an RDA, an AI is usually developed. For healthy breast-fed infants, an AI is the mean intake. The AI for other life stage and gender groups is believed to cover the needs of all healthy individuals in the groups, but lack of data or uncertainty in the data prevent being able to specify with confidence the percentage of individuals covered by this intake.

pigmented skin.[73] Human milk vitamin D content and subsequent infant serum 25(OH)D concentrations are associated with maternal stores. Vitamin D in human milk also comes from maternal dietary intake as well as sunlight exposure during pregnancy and postpartum.[76] Vitamin D uptake into human milk is minimal, providing roughly 15 IU/day to the exclusively breastfed infant.[68] Maternal obesity also appears to be negatively correlated with vitamin D in human milk.[62] As a precaution, the National Academy of Medicine and the American Academy of Pediatrics recommend that exclusively breastfed infants receive 400 IU of supplemental vitamin D daily.[77] Due to poor tolerance and compliance in treating infants, maternal supplementation of high doses of vitamin D as an alternative to direct infant supplementation was tested.[78,79] Hollis et al. concluded that infants 25(OH) D status did not differ between those who received 400 IU cholecalciferol directly and those whose mothers took 6400 IU daily for 7 months during breastfeeding.[78] However, the Academy of Nutrition and Dietetics position paper states that there is currently insufficient evidence that maternal supplementation of vitamin D could replace the need for infant supplementation.[80]

Colostrum is rich in retinol, and the concentration declines as milk matures, until weeks 2 and 4 at which time the level is stabilized. The lipid composition of human milk along with maternal intake of retinol has been associated with the retinol content of human milk.[60,64] Supplementation with β-carotene improves retinol concentrations in human milk of vitamin A–deficient women but does not have the same effect in well-nourished women, whereas preformed retinol supplementation during pregnancy may increase retinol in colostrum in well-nourished women.[68] Lactating women supplemented with one dose of 200,000 IU retinyl palmitate, postpartum saw increases in colostrum retinol concentration[81] but not in mature milk, and α-tocopherol bioavailability was decreased as an unintended side effect.[82] Carotenoid compounds in milk, including lycopene, lutein, zeaxanthin, and β-carotene, are positively correlated with maternal dietary intake. Maternal obesity appears to have a negative impact on lutein and zeaxanthin in human milk.[83]

Colostrum is rich in α-tocopherol, the predominant form of vitamin E in human milk. α-Tocopherol declines within the first month of lactation and appears to remain stable from month 3 through 6. Studies examining the effect of diet on the vitamin E concentration in human milk have conflicting results. In some studies, the overall lipid content of human milk appears to influence vitamin E content, while in others, there was no impact of maternal food or supplement intake on vitamin E in human milk.[84,85] In further studies using vitamin E supplementation, an increase was seen in colostrum and transitional milk with natural forms of vitamin E having a greater effect than synthetic forms. This contrasts with findings that demonstrate vitamin E concentration did not increase in mature milk after supplementation.[86,87]

Water-soluble vitamins; Vitamin B concentrations are higher in transitional and mature milk than in colostrum.[64,88,89] While maternal dietary intake of thiamine influences human milk concentrations,[90] it appears to only increase thiamine in the breast milk of thiamine deficient mothers.[91] Infants who are exclusively breastfed have lower vitamin B12 concentrations at 4–6 months than those who drink cow milk or infant formula. Both maternal diet and maternal vitamin B12 status correlated with human milk concentration.[89] Infants whose mothers are chronically deficient or have malabsorption of vitamin B12 are at increased risk for deficiency, as are the infants of mothers who consume a macrobiotic or vegetarian diet.[60] Human milk vitamin B12 concentration responds to supplementation in mothers who are deficient but does not appear to increase B12 in those who are well nourished.[67] If symptoms of deficiency appear, both mother and infant should be treated with vitamin B12 intramuscularly.[89] While maternal supplementation with riboflavin increases the concentration in human milk in the short term, it does not have the same effect long term.[67] Both riboflavin[92] and vitamin A[93] are susceptible to photodegradation. To prevent the loss of these vitamins in human milk, expressed human milk should be stored in an opaque container in the refrigerator or freezer.[94]

Maternal folate intake recommendation during lactation only increases by about 25%, despite high infant folate needs. Folate concentrations in human milk are higher than in maternal plasma, which may be the result of increased transport of folate into human milk. Folate concentrations are higher in mature milk than colostrum,[95] and folate in human milk is in the form 5-methyltetrahydrofolate. Studies of folic acid supplementation versus food intake of folate have no increase in milk folate.[96,97] Vitamin B6 increases in human milk over the first few weeks of lactation and then declines gradually and may not be able to meet infant needs after 6 months.[67] Human milk concentration of vitamin B6 is highly affected by maternal food intake and supplementation.[98]

Vitamin C, which is involved in immune function, is more concentrated in colostrum than mature milk.[99] However, its concentration varies depending on maternal diet and supplementation appears to have the greatest impact in deficient mothers.[78,88,100,101] Refrigeration and freezing substantially decrease vitamin C concentration in expressed human milk and should be considered if expressed human milk is the primary form of nutrition for an infant.[102] Smoking and diabetes are also negatively associated with human milk vitamin C concentrations.[60]

Due to rapid growth, infants require large amounts of choline,[103] and choline concentration doubles in human milk by 6–7 days after birth and in maternal serum 12–28 days postpartum.[103,104] Maternal intake influences the amount of choline in human milk, and genetic polymorphisms may increase the maternal or infant requirement for choline.[105]

Minerals; Though human milk is low in iron, it is highly bioavailable. Human milk is also rich in vitamin C, (if maternal intake is sufficient) further increasing iron bioavailability. Exclusive breastfeeding elongates the duration of postpartum amenorrhea, which allows the mother to retain more of her own iron stores. Amenorrhea decreases iron needs in the mother until menstruation resumes.[25,106] Since iron in human milk is low, infant iron status relies more on fetal stored iron accumulated during gestation.[67] If the infant is found to be deficient in iron, supplementation may be indicated, as is often the case in infants whose mothers were deficient during pregnancy, in developing countries and in some premature or low-birth weight infants. Maternal intakes of iron, both dietary and supplemental, postpartum appear to not affect the iron content of milk.[60,66] As infant iron stores accumulate in the third trimester of pregnancy, low maternal stores result in an early infant deficit. Iron concentrations in both mother and infant decrease with age.[107]

Calcium, phosphorus, magnesium, copper, zinc, fluorine, and sulfur levels also appear to be stable in human milk despite varying levels in maternal dietary intake.[25,63,66,108] Maternal urinary calcium excretion decreases during lactation and mobilization from bone increases, allowing maternal dietary need for calcium to remain the same as a nonlactating female adult.[25] A study comparing two different culturally based food patterns in Ethiopia determined that maternal diets richer in calcium resulted in human milk that was higher in calcium,[66] while Daniels et al. found that concentrations were consistent in human milk despite less than AIs by Indonesian women.[64] However, human milk calcium and zinc concentration does decline when milk volume is less than 300 mL per day.[62]

Sodium, potassium, and chloride concentrations in human milk are regulated by the mammary secretory cell across an electrical potential gradient. However, sodium concentration increases in milk when the daily volume decreases.[62] Phosphorus content of human milk is lower than in other mammals.

Maru et al. found that copper concentrations in milk appeared to correlate with maternal diet. The researchers concluded that decreased copper in human milk may be more likely attributed to prolonged diarrhea in addition to poor dietary intake rather than diet alone in areas of the world where medical resources are scarce and diarrhea is common.[66] Selenium and iodine concentrations in human milk are related to maternal dietary intakes and are usually associated with soil mineral content in the region.[27,109] Low maternal intake of selenium can result in clinical deficiency in the exclusively breastfed infant.[67] The mammary gland has preferential uptake for iodine, suggesting that iodine moves into human milk preferentially at the expense of the mother's iodine status and may not decline in milk until maternal intakes have been decreased for a long period of time.[110] Maternal smoking decreases iodine in human milk.[111] Maternal smoking increases the concentration of serum levels of thiocyanate. The decrease of iodine in human milk may be due to the competitive inhibition of the sodium–iodide symporter in the lactating mammary gland by thiocyanate responsible for iodide transport.[111]

Given the varying effectiveness of vitamin and mineral supplementation on human milk composition, and micronutrient concentration as compared to absorption from food, a nutrient-dense maternal dietary pattern through moderate intake of a wide variety of food best supports maternal health and boosts the nutritional quality of human milk.[64,86,97]

Issues of concern

Bariatric surgery; Gastric bypass surgery has increased from an estimated 113,000 in 2007[112] to 228,000 in 2017.[113] Women of childbearing age, 18–45 years of age, make up 50%[114] or more[115] of the patients undergoing bariatric surgery, and this is not a contraindication for breastfeeding. Jans et al.[116] report that the milk of postbariatric surgery patients is adequate in energy, macronutrients, and vitamin A for at least the first 6 weeks of breastfeeding. Patients should be monitored for nutritional deficiencies including B12 as maternal B12 deficiency can result in infant deficiency in an exclusively breastfed infant.[117] As limited data are available in this population, regular nutritional screening is advisable.

Substances of concern; Some common substances in maternal diets may be cause for concern in lactating women. Caffeine, chocolate, and alcohol transfer into human milk, with caffeine in human milk peaking at 1–2 h after ingestion.[118] Coffee and chocolate consumption has not been proven to impact infant sleep patterns, but caffeine metabolism in infants is slower than in adults.

Maternal intake of coffee and chocolate has been associated with colic in infants.[119] The recommendation for maternal caffeine intake is less than three cups of coffee per day (<450 mg caffeine/day), although research suggests that most infants are not affected by caffeine intake less than 750 mg/day (about five5 cups of coffee equivalents).[120] The AAP recommends no more than 450 mg of caffeine a day.[1] Typical servings of coffee contain 150 mg of caffeine per serving, tea varies between 6 and 110 mg per serving, and soda can vary by brand. Caffeine content varies greatly between coffees, depending on the brand and strength of the brew. For example, an eight-ounce cup of coffee can range from 95 to 200 mg of caffeine.

C. Other Guidance

Exercise

Moderate exercise is health promoting for lactating women[121] and does not adversely affect milk production or composition,[122] nor does it negatively impact infant growth.[123] Exercise can improve the mother's overall health and sense of well-being.[124] Elite athletes have been reported to breastfeed for longer durations and at higher rates than members of the general public.[125] At the other end of the weight spectrum, lactating women who are obese decreased their health risks after a twelve-week structured food and exercise routine. The improved health parameters that persisted up to the one-year follow-up included fasting insulin, total cholesterol, LDL cholesterol, and waist circumference persisted at the 1 year follow-up.[126]

While mothers will seek out nutrition information, among low-income mothers most were interested in seeking information on the Internet for infant health information.[127] Often, the information women found on the Internet was incomplete or wrong.[128] Health professionals stated that a centralized website could help mothers by providing information on feeding/breastfeeding, the infant's needs, and "baby blues,"[128] indicating that these mothers may be more interested in nutrition information with a focus on the mother–infant dyad rather than solely on maternal health.

Allergies and food sensitivities

The prevalence of food allergy is increasing in both developed and developing countries in the decade.[129] Rates as high as approximately 10% have been reported.[130] It is predicted that there will be a continued increase in food allergy prevalence until effective treatment is identified.[131] Unless a specific food allergy is already identified, no maternal dietary restrictions are required during lactation. Healthy, balanced maternal food routines inclusive of fruits, vegetables, and vitamins may play an important role in the prevention of infant allergies[132] and have myriad advantages to general health and well-being of the mother. The reason posited for the upsurge in prevalence of food allergies is "modern lifestyle," which is poorly understood.[133] There remains a need for large-scale randomized controlled trials for all other nutritional interventions in the hope that more can be done for the primary prevention of allergies in the future.[134]

It is not recommended that lactating women follow food routines that exclude specific foods as it increases the risk of inadequate nutrient intakes needed to support maternal and infant health.[25] No significant differences have been found between mothers on restricted and unrestricted food routines on the development of their breastfed infants developing asthma as children.[135,136]

Weight loss supplements

It is not recommended that lactating women use weight loss aids, either over-the-counter medications or food supplements designed for weight loss. One such weight loss aid is Orlistat. This over-the-counter drug prevents the digestion and absorption of lipids from food. Orlistat blocks the action of the lipase enzyme and thereby stops the digestion of some of dietary lipids.[137] Orlistat blocks about 25% of the lipid in a meal. The unabsorbed lipid is excreted in the stool. While it is possible that an extremely low level of Orlistat gets into maternal circulation, it can interfere with the absorption of lipid-soluble vitamins, A, D, E, and K in the gastrointestinal tract.[138]

RESEARCH GAPS

Future directions and gaps in knowledge

Insufficient research has been conducted to evaluate the impact of maternal diet on the composition of human milk. More needs to be known about the direct and indirect relationship between maternal intake and availability of nutrients in human milk. Additionally, the relationship between mother–infant interaction at the breast with the movement of infant saliva into the breast is thought to change the microRNA, which may play a role in regulating infant health.[139] It is speculated that maternal high-lipid food intake impacts the regulation of some microRNAs.[140] More research is needed to decipher the impact on infant short- and long-term health outcomes, as well as potential impact on maternal health.

The use and the impact of cannabis sativa (marijuana), tetrahydrocannabinol (THC), and cannabidiol by lactating women is a new area of study. The active ingredients in marijuana pass into human milk and result in infant exposure.[141] THC has been shown to be present in measurable amounts in human milk up to 6 days after maternal use.[142] Breastfeeding women in locations with legalized recreational use of cannabis self-report that approximately 5% were using cannabis while breastfeeding in the early postpartum.[143] With little published evidence in the medical literature, changes in cultural belief, the legality of use, and no consensus in professional guidelines, more information is needed.[144,145]

Microbiome

The intestinal microbiota is strongly personalized and influenced by environmental factors, especially dietary intake patterns. While dietary intake influences organism variety, plenty, and function,[146] the impact of the maternal microbiota on health and well-being based on nutritional and infant interaction is not well defined. Very little is understood about the mechanisms involved in the regulation of microbiome organism populations, and there is increasing evidence that suggests that maternal overnutrition or poor food patterns can influence the development and variety of organisms in the infant gut microbiome.[147] The lactating breast microbiome has yet to be completely characterized. A major role for breast microbiome and the human milk microbiome inoculum for the infant gut has been proposed. Women with obesity have lower microbial diversity, increased abundance of opportunistic pathogens, and depletion of commensal obligate anaerobes, and how this is related to maternal health, human milk, and infant health is unknown.[148] The human milk microbiome is a part of the physiology of the maternal mammary tissue and a predictor for the infant gut microbiome.[148] There are suggested potential health benefits and an emerging connection between the human milk microbiome and mammary gland physiology and lactation.[149]

Acknowledgments

This chapter is an update of the chapter titled "39. Maternal Nutrient Metabolism and Requirements in Pregnancy and Lactation" by Lindsay H. Allen, in Present Knowledge in Nutrition, 10th Edition, edited by Erdman JW, Macdonald IA, and Zeisel SH and published by Wiley-Blackwell. © 2012 International Life Sciences Institute. Portions of this update are from the previously published chapter and the contributions of previous authors are acknowledged.

V. REFERENCES

1. Pediatrics TAA of Policy Statement. Breastfeeding and the use of human milk. *Pediatrics*. 2012;129(3):e827–e841. https://doi.org/10.1542/peds.2011-3552.
2. Lee S, Kelleher SL. Biological underpinnings of breastfeeding challenges: the role of genetics, diet, and environment on lactation physiology. *Am J Physiol Endocrinol Metab*. 2016;311(2):E405–E422. https://doi.org/10.1152/ajpendo.00495.2015.
3. Bergmann RL, Bergmann KE, Von Weizsäcker K, Berns M, Henrich W, Dudenhausen JW. Breastfeeding is natural but not always easy: intervention for common medical problems of breastfeeding mothers - a review of the scientific evidence. *J Perinat Med*. 2014;42(1). https://doi.org/10.1515/jpm-2013-0095.
4. Tahir MJ, Haapala JL, Foster LP, et al. Higher maternal diet quality during pregnancy and lactation is associated with lower infant weight-for-length, body fat percent, and fat mass in early postnatal life. *Nutrients*. 2019;11(3). https://doi.org/10.3390/nu11030632.
5. Kent JC, Mitoulas LR, Cregan MD, Ramsay DT, Doherty DA, Hartmann PE. Volume and frequency of breastfeedings and fat content of breast milk throughout the day. *Pediatrics*. 2006;117(3). https://doi.org/10.1542/peds.2005-1417.
6. Walters-Bugbee SE, McClure KS, Kral TVE, Sarwer DB. Maternal child feeding practices and eating behaviors of women with extreme obesity and those who have undergone bariatric surgery. *Surg Obes Relat Dis*. 2012;8(6):784–791. https://doi.org/10.1016/j.soard.2012.07.016.
7. Center for Disease Control. *Breastfeeding FAQ*; 2019. https://www.cdc.gov/nccdphp/dnpao/index.html. Accessed October 2, 2019.
8. Sobhy SI, Mohame NA. The effect of early initiation of breast feeding on the amount of vaginal blood loss during the fourth stage of labor. *J Egypt Public Health Assoc*. 2004;79(1–2):1–12. http://www.ncbi.nlm.nih.gov/pubmed/16916046.
9. Chowdhury R, Sinha B, Sankar MJ, et al. Breastfeeding and maternal health outcomes: a systematic review and meta-analysis. *Acta Paediatr*. 2015;104(467):96–113. https://doi.org/10.1111/apa.13102.
10. Larson-Meyer DE, Schueler J, Kyle E, Austin KJ, Hart AM, Alexander BM. Do lactation-induced changes in ghrelin, glucagon-like peptide-1, and peptide YY influence appetite and

body weight regulation during the first postpartum year? *J Obes*. 2016;2016. https://doi.org/10.1155/2016/7532926.

11. Mosca F, Giannì ML. Human milk: composition and health benefits. *La Pediatr Medica e Chir*. 2017;39(2). https://doi.org/10.4081/pmc.2017.155.
12. Li D-P, Du C, Zhang Z-M, et al. Breastfeeding and ovarian cancer risk: a systematic review and meta-analysis of 40 epidemiological studies. *Asian Pac J Cancer Prev*. 2014;15(12):4829–4837. https://doi.org/10.7314/apjcp.2014.15.12.4829.
13. Wang L, Li J, Shi Z. Association between breastfeeding and endometrial cancer risk: evidence from a systematic review and meta-analysis. *Nutrients*. 2015;7(7):5697–5711. https://doi.org/10.3390/nu7075248.
14. Stuebe AM, Schwarz EB, Grewen K, et al. Duration of lactation and incidence of maternal hypertension: a longitudinal cohort study. *Am J Epidemiol*. 2011;174(10):1147–1158. https://doi.org/10.1093/aje/kwr227.
15. Wu Y, Zhao P, Li W, Cao MQ, Du L, Chen JC. The effect of remote health intervention based on internet or mobile communication network on hypertension patients: protocol for a systematic review and meta-analysis of randomized controlled trials. *Medicine*. 2019;98(9):e14707. https://doi.org/10.1097/MD.0000000000014707.
16. Hughes O, Mohamad MM, Doyle P, Burke G. The significance of breastfeeding on sleep patterns during the first 48 hours postpartum for first time mothers. *J Obstet Gynaecol*. 2018;38(3):316–320. https://doi.org/10.1080/01443615.2017.1353594.
17. Bartick M, Reinhold A. The burden of suboptimal breastfeeding in the United States: a pediatric cost analysis. *Pediatrics*. 2010;125(5):e1048–e1056. https://doi.org/10.1542/peds.2009-1616.
18. Mass SB. Supporting breastfeeding in the United States: the surgeon general's call to action. *Curr Opin Obstet Gynecol*. 2011;23(6):460–464. https://doi.org/10.1097/GCO.0b013e32834cdcb3.
19. Butte NF, King JC. Energy requirements during pregnancy and lactation. *Public Health Nutr*. 2005;8(7A):1010–1027. http://www.ncbi.nlm.nih.gov/pubmed/16277817.
20. Truchet S, Honvo-Houéto E. Physiology of milk secretion. *Best Pract Res Clin Endocrinol Metabol*. 2017;31(4):367–384. https://doi.org/10.1016/j.beem.2017.10.008.
21. Pang WW, Hartmann PE. Initiation of human lactation: secretory differentiation and secretory activation. *J Mammary Gland Biol Neoplasia*. 2007;12(4):211–221. https://doi.org/10.1007/s10911-007-9054-4.
22. Kobayashi K, Tsugami Y, Matsunaga K, Oyama S, Kuki C, Kumura H. Prolactin and glucocorticoid signaling induces lactation-specific tight junctions concurrent with β-casein expression in mammary epithelial cells. *Biochim Biophys Acta*. 2016;1863(8):2006–2016. https://doi.org/10.1016/j.bbamcr.2016.04.023.
23. Santoro W, Martinez FE, Ricco RG, Jorge SM. Colostrum ingested during the first day of life by exclusively breastfed healthy newborn infants. *J Pediatr*. 2010;156(1):29–32. https://doi.org/10.1016/j.jpeds.2009.07.009.
24. Ballard O, Morrow AL. Human milk composition. Nutrients and bioactive factors. *Pediatr Clin N Am*. 2013. https://doi.org/10.1016/j.pcl.2012.10.002.
25. Marangoni F, Cetin I, Verduci E, et al. Maternal diet and nutrient requirements in pregnancy and breastfeeding. An Italian consensus document. *Nutrients*. 2016;8(10). https://doi.org/10.3390/nu8100629.
26. Neville MC, Keller R, Seacat J, et al. Studies in human lactation: milk volumes in lactating women during the onset of lactation and full lactation. *Am J Clin Nutr*. 1988;48(6):1375–1386. https://doi.org/10.1093/ajcn/48.6.1375.
27. Parr RM, DeMaeyer EM, Iyengar VG, et al. Minor and trace elements in human milk from Guatemala, Hungary, Nigeria, Philippines, Sweden, and Zaire. Results from a WHO/IAEA joint project. *Biol Trace Elem Res*. 1991;29(1):51–75. http://www.ncbi.nlm.nih.gov/pubmed/1711362.
28. Ndikom CM, Fawole B, Ilesanmi RE. Extra fluids for breastfeeding mothers for increasing milk production. *Cochrane Database Syst Rev*. 2014;6. https://doi.org/10.1002/14651858.CD008758.pub2.
29. Lessen RDIBCLCLDNRM, Kavanagh KLDNKR. From the academy position paper position of the academy of nutrition and dietetics: promoting and supporting breastfeeding position statement. *J Acad Nutr Diet*. 2015;115:444–449. https://doi.org/10.1016/j.jand.2014.12.014.
30. McKenzie AL, Muñoz CX, Ellis LA, et al. Urine color as an indicator of urine concentration in pregnant and lactating women. *Eur J Nutr*. 2017;56(1):355–362. https://doi.org/10.1007/s00394-015-1085-9.
31. McKenzie AL, Armstrong LE. Monitoring body water balance in pregnant and nursing women: the validity of urine color. *Ann Nutr Metab*. 2017;70(Suppl 1):18–22. https://doi.org/10.1159/000462999.
32. Butte NF, King JC. Energy requirements during pregnancy and lactation. *Public Health Nutr*. 2005;8(7A):1010–1027. http://www.ncbi.nlm.nih.gov/pubmed/16277817.
33. Butte NF, Wong WW, Hopkinson JM. Energy requirements of lactating women derived from doubly labeled water and milk energy output. *J Nutr*. 2001;131(1):53–58. https://doi.org/10.1093/jn/131.1.53.
34. Flidel-Rimon O, Shinwell ES. Breast feeding twins and high multiples. *Arch Dis Child Fetal Neonatal Ed*. 2006;91(5). https://doi.org/10.1136/adc.2005.082305.
35. Kominiarek MA, Rajan P. Nutrition recommendations in pregnancy and lactation. *Med Clin N Am*. 2016;100(6):1199–1215. https://doi.org/10.1016/j.mcna.2016.06.004.
36. Boada LD, Henríquez-Hernández LA, Luzardo OP. The impact of red and processed meat consumption on cancer and other health outcomes: epidemiological evidences. *Food Chem Toxicol*. 2016;92:236–244. https://doi.org/10.1016/j.fct.2016.04.008.
37. Ko GJ, Obi Y, Tortorici AR, Kalantar-Zadeh K. Dietary protein intake and chronic kidney disease. *Curr Opin Clin Nutr Metab Care*. 2017;20(1):77–85. https://doi.org/10.1097/MCO.0000000000000342.
38. Agnoli C, Baroni L, Bertini I, et al. Position paper on vegetarian diets from the working group of the Italian Society of Human Nutrition. *Nutr Metab Cardiovasc Dis*. 2017;27(12):1037–1052. https://doi.org/10.1016/j.numecd.2017.10.020LK-. http://limo.libis.be/resolver?&sid=EMBASE&issn=15903729&id=doi:10.1016%2Fj.numecd.2017.10.020&atitle=Position+paper+on+vegetarian+diets+from+the+working+group+of+the+Italian+Society+of+Human+Nutrition&stitle=Nutr.+Metab.+Cardiovasc.+Dis.&title=Nutrition%2C+Metabolism+and+Cardiovascular+Diseases&volume=27&issue=12&spage=1037&epage=1052&aulast=Agnoli&aufirst=C.&auinit=C.&aufull=Agnoli+C.&coden=&isbn=&pages=1037-1052&date=2017&auinit1=C&auinitm=.
39. Rizzo G, Laganà AS, Rapisarda AMC, et al. Vitamin B12 among vegetarians: status, assessment and supplementation. *Nutrients*. 2016;8(12). https://doi.org/10.3390/nu8120767.
40. Dickton D, Francis J. Case review: food pattern effects on milk lipid profiles. *J Nutr Heal Food Eng*. 2018;8(6):467–470. https://doi.org/10.15406/jnhfe.2018.08.00311.
41. Bzikowska-Jura A, Czerwonogrodzka-Senczyna A, Jasińska-Melon E, et al. The concentration of omega-3 fatty acids in human milk is related to their habitual but not current intake. *Nutrients*. 2019;11(7):1585. https://doi.org/10.3390/nu11071585.
42. Park JE, Miller M, Rhyne J, Wang Z, Hazen SL. Differential effect of short-term popular diets on TMAO and other cardio-metabolic risk markers. *Nutr Metab Cardiovasc Dis*. 2019;29(5):513–517. https://doi.org/10.1016/j.numecd.2019.02.003.
43. Nnodum BN, Oduah E, Albert D, Pettus M. Ketogenic diet-induced severe ketoacidosis in a lactating woman: a case report and review of the literature. *Case Rep Nephrol*. 2019;2019:1214208. https://doi.org/10.1155/2019/1214208.

44. Hernandez LL, Grayson BE, Yadav E, Seeley RJ, Horseman ND. High fat diet alters lactation outcomes: possible involvement of inflammatory and serotonergic pathways. *PLoS One*. 2012;7(3): e32598. https://doi.org/10.1371/journal.pone.0032598.
45. National Center for Biotechnology Information. *Linolenic Acid*. PubChem Database; 2019. https://pubchem.ncbi.nlm.nih.gov/compound/Linolenic-acid. Accessed October 13, 2019.
46. National Center for Biotechnology Information. Linoleic Acid. PubChem Database.
47. Burns-Whitmore, Froyen, Heskey, Parker, San Pablo. Alpha-linolenic and linoleic fatty acids in the vegan diet: do they require dietary reference intake/adequate intake special consideration? *Nutrients*. 2019;11(10):2365. https://doi.org/10.3390/nu11102365.
48. Hishikawa D, Valentine WJ, Iizuka-Hishikawa Y, Shindou H, Shimizu T. Metabolism and functions of docosahexaenoic acid-containing membrane glycerophospholipids. *FEBS Lett*. 2017; 591(18):2730–2744. https://doi.org/10.1002/1873-3468.12825.
49. Innis SM. Impact of maternal diet on human milk composition and neurological development of infants. *Am J Clin Nutr*. 2014; 99(3). https://doi.org/10.3945/ajcn.113.072595, 734S–41S.
50. Lovegrove JA, Griffin BA. The acute and long-term effects of dietary fatty acids on vascular function in health and disease. *Curr Opin Clin Nutr Metab Care*. 2013;16(2):162–167. https://doi.org/10.1097/MCO.0b013e32835c5f29.
51. Biasucci LM, La Rosa G, Pedicino D, D'Aiello A, Galli M, Liuzzo G. Where does inflammation fit? *Curr Cardiol Rep*. 2017; 19(9). https://doi.org/10.1007/s11886-017-0896-0.
52. Richard C, Lewis ED, Field CJ. Evidence for the essentiality of arachidonic and docosahexaenoic acid in the postnatal maternal and infant diet for the development of the infant's immune system early in life. *Appl Physiol Nutr Metabol*. 2016;41(5):461–475. https://doi.org/10.1139/apnm-2015-0660.
53. Guesnet P, Alessandri JM. Docosahexaenoic acid (DHA) and the developing central nervous system (CNS) – implications for dietary recommendations. *Biochimie*. 2011;93(1):7–12. https://doi.org/10.1016/j.biochi.2010.05.005.
54. Koletzko B, Cetin I, Thomas Brenna J, et al. Dietary fat intakes for pregnant and lactating women. *Br J Nutr*. 2007;98(5):873–877. https://doi.org/10.1017/S0007114507764747.
55. Cetin I, Koletzko B. Long-chain ω-3 fatty acid supply in pregnancy and lactation. *Curr Opin Clin Nutr Metab Care*. 2008;11(3): 297–302. https://doi.org/10.1097/MCO.0b013e3282f795e6.
56. Helland IB, Smith L, Saarem K, Saugstad OD, Drevon CA. Maternal supplementation with very-long-chain n-3 fatty acids during pregnancy and lactation augments children's IQ at 4 years of age. *Pediatrics*. 2003;111(1):e39–44. https://doi.org/10.1542/peds.111.1.e39.
57. Bergmann RL, Haschke-Becher E, Klassen-Wigger P, et al. Supplementation with 200 mg/day docosahexaenoic acid from mid-pregnancy through lactation improves the docosahexaenoic acid status of mothers with a habitually low fish intake and of their infants. *Ann Nutr Metab*. 2008;52(2):157–166. https://doi.org/10.1159/000129651.
58. Wroble KA, Trott MN, Schweitzer GG, Rahman RS, Kelly PV, Weiss EP. Low-carbohydrate, ketogenic diet impairs anaerobic exercise performance in exercise-trained women and men: a randomized-sequence crossover trial. *J Sports Med Phys Fitness*. 2019;59(4):600–607. https://doi.org/10.23736/S0022-4707.18.08318-4.
59. Mata F, Valenzuela PL, Gimenez J, et al. Carbohydrate availability and physical performance: physiological overview and practical recommendations. *Nutrients*. 2019;11(5). https://doi.org/10.3390/nu11051084.
60. Dror DK, Allen LH. Overview of nutrients in human milk. *Adv Nutr*. 2018;9(suppl_1):278S–294S. https://doi.org/10.1093/advances/nmy022.
61. Khambalia A, Latulippe ME, Campos C, et al. Milk folate secretion is not impaired during iron deficiency in humans. *J Nutr*. 2006;136(10):2617–2624. https://doi.org/10.1093/jn/136.10.2617.
62. Wu X, Jackson RT, Khan SA, Ahuja J, Pehrsson PR. Human milk nutrient composition in the United States: current knowledge, challenges, and research needs. *Curr Dev Nutr*. 2018;2(7). https://doi.org/10.1093/cdn/nzy025.
63. Björklund KL, Vahter M, Palm B, Grandér M, Lignell S, Berglund M. Metals and trace element concentrations in breast milk of first time healthy mothers: a biological monitoring study. *Environ Health*. 2012;11(1). https://doi.org/10.1186/1476-069X-11-92.
64. Daniels L, Gibson RS, Diana A, et al. Micronutrient intakes of lactating mothers and their association with breast milk concentrations and micronutrient adequacy of exclusively breastfed Indonesian infants. *Am J Clin Nutr*. 2019. https://doi.org/10.1093/ajcn/nqz047.
65. McKenzie AL, Perrier ET, Guelinckx I, et al. Relationships between hydration biomarkers and total fluid intake in pregnant and lactating women. *Eur J Nutr*. 2017;56(6):2161–2170. https://doi.org/10.1007/s00394-016-1256-3.
66. Maru M, Birhanu T, Tessema DA. Calcium, magnesium, iron, zinc and copper, compositions of human milk from populations with cereal and "enset" based diets. *Ethiop J Health Sci*. 2013;23(2): 90–97. http://www.ncbi.nlm.nih.gov/pubmed/23950625%0Ahttp://www.pubmedcentral.nih.gov/articlerender.fcgi?artid=PMC3742886.
67. Allen LH, Donohue JA, Dror DK. Limitations of the evidence base used to set recommended nutrient intakes for infants and lactatingwomen. *Adv Nutr*. 2018;9:295S–312S. https://doi.org/10.1093/advances/nmy019.
68. Dror DK, Allen LH. Retinol-to-fat ratio and retinol concentration in humanmilk show similar time trends and associations with maternal factors at the population level: a systematic review and meta-analysis. *Adv Nutr*. 2018;9:332S–346S. https://doi.org/10.1093/advances/nmy021.
69. Greer FR, Marshall S, Cherry J, Suttie JW. Vitamin K status of lactating mothers, human milk, and breast-feeding infants. *Pediatrics*. 1991;88(4):751–756. http://www.ncbi.nlm.nih.gov/pubmed/1896278.
70. Canfield LM, Hopkinson JM, Lima AF, Silva B, Garza C. Vitamin K in colostrum and mature human milk over the lactation period–a cross-sectional study. *Am J Clin Nutr*. 1991;53(3):730–735. https://doi.org/10.1093/ajcn/53.3.730.
71. Kojima T, Asoh M, Yamawaki N, Kanno T, Hasegawa H, Yonekubo A. Vitamin K concentrations in the maternal milk of Japanese women. *Acta Paediatr*. 2004;93(4):457–463. http://www.ncbi.nlm.nih.gov/pubmed/15188971.
72. Dawodu A, Tsang RC. Maternal vitamin D status: effect on milk vitamin D content and vitamin D status of breastfeeding infants. *Adv Nutr*. 2012;3(3):353–361. https://doi.org/10.3945/an.111.000950.
73. Parva NR, Tadepalli S, Singh P, et al. Prevalence of vitamin D deficiency and associated risk factors in the US population (2011–2012). *Cureus*. 2018. https://doi.org/10.7759/cureus.2741.
74. Zhao G, Ford ES, Tsai J, Li C, Croft JB. Factors associated with vitamin D deficiency and inadequacy among women of childbearing age in the United States. *ISRN Obstet Gynecol*. 2012;2012: 691486. https://doi.org/10.5402/2012/691486.

75. Ginde AA, Sullivan AF, Mansbach JM, Camargo CA. Vitamin D insufficiency in pregnant and nonpregnant women of childbearing age in the United States. *Am J Obstet Gynecol*. 2010; 202(5). https://doi.org/10.1016/j.ajog.2009.11.036, 436.e1-8.
76. Li K, Jiang J, Xiao H, et al. Changes in the metabolite profile of breast milk over lactation stages and their relationship with dietary intake in Chinese women: HPLC-QTOFMS based metabolomic analysis. *Food Funct*. 2018;9(10):5189–5197. https://doi.org/10.1039/c8fo01005f.
77. Wagner CL, Greer FR. Prevention of rickets and vitamin D deficiency in infants, children, and adolescents. *Pediatrics*. 2008; 122(5):1142–1152. https://doi.org/10.1542/peds.2008-1862.
78. Hollis BW, Wagner CL, Howard CR, et al. Maternal versus infant Vitamin D supplementation during lactation: a randomized controlled trial. *Pediatrics*. 2015;136(4):625–634. https://doi.org/10.1542/peds.2015-1669.
79. Wheeler BJ, Taylor BJ, Herbison P, et al. High-dose monthly maternal cholecalciferol supplementation during breastfeeding affects maternal and infant vitamin D status at 5 Months postpartum: a randomized controlled trial. *J Nutr*. 2016;146(10): 1999–2006. https://doi.org/10.3945/jn.116.236679.
80. Melina V, Craig W, Levin S. Position of the Academy of nutrition and Dietetics: vegetarian diets. *J Acad Nutr Diet*. 2016;116(12): 1970–1980. https://doi.org/10.1016/j.jand.2016.09.025.
81. Grilo EC, Lima MSR, Cunha LRF, Gurgel CSS, Clemente HA, Dimenstein R. Effect of maternal vitamin A supplementation on retinol concentration in colostrum. *J Pediatr*. 2015;91(1):81–86. https://doi.org/10.1016/j.jped.2014.05.004.
82. Grilo EC, Medeiros WF, Silva AGAA, Gurgel CSSS, Ramalho HMMM, Dimenstein R. Maternal supplementation with a megadose of vitamin A reduces colostrum level of α-tocopherol: a randomised controlled trial. *J Hum Nutr Diet*. 2016; 29(5). https://doi.org/10.1111/jhn.12381.
83. Zielinska MA, Hamulka J, Wesolowska A. TitleCartenoid content in breastmilk in the 3rd and 6th month of lactation and ist association with maternal dietary intake and anthropometric characteristics. *Nutrients*. 2019;11(1). https://doi.org/10.3390/nu11010193.
84. Antonakou A, Chiou A, Andrikopoulos NK, Bakoula C, Matalas A-LL. Breast milk tocopherol content during the first six months in exclusively breastfeeding Greek. *Eur J Nutr*. 2011; 50(3):195–202. https://doi.org/10.1007/s00394-010-0129-4.
85. Martysiak-Zurowska D, Szlagatys-Sidorkiewicz A, Zagierski M, et al. Concentrations of alpha- and gamma-tocopherols in human breast milk during the first months of lactation and in infant formulas. *Matern Child Nutr*. 2013;9(4). https://doi.org/10.1111/j.1740-8709.2012.00401.x.
86. Clemente HA, Ramalho HMM, Lima MSR, Grilo EC, Dimenstein R. Maternal supplementation with natural or synthetic vitamin E and its levels in human colostrum. *J Pediatr Gastroenterol Nutr*. 2015;60(4):533–537. https://doi.org/10.1097/MPG.0000000000000635.
87. Pires Medeiros JF, Ribeiro KDDS, Lima MSR, et al. α-Tocopherol in breast milk of women with preterm delivery after a single postpartum oral dose of vitamin e. *Br J Nutr*. 2016;115(8):1424–1430. https://doi.org/10.1017/S0007114516000477.
88. Keikha M, Bahreynian M, Saleki M, Kelishadi R. Macro- and micronutrients of human milk composition: are they related to maternal diet? A comprehensive systematic review. *Breastfeed Med*. 2017;12(9):517–527. https://doi.org/10.1089/bfm.2017.0048.
89. Neumann CG, Oace SM, Chaparro MP, Herman D, Drorbaugh N, Bwibo NO. Low vitamin B12 intake during pregnancy and lactation and low breastmilk vitamin 12 content in rural Kenyan women consuming predominantly maize diets. *Food Nutr Bull*. 2013;34(2): 151–159. https://doi.org/10.1177/156482651303400204.
90. Ortega RM, Martínez RM, Andrés P, Marín-Arias L, López-Sobaler AM. Thiamin status during the third trimester of pregnancy and its influence on thiamin concentrations in transition and mature breast milk. *Br J Nutr*. 2004;92(1):129–135. https://doi.org/10.1079/bjn20041153.
91. Hampel D, Shahab-Ferdows S, Adair LS, et al. Thiamin and riboflavin in human milk: effects of lipid-based nutrient supplementation and stage of lactation on vitamer secretion and contributions to total vitamin content. *PLoS One*. 2016;11(2). https://doi.org/10.1371/journal.pone.0149479.
92. Francis J. Effects of light on riboflavin and ascorbic acid in freshly expressed human milk. *J Nutr Heal Food Eng*. 2015;2(6):2–4. https://doi.org/10.15406/jnhfe.2015.02.00083.
93. Mestdagh F, De Meulenaer B, De Clippeleer J, Devlieghere F, Huyghebaert A. Protective influence of several packaging materials on light oxidation of milk. *J Dairy Sci*. 2005;88(2):499–510. https://doi.org/10.3168/jds.S0022-0302(05)72712-0.
94. Francis J, Rogers K, Dickton D, Twedt R, Pardini R. Decreasing retinol and α-tocopherol concentrations in human milk and infant formula using varied bottle systems. *Matern Child Nutr*. 2012;8(2): 215–224. https://doi.org/10.1111/j.1740-8709.2010.00279.x.
95. Mackey AD, Picciano MF. Maternal folate status during extended lactation and the effect of supplemental folic acid. *Am J Clin Nutr*. 1999;69(2):285–292. https://doi.org/10.1093/ajcn/69.2.285.
96. Houghton LA, Yang J, O'Connor DL. Unmetabolized folic acid and total folate concentrations in breast milk are unaffected by low-dose folate supplements. *Am J Clin Nutr*. 2009;89(1): 216–220. https://doi.org/10.3945/ajcn.2008.26564.
97. West AA, Yan J, Perry CA, Jiang X, Malysheva OV, Caudill MA. Folate-status response to a controlled folate intake in nonpregnant, pregnant, and lactating women. *Am J Clin Nutr*. 2012;96(4): 789–800. https://doi.org/10.3945/ajcn.112.037523.
98. Kang-Yoon SA, Kirksey A, Giacoia G, West K. Vitamin B–6 status of breast-fed neonates: influence of pyridoxine supplementation on mothers and neonates. *Am J Clin Nutr*. 1992;56(3):548–558. https://doi.org/10.1093/ajcn/56.3.548.
99. Ahmed L, Islam S, Khan N, Nahid S. Vitamin C content in human milk (colostrum, transitional and mature) and serum of a sample of bangladeshi mothers. *Malays J Nutr*. 2004;10(1):1–4. http://www.ncbi.nlm.nih.gov/pubmed/22691742.
100. Bates CJ, Prentice AM, Prentice A, Paul AA, Whitehead RG. Seasonal variations in ascorbic acid status and breast milk ascorbic acid levels in rural Gambian women in relation to dietary intake. *Trans R Soc Trop Med Hyg*. 1982;76(3):341–347. https://doi.org/10.1016/0035-9203(82)90185-7.
101. Daneel-Otterbech S, Davidsson L, Hurrell R. Ascorbic acid supplementation and regular consumption of fresh orange juice increase the ascorbic acid content of human milk: studies in European and African lactating women. *Am J Clin Nutr*. 2005; 81(5):1088–1093. https://doi.org/10.1093/ajcn/81.5.1088.
102. Buss IH, McGill F, Darlow BAB, Winterbourn CCC. Vitamin C is reduced in human milk after storage. Acta Paediatr 90(7):813-815. doi:10.1111/j.1651-2227.2001.tb02810.x.
103. Ilcol YO, Ozbek R, Hamurtekin E, Ulus IH. Choline status in newborns, infants, children, breast-feeding women, breast-fed infants and human breast milk. *J Nutr Biochem*. 2005;16(8):489–499. https://doi.org/10.1016/j.jnutbio.2005.01.011.
104. Holmes HC, Snodgrass GJ, Iles RA. Changes in the choline content of human breast milk in the first 3 weeks after birth. *Eur J Pediatr*. 2000;159(3):198–204. https://doi.org/10.1007/s004310050050.
105. Fischer LM, Da Costa KA, Galanko J, et al. Choline intake and genetic polymorphisms influence choline metabolite concentrations in human breast milk and plasma. *Am J Clin Nutr*. 2010;92(2): 336–346. https://doi.org/10.3945/ajcn.2010.29459.

106. Dewey KG, Cohen RJ, Brown KH, Rivera LL. Effects of exclusive breastfeeding for four versus six months on maternal nutritional status and infant motor development: results of two randomized trials in Honduras. *J Nutr.* 2001;131(2):262–267. https://doi.org/10.1093/jn/131.2.262.
107. Özden TA, Gökçay G, Cantez MS, et al. Copper, zinc and iron levels in infants and their mothers during the first year of life: a prospective study. *BMC Pediatr.* 2015;15(1). https://doi.org/10.1186/s12887-015-0474-9.
108. Hannan MA, Faraji B, Tanguma J, Longoria N, Rodriguez RC. Maternal milk concentration of zinc, iron, selenium, and iodine and its relationship to dietary intakes. *Biol Trace Elem Res.* 2009;127(1):6–15. https://doi.org/10.1007/s12011-008-8221-9.
109. Dorea JG. Selenium and breast-feeding. *Br J Nutr.* 2002;88(5):443–461. https://doi.org/10.1079/BJN2002692.
110. Azizi F, Smyth P. Breastfeeding and maternal and infant iodine nutrition. *Clin Endocrinol.* 2009;70(5):803–809. https://doi.org/10.1111/j.1365-2265.2008.03442.x.
111. Laurberg P, Nøhr SB, Pedersen KM, Fuglsang E. Iodine nutrition in breast-fed infants is impaired by maternal smoking. *J Clin Endocrinol Metab.* 2004;89(1):181–187. https://doi.org/10.1210/jc.2003-030829.
112. Livingston EH. The incidence of bariatric surgery has plateaued in the U.S. *Am J Surg.* 2010;200(3):378–385. https://doi.org/10.1016/j.amjsurg.2009.11.007.
113. Surgery AS for M and B. *Estimate of Bariatric Surgery Numbers, 2011–2017. WwwAsmbsOrg;* June 2018:24–27. https://asmbs.org/resources/estimate-of-bariatric-surgery-numbers.
114. Center SCEP, Shekelle PG, Newberry S, et al. Bariatric surgery in women of reproductive age: special concerns for pregnancy. *Evid Rep Technol Assess.* 2008;169:1–51. http://www.ncbi.nlm.nih.gov/pubmed/20731480.
115. Edison E, Whyte M, van Vlymen J, et al. Bariatric surgery in obese women of reproductive age improves conditions that underlie fertility and pregnancy outcomes: retrospective cohort study of UK national bariatric surgery registry (NBSR). *Obes Surg.* 2016;26(12):2837–2842. https://doi.org/10.1007/s11695-016-2202-4.
116. Jans G, Devlieger R, De Preter V, et al. Bariatric surgery does not appear to affect women's breast-milk composition. *J Nutr.* 2018;148(7):1096–1102. https://doi.org/10.1093/jn/nxy085.
117. Rottenstreich A, Elazary R, Goldenshluger A, Pikarsky AJ, Elchalal U, Ben-Porat T. Maternal nutritional status and related pregnancy outcomes following bariatric surgery: a systematic review. *Surg Obes Relat Dis.* 2019;15(2):324–332. https://doi.org/10.1016/j.soard.2018.11.018.
118. Berlin CM, Denson HM, Daniel CH, Ward RM. Disposition of dietary caffeine in milk, saliva, and plasma of lactating women. *Pediatrics.* 1984;73(1):59–63. http://www.ncbi.nlm.nih.gov/pubmed/6691042.
119. Aimee M, Sumedha B, Lucy B, James SS, Yen-Fu C. Effects of maternal caffeine consumption on the breastfed child: a systematic review. *Swiss Med Wkly.* 2018;148:39–40. https://doi.org/10.4414/smw.2018.14665.
120. Temple JL, Bernard C, Lipshultz SE, Czachor JD, Westphal JA, Mestre MA. The safety of ingested caffeine: a comprehensive review. *Front Psychiatr.* 2017;8:80. https://doi.org/10.3389/fpsyt.2017.00080.
121. Bane SM. Postpartum exercise and lactation. *Clin Obstet Gynecol.* 2015;58(4):885–892. https://doi.org/10.1097/GRF.0000000000000143.
122. Lovelady C. Balancing exercise and food intake with lactation to promote post-partum weight loss. *Proc Nutr Soc.* 2011;70(2):181–184. https://doi.org/10.1017/S002966511100005X.
123. Lovelady CA. The impact of energy restriction and exercise in lactating women. *Adv Exp Med Biol.* 2004;554:115–120. https://doi.org/10.1007/978-1-4757-4242-8_11.
124. Harrison CL, Brown WJ, Hayman M, Moran LJ, Redman LM. The role of physical activity in preconception, pregnancy and postpartum health. *Semin Reprod Med.* 2016;34(2):e28–37. https://doi.org/10.1055/s-0036-1583530.
125. Giles AR, Phillipps B, Darroch FE, McGettigan-Dumas R. Elite distance runners and breastfeeding. *J Hum Lactation.* 2016;32(4):627–632. https://doi.org/10.1177/0890334416661507.
126. Brekke HK, Bertz F, Rasmussen KM, Bosaeus I, Ellegård L, Winkvist A. Diet and exercise interventions among overweight and obese lactating women: randomized trial of effects on cardiovascular risk factors. *PLoS One.* 2014;9(2). https://doi.org/10.1371/journal.pone.0088250.
127. Slomian J, Bruyère O, Reginster JY, Emonts P. The internet as a source of information used by women after childbirth to meet their need for information: a web-based survey. *Midwifery.* 2017;48:46–52. https://doi.org/10.1016/j.midw.2017.03.005.
128. Slomian J, Emonts P, Erpicum M, Vigneron L, Reginster JY, Bruyère O. What should a website dedicated to the postnatal period contain? A Delphi survey among parents and professionals. *Midwifery.* 2017;53:9–14. https://doi.org/10.1016/j.midw.2017.07.004.
129. Loh W, Tang MLK. The epidemiology of food allergy in the global context. *Int J Environ Res Public Health.* 2018;15(9). https://doi.org/10.3390/ijerph15092043.
130. Sicherer SH, Sampson HA. Food allergy: a review and update on epidemiology, pathogenesis, diagnosis, prevention, and management. *J Allergy Clin Immunol.* 2018;141(1):41–58. https://doi.org/10.1016/j.jaci.2017.11.003.
131. Tang MLK, Mullins RJ. Food allergy: is prevalence increasing? *Intern Med J.* 2017;47(3):256–261. https://doi.org/10.1111/imj.13362.
132. Neerven RJJ van, Savelkoul H. Nutrition and allergic diseases. *Nutrients.* 2017;9(7):762. https://doi.org/10.3390/nu9070762.
133. Allen KJ, Koplin JJ. The epidemiology of IgE-mediated food allergy and anaphylaxis. *Immunol Allergy Clin N AM.* 2012;32(1):35–50. https://doi.org/10.1016/j.iac.2011.11.008.
134. Perkin MR, Logan K, Tseng A, et al. Randomized trial of introduction of allergenic foods in breast-fed infants. *N Engl J Med.* 2016;374(18):1733–1743. https://doi.org/10.1056/NEJMoa1514210.
135. Netting MJ, Middleton PF, Makrides M. Does maternal diet during pregnancy and lactation affect outcomes in offspring? A systematic review of food-based approaches. *Nutrition.* 2014;30(11–12):1225–1241. https://doi.org/10.1016/j.nut.2014.02.015.
136. Fujimura T, Lum SZC, Nagata Y, Kawamoto S, Oyoshi MK. Influences of maternal factors over offspring allergies and the application for food allergy. *Front Immunol.* 2019;10:1933. https://doi.org/10.3389/fimmu.2019.01933.
137. Heck AM, Yanovski JA, Calis KA. Orlistat, a new lipase inhibitor for the management of obesity. *Pharmacotherapy.* 2000;20(3):270–279. https://doi.org/10.1592/phco.20.4.270.34882.
138. Zhi J, Melia AT, Eggers H, Joly R, Patel IH. Review of limited systemic absorption of Orlistat, a lipase inhibitor, in healthy human volunteers. *J Clin Pharmacol.* 1995;35(11):1103–1108. https://doi.org/10.1002/j.1552-4604.1995.tb04034.x.
139. Cui J, Zhou B, Ross SA, Zempleni J. Nutrition, microRNAs, and human health. *Adv Nutr.* 2017;8(1):105. https://doi.org/10.3945/an.116.013839.Exosomes.
140. Munch EM, Harris RA, Mohammad M, et al. Transcriptome profiling of microRNA by next-gen deep sequencing reveals known and novel miRNA species in the lipid fraction of human breast milk. *PLoS One.* 2013;8(2):1–13. https://doi.org/10.1371/journal.pone.0050564.
141. Metz TD, Borgelt LM. Marijuana use in pregnancy and while breastfeeding. *Obstet Gynecol.* 2018;132(5):1198–1210. https://doi.org/10.1097/AOG.0000000000002878.

142. Bertrand KA, Hanan NJ, Honerkamp-Smith G, Best BM, Chambers CD. Marijuana use by breastfeeding mothers and cannabinoid concentrations in breast milk. *Pediatrics*. 2018; 142(3). https://doi.org/10.1542/peds.2018-1076.
143. Crume TL, Juhl AL, Brooks-Russell A, Hall KE, Wymore E, Borgelt LM. Cannabis use during the perinatal period in a state with legalized recreational and medical marijuana: the association between maternal characteristics, breastfeeding patterns, and neonatal outcomes. *J Pediatr*. 2018;197:90–96. https://doi.org/10.1016/j.jpeds.2018.02.005.
144. Miller J. Ethical issues arising from marijuana use by nursing mothers in a changing legal and cultural context. *HEC Forum*. 2019;31(1):11–27. https://doi.org/10.1007/s10730-018-9368-1.
145. Mourh J, Rowe H. Marijuana and breastfeeding: applicability of the current literature to clinical practice. *Breastfeed Med*. 2017; 12(10):582–596. https://doi.org/10.1089/bfm.2017.0020.
146. Chu DM, Antony KM, Ma J, et al. The early infant gut microbiome varies in association with a maternal high-fat diet. *Genome Med*. 2016;8(1). https://doi.org/10.1186/s13073-016-0330-z.
147. Mulligan CM, Friedman JE. Maternal modifiers of the infant gut microbiota: metabolic consequences. *J Endocrinol*. 2017;235(1): R1–R12. https://doi.org/10.1530/JOE-17-0303.
148. Sakwinska O, Bosco N. Host microbe interactions in the lactating mammary gland. *Front Microbiol*. 2019;10:1863. https://doi.org/10.3389/fmicb.2019.01863.
149. Williams JE, Carrothers JM, Lackey KA, et al. Human milk microbial community structure is relatively stable and related to variations in macronutrient and micronutrient intakes in healthy lactating women. *J Nutr*. 2017;147(9):1739–1748. https://doi.org/10.3945/jn.117.248864.

CHAPTER

5

NUTRITION, AGING, AND REQUIREMENTS IN THE ELDERLY

Ibrahim Elmadfa, PhD
Alexa L. Meyer, PhD
Nutritional Sciences, Faculty of Life Sciences, University of Vienna, Vienna, Austria

SUMMARY

Aging has profound effects on body functions and health influencing the nutritional needs and choice of food of older persons. Most notable are the changes in body composition leading to a decrease in lean body and particularly muscle mass and a decline in organ tissue and bone mineral density while body fat content is increasing. The associated loss of active cell mass causes a reduction of resting energy expenditure. However, the requirements of most nutrients are not or only minimally changed so that the diet has to be more nutrient-dense to ensure a sufficient supply of essential nutrients. Moreover, some nutrients have special preventive and additional health effects such as protein, vitamin D, and calcium with regard to bone and muscle function and antioxidants and n-3 PUFAs that protect against oxidative stress and inflammatory diseases. Therefore, a balanced diet and regular physical activity should be adopted to support healthy aging.

Keywords: Anorexia of aging; Body composition and aging; Chronic inflammation; Immunosenescence; Nutrient density; Sarcopenia.

I. INTRODUCTION

All over the world, populations are getting older, most notably in the industrialized high-income countries but increasingly also in middle- and low-income countries. In 2017, the global number of persons aged 60 years or more was estimated to 962 million and thus has more than doubled since 1980 when 382 million persons were at least 60 years old. This number will further increase and is predicted to reach over 2 billion by 2050.[1] While a rising life expectancy is the main driver of this growth, it is not necessarily associated with better health in later life. Against this background, the maintenance of good health in older age is of great importance. The WHO has recently defined healthy aging as "the process of developing and maintaining the functional ability that enables well-being in older age."[2] Adequate healthy nutrition is an essential contributor to this goal. Aging has profound effects on the physiology and functions of the body that in turn influence the nutritional requirements of elderly persons. Although it is a continuous process and begins as early as in the third life decade, manifest effects of aging generally start appearing with the onset of menopause in women and at about 60–65 years in men. Generally, the group defined as elderly is very heterogeneous, more so than other population groups, due to the individual variability of the progression of aging and the health and fitness state.[2] These factors also influence the nutritional needs of older persons.

II. PHYSIOLOGICAL DEMANDS OF OLDER PERSONS

A. Age-Related Changes in Body Composition and Functions

Aging is associated with a number of physiological changes that determine the functionality and performance of the body. These changes also influence the body's

https://doi.org/10.1016/B978-0-12-818460-8.00005-8

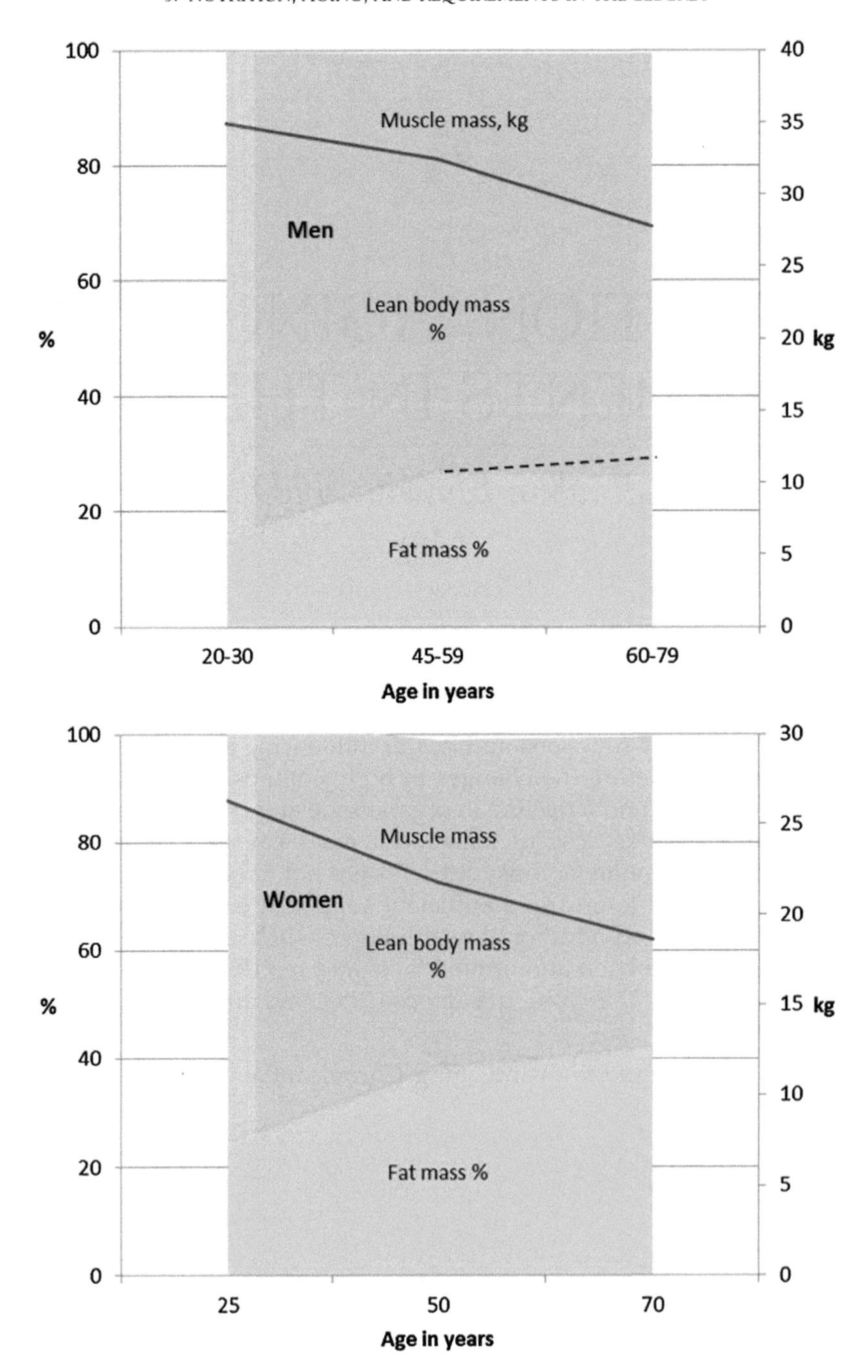

FIGURE 5.1 Age-associated changes in body composition and muscle mass. The dotted line indicates the trend in fat mass increase observed in three other studies.[3,4,10] *Based on data from Ref. 5.*

requirement for energy and nutrients. Overall, the last third of life is characterized by the decline of body functions and tissue mass. The onset of this gradual process varies by function and tissue as well as individually (Fig. 5.1).

Most notable is the decrease of lean body mass (LBM), mostly in the form of muscle, and of bone mass.[5,6,7] This loss of LBM is characterized by a decline in the cell fraction.[8] Between the ages of 20 and 80 years, on average about 40% of the muscle mass are lost.[9] In turn, body fat content increases until the age of 70–80 years with a slight decrease thereafter.[3,4,10] These changes often lead to maintenance of total body weight. Due to the fact that body height is often reduced, the body mass index (kg/m^2) does also not change markedly. However, due to the greater loss of LBM, the relative fat content increases continually.[8,4,11,7,12,10] The accretion of body fat occurs predominantly in the abdominal area where it is associated with insulin resistance and cardiovascular risk factors.[13,14] Furthermore, fat is also accumulated ectopically in organs, muscle, and bone.[11]

Sarcopenia

Loss of muscle mass is a normal age-associated phenomenon, also known as sarcopenia (derived from Greek σάρξ [sárx] meaning flesh and πενία [*penia*] meaning poverty) that, in addition to a quantitative reduction of muscle mass, involves a qualitative loss of muscle function. The reduction of muscle mass begins in the third decade life significantly manifesting from the fifth decade onwards and is of the order of 6% per decade resulting in a loss of about 25% of muscle mass between the ages of 45 and 85 years.[15,16] Sarcopenia is defined as a loss of muscle mass combined with low muscle function as evidenced by decreased muscle strength and/or physical performance.[17] Motor units, i.e., bundles of muscle fibers innervated by a motor neuron, contain exclusively one type of fiber. Fast-twitching type II motor units are characterized by a higher number of fibers with a larger cross-sectional area and higher contractile velocity giving them greater force, even though they tire more easily and have a lower endurance than slow-twitching type I motor units. Aging, and sarcopenia in particular, is associated with a reduction of both slow and fast muscle motor units, but the loss of fast motor units is more pronounced. Moreover, there is a conversion of fast-contracting type II myosin fibers to slow-contracting type I fibers causing a loss of muscle power needed for fast movements such as standing up or climbing stairs. This loss is accompanied by atrophy of type II fibers resulting in a decline in muscle cross-sectional area and the denervation of motor units. Motor neurons and nerve fibers are lost and neuromuscular junctions are altered.[18,19,20] Muscle strength was shown to decline by 50%–60% between the third and the ninth decade of life in men.[21] The synthesis of muscle protein decreases due to a lower secretion of hormonal stimulators such as insulin-like growth factor 1 and growth hormone and the increase in proinflammatory mediators (especially tumor necrosis factor alpha and interleukin 6) that promote protein degradation and apoptosis of muscle cells.[20] Moreover, aging muscle is increasingly infiltrated by fat tissue with a two fold to threefold rise in the content of noncontractile elements between 25–45 and 65–85 years of age.[22] The replacement of muscle tissue by fat leads to the development of sarcopenic obesity causing further declines of muscle quality and performance.[17] Sarcopenia is associated with a higher risk for frailty and disability and hence a loss of independence[16] (Fig. 5.2).

Changes due to decreased organ function

There is also a loss of organ mass that results in reduced organ-related functions and metabolic processes. A good example is the kidney that shows an age-related occurrence of functional and structural alterations that can be studied in detail in the frame of the health examinations of kidney donors. It was found that degenerative macrostructural changes occur in the human kidney even in the absence of comorbidities. Starting at about 50 years, the kidney volume decreases at a rate of about 20 cm^3 per decade. This decline is due to a loss of cortical volume, while medullary volume increases between 30 and 50 years. Age-related microanatomical changes include nephrosclerosis, consisting of arteriosclerosis of the kidney arteries and arterioles,

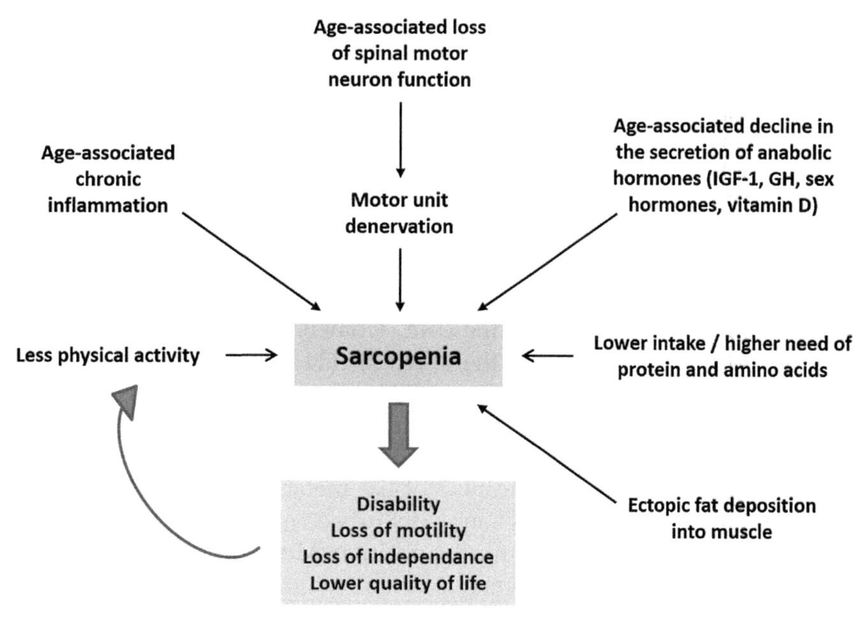

FIGURE 5.2 Causes for the development and progression of sarcopenia.

glomerulosclerosis, tubule atrophy, and fibrosis. This is accompanied by a loss of nephrons and a compensatory hypertrophy of the remaining nephrons.[23,24] After 40 years of age, glomerular filtration rate starts to decrease by about 8–10 mL/min per decade[25] and in elderly often falls below the threshold of <60 mL/min/1.73 m^2 used to define chronic kidney disease. However, a moderate reduction is not generally associated with higher mortality, and the threshold may not apply to older individuals.[23]

The functional changes of the kidney decrease its capacity to concentrate the urine associated with higher obligatory urine volumes. The resulting greater fluid loss is compensated by lower nonrenal water losses such as reduced sweating, especially in elderly men, and by higher fluid intake.[26] However, the hydration balance in older persons can be disturbed by exposure to high temperatures as well as by impaired thirst perception with a lower compensatory fluid intake.[27,28]

Alongside LBM, total body water also shows a decrease with aging, falling from over 55% in young men and just under 50% in young women (<30 years) to well below 50% in elderly persons.[29,30,31] However, this decline is entirely due to the decrease in LBM as the hydration level of the fat-free mass remains constant or even slightly increases, amounting to about 73% on average.[31] The decrease of body water mostly occurs in the intracellular compartment in accordance with the loss of cell mass.[29]

B. Effect of Aging on Bone Mass and Mineral Density

Aging is associated with a loss of bone mass and a decrease in bone mineral content, referred to as osteopenia. This process begins shortly after the end of the period of growth when peak bone mass is reached, by the age of 15–30 years depending on bone site.[79,33,34] However, this early degradation is slow and mostly due to a reduced bone formation.[35] In women, a significant increase in bone loss occurs with the onset of menopause when the rate of bone mineral loss rises from ≤10% per decade to 40% per decade and more.[36] Despite differences between individual bone sites, the loss of bone mass is more pronounced for the trabecular bone, i.e., the inner spongy part of a bone, than for the dense and solid cortical bone.[36] Overall, between the ages of 20 and 90 years, trabecular bone mineral density at central sites has been reported to decrease by 55% and 46% in women and men, respectively, while the decline was smaller at peripheral sites, and showed no significant differences between sexes (−24% in women vs. −26% in men). A smaller decrease was also seen in cortical mineral density that was larger in women than in men (about −25% vs. −18%, respectively).[37] The higher loss in women has been linked to a greater decline in periosteal apposition (the deposition of new bone material from the outside) in women than in men.

The decrease in bone mass and mineral content can ultimately lead to osteoporosis. Osteoporosis is characterized by a loss of bone mass and a microstructural deterioration that exceeds the normal aged-related decline and is due to an imbalance between bone resorption and formation. This alteration of bone structure reduces the density and strength of bone and is associated with a high fracture risk.[38] Although affecting both sexes especially in later life, osteoporosis is more common in women with the onset of menopause because estrogen has a stimulatory effect on bone-building osteoblasts by promoting the release of growth factors and through antiinflammatory effects, and it inhibits the generation and activation of osteoclasts.[39] Estrogen deficiency shifts the balance between bone formation and bone resorption toward the latter. Besides hormonal deficiency, the proinflammatory status associated with aging as well as certain medications that are frequently used by older persons promotes the development of osteoporosis.[39] However, nutrition and lifestyle are also important determinants of bone metabolism and can thus influence the development of osteoporosis.[39]

C. Age-Related Changes in Energy Expenditure—Effects of Body Composition and Physical Activity

The changes in body composition during aging have effects on the energy expenditure. The decrease in LBM and metabolically active organ tissue entails a decline of resting energy expenditure (REE) that has been found to be about 1%–3% per decade.[40] Together with a generally lower physical activity, this leads to a reduction in total energy expenditure. However, the decrease in REE cannot be fully explained by the loss in LBM. In a study in German elderly persons (aged ≥ 60 years) combining cross-sectional and longitudinal data over a period of 10 years, the decline of REE was greater than predicted by the changes in body composition and higher in men than in women. In addition to fat-free body mass, age was a significant predictor of REE, and a decrease of 1.5%–2% and 4.1%–5.2% per decade was observed in women and men, respectively, corresponding to 100 kJ (24 kcal) per decade in women and 300 kJ (70 kcal) per decade in men, regardless of body composition.[41] Among the factors underlying the observed discrepancies are decreases in the cell fraction of LBM and of the metabolic activity of various organs[42] as well as disturbed organ function following ectopic fat deposition. Moreover, a reduction of 50% in the mitochondrial oxidative performance in elderly (65–80 years) compared to younger adults (25–48 years) was reported[43] as well as a decrease in Na–K pump activity[44] that would contribute to the decline in REE.

In addition to the lower REE, a lower physical activity level in older persons contributes to a decrease in total energy expenditure, as with increasing age, the rate of inactivity rises.[45,46,47,48]

D. Changes in the Immune Function: Chronic Low-Grade Inflammation and its Consequences

Aging has profound effects on the immune system, which are summarized under the term immunosenescence or senescent immune remodeling. While immunosenescence affects all immune cell populations, the most serious effects are observed in T lymphocytes. The age-related changes are characterized by the involution, i.e., the shrinking of the thymus that begins early in the newborn progressing at a rate of about 3%/year until middle age and at about 1%/year henceforth, and lead to a loss of thymopoietic epithelial tissue and an increase in adipocytes.[49] As a result, the output of naïve T cells is reduced and is compensated by an increase in memory T cells. Age-specific functional changes in T cells include impaired T-cell receptor (TCR)–mediated proliferation and IL-2 production[50] and the loss of the costimulatory CD28 antigen.[51] These age-related changes are more pronounced in cytotoxic $CD8^+$ T cells.[52] The decrease in naïve T cells is associated with a lower TCR diversity and thus a reduced capacity to recognize and respond to antigens. This decline of TCR diversity occurs abruptly between the ages of 65 and 75 years.[53] Immunosenescence is also characterized by impaired cell proliferation due to telomere erosion and accumulated DNA damage, metabolic dysfunction, alterations in cell signaling, increased secretion of proinflammatory cytokines, and a tendency toward autoreactivity, promoting inflammatory diseases like rheumatoid arthritis, atherosclerosis, and neuro- and other degenerative diseases.[54,55,52]

In addition to T cells, other immune cells are affected by aging. Impaired B-cell development leads to a decline in the number of B cells and a lower diversity of B-cell receptors and ultimately to diminished responses to infection and vaccination and decreased humoral immunity.[56] Age-associated changes have also been reported in the innate immune system, including an increase in the number of natural killer cells accompanied by a disturbed cytotoxic activity of this cell population, and in macrophages where reduced phagocytosis, a lower production of inflammatory cytokines, and a lower respiratory burst in response to mitogens have been noted,[57,58] as well as defects in neutrophil functions.[59]

Generally, aging is associated with a state of chronic low-grade inflammation. Besides age-related changes of the immune function itself, the accumulation of garbage structures in the form of cellular debris and dysfunctional self-molecules over time due to disturbed disposal has been suggested as an underlying cause. The recognition of these disposed particles by immune cells triggers inflammatory responses.[60,61] The increase in visceral adipose tissue as well as ectopic fat has also been suggested as a factor contributing to chronic inflammation as visceral fat is a source of adipokines and certain cytokines acting as mediators of inflammation.[62] Moreover, aging has also been associated with changes in the gut microbiota leading to increased secretion of proinflammatory cytokines and gut permeability that drive the development of chronic inflammation.[63] Alterations in the gut microbiota associated with negative effects show an inverse correlation with biological age but not with chronological age.[64]

E. Age-Associated Diseases

Aging is also associated with a higher risk and prevalence of many chronic diseases, including cardiovascular diseases, hypertension, impaired glucose tolerance and diabetes mellitus type 2, cancer, and various degenerative diseases such as cognitive impairment. These diseases often occur together, contributing to multimorbidity.[2] The increased inflammatory activity seen in the elderly entails higher oxidative stress and thereby acts as one promoter of the development and progression of these diseases. However, lifestyle and nutritional factors also influence these conditions. Thus hyperhomocysteinemia related to the marginal status of the B vitamins B_{12}, folate, B_6, and riboflavin (B_2) is an important risk factor of cardiovascular diseases[65,66] and cognitive dysfunction.[67] Specific dietary fatty acids have effects on the blood lipids and modulate inflammatory responses in their own right.[68,69,70] In turn, chronic diseases also determine the nutritional needs of those affected by them and have to be taken into account when it comes to making food choices. Moreover, certain drugs commonly prescribed to older persons can have effects on the absorption and metabolism of nutrients as well (Table 5.1).[71,72] This is particularly relevant in considering the effects of aging on the metabolism, disposal, and excretion of drugs due to metabolic changes and declines in kidney function.[73]

III. NUTRITIONAL REQUIREMENTS OF OLDER PERSONS

A. Basis for Key Nutrient Recommendations

While energy needs decrease with age, the recommended intakes of most nutrients do not or only minimally change (see Table 5.2). In the case of iron,

TABLE 5.1 Drugs commonly prescribed to older persons that influence micronutrient status.

Drug	Indication	Nutrients affected	Effects	Mechanism(s)
Proton-pump inhibitors	Gastroesophageal reflux disease	Vitamin B_{12}, Zn,	Impaired absorption	Vitamin B_{12}, Zn: Lower secretion of hydrochloric acid and pepsin, increase in gastric pH
		Vitamin C, Mg^{++}, Ca^{++}		Other nutrients: Unknown
Metformin	Non–insulin-dependent diabetes mellitus	Vitamin B_{12}	Impaired absorption	Mostly likely disturbance of the Ca-mediated binding of the IF–Cbl complex to its membrane receptor
Laxatives	Constipation	Electrolytes (K^+, Mg^{++})	Reduced absorption, increased losses with the stools	Diuretic diarrhea, shortened intestinal passage
Nonsteroidal antiinflammatory drugs (aspirin)	Inflammatory conditions	Vitamin C, iron	Lower status of vitamin C (plasma, leukocytes, platelets) and of iron (Hb, ferritin)	Disturbed cellular uptake of vitamin C Mucosal damage associated with blood loss
Diuretics (thiazides, triamterene)	Hypertension	K^+, Mg^{++}, thiamin	Higher excretion	Inhibited renal reabsorption, stimulated excretion of K^+ in the urine
		Folate	Lower folate status	Competitive inhibition of dihydrofolate reductase by triamterene
		Ca^{++}	Higher serum Ca^{++} levels	Renal reabsorption of Ca^{++}
Angiotensin-converting enzyme (ACE) inhibitors	Hypertension	Zn^{++}	Higher excretion	Chelation of Zn^{++}
		K^+	Hyperkalemia	Renal retention of K
Statins	Hypercholesterolemia	Vitamin E β-Carotene	Possibly lower status	Vitamin E, β-carotene: Possibly through decrease in lipoproteins
Glucocorticosteroids	Inflammatory diseases (e.g., rheumatoid arthritis, asthma)	Vitamin D, Ca^{++}	Decreased renal and intestinal absorption	Suppressed transcription of calcium transporters, counteracting vitamin D
		Na^+, K^+	Increased Na^+ retention; K^+ excretion	Na^+/K^+: Unclear mechanisms

Based on Ref. 93.

TABLE 5.2 Recommended daily intake of selected micronutrients for younger and older adults from different countries and the WHO/FAO.

	WHO/FAO[154]				IOM (US & Canada)[56]				EFSA (European Union)[38]				Australia/New Zealand[11]			
	19–65 y		≥65 y		19–30 y		≥51 y		18–59 y		≥60 y		19–30 y		>70 y	
Nutrient	M	F	M	F	M	F	M	F	M	F	M	F	M	F	M	F
Ca (mg)	1000	1000	1300	1300	1000	1000	1000–1200	1200	950–1000[a]	950–1000[a]	950	950	1000	1000	1300	1300
Mg (mg)	260	220	224	190	400	310	420	320	350	300	350	300	400	310	420	320
Na (mg)	<2000	<2000	<2000	<2000	2300	2300	2300	2300	tbd	tbd	tbd	tbd	460–920	460–920	460–920	460–920
Fe (mg)	9.1–27.4[b]	19.6–58.8[b]	9.1–27.4[b]	7.5–22.6[b]	8	18	8	8	11	16	11	16	8	18	8	8
Zn (mg)	4.2–14.0[b]	3.0–9.8[b]	4.2–14.0[b]	3.0–9.8[b]	11	8	11	8	9.4–16.3[b]	7.5–12.7[b]	9.4–16.3[b]	7.5–12.7[b]	14	8	14	8
Se (μg)	34	26	33	25	55	55	55	55	70	70	70	70	70	60	70	60
Vitamin D (μg)	5–10	5–10	15	15	15	15	15–20[c]	15–20[c]	15	15	15	15	5	5	15	15
Vitamin E (mg)	n.d.	n.d.	n.d.	n.d.	15	15	15	15	13	11	13	11	10	7	10	7
Vitamin K (μg)	65	55	65	55	120	90	120	90	70	70	70	70	70	60	70	60
Thiamin (mg)	1.2	1.1	1.2	1.1	1.2	1.1	1.2	1.1	0.1 mg/MJ[d]	0.1 mg/MJ[d]	0.1 mg/MJ[d]	0.1 mg/MJ[d]	1.2	1.1	1.2	1.1
Riboflavin (mg)	1.3	1.1	1.3	1.1	1.3	1.1	1.3	1.1	1.6	1.6	1.6	1.6	1.3	1.1	1.6	1.3
Vitamin B_6 (mg)	1.3	1.3	1.7	1.5	1.3	1.3	1.7	1.5	1.7	1.6	1.7	1.6	1.3	1.3	1.7	1.5
Vitamin B_{12} (μg)	2.4	2.4	2.4	2.4	2.4	2.4	2.4	2.4	4.0	4.0	4.0	4.0	2.4	2.4	2.4	2.4
Folate (μg)	400	400	400	400	400	400	400	400	330	330	330	330	400	400	400	400

	NNR (Nordic)[103]				D-A-CH (Germanic)[32]				CNS (Chinese)[25]			
	18–60 y		>60 y		19–25 y		≥65 y		18–49 y		≥65 y	
Nutrient	M	F	M	F	M	F	M	F	M	F	M	F
Ca (mg)	800/900[e]	800/900[e]	800	800	1000	1000	1000	1000	800	800	1000	1000
Mg (mg)	350	280	350	280	350	300	350	300	330	330	310/320[f]	310/320[f]
Na (mg)	≤2400	≤2400	≤2400	≤2400	1500	1500	1500	1500	1500	1500	1400	1400
Fe (mg)	9	9/15[g]	9	9	10	15	10	10	12	20	12	12
Zn (mg)	10	7	10	7	9	7	9	7	12.5	7.5	12.5	7.5
Se (μg)	60	50	60	50	70	60	70	60	60	60	60	60
Vitamin D (μg)	10	10	10/20[h]	10/20[h]	20[i]	20[i]	20[i]	20[i]	10	10	15	15
Vitamin E (mg)	10	8	10	8	14/15[j]	12	12	11	14	14	14	14

Continued

TABLE 5.2 Recommended daily intake of selected micronutrients for younger and older adults from different countries and the WHO/FAO.—cont'd

	NNR (Nordic)[103]				D-A-CH (Germanic)[32]				CNS (Chinese)[25]			
	18–60 y		>60 y		19–25 y		≥65 y		18–49 y		≥65 y	
Nutrient	M	F	M	F	M	F	M	F	M	F	M	F
Vitamin K (μg)	n.d.	n.d.	n.d.	n.d.	70	60	80	65	80	80	80	80
Thiamin (mg)	1.3/1.4[k]	1.1	1.2	1.0	1.2/1.3[j]	1.0	1.1	1.0	1.4	1.2	1.4	1.2
Riboflavin (mg)	1.5/1.6[k]	1.2–1.3[k]	1.3/1.4[l]	1.2	1.4	1.1	1.3	1.0	1.4	1.2	1.4	1.2
Vitamin B6 (mg)	1.5	1.2	1.5	1.3	1.5	1.2	1.4	1.2	1.4	1.4	1.4	1.4
Vitamin B12 (μg)	2.0	2.0	2.0	2.0	4.0	4.0	4.0	4.0	2.4	2.4	2.4	2.4
Folate (μg)	300	300/400[k]	300	300	300	300	300	300	400	400	400	400

n.d, not defined; *tbd*, to be defined.
[a] *1000 mg for < 25 y.*
[b] *Depending on bioavailability from the diet (phytate content).*
[c] *20 μg for ≥71 y.*
[d] *MJ = Megajoules; equivalent 0.4 mg/1000 kcal.*
[e] *900 for 18–20 y.*
[f] *310 mg for ≥80 y.*
[g] *15 mg premenopausal.*
[h] *20 μg for ≥75 y.*
[i] *In the absence of endogenous synthesis.*
[j] *Higher values for <25 y.*
[k] *Higher values for ≤30 y.*
[l] *Higher values for <75 y.*

women after menopause have lower needs that are the same as in men. However, adequate iron supply is important to prevent the development of anemia that is a common problem in aged adults, especially with low-grade inflammation, and is associated with increased disability and frailty, higher risk of falls, cardiovascular diseases, and cognitive decline, as well as a higher mortality.[81,82]

Moreover, for some nutrients, a higher intake is recommended to compensate for impaired absorption or because these nutrients have been specifically associated with the maintenance of physiological function. The latter is the case for protein. Metaanalyses of nitrogen balance studies do not suggest significant differences in the protein requirements of older and younger adults so that the Estimated Average Requirement of 0.66 g high-quality protein per kg body weight and accordingly the recommended intake of 0.83 g protein per kg body weight are valid for adults of all ages.[83,84,85] However, a number of studies found that a higher protein intake (≥1.2 g/kg body weight) was associated with a better maintenance of LBM and body functions related to mobility and strength as well as a lower risk of frailty.[86,87,88,89] Moreover, it was shown that the synthesis of muscle protein declines with aging.

Protein

There is evidence that a higher protein intake is required to stimulate the maximal anabolic response.[90] In 2013, the PROT-AGE Study Group, made up of the European Union Geriatric Medicine Society, the International Association of Gerontology and Geriatrics-European Region, the International Association of Nutrition and Aging, and the Australian and New Zealand Society for Geriatric Medicine, recommended a daily protein intake of 1.0–1.2 g/kg body weight for older adults to maintain physical function, suggesting an even higher intake level of 1.2–1.5 g/kg for older persons suffering from acute or chronic diseases and up to 2.0 g/kg for malnourished or severely ill individuals.[91] These recommendations were endorsed by the European Society for Clinical Nutrition and Metabolism (ESPEN).[92] The evidence on higher protein requirements of older adults are also reflected in the recommendations for protein intake of some countries that set higher values for older adults ranging from 1.0 to 1.3 g/kg normal body weight (see Table 5.3).

Micronutrients

Although the basic requirements of most micronutrients may not differ between older and younger adults, higher intake levels have been recommended in light of a relatively lower intestinal absorption. For instance, the increased use with age of certain drugs is associated with disturbed absorption and also with altered metabolism of some nutrients and can thus cause deficiencies of these nutrients[71,72] (see Table 5.1).

Malabsorption has a particular impact on the status of vitamin B_{12} in older adults as this vitamin must be released from its tight binding to proteins in foods by the action of hydrochloric acid and pepsin in the stomach. Atrophic gastritis is a common condition in older persons leading to a reduced secretion of hydrochloric acid and pepsin and thereby a lower bioavailability of dietary vitamin B_{12}. The resulting cobalamin malabsorption is further aggravated by the use of proton pump inhibitors to reduce gastric acid secretion that is also higher in the older population due to the age-associated occurrence of gastroesophageal reflux disease.[93] A less common cause of cobalamin malabsorption is the lack of intrinsic factor (IF) that acts as a carrier for cobalamin in the small intestine and enables its receptor-mediated uptake in the distal ileum. IF can become the target of an autoimmune reaction leading to pernicious anemia that occurs more often in older persons.[94] Malabsorption of vitamin B_{12} has also been observed with the application of the drug metformin that is widely used in the treatment of diabetes mellitus type 2, most likely by

TABLE 5.3 Recommended daily intake of protein for younger and older adults from different countries and the WHO/FAO.

	Age group (men/women as applicable)		Difference between age groups
WHO/FAO[154]	≥18 y: 0.83 g/kg BW		–
IOM (US & Canada)[56]	≥19 y: 0.8 g/kg BW		–
EFSA (European Commission)[38]	≥18 y: 0.83 g/kg BW		–
COMA (United Kingdom)[27]	≥18 y: 0.75 g/kg BW		–
AUS/NZ[11]	19–70 y: 0.84/0.75 g/kg BW	>70 y men: 1.07/0.94 g/kg BW	+27/+25%
D-A-CH (Germanic)[121]	19–64 y: 0.8 g/kg BW	≥65 y: 1.0 g/kg BW	+25%
NNR (Nordic)[103]	18–64 y: 0.8–1.5 g/kg BW (10–20% of energy)	≥65 y: 1.1–1.3 g/kg BW (15%–20% of energy)	Up to +60%
AFSSA (France)[1]	19–60 y: 0.83 g/kg BW	>60 y: 1.0 g/kg BW	+20%

BW, Body weight.

interfering with the calcium-mediated binding of the IF—vitamin B_{12} complex to its receptor.[98]

Along with folate and vitamin B_6, vitamin B_{12} also deserves special attention in relation to its role in cognitive performance and neuronal functions. This is due to the involvement of these vitamins in one-carbon metabolism that supplies methyl groups for methylation reactions. Vitamin B_{12} and folate act together in the conversion of homocysteine (HCys) to methionine. In the brain and nerve tissue, S-adenosylmethionine serves as the methyl group donor in the synthesis of neurotransmitters, phospholipids, and myelin. A deficiency of folate or vitamin B_{12} has been associated with cognitive decline,[67] brain lesions,[67] and a higher risk for cerebral infarcts[67] and Alzheimer's disease.[67] This seems in part related to increased concentrations of HCys which has shown vasotoxic and neurotoxic effects in animal studies, although the exact mechanisms are unclear and probably multifaceted. In this context, the balance between folate and vitamin B_{12} is of great importance as folate can exacerbate the neurological symptoms of vitamin B_{12} deficiency and also mask this latter by correcting the megaloblastic anemia that is caused by both, folate and vitamin B_{12} deficiency.[99] In light of the high risk of vitamin B_{12} deficiency in older adults, fortification of staple foods like wheat flour with folic acid as it is practiced in several countries worldwide may present a problem in this group if vitamin B_{12} is not also supplied sufficiently.[67,99]

Considering the lower energy requirements in elderly, the requirements for micronutrients involved in the metabolism of energy and macronutrients, such as the B vitamins thiamin, riboflavin, niacin, and pyridoxal, would also be reduced in this age group. This approach was chosen by the Nutrition Societies of the German-speaking countries (D-A-CH) in their 2016 revisions of reference values for thiamin, riboflavin, niacin, and vitamin B_6 in which the recommended intakes decreased with age, especially in men.[100] However, there is evidence, albeit from a small number of studies, for a slightly higher requirement of vitamin B_6 in elderly to maintain an adequate status.[101,65,102,103] Lower status of vitamin B_6 has been repeatedly observed in older individuals, even when recommended dietary reference intakes were met. In addition, adequate riboflavin intake is required to generate the bioactive form of vitamin B_6, pyridoxal 5′-phosphate, by the FMN-dependent pyridoxine 5′-phosphate oxidase.[103] A higher catabolism or an effect of certain drugs has been suggested as factors contributing to lower vitamin B_6 status in older adults.[103,104,105] Accordingly, the Institute of Medicine (IOM) in 1998 and the WHO/FAO in 2004 set higher recommended intakes for adults aged $\geq$51 and $\geq$65 years, respectively, compared to younger adults (1.7 mg/d vs. 1.3 mg/d for men and 1.5 mg/d vs. 1.3 mg/d for women),[106,74] while the European Food Safety Agency recommends the higher intake levels for all adults $\geq$18 years.[107] The recommended intake for vitamin B_6 set by the French Food Safety Agency (ANSES) in 2001 for persons $\geq$75 years of both sexes was even higher at 2.2 mg/d.[108]

Nutrients in bone health: Calcium, vitamin D, vitamin K

Considering the loss of bone mass and the increased risk of osteoporosis in elderly, a higher intake of calcium and vitamin D is widely recommended. Aging is associated with a lower endogenous synthesis of vitamin D_3 in the skin and the kidneys. The production of pre-vitamin D_3 from its precursor 7-dehydrocholesterol in the epidermis and dermis showed a steady decline with age, and in persons aged over 70 years, it was only 40% of that in 8 year old children.[109] The epidermal concentration of 7-dehydrocholesterol also decreases with age,[109] and in rats, the hydroxylation of 25(OH)-vitamin D_3 to its active form 1,25$(OH)_2$-vitamin D_3 in the kidneys also showed a decline with age due to a lower activity of the catalyzing enzyme 1α-hydroxylase and a lower number of mitochondria. In turn, the production of the catabolite 24,25$(OH)_2$-vitamin D_3 increases with age.[110,111] In accordance with the lower circulating concentrations of vitamin D_3, aging also causes a reduction in the intestinal absorption of calcium[112] and reduced adaptation to low calcium intakes,[113] and this decline is further promoted by the development of a resistance to vitamin D_3 in the intestine that is associated with a lower absorption of calcium.[114,115] Overall, older, postmenopausal women are more at risk of becoming vitamin D—deficient than their male counterparts, and they also have a higher risk of osteoporosis. Especially with the decrease of vitamin D—mediated transcellular calcium absorption, passive paracellular absorption may be promoted by higher dietary calcium intake.[116]

Another nutrient playing an important role for bone health is vitamin K, a cofactor of the enzyme γ-glutamyl-carboxylase that catalyzes the γ-carboxylation of glutamic acid in osteocalcin, a protein required for bone mineralization. This step activates osteocalcin. Vitamin K status has been positively associated with higher bone mineral density and better function of the lower extremities in elderly[117,118] while deficiency was highly prevalent in older adults with hip fractures.[119] It has also shown independent antiinflammatory effects.[117] As vitamin K is in part supplied by the gut microbiota in form of menaquinones (vitamin K_2), prolonged use of antibiotics can lead to deficiency.[120] Intestinal malabsorption is also a contributing factor. This has prompted the recommendation of slightly higher daily intake levels for older adults (>50 years) by the nutrition societies of the German-speaking countries[79] (see Table 5.2) even though the benefits of vitamin K supplementation in aged persons are still equivocal.[117]

B. Dietary Guidance

Reduced energy requirements call for a higher nutrient density

To comply with the lower energy requirements and the unchanged or even higher requirements of different nutrients, the diet for older persons must include nutrient-dense foods. Vegetables and fruits, pulses, and wholegrain cereals are the optimal choices all the more, as they are also good sources of dietary fiber to prevent constipation or its more intractable form, obstipation, to maintain a healthy gut microflora and to provide secondary plant compounds with antioxidant and other bioactive effects. These foods are also major sources of various vitamins of the B group including folate and of vitamin C and carotenoids. Nuts, seeds, and plant oil of good quality supply vitamin E and essential PUFAs. However, moderate amounts of animal foods in the form of low fat milk products, eggs, fish, and lean meat should be consumed to ensure the adequate supply of high-quality protein and the critical micronutrients iron, zinc, calcium, and vitamin B_{12} that these foods contain in a highly bioavailable form. Especially during the winter at high geographical latitudes or when sun exposure is low, vitamin D should be supplemented.

Beneficial effects of nutrients on immune function

A higher intake of certain nutrients can support the therapy of some age-associated diseases. For instance, the proinflammatory state in rheumatoid arthritis causes oxidative stress through the generation of reactive oxygen and nitrogen species, and antioxidant micronutrients such as the vitamins C and E, carotenoids, and nonnutritive polyphenolic compounds have been successfully employed as a complement to drug therapy to alleviate symptoms and prevent oxidative stress.[121,122] Antioxidants have also been shown to restore macrophage function against pathogenic challenge.[57] Lower oxidative stress also reduces the risk of age-associated noncommunicable diseases such as cardiovascular diseases, diabetes mellitus, and cancer.

Moreover, increased oxidative stress is encountered in patients with impaired cognitive performance and dementia, justifying a higher intake or supplementation of antioxidative nutrients such as vitamin C and E to maintain cognitive function and prevent cognitive decline.[123]

Nutrients can also boost immune functions and thus counteract the effects of immunosenescence. This has been shown for vitamin E, which enhances the proliferation and response of T lymphocytes to mitogen stimulation when supplemented in doses above the recommended daily intake levels.[124] Vitamin E inhibits the production of the T cell–suppressive eicosanoid PGE_2, the production of which is upregulated with aging. Vitamin E also has other direct effects on T cells by increasing the secretion of the stimulatory IL-2 and by modulating signal transduction.[124,125,126]

Other food components with particular relevance for immune function in older age are n-3 PUFAs that act as precursors for mediators of inflammatory and other immune responses such as the eicosanoids in the case of eicosapentaenoic acid (EPA) and resolvins in the case of docosahexaenoic acid (DHA). n-3 PUFAs have a less proinflammatory profile than their n-6 counterparts. EPA and DHA found in fatty fish, particularly of marine and to a lesser extent of freshwater origin, and microorganisms, especially algae, are the actual active precursors and fish oil is the best source for these PUFAs, while there is some controversy about the extent of conversion of the plant-derived α-linolenic acid to EPA and DHA.[127] A number of studies support antiinflammatory effects of n-3 PUFAs in rheumatoid arthritis with most evidence available for EPA and DHA.[128] In the context of inflammation, fatty acids also differentially modulate proinflammatory signaling pathways via their interaction with Toll-like receptors. Saturated fatty acids, for example, palmitic acid, activate this pathway and induce the secretion of IL-1β, whereas DHA inhibits it.[70]

Beneficial effects of nutrients on muscle and bone

More recently, n-3 PUFAs, especially EPA and DHA, have also been studied with regard to their beneficial effects on the musculoskeletal system. Evidence for the anabolic properties of n-3 PUFAs comes from a number of studies in animals, humans, and in vitro showing a stimulation of muscle protein synthesis, better muscle function, and greater strength. These effects have been attributed to the antiinflammatory properties of n-3 PUFAs and also to a direct activation of the mTOR (mammalian target of rapamycin) signaling pathway.[129,130] A higher intake of PUFAs in general, of the n-3 and the n-6 families, has also been associated with positive effects on bone mineral density and a lower fracture risk.[131] However, even stronger effects were seen for fish intake that also supplies other nutrients with relevance to bone health, such as vitamin D and protein.[131]

Beneficial effects of nutrients on cardiovascular risk factors

Another important role for PUFAs in the diet of older adults arises from their effect on blood lipids and lipoproteins. n-3 PUFAs have repeatedly shown positive effects of reducing LDL cholesterol and triglyceride levels in the plasma and increasing HDL cholesterol and are associated with reduced cardiovascular risk.[132,68]

Beneficial effects of fiber

Considering the high prevalence of constipation in older adults, the diet should contain sufficient dietary fiber. Dietary interventions in geriatric care institutions have shown that dietary fiber can be easily introduced into the daily diet and that it improves bowel function and reduces the use of laxatives of older test populations.[133,134] Higher dietary fiber intake in the form of oat bran also resulted in small, nonsignificant improvements in the status of folate, vitamin B_6, and cobalamin and a reduction of HCys, probably through its beneficial effects on the gut microbiota.[135]

C. Factors Contributing to Malnutrition in Older Adults

While the decreasing REE may initially promote weight gain in middle-aged and older adults, with increasing age, the incidence of malnutrition in the sense of undernutrition rises due to an overall decline in food consumption leading to an inadequate intake of energy and essential nutrients. This malnutrition is an important risk factor for frailty, morbidity, and mortality in elderly and is particularly prevalent among persons living in institutions: it may affect over 50% of those in geriatric care institutions or hospitals.[136] However, community-living elderly are also at significant risk as shown by a study from 12 mostly high-income countries reporting that 52.6% of men aged $\geq$65 years were at risk of malnutrition and 9.5% were malnourished.[137]

Lowered food intake

A number of factors contribute to the lower food intake in elderly, including the frequently observed loss of appetite, termed anorexia of aging. Age-associated changes of gastrointestinal function include a reduction of esophageal and gastric motility that can lead to slower gastric emptying and greater and longer postprandial fullness and satiation.[138,139] Alterations in the secretion of satiety hormones and mediators in older persons have also been reported, particularly a higher secretion of the anorexigenic cholecystokinin, while the release and the sensitivity to orexigenic hormones and neuropeptides such as ghrelin and NPY appear to be reduced in older animals and humans.[140,141] Inflammatory processes that are often enhanced in older persons also reduce appetite through the action of proinflammatory cytokines.[142]

Other factors leading to anorexia

Food intake is also impaired by dysphagia, i.e., a difficulty swallowing that is common in elderly, mostly driven by comorbidities and the use of certain drugs.[143,139] Dental problems, for example, loss of teeth and dental function, are another risk factor for malnutrition and have a strong effect on food choice. Better dental quality was related to higher diet quality and better nutrient supply.[144,145] Moreover, aging is associated with impaired taste sensation. Older adults have higher thresholds for the recognition of four basic tastes (sweet, salty, sour, and bitter) than their younger counterparts and an impaired ability to discriminate between tastes.[146,147]

Food intake can also be influenced by certain drugs that are frequently taken by older persons such as metformin, antihypertensives, antidepressants, and statins through their effects on appetite, orosensory perception, or gastrointestinal function.[71,72]

Besides age-related physiological changes, insufficient food intake in older persons is also promoted by psychological and sociodemographic factors (see Table 5.4). Age-related disability and impaired mobility and also low socioeconomic status make access to adequate food difficult. Depression is a common condition in older persons, especially after the loss of a partner or in the presence of health problems and chronic disease, and is associated with inadequate food consumption.[148]

Malnutrition is a determinant of frailty, morbidity, and mortality in older persons. The protective effect of a higher body weight is thought to be the underlying cause of the so called "obesity paradox," i.e., the observation that older persons with a BMI in the overweight or obese range have a lower risk for many chronic diseases such as those of the cardiovascular system and a lower mortality.[149] However, the causality behind this phenomenon is unclear, and it is probable that serious health conditions lead to a lower body weight. Moreover, body composition has to be taken into account, and a high level of visceral fat has shown the same negative effects in older

TABLE 5.4 Causes of malnutrition in older persons.

Primary causes	Secondary causes
Panmalnutrition/low food security	Lack of knowledge about healthy nutrition
Unfavorable eating habits	Isolation
Lack of appetite (anorexia of aging)	Loneliness
Dental problems	Depression
Higher nutrient requirements	Physical disability
Malabsorption	Mental disorders
Alcoholism	Disturbed memory
Drug (ab)use	Poverty
Chronic diseases	

as in younger adults.[149] Nevertheless, based on findings that a BMI above the range recommended by the World Health Organization (i.e., 18.5–24.9 kg/m^2)[150] is associated with lower mortality in older adults, a higher BMI range might be advisable for this population group.[151]

Overall, the adoption of a healthy diet pattern like the Mediterranean diet, the Healthy Nordic, or any other with the focus on plant foods and rich in vegetables, fruits, pulses, wholegrain cereals complemented with moderate amounts of animal products, especially dairy products and fish, and fat of good quality, is also the best option for older adults.

D. Other Guidance

In addition to adequate nutrition, regular physical activity that is adapted to an individual's physical capacities is an important contributor to health and well-being in older adults. Maintaining an adequate level of physical activity increases the total energy expenditure and the amount of food consumed, thereby facilitating a sufficient intake of essential nutrients. Physical activity was associated with better energy balance in older adults.[152] Most importantly, adequate physical activity can slow the loss of muscle mass, particularly when combined to higher protein intake.[92] It counteracts the reduction in bone mineral density, the development of frailty, and osteoporosis[153,154,155,156] and has also shown positive effects on cognitive function and can contribute to the prevention of dementia.[157] Additionally, regular outdoor physical activity offers an opportunity for sunlight exposure to improve vitamin D status. Despite lower endogenous synthesis, daily sunlight exposure was an important contributor to 25(OH)-vitamin D_3 serum levels in older adults.[158] Thus regular physical activity is essential for maintaining physical and mental function and independence in older adults and should be promoted in this population group.[2]

RESEARCH GAPS

- Most values for recommended nutrient intakes in elderly are derived from younger adults. There is a need for studies on the specific nutritional needs of the elderly population.
- Data are also needed for very old populations.
- It is important to study differences within the aged population group based on fitness and activity level.
- Effects of interventions with specific nutrients in older adults should be determined.
- Additional insights are needed regarding the impact of diseases and of drug use on nutritional status in elderly.

IV. REFERENCES

1. WHO (World Health Organization). *World Population Ageing 2017. Highlights*. Geneva, Switzerland: World Health Organization; 2017.
2. WHO (World Health Organization). *World Report on Ageing and Health*. Geneva, Switzerland: World Health Organization; 2015.
3. Ravaglia G, Forti P, Maioli F, et al. Measurement of body fat in healthy elderly men: a comparison of methods. *J Gerontol A Biol Sci Med Sci*. 1999;54(2):M70–M76.
4. Ito H, Ohshima A, Ohto N, et al. Relation between body composition and age in healthy Japanese subjects. *Eur J Clin Nutr*. 2001;55: 462–470.
5. Proctor DN, O'Brien PC, Atkinson EJ, Nair KS. Comparison of techniques to estimate total body skeletal muscle mass in people of different age groups. *Am J Physiol*. 1999;277(3):E489–E495.
6. Krems C, Luhrmann PM, Strassburg A, et al. Lower resting metabolic rate in the elderly may not be entirely due to changes in body composition. *Eur J Clin Nutr*. 2005;59:255–262.
7. St-Onge M-P, Gallagher D. Body composition changes with aging: The cause or the result of alterations in metabolic rate and macronutrient oxidation? *Nutrition*. 2010;26(2):152–155.
8. Kyle UG, Genton L, Hans D, et al. Age-related differences in fat-free mass, skeletal muscle, body cell mass and fat mass between 18 and 94 years. *Eur J Clin Nutr*. 2001;55:663–672.
9. Padilla Colón CJ, Molina-Vicenty IL, Frontera-Rodríguez M, et al. Muscle and bone mass loss in the elderly population: Advances in diagnosis and treatment. *J Biomed*. 2018;3:40–49.
10. Amdanee N, Di W, Liu J, et al. Age-associated changes of resting energy expenditure, body composition and fat distribution in Chinese Han males. *Phys Rep*. 2018;6(23):e13940.
11. Cartwright MJ, Tchkonia T, Kirkland JL. Aging in adipocytes: potential impact of inherent, depot-specific mechanisms. *Exp Gerontol*. 2007;42(6):463–471.
12. Imboden MT, Swartz AM, Finch HW, et al. Reference standards for lean mass measures using GE dual energy X-ray absorptiometry in Caucasian adults. *PLoS One*. 2017;12(4):e0176161.
13. Hunter GR, Gower BA, Kane BL. Age related shift in visceral fat. *Int J Body Compos Res*. 2010;8(3):103–108.
14. Matsuzawa Y. Obesity and metabolic syndrome: the contribution of visceral fat and adiponectin. *Diabetes Manag*. 2014;4(4):391–401.
15. Janssen I, Heymsfield SB, Wang Z, Ross R. Skeletal muscle mass and distribution in 468 men and women aged 18–88 yr. *J Appl Physiol*. 2000;89:81–88.
16. Janssen I, Ross R. Linking age-related changes in skeletal muscle mass and composition with metabolism and disease. *J Nutr Health Aging*. 2005;9(6):408–419.
17. Cruz-Jentoft AJ, Baeyens JP, Bauer JM, et al. Sarcopenia: European consensus on definition and diagnosis. *Age Ageing*. 2010;39: 412–423.

18. Nikolić M, Malnar-Dragojević D, Bobinac D, et al. Age-related skeletal muscle atrophy in humans: An immunohistochemical and morphometric study. *Coll Antropol*. 2001;25(2):545–553.
19. Lee WS, Cheung WH, Qin L, et al. Age-associated decrease of type IIA/B human skeletal muscle fibers. *Clin Orthop Relat Res*. 2006; 450:231–237.
20. Lang T, Streeper T, Cawthon P, et al. Sarcopenia: etiology, clinical consequences, intervention, and assessment. *Osteoporos Int*. 2010; 21:543–559.
21. Kostka T. Quadriceps maximal power and optimal shortening velocity in 335 men aged 23–88 years. *Eur J Appl Physiol*. 2005;95:140–145.
22. Kent-Braun JA, Ng AV, Young K. Skeletal muscle contractile and noncontractile components in young and older women and men. *J Appl Physiol*. 2000;88:662–668.
23. Denic A, Glassock RJ, Rule AD. Structural and functional changes with the aging kidney. *Adv Chron Kidney Dis*. 2016;23(1):19–28.
24. Hommos MS, Glassock RJ, Rule AD. Structural and functional changes in human kidneys with healthy aging. *J Am Soc Nephrol*. 2017;28(10):2838–2844.
25. Silva FG. The aging kidney: A review – Part I. *Int Urol Nephrol*. 2005;37:185–205.
26. Manz F, Johner SA, Wentz A, et al. Water balance throughout the adult life span in a German population. *Br J Nutr*. 2012;107(11): 1673–1681.
27. Stachenfeld NS, DiPietro L, Nadel ER, Mack GW. Mechanism of attenuated thirst in aging: role of central volume receptors. *Am J Physiol 272 (Regulatory Integrative Comp. Physiol*. 1997;41: R148–R157.
28. Kenney WL, Chiu P. Influence of age on thirst and fluid intake. *Med Sci Sports Exerc*. 2001;33(9):1524–1532.
29. Aloia JF, Vaswani A, Flaster E, Ma R. Relationship of body water compartments to age, race, and fat-free mass. *J Lab Clin Med*. 1998; 132(6):483–490.
30. Chumlea WC, Guo SS, Zeller CM, et al. Total body water data for white adults 18 to 64 years of age: The Fels Longitudinal Study. *Kidney Int*. 1999;56:244–252.
31. Ritz P. Body water spaces and cellular hydration during healthy aging. *Ann N Y Acad Sci*. 2000;904:474–483.
32. Ott SM. Editorial: Attainment of peak bone mass. *J Clin Endocrinol Metab*. 1990;71(5), 1082A–1082C.
33. Matkovic V, Jelic T, Wardlaw GM, et al. Timing of peak bone mass in Caucasian females and its implication for the prevention of osteoporosis. Inference from a cross-sectional model. *J Clin Invest*. 1994;93:799–808.
34. Baxter-Jones ADG, Faulkner RA, Forwood MR, et al. Bone mineral accrual from 8 to 30 years of age: an estimation of peak bone mass. *J Bone Miner Res*. 2011;26(8):1729–1739.
35. Seeman E, Delmas PD. Bone quality — The material and structural basis of bone strength and fragility. *N Engl J Med*. 2006;354: 2250–2261.
36. O'Flaherty EJ. Modeling normal aging bone loss, with consideration of bone loss in osteoporosis. *Toxicol Sci*. 2000;55: 171–188.
37. Riggs BL, Melton LJ, Robb RA, et al. Population-based study of age and sex differences in bone volumetric density, size, geometry, and structure at different skeletal sites. *J Bone Miner Res*. 2004;19: 1945–1954.
38. Cooper C, Dere W, Evans W, et al. Frailty and sarcopenia: Definitions and outcome parameters. *Osteoporos Int*. 2012;23:1839–1848.
39. Pietschmann P, Resch H, Peterlik M. Etiology and pathogenesis of osteoporosis. In: Yuehuei HA, ed. *Orthopaedic Issues in Osteoporosis*. Boca Raton, FL: CRC Press; 2002:3–18.
40. Food and Agriculture Organization of the United Nations (FAO), United Nations University (UNU), World Health Organization (WHO). *Human Energy Requirements. Report of a Joint FAO/WHO/UNU Expert Consultation, Rome, 17-24 October 2001*. In: *FAO Food and Nutrition Technical Report Series 1*. Rome: FAO; 2004, 2004.
41. Lührmann PM, Edelmann-Schäfer B, Neuhauser-Berthold M. Changes in resting metabolic rate in an elderly German population: cross-sectional and longitudinal data. *J Nutr Health Aging*. 2010;14(3):232–236.
42. Wang Z, Ying Z, Bosy-Westphal A, et al. Specific metabolic rates of major organs and tissues across adulthood: evaluation by mechanistic model of resting energy expenditure. *Am J Clin Nutr*. 2010; 92:1369–1377.
43. Conley KE, Jubrias SA, Esselman PC. Oxidative capacity and ageing in human muscle. *J Physiol*. 2000;526(Pt 1):203–210.
44. Poehlman ET, Toth MJ, Webb GD. Sodium-potassium pump activity contributes to the age-related decline in resting metabolic rate. *J Clin Endocrinol Metab*. 1993;76(4):1054–1057.
45. Rothenberg EM, Bosaeus IG, Westerterp KR, Steen BC. Resting energy expenditure, activity energy expenditure and total energy expenditure at age 91–96 years. *Br J Nutr*. 2000;84(3): 319–324.
46. Evenson KR, Buchner DM, Morland KB. Objective measurement of physical activity and sedentary behavior among US adults aged 60 years or older. *Prev Chronic Dis*. 2012;9:110109.
47. Cooper JA, Manini TM, Paton CM, et al. Longitudinal change in energy expenditure and effects on energy requirements of the elderly. *Nutr J*. 2013;12:73.
48. European Commission. *Special Eurobarometer 472. Sports and Physical Activity*. Report. Wave EB88.4. Brussels: TNS opinion & social; 2017.
49. Lynch HE, Goldberg GL, Chidgey A, et al. Thymic involution and immune reconstitution. *Trends Immunol*. 2009;30(7):366–373.
50. Sato K, Kato A, Sekai M, et al. Physiologic thymic involution underlies age-dependent accumulation of senescence-associated CD4+ T cells. *J Immunol*. 2017;199:138–148.
51. Weng N, Akbar AN, Goronzy J. CD28⁻ T cells: their role in the age-associated decline of immune function. *Trends Immunol*. 2009; 30(7):306–312.
52. Weyand CM, Goronzy J. Aging of the immune system. Mechanisms and therapeutic targets. *Ann Am Thorac Soc*. 2016;13(Suppl 5):S422–S428.
53. Naylor K, Li G, Vallejo AN, et al. The influence of age on T cell generation and TCR diversity. *J Immunol*. 2005;174:7446–7452.
54. Fulop T, Le Page A, Fortin C, et al. Cellular signaling in the aging immune system. *Curr Opin Immunol*. 2014;29:105–111.
55. Akbar AN, Henson SI, Lanna A. Senescence of T lymphocytes: implications for enhancing human immunity. *Trends Immunol*. 2016; 37(12):866–876.
56. Cancro MP, Hao Y, Scholz JL, et al. B cells and aging: molecules and mechanisms. *Trends Immunol*. 2009;30(7):313–318.
57. Stout RD, Suttles J. Immunosenescence and macrophage functional plasticity: dysregulation of macrophage function by age-associated microenvironmental changes. *Immunol Rev*. 2005;205: 60–71.
58. Panda A, Arjona A, Sapey E, et al. Human innate immunosenescence: causes and consequences for immunity in old age. *Trends Immunol*. 2009;30(7):325–333.
59. Drew W, Wilson DV, Sapey E. Inflammation and neutrophil immunosenescence in health and disease: Targeted treatments to improve clinical outcomes in the elderly. *Exp Gerontol. 2018; 105:70–77.*
60. Lasry A, Ben-Neriah Y. Senescence-associated inflammatory responses: Aging and cancer perspectives. *Trends Immunol*. 2015; 36(4):217–228.
61. Franceschi C, Garagnani P, Vitale G, et al. Inflammaging and 'Garb-aging'. *Trends Endocrinol Metab*. 2017;28(3):199–212.
62. Alexopoulos N, Katritsis D, Raggi P. Visceral adipose tissue as a source of inflammation and promoter of atherosclerosis. *Atherosclerosis*. 2014;233:104–112.

63. Thevaranjan N, Puchta A, Schulz C, et al. Age-associated microbial dysbiosis promotes intestinal permeability, systemic inflammation, and macrophage dysfunction. *Cell Host Microbe.* 2017;21(4): 455–466.e4.
64. Kim S, Jazwinski SM. The gut microbiota and healthy aging: a mini-review. *Gerontol.* 2018;64:513–520.
65. Selhub J, Jacques PF, Wilson PW, et al. Vitamin status and intake as primary determinants of homocysteinemia in an elderly population. *J Am Med Assoc.* 1993;270(22):2693–2698.
66. Selhub J. Public health significance of elevated homocysteine. *Food Nutr Bull.* 2008;29(2, suppl.):S116–S125.
67. Selhub J, Troen A, Rosenberg IH. B vitamins and the aging brain. *Nutr Rev.* 2010;68(Suppl. 2):S112–S118.
68. Ooi EMM, Watts GF, Ng TWK, Barrett HR. Effect of dietary Fatty acids on human lipoprotein metabolism: A comprehensive update. *Nutrients.* 2015;7(6):4416–4425.
69. Calder PC. Polyunsaturated fatty acids and inflammatory processes: New twists in an old tale. *Biochimie.* 2009;91:791–795.
70. Snodgrass RG, Huang S, Choi IW, et al. Inflammasome-mediated secretion of IL-1β in human monocytes through TLR2 activation. Modulation by dietary fatty acids. *J Immunol.* 2013;191(8):4337–4347.
71. van Zyl M. The effects of drugs on nutrition. *S Afr J Clin Nutr.* 2011;24(3):S38–S41.
72. Mohn ES, Kern HJ, Saltzman E, et al. Evidence of drug–nutrient interactions with chronic use of commonly prescribed medications: an update. *Pharmaceutics.* 2018;10:36.
73. Turnheim K. When drug therapy gets old: pharmacokinetics and pharmacodynamics in the elderly. *Exp Gerontol.* 2003;38:843–853.
74. (WHO) World Health Organization and Food and (FAO) Agriculture Organization of the United Nations. *Vitamin and Mineral Requirements in Human Nutrition: Report of a Joint FAO/WHO Expert Consultation, Bangkok, Thailand, 21–30 September 1998.* Geneva, Switzerland: World Health Organization; 2004.
75. IOM (Institute of Medicine). IOM (Institute of Medicine). Dietary Reference Intakes for Energy, Carbohydrate, Fiber, Fat, Fatty Acids, Cholesterol, Protein, and Amino Acids. Washington, D.C.: National Academies Press; 2002/2005.
76. EFSA (European Food Safety Authority) Panel on Dietetic Products, Nutrition and Allergies (NDA). Scientific Opinion on dietary reference values for protein. *EFSA J.* 2012;10(2):2557.
77. Australian National Health and Medical Research Council (NHMRC), Australian Government Department of Health, and New Zealand Ministry of Health (NZ MoH). Nutrient Reference Values for Australia and New Zealand. https://www.nrv.gov.au/nutrients. Updated April 09, 2014. Accessed April 3, 2019.
78. Nordic Cooperation (NNR). *Nordic Nutrition Recommendations 2012: Integrating Nutrition and Physical Activity.* 5th ed. Copenhagen, Denmark: Nordic Council of Ministers; 2014.
79. D-A-CH (German Nutrition Society, Austrian Nutrition Society, Swiss Nutrition Society). *Reference Values for Nutrient Intake.* 2nd ed. 4th updated release. Bonn: Umschau/Braus; 2018.
80. Chinese Nutrition Society (CNS). *Dietary Reference Intakes for China.* https://www.cnsoc.org/drpostand/page1.html (in Chinese). (Accessed August 27, 2019).
81. Chaves PH. Functional outcomes of anemia in older adults. *Semin Hematol.* 2008;45(4):255–260.
82. Ferrucci L, Balducci L. Anemia of aging: the role of chronic inflammation and cancer. *Semin Hematol.* 2008;45(4):242–249.
83. Rand WM, Pellett PL, Young VR. Meta-analysis of nitrogen balance studies for estimating protein requirements in healthy adults. *Am J Clin Nutr.* 2003;77:109–127.
84. Joint FAO/WHO/UNU Expert Consultation on Protein and Amino Acid Requirements in Human Nutrition (2002: Geneva, Switzerland), Food and Agriculture Organization of the United Nations, World Health Organization, and United Nations University. *Protein and Amino Acid Requirements in Human Nutrition: Report of a Joint FAO/WHO/UNU Expert Consultation.* Geneva: World Health Organization; 2007.
85. Li M, Sun F, Piao JH, Yang XG. Protein requirements in healthy adults: a meta-analysis of nitrogen balance studies. *Biomed Environ Sci.* 2014;27(8):606–613.
86. Beasley JM, Wertheim BC, LaCroix AZ, et al. Biomarker-calibrated protein intake and physical function in the Women's Health Initiative. *J Am Geriatr Soc.* 2013;61(11):1863–1871.
87. Lemieux FC, Filion ME, Barbat-Artigas S, et al. Relationship between different protein intake recommendations with muscle mass and muscle strength. *Climacteric.* 2014;17(3):294–300.
88. Isanejad M, Mursu J, Sirola J, et al. Dietary protein intake is associated with better physical function and muscle strength among elderly women. *Br J Nutr.* 2016;115(7):1281–1291.
89. McLean RR, Mangano KM, Hannan MT, et al. Dietary protein intake is protective against loss of grip strength among older adults in the Framingham Offspring Cohort. *J Gerontol A Biol Sci Med Sci.* 2016;71(3):356–361.
90. Shad BJ, Thompson JL, Breen L. Does the muscle protein synthetic response to exercise and amino acid-based nutrition diminish with advancing age? A systematic review. *Am J Physiol Endocrinol Metab.* 2016;311:E803–E817.
91. Bauer J, Biolo G, Cederholm T, et al. Evidence-based recommendations for optimal dietary protein intake in older people: A position paper from the PROT-AGE Study Group. *JAMDA.* 2013;14: 542–559.
92. Deutz NEP, Bauer JM, Barazzoni R, et al. Protein intake and exercise for optimal muscle function with aging: Recommendations from the ESPEN Expert Group. *Clin Nutr.* 2014;33:929–936.
93. Bashashati M, Sarosiek I, McCallum RW. Epidemiology and mechanisms of gastroesophageal reflux disease in the elderly: A perspective. *Ann NY Acad Sci.* 2016;1380:230–234.
94. Hughes CF, Ward M, Hoey L, McNulty H. Vitamin B_{12} and ageing: current issues and interaction with folate. *Ann Clin Biochem.* 2013;50(4):315–329.
95. Committee on Medical Aspects of Food Policy (COMA), Panel on Dietary Reference Values, Department of Health (UK). *Dietary Reference Values for Food Energy and Nutrients for the United Kingdom.* London: TSO; 1991.
96. Richter M, Baerlocher K, Bauer JM, et al. Revised reference values for the intake of protein. *Ann Nutr Metab.* 2019;74:242–250.
97. AFSSA (Agence française de sécurité sanitaire des aliments). *Apport en protéines: consommation, qualité, besoins et recommandations.* Maisons-Alfort: AFSSA; 2007.
98. Mazokopakis EE, Starakis IK. Recommendations for diagnosis and management of metformin-induced vitamin B_{12} (Cbl) deficiency. *Diabetes Res Clin Pract.* 2012;97:359–367.
99. Selhub J, Rosenberg IH. Excessive folic acid intake and relation to adverse health outcome. *Biochimie.* 2016;126:71–78.
100. Strohm D, Bechthold A, Isik N, Leschik-Bonnet E, Heseker H, German Nutrition Society (DGE). Revised reference values for the intake of thiamin (vitamin B_1), riboflavin (vitamin B_2), and niacin. *NFS Journal.* 2016;3:20–24.
101. Ribaya-Mercado JD, Russell RM, Sahyoun N, et al. Vitamin B_6 requirements of elderly men and women. *J Nutr.* 1991;121:1062–1074.
102. Pannemans DLE, van den Berg H, Westerterp KR. The Influence of protein intake on vitamin B_6 metabolism differs in young and elderly humans. *J Nutr.* 1994;124(8):1207–1214.
103. Madigan SM, Tracey F, McNulty H, et al. Riboflavin and vitamin B_6 intakes and status and biochemical response to riboflavin supplementation in free-living elderly people. *Am J Clin Nutr.* 1998; 68:389–395.
104. Bates CJ, Pentieva KD, Prentice A, et al. Plasma pyridoxal phosphate and pyridoxic acid and their relationship to plasma homocysteine in a representative sample of British men and women aged 65 years and over. *Br J Nutr.* 1999;81:191–201.

105. Ueland PM, Ulvik A, Rios-Avila L, et al. Direct and functional biomarkers of vitamin B6 status. *Annu Rev Nutr*. 2015;35:33–70.
106. IOM (Institute of Medicine). Dietary Reference Intakes for Thiamin, Riboflavin, Niacin, Vitamin B6, Folate, Vitamin B12, Pantothenic Acid, Biotin, and Choline. Washington, D.C.: National Academy Press; 1998.
107. EFSA NDA Panel. Dietary reference values for vitamin B_6. *EFSA J*. 2016;14(6):4485.
108. ANSES (Agence nationale de sécurité sanitaire de l'alimentation, de l'environnement et du travail). *Apports Nutritionnels Conseillés*. Paris: Tec et Doc. Lavoisier; 2001.
109. MacLaughlin J, Holick MF. Aging decreases the capacity of human skin to produce vitamin D_3. *J Clin Invest*. 1985;76:1536–1538.
110. Armbrecht HJ, Zenser TV, Davis BB. Effect of age on the conversion of 25-hydroxyvitamin D_3 to 1,25-dihydroxyvitamin D_3 by kidney of rat. *J Clin Invest*. 1980a;66:1118–1123.
111. Ishida M, Bulos B, Takamoto S, Sacktor B. Hydroxylation of 25-hydroxyvitamin D_3 by renal mitochondria from rats of different ages. *Endocrinology*. 1987;121:443–448.
112. Ireland P, Fordtran JS. Effect of dietary calcium and age on jejunal calcium absorption in humans studied by intestinal perfusion. *J Clin Invest*. 1973;52:2672–2681.
113. Armbrecht HJ, Zenser TV, Gross CJ, Davis BB. Adaptation to dietary calcium and phosphorus restriction changes with age in the rat. *Am J Physiol*. 1980b;239(5):E322–E327.
114. Wood RJ, Fleet JC, Cashman K, et al. Intestinal calcium absorption in the aged rat: Evidence of intestinal resistance to $1,25(OH)_2$ vitamin D. *Endocrinology*. 1998;139:3843–3848.
115. Pattanaungkul S, Riggs BL, Yergey AL, et al. Relationship of intestinal calcium absorption to 1,25-dihydroxyvitamin D [1,25(OH) 2D] levels in young versus elderly women: evidence for age-related intestinal resistance to 1,25(OH)2D action. *J Clin Endocrinol Metab*. 2000;85:4023–4027.
116. Hoenderop JGJ, Nilius B, Bindels RJM. Calcium absorption across epithelia. *Physiol Rev*. 2005;85:373–422.
117. Harshman SG, Shea MK. The role of vitamin K in chronic aging diseases: inflammation, cardiovascular disease, and osteoarthritis. *Curr Nutr Rep*. 2016;5:90–98.
118. Shea MK, Loeser RF, Hsu FC, et al. Vitamin K status and lower extremity function in older adults. The Health Aging and Body Composition Study. *J Gerontol Series A*. 2016;71(10):1348–1355.
119. Bultynck C, Munim N, Harrington DJ, et al. Prevalence of vitamin K deficiency in older people with hip fracture. *Acta Clin Belg*. 2019; Jan 8:1–5. https://doi.org/10.1080/17843286.2018.1564174. [Epub ahead of print].
120. Shevchuk YM, Conly JM. Antibiotic-associated hypoprothrombinemia: a review of prospective studies, 1966–1988. *Rev Infect Dis*. 1990;12(6):1109–1126.
121. Rennie KL, Hughes J, Lang R, Jebb SA. Nutritional management of rheumatoid arthritis: a review of the evidence. *J Hum Nutr Diet*. 2003;16(3):97–109.
122. Bala A, Mondal C, Haldar PK, Khandelwal B. Oxidative stress in inflammatory cells of patient with rheumatoid arthritis: clinical efficacy of dietary antioxidants. *Inflammopharmacology*. 2017; 25(6):595–607.
123. Alavi Naeini AM, Elmadfa I, Djazayery A, et al. The effect of antioxidant vitamins E and C on cognitive performance of the elderly with mild cognitive impairment in Isfahan, Iran: A double-blind, randomized, placebo-controlled trial. *Eur J Nutr*. 2014;53: 1255–1262.
124. Meydani SN, Han SN, Wu D. Vitamin E and immune response in the aged: molecular mechanisms and clinical implications. *Immunol Rev*. 2005;205:269–284.
125. Marko MG, Ahmed T, Bunnell SC, et al. Age-associated decline in effective immune synapse formation of $CD4^+$ T cells is reversed by vitamin E supplementation. *J Immunol*. 2007;178:1443–1449.
126. Molano A, Meydani SN. Vitamin E, signalosomes and gene expression in T cells. *Mol Aspect Med*. 2012;33(1):55–62.
127. Williams CM, Burdge G. Long-chain n-3 PUFA: plant v. marine sources. *Proc Nutr Soc*. 2006;65:42–50.
128. Navarini L, Afeltra A, Afflitto GG, Margiotta DPE. Polyunsaturated fatty acids: any role in rheumatoid arthritis? *Lipids Health Dis*. 2017;16:197.
129. Smith GI. The effects of dietary omega-3s on muscle composition and quality in older adults. *Curr Nutr Rep*. 2016;5:99–105.
130. Dupont J, Dedeyne L, Dalle S, et al. The role of omega-3 in the prevention and treatment of sarcopenia. *Aging Clin Exp Res*. 2019 [Epub ahead of print].
131. Longo AB, Ward WE. PUFAs, Bone mineral density, and fragility fracture: Findings from human studies. *Adv Nutr*. 2016;7(2): 299–312.
132. Mozaffarian D, Micha R, Wallace S. Effects on coronary heart disease of increasing polyunsaturated fat in place of saturated fat: A systematic review and meta-analysis of randomized controlled trials. *PLoS Med*. 2010;7(3):e1000252.
133. Khaja M, Thakur CS, Bharathan T, et al. Fiber 7′ supplement as an alternative to laxatives in a nursing home. *Gerodontology*. 2005; 22(2):106–108.
134. Sturtzel B, Mikulits C, Gisinger C, Elmadfa I. Use of fiber instead of laxative treatment in a geriatric hospital to improve the wellbeing of seniors. *J Nutr Health Aging*. 2009;13(2): 136–139.
135. Sturtzel B, Dietrich A, Wagner K-H, et al. The status of vitamins B_6, B_{12}, folate, and of homocysteine in geriatric home residents receiving laxatives or dietary fiber. *J Nutr Health Aging*. 2010; 14(3):219–223.
136. Agarwal E, Miller M, Yaxley A, Isenring E. Malnutrition in the elderly: a narrative review. *Maturitas*. 2013;76:296–302.
137. Kaiser MJ, Bauer JM, Rämsch C, et al. Frequency of malnutrition in older adults: a multinational perspective using the Mini Nutritional Assessment. *J Am Geriatr Soc*. 2010;58:1734–1738.
138. Parker BA, Chapman IM. Food intake and ageing—the role of the gut. *Mech Ageing Dev*. 2004;125:859–866.
139. Dumic I, Nordin T, Jecmenica M, et al. Gastrointestinal tract disorders in older age. *Chin J Gastroenterol Hepatol*. 2019;2019: 6757524.
140. Kmiec Z. Central regulation of food intake in ageing. *J Physiol Pharmacol*. 2006;57(Supp 6):7–16.
141. Moss C, Dhillo WS, Frost G, Hickson M. Gastrointestinal hormones: the regulation of appetite and the anorexia of ageing. *J Hum Nutr Diet*. 2012;25:3–15.
142. Morley JE. Anorexia of aging: physiologic and pathologic. *Am J Clin Nutr*. 1997;66:760–773.
143. Grande L, Lacima G, Ros E, et al. Deterioration of esophageal motility with age: a manometric study of 79 healthy subjects. *Am J Gastroenterol*. 1999;94:1795–1801.
144. Hildebrandt GH, Dominguez BL, Schork MA, Loesche WJ. Functional units, chewing, swallowing, and food avoidance among the elderly. *J Prosthet Dent*. 1997;77:588–595.
145. Walls AWG, Steele JG. The relationship between oral health and nutrition in older people. *Mech Ageing Dev*. 2004;125:853–857.
146. Nordin S, Razani LJ, Markison S, Murphy C. Age-associated increases in intensity discrimination for taste. *Exp Aging Res*. 2003; 29(3):371–381.
147. Fukunaga A, Uematsu H, Sugimoto K. Influences of aging on taste perception and oral somatic sensation. *J Gerontol Med Sci*. 2005;60A(1):109–113.
148. Porter Starr KN, McDonald SR, Bales CW. Nutritional vulnerability in older adults: A continuum of concerns. *Curr Nutr Rep*. 2015;4(2):176–184.
149. Lechi A. The obesity paradox: is it really a paradox? Hypertension. *Eat Weight Disord*. 2017;22:43–48.

150. WHO. Body Mass Index (BMI) classifications. Global Database on Body Mass Index, World Health Organization website. http://apps.who.int/bmi/index.jsp?introPage=intro_3.html. Accessed August 25, 2019.
151. Winter JE, MacInnis RJ, Wattanapenpaiboon N, Nowson CA. BMI and all-cause mortality in older adults: A meta-analysis. *Am J Clin Nutr.* 2014;99:875–890.
152. Van Walleghen EL, Orr JS, Gentile CL, et al. Habitual physical activity differentially affects acute and short-term energy intake regulation in young and older adults. *Int J Obes.* 2007;31: 1277–1285.
153. Marques EA, Mota J, Carvalho J. Exercise effects on bone mineral density in older adults: a meta-analysis of randomized controlled trials. *AGE.* 2012;34:1493–1515.
154. Muir JM, Ye C, Bhandari M, et al. The effect of regular physical activity on bone mineral density in post-menopausal women aged 75 and over: A retrospective analysis from the Canadian multicentre osteoporosis study. *BMC Muscoskel Disord.* 2013;14: 253.
155. Chastin SFM, Mandrichenko O, Helbostadt JL, Skelton DA. Associations between objectively-measured sedentary behaviour and physical activity with bone mineral density in adults and older adults, the NHANES study. *Bone.* 2014;64:254–262.
156. McPhee JS, French DP, Jackson D, et al. Physical activity in older age: perspectives for healthy ageing and frailty. *Biogerontology.* 2016;17:567–580.
157. Blondell SJ, Hammersley-Mather R, Veerman JL. Does physical activity prevent cognitive decline and dementia?: a systematic review and meta-analysis of longitudinal studies. *BMC Publ Health.* 2014;14:510.
158. Brouwer-Brolsma EM, Vaes AMM, van der Zwaluw NL, et al. Relative importance of summer sun exposure, vitamin D intake, and genes to vitamin D status in Dutch older adults: the B-PROOF study. *J Steroid Biochem Mol Biol.* 2016;164:168–176.

CHAPTER

6

NUTRITION FOR SPORT AND PHYSICAL ACTIVITY

Louise M. Burke[1], *OAM, PhD, APD, FACSM*
Melinda M. Manore[2], *PhD, RD, CSSD, FACSM*
[1]**Australian Institute of Sport, Belconnen, ACT, Australia**
[2]**Oregon State University, Corvallis, OR, United States**

SUMMARY

Athletes and active individuals have energy and nutrient needs that differ from their sedentary counterparts. These needs will depend on exercise training intensity, duration, frequency, and mode and environmental conditions. Energy intake should be adequate to support exercise performance, prevent injury, and maintain health but will change over time depending on the exercise-training schedule and weight goals. Carbohydrate and protein needs are typically higher in active individuals, especially in competitive athletes. Carbohydrate is required for fuel and glycogen replacement, while protein is needed for growth, repair, and muscle adaptations, and selected foods must supply the additional requirements for micronutrients. Exercise/sport events are physiological challenging and require individualized food and fluid recommendations before, during, and after exercise, to reduce/delay fatigue and allow for optimal performance. Postexercise recovery nutrition should restore fuel and fluids homeostasis. Exercise training/competitions also create practical challenges, including accessibility of suitable foods and fluids at the right time around exercise and making good choices regarding supplements and sport foods.

Keywords: Athlete; Carbohydrate; Energy intake; Exercise; Protein; Recovery nutrition; Sport foods; Supplements.

I. OVERVIEW

Despite the range of physiological challenges and practical considerations that arise between and within sports and types of physical activity in which people are engaged, there are some common themes shared by all athletes and fitness enthusiasts. During training, the athlete needs to eat to achieve an ideal physique for their event, to stay healthy and injury free, and to be able to train hard and recover optimally from each session. Each competitive event involves a physiological challenge; in many cases, nutritional strategies undertaken before and during the event, or in the recovery between games or heats and the final, can help to reduce or delay fatigue and allow the athlete to perform optimally. The practical needs of sports also create special challenges: these include finding opportunities to eat well while traveling, having access to suitable foods and fluids at the strategic times around workouts or competition, and making good decisions regarding supplements and sports foods.

The nutrition recommendations, strategies, and approaches used by the fitness enthusiast or recreational athlete may need to be modified from those suited to the elite athlete, according to the individual's goals and overall training load. For example, individuals who embark on a campaign to complete a marathon or Ironman race will benefit from similar nutrition strategies to those recommended to the high performance athlete to support a commitment to daily training and a fuel-demanding race. However, these are unnecessary for an individual who is beginning a fitness program for

Present Knowledge in Nutrition, Volume 2
https://doi.org/10.1016/B978-0-12-818460-8.00006-X

weight or chronic disease management, where the daily energy expenditure involved in exercise is modest. It is important that each individual understands the energy and nutrient costs of exercise and the likely value of implementing special nutrition strategies.

II. INTRODUCTION

The demands of sport vary greatly according to the type of event, the phase of training or competition, and the individual characteristics of each athlete or fitness enthusiast. However, there are some common threads to the nutritional goals of sport. The aim of this chapter is to provide a summary of these key goals of sports nutrition and to provide recommendations and strategies that will help athletes of all levels—elite to recreational—achieve some of these goals. It will also identify emerging or controversial ideas in sports nutrition from which new recommendations in sports nutrition will evolve. Given the breadth of topics covered, it is impossible to provide the depth of information that would allow adequate coverage of any single area. To counter this problem, recent papers are cited giving a more sophisticated review of the current knowledge on a specific area, with particular reference to applications in sport. This is not meant to show disrespect to the pioneers of sports nutrition and the original or seminal papers, rather the aim is to provide a connection to literature from which both the historical and current perspectives can be gained.

III. FUELING FOR SPORT AND PHYSICAL ACTIVITY

A. Matching Energy Intake Changes in Energy Demands

Energy intake provides an important focus for an active individual's training diet since it must provide the carbohydrate cost of training and recovery, protein needs for growth, repair, and adaptation, and sufficient foods to supply any additional requirements for micronutrients and phytonutrients that arise from the commitment to daily exercise. It also plays a direct role in physique changes and can influence health and injury risks.

Energy requirements vary among sports, among athletes in the same sport, and across various times in an individual athlete's periodized training program. A periodized training program refers to how an active individual's training schedule might change over the year based on their exercise goals or the exercise events for which they are training. Extremes in energy intake and energy demand vary greatly. The low end of the energy spectrum includes athletes in sports or activities focused on brief moments of skill/technique rather than prolonged movement (e.g., archery or shooting), those who need to achieve or maintain a low body mass/fat level (e.g., athletes in weight-division sports or physique-conscious sports), and those which combine these two characteristics (e.g., gymnastics, dance, diving). At the high end of the energy range are athletes or active individuals in sports or events involving prolonged sessions of high-intensity exercise (e.g., cyclists undertaking a stage race, runners doing interval training), those supporting growth, large muscle mass, or intentional muscle-gain programs (e.g., adolescent basketball players, American football players), and combinations of these (e.g., heavy-weight rowers or wrestlers).

High energy needs often require both elite and recreational athletes to consume energy in greater amounts than would be provided in culturally determined eating patterns, or dictated by their appetite and hunger. They may also need to consume energy during and after exercise when the availability of foods and fluids, or opportunities to consume them, is limited. Practical issues interfering with the achievement of energy intake goals during postexercise recovery include loss of appetite and fatigue, poor access to suitable foods, and distraction by other activities. Specialized advice from a sports dietitian is useful in the development of a plan to address the energy intake challenges faced by any active individual. Valuable strategies include a pattern of frequent eating occasions, good organization in order to ensure access to suitable foods and drinks in a busy day, and a focus on choices that are low in bulk and high in energy density including high-energy fluids and specialized sports foods.[1] Alternatively, the athlete or fitness enthusiast with reduced energy needs face their own practical challenges to meet their nutritional goals and appetite with a smaller energy budget. General principles that may assist in this scenario include behavior modification to reduce unnecessary eating, focus on choices that are high in bulk or satiety, and choosing nutrient-rich foods that can meet nutritional goals with a lower energy cost.[1]

Recent updates to sports nutrition guidelines include the recognition that an active individual's energy requirements change from day-to-day and across various parts of the sporting calendar, particularly with changes in the energy demands of a training (or competition) program or strategies to alter physique. There are several advantages in trying to track energy intake with energy needs. For example, a consistently high-energy intake is needed during periods of extremely high-energy demands since it may be beyond the absorptive capacity of the gut to play "catchup" once a significant energy deficit has accumulated.[2] Furthermore, a new concept of energy availability has been developed to assess the suitability of an athlete's energy intake.

Energy availability is defined operationally as the energy cost of the athlete or active individual's exercise program subtracted from their total energy intake, which then provides an approximation of the amount of energy remaining to support other functions of the body required for good health.[3] Energy availability may be low when an athlete restricts their energy intake to achieve or maintain a light or lean physique or when they fail to increase their energy intake sufficiently to meet a strenuous exercise load. When energy availability drops below about 30 kcal (125 kJ)/kg fat-free mass for as little as 5 days, there is metabolic suppression and impairment of homeostasis and function, including impaired hormone and bone function.[4] The actual level of energy availability below which an athlete experiences metabolic abnormalities may vary for each athlete. Cialdella-Kam et al.[5] reported the mean energy availability of their amenorrheic female athletes was 36.7 ± 10.2 kcal, and athletes had to increase energy take to 45.4 ± 14.7 kcal before menses and ovulation returned. This is the basis of the syndromes known as Female Athlete Triad and Relative Energy Deficiency in Sport (RED-S) that are discussed in Commentary 3 in Section VII below.

Therefore, it makes sense for the elite or highly active recreational athlete to adjust their daily energy intake in reasonable harmony with fluctuations in training load. A strategy that can assist with this goal is to consume food and drinks before, during, and after each exercise session. As will be discussed under Section IV, this will help to support performance and recovery around the workout or event. However, it is also a practical way to allow energy intake to increase when training sessions are increased in duration or frequency and to remove unnecessary intake when the training load is reduced, especially during injuries or the off-season.

B. Management of Body Weight and Composition for Optimal Performance

Physical characteristics such as height, body weight (BW), lean body weight (LBW), and body fat play a role in the performance of many sports.[6] For example, a large BW and LBW are linked with strength, power, and momentum and are important in football, throwing and lifting events, rowing, and track cycling. By contrast, low BW and body fat levels offer biomechanical and "power-to-weight" advantages to allow athletes to move their bodies over distances, against gravity, or in a small space (e.g., distance running, uphill cycling, diving, and gymnastics). Esthetic considerations are important for the subjectively biased outcomes of sports such as gymnastics, figure skating, diving, and bodybuilding; however, many individuals are also motivated by a personal desire to look good in a skimpy or figure-hugging sporting uniform. In combative events (e.g., boxing, wrestling, judo), weight-lifting, and light-weight rowing, athletes compete in weight divisions that attempt to match competitors based on size, strength, and reach. Eligibility for competition is decided at a weigh-in undertaken just before the event, according to specific rules of the sport.[7,8]

Elite competitors typically reach the optimal physique for their event via the genetic predispositions that have helped to determine their sporting interests and the conditioning effects of nutrition and training. While some appear to achieve this physique easily, others need to manipulate their training and dietary programs to achieve their desired size and shape. Unfortunately, some athletes, regardless of competitive level, embark on extreme weight-loss schemes, often involving excessive training, chronic low energy availability, suboptimal nutrient intake, and psychological distress.[9,10] Problems arising from these activities include fatigue, micronutrient deficiencies (especially iron and calcium), reduced immune status, altered hormonal balance, disordered eating, and poor body image. "Making weight" is another common activity undertaken in weight-division sports, whereby athletes, many of whom are already lean, shed kilograms in the hours or days prior to the weigh-in to qualify for a division lighter than their normal BW.[9,10] Although this strategy is used to gain advantage in strength or reach over a smaller opponent, it brings disadvantages in terms of dehydration or suboptimal nutritional status resulting from rapid weight-loss techniques. Medical committees and governing organizations have issued guidelines warning against extreme "making weight" activities.[11]

Targets for "ideal" BW and body fat should be set in terms of ranges, with each individual setting targets that are compatible with long-term health and performance, rather than short-term benefits alone. Where loss of body fat is warranted, it should be achieved by a gradual program of sustained and moderate energy deficit. Furthermore, there is good evidence that a higher protein intake (e.g., 1.6–2.4 g/kg/d) may support body composition manipulation by maintaining or even increasing lean body mass during periods of energy deficit/BW loss.[12,13] Each individual, regardless of activity level, should be able to achieve targets while eating a diet adequate in energy and nutrients, and free of unreasonable food-related stress.[10] Most importantly, the characteristics of elite athletes should not be considered natural or necessary for recreational and subelite performers; furthermore, chronic achievement of minimal body fat levels is neither necessary nor healthy for any athlete. Indeed, most elite athletes periodize their body mass and body fat levels, achieving their "race weight" only for times they are at their competition peak. This concept of deliberate manipulation of energy intake and body fat at different phases of the yearly training plan is well-illustrated in a recent case history of an international-level female middle-distance runner.[14] Special nutrition support should be given to athletes in weight-making sports to assist them to choose an appropriate weight division and to adopt the diet and exercise strategies that achieve their weigh-in targets with minimal negative effects.[7,8]

Athletes or fitness enthusiasts who wish to gain muscle mass are at the other end of the spectrum. These individuals often focus dietary interests on excessive protein intake and special supplements that make extravagant claims. However, emerging evidence suggests that the key nutritional support for a resistance-training program is adequate energy intake and well-timed intake of protein over the day.[15,16] Protein for recovery will be addressed further in the later Section V.

C. Eating for Health and Injury Prevention

Staying healthy and injury free is a key ingredient in a sporting career, or for any individual wishing to maintain a high level of fitness, since it supports consistent training and ensures that the athlete can be at their peak for important competitions. However, the intensive exercise programs undertaken by many athletes straddle the fine line between providing the maximum stimulus for performance improvements and increasing the risk of illness and injury. Although we do not have sufficient evidence to set recommendations for nutritional practices that will guarantee good health and minimum downtime due to injury, some nutritional risk factors for the opposite outcome can be identified.

There is a general belief that athletes or fitness enthusiasts are at increased risk of succumbing to infectious illnesses, particularly upper respiratory tract infections, during periods of high-volume training, or after strenuous competitive events.[17] However, there is evidence of suppression of markers of acquired immune function during the acute response to a bout of exercise, and it is intuitive that an exacerbation of the duration or severity of such effects could lead to chronic immunosuppression and compromised resistance to common infections.[17] Nutritional factors that may exacerbate this risk include inadequate fueling (low carbohydrate availability) around exercise sessions and poor energy availability. Athletes or any active individual are advised to follow nutritional practices that avoid such deficiencies. Meanwhile, nutritional supplements have been promoted to offer protection with mixed support; there is limited evidence of benefits from supplementation with vitamin C, and from herbal products such as echinacea and glutamine, mixed support for colostrum and probiotics, and some apparent potential associated with polyphenolic compounds such as quercetin.[18]

Injuries generally occur via two mechanisms: acute problems occurring following a collision or contact impact or chronic problems that arise from inadequate resilience to continual high levels of exercise or over training. Nutritional factors may be indirectly involved with some aspects of acute injury if inadequate nutrition contributes to the fatigue that facilitates poor concentration and technique or an increased risk of accidents.[19] Nutritional factors are often involved in the development of stress fractures since low bone density is a risk factor in the development of this chronic injury.[20] Reduced bone density in athletes seems contradictory, since exercise is an important protector of bone health. However, many athletes suffer from either direct loss of bone density or failure to optimize the gaining of peak bone mass that should occur during the 10–15 years after the onset of puberty.[21] The involvement of poor bone health in the Female Athlete Triad and RED-S underpinned by low energy availability is discussed further in the Section VII.

In addition to an environment of adequate availability of energy, healthy bones required adequate bone building nutrients, and potentially, carbohydrate. Adequate calcium intake in necessary. Calcium recommendations for females with impaired menstrual function is 1300–1500 mg/day, the same as the recommendation for postmenopausal women.[21] Where adequate calcium intake cannot be met through dietary means, usually through use of low-fat dairy foods or calcium-enriched soy alternatives, a calcium supplement may be considered. Although low bone density was first identified in female athletes, it is also seen in male athletes. High-risk groups include elite cyclists; this presumably results from the low energy availability associated with heavy energy expenditure and a desire for low body fat levels but may be exacerbated by the lack of bone loading during cycling activities.[22]

Vitamin D deficiency or insufficiency is now recognized as a community health problem with consequences including impairment of bone health, muscle function, and immune status. Education campaigns target people at high risk to seek assessment and reversal of inadequate vitamin D status. Some athletes and active individuals may be vulnerable to such problems.[23] Individuals at greatest risk are those doing indoor training (e.g., gymnasts, swimmers), residing at latitudes greater than 35 degrees, training in the early morning or late evening, thus avoiding sunlight exposure, wearing protective clothing or sunscreen, and consuming a diet low in vitamin D. Individuals with these characteristics should seek professional advice and have their vitamin

D status monitored. Although there is dispute over optimal vitamin D status, vitamin D supplementation may be required to prevent or treat insufficiency.[23,24]

IV. EATING BEFORE/DURING EXERCISE TO REDUCE/DELAY FATIGUE

To achieve optimal performance, an athlete or fitness enthusiast should identify potentially preventable factors that contribute to fatigue during an exercise task and undertake nutritional strategies before, during, and after exercise that minimize or delay the onset of this fatigue. This is obviously important during competition, but active individuals should also practice such strategies during key training sessions, both to support technique and intensity during the workout and to fine-tune the nutritional plan for a specific event. The nutritional challenges of competition vary according to length and intensity of the event, the environment, and factors that influence the recovery between events or the opportunity to eat and drink during the event itself (see Table 6.1).

Carbohydrate reserves for the muscle and central nervous system limit the performance of prolonged (>90 min) submaximal or intermittent high-intensity exercise and play a permissive role in the performance of brief or sustained high-intensity work.[25] Competition eating should target strategies to consume carbohydrate before and during such events to meet these fuel needs (described as achieving high carbohydrate availability). Carbohydrate should be consumed over the day(s) leading up to a competitive event commensurate with the muscle glycogen requirements of the task (e.g., marathon vs. ½ marathon or 10K fun run). The trained muscle is able to normalize its high resting glycogen stores within 24 h of rest and carbohydrate intake (see Table 6.2). If an individual can extend the time and carbohydrate ingestion to 24–48 h, they can achieve a supercompensation of muscle glycogen, commonly known as carbohydrate loading, and improve performance of events of more than 90 min duration.[26] Carbohydrate eaten in the hours prior to an event can also ensure adequate liver glycogen, especially for events undertaken after an overnight fast.[27] Although general fuel targets can be provided for the preevent meal (Table 6.2), the type, timing, and amount of carbohydrate-rich foods and drinks should be chosen with consideration of practical issues such as gastrointestinal comfort, individual preferences, and catering arrangements in the competition environment. Sustained-release (low glycemic index) carbohydrate sources or foods consumed just prior to the start of the competition will also provide an ongoing source of glucose from the gut during exercise.[28]

According to the specific logistics and culture of a sport, athletes and fitness enthusiasts can continue to consume carbohydrate during exercise from a range of specialized sports products (e.g., carbohydrate–electrolyte sports drinks, gels, bars) or everyday foods (soft drinks, fruit, confectionery). Until recently, refueling recommendations for athletes during exercise encouraged the development of a personalized nutrition plan for events of >60 min that combined carbohydrate intake of 30–60 g/h and adequate rehydration with the practical opportunities for intake during the session.[29] Opportunities for a more systematic approach to specific carbohydrate needs for different types of situations were, however, discouraged by a number of prevailing beliefs. These included the idea that the oxidation rate of exogenous carbohydrate was capped at 60 g/h, the concern that larger intakes might cause gastrointestinal distress, and the lack of evidence that more carbohydrate was better for some events.[30] New information has allowed a differentiation of strategies for both nonendurance (45–75 min) and ultraendurance (>3–4 h) events.

There is now robust evidence that intestinal absorption limits the ability to supply the working muscle with exogenous carbohydrate. This limitation can be overcome by consuming a mixture of carbohydrate sources that use different intestinal transport mechanisms, such as fructose and glucose.[31] Such mixes allow better gastrointestinal comfort and higher rates of oxidation of ingested carbohydrate with higher rates of intake. The evidence of a dose response between carbohydrate intake and performance benefits in ultraendurance exercise[32,33] has led to separate recommendations for such events (see Table 6.2). The optimal feeding rates may be up to 80–90 g/h, using carbohydrate mixtures, with these targets being provided in absolute amounts rather than g/kg BW, since the absorptive capacity of the gut appears to be independent of body size.[31] Athletes of all levels are also encouraged to practice intake during training sessions, since this may also be associated with an adaptation of the gut to promote greater exogenous fuel use[34] and further enhance performance.[35]

Events of ~60 min duration are not associated with limitations of muscle fuel supply when adequate preparation has occurred. However, new research has shown that intake of small amounts of carbohydrate, even in the form of frequent rinsing of the mouth with a carbohydrate solution, are associated with better performance in such protocols.[36] It appears that there is communication between receptors in the mouth/throat and centers of reward and motor control in the central nervous system.[37] These findings have been incorporated into new recommendations for athletes and active individuals (Ref. 38; Table 6.2), and although the magnitude of the effect is smaller when a preevent carbohydrate-rich meal has been consumed, a detectable benefit is still evident.[39]

TABLE 6.1 Factors related to nutrition that could produce fatigue or suboptimal performance during sports competition or intense training.[40]

Factor	Description	Examples of high-risk/common occurrence in sports
Dehydration	Mismatch between sweat losses and fluid intake during an event. May be exacerbated if an athlete begins the event in fluid deficit.	Events undertaken in hot conditions, particularly involving high-intensity activity patterns and/or heavy protective garments. Repeated competitions (e.g., tournaments) may increase risk of compounding dehydration from one event to the next. Athletes in weight-making sports may deliberately dehydrate themselves to achieve their weigh-in target, with insufficient time between weigh-in and the start of their event to restore fluid levels.
Muscle glycogen depletion	Depletion of key muscle fuel due to high utilization in a single event and/or poor recovery of stores from previous activity/ event. Typically occurs in events longer than 90 min of sustained or intermittent high-intensity exercise.	Occurs in endurance events such as marathon and distance running, road cycling, and Ironman triathlons. May occur in some team sports in "running" players with large total distances covered at high intensities (e.g., midfield players in soccer, Australian rules football). Repeated competitions (e.g., tournaments) may increase risk of poor refueling from one match to the next.
Hypoglycemia	Reduction in blood glucose concentrations due to poor carbohydrate availability. However, not all athletes are susceptible to feeling fatigue when blood glucose concentrations become low. Note that even when the central nervous system is not fuel deprived, intake of carbohydrate can promote a "happy brain," allowing the muscle to work at a higher power output	Low blood glucose concentrations may occur in athletes with high carbohydrate requirements (see above) who fail to consume carbohydrate during their event. Events lasting 45–75 min may benefit from intake of even small amounts of carbohydrate that stimulate the brain and central nervous system. This includes half marathons, 40-km cycling time trial, and many team sports.
Disturbance of muscle acid– base balance	High rates of H+ production via anaerobic glycolytic power system.	Prolonged high-intensity activities lasting 1–8 min, e.g., rowing events, middle-distance running, 200–800 m swimming, and track cycling team pursuit. May also occur in events with repeated sustained periods of high-intensity activity—perhaps in some team games or racquet sports.
Depletion of phosphocreatine	Inadequate recovery of phosphocreatine system of ATP regeneration leading to gradual decline in power output in subsequent efforts.	Occurs in events with repeated efforts of high-intensity activity with short recovery intervals—perhaps in some team games or racquet sports.
Gastrointestinal disturbances	These include vomiting and diarrhea which directly reduce performance and interfere with nutritional strategies aimed at managing fluid and fuel status.	Poorly chosen intake of food and fluid before and/or during an event. Risks included consuming a large amount of fat or fiber in preevent meal, consuming excessive amounts of single carbohydrates during the event, or becoming significantly dehydrated.
Water intoxication/ hyponatremia (low blood sodium)	Excessive intake of fluids leading to hyponatremia ranging from mild (often asymptomatic) to severe (can be fatal). While this problem is more of a medical concern than a cause of fatigue, symptoms can include headache and disorientation, which can be mistaken as signs of dehydration.	Athletes with low sweat losses (e.g., low-intensity exercise in cool weather) who overzealously consume fluid before and during an event. This has most often been seen during marathons, ultraendurance sports, and hiking.

TABLE 6.2 Summary of recommendations for carbohydrate intake for athletes and fitness enthusiasts.

Training situation	Carbohydrate targets		Comments on type and timing of carbohydrate intake
Daily needs for fuel and recovery: 1. The following targets are intended to provide high carbohydrate availability (i.e., to meet the carbohydrate needs of the muscle and central nervous system) for different exercise loads in situations where exercise is high quality and/or at high intensity. These general recommendations should be fine-tuned with individual consideration of total energy needs, specific training protocols, and feedback from training performance. 2. On other occasions, when exercise quality or intensity is less important, it may be less important to achieve these carbohydrate targets or to arrange carbohydrate intake over the day to optimize availability for specific sessions. In these cases, carbohydrate intake should meet energy goals and food preferences or availability. 3. In some scenarios, when the focus is on enhancing the training stimulus or adaptive response, low carbohydrate availability may be deliberately achieved by reducing total carbohydrate intake or by manipulating carbohydrate intake related to training sessions (e.g., training in a fasted state, undertaking a second session of exercise without adequate opportunity for refueling after the first session).			
Light	• Low-intensity or skill-based activities	3–5 g/kg body weight (BM)/d	• Timing of carbohydrate intake over the day may be manipulated to promote high carbohydrate availability for a specific training session by consuming carbohydrate before or during the session or in recovery from a previous session. • As long as total fuel needs are met, the pattern of carbohydrate intake may simply be guided by convenience and individual choice. • Athletes should choose nutrient-rich carbohydrate sources to allow overall nutrient needs to be met.
Moderate	• Moderate exercise program (e.g., ~1 h per day)	5–7 g/kg BM/d	
High	• Endurance program (e.g., 1–3 h/d moderate- to high-intensity exercise)	6–10 g/kg BM/d	
Very high	• Extreme commitment e.g., >4–5 h/d moderate- to high-intensity exercise	8–12 g/kg BM/d	
Acute fueling strategies: These guidelines promote high carbohydrate availability to fuel optimal performance in competition or key training sessions.			
General fueling	• Preparation for events <90 min exercise	7–12 g/kg BW per 24 h as for d aily fuel needs	• Athletes may choose carbohydrate-rich sources that are low in fiber/residue and easily consumed to ensure that fuel targets are met and to meet goals for gut comfort or lighter "racing weight."
Carbohydrate loading	• Preparation for events >90 min of sustained/intermittent exercise	36–48 h of 10–12 g/kg BW per 24 h	
Speedy refueling	• < 8 h recovery between two fuel-demanding sessions	1–1.2 g/kg BW/h for first 4 h then resume daily fuel needs	• Small regular snacks may help refueling during short periods. • Carbohydrate-rich foods and drink may help to ensure that fuel targets are met.
Pre-event fueling	• Before exercise >60 min	1–4 g/kg consumed 1–4 h before exercise	• Timing, amount and type of carbohydrate foods and drinks should be chosen to suit the practical needs of the event and individual preferences/experiences. • Foods high in fat, protein, or fiber may need to be avoided to reduce risk of gastrointestinal issues during the event. • Low glycemic index food choices may provide a more sustained source of fuel for situations where carbohydrate cannot be consumed during exercise.

Continued

TABLE 6.2 Summary of recommendations for carbohydrate intake for athletes and fitness enthusiasts.—cont'd

Training situation	Carbohydrate targets		Comments on type and timing of carbohydrate intake
During brief exercise sessions	• < 45 min	Not needed	
During sustained high-intensity exercise	• 45–75 min	Small amounts including mouth rinse	• A range of drinks and sport food products can provide easily consumed carbohydrate. • The frequent contact of carbohydrate with the mouth and oral cavity can stimulate parts of the brain and central nervous system to enhance perceptions of well-being and increase self-chosen work outputs.
During endurance exercise, including "stop and start" sports	• 1–2.5 h	30–60 g/h	• Carbohydrate intake provides a source of fuel for the muscles to supplement endogenous stores. • Opportunities to consume foods and drinks vary according to the rules and nature of each sport. • A range of everyday food choices and specialized sport foods and products ranging in from liquid to solid may be useful. • The athlete should practice to find a refueling plan that suits their individual goals, including hydration needs and gut comfort.
During ultraendurance exercise	• > 2.5–3 h	Up to 90 g/h	• As above. • Higher intakes of carbohydrate are associated with better performance. • Products providing multiple transportable carbohydrates (glucose: fructose mixtures) achieve high rates of oxidation of carbohydrate consumed during exercise.

Reproduced with permission from Ref. 41.

Other major nutritional strategies during exercise involve replacement of the fluid and electrolytes lost in sweat (see Fig. 6.1). Sweat losses vary during exercise based on the duration and intensity of exercise, environmental conditions, and the acclimatization of the individual, but typically range between 500 and 2000 mL/h[29]. As fluid deficit increases, so does the stress associated with exercise, such as the drifting increase in heart rate and perception of effort.[42] The point at which this causes a noticeable or significant impairment of exercise capacity and performance will depend on the individual, their response to the environmental conditions (effects are greater in the heat or at altitude), and the type of exercise.[43] If exercise lasts longer than ~45 min, there may be advantages associated with consuming fluids during the session. The general recommendations are that active individuals use the refueling and beverage opportunities that are specific to their sport to replace as much of their sweat loss as is practical during the event,[44] and particularly to keep the fluid deficit below ~2% of body mass in stressful environments.[29,45] Depending on the event, there may be opportunities to drink during breaks in play (i.e., half-time, substitutions or time-outs in team games) or during the exercise itself (from aid stations, handlers, or self-carried supplies). Checking body mass before and after the session, then accounting for the weight of drinks and foods consumed during the session, will allow the athlete to calculate sweat rates, rates of fluid replacement, and the total sweat deficit over the session.[46] This can be useful in developing and fine-tuning an individualized hydration plan that is specific to an event and its conditions.[43,47]

Fluid mismatches during competitive events mostly err on the side of a fluid deficit.[44] However, it is possible for some athletes to overhydrate if they drink excessively during events, especially when sweat rates are low.[48] This situation can be dangerous if it leads to the potentially fatal condition of hyponatremia (low blood sodium concentration; often known as water intoxication).[49,50] The recognition of this problem and the justifiable publicity surrounding deaths in some recreational sporting events has led some sports scientists to blame guidelines for fluid intake or the marketing of sports drinks as a contributing cause.[51,52] Indeed, there has been an evolution of recommendations for fluid intake during exercise over the past 30 years. We now know that prescriptive fluid advice may be unsuitable, and the implication from previous guidelines that athletes should drink as much as possible during exercise is unnecessary and potentially harmful.[29,53] As stated above, the current fluid guidelines warn against overdrinking but encourage an individualized fluid plan that keeps the fluid deficit to an acceptable level.[54]

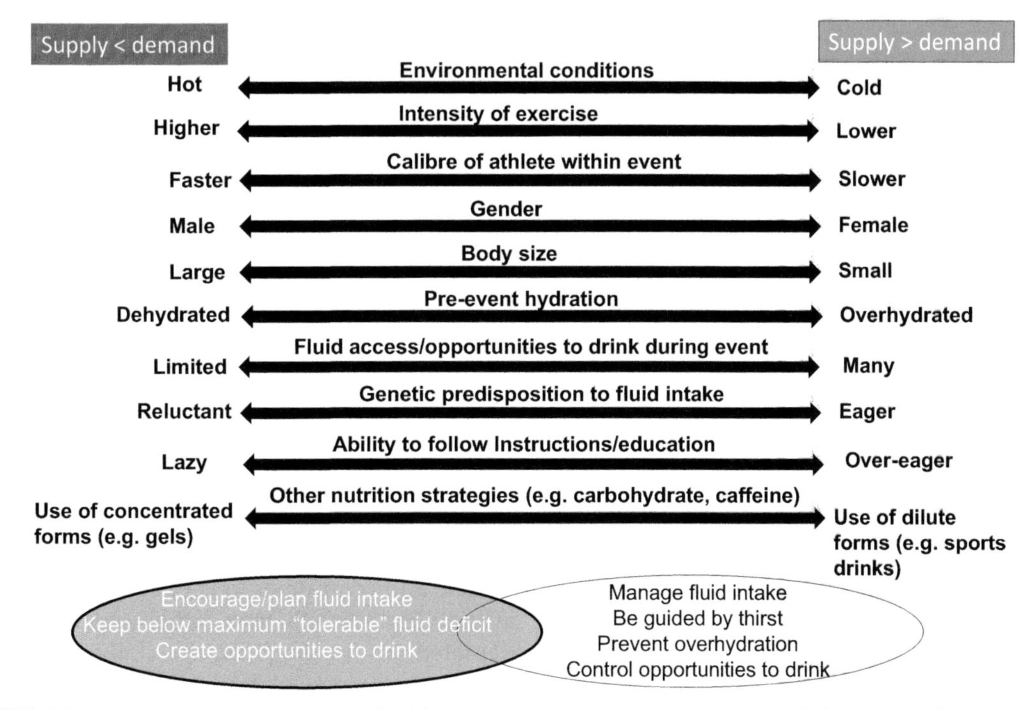

FIGURE 6.1 Considerations for managing fluid balance during an exercise session of >1 h duration. *Adapted from Ref. 55.*

It should be noted that even the above fluid recommendations have been criticized as being unnecessary and complicated and still capable of leading to hyponatremia.[49,52] Instead, it has been argued that athletes and fitness enthusiasts should simply drink according to their thirst.[52,54] The opinion of these authors is that thirst or ad libitum intake of fluid provides a reasonable starting point for developing a fluid plan for an active individual; however, there are often good reasons to improve on these subjective dictates. As illustrated in Fig. 6.1, there are situations where usual circumstances results in large fluid deficits and a more proactive fluid plan would be of benefit. For example, in sports where opportunities for fluid intake are limited (e.g., endurance running, swimming, or cross-country skiing), the athlete may need to drink at the available opportunities early in an event (i.e., "ahead of their thirst") to better pace total fluid intake over the session. Conversely, other events allow athletes to drink at greater frequencies, allowing a better match between fluid intake to sweat losses. Finally, some individuals have poor judgment and may need guidance to drink more appropriate (lower) fluid volumes despite their perceived thirst. Cases of symptomatic hyponatremia include scenarios where excessive fluid intake has occurred when an athlete claimed to be "drinking ad libitum" or "to thirst."[56]

The need to replace sodium losses during exercise is also debated. The inclusion of modest amounts of salt in commercial carbohydrate–electrolyte beverages (sports drinks) improves the taste and voluntary intake of a beverage. Large salt losses are documented in the case of athletes who experience large losses of sweat during prolonged sessions of exercise in the heat[57] and/or excrete "salty sweat."[58] There is anecdotal evidence that proactive replacement of salt during and between exercise sessions may prevent the development of whole body cramps during exercise in the heat in some individuals,[59] but this hypothesis is disputed by others[60] and research evidence is not strong. Similarly, the contribution of large salt losses to the development of hyponatremia or low plasma salt concentrations is controversial. Modeling of salt and fluid changes during exercise shows that sodium losses can contribute to a worsening of plasma sodium homeostasis for any given level of dehydration/fluid replacement.[61] However, since the primary risk factor for the development of hyponatremia is excessive intake of fluids compared with fluid losses, more focus is needed on this aspect rather than sodium supplementation.

Other strategies to attenuate the physiological factors causing fatigue during sport include the use of ergogenic aids such as caffeine, the buffering agents beta-alanine and bicarbonate, beetroot juice/nitrate, and creatine (discussed under Section VI).

V. RECOVERY NUTRITION

A. Eating for Optimal Recovery

Recovery is a major challenge for the elite athlete, who undertakes two or even three workouts each day during certain phases of the training cycle with 4–24 h between each session. However, recovery can also be a concern for the recreational athlete who trains once or twice a day in preparation for a special endurance event such as a marathon or triathlon. Recovery may also be important in determining the outcome of multibout or multiday competitions such as tournaments, stage races, and events with heats and finals. Recovery involves a complex range of processes of restoration of homeostasis and adaptation to the physiological stress of exercise, including factors related to the maintenance of health and function covered in Section IV. Other recovery goals include the restoration of fluid balance following the loss of fluid and electrolytes in sweat,[45,62] replacement of fuel stores including muscle and liver glycogen and intramuscular triglycerides,[30,63] and the synthesis of new protein for muscular development, adaptation, and repair.[16] Extensive research allows recommendations to be provided for each of these goals. Recovery eating strategies need to individualized based on the nutritional stress or challenges of the specific exercise session, the recovery period until the next session, and the "bigger picture" nutrition goals, such as physique management. In all cases, there may be practical impediments to consuming the foods and drinks needed to achieve recovery eating goals, such as loss of appetite after intense exercise, lack of availability of suitable choices, and distraction from other postcompetition activities (e.g., team events, travel schedules, performance debriefs, drug tests, equipment management, and media commitments).

Recommendations for carbohydrate intake in the everyday diets and specific recovery eating strategies of athletes and fitness enthusiasts have evolved over the past decade. While early sports nutrition recommendations proposed a seemingly ubiquitous "high carbohydrate diet" for athletes,[64] later refinements discouraged the terminology of expressing carbohydrate intake as a percentage of total energy intake in favor of guidelines scaled to the size of the athlete and the fuel cost of their exercise program.[63] An elite or recreational athlete's carbohydrate status is best considered in terms of whether daily carbohydrate intake or timing of intake maintains an adequate supply of carbohydrate substrate for the muscle and central nervous system ("high carbohydrate availability") or whether carbohydrate fuel sources are depleted or limiting for the daily exercise program ("low carbohydrate availability").[30] While high carbohydrate availability is important for situations where the athlete needs to perform optimally, especially with exercise of high intensities, in real life, there may be practical reasons why active individuals undertake some training sessions with low carbohydrate availability. Whether there may be some advantages gained by deliberately training in this way is a topical question (see Section VI).

Table 6.2 summarizes the current recommendations for carbohydrate intake in the athlete's everyday recovery diet including strategies to enhance postexercise refueling by commencing intake soon after the completion of the exercise bout. An active individual's carbohydrate intake is not static but changes according the daily, weekly, or seasonal goals and exercise commitments within a training program.[30] It can be useful to adjust carbohydrate intake by strategically consuming meals/snacks providing carbohydrate and other nutrients around important exercise sessions. This allows nutrient and energy intake to track with the needs of the individual's exercise commitments and promotes high carbohydrate availability to enhance performance and recovery.[30]

Recommendations regarding rehydration and consumption of protein to promote muscular development, adaptation, and repair are provided in Table 6.3. Current sport nutrition research has provided new insights into protein needs in response to exercise. Many of the adaptations to training result from the synthesis of new proteins during the recovery from each exercise bout with the various types of protein being determined by the type of exercise that was just undertaken.[65] To maximize the functional output of training (i.e., growth in muscle size and strength, enhancement of aerobic or anaerobic metabolism), the athlete and fitness enthusiast needs to enhance the protein synthetic response to the exercise stimulus. Recent resistance exercise studies show that muscle protein synthesis is optimized with the intake

TABLE 6.3 Recommendations for rehydration and repair/adaptations following exercise.

Issue	Summary of current recommendations

Rehydration	• Fluid intake equal to 125%–150% of a postexercise fluid deficit will be needed to accommodate further sweat and urine losses and restore fluid balance.
	• Thirst may not guarantee adequate fluid intake: when the fluid deficit is >2% body mass, an athlete should have a fluid plan and access to a supply of palatable beverages.
	  • Sweetened, cool drinks encourage voluntary intake of fluids.
	• Rehydration requires replacement of the electrolytes lost in sweat, especially sodium. Fluid intake in the absence of electrolyte replacement will reduce plasma osmolarity and result in large urine losses.
	  • Sodium can be replaced via special drinks such as oral rehydration solutions (50–80 mmol/L) or higher salt-containing sports drinks (30–35 mmol/L).
	  • Alternatively, sodium can be consumed in foods or added to the meals eaten in conjunction with fluid intake.
	• The intake of protein-containing fluids postexercise, such as dairy choices, may also assist with fluid retention and contribute to other recovery goals.
	• Where possible, it is better to space fluid intake over a period rather than consuming large volumes at a single time: this pattern will reduce urine losses and maximize fluid retention.

Repair and adaptation (protein synthesis)	• Protein should be consumed soon after an exercise session to promote the synthesis of new proteins as dictated by the specific exercise stimulus.
	  • An intake of 0.3–0.4 kg BM (20–30 g) of protein is sufficient to optimize the response to exercise.
	  • Protein intake should include high-quality proteins such as animal sources (e.g., dairy, eggs, meat). Alternatively, plant sources could include soy milk or other soy or pea protein products.
	• Although previous discussions on increased protein requirements for athletes remain unresolved, it is likely that all needs can be met from intake of 1.2–1.6 g/kg BW/day. Protein needs during targeted weight-loss periods, where the retention of lean body mass (LBM) is a priority, may require protein intakes of 1.6–2.4 g/kg BW/d.
	• To maximize muscle protein synthesis over the 24 h cycle, protein intake should be spread every 3–5 h over the day. In addition to traditional meals, a postexercise snack and a prebed protein boost represent other strategic occasions for intake.

of modest amounts (0.3–0.4 g/kg BW; ~ 20–30 g) of high-quality protein, spread over meals and snacks every 3–5 h over the day. Protein intake is especially important during the recovery period after exercise[66] and, potentially, just before sleep.[67] Recommendations for the total daily intake of protein for athletes and fitness enthusiasts undertaking heavy training loads, regardless of mode or training or goals around BW gain, are now set at 1.2–1.6 g/kg/d.[13] Although this amount of protein represents a doubling or tripling of the Recommended Dietary Allowance reference values for the general population (~0.8 g/kg BW/d), these protein needs are generally met within the high-energy intakes typical of athletes undertaking heavy training.[68] Meanwhile, carbohydrate may be needed to fuel training sessions and recovery, and both fat and carbohydrate might contribute to the energy surplus needed to promote optimal gain in BW or general growth.[15]

VI. SPORT FOODS AND SUPPLEMENTS: ARE THEY NECESSARY?

A. Use of Sports Foods and Supplements

Given that the podium places at important sporting competitions are decided by milliseconds and millimeters, it is understandable that elite athletes are in constant search for any product or intervention that might improve performance by even a small margin. However, even recreational athletes are seduced by the promises of the multitude of sports foods and supplements that represent a multi-billion dollar industry. The crowded and creative commercial market for these products provides a challenge to stay abreast of the number of products, the marketing claims, and the evidence base for their real contribution to an athlete's sporting goals. Products used by athletes and fitness enthusiasts fall into three different categories[69]: (1) sports foods providing energy or nutrients when it is impractical to consume everyday foods (e.g., sports drinks, protein supplements); (2) nutrient supplements for treatment or prevention of deficiencies (e.g., iron, vitamin D); (3) performance supplements that directly enhance exercise capacity and (4)supplements that provide indirect benefits through recovery, body composition management, and other goals.

Despite earlier reluctance, many expert groups, including the International Olympic Committee, now pragmatically accept the use of supplements passing a risk: benefit analysis of being safe, effective, legal, and appropriate to an athlete's age and maturation in their sport.[69] The Sports Supplement Framework of the Australian Institute of Sport also provides cautious support for the appropriate use of sports foods and the few performance supplements that enjoy robust evidence of efficacy.[70] These include caffeine,[71,72] bicarbonate,[73,74] and β-alanine[75] as extracellular buffering agents and creatine[76] and nitrate/beetroot juice as intracellular buffering agents.[77,78] Athletes and coaches should, however, be aware that these benefits are limited to specific situations (Fig. 6.2).

Any benefits associated with supplement use must be balanced against the expense, the potential for adverse outcomes due to poor protocols of use (e.g., excessive doses, interactions with other supplements), and the dangers inherent with products whose manufacture and marketing is less regulated than that of foods or pharmaceutical goods. Elite athletes also need to consider the danger that supplements have been found to contain contaminants or undeclared ingredients that are prohibited by the antidoping codes under which they compete[79]; these include stimulants, anabolic agents, selective androgen receptor modulators, diuretics, anorectics, and β2 agonists.[69] Strict liability codes mean that a positive urine test can trigger a doping rule violation with potentially serious impact on the athlete's career, livelihood, and reputation, despite unintentional intake or minute (ineffective) doses. Third-party auditing of products can help elite athletes to make informed choices about supplement use but cannot provide an absolute guarantee of product safety.[69] Active individuals are encouraged to make a well-considered decision, based on consideration of their specific situation and issues (see Fig. 6.3).

VII. CURRENT ISSUES IN SPORTS NUTRITION: COMMENTARIES ON TOPICAL CONTROVERSIES IN SPORTS NUTRITION

A. Commentary 1: "Train Low" for Optimal Training Adaptations: When Less is More

Although current recommendations promote exercise under conditions of optimal nutritional support (e.g., adequate fluid and macronutrients) to enhance performance, recently sport practices have focused on the potential advantages of training with "low" nutrient availability. Scientific techniques now allow us to study the cellular responses to exercise and nutrient stimuli. Such techniques have provided the insight that the provision of nutrient support promotes optimal function and then quickly restores homeostasis and exercise capacity in the postexercise period ("train harder" strategies). Meanwhile, the absence or deliberate withdrawal of nutritional support may increase the exercise stress/stimuli and enhance or prolong signaling pathways

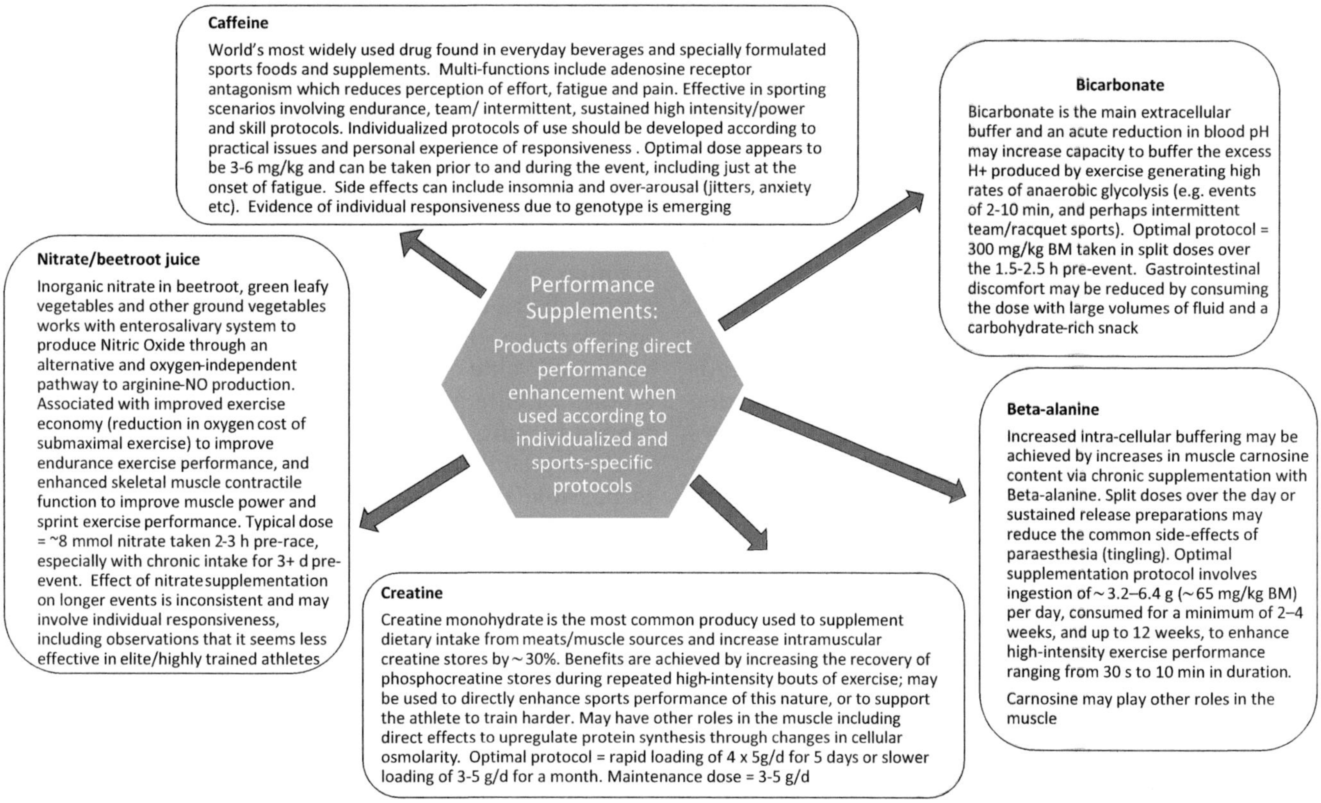

Caffeine
World's most widely used drug found in everyday beverages and specially formulated sports foods and supplements. Multi-functions include adenosine receptor antagonism which reduces perception of effort, fatigue and pain. Effective in sporting scenarios involving endurance, team/ intermittent, sustained high intensity/power and skill protocols. Individualized protocols of use should be developed according to practical issues and personal experience of responsiveness . Optimal dose appears to be 3-6 mg/kg and can be taken prior to and during the event, including just at the onset of fatigue. Side effects can include insomnia and over-arousal (jitters, anxiety etc). Evidence of individual responsiveness due to genotype is emerging
Bicarbonate
Bicarbonate is the main extracellular buffer and an acute reduction in blood pH may increase capacity to buffer the excess H+ produced by exercise generating high rates of anaerobic glycolysis (e.g. events of 2-10 min, and perhaps intermittent team/racquet sports). Optimal protocol = 300 mg/kg BM taken in split doses over the 1.5-2.5 h pre-event. Gastrointestinal discomfort may be reduced by consuming the dose with large volumes of fluid and a carbohydrate-rich snack
Nitrate/beetroot juice
Inorganic nitrate in beetroot, green leafy vegetables and other ground vegetables works with enterosalivary system to produce Nitric Oxide through an alternative and oxygen-independent pathway to arginine-NO production. Associated with improved exercise economy (reduction in oxygen cost of submaximal exercise) to improve endurance exercise performance, and enhanced skeletal muscle contractile function to improve muscle power and sprint exercise performance. Typical dose = ~8 mmol nitrate taken 2-3 h pre-race, especially with chronic intake for 3+ d pre-event. Effect of nitrate supplementation on longer events is inconsistent and may involve individual responsiveness, including observations that it seems less effective in elite/highly trained athletes
Performance Supplements:
Products offering direct performance enhancement when used according to individualized and sports-specific protocols
Beta-alanine
Increased intra-cellular buffering may be achieved by increases in muscle carnosine content via chronic supplementation with Beta-alanine. Split doses over the day or sustained release preparations may reduce the common side-effects of paraesthesia (tingling). Optimal supplementation protocol involves ingestion of ~ 3.2–6.4 g (~ 65 mg/kg BM) per day, consumed for a minimum of 2–4 weeks, and up to 12 weeks, to enhance high-intensity exercise performance ranging from 30 s to 10 min in duration.
Carnosine may play other roles in the muscle
Creatine
Creatine monohydrate is the most common producy used to supplement dietary intake from meats/muscle sources and increase intramuscular creatine stores by ~ 30%. Benefits are achieved by increasing the recovery of phosphocreatine stores during repeated high-intensity bouts of exercise; may be used to directly enhance sports performance of this nature, or to support the athlete to train harder. May have other roles in the muscle including direct effects to upregulate protein synthesis through changes in cellular osmolarity. Optimal protocol = rapid loading of 4 x 5g/d for 5 days or slower loading of 3-5 g/d for a month. Maintenance dose = 3-5 g/d

FIGURE 6.2 Performance supplements: products offering direct performance enhancement when used according to individualized and sports-specific protocols. *Taken with permission from Ref. 80.*

Making good decisions about performance supplements:
The decision tree approach
Age/maturation/experience? Resources? Sporting Goals? Other items ticked off, medical indications....
Is it the right time for me to consider?
Yes
No
Don't use
Is there scientific evidence that it Works for my event? Do I know the Right protocol? Have I trialed it?
Does it work?
Yes
No
Don't use
Are there any side effects from using this product? Will it interact with anything else I am doing?
Is it safe?
Yes
No
Don't use
Does it contain banned substances? Has it been tested for banned substances? Is it otherwise low risk?
Is it permitted?
Yes
No
Don't use
Consider use

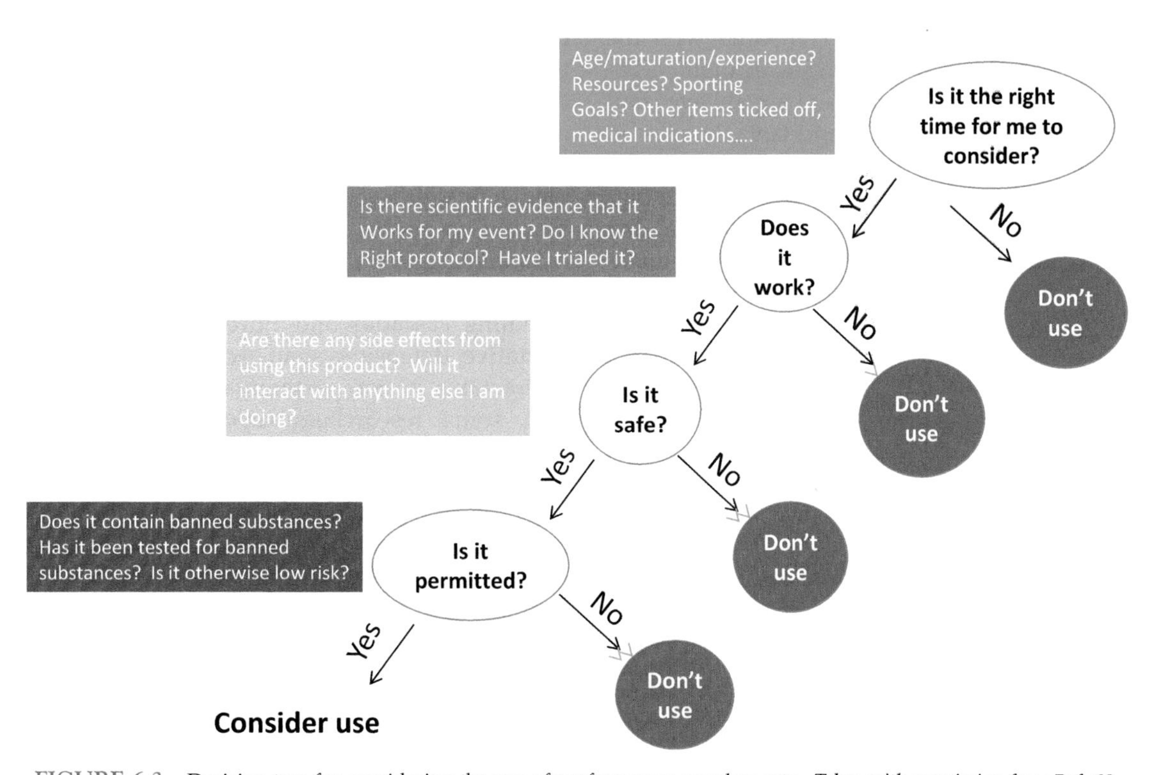

FIGURE 6.3 Decision tree for considering the use of performance supplements. *Taken with permission from Ref. 69.*

that remodel the muscle and other physiological systems to enhance the training response (a "train smarter" approach). There is evidence that although fluid intake enhances endurance performance in the heat, deliberate exposure to dehydration during an exercise session may enhance the physiological and cardiovascular processes of acclimatization.[81] Nevertheless, the area in which most investigation has been undertaken around the theme of strategic addition or withholding of nutritional support involves the manipulation of carbohydrate availability.

In addition to its contribution to the substrate needs of exercise, glycogen plays important roles in regulating the cellular activities that underpin the muscle's response to exercise.[82] Specifically, undertaking a bout of endurance exercise with low muscle glycogen stores produces a coordinated upregulation of key signaling and regulatory proteins in the muscle to enhance the adaptive processes following the exercise session.[83] Strategies that restrict exogenous carbohydrate availability (e.g., training in a fasted state) also promote an improved signaling response, although of a lower magnitude than is the case for exercise with low glycogen stores.[83] These strategies (summarized in Table 6.4) enhance the cellular outcomes of endurance training such as increased maximal mitochondrial enzyme activities and/or mitochondrial content and increased rates of lipid oxidation.

Studies in subelite athletes (e.g., highly fit individuals), in which these protocols have been superimposed on most workouts in a training block, show evidence of enhanced cellular adaptation.[84,85] Somewhat curiously, however, these "muscle advantages" have not transferred to superior performance outcomes compared with the improvements seen following training with high carbohydrate availability.[84,85] Although there are always challenges in measuring small but important changes in sports performance, the most likely explanation for the "disconnect" between mechanistic and performance outcomes is that training with low carbohydrate availability increases the perception of effort and reduces the intensity of the training sessions.[84,85] In other words, although metabolic benefits were achieved, they were negated by the interference to training quality. This suggests that "train low" strategies need to be carefully integrated into the periodized training program to match the specific goal of the session and the larger goals of the training period; this concept is described as "fueling for the work required."[86]

More recently, the withholding of carbohydrate during early recovery to delay glycogen resynthesis has been shown to upregulate markers of mitochondrial biogenesis and lipid oxidation during the recovery phase without interfering with the quality of the session (see Refs. 83,86). The practical application of this new strategy is that it allows the sequencing of (1) a "train high" high-quality training session, (2) overnight or within day carbohydrate restriction ("sleep low"), and (3) a moderate-intensity workout undertaken without carbohydrate intake ("train low") (see Table 6.4). The integration of several cycles of such periodized carbohydrate availability into the weekly training programs of subelite athletes has been shown to improve performance, whereas such benefits were not observed in a control group who undertook similar training with a similar intake of carbohydrate that was evenly distributed within and between days.[87] Such an approach has also been described in the real-life preparation of elite endurance athletes.[88] Nevertheless, studies of elite athletes appear to show fewer performance benefits from strategies to periodize carbohydrate availability than seen in subelite athletes.[89,90] It is possible that elite athletes have a reduced ceiling for improvements making differences harder to detect, or they have an ability to undertake training of such intensity and volume that the stimulus already maximizes the adaptive response. Further investigation is merited, but it is likely that most highly trained athletes already integrate some form of periodization of carbohydrate availability within their schedules, either by design or practicality. The challenge for sports science will be to improve on what athletes achieve through trial and error.

Finally, exercise is known to increase the production of free oxygen and nitrogen radical species (RNOS), which in excess are thought to contribute to acute impairment of the muscle's ability to produce force and long-term inflammation, damage, and soreness.[91] While increasing cellular antioxidant capacity via antioxidant supplementation seems logical to counteract the negative effects of RNOS on muscle force capability, the research examining antioxidant supplementation in acute or chronic exercise models is equivocal with respect to muscle damage or performance outcomes.[92,93] Newer insights indicate that only excessive oxidative damage is problematic and that small and confined oxidative changes in the muscle fulfill an important role in the adaptation to exercise. For example, inducing signaling cascades and upregulating the endogenous oxidative defense system, which consists of complex interactions of compartmentalized antioxidants.[65,93] In fact, some researchers report that supplementation with isolated antioxidants such as vitamin C and/or E can actually reduce the benefits of exercise training.[94,95]

The most recent dietary recommendations for athletes and active individuals promote the benefits of a varied diet including a range of antioxidant- and phytochemical-containing fruits and vegetables. Nevertheless, research continues to investigate potential benefits from the consumption of specific food phytochemicals, including polyphenols,[96] which may contribute a range of functions including effects on the immune system, the antiinflammatory response, and mitochondrial biogenesis.

TABLE 6.4 Dietary strategies for training with low carbohydrate availability.

"Train Low" strategies undertaken to increase the exercise stimulus and/or to enhance the adaptive response to an exercise bout (see 102)	
Strategy	**Protocol**
Acute (session-by-session) exposure to low carbohydrate availability	
Acute low carbohydrate availability training ("train low")—endogenous	• Undertaking prior bout of prolonged sustained or intermittent exercise followed by restricted intake of carbohydrate to limit glycogen resynthesis during recovery phase. Note that it is the second session that is done as a "train low" session, and the between session recovery phase can be brief (1–2 h) or prolonged (e.g., overnight or full day)
Acute low carbohydrate availability training ("train low")—exogenous	• Undertaking workout in the morning in a fasted state and without any carbohydrate intake during the session. • (Note: Could also be done for a session later only water during the session)
Acute postexercise low carbohydrate availability ("recover low" or "sleep low"—if overnight)	• Restricting carbohydrate intake in the hours after a key workout to delay glycogen resynthesis.
Strategic sequencing or periodization of carbohydrate availability	
"Sleep low sequencing"	• A practical application of this new strategy is that it allows the sequencing of (1) a "train high" high-quality training session, (2) overnight or within day carbohydrate restriction ("sleep low"), and (3) a moderate-intensity workout undertaken without carbohydrate intake ("train low").
Chronic adaptation to low carbohydrate availability (e.g. FAT ADAPTATION)	
Chronic low carbohydrate availability (achieves low endogenous and exogenous carbohydrate availability)	• Ketogenic low-carbohydrate, high-fat (LCHF) diet (< 50 g/day carbohydrate; ~ 80% energy as fat) • Non-ketogenic LCHF diet (15%–20% energy as carbohydrate; 60%–65% energy as fat)

B. Commentary 2. The Resurgence of Ketogenic Low-Carbohydrate, High-Fat Diets for Endurance Performance

In many events, success is determined by the muscle's ability to optimize the production of adenosine triphosphate (ATP) to meet the requirements of the exercise task. This reflects both the size of the available fuel stores and the muscle's ability to efficiently use these fuels. It has been hypothesized that strategies that improve an individual's capacity to utilize their larger fat stores will spare the muscle glycogen stores and enhance endurance performance.[97] Although training achieves this outcome, the use of fat as a muscle fuel can be further increased by adapting to a low-carbohydrate, high-fat (LCHF) diet. Indeed, short-term (~5 d) exposure to a diet providing <20% energy from carbohydrate and > 60% from fat while undertaking both high-volume and high-intensity training sessions achieves a robust retooling of the muscle to increase the mobilization, transport, and oxidation of fat during exercise.[98] If this high-fat diet is further restricted in carbohydrate (<50 g/day) with 75%–80% energy provided by fat, additional benefits from exposure to high levels of circulating ketone bodies are also claimed; this ketogenic LCHF diet has recently resurfaced in popular interest.[97] Despite considerable discussion about this diet being "the future of elite endurance sport" in lay and social media, there is no evidence that it enhances the performance of high-performance endurance athletes. Chronic (>3–4 weeks) adaptation to the ketogenic LCHF clearly increases the muscle's capacity for fat oxidation during exercise, providing effective fuel support for moderate-intensity exercise.[99] However, a recent study[89] that adapted elite race walkers to the LCHF over this time period provided a reminder of an important biochemical fact: the oxygen demand of fat oxidation to produce a given amount of ATP is greater than that of carbohydrate. Although the group of highly trained to world class race walkers was observed to achieve the highest rates of fat oxidation ever reported in the literature across a range of speeds relevant to the races on the Olympic program, this was associated with a loss of economy (a greater oxygen was required to walk at the same speed). In contrast to a control group of athletes who improved their performance of a real-life 10,000 km track race by ~ 6% following a 3 week training block supported by strategic or chronic carbohydrate availability, the LCHF made no performance gains despite improving their aerobic capacity to a similar extent.[89] These results were attributed, at least partially, to reduced walking economy and a limit on the intensity of exercise that can be supported by fat oxidation due to the limits of the muscle's oxygen supply. This suggests that adaptation to LCHF may be suited to athletes who compete in events conducted entirely at moderate intensities. However, LCHF may provide a disadvantage to endurance sports and ultraendurance sports involving critical passages of high-intensity work, where success is determined by the ability to exercise as economically as possible at the highest sustainable intensity.

C. Commentary 3. Low Energy Availability, Female Athlete Triad, and Relative Energy Deficiency in Sport

The term Female Athlete Triad was first coined in the 1990s to describe the coincidental presence of eating disorders, amenorrhea, and osteoporosis in female athletes and the relationships among these problems.[100] Later, the syndrome was updated to describe the interrelatedness of three issues of energy availability, menstrual health, and bone health in female athletes with each of these factors existing in a continuum between optimal function and a clinical disorder.[101] Female athletes were encouraged to regard movement toward the negative end of any of these spectra as unwelcome and to seek early intervention for such changes. A major change involved the recognition that low energy availability rather than eating disorders per se provided a key dietary input. A mismatch between energy intake, energy committed to exercise, and the energy cost of healthy body function can certainly occur in athletes with disordered eating, representing psychological issues. However, other causes could be considered simply misguided (e.g., an overzealous weight-loss campaign to achieve a justified change in body composition) or inadvertent (failure to recognize or respond to a sudden increase in training volume).[3] Indeed, other very specific causes have been identified in special populations, such as food insecurity due to poor finances among East African distance runners.[102]

Further research and real-life observations have led to a continual evolution of our knowledge and messaging about the causes and effects of low energy availability. This includes recognition that the relationships between the variables in the Female Athlete Triad are not as predictable or tightly associated as previously indicated. Indeed, both the errors and resources involved in undertaking an assessment of energy availability in free-living populations make it useful as a concept rather than a strict diagnostic tool.[103] Furthermore, although original research had suggested that there were bands or thresholds that could predict the likely healthy and unhealthy ranges of energy availability (see Table 6.5), recent research suggests that these thresholds should be used as a very general guide only.[104] Although such research suggests that the likelihood of health problems increases with the reduction in

TABLE 6.5 Illustrating different levels of energy availability in sport.

Situation	Energy availability (energy intake − energy cost of exercise[a]) relative to the athlete's fat-free mass (FFM)	Examples
Weight gain, growth, hypertrophy	>45 kcal (189 kJ) per kg FFM	Swimmer A: 65 kg (20% body fat = 80% FFM); weekly training = 5600 kcal (23.5 MJ); daily energy intake = 3520 kcal (14.7 MJ) Energy availability = (3520 − 800 kcal)/(0.8 * 65) = 52 kcal/kg FFM (219 kJ)
Weight/physique maintenance and optimal health and function	~45 kcal (189 kJ) per kg FFM	Swimmer B: 65 kg (15% body fat = 85% FFM); weekly training = 5600 kcal (2.35 MJ); daily energy intake = 3285 kcal (13.8 MJ) Energy availability = (3285−800 kcal)/(0.85 * 65) = 45 kcal/kg FFM (189 kJ)
Healthy weight loss (or weight maintenance at reduced metabolic rate)	30−45 kcal (125−189 kJ) per kg FFM Note that this range of energy availability is no longer considered free of risk of suboptimal function of all body systems, and other factors may interact with energy availability to protect against or exacerbate health outcomes.	Runner C: 55 kg (20% body fat = 80% FFM); weekly training = 5600 kcal (23.5 MJ); daily energy intake = 2340 kcal (9.8 MJ) Energy availability = (2340 − 800 kcal)/(0.8 * 55) = 35 kcal/kg FFM (164 kJ)
Low energy availability—health implications	<30 kcal (125 kJ) per kg FFM Note that although there may not be an exact threshold below which the effects of low energy availability are observed, a greater risk of various problems is found as energy availability is reduced.	Runner D: 55 kg (25% body fat = 75% FFM); weekly training = 5600 kcal (2.35 MJ); daily energy intake = 1880 kcal (7.9 MJ) Energy availability = (1880−800 kcal)/(0.75 * 55) = 26 kcal/kg FFM (110 kJ)

[a]*Note that the energy expenditure associated with training should only include the energy cost above that of resting metabolic rate that is incurred due to the exercise.*

energy availability, neither thresholds nor universal relationships between the three axes of the Female Athlete Triad are always seen.[104]

The recognition that a larger range of health problems can occur in association with low energy availability, and are also observed in males, led to the development of a larger umbrella term to describe this syndrome: RED-S. RED-S recognizes that low energy deficiency is associated with increased risk of illness and injury, cardiovascular complications, gastrointestinal disturbances, and reduced performance.[105] While further work is needed to better harmonize the positioning of syndromes, the greater need is for evolution in the science and practice of prevention and treatment of the problems associated with low energy availability.

VIII. CONCLUSION

Athletes and active individuals have different energy, nutrient, and fluid needs compared to their sedentary peers. First, they need to consume adequate energy to meet the energy demands of exercise training and competition, normal energy costs of daily living, and growth, tissue building and repair, and reproduction needs. These energy needs will change over time depending on the training or exercise schedule maintained, competition times, and physique goals. Carbohydrate needs increase to provide fuel and replace glycogen, while protein requirements increase to meet muscle adaptations, building, and repair. Second, athletes and active individuals need to maintain a body size and composition that maximizes sport performance, yet it is achievable without increasing the risk of disordered eating or low energy availability and its consequences. Third, to stay healthy and injury free, an active individual needs to be adequately fueled, with a diet that meets macro- and micronutrient needs. Fourth, training and competitive events are physiological demanding and require individualized food and fluid recommendations before, during, and after exercise, to reduce/delay fatigue and allow for optimal performance. Postexercise recovery nutrition should restore fuel and fluids homeostasis, preparing the body for the next exercise event. Finally, exercise training and competitive events create practical challenges, including accessibility of suitable foods and fluids at the right time around exercise and making good choices regarding supplements and sport foods.

RESEARCH GAPS

- Energy and nutrient needs of active growing individuals
- Precise tools for assessing energy availability and making a diagnosis of low energy availability in female and male athletes and active individuals
- Differences in the susceptibility to outcomes related to low energy availability within and between active males and females
- The effect of the caliber of the athlete (e.g., elite vs. recreational) and the level of training (highly and specifically trained vs. generally active) on the effectiveness of various nutrition strategies (e.g., fueling for events, performance supplements)
- The use of evidence-based performance supplements as it often needs to be implemented in real-life sport (e.g., use of several supplements at the same time, whether they can be used more than once in a certain time frame such as the heats and finals of an event in the same day)
- Whether strategies that create positive changes in a muscle cell (e.g., training with low glycogen) transfer to a change in sports performance
- Whether genetic differences in individuals lead to different responses to sports nutrition strategies and require a "personalized nutrition" approach
- Safe and effective ways to change body composition to reduce body fat while maximizing lean mass (or minimizing its loss)
- The effect of exercise and sports participation on the microbiome
- Strategies to address the gut dysfunction and damage that occurs in some sporting activities to improve health and comfort during exercise, as well as allow
- Whether special diets (e.g., ketogenic LCHF, vegan, paleo) offer any advantages to the athletes or active individual. Which types of sporting activities or issues may benefit and which may be harmed? Which aspects of a diet might be useful for health and performance and which should be ignored?

IX. REFERENCES

1. Burke LM. Energy needs of athletes. *Can J Appl Physiol.* 2001;26:S202–S219.
2. Saris WHM, Van Erp-Baart MA, Brouns F, et al. Study on food intake and energy expenditure during extreme sustained exercise: the Tour de France. *Int J Sports Med.* 1989;10:S26–S31.
3. Loucks AB. Energy balance and body composition in sports and exercise. *J Sports Sci.* 2004;22:1–14.
4. Loucks AB, Verdun M, Heath EM. Low energy availability, not stress of exercise, alters LH pulsatility in exercising women. *J Appl Physiol.* 1998;84:37–46.
5. Cialdella-Kam L, Guebels CP, Maddalozzo GF, Manore MM. Dietary intervention restored menses in female athletes with exercise-associated menstrual dysfunction with limited impact on bone and muscle health. *Nutrients.* 2014;6:3018–3039.
6. O'Connor H, Olds T, Maughan RJ. Physique and performance for track and field events. *J Sports Sci.* 2007;25(Suppl 1):49S–60S.
7. Reale R, Slater G, Burke LM. Individualized dietary strategies for Olympic combat sports: acute weight loss, recovery and competition nutrition. *Eur J Sport Sci.* 2017;17:727–740.
8. Walberg Rankin J, Gibson J. Making weight. In: Burke L, Deakin V, eds. *Clinical Sports Nutrition.* 5th ed. Sydney, AU: McGraw-Hill; 2015:191–233.
9. Jeacocke NA, Beals KA. Eating disorders and disordered eating in athletes. In: Burke L, Deakin V, eds. *Clinical Sports Nutrition.* 5th ed. Sydney, AU: McGraw-Hill; 2015:213–233.
10. O'Connor H, Honey A, Caterson I. Weight loss and the athlete. In: Burke L, Deakin V, eds. *Clinical Sports Nutrition.* 5th ed. Sydney, AU: McGraw-Hill; 2015:164–190.
11. Burke LM. Weight-making sports. In: *Practical Sports Nutrition.* Champaign, IL: Human Kinetics; 2007:289–312.
12. Hector AJ, Phillips SM. Protein recommendations for weight loss in elite athletes: a focus on body composition and performance. *Int J Sport Nutr Exerc Metabol.* 2018;28:170–177.
13. Witard OC, Garthe I, Phillips SM. Dietary protein for training adaptation and body composition manipulation in track and field athletes. *Int J Sport Nutr Exerc Metabol.* 2019;29:165–174.
14. Stellingwerff T. Case study: body composition periodization in an Olympic-level female middle-distance runner over a 9-year career. *Int J Sport Nutr Exerc Metabol.* 2018;28:428–433.

15. Slater GJ, Dieter BP, Marsh DJ, et al. Is an energy surplus required to maximize skeletal muscle hypertrophy associated with resistance training. *Front Nutr.* 2019;6:131. https://doi.org/10.3389/fnut.2019.00131.
16. Burd NA, Tang JE, Moore DR, et al. Exercise training and protein metabolism: influences of contraction, protein intake, and sex-based differences. *J Appl Physiol.* 2009;106:1692–1701.
17. Walsh NP, Gleeson M, Shephard RJ, et al. Position statement part one: immune function and exercise. *Exerc Immunol Rev.* 2011;17:6–63.
18. Walsh NP, Gleeson M, Pyne DB, et al. Position statement part two: maintaining immune health. *Exerc Immunol Rev.* 2011;17:64–103.
19. Brouns FJPH, Saris WHM, Ten Hoor F. Dietary problems in the case of strenuous exertion. *J Sports Med.* 1986;26:306–319.
20. Bennell KL, Malcolm SA, Wark JD, et al. Models for the pathogenesis of stress fractures in athletes. *Br J Sports Med.* 1996;30:200–204.
21. Kerr D, Khan K, Bennell K. Bone, exercise and nutrition. In: Burke L, Deakin V, eds. *Clinical Sports Nutrition.* 4th ed. Sydney, AU: McGraw-Hill; 2010:200–221.
22. Campion F, Nevill AM, Karlsson MK, et al. Bone status in professional cyclists. *Int J Sports Med.* 2010;31:511–515.
23. Larson-Meyer DE, Willis KS. Vitamin D and athletes. *Curr Sports Med Rep.* 2010;9:220–226.
24. Owens DJ, Allison R, Close GL. Vitamin D and the athlete: current perspectives and new challenges. *Sports Med.* 2018;48(Suppl 1):3–16.
25. Coyle EF. Fluid and fuel intake during exercise. *J Sports Sci.* 2004;22:39–55.
26. Hawley JA, Schabort EJ, Noakes TD, et al. Carbohydrate-loading and exercise performance: an update. *Sports Med.* 1997;24:73–81.
27. Hargreaves M, Hawley JA, Jeukendrup AE. Pre-exercise carbohydrate and fat ingestion: effects on metabolism and performance. *J Sports Sci.* 2004;22:31–38.
28. O'Reilly J, Wong SH, Chen Y. Glycemic index, glycemic load and exercise performance. *Sports Med.* 2010;40:27–39.
29. Sawka MN, Burke LM, Eichner ER, et al. American college of sports medicine position stand. Exercise and fluid replacement. *Med Sci Sports Exerc.* 2007;39:377–390.
30. Burke LM, Hawley JA, Wong S, et al. Carbohydrates for training and competition. *J Sports Sci.* 2011;29(Supp 1):S17–S27.
31. Jeukendrup AE. Carbohydrate and exercise performance: the role of multiple transportable carbohydrates. *Curr Opin Clin Nutr Metab Care.* 2010;13:452–457.
32. Pfeiffer B, Stellingwerff T, Hodgson AB, et al. Nutritional intake and gastrointestinal problems during competitive endurance events. *Med Sci Sports Exerc.* 2012;44(2):344–351. https://doi.org/10.1249/MSS.0b013e31822dc809.
33. Smith JW, Pascoe DD, Passe DH. Curvilinear dose-response relationship of carbohydrate (0-120 g.h(-1)) and performance. *Med Sci Sports Exerc.* 2013;45(2):336–341.
34. Cox GR, Clark SA, Cox AJ, et al. Daily training with high carbohydrate availability increases exogenous carbohydrate oxidation during endurance cycling. *J Appl Physiol.* 2010;109:126–134.
35. Costa RJS, Miall A, Khoo A. Gut-training: the impact of two weeks repetitive gut-challenge during exercise on gastrointestinal status, glucose availability, fuel kinetics, and running performance. *Appl Physiol Nutr Metab.* 2017;42(5):547–557.
36. Jeukendrup AE, Chambers ES. Oral carbohydrate sensing and exercise performance. *Curr Opin Clin Nutr Metab Care.* 2010;13:447–451.
37. Chambers ES, Bridge MW, Jones DA. Carbohydrate sensing in the human mouth: effects on exercise performance and brain activity. *J Physiol.* 2009;587:1779–1794.
38. Burke LM, Maughan RJ. The Governor has a sweet tooth -mouth sensing of nutrients to enhance sports performance. *Eur J Sport Sci.* 2015;15(1):29–40.
39. Lane SC, Bird SR, Burke LM, et al. Effect of a carbohydrate mouth rinse on simulated cycling time-trial performance commenced in a fed or fasted state. *Appl Physiol Nutr Metab.* 2013;38(2):134–139.
40. Burke LM. Nutrition for competition. In: Stear S, Shirreffs SM, eds. *Sport and Exercise Nutrition.* London, UK: Wiley Publishers; 2011:200–216.
41. Thomas DT, Erdman KA, Burke LM. American College of Sports Medicine joint position statement. Nutrition and athletic performance. *Med Sci Sports Exerc.* 2016;48(3):543–568.
42. Montain SJ, Coyle EF. Influence of graded dehydration on hyperthermia and cardiovascular drift during exercise. *J Appl Physiol.* 1992;73:1340–1350.
43. Cheuvront SN, Kenefick RW. Dehydration: physiology, assessment, and performance effects. *Compr Physiol.* 2014;4(1):257–285.
44. Garth A, Burke L. What do athletes drink during competitive sporting activities? *Sports Med.* 2013;43:539–564.
45. Shirreffs SM, Sawka MN. Fluid needs during and after exercise. *J Sports Sci.* 2011;29:39–46.
46. Maughan RJ, Shirreffs SM. Development of individual hydration strategies for athletes. *Int J Sport Nutr Exerc Metabol.* 2008;18:457–472.
47. Kenefick RW. Drinking strategies: planned drinking versus drinking to thirst. *Sports Med.* 2018;48(Suppl 1):31–37.
48. Almond CSD, Shin AY, Fortescue EB, et al. Hyponatremia among runners in the Boston marathon. *N Engl J Med.* 2005;352:1550–1556.
49. Noakes TD. Overconsumption of fluid by athletes. *Br Med J.* 2003;327:113–114.
50. Noakes TD, Speedy DB. The aetiology of exercise-associated hyponatraemia is established and is not "mythical". *Br J Sports Med.* 2007b;41:111–113.
51. Noakes TD, Speedy DB. Lobbyists for the sports drink industry: an example of the rise of "contrarianism" in modern scientific debate. *Br J Sports Med.* 2007a;41:107–109.
52. Noakes TD, Speedy DB. Time for the American College of Sports Medicine to acknowledge that humans, like all other earthly creatures, do not need to be told how much to drink during exercise. *Br J Sports Med.* 2007c;41:109–111.
53. Casa DJ, Armstrong LE, Hillman SK, et al. National Athletic Trainers' Association position statement: fluid replacement for athletes. *J Athl Train.* 2000;35:212–224.
54. Goulet EDB. Comment on "drinking strategies: planned drinking versus drinking to thirst". *Sports Med.* 2018;49(4):631–633. https://doi.org/10.1007/s40279-018-0973-6.
55. Burke LM, Cox G. *The Complete Guide to Food for Sports Performance.* 3rd ed. Sydney, AU: Allen and Unwin; 2011.
56. Hew-Butler T, Rosner MH, Fowkes-Godek S, et al. Statement of the 3rd International Exercise-Associated Hyponatremia Consensus Development Conference, Carlsbad, California, 2015. *Br J Sports Med.* 2015;49(22):1432–1446.
57. Godek SF, Bartolozzi AR, Godek JJ. Sweat rate and fluid turnover in American football players compared with runners in a hot and humid environment. *Br J Sports Med.* 2005;39:205–211.
58. Godek SF, Peduzzi C, Burkholder R, et al. Sweat rates, sweat sodium concentrations, and sodium losses in 3 groups of professional football players. *J Athl Train.* 2010;4:364–371.
59. Eichner ER. The role of sodium in "heat cramping". *Sports Med.* 2007;37:368–370.
60. Schwellnus MP. Cause of exercise associated muscle cramps (EAMC)–altered neuromuscular control, dehydration or electrolyte depletion? *Br J Sports Med.* 2009;43:401–408.
61. Montain SJ, Cheuvront SN, Sawka MN. Exercise associated hyponatraemia: quantitative analysis to understand the aetiology. *Br J Sports Med.* 2006;40:98–105.

62. Shirreffs SM, Armstrong LE, Cheuvront SN. Fluid and electrolyte needs for preparation and recovery from training and competition. *J Sports Sci.* 2004;22:57–63.
63. Burke LM, Kiens B, Ivy JL. Carbohydrates and fat for training and recovery. *J Sports Sci.* 2004;22:15–30.
64. Coyle EF. Timing and method of increased carbohydrate intake to cope with heavy training, competition and recovery. *J Sports Sci.* 1991;9:29–52.
65. Hawley JA, Burke LM, Phillips SM, et al. Nutritional modulation of training-induced skeletal muscle adaptation. *J Appl Physiol.* 2011;110:834–845.
66. Moore DR, Robinson MJ, Fry JL, et al. Ingested protein dose response of muscle and albumin protein synthesis after resistance exercise in young men. *Am J Clin Nutr.* 2009;89:161–168.
67. Res PT, Groen B, Pennings B, et al. Protein ingestion before sleep improves postexercise overnight recovery. *Med Sci Sports Exerc.* 2012;44(8):1560–1569.
68. Gillen JB, Trommelen J, Wardenaar FC, et al. Dietary protein intake and distribution patterns of well-trained Dutch athletes. *Int J Sport Nutr Exerc Metabol.* 2017;27:105–114.
69. Maughan RJ, Burke LM, Dvorak J, et al. IOC Consensus Statement: dietary supplements and the high-performance athlete. *Br J Sports Med.* 2018;52:439–455.
70. Peeling P, Binnie MJ, Goods PSR, et al. Evidence-based supplements for the enhancement of athletic performance. *Int J Sport Nutr Exerc Metabol.* 2018;28:178–187.
71. Burke LM. Caffeine and sports performance. *Appl Physiol Nutr Metab.* 2008;33:1319–1334.
72. Pickering C, Grgic J. Caffeine and exercise: what next? *Sports Med.* 2019;49(7):1007–1030.
73. Carr AJ, Hopkins WG, Gore CJ. Effects of acute alkalosis and acidosis on performance: a meta-analysis. *Sports Med.* 2011;41(10):801–814.
74. Hadzic M, Eckstein ML, Schugardt M. The impact of sodium bicarbonate on performance in response to exercise duration in athletes: a systematic review. *J Sports Sci Med.* 2019;18(2):271–281.
75. Saunders B, Elliott-Sale K, Artioli GG, et al. βeta-alanine supplementation to improve exercise capacity and performance: a systematic review and meta-analysis. *Br J Sports Med.* 2017;51(8):658–669.
76. Kreider RB, Kalman DS, Antonio J, et al. International Society of Sports Nutrition position stand: safety and efficacy of creatine supplementation in exercise, sport, and medicine. *J Int Soc Sports Nutr.* 2017;14:18. https://doi.org/10.1186/s12970-017-0173-z.
77. Jones AM. Influence of dietary nitrate on the physiological determinants of exercise performance: a critical review. *Appl Physiol Nutr Metab.* 2014;39(9):1019–1028.
78. Van De Walle GP, Vukovich MD. The effect of nitrate supplementation on exercise tolerance and performance: a systematic review and meta-analysis. *J Strength Cond Res.* 2018;32(6):1796–1808.
79. Geyer H, Parr MK, Koehler K, et al. Nutritional supplements cross-contaminated and faked with doping substances. *J Mass Spectrom.* 2008;43:892–902.
80. Burke LM. Supplements for optimal sports performance. *Curr Opin Physiol.* 2019;10:156–165.
81. Garrett AT, Goosens NG, Rehrer NJ, et al. Short-term heat acclimation is effective and may be enhanced rather than impaired by dehydration. *Am J Human Biol.* 2014;26(3):311–320.
82. Philp A, Hargreaves M, Baar K. More than a store: regulatory roles for glycogen in skeletal muscle adaptation to exercise. *Am J Physiol Endocrinol Metab.* 2012;302(11). E1343–1351.
83. Bartlett JD, Hawley JA, Morton JP. Carbohydrate availability and exercise training adaptation: too much of a good thing? *Eur J Sport Sci.* 2015;15(1):3–12.
84. Hulston CJ, Venables MC, Mann CH, et al. Training with low muscle glycogen enhances fat metabolism in well-trained cyclists. *Med Sci Sports Exerc.* 2010;42(11):2046–2055.
85. Yeo WK, Paton CD, Garnham AP, et al. Skeletal muscle adaptation and performance responses to once a day versus twice every second day endurance training regimens. *J Appl Physiol.* 2008;105(5):1462–1470.
86. Impey SG, Hearris MA, Hammond KM, et al. Fuel for the work required: a theoretical framework for carbohydrate periodization and the glycogen threshold hypothesis. *Sports Med.* 2018;48(5):1031–1048.
87. Marquet LA, Brisswalter J, Louis J, et al. Enhanced endurance performance by periodization of carbohydrate intake: "sleep low" strategy. *Med Sci Sports Exerc.* 2016;48:663–672.
88. Stellingwerff T. Contemporary nutrition approaches to optimize elite marathon performance. *Int J Sports Physiol Perform.* 2013;8:573–578.
89. Burke LM, Ross ML, Garvican-Lewis LA. Low carbohydrate, high fat diet impairs exercise economy and negates the performance benefit from intensified training in elite race walkers. *J Physiol.* 2017;595(9):2785–2807.
90. Gejl KD, Thams L, Hansen M, et al. No superior adaptations to carbohydrate periodization in elite endurance athletes. *Med Sci Sports Exerc.* 2017;49(12):2486–2497.
91. Konig D, Wagner KH, Elmadfa I, et al. Exercise and oxidative stress: significance of antioxidants with reference to inflammatory, muscular, and systemic stress. *Exerc Immunol Rev.* 2001;7:108–133.
92. Fisher-Wellman K, Bloomer RL. Acute exercise and oxidative stress: a 30 year history. *Dyn Med.* 2009;8:1. https://doi.org/10.1186/1476-5918-8-1.
93. Merry TL, Ristow M. Do antioxidant supplements interfere with skeletal muscle adaptation to exercise training? *J Physiol.* 2016;594(18):5135–5147.
94. Gomez-Cabrera MC, Domenech E, Romagnoli M. Oral administration of vitamin C decreases muscle mitochondrial biogenesis and hampers training-induced adaptations in endurance performance. *Am J Clin Nutr.* 2008;87:142–149.
95. Ristow M, Zarse K, Oberbach A, et al. Antioxidants prevent health promoting effects of physical exercise in humans. *Proc Natl Acad Sci Unit States Am.* 2009;106:8665–8670.
96. Bowtell J, Kelly V. fruit-derived polyphenol supplementation for athlete recovery and performance. *Sports Med.* 2019;49(Suppl 1):3–23.
97. Volek JS, Noakes T, Phinney SD. Rethinking fat as a fuel for endurance exercise. *Eur J Sport Sci.* 2015;15(1):13–20.
98. Burke LM. Re-examining high-fat diets for sports performance: did we call the "nail in the coffin" too soon? *Sports Med.* 2015;15(Suppl 1):S33–S49.
99. Phinney SD, Bistrian BR, Evans WJ, et al. The human metabolic response to chronic ketosis without caloric restriction: preservation of submaximal exercise capability with reduced carbohydrate oxidation. *Metabolism.* 1983;32(8):769–776.
100. Otis CL, Drinkwater B, Johnson M, et al. American College of Sports Medicine position stand. The female athlete triad. *Med Sci Sports Exerc.* 1997;29:i–ix.
101. Nattiv A, Loucks AB, Manore MM, et al. American College of Sports Medicine position stand. The female athlete triad. *Med Sci Sports Exerc.* 2007;39:1867–1882.
102. Burke LM, Close GL, Lundy B, et al. Relative energy deficiency in sport in male athletes: a commentary on its presentation among selected groups of male athletes. *Int J Sport Nutr Exerc Metabol.* 2018;28(4):364–374.
103. Burke LM, Lundy B, Fahrenholtz IL, et al. Pitfalls of conducting and interpreting estimates of energy availability in free-living athletes. *Int J Sport Nutr Exerc Metabol.* 2018;28(4):350–363.
104. Lieberman JL, De Souza MJ, Wagstaff DA, et al. Menstrual disruption with exercise is not linked to an energy availability threshold. *Med Sci Sports Exerc.* 2018;50(3):551–561.
105. Mountjoy M, Sundgot-Borgen JK, Burke LM, et al. IOC consensus statement on relative energy deficiency in sport (RED-S): 2018 update. *Br J Sports Med.* 2018;52(11):687–697.

CHAPTER

7

A RATION IS NOT FOOD UNTIL IT IS EATEN: NUTRITION LESSONS LEARNED FROM FEEDING SOLDIERS

Karl E. Friedl[1], *PhD*
E. Wayne Askew[2], *PhD*
David D. Schnakenberg[3], *PhD*

[1]US Army Research Institute of Environmental Medicine, Natick, MA, United States
[2]Department of Nutrition and Integrative Physiology, College of Health, University of Utah, Salt Lake City, UT, United States
[3]Historian of Military Nutrition Science, Vienna, VA, United States

SUMMARY

Nutrition science in the United States has been shaped by national security needs, specifically the need to feed armies to sustain their performance in the face of adversity. In the 20th century, Army nutrition research provided foundational data on metabolic requirements of healthy men and women, developed important methodologies for laboratory and field nutrition surveys, and led national efforts on performance in extreme environments. The study of human metabolism in challenging environments has proven to be an enduring need for the Army, and this requires unique capabilities with embedded soldier-scientists conducting credible studies in relevant field environments. Support for military nutrition research periodically surged during the 20th century, including reincarnations in the 1940 and 1980s when nutritional physiologists were colocated with food developers. Major findings repeatedly centered on the challenges of inadequate energy intakes in all extreme environments rather than identifying any unique needs for specific ration components.

Keywords: 20th century; Dietary supplements; Energy metabolism; Federally funded research; Military rations; Return on research investment; Scientometrics.

I. INTRODUCTION

Dr. Ancel Keys had preceded us in the desert. He reported favorably on K-rations. But we followed the path of a maneuvering unit by the trail of discarded K biscuits. Even small desert rodents avoided them. Experts who designed the ration must have thought in terms of animal husbandry. They concluded that each ration each day should have the liberal allowance of vitamins, etc., recommended by the Food and Nutrition Board. To get such constituents within the physical requirements for an emergency ration, brewer's yeast, soybean flour, and liver extract had to be added. This was not what one would recommend offhand for flavor. The Surgeon General of the Army commanded me to write a critique of Army emergency rations.

The resulting document had all the earmarks of genius ... First, a ration is no good if it is not eaten ... The second radical discovery was that soldiers are people and eat things they are familiar with more readily than exotic ones, and variation, not monotony, encourages eating. ***William B. Bean, 1968.***[1]

William Bean was one of the many young medical researchers whose career paths were abruptly diverted to solve problems of soldier health and performance to help win World War II. Almost overnight, task-organized labs were assembled, with multidisciplinary expertise representing medicine, physiology, engineering, chemistry, public health, and any other specialty that was available

https://doi.org/10.1016/B978-0-12-818460-8.00007-1

and might be useful. Bean was assigned to the Armored Medical Research Laboratory, in Fort Knox, Kentucky, where the "science war" forged a new generation of biomedical scientists. Allied successes relied heavily on technological advances, ranging from development of antibiotics to nuclear weapons.[1,2] It also produced a new generation of nutrition scientists for the nation.[3]

Nutrition research is a national security priority because of the need to fuel an army of soldiers, sustain their morale with palatable rations, and ensure that they are metabolically fit and ready for unpredictable challenges in the widest possible range of environments. This is an enduring need because the army that discovers a way to fuel their soldiers more effectively has the advantage of greater lethality through more capable warfighters. Problem-solving for the US Army also typically has broader benefits in the form of "dual use" applications. The often-cited development of canning technology to preserve rations for Napoleon's army is just one example of how military technology advances have impacted society. In World War I, concern about military food waste led to studies that provided substantive data on the energy requirements of active, young men who are still valid today, confirmed with doubly labeled water and other techniques in free-living individuals.[4,5] General concepts that now seem obvious also emerged from Army research needs, such as the seminal World War II studies on "man in the desert" that highlighted the importance of maintaining hydration instead of trying to train the body to water restriction.[6,7] National defense needs were the motivation for Congress to enact legislation to establish the School Lunch Program after World War II, based on the observation that too many American children were chronically malnourished and would not be qualified for military service.[8] The Army Office of the Surgeon General sponsored Ancel Keys' classic Minnesota Starvation Study to understand how to refeed semistarved soldiers returning from prisoner-of-war camps and starving postwar civilian populations. Researchers today still use the published data from this truly unique experiment to test and validate human metabolic models.[9] The concept and methodological foundation of the National Health and Nutrition Examination Survey (NHANES) is directly traceable to the international nutrition survey assistance programs conducted by the Army in the postwar period and later efforts organized under the Interdepartmental Committee of Nutrition for National Defense (ICNND).[10–12] The military nutritional surveys drove advances in understanding micronutrient deficiencies and the substantial elimination of previously common diseases such as scurvy, pellagra, and beriberi in this country and others.[13] Military research produced the methods for body composition assessment used routinely in nutrition science, initially driven by the need to assess body fat and dissolved nitrogen stores in military divers.[14–16] Fundamental advances in the role of nutrition and immune function came out of military infectious disease research, where Colonel William Beisel identified the role of interleukin-1 in the effect of multiple stressors on reduced disease resistance and in disease-mediated loss of muscle mass.[17,18] Many modern food preservation technologies to extend nutrient shelf life in extreme conditions, and where the food will still be relatively appetizing and palatable, have come out of the developmental efforts of Army food technology and packaging experts.[19,20]

The Army conducts and supports operational medicine research to expand performance capabilities and sustain soldier health, with clear spin-off benefits to society. This review and analysis of the 20th century military nutrition research program considers the advances that were made and the organizational factors and opportunities that permitted these advances in nutrition science. Key accomplishments of the program were foundational data on metabolic requirements of healthy, young men and women, new methodologies for laboratory and field studies, and national leadership of research on performance in extreme environments.

II. MILITARY RESEARCH PRIORITIES

A. Soldier Provisioning in the Public Eye

The Army is reactive by nature, responding to issues of national security as they arise. This reactive response to emerging threats also affects military research programs. The galvanizing issues in military nutrition research have typically centered on national outcries about the quality of field rations when America's young men and women have been sent into harm's way. Along with providing better protection and equipment, providing better food to soldiers in combat is one of the tangible opportunities for Americans to voice their support for the troops. In the Spanish American war, a very public debate questioned the appropriateness of a high-fat ration for soldiers fighting in hot, humid conditions in the Philippines.[21,22] In World War I, public concern focused on wasted food at Army camps during a time when the country was sacrificing for the war effort.[23] In World War II, Keys' nutritionally balanced "K rations" were scientifically constructed but unpalatable emergency rations; however, by the end of the war, the new canned "C ration" was considered a huge improvement.[24,25] At the start of the 1990–91 Persian Gulf War, some field units ate only the Meal, Ready-to-Eat (MRE) packaged ration for several months without supplementation with fresh foods.[26] This contributed to very public complaints about the adequacy of field rations (specifically, palatability and resulting inadequate energy intake) that led to a successful ration improvement program that continues today.[20,27] Later, soldiers in Iraq were provided with so much high-quality food in garrison that there was a backlash about the excess.[28] Each issue has provoked new science related to soldier feeding strategies and policies.

B. Nutritional Health Diplomacy

Military biomedical initiatives also serve diplomatic goals and advance peacekeeping efforts, offering low-risk humanitarian, bridge-building opportunities.[10] The methodologies developed to assess the nutrition of troops in the South Pacific were subsequently applied in civilian postwar reconstruction efforts in Germany and Japan.[11,29] The ICNND program, led by the Department of Defense (DoD) Assistant Secretary for Health Affairs, conducted nutritional surveys to establish vital health status and improve micronutrient intakes in 37 allied countries for more than a decade (1955–67).[30] This nutrition status methodology, using anthropometry, biochemical assessments, and clinical examinations, later formed the basis of the NHANES program for nutritional surveys within the United States.[12] In parallel, the methodologies were adapted to evaluate nutrient intakes of military populations through extensive field ration tests and in dining facilities.[31,32]

C. Military Organizational Priorities

In addition to the ever-present need for nutritious and palatable rations, more specific organizational needs have driven Army nutrition science. The main efforts can be roughly categorized around four eras of military nutrition research in the 20th century (Table 7.1). In 1917, Herbert Hoover (in his role in charge of Food Administration) and General William C. Gorgas (the Army Surgeon General) asked Major John Murlin to establish a nutrition research team, based in Washington DC, to conduct field studies with soldiers "to determine ration suitability and requirement."[33] The purpose was to scientifically define the metabolic requirements of soldiers and advise the Quartermaster Corps on field and garrison rations.[34]

The nutrition questions changed in World War II. Operations were faster paced and took place in a wide range of environmental extremes around the world, including "steaming tropics, dry desert, cold and windy islands, and frigid subarctic."[3] There was concern that "the newer knowledge of nutrition had not had a marked effect on the kind and amount of food eaten in the Army since World War I."[35] The Armored Medical Research Laboratory was established (1942–61), and the lab fielded teams around the world to study nutritional needs in the context of environmental physiology.[1] At the same time, a team of nutritional physiologists was moved from Washington DC to a new Medical Nutrition Laboratory (1944–51) colocated with food developers in the Quartermaster Subsistence Research and Development Laboratory in Chicago. Their role was to advance nutrition science, particularly as it related to the composition of rations and their actual use in the field.[3,36] After the end of the war, recurrent recommendations by the Quartermaster Corps to disestablish nutrition research were finally successful, although a small element of the Medical Nutrition Laboratory was saved and moved to Fitzsimons Army Hospital in Colorado to address new questions about the role of nutrition on soldier health and readiness.[3]

In 1958, the US Army Medical Research and Nutrition Laboratory (USAMRNL) was established.[3] In 1974, the lab was moved and consolidated with other biomedical research components in the new Letterman Army Institute of Research (LAIR) at the Presidio of San Francisco, permitting new synergies with other research departments and a major medical center.[37] During a 30-year period (1958–78), nutrition research by USAMRNL and, later, LAIR supported international studies on micronutrient deficiencies and explored nutritional health- and performance-related questions, reported in over 2000 publications.[38–41]

In 1978, the Army divested itself of nutrition research after a determination that micronutrient deficiencies had been largely addressed, soldier-specific research requirements were not well identified, and other federal agencies were now heavily invested in nutrition science.[37,42] The Army nutrition research division at LAIR was closed, and nutrition research assets were transferred to the Western Human Nutrition Research Center of the US Department of Agriculture (USDA).[42] Research on the nutritional consequences of infection was also shut down at the US Army Research Institute of Infectious Diseases.[42] The LAIR project "Evaluation of the MCI and MRE Rations as the Sole Subsistence for an Extended Period" was terminated before data collection ever began. However, the proposed reliance on the USDA to address future Army needs in this area lasted only until the realization that field studies for this new class of rations, the MRE, required a capability that no longer existed, and testing the new MRE with college students using microwave ovens in their dorm rooms was hardly a soldier-relevant test environment.[20,43]

The Army directed the reestablishment and funding of an intramural biomedical research capability that would support field ration development and resume research on nutritional strategies for soldier performance enhancement, including "performance of cognitive, psychomotor, and physical tasks during sustained periods *under all environmental extremes*."[44] This was again colocated with the food developers, who had moved from Chicago to Natick, Massachusetts.

TABLE 7.1 Timeline of key military nutrition research activities of the past century.

1917	Establishment of the Nutrition Division in the Office of the Surgeon General under the leadership of Major John Murlin, Sanitary Corps, for purposes of "safeguarding the nutritional interests of the Army."
1918	Establishment of an expert advisory panel, the Food and Nutrition Board, including widely recognized founders of the science of nutrition research: C.I. Alsberg, F.G. Benedict, Graham Lusk, L.B. Mendel, E.V. McCollum, and A.E. Taylor.
1919	Surgeon General William Gorgas orders Nutrition Division to examine food wastage in World War I Army training camps. Survey concluded that too much food was provided, meals were not nutritionally balanced for mineral salts, and there was an excess of fat.
1942	Establishment of the Armored Medical Research Laboratory at Fort Knox, Kentucky, charged with conducting lab and field studies on physiology of the soldier in tanks and in extreme environments, including nutritional physiology. Closed in 1961 and reestablished as the US Army Research institute of Environmental Medicine (USARIEM) in Natick, Massachusetts.
1942	Reestablishment of military nutrition research capabilities, with commissioned nutrition officers and a lab under the director of laboratories, Army Medical School, Washington DC, led by Major George Berryman, Sanitary Corps, and Robert E. Johnson as Scientific Advisor.
1944	Medical Nutrition Laboratory aligns with Quartermaster subsistence R&D Laboratory in Chicago, with mission to investigate nutritional health of troops in all environments (including a large number of field ration surveys); prevent and treat disease and damage by nutritional and metabolic means; and observe and make recommendations on nutrition and health of civil populations under military control.
1945-46	Development of procedures for anthropometric, biochemical, and clinical examination methodologies to assess nutritional status of military and civilian populations, studying troops in the South Pacific and in studies of civilian populations in Germany and Japan.
1945	Ancel Keys' team conducts Minnesota Starvation Study for the Department of Defense (DoD) in order to discover responses to starvation and explore refeeding strategies.
1955–67	Interdepartmental Committee of Nutrition for National Defense (ICNND) conducted studies in 37 countries, improving international nutritional health and refining nutrition assessment survey methodologies, providing foundation for later NHANES.
1958	US Army Medical Research and Nutrition Laboratory (USAMRNL—the "nut lab") formed at Fitzsimmons General Hospital from the US Army Research and Development Unit, previously engaged in tuberculosis and chest surgery research and the Medical Nutrition Laboratory; COL John Youmans becomes tech director of USAMRDC (1948–50).
1974	USAMRNL moved from Denver to San Francisco and integrated into Department of Nutrition and Department of Medicine of Letterman Army Institute of Research (LAIR).
1980	Disestablishment of Army nutrition research and transfer of some elements to US Department of Agriculture.
1982	Reestablishment of a new Army medical nutrition research program at the US Army Research institute of Environmental Medicine, Natick, ordered by General Maxwell Thurman in response to critical need to evaluate nutritional adequacy of field feeding and operational rations.
1984–2012	Establishment of the standing Committee on Military Nutrition Research (CMNR, Food and Nutrition Board, institute of Medicine) to provide authoritative advice to the DoD.
1985	Combat Field Feeding System (CFFS) Test established health and performance relationships to new feeding systems and began a new era of continuous improvement and optimization of rations for use in austere environments.
1987	First congressional special funding to help establish Army nutrition research capability in Baton Rouge, Florida, in partnership with "Doc" Pennington Foundation.
1985–2000	Field ration testing program evaluates a large number of field rations with soldiers in a wide range of extreme environments and mission profiles.
1994–99	First nutrition research Science and Technology Objective (STO) initiative on performance-enhancing ration components concludes that caffeine and carbohydrate each contribute at least an additional 15% endurance time to exhaustion. This tech base research provided the science basis for the formulation of components in the First Strike Ration.

Derived from Schnakenberg, "A Brief History of Military Nutrition Research,"[37].

III. A NEW RESEARCH ORGANIZATIONAL STRATEGY

A. Modern Army Nutrition Science Research

The program restart in the 1980s was accomplished by Colonel David Schnakenberg[42] (Fig. 7.1). He had the influential backing of Lieutenant General Maxwell Thurman to establish a modern nutrition science program, and he was able to do it as he moved through a succession of key military positions. He led the Natick-based US Army Research Institute of Environmental Medicine (USARIEM) laboratory, where he built the new Nutrition Research Division, coordinated new nutrition directives at medical headquarters, and then planned and programmed long-term funding as the head of the Army operational medicine research program.[43] At USARIEM, Schnakenberg inserted Colonel E. Wayne Askew as the chief of the new Nutrition Research Division and devised a research program with interrelated elements. These included a synergistic colocation with food developers at Natick labs; establishment of the Committee on Military Nutrition Research (CMNR), a new standing committee from the Institute of Medicine's (IOM's) Food and Nutrition Board; military representation at federal nutrition coordinating committees, such as the congressionally mandated Interagency Committee on Human Nutrition Research; and a newly established extramural partnership with a semiautonomous nutrition center, the Pennington Biomedical Research Center (PBRC) (Fig. 7.2).

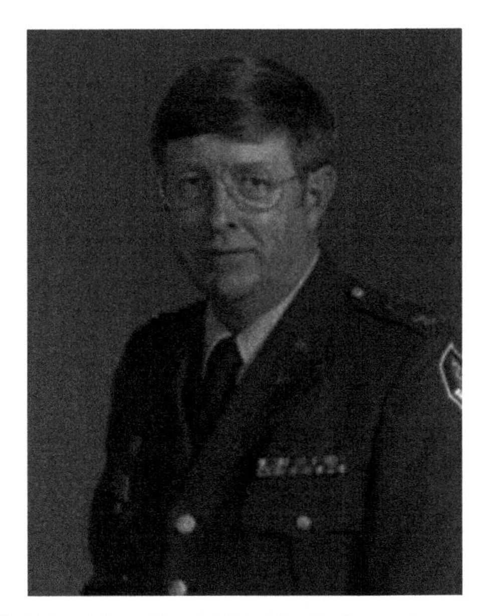

FIGURE 7.1 Colonel David D. Schnakenberg, Army nutritional biochemist. His extraordinary vision for a modern military nutrition research program formed the basis of the nutrition science program that continues today.

B. Colocation of Food Technology and Nutrition Science

In 1984, the Army was assigned executive agency responsibility for nutrition research to address the needs of all the military services.[45] Later, in Army medical headquarters, Schnakenberg established a permanent Army funding line for ration sustainment testing that provided support to annual studies involving ration improvement and addressed issues about garrison feeding. These funds permitted collaborative investigations with ration developers that included scientists focused on nutrition *before* it entered the mouth, including food psychology (Natick Soldier Systems Center), and those focused on the effects on humans *after* it entered the mouth (USARIEM), in distinctly different and complimentary "skin out" and "skin in" research missions.[46] These collaborations contributed to a highly productive, science-based ration development program (Table 7.2).

C. Partnership With the Pennington Biomedical Research Center (PBRC)

A cornerstone of the revised USARIEM nutrition research program was a special collaboration with the PBRC in Baton Rouge, Louisiana. PBRC augmented the Army nutrition research capabilities, permitting major research studies that would not have otherwise been possible. This research partnership began in 1989 through special congressional funding to the Army for nutrition research, only to be conducted in the newly established $125M center built in Baton Rouge by a local benefactor, C.B. Pennington.[47] While a congressional earmark through the USDA provided equipment for the laboratory ($9.4M), Schnakenberg strategically leveraged the directed Army funding to support and extend the objectives of the newly established military nutrition research program. Schnakenberg recalls his first visit to an empty new building with only a security guard and his opportunity to point out the Army's desires: a stable isotope lab, food composition lab, and metabolic chambers (David D. Schnakenberg, oral communication, October 2003). This initial 1989 grant, championed by the Speaker of the House, Congressman Bob Livingston, became a regular congressional special interest appropriation added to the DoD budget. This supplemental budget item, deemed essential to support Army nutrition research, continued through the 2010 defense appropriations.

Over $60M from the DoD provided a PBRC capability that supported field studies with direct laboratory and field staff resources for 103 major studies and more than 100 significant peer-reviewed publications (Summary accomplishments, Table 7.2). PBRC scientists, under the scientific leadership of Donna Ryan (for the Army studies), helped design and lead nutrition field

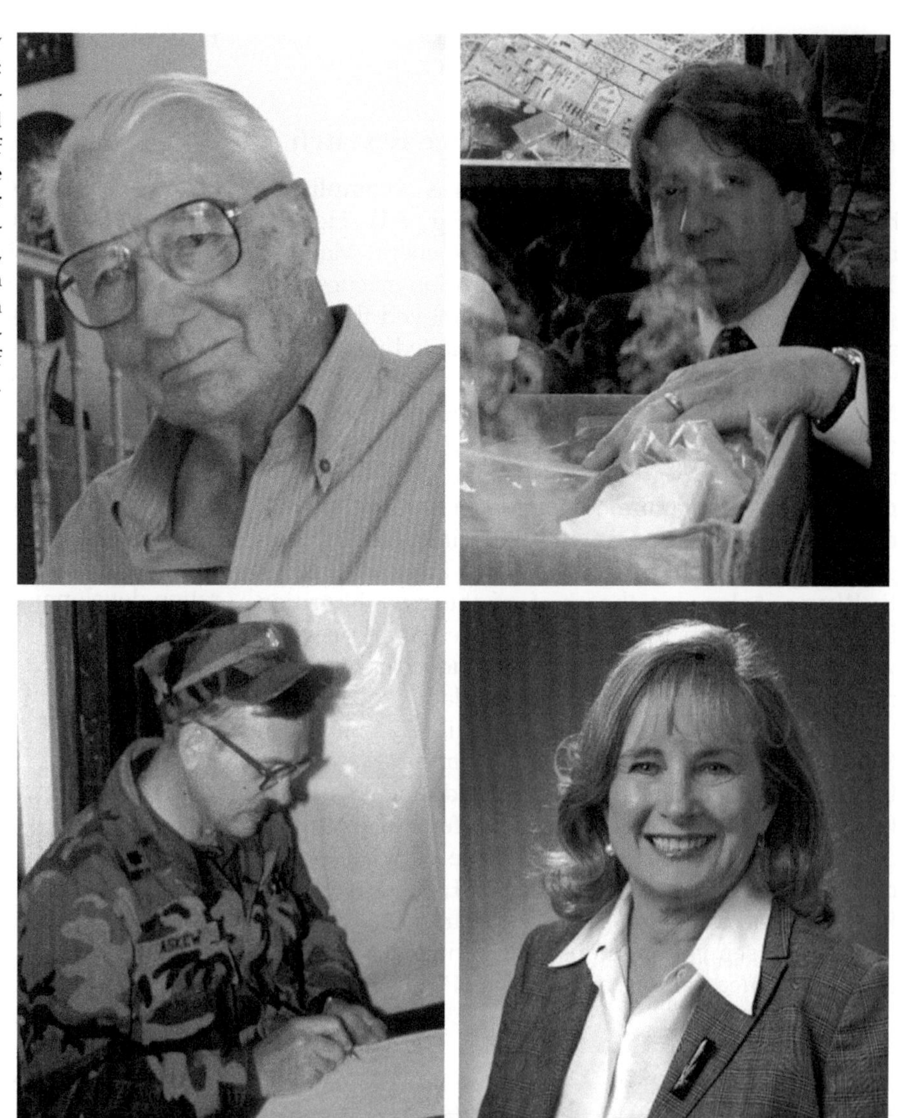

FIGURE 7.2 Key leaders of modern Army nutrition science. Clockwise from upper left: Robert O. Nesheim, PhD, chair of the Committee on Military Nutrition Research, Food and Nutrition Board, National Academy of Sciences; Gerald (Gerry) Darsch, head of the Combat Feeding Directorate, Natick Soldier Center (demonstrating a chemical ration heater); Donna Ryan, MD, Principal Investigator, Army nutrition research grants, Pennington Biomedical Research Center; and Eldon (Wayne) Askew, PhD, Chief of Military Nutrition Division, US Army Research Institute of Environmental Medicine (collecting field data).

and laboratory studies alongside USARIEM researchers (Fig. 7.2). The PBRC Army research ranged from housing Special Forces soldiers for intensive laboratory studies at the Pennington Center to supervising modification of the Army master menu with studies at Fort Polk, Louisiana[48,49](Table 7.2). PBRC also designed and led large field studies on weight management data with Fort Bragg units in North Carolina, Army Reserves in the Northeastern United States, and the entire Louisiana National Guard.[50–53] In turn, this Army investment helped PBRC establish common capabilities that supported civilian and other governmental agency-funded projects in metabolism, obesity, and nutritional supplement research. Today, these PBRC projects include over $55M in annual core operating costs, with major grants from National Institutes of Health (NIH) and the USDA, and PRBC continues collaborative research with the Army through new competitive grants. The PBRC has contributed essential capabilities and expertise to address the Army's research priorities in soldier nutrition (Table 7.3).

D. Authoritative Advice From the Committee on Military Nutrition Research (CMNR)

Another key feature of the program was the formation of an authoritative external advisory board. Following earlier models,[34] the standing CMNR was established within the Food and Nutrition Board of the IOM in October 1982. Major General Garrison Rapmund needed the wide-ranging expertise of this group to provide mainstream, national nutritional science advice to

TABLE 7.2 Major studies related to adequacy of military rations (1985–2000). Each field ration test provided the opportunity to address research questions concerning the role of nutrition in sustaining or enhancing soldier performance in extreme environments.

1985	Prolonged feeding of the MRE (CFFS study)[88]
1986	Weight effects and A-ration feeding in the field
1987	Dietary carbohydrate supplement during exercise at altitude[141]
1987	Ration, lightweight 30-day feeding[87]
1987	Ration, Cold Weather (RCW) and MRE feeding with Special Forces for 10-day cold weather field training exercise
1988	MRE, RCW, and LRP in 11-day cold weather training at Marine Mountain warfare Center
1990	Minimal ration energy requirements in high-risk training environments[70]
1991	High-altitude nutritional intake and energy expenditure[98]
1992	Eighteen-man Arctic Tray Pack Ration Module with MRE or Long Life Ration Packet during a cold-weather field training exercise[101]
1992	Food packet, survival, general purpose aircrew simulated survival scenario[115]
1994	Unitized Group Ration (UGR) test in US Marine Corps hot-weather training
1995	Ration adequacy in Special Forces Assessment and Selection course study[62]
1995	Thirty-day continuous feeding of the MRE[110]
1997	Hot-weather feeding of the UGR and carbohydrate beverage[97]
2000	Sixty-day Tray ration consumption (Great Inagua Island, Bahamas)[111]

TABLE 7.3 Top 10 military contributions from Pennington Biomedical Research Center, in a research partnership augmenting Army intramural capabilities.

- Measured total daily energy expenditure (TDEE) of healthy, young men and women across a full range of field settings and occupational tasks using the doubly labeled water technique
- Participated in field studies of soldier nutrition and ration development in extreme environments including extreme cold, hot-dry, high-altitude, and high-intensity training
- Evaluated adequacy of a wide range of new and specialized operational ration concepts, providing biochemical analyses of rations and soldier samples for a wide range of rations and ration concepts in field feeding
- Supported studies on health and performance of female soldiers in basic training, through pregnancy and lactation, and in other specialized settings in Officer's Basic Course, on ships, and in the field
- Conducted military food studies with master menu analyses for health, soldier acceptance, and logistical feasibility and supported periodic assessments of service dining facilities
- Developed food databases based on food composition analyses as a significant tool for military and civilian food scientists and dieticians
- Conducted laboratory studies on performance enhancing ration components including carbohydrate to extend endurance performance, tyrosine for sleep and cognition, and supported field studies on creatine, caffeine, hyperhydration with glycerol, sodium depletion, and zinc to prevent diarrheal disease
- Collaborated on extensive series of studies on soldier mineral metabolism status for iron, salt, and other minerals and vitamins
- Led Army weight management studies, pioneering epidemiological data acquisition and technologies and internet-based computational tools (H.E.A.L.T.H.) and conducted large Army epidemiological studies at Fort Bragg, New England RRC, and Louisiana Army National Guard
- Supported a wide range of specialized military studies for biochemical and metabolic balance studies, including disabled submarine, amino acid supplementation, and nutritional requirements of military women

respond to an increasing number of nutrition issues that arose as the Army moved to a radically different Combat Field Feeding System (CFFS) (David D. Schnakenberg, oral communication, October 2003). This committee was available to provide authoritative advice to the Army as important issues and nutrition policy questions arose.[54,55] The first CMNR meeting evaluated and reviewed nutritional influences on physical and cognitive performance, and this watershed symposium provided impetus to the core program for years to come.[56] For 30 years, the CMNR provided specific endorsements of military nutrition policy issues and influenced Army nutrition science (Table 7.4). Many of these recommendations also influenced extramural researchers to work on problems of importance to the military in their own research programs. In several cases, special reviews were conducted to address urgent questions from the Army medical leadership, such as antioxidant nutrition, iron deficiency status in military women, and use of high-fat rations, with the committee chair, Bob Nesheim, Ph.D., providing authoritative recommendations to senior leaders (Table 7.4). The CMNR conducted periodic site reviews of the PBRC program's support to Army nutrition, with constructive suggestions to the Army on how to get the best synergy in the research partnership (Table 7.4). The DoD discontinued the CMNR in 2012, in response to a priority need to increase funding for military psychological health.

IV. ENERGY REQUIREMENTS FOR ACTIVE, HEALTHY INDIVIDUALS

Urgent dispatches by George Washington during the Revolutionary War highlighted critical tactical failings that resulted from nutritional deficiencies and underfeeding of his soldiers.[3] The important relationship between energy metabolism and soldier performance was well studied through the 20th century, and this included extending upper limits of energy expenditure

TABLE 7.4 National Academy of Sciences and Committee on Military Nutrition Research (CMNR) workshops and reviews.

1984	Cognitive testing methodologies for military nutrition research
1984	Predicting decrements in military performance due to inadequate nutrition
1986	*Ration, Lightweight 30-Day*[b] (Camp Ethan Allan, Vermont)
1987	*Calorie-dense rations*[b]
1987	*Ration, Lightweight 30-Day and Nuclear, Biological, and Chemical (NBC) nutrient solution*[b]
1988	*Review of nutrition research concepts for the Pennington Biomedical Research Center*[b]
1989	Fluid replacement and heat stress
1989	*Sodium intake in soldiers*[b]
1989	*Military nutrition initiatives*[b] (NAS, Washington DC)
1990	The relationship of soldier body composition to physical performance
1990	*The Long Life Ration Packet*[b]
1991	Nutritional needs in hot environments
1992	*Review of three research proposals from the Pennington Biomedical Research Center*[b]
1992	Can food components be used to enhance soldier performance?
1992	*A nutritional assessment of US Army Ranger Training Class 11/91*[a]
1993	Not eating enough, overcoming underconsumption of military operational rations
1993	*Review of the results of Nutritional Intervention, Ranger Training Class 11/92 (Ranger II)*[a]
1994	Nutritional needs in cold and in high-altitude environments
1995	Emerging technologies for nutrition research: assessing military performance capability
1995	*Medical Services Nutrition Allowances, Standards, and Education (AR 40–25, 1985)*[b]
1995	*Review of issues related to iron status in women during US Army Basic Combat Training*[b]
1996	Nutritional sustainment of immune function in the field
1996	*Pennington Biomedical Research Center September 1996 Site Visit*[b]
1996	Assessing readiness in military women (BCNH)
1997	Protein requirements for operational environments
1997	Reducing stress fractures in physically active military women (BCNH)
1998	*Antioxidants and oxidative stress in military personnel*[b]
1999	Caffeine for sustainment of mental task performance: formulations for military operations
1999	Weight management: State of the science and opportunities for military programs
2000	Dietary Reference Intakes for vitamin C, vitamin E, selenium, and carotenoids (DRI feds)
2002	High-energy, nutrient-dense emergency relief food product
2003	Metabolic monitoring technologies for military field applications (Brooks Air Force Base)
2004	Nutrient composition of rations for short-term, high-intensity combat operations
2005	Mineral dietary requirements for military personnel
2007	Dietary supplement use by military personnel (supported by TATRC and Samueli Institute)
2010	Nutrition and traumatic brain injury
2011	Dietary Reference Intakes for calcium and vitamin D (DRI feds)

Notes: Unless otherwise annotated in italics, all of the listed reviews involved workshops with subject matter experts and resulted in books published by the National Academy Press; BCNH, Body composition, Nutrition, and Health Committee, cochaired with CMNR; DRI feds, Army nutrition program was a significant contributor to the federal DRI consortium.
[a]*Brief reports.*
[b]*Letter reports.*

in prolonged, exhaustive military operations. The studies of American chemist, physiologist, and nutritionist Francis Gano Benedict provided a foundation for modern metabolic research, and he was part of a small team of external scientific steering committee members, who guided the Army nutrition program in World War I.[34,57] Subsequent energy metabolism research has had a close relationship with the Army. By the end of the 20th century, collaborative studies led by Reed Hoyt, Ph.D., applied modern tools with stable isotope tracers and wearable physiological monitoring to address soldier issues. Efforts to apply emerging technologies, such as wearable physiological monitoring, to practical field metabolic measurement continue today.[58–60] The NIH encouraged and cofunded Hoyt's field studies because of the paucity of data on energy requirements of healthy, active Americans at the time (Van Hubbard, unpublished).

A. Total Daily Energy Expenditure Requirements

In World War I, there was an urgent need to address a perception of food wastage at military camps, as the war effort was being supported by nationwide rationing and restrictions. Murlin's new military nutrition team set out to determine the actual intakes and requirements for young men in training and in garrison.[4] The team produced remarkably detailed energy balance studies based on estimated intakes, food waste, and weight balance–based measurements made in 427 Army messes with 135,000 men.[61] Murlin determined that healthy, young men engaged in high levels of physical activity sustained a total daily energy expenditure (TDEE) of 4000 kcal/day, while average soldier requirements were 3600 kcal/d for an ad libitum diet.[61] The findings are remarkably comparable to values obtained in a subsequent World War II survey of messes, and this value has again been confirmed in studies using doubly labeled water.[5,62] The value of 4000 kcal/d for male requirements appears to represent a ceiling for sustainable energy expenditure by men for an extended period of time (weeks), including Special Forces trainees fed ad libitum and Ranger course trainees on restricted diets, for a Physical Activity Level of about 2.25.[63,64] This TDEE has been the basis for an adequate field ration, including the current MRE (3 meals/day = 4000 kcal). Values for Military Dietary Reference Allowance that are more recent recommend 3600 kcal as an upper bound for men and 2800 kcal for women.[65]

In a large series of studies across a wide range of military activities where men and women had equal participation, Hoyt and James DeLany, Ph.D., demonstrated that TDEE measured using the doubly labeled water technique is proportionately lower for typically smaller-bodied women than for men.[66] In a review of body composition, health, and nutrition of military women, the IOM noted that despite this fact, there was no "pink ration" to provide a nutritionally balanced, lower-energy ration for women. However, because of the IOM review, nutritional information was added to the individual ration packets to guide women in their selection of a balanced diet from the entire ration.[67]

B. Not Eating Enough

Inadequate energy intake by soldiers in the field was the single most important finding of the many nutrition studies conducted during World War II, and this observation has been repeated in nearly every field study since.[5,13,25,26] Generally, it was viewed as a simple problem of weight loss that could later be easily restored. In a carefully controlled field study, acute food restriction for up to 10 days during patrolling activities in the Panamanian jungle produced weight loss and negative nitrogen balance but no appreciable performance decrements.[41] However, chronically underfed individuals demonstrate an attenuated work capacity or a ceiling effect imposed by a limited energy intake.[68] Other studies have demonstrated that ensuring an adequate energy intake supports prolonged high-intensity work in extreme environments with no appreciable breakdown of muscle mass or performance decrements ("overtraining").[69]

Analysis of a large series of field feeding studies, using doubly labeled water measurement of energy expenditure, demonstrated a typical underconsumption of food energy by approximately one quarter of measured energy expenditure.[5] A 1993 CMNR workshop hosted at USARIEM on the theme of "Not Eating Enough" examined likely explanations for field ration underconsumption and reviewed data on consequences of underfeeding, including reduced work capacity, increased susceptibility to infection, and effects on decision-making.[26] The CMNR concluded that a "food discipline" policy, similar to water consumption policies, was important to encourage adequate intakes of both water and energy in the field and suggested that this is a leadership issue. A range of ration improvements to improve variety and other adjustments to feeding policy that might encourage eating were also made based on the 1995 report.[26]

C. Physiology of Semistarvation

The Army has well-studied chronic energy deficiency in healthy individuals, including during Keys' 1945 Minnesota Starvation Study and in more recent studies of high-intensity training with deliberate food restriction.[9] In the Keys study, young men on an energy-restricted diet lost 24% of body weight over 24 weeks, with a controlled refeeding period involving several different diet groups. In Robert Moore's 1990 study of Ranger students, healthy, young males also lost most of their available fat energy stores, with weight losses ranging between 15% and 25% over 8 weeks, and lost sizable amounts of lean mass and strength. However, as with the Keys study, everyone was fully recovered within a few months of refeeding.[70] This seemingly remarkable resilience belied a compromised immune function and increased susceptibility to infection.[9,71,72] At the start of his two-volume report on the Minnesota Starvation Study, Keys noted that inadequate nutrition and susceptibility to infectious disease was a consistent outcome of major wars and, specifically, that increasing incidence and virulence of diseases was related to the state of undernutrition.[9] These data paralleled results of comprehensive nutritional status monitoring of postwar German and Japanese civilian populations (1945–51) that demonstrated continuing weight losses during protracted periods of restricted food availability, usually less than 1500 kcal/d/person over several years in these countries.[3] Years later, separate CMNR reviews of Ranger training,[73] inadequate energy intake of soldiers,[26] nutritional influences on immune function,[74] and refeeding refugee populations[75] consistently reiterated the conclusion that relatively modest energy supplements could be effective in preserving disease resistance in high-stress conditions.

Subsequent field studies to examine antioxidants and other specific nutrients to boost immune function in stressful field conditions were unsuccessful in identifying any simple nutrient or vitamin supplementation shortcut to the effect of energy deficit.[76] These data are meaningful in the context of protection of soldiers in their worldwide deployments and in the susceptibility of populations in third world countries facing regional epidemics. These studies provided a basis for recommendations on the composition of humanitarian rations following a CMNR symposium cosponsored by the Army and US Agency for International Development.[75]

Similar energy deficits of 1000 kcal/d produced hypogonadism in men and women and increasing risk of bone loss, in addition to other tissue loss.[77–79] Hoyt described the metabolic differences between fit, young men and women conducting high-intensity work in the field for a week with no food and no organized sleep, highlighting the apparent advantage of estrogen-enhanced lipid metabolism in preserving lean mass stores in these conditions of high metabolic stress.[80] Subjective observations in these studies suggest that women, perhaps because of the better metabolic access to and utilization of lipid stores, have better physical and mental endurance, a concept that has been demonstrated elsewhere when male subjects were provided with low-dose estrogen.

D. Macronutrition

The macronutrient intakes of soldiers have typically been about one-third of calories from fat energy, and the best accepted rations tended to reflect those preferences.[61,62,81] In Murlin's World War I study, soldiers were consuming an average of 485 g of carbohydrate, 123 g of fat, and 122 g of protein.[61] Murlin noted that protein was the most expensive part of the diet, and since muscular work was derived most economically from carbohydrate and fat, "a relatively small amount of protein or meat in the diet would be sufficient for muscular work."[34] However, he was not prepared to recommend a reduction in the meat intake, which was ¾ lb/soldier/day. He noted that "we certainly desire that the American soldier shall have plenty of 'punch' to his fight, and if a high protein diet will insure this punch, nobody, I am sure, will grudge him all the meat he feels like eating."[34] In the first Gulf War, soldiers complained that the main course of the MRE was unsatisfactory; as part of the ration improvement plan, the portion size was promptly doubled from 5 to 8 ounces.[82] Thus, protein composition of US rations has also reflected a morale factor related to giving soldiers what they like to eat. The actual protein content of the MRE has remained at similar levels since the assessment of average intakes of young male soldiers in World War I and World War II messes (125 g/d).[4,61,62]

A recurring concept of nutrition tailored to individual metabolic profiles has been tested, and the findings typically demonstrate that human metabolism is more the same than different, at least in terms of fine-tuning macronutrient composition between individuals.[83,84] Nevertheless, hedonic aspects of food preference may be quite individualistic, as previously noted by Murlin, Bean, and many earlier nutrition scientists.

V. TEST AND EVALUATION OF FIELD RATIONS: NUTRITIONAL REQUIREMENTS IN EXTREME ENVIRONMENTS

A. Ration Technology Development

Operational rations were developed for use in the field when kitchen services were not available. In World War I, the Trench ration served this purpose (4000 kcal/d)[59]; in World War II, a broader range of rations included the C-ration (3200 kcal/d, limited to 21 days of continuous use), the K-ration (2700 kcal, intended for no longer than 5 days), and the D-ration (survival use).[29] Other special purpose rations were devised for various environments, such as the mountain and jungle rations, and unit rations were also created (e.g., 10-in-1 ration, larger field rations intended to feed 10 men for 1 day).[3,29] In the last quarter of the century, the C-ration was replaced by the MRE, and new versions of special purpose rations were developed.

Presenting palatable food to soldiers in the field, where fresh food was not available, has been an enduring challenge for food technologists.[83] Murlin had already noted in 1918 that "one the most important factors in the diet for the maintenance of morale is variety."[4] The food must also have a long shelf life, without significant loss of nutritional value during storage in extreme environments; and the packages must withstand air delivery and be able to be decontaminated after chemical, radiological, and biological attack. Due to technological advances in Army food research and a better understanding of underlying biochemical processes, researchers were able to find a way to biochemically stabilize egg products for packaged rations.[83] Other major advances occurred with the development of the MRE, especially after the MRE enhancement program following the first Gulf War and under the leadership of Gerald Darsch of the Food Engineering Directorate of Natick Laboratories (Fig. 7.2).[82,83] Improvements included increasing menu diversity and portion sizes and adding chemical heaters. These changes, along with paying attention to soldiers' tastes in the field, all contributed to soldiers' increased acceptability of these later-generation field rations.[20,82,83,85]

It must be emphasized that products intended for use by soldiers must be studied in the relevant environments with soldiers because the end users will come up with surprising innovations. As one example, the addition of small 1/8 oz bottles of hot sauce to the ration was a welcomed novelty, but shortly after the new rations circulated, the chief dietician of the Army received an urgent inquiry about the risk of corneal ulceration from hot sauce in the eye. Soldiers going through high-intensity training without access to coffee had discovered that dripping hot sauce into the eye had a stimulant effect, and this had become a new trend.

B. Field Ration Studies

Along with food technology improvements, there was a critical need to ensure that the rations would support soldier health and performance in field environments. Not all rations passed this test. Such rations included the K-ration, which was deficient in energy and vitamins, yet had already been relied on for extended feeding; a high-fat, low-carbohydrate pemmican ration that rendered soldiers ineffective after 3 days of a high-intensity field training exercise; and the extended use of rations limited in energy and protein, such as the Ration, Lightweight.[13,86,87] It was vitally important to make these discoveries prior to fielding a ration for actual mission use. Robert Ryer summarized at least 15 major field nutrition surveys conducted by the Military Nutrition Lab (1942–48), including desert feeding; cold weather feeding in arctic, subarctic, and mountains; evaluation of the B and E rations; nutritional status in hot tropics in the Pacific; and survival rations in cold weather conditions.[3] Results of these surveys formed the basis for further research by the Medical Department, with problems prioritized by "their importance to military operations and the resources that can be applied to their solution."[3]

Conducting physiological studies in the field was not a trivial task, as discovered by the civilian researchers called to active duty to solve soldier problems during World War II. John Youmans, formerly the Chief of the Nutrition Division in the Office of the Surgeon General, wrote the most definitive account of wartime soldier and civilian feeding challenges, research, and solutions. His account also included important observations on the parallel strategies of seeking solutions through extramural academic research organized by the Office of Scientific Research and Development and more immediate solutions that could be obtained through military research organizations.[13] As a member of the latter group of Army "embedded" field researchers, Bean summarized lessons learned for an effective Army field study, factors often not immediately appreciated by extramural researchers (Table 7.5). Bean had been involved in some very large ration field studies, including Operation Topside involving 1000 soldiers in Pike National Forest in Colorado, where the K-ration, C-ration, 10-in-1 ration, and Canadian Army Mess Tin Ration were tested in an 8-week tactical simulation, with extensive chemistries, fitness tests, clinical evaluations, acceptability testing, and movie documentation.[24]

In the 1980s, the Army adopted an entirely new approach to combat field feeding based on new mobility requirements and new food processing and packaging technologies. The concept was to provide one to two hot meals per day with minimal preparation or refrigeration requirements; the system was estimated to cut food-staffing needs in half and to save 2 million gallons of water and 200,000 gallons of fuel per day.[88] As described earlier in this chapter, the USARIEM nutrition task force was established to ensure the adequacy of the new MRE, which was being phased in to replace the previous generation of C-rations, as part of this new field feeding system. Marilyn (Teves) Sharp was a research leader in the largest field nutrition study ever conducted, the CFFS study. Her study compared body composition, strength, and aerobic performance in six groups of soldiers sustained for 44 days in the field on the new MRE, tray ration, and fresh rations, and it included a male and female group comparison.[88] A preliminary study had indicated that MREs caused an unacceptable weight loss. Sharp was able to demonstrate that there was only a modest reduction, primarily in fat mass, clearing the way for further development of the new generation rations.[88] This watershed study was followed by the establishment of a formal research team within USARIEM to conduct nutritional studies, including a long series of field ration evaluations, revisiting issues raised in World War II research on requirements for specialized uses and environments.

TABLE 7.5 Lessons learned from World War II field ration studies.[24]

- Design the smallest possible research footprint with minimal interference in military operations
- Evaluate rations in the normal military field activities for which they were designed
- Gain full buy-in and cooperation of the line and noncommissioned officers to conduct the studies and obtain their constructive evaluations
- Conduct operational evaluations as close to combat front lines as possible
- Isolate test units from outside food contamination
- Prohibit conflicts of interest in testing by vendors and ration developers
- Design an adequate test duration and sample size
- Have a clear plan for implementation of the results

C. Hot Weather Rations

Consideration to soldier nutrient requirements in extreme environments has been an elusive research goal since the Spanish American war with early concerns about the optimal macronutrient mix to sustain health and performance in hot, tropical environments.[21] However, a key conclusion from World War II studies was that there was no special food requirement that could be identified for hot, humid environments.[25,29,89] World War II research examined and rejected popular notions of "tropical deterioration" and the need for a specifically designed tropical ration.[90] Research conducted through the Vietnam era focused on requirements for activities in hot, humid jungle environments, including metabolic acclimation, but still failed to identify unique feeding requirements or a greater need for any specific nutrient component.[41] C. Frank Consolazio demonstrated an increasing energy requirement for hard work in hot weather, ranging as high as 11% −13%, perhaps due to metabolic cost of sweating and increased ventilatory rates, but tolerable work rates are also reduced in very hot conditions.[91]

Nearly a decade before the start of the 1990 Persian Gulf War, Roger Hubbard at USARIEM resuscitated the World War II concept of "water as a tactical weapon." He identified problems of factors related to adequate water intake learned in World War II and already forgotten.[92] Extensive studies during World War II debunked several myths, including that individuals could readily develop a tolerance to dehydration and that a person would completely replenish their water needs based on thirst alone. This came out of studies during 1942–45, led by E.F. Adolph and the Rochester Desert Unit.[6,7] These vitally important physiological advances altered Army policies. Among their many important findings was the observation that much of a normal day's water loss would be replaced during the consumption of a meal. Men would voluntarily dehydrate 3%–5% and fail to drink enough to replace sweat losses unless rehydration was enhanced with regular meal discipline.[6,93,94] There was generally no need for salt supplementation in men with normal food intakes.[6,95] Later attempts to water load individuals, a concept promoted by the accounts of T.E. Lawrence and other desert-experienced soldiers, proved ineffective. A series of lab studies with a glycerol supplement provided some total volume expansion but did not appear to provide a significant advantage for work in the heat.[96]

Hot weather field feeding was again tested with Marines working hard in hot, dry desert conditions, and a main finding was that energy deficits could also be improved by intake of a carbohydrate drink.[97] Similar benefits to water and energy balance were demonstrated with a carbohydrate drink at high altitude in a study of Army engineers building an airstrip in Bolivia.[98] A very careful and detailed USARIEM laboratory study on salt balance concluded that 4 g NaCl per day, compared to a normal US intake of 8 g NaCl per day, did not compromise subjects for water balance or other physiological parameters.[99] Researchers also extensively studied mineral and water losses from increased sweat rates, and new data did not suggest a need for any special replacement strategy, other than what would be provided in existing rations.[100]

D. Cold Weather Rations

There is a higher energy requirement for individuals in military operations in cold environments. This was repeatedly demonstrated in World War II studies, such as Operation "Musk Ox" and other studies in Alaska and Canada, and it was confirmed with later studies using doubly labeled water in troops in Alaska during tests of the Ration, Cold Weather (RCW), with TDEE between 4000 and 5000 kcal/d.[58,101,102] Between 1986 and 1991, at least six different ration tests in the cold estimated energy requirements in excess of 4000 kcal/d.[103] Robert Johnson and Robert Kark demonstrated that voluntary energy intake in the field was inversely proportional to the ambient temperature.[104] There is indeed an increased energy cost for subjects actually exposed to cold temperatures to support both shivering and nonshivering thermogenesis, but soldiers operating in the cold with adequate cold weather protective clothing incur increased costs from the difficulty of moving in snow and as much as an additional 10% cost from the hobbling effects of cold weather clothing.[103,105]

Attempts to reduce the bulk and weight of rations, to satisfy higher energy requirements in cold environments, have met with limited success. Dehydrated rations, such as the RCW, provide special challenges in cold environments where water may be frozen and not readily available and where hypohydration is already a problem for soldiers.[102,103] Increasing fat content of the ration has also been challenging.[106] There may be a specific thermogenic benefit from the high fat and protein in traditional diets of cold-weather dwellers. Native cold-weather dwellers eat these foods because they are available in very cold regions, but there is also some evidence of adaptation of native cold dwellers to this diet, with a metabolic shift to increased heat production. Nevertheless, high-fat (~70%) diets have not been successful in previous soldier feeding studies.[107] One World War II era pemmican study with soldiers left the men incapacitated by the third day on this diet.[86] In 1946, Operation "Musk Ox," a United States–Canadian mechanized snowmobile expedition across 3400 miles of Arctic terrain determined that soldiers consumed more calories in the cold, and 40% of calories from fat were accepted. However, along with other surveys of food intake in cold weather Army posts, there was no increased appetite for fat.[108,109] In later years, similar tests of a cold weather field ration in Alaskan troops conducting operations in subzero temperatures confirmed earlier findings of the adequate nutritional support provided by several different ration formulations with 35% energy content from fat.[103] There is a thermogenic benefit from frequent eating in a cold environment, explained by the thermic effect of feeding. The significance of macronutrient balance to performance in the heat and cold appears to be directly related to palatability and total energy intake, but it deserves further investigation with newer tracer isotope methods and refined techniques for assessment of outcomes.[58–60]

E. Continuous Ration Feeding

An important, recurring question is how long health and performance can be sustained with rations not supplemented with fresh foods. Improvements in packaged field rations tend to lure leaders into an overreliance on extended duration ration feeding. This problem was identified in World War II, and the triservice regulation on nutrition specifically noted that field rations were only approved for 10 days of continuous use.[29] Johnson and Kark conducted a comprehensive analysis of World War II US and Canadian field feeding study results. They concluded that the field rations were generally inadequate, especially at the start of the war; that inadequate intake of water and food calories sometimes impaired operational fitness of fighting units; and that there was an overreliance on packaged rations when better methods of feeding were available.[25] In the 1990 Gulf War, reports that soldiers were subsisting on MREs alone for 6-month periods led to a series of detailed field studies designed to determine the nutrition adequacy (and acceptance) of rations eaten continuously for 30 days.[87,110,111] Modern day rations were found to be nutritionally adequate to meet the nutrient requirements of active soldiers, provided they are consumed to energy requirements. The consistent challenge was, and always has been, getting soldiers to eat enough to meet their energy requirements, due to appetite suppression, preoccupation with the events of a field training exercise, and palate fatigue with the field ration menus. Even with inadequate consumption, World War II troops were generally well nourished, with no significant vitamin deficiencies detected by the cadre of nutritionally trained physician examiners who were looking for evidence of deficiency.[25,112] It was still surprising that no biochemical or physical clinical signs of micronutrient deficiency were detected in modern day Ranger students, even with restriction to only one MRE meal per day (or to combat engineers tested with only MREs for 30 days). This was because the rations were so well fortified with nutrients and because the soldiers began with an excellent nutritional status.[70,110,113]

F. Limited Use Rations

The special needs of the military for compact, lightweight rations have been a recurring consideration, extending back to the hard tack ration used in the Revolutionary War. The science behind special purpose rations for long-range patrols has evolved from the K-ration to today's First Strike Ration.[114] Survival and emergency rations are a special class of their own with special life support characteristics that have not changed a great deal between World War II and the end of the century.[115]

Keys originally developed the K-ration, intended as a pocket-sized emergency ration or "paratrooper ration," with off-the-shelf items in a local grocery store that he put together for a prototype meal and tested with six soldiers, who concurred that it might be okay if no other food was available. Further development resulted in a ration that provided about 2700 kcal/day, and a limited 3-day test at Fort Benning determined this to be "adequate." The Quartermaster Corps liked it because it was cheaper and easier to manage than the more expensive specialty rations, like the mountain and jungle rations, which were swiftly phased out. The K-ration ended up being used for extended periods of time and was repeatedly cited as one of the key problems in deteriorating soldier effectiveness in remote areas where alternate sources of food were not readily available and when men refused to eat the ration.[3,29] This highlighted another myth identified by World War II nutrition researchers; it was not true that a hungry soldier will eat anything. The K-ration was phased out immediately after the end of World War II, in favor the canned C-ration.

Periodic efforts to provide a compact ration with high fat have failed because of the gastrointestinal upset and reduction in soldier effectiveness that comes from this unaccustomed diet. This was demonstrated in pemmican feeding studies, such as the Prince Albert trials where soldiers had deteriorated to "ineffective" within 3 days on this diet.[86] In contrast to high-fat diets, studies with Special Forces soldiers at the PBRC demonstrated a 15% improvement in endurance march times with carbohydrate supplementation during the work.[47] Field studies confirmed the value of increased energy intake, observed with carbohydrate supplements in food bar and drink forms with soldiers on patrol and in extreme environments, such as at altitude and in the cold.[98,101]

These findings contributed to the design of the First Strike Ration, which includes high-carbohydrate snacks that soldiers can eat on the move. Although the ration does not provide the full amount of energy required, it was intended to solve the problem of soldiers stripping MRE rations for a few random items when the volume and weight was impractical for a patrol mission. A key difference between this limited energy ration and the K-ration was that the components of the ration were items that soldiers actually asked for, the composition was nutritionally balanced (except for adequate total energy), and the items were selected for the convenience of an eat-as-you-move ration.[114,116]

From his experience with ration studies in the Panamanian jungle and in early Ranger student studies, Herman Johnson concluded that restricted-intake rations for short military missions (<2 weeks) should include at least 50% of energy requirements, at least 150 g of carbohydrate, 50 g of protein, close to the RDA for vitamins and minerals, and adequate supplies of water.[41,117,118] He also highlighted a major remaining question: psychological stressors of combat affect food intake and nutritional balance but cannot be quantified because they cannot be readily simulated.

VI. PERFORMANCE-ENHANCING RATION COMPONENTS AND TRYING TO PROTECT SOLDIERS FROM BAD IDEAS

The NIH leads the nation in the science of nutritional supplements, and the Office of Dietary Supplements (ODS) was created as part of the Dietary Supplement Health and Education Act of 1994 (DSHEA) legislation to specifically address this topic area. While ODS is focused on health benefits, it has fallen to the Army to address claims about performance effects. Nutrition and dietary supplements offer some promising opportunities to enhance soldier performance, and as the primary human performance research capability in the federal government, the Army program serves an important national role in the investigation of performance-enhancing nutrition components.[119] For healthy, young men and women who are primary targets of sports supplement advertising, it has been just as important to protect soldiers from harmful dietary supplements as it is to promote those that are effective.[120]

A. Supplements

With the emerging discoveries in vitamins and other nutrients in the World War II era, numerous studies examined the question of a continuum of effects, where more might be better, especially with some kind of performance enhancement effect in soldiers. Empirical studies with vitamins, creatine, and even creatine combined with oral androgens yielded little effect on simple performance measures.[121–125] With greater understanding of mechanisms and testing methodologies by the 1980s, it seemed that, outside of deficiency conditions, there were actually few dietary supplements with specific effects on human physical and mental performance. If this were not true, human physiology might run amok with every meal. Nevertheless, there are performance-enhancing substances in some foods that, especially when concentrated beyond normal food composition, provide a performance advantage. A clear example is creatine, well studied for its benefit to high-intensity exercise. Ingestion of 20 g/d for several days (each dose equivalent to that found in several kilograms of red meat) increases muscle phosphocreatine and supports short-burst glycolytic energy requirements. In field exercises with US Army Rangers, this type of enhanced performance provided no measureable advantage, as the typical limit to soldier performance is endurance and not explosive strength.[126]

B. Performance-Enhancing Ration Components

In 1994, all Army research funding was reorganized to center on defined science and technology objectives (STOs); one of these first STO initiatives was a multiyear effort to develop performance-enhancing ration components that would demonstrate at least a 15% improvement in militarily relevant performance measures. Investigating the benefits of creatine was one of the objectives of these field studies, which researchers conducted on a range of promising components that used practical delivery methods, such as snack bars and beverages.[119] Tyrosine was proven to provide benefits as a rate-limiting substrate in very high-stress conditions in animals where brain microdialysis studies indicated diminished levels of catecholamines.[127] The cognitive performance benefits have been more difficult to demonstrate in humans because of ethical constraints in creating very high-stress conditions in which to test the intervention. However, 150 mg/kg of tyrosine in a food bar improved mood and performance in a human hypothermia model, suggesting potential value as a component in a future "performance under stress" bar.[128,129] Soldier performance benefits could not be proven for other components such as choline and creatine.[126,130] B vitamins have been reexamined for mood and performance benefits but seem to provide limited effects. Ultimately, new Army research data led to incorporating caffeine and carbohydrate formulations into soldier feeding systems as proven performance enhancers.

C. Caffeine

Coffee and soldiering has a long history, and the Army has repeatedly attempted to evaluate its specific benefits to performance. A research team included coffee use in a structured interview with soldiers, following forced marches to Gettysburg in 1863.[131] Later researchers found that caffeine, especially in higher doses than obtained in a normal cup of coffee (250 mg), could effectively sustain work performance in sleep-deprived soldiers in World War II studies, and this was superior to the effects of amphetamine in side-by-side studies.[132] Findings from a wide range of studies in recent decades have repeatedly demonstrated the benefits of caffeine, including sustained attention during sentry duty in well-rested soldiers,[133] cognitive performance during high-intensity training,[134] and temporary restoration of alertness and cognitive performance in sleep deprivation.[135,136] Studies in the 1990s well defined the advantages of high-dose caffeine over amphetamine and modafinil for most applications, evincing effects to extend muscular and mental fatigue limits versus effects largely centered on perception and motivation.[137] Most importantly for soldiers, caffeine helped to reverse diminishing judgment and decision-making in sleep-deprived subjects, while amphetamine appeared to increase the willingness to take risks.[138] An important study of the pharmacodynamics of a caffeinated gum demonstrated 5 min to peak absorption from oral mucosal absorption and a rapid elimination period, making this a suitable countermeasure for sleep inertia in sentry duty and other military settings.[139] A CMNR review of performance effects of caffeine and on safe upper limits supported Army decisions to field caffeine gum as part of the First Strike Ration.[114,139]

D. Carbohydrates

The benefits of carbohydrates during work to extend performance have been well-described.[47,140] In a definitive military study, Special Forces soldiers performed a study at PBRC that demonstrated a 15% extension of time to exhaustion.[47] A study at altitude with Army engineers building a runway in Bolivia showed a beneficial effect of a carbohydrate drink to increasing energy intake, despite the anorexic influences typically seen at altitude.[98] Carbohydrate supplements have been shown to be useful in enhancing or preventing performance decrements in a variety of military training scenarios, including work at moderate altitude, load bearing work, and other high-intensity field training exercises.[98,141,142]

E. Antioxidants

Antioxidant nutrition could be beneficial in reversing the biochemical stress observed in high-intensity military operations, especially in hypoxic environments such as troops performing at altitude, but near-term benefits of supplemental antioxidants have been difficult to demonstrate.[143,144] An Army Surgeon General believed that soldiers were at special risk for greater than average oxidative stress because of the nature of military occupations and would derive health benefits from antioxidant nutrition provided in another shaker next to the salt and pepper on every table in Army dining facilities. The CMNR was asked to evaluate and endorse this concept. After considering all available evidence of soldier activities and exposures (e.g., blast overpressure, toxicological exposures, high work rates, etc.), the committee recommended there was little reason to believe that soldiers were typically operating at levels of oxidative stress sufficient to justify special supplementation of their intakes.[145] This, of course, does not negate the potential mitigation of long-term health outcomes by antioxidant nutrition, including from greater chronic stress exposure in military occupations. These long-term associations are difficult to test.

F. Mineral/Micronutrients

Most recently, micronutrient deficiencies in the military have focused on iron status and vitamin D, primarily for women, and especially after a 1994 change in military policy on allowing more women in the services. Through a series of experiments, James McClung, Ph.D., led a team that substantially resolved the issues of poor iron status during initial entry training for women and provided a solution to reduce stress fracture rates. Iron status deteriorates during initial entry training, particularly for women, and this affects a wide range of outcomes related to health and performance.[146,147] The explanation for a progressive deterioration only during this training phase appears to be related to a stress response, likely involving activation of hepcidin, which reduces iron uptake in the gut.[148] Voluntary supplementation with prenatal vitamins high in iron was shown to improve 2-mile run times in recruits with iron deficiency anemia by an average drop of 2 min.[149]

A 1994 randomized controlled study with calcium and vitamin D supplementation of midshipmen (women) in Navy basic training demonstrated a marked reduction in stress fracture rates.[150] In a series of studies, the benefit of a modest vitamin D supplement during this period of extraordinary bone remodeling was further characterized, and a supplemental "nighttime snack" bar was recently developed for recruits that included supplemental vitamin D.[151] The one group identified as likely deficient in vitamin D by the IOM review of vitamin D and calcium Dietary Reference Intakes was, in fact, young women of military age.[152]

VII. BODY COMPOSITION AND READINESS STANDARDS

A. Body Composition Methodologies Development

The military has been a pacesetter in body composition studies and development of methodologies that have been vital to modern nutrition research. US Navy divers faced specific problems such as decompression sickness, in which nitrogen is sequestered in the body if individual diving table calculations are not correct. Solving this problem in diving medicine required new methods in body fat composition analysis. Modern-day body composition tools came from these programs. Captain Albert Behnke and his dive researchers evolved underwater weighing to estimate the fat compartment, and Commander Nello Pace developed the body water dilutional techniques as another approach.[14–16] A watershed symposium at Natick Army Labs in 1959 produced recommendations for standardized body composition techniques, including two- and three-compartment models using underwater weighing and body water determination.[153] Later efforts provided the foundation for air-displacement plethysmography methods[154]; four-compartment model estimates, including estimated bone content[155]; and methods specifically estimating total nitrogen and muscle mass components, such as K40 in soldiers at Fort Carson.[156] Nutritional surveys relied heavily on anthropometric measures, and these methodologies were substantially advanced in applications by military researchers, including Behnke and Consolazio.[15,16,157]

B. Body Fat Standards

In the World War II era, underweight status was still a key marker for chronically malnourished and diseased (e.g., tuberculosis) recruits and a common cause for rejection. In subsequent years, with improved medicine and nutrition, the military began to focus on overweight and obesity for force readiness. Even in the World War II era, body weight was recognized as an inappropriate basis to assess obesity and poor military readiness because it did not distinguish between fat and muscular, large individuals. Captain Albert Behnke published observations from a group of football players, who would have failed to meet military weight standards of the time but, in fact, had a high total body density and were, therefore, very lean and muscular.[158] The Marines adopted a body composition standard using a body fat estimation method derived from a waist circumference equation originally developed by Behnke and Wilmore.[16,159] Following a 1980 review of fitness in the services that were ordered by President Carter, waist circumference–based body fat standards were mandated for all military members. The current DoD Instruction directs the services to a common method of measurement using simple robust male and female equations developed by the Naval Health Research Center.[160] Obesity in the services had risen to public attention, especially following a national commentary by television newscasters when cameras panned across the ample potbellies of the honor guard members during a ceremony in Washington DC in the late 1970s (David Schnakenberg, unpublished observations). The development of field expedient assessments came from large Navy and Army data collection efforts, with cross-validation of a range of techniques and equations on each data set.[161] Bioelectrical impedance and other technologically sophisticated techniques were too inconsistent for individual standards testing, and ultimately, the simplest circumference-based equations developed by the Navy were determined to be the best.[162] Waist circumference–based body fat standards are an important part of military readiness standards today, and failure to meet the standard can result in discharge from the military.[161] Only Japan has a comparable standard applied across a large population, using mandatory waist circumferences in men and women over age 50 in an effort to stem the rising tide of type 2 diabetes and other obesity-related diseases. The evolution and science of military body composition standards are reviewed elsewhere.[163]

C. Soldier Readiness and Weight Management

Once enforceable standards were in place, it became important to improve methods to assist soldiers in meeting those body composition standards. A wide range of garrison feeding studies were conducted, with research dieticians focusing on food preparation, food selection, and food consumption in service dining facilities, including service academies, special operations soldiers, and regular facilities. This was not a new emphasis in 1980, as it had been one of the primary mission objectives of Murlin's group in World War I and for each new incarnation of Army nutrition research since then.[33] The main goal has been to adjust Army master menus to meet the nutritional needs of active, young men and women. A wide range of dining facility studies were conducted in the 20th century to ensure that garrison feeding of soldiers optimized performance and military readiness.[31,164,165] This included efforts to modify individual soldiers' food choices in "performance nutrition" programs.[166]

A series of three major efforts led by the PBRC, in collaboration with USARIEM, focused on monitoring and managing soldier body composition and fitness. Although large in scale, each started as seemingly simple projects that quickly devolved to difficulties that each highlighted specific challenges of conducting field studies. This included reorganization of the military unit midstudy (Army Reservists in the 95th RRC), unpredictable massive deployment of the units under study (units within a major Army base, Fort Bragg, NC), and unresolvable geographic mixing of randomized study groups following statewide response to a natural disaster (the Louisiana Army National Guard, randomized by parish).[50–52] Despite disruption of each study, the efforts provided foundational data for developing future comprehensive and integrated health readiness programs.

VIII. CONCLUSIONS

Military nutrition research in the 20th century applied science to the feeding of soldiers and advanced science about the metabolic basis of human performance. Energy requirements to sustain performance were defined, with short-term deficits well tolerated, but long-term deficits compromising soldier performance and physiological resilience (e.g., resistance to infectious disease). A significant finding concerning metabolism in extreme environments was that soldiers do not eat enough calories to counteract the heightened environmental influences of heat, cold, or altitude on energy expenditures during field operations. Another significant finding was that rations could be tailored to individuals and to specific environmental extremes, but these are related to taste preferences and not because of differences in metabolic requirements. In other words, individual metabolism was more the same than different, and there were no specific differences in nutrient requirements for performance in a wide range of extreme environments. Also, few dietary supplements were actually found to be effective for soldier performance enhancement, with the notable exceptions of caffeine, carbohydrates, and tyrosine. The reestablishment of Army nutrition research in the 1980s is a model of federal government research organization. It included colocating with the intended users, the ration developers; leveraging limited resources by partnering with a very strong academic partner, the PBRC; accessing authoritative advice on nutrition research directions and interpretations from the Food and Nutrition Board; and closely coordinating with other federal agencies involved in nutrition science.

RESEARCH GAPS

- TDEE of fit young men and women has been well investigated, and further research is not likely to alter the conclusions derived from a century of work on this topic; however, further resolution of protein requirements to sustain and increase muscle mass in healthy active individuals is still needed
- There is no basis in science established for "arctic" or "tropical" rations based on any measureable differences in substrate oxidation (i.e., fat and carbohydrate oxidation), but further investigation of strategies to increase soldier field consumption of carbohydrate energy is needed
- The metabolic and performance advantages of special "performance" diets such as ketogenic diet and tolerance of such diets are unknown, and the impact of a critical deficiency in carbohydrate intake has not been well defined
- Other than caffeine and carbohydrate supplements, no specific performance enhancing food components have been put into practical use (e.g., tyrosine)
- Bioenergetics of individuals within specialized job functions such as Army divers, long-range surveillance detachments, specialized arctic teams, etc., require further investigation (e.g., relative importance of brown adipose tissue)
- The interrelationships between field nutrition and sleep affecting immune–host response have not been addressed, nor has the distinction between acute phase responses and sustained health and performance in field operations
- The interaction between sleep and nutrition in effective weight management and metabolic flexibility has not been addressed for fit and active soldiers
- The neurobiology of food preferences and presentation and the effects on mental status and mood, nutrient absorption, and gut microbiota bear further research

Acknowledgment

The authors gratefully acknowledge the editing support by Ms. Mallory Roussel.

Disclaimer

The opinions and assertions in this article are those of the author and do not necessarily represent the official views or policies of the US Army.

IX. REFERENCES

1. Bean WB. President's address: the ecology of the soldier in World War II. *Trans Am Clin Climatol Assoc*. 1968;79:1–12.
2. Rasmussen N. Of 'small men', big science and bigger business: the second world war and biomedical research in the United States. *Minerva*. 2002;40:115–146.
3. Ryer R. Chapter XIII: laboratory specialties, section 9: nutrition. In: The History of the US Army Medical Service Corps. Washington

DC: Office of the Surgeon General and Center of Military History, US Army. (in press).
4. Murlin JR, Hildebrant FM. Average food consumption in the training camps of the United States. *Am J Physiol.* 1919;49:531–556.
5. Tharion WJ, Lieberman HR, Montain SJ, et al. Energy requirements of military personnel. *Appetite.* 2005;44:47–65.
6. Adolph EF, Dill DB. Observations on water metabolism in the desert. *Am J Physiol.* 1938;123:369–378.
7. Adolph EF. *Physiology of Man in the Desert.* New York: Interscience Publishers, Inc; 1947.
8. *National School Lunch Act, Pub L No. 79-396, 60 Stat 230.* 1946.
9. Keys A, Brožek J, Henschel A, Mickelsen O, Taylor HL. *The Biology of Human Starvation.* Vols. 1–2. Minneapolis, MN: University of Minnesota Press; 1950.
10. Schaefer AE. Interdepartmental committee on nutrition for national defense. *Nutr Rev.* 1958;16:193–196.
11. Berry FB, Schaefer A. Nutrition surveys in the near and far east: report of the interdepartmental committee on nutrition for national defense. *Am J Clin Nutr.* 1958;6:342–353.
12. Wilson CS, Schaefer AE, Darby WJ, et al. A review of methods used in nutrition surveys conducted by the Interdepartmental Committee on Nutrition for National Defense (ICNND). *Am J Clin Nutr.* 1964;15:29–44.
13. Youmans JB. Malnutrition and deficiency diseases. In: Coates Jr JB, Hoff EC, eds. *Personal Health Measures and Immunization.* Washington DC: Office of the Surgeon General, Department of the Army; 1955:159–170. Preventive Medicine in World War II; Vol. 3.
14. Behnke AR. Physiologic studies pertaining to deep sea diving and aviation, especially in relation to the fat content and composition of the body: the Harvey lecture, March 19, 1942. *Bull N Y Acad Med.* 1942;18(9):561–585.
15. Behnke AR, Feen BG, Welham WC. The specific gravity of healthy men: body weight ÷ volume as an index of obesity. *J Am Med Assoc.* 1942;118(7):495–498.
16. Pace N, Rathbun EN. Studies on body composition: III. the body water and chemically combined nitrogen content in relation to fat content. *J Biol Chem.* 1945;158:685–691.
17. Beisel WR. Magnitude of the host nutritional responses to infection. *Am J Clin Nutr.* 1977;30:1236–1247.
18. Pekarek RS, Wannemacher Jr RW, Beisel WR. The effect of leukocytic endogenous mediator (LEM) on the tissue distribution of zinc and iron. *Proc Soc Exp Biol Med.* 1972;140:685–688.
19. Floros JD, Newsome R, Fisher W, et al. Feeding the world today and tomorrow: the importance of food science and technology. *Compr Rev Food Sci Food Saf.* 2010;9(5):572–599.
20. Hirsch ES, Kramer FM, Meiselman HL. Effects of food attributes and feeding environment on acceptance, consumption and body weight: lessons learned in a twenty-year program of military ration research (Part 2). *Appetite.* 2005;44:33–45.
21. Bacon as soldiers' food: col. Woodruff and Dr. Edson give their opinions anent its value. widely divergent views the Assistant Commissary General favors fat food for the tropics, and the physician holds that it is unsuitable. *N Y Times.* July 31, 1898:10.
22. Woodruff CE. The US Army ration and military food. *J Am Med Assoc.* 1892;19:651–663.
23. Kellogg V. The food problem. In: Yerkes RM, ed. *The New World of Science: Its Development during the War.* New York: The Century Co; 1920:273.
24. Bean WB. Field testing of army rations. *J Appl Physiol.* 1948;1: 448–457.
25. Johnson RE, Kark RM. *Feeding Problems in Man as Related to Environment: An Analysis of United States and Canadian Army Ration Trials and Surveys, 1941-1946.* Boston, MA: Harvard Fatigue Laboratory; 1946:93.
26. Committee on Military Nutrition Research, Food and Nutrition Board, Marriott BM, eds. *Not Eating Enough: Overcoming under Consumption of Military Operational Rations.* Washington DC: National Academy Press; 1995.
27. Meiselman HL, Schutz HG. History of food acceptance research in the US Army. *Appetite.* 2003;40:199–216.
28. Los Angeles Times. *Iraq Chow Can Be Too Hearty.* Baltimore Sun; July 15, 2007. https://www.baltimoresun.com/news/bs-xpm-2007-07-15-0707140314-story.html. Accessed June 25, 2019.
29. Youmans JB. Chapter IV: nutrition. In: Coates Jr JB, Hoff EC, eds. *Preventive Medicine in World War II.* Washington DC: Office of the Surgeon General, Department of the Army; 1955:85–158. Personal Health Measures and Immunization; Vol. 3.
30. Sandstead HH. Origins of the interdepartmental committee on nutrition for national defense, and a brief note concerning its demise. *J Nutr.* 2005;135:1257–1262.
31. Szeto EG, Carlson DE, Dugan TB, Buchbinder JC. *A Comparison of Nutrient Intakes between a Ft.* Riley Contractor-Operated and a Ft. Lewis Military-Operated Garrison Dining Facility. Natick, MA: US Army Research Institute of Environmental Medicine; 1987.
32. Klicka MV, King N, Lavin PT, Askew EW. Assessment of dietary intakes of cadets at the US military Academy at west point. *J Am Coll Nutr.* 1996;15(3):273–282.
33. Murlin JR. Origin of the food and nutrition division [letter to Lieutenant K.P. McConnell, october 26, 1943]. Quoted by: Ryer R. Chapter XIII: laboratory specialties, section 9: nutrition. In: History of the US Army Medical Service Corps. Washington DC: Office of the Surgeon General and Center of Military History, US Army. (in press):12-16.
34. Murlin JR. Some problems of nutrition in the Army. *Science.* 1918; 47(1221):495–508.
35. Howe PE. The effect of recent developments in nutrition on the rationing of the Army. *Conn State Med J.* 1942;6:157.
36. Johnson RE. The Army's medical nutrition laboratory. *Nutr Rev.* 1949;7:65–66.
37. Schnakenberg DD. *Military Nutrition Research: A Brief History, 1917-1980. Military History Notes.* No. 25, Spring 1986. Nashville, TN: Vanderbilt Medical Center Library; 1986:1–4.
38. Kuemmerlin AJ, Wilson BL, Rhodes YM, Canham JZ. *Three Decades of Endeavor – A Bibliography: 1944-1974.* Denver, CO: US Army Medical Research and Nutrition Laboratory, Fitzsimmons Army Medical Center; 1974:172. Laboratory Report No. 345. AD A7820977.
39. Omaye ST, Turnbull JD, Sauberlich HE. Selected methods for the determination of ascorbic acid in animal cells, tissues, and fluids. *Methods Enzymol.* 1979;62:3–11.
40. Baker EM, Canham JE, Nunes WT, Sauberlich HE, McDowell ME. Vitamin B6 requirement for adult men. *Am J Clin Nutr.* 1964;15(2): 59–66.
41. Consolazio CF, Johnson HL, Nelson RA, Dowdy R, Krzywicki HJ. *The Relationship of Diet to the Performance of the Combat Soldier: Minimal Calorie Intake during Combat Patrols in a Hot Humid Environment (Panama).* Technical Report No. 76. San Francisco, CA: Letterman Army Institute of Research; 1979. Presidio of San Francisco; AD A078695.
42. Schnakenberg DD. *Military Nutrition Research: Goals and Directions for the Future.* Paper Presented at: Annual Meeting of R&D Association. 1981 (Chicago, IL).
43. Hollis W. *Out of Cycle Manpower Request for USARIEM memorandum for General Maxwell Thurman.* March 19, 1987.
44. *Army Studies Nutritional Needs of the Future [press release].* Fort Detrick, MD: US Army Medical Research and Development Command Public Affairs Office; September 7, 1984.
45. Department of Defense Directive 3235.2-R. *Food and Nutrition Research and Engineering Program.* April 27, 1984.

46. Friedl KE, Allan JH. USARIEM: physiological research for the warfighter. *Army Med Dep J*. 2004:33–43.
47. Ryan DH, Bray GA. Philanthropy refocuses nutrition thinking. *J La State Med Soc*. 1990;142(2):22–24.
48. Murphy TC, Hoyt RW, Jones TE, Gabaree CL, Askew EW. *Performance Enhancing Ration Components Program: Supplemental Carbohydrate Test*. Natick, MA: US Army Research Institute of Environmental Medicine; 1994.
49. Champagne CM, Hunt AE, Cline AD, Patrick K, Ryan DH. Incorporating new recipes into the Armed Forces recipe file: determination of acceptability. *Mil Med*. 2001;166(2):184–190.
50. Williamson DA, Bathalon GP, Sigrist LD, et al. Military services fitness database: development of a computerized physical fitness and weight management database for the US Army. *Mil Med*. 2009;174(1):1–8.
51. Williamson DA. *Weight Measurements and Standards for Soldiers*. Baton Rouge, LA: Pennington Biomedical Research Center; 2009.
52. Newton Jr RL, Han H, Stewart TM, Ryan DH, Williamson DA. Efficacy of a pilot internet-based weight management program (HEALTH) and longitudinal physical fitness data in Army Reserve soldiers. *J Diabetes Sci Technol*. 2011;5(5):1255–1262.
53. Stewart T, Beyl R, Switzer M, et al. HEALTH (Healthy Eating, Activity, Lifestyle Training Headquarters) internet/mobile weight management program for the US Army: outcomes and future directions. *J Sci Med Sport*. 2017;20:S34–S35.
54. Marriott BM, Earl R. *Committee on Military Nutrition Research Activity Report 1986-1992*. Washington DC: National Academy of Sciences, National Academies Press; 1992.
55. Poos MI, Costello R, Carlson-Newberry SJ. *Committee on Military Nutrition Research Activity Report December 1, 1994 through May 31, 1999*. Washington DC: National Academy of Sciences, National Academies Press; 1999.
56. Committee on Military Nutrition Research, Food and Nutrition Board, National Academy of Sciences. *Predicting Decrements in Military Performance Due to Inadequate Nutrition*. Washington DC: National Academies Press; 1986.
57. Benedict FG. *A Study of Prolonged Fasting*. Carnegie Institute Publication No. 203. Washington DC: Carnegie Institute of Washington; 1915:418.
58. Hoyt RW, Jones TE, Stein TP, et al. Doubly labeled water measurement of human energy expenditure during strenuous exercise. *J Appl Physiol*. 1991;71(1):16–22.
59. Hoyt RW, Buller MJ, Santee WR, Yokota M, Weyand PG, Delany JP. Total energy expenditure estimated using foot–ground contact pedometry. *Diabetes Technol Ther*. 2004;6(1):71–81.
60. Hoyt RW, Buller MJ, DeLany JP, Stultz D, Warren K. *Warfighter Physiological Status Monitoring (WPSM): Energy Balance and Thermal Status during a 10-Day Cold Weather US Marine Corps Infantry Officer Course Field Exercise*. Natick, MA: US Army Research Institute of Environmental Medicine; 2001.
61. Murlin JR, Miller CW. Preliminary results of nutrition surveys in United States Army Camps. *Am J Public Health*. 1919;9:401–413.
62. Howe PE, Berryman GH. Average food consumption in the training camps of the United States Army (1941–43). *Am J Physiol-Legacy Content*. 1945;144(4):588–594.
63. Hoyt RW, Friedl KE. Field studies of exercise and food deprivation. *Curr Opin Clin Nutr Metab Care*. 2006;9(6):685–690.
64. Fairbrother B, Shippee R, Kramer T, et al. *Nutritional and Immunological Assessment of Soldiers during the Special Forces Assessment and Selection Course*. Technical Report T95-22. Natick, MA: Army Research Institute of Environmental Medicine; 1995. AD A299 556.
65. Nesheim RO [Committee on Military Nutrition Research]. *Letter Report: Review of the Revision of the Medical Services Nutrition Allowances, Standards, and Education*. Army Reg 40-25 (1985) [report for Brigadier General Russ Zajtchuk. US Army Medical Research and Materiel Command; October 26, 1995.
66. Friedl KE, Ness JW. *Upper Limits of Energy Expenditure for Men and Women in Military Operational Settings: Does Female Fat Metabolism Provide a Performance Advantage*. Paper Presented at: NATO HFM Symposium-Impacts of Gender Differences on Conducting Operational Activities. 2008.
67. Grumstrup-Scott J, Marriott BM, eds. *Body Composition and Physical Performance: Applications for the Military Services*. Washington DC: The National Academies Press; 1992.
68. Spurr GB. Physical work performance under conditions of prolonged hypocaloria. In: *Predicting Decrements in Military Performance Due to Inadequate Nutrition*. Washington DC: Committee on Military Nutrition Research, Food and Nutrition Board, National Academy of Sciences, National Academies Press; 1986: 99–135.
69. Frykman PN, Harman EA, Opstad PK, Hoyt RW, DeLany JP, Friedl KE. Effects of a 3-month endurance event on physical performance and body composition: the G2 trans-Greenland expedition. *Wild Environ Med*. 2003;14(4):240–248.
70. Moore RJ, Friedl KE, Kramer TR, Martinez-Lopez LE, Hoyt RW. *Changes in Soldier Nutritional Status and Immune Function during the Ranger Training Course*. Natick, MA: Army Research Institute of Environmental Medicine; 1992.
71. Martinez-Lopez LE, Friedl KE, Moore RJ, Kramer TR. A longitudinal study of infections and injuries of ranger students. *Mil Med*. 1993;158(7):433–437.
72. Kramer TR, Moore RJ, Shippee RL, et al. Effects of food restriction in military training on T-lymphocyte responses. *Int J Sports Med*. 1997;18(S 1):S84–S90.
73. Kinney JM. Weight loss and malnutrition in ranger trainees. In: Marriott BM, ed. *Review of the Results of Nutritional Intervention, Ranger Training Class 11/92 (Ranger II)*. Washington DC: Committee on Military Nutrition Research, Food and Nutrition Board, Institute of Medicine; 1993:215–226.
74. Beisel WR, Blackburn GL, Feigin RD, Keusch GT, Long CL, Nichols BL. Proceedings of a workshop: impact of infection on nutritional status of the host. *Am J Clin Nutr*. 1977;30:1203.
75. Committee on Military Nutrition Research. *High-Density, Nutrient-Dense Emergency Relief Food Product*. Washington DC: National Academy Press; 2002.
76. Friedl KE. Military studies and nutritional immunology. In: *Diet and Human Immune Function*. Totowa, NJ: Humana Press; 2004: 381–396.
77. Loucks AB, Thuma JR. Luteinizing hormone pulsatility is disrupted at a threshold of energy availability in regularly menstruating women. *J Clin Endocrinol Metab*. 2003;88(1):297–311.
78. Ihle R, Loucks AB. Dose-response relationships between energy availability and bone turnover in young exercising women. *J Bone Miner Res*. 2004;19:1231–1240.
79. Friedl KE, Moore RJ, Hoyt RW, Marchitelli LJ, Martinez-Lopez LE, Askew EW. Endocrine markers of semi-starvation in healthy lean men in a multi-stressor environment. *J Appl Physiol*. 2000;88: 1820–1830.
80. Hoyt RW, Opstad PK, Haugen AH, DeLany JP, Cymerman A, Friedl KE. Negative energy balance in male and female rangers: effects of 7 d of sustained exercise and food deprivation. *Am J Clin Nutr*. 2006;83:1068–1075.
81. Friedl KE, Hoyt RW. Development and biomedical testing of military operational rations. *Annu Rev Nutr*. 1997;17:51–75.
82. Davenport C. Military rations take gourmet turn. *Seattle Times (WA)*; November 2, 2011. https://www.seattletimes.com/nation-world/military-rations-take-gourmet-turn/. Accessed June 25, 2019.
83. Feeney RE, Askew EE, Jezior DA. The development and evolution of US Army field rations. *Nutr Rev*. 1995;53:221–225.

84. Gabaree CL, Jones TE, Murphy TC, Brooks E, Tulley RT. *Assessment of Intra- and Inter-individual Metabolic Variation in Special Operations Forces (SOF) Soldiers*. Natick, MA: Army Research Institute of Environmental Medicine; 1995.
85. Bell R, Johnson JL, Kramer FM, DeGraaf C, Lesher LL. *A Qualitative Study of Soldier Perceptions of the Relative Importance of MRE Portion Size and Variety.* Natick, MA: Army Soldier and Biological Chemical Command, Soldier Systems Center; 1999.
86. Kark RM, Johnson RE, Lewis JS. Defects of pemmican as an emergency ration for infantry troops. *War Med.* 1945;7:345–352.
87. Askew EW, Munro I, Sharp MA, et al. *Nutritional Status and Physical and Mental Performance of Special Operations Soldiers Consuming the Ration, Lightweight, or the Meal, Ready-To-Eat Military Field Ration during a 30-Day Field Training Exercise*. Natick, MA: Army Research Institute of Environmental Medicine; 1987.
88. Teves MA, Vogel JA, Carlson DE, Schnakenberg DD. *Body Composition and Muscle Performance Aspects of the 1985 CFFS Test.* Technical Report No. T12/86. Natick, MA: US Army Research Institute of Environmental Medicine; 1986. AD A172 752.
89. Bean WB. Nutrition survey of American troops in the Pacific. *Nutr Rev.* 1946;4:257–259.
90. Kark RM, Aiton HF, Pease ED, et al. Clinical and biochemical observations on troops. *Medicine*. 1947;26(1):1–40.
91. Consolazio CF, Shapiro R, Masterson JE, McKinzie PS. Energy requirements of men in extreme heat. *J Nutr.* 1961;73(2):126–134.
92. Hubbard RW, Mager M, Kerstein M. *Water as a Tactical Weapon: A Doctrine for Preventing Heat Casualties*. Technical Report No. M18/82. Natick, MA: US Army Research Institute of Environmental Medicine; 1982. AD A113 477.
93. Szlyk PC, Sils IV, Francesconi RP, Hubbard RW, Armstrong LE. Effects of water temperature and flavoring on voluntary dehydration in men. *Physiol Behav.* 1989;45:639–647.
94. Szlyk PC, Sils IV, Francesconi RF, Hubbard RW. Patterns of human drinking: effects of exercise, water temperature, and food consumption. *Aviat Space Environ Med*. 1990;61:43–46.
95. Marriott BM. *Nutritional Needs in Hot Environments – Applications for Military Personnel in Field Operations*. Washington DC: Committee on Military Nutrition Research, Food and Nutrition Board, National Academy Press; 1993.
96. Latzka WA, Sawka MN, Montain SJ, et al. Hyperhydration: thermoregulatory effects during compensable exercise-heat stress. *J Appl Physiol*. 1997;83(3):860–866.
97. Tharion W, Cline A, Hotson N, et al. *Nutritional Challenges for Field Feeding in a Desert Environment: Use of the Unitized Group Ration (UGR) and a Supplemental Carbohydrate Beverage*. Natick, MA: Army Research Institute of Environmental Medicine; 1997:191. AD A328 882.
98. Edwards JS, Askew EW, King N, Fulco CS. Nutritional intake and carbohydrate supplementation at high altitude. *J Wilderness Med.* 1994;5(1):20–33.
99. Armstrong LE, Hubbard RW, Askew EW, et al. Responses to moderate and low sodium diets during exercise-heat acclimation. *Int J Sport Nutr.* 1993;3:207–221.
100. Montain SJ, Shippee RL, Tharion WJ, Kramer TR. *Carbohydrate-Electrolyte Solution during Military Training: Effects on Physical Performance, Mood State and Immune Function.* Technical Report T95-13. Natick, MA: Army Research Institute of Environmental Medicine; 1995.
101. Edwards JS, Roberts DE. The influence of a calorie supplement on the consumption of the meal, ready-to-eat in a cold environment. *Mil Med.* 1991;156:466–471.
102. Edwards JSA, Roberts DE, Mutter SH. Rations for use in a cold environment. *J Wilderness Med.* 1992;3(1):27–47.
103. Edwards JS, Askew EW, King N. Rations in cold Arctic environments: recent American military experiences. *Wilderness Environ Med.* 1995;6(4):407–422.
104. Johnson RE, Kark RM. Environment and food intake in man. *Science*. 1947;105:378–379.
105. Consolazio CF, Schnakenberg DD. Nutrition and the responses to extreme environments. *Fed Proc.* 1977;36:1673–1677.
106. Lazen AG [Committee on Military Nutrition Research]. *Letter Report: Calorie-Dense Rations, September 1987 [report for Major General Philip Russell.* US Army Medical Research and Development Command; September 30, 1987.
107. Consolazio FC, Forbes WH. The effects of a high fat diet in a temperate environment. *J Nutr.* 1946;32:195–211.
108. Kark RM, Croome RR, Cawthorpe J, et al. Observations on a mobile Arctic force: the health, physical fitness and nutrition of exercise "musk ox", February-May 1945. *J Appl Physiol.* 1948;1:73–92.
109. Swain HL, Toth FM, Consolazio FC, Fitzpatrick WH, Allen DI, Koehn CJ. Food consumption of soldiers in a subarctic climate (Fort Churchill, Manitoba, Canada, 1947–1948). *J Nutr.* 1949;38:63–72.
110. Thomas CD, Friedl KE, Mays MZ, et al. *Nutrient intakes and nutritional status of soldiers consuming the meal, ready-to-eat (MRE XII) during a 30 day field training exercise*. Technical Report T95-6. Natick, MA: U.S. Army Research Institute of Environmental Medicine; January 1995. AD A297339.
111. Tharion WJ, Baker-Fulco CJ, McGraw S, et al. The effects of 60 Days of tray ration consumption. In: *Marine Combat Engineers while Deployed on Great Inagua Island, Bahamas.* Natick, MA: Army Research Institute of Environmental Medicine; 2000.
112. Bean WB. An analysis of subjectivity in the clinical examination in nutrition. *J Appl Physiol.* 1948;1:458–468.
113. Moore RJ, Friedl KE, Tulley RT, Askew EW. Maintenance of iron status in healthy men during an extended period of stress and physical activity. *Am J Clin Nutr.* 1993;58:923–927.
114. Montain SJ, Koenig C, McGraw S. *First Strike Ration Acceptability: Dismounted Combat Soldiers in Afghanistan*. Technical Report T06-02. Natick, MA: Army Research Institute of Environmental Medicine; 2005:33. AD A444 070.
115. Jones TE, Mutter SH, Aylward JM, et al. *Nutrition and Hydration Status of Aircrew Members Consuming the Food Packet, Survival, General Purpose, Improved during a Simulated Survival Scenario.* Natick, MA: Army Research Institute of Environmental Medicine; 1992.
116. Erdman JW, Bistrian BR, Clarkson PM, et al. *Nutrient Composition of Rations for Short-Term, High-Intensity Combat Operations.* Washington DC: Committee on Military Nutrition Research, Food and Nutrition Board, National Academy Press; 2006.
117. Johnson HL, Krzywicki HJ, Canham JE, et al. *Evaluation of Calorie Requirements for Ranger Training at Fort Benning, Georgia.* Institute Report No. 34. San Francisco, CA: Letterman Army Institute of Research; 1976. Presidio of San Francisco; AD A070 880.
118. Johnson HL. Practical military implications of fluid and nutritional imbalances for performance. In: *Predicting Decrements in Military Performance Due to Inadequate Nutrition.* Washington DC: Committee on Military Nutrition Research, Food and Nutrition Board, National Academy of Sciences, National Academy Press; 1986:55–68.
119. Committee on Military Nutrition Research, Food and Nutrition Board, National Academy of Science, Marriott BM, eds. *Food Components to Enhance Performance: An Evaluation of Potential Performance-Enhancing Food Components for Operational Rations.* Washington DC: National Academy Press; 1994.
120. Friedl KE, Moore RJ, Marchitelli LJ. Nutrition: steroid replacers - let the athlete beware. *Strength Cond J.* 1992;14:14–19.
121. Friedl KE. US Army research on pharmacological enhancement of soldier performance: stimulants, anabolic hormones, and blood doping. *J Strength Cond Res.* 2015;29:S71–S76.
122. Ryer III R, Grossman M, Friedemann T, et al. The effect of vitamin supplementation on soldiers residing in a cold environment: 2.

psychological, biochemical and other measurements. *J Clin Nutr.* 1954;2:179–194.
123. Samuels LT, Henschel AF, Keys A. Influence of methyl testosterone on muscular work and creatine metabolism in normal young men. *J Clin Endrocrinol.* 1942;2:649–654.
124. Keys A, Henschel AF. Vitamin supplementation of US Army rations in relation to fatigue and the ability to do muscular work. *J Nutr.* 1942;23:259–269.
125. Friedl KE. Influence of dietary supplements on body composition. In: Lukaski H, ed. *Body Composition: Health and Performance in Exercise and Sport.* Boca Raton, FL: CRC Press, Taylor & Francis Group; 2017:343–356.
126. Warber JP, Tharion WJ, Patton JF, Champagne CM, Mitotti PE, Lieberman HR. The effect of creatine monohydrate supplementation on obstacle course and multiple bench press performance. *J Strength Cond Res.* 2002;16:500–508.
127. Rauch TM, Lieberman HR. Tyrosine pretreatment reverses hypothermia-induced behavioral depression. *Brain Res Bull.* 1990;24:147–150.
128. Shurtleff D, Thomas JR, Schrot J, Kowalski K, Harford R. Tyrosine reverses a cold-induced working memory deficit in humans. *Pharmacol Biochem Behav.* 1994;47:935–941.
129. Mahoney CR, Castellani J, Kramer FM, Young A, Lieberman HR. Tyrosine supplementation mitigates working memory decrements during cold exposure. *Physiol Behav.* 2007;92:575–582.
130. Warber JP, Patton JF, Tharion WJ, et al. The effects of choline supplementation on physical performance. *Int J Sport Nutr Exerc Metab.* 2000;10(2):170–181.
131. Gould BA. *Investigations in the Military and Anthropological Statistics of American Soldiers.* New York: US Sanitary Commission, Hurd and Houghton; 1869.
132. Foltz EE, Ivy AC, Barborka CJ. The influence of amphetamine (benzedrine) sulfate, d-desoxyephedrine hydrochloride (pervitin), and caffeine upon work output and recovery when rapidly exhausting work is done by trained subjects. *J Lab Clin Med.* 1943;28:603–606.
133. Johnson RF, Merullo DJ. Caffeine, gender, and sentry duty: effects of a mild stimulant on vigilance and marksmanship. *Penningt Cent Nutr Ser.* 2000;10:272–289.
134. Lieberman HR, Tharion WJ, Shukitt-Hale B, Speckman KL, Tulley R. Effects of caffeine, sleep loss, and stress on cognitive performance and mood during US Navy SEAL training. *Psychopharmacology.* 2002;164(3):250–261.
135. Wesensten NJ, Killgore WD, Balkin TJ. Performance and alertness effects of caffeine, dextroamphetamine, and modafinil during sleep deprivation. *J Sleep Res.* 2005;14(3):255–266.
136. Waters WF, Magill RA, Bray GA, et al. *Effects of Tyrosine, Phentermine, Caffeine, D-Amphetamine, and Placebo during Sleep Deprivation: I. Sleep Drive, Quantity and Quality.* Pennington Center Nutrition Series; 1999:10.
137. Committee on Military Nutrition Research, Food and Nutrition Board, Institute of Medicine. *Caffeine for the Sustainment of Mental Task Performance: Formulations for Military Operations.* Washington DC: National Academy Press; 2001.
138. Penetar D, McCann U, Thorne D, et al. Caffeine reversal of sleep deprivation effects on alertness and mood. *Psychopharmacology.* 1993;112(2–3):359–365.
139. Kamimori GH, Karyekar CS, Otterstetter R, et al. The rate of absorption and relative bioavailability of caffeine administered in chewing gum versus capsules to normal healthy volunteers. *Int J Pharm.* 2002;234(1–2):159–167.
140. Consolazio CF, Johnson HL. Dietary carbohydrate and work capacity. *Am J Clin Nutr.* 1972;25(1):85–90.
141. Askew EW, Claybaugh JW, Hashiro GM, Stokes WS, Sato A, Cucinell SA. *Mauna Kea III: Metabolic Effects of Dietary Carbohydrate Supplementation during Exercise at 4100 M Altitude.* Natick, MA: Army Research Institute of Environmental Medicine; 1987.
142. Marsh ME, Murlin JR. Muscular efficiency on high carbohydrate and high fat diets. *J Nutr.* 1928;1(2):105–137.
143. Askew EW. Work at high altitude and oxidative stress: antioxidant nutrients. *Toxicology.* 2002;180(2):107–119.
144. Chao WH, Askew EW, Roberts DE, Wood SM, Perkins JB. Oxidative stress in humans during work at moderate altitude. *J Nutr.* 1999;129(11):2009–2012.
145. Vanderveen JE [Committee on Military Nutrition Research]. *Letter Report: Antioxidants and Oxidative Stress in Military Personnel [report for Major General John Parker.* US Army Medical Research and Materiel Command, and Lieutenant General Ronald Blanck, Army Surgeon General; February 12, 1999.
146. Friedl KE, Marchitelli LJ, Sherman DE, Tulley R. *Nutritional Assessment of Cadets at the US Military Academy: Part 1. Anthropometric and Biochemical Measures.* Natick, MA: Army Research Institute of Environmental Medicine; 1990.
147. McClung JP, Karl JP, Cable SJ, Williams KW, Young AJ, Lieberman HR. Longitudinal decrements in iron status during military training in female soldiers. *Br J Nutr.* 2009;102(4): 605–609.
148. Karl JP, Lieberman HR, Cable SJ, Williams KW, Young AJ, McClung JP. Randomized, double-blind, placebo-controlled trial of an iron-fortified food product in female soldiers during military training: relations between iron status, serum hepcidin, and inflammation. *Am J Clin Nutr.* 2010;92(1):93–100.
149. McClung JP, Karl JP, Cable SJ, et al. Randomized, double-blind, placebo-controlled trial of iron supplementation in female soldiers during military training: effects on iron status, physical performance, and mood. *Am J Clin Nutr.* 2009;90(1):124–131.
150. Lappe J, Cullen D, Haynatzki G, Recker R, Ahlf R, Thompson K. Calcium and vitamin D supplementation decreases incidence of stress fractures in female navy recruits. *J Bone Miner Res.* 2008; 23(5):741–749.
151. Gaffney-Stomberg ER, McClung JP. Nutrition, genetics, and human performance during military training. In: Matthews MD, Schnyer DM, eds. *Human Performance Optimization: The Science and Ethics of Enhancing Human Capabilities.* New York: Oxford University Press; 2018:45–61.
152. Institute of Medicine, Del Valle HB, Yaktine AL, Taylor CL, Ross AC, eds. *Dietary Reference Intakes for Calcium and Vitamin D.* Washington DC: National Academies Press; 2011.
153. Siri WE. Body composition from fluid spaces and density: analysis of methods. In: Brozek J, Henschel A, eds. *Techniques for Measuring Body Composition.* Washington DC: National Academy of Sciences; 1961:223–244.
154. Allen TH. Measurement of human body fat: a quantitative method suited for use by aviation medical officers. *Aero Med.* 1963;34:907–909.
155. Allen TH, Welch BE, Trujillo TT, Roberts JE. Fat, water and tissue solids of the whole body less its bone mineral. *J Appl Physiol.* 1959; 14:1009–1012.
156. Krzywicki HJ, Ward GM, Rahman DP, Nelson RA, Consolazio CF. A comparison of methods for estimating human body composition. *Am J Clin Nutr.* 1974;27(12):1380–1385.
157. Consolazio CF, Shapiro R, Isaac GJ, Hursh L, Birchler VR, Coman GR. Nutritional evaluation of a selected military population. *Am J Clin Nutr.* 1962;11:577–585.
158. Welham WC, Behnke AR. The specific gravity of healthy men: body weight ÷ volume and other physical characteristics of exceptional athletes and of naval personnel. *J Am Med Assoc.* 1942;118(7):498–501.
159. Taylor WL, Behnke AR. Anthropometric comparison of muscular and obese men. *J Appl Physiol.* 1961;16(6):955–959.

160. Friedl KE. Mathematical modeling of anthropometrically-based body fat for military health and performance applications. In: Lukaski H, ed. *Body Composition: Health and Performance in Exercise and Sport*. Boca Raton, FL: CRC Press, Taylor & Francis Group; 2017:285–305.
161. Hodgdon JA, Friedl K. *Development of the DoD Body Composition Estimation Equations*. San Diego, CA: Naval Health Research Center; 1999.
162. Segal KR, Van Loan M, Fitzgerald PI, Hodgdon JA, Van Itallie TB. Lean body mass estimation by bioelectrical impedance analysis: a four-site cross-validation study. *Am J Clin Nutr*. 1988; 47(1):7–14.
163. Friedl KE. Body composition and military performance—many things to many people. *J Strength Cond Res*. 2012;26:S87–S100.
164. Schnakenberg DD, Hill TM, Morris MS, Consolazio CF, Canham JE. *Nutrient Intakes of NAS/Alameda Personnel Before and After Conversion to a Cash a la Carte Food Service System*. San Francisco, CA: Letterman Army Institute of Research; 1978.
165. Kretsch MJ, Conforti PM, Sauberlich HE. *Nutrient Intake Evaluation of Male and Female Cadets at the United States Military Academy*. West Point, New York. San Francisco, CA: Letterman Army Institute of Research; 1986.
166. Thomas CD, Baker-Fulco CJ, Jones TE, King N, Jezior DA. *Nutrition for Health and Performance: Nutritional Guidance for Military Operations in Temperate and Extreme Environments*. Natick, MA: Army Research Institute of Environmental Medicine; 1993.

CHAPTER

8

ENERGY BALANCE: IMPACT OF PHYSIOLOGY AND PSYCHOLOGY ON FOOD CHOICE AND EATING BEHAVIOR

Alexandra M. Johnstone, PhD
Sylvia Stephen, MSc
The Rowett Institute, University of Aberdeen, Aberdeen, United Kingdom

SUMMARY

Food choice and eating behavior is influenced by a complex array of physiological and psychological processes. Culture, social surroundings, environmental factors, mood and emotion, and economics have strong influences over our dietary habits. The food choices we make also have a major impact on our health. Not all calories are equal, and our food choices have a direct influence on subsequent appetite and energy balance. For example, diets with a high- energy density can lead to passive overconsumption with little or no mechanism for defense. Moreover, in an increasingly obesogenic environment, it is extremely difficult to maintain energy balance. Further research is required to develop an integrated approach across health and technological disciplines to advance our understanding of the complex issue of food choice and eating behavior.

Keywords: Appetite; Body composition; Body weight; Energy balance; Food choice; Obesity.

I. INTRODUCTION

A. Background

The study of human eating behavior is undertaken by researchers in various disciplines including health psychology, business, and medicine. Eating fulfills a biological need, but is also a source of pleasure and comfort, and reflects economic, social, and cultural realities and perceptions.[1] Eating behavior can be thought of as "actions" or "things we do" and is influenced by both physiology and psychology. Daily food intake choices influence health, and poor diet choices can lead to an increased risk of noncommunicable disease (NCD). NCDs are chronic diseases, deriving from a combination of genetic, physiological, environmental, and behavioral factors and include cardiovascular disease, cancers, chronic respiratory diseases, and diabetes.[2]

In the developed world, our eating environment delivers a plentiful supply of energy-dense and cheap food, often resulting in overeating relative to requirements. Subsequent weight gain means that excess energy is stored as body fat. Obesity, however, is a complex issue. In 2007, the United Kingdom (UK) Foresight Report[3] described this disease as a "complex web of societal and biological factors that have, in recent decades, exposed our inherent human vulnerability to weight gain." This report produced an obesity system map, with energy balance at its center, identifying over 100 variables that are thought to directly or indirectly influence energy balance. The complexity of obesity as a disease creates both challenges and opportunities! In this era of novel "big data," we have access to information that can enhance our understanding of the role of food in medicine and public health arenas.[4] For

Present Knowledge in Nutrition, Volume 2
https://doi.org/10.1016/B978-0-12-818460-8.00008-3

example, data on our movement (via Global Positioning System and smart devices), shopping behavior and location, transport on motorways, interaction on social media, and purchase patterns from in-store loyalty cards have been shown to offer fruitful research opportunities, contributing in ways where traditionally sourced research data perhaps could not. For example, by utilizing both traditional diet survey data and the "big data" approach to analyze in-store purchase patterns, a UK collaborative study between academics and the food sector identified that the aging UK population fails to consume adequate protein to maintain muscle strength and function into later life.[5] This type of data can be used to assess how our eating environment can be adapted to tackle obesity[6] by combining both traditional laboratory-based data with novel biobank data and longitudinal cohort studies for identification and prioritizing of future research for societal and health benefits.

B. Key Issues

Individual differences in food likes and desires develop throughout the life course because of differing food experiences and attitudes[7] within our cultural experiences. We learn eating as a form of behavior, similar to physical activity. Over the last 30 years, major theories have dominated the study of the behavioral and cognitive aspects of eating style in relation to obesity and weight control, relating to the influence of dietary restraint, disinhibition, emotional eating, and external influences. Further, the role of nutritional and non-nutritional factors that influence our eating habits and food choices will be discussed in the context of influencing energy balance. The impact of diet composition on appetite is introduced as a theme, where "all calories are not equal." Furthermore, the energy density (ED) of the diet, as the amount of energy per gram of food (kcal/g), can act as a constraint or enhancer to calorie intake and feeding behavior. Governments can use policies to apply fiscal or choice-editing regulation to bias our food choices toward healthier and sustainable patterns. We will explore the role of portion size via plate size or meal size to influence how much we eat. Also, how do your emotions influence food choice, do you eat more or less when stressed? Do you reach for a biscuit when challenged by daily stresses and hassles? We will explore what is meant by the food addiction phenomenon and investigate whether there is evidence to support its existence.

Our brain is considered the "control center" where all information on food intake is processed. There are many biological signals related to satiety and regulation of energy balance that give us information about our nutritional needs or requirements, and the classical pathways of energostatic and hedonistic physiology pathways are discussed in relation to influencing food choice. The satiety cascade is mentioned in the context as a target for obesity therapy—to design foods to feel fuller for longer and control calorie intake and how food can influence energy balance through impact on gut microbiota via the food–gut–brain axis. Finally, body composition assessment of body stores is described, since the efficacy of any dietary approach will be assessed as a change in energy balance. We can achieve this though body composition assessment to monitor changes in body stores. The energy cost of weight gain and weight loss (WL) are also outlined in the context of energy balance.

II. PSYCHOLOGY OF FOOD CHOICE—WHY WE EAT WHAT WE EAT

We can think of eating as a behavior, and behaviors are actions or things we do.[8] The question "why do we eat?" is simple—people engage in eating behavior as a matter of survival, normally every day. Eating gives us great pleasure but can be perturbed leading to undernutrition, overnutrition, and eating disorders. People generally make choices about what to eat, when, and how much to eat, dependent on social, culture, or habitual aspects of their diet. In the developed world, food is abundant, cheap, and available in great variety, which is often linked to overconsumption. Eating is a fundamentally rewarding behavior, intrinsically linked with mood and emotion—we do not just eat for hunger, but rather it is an enjoyable process linked to emotions such as boredom, stress, or work routine. Similarly, there may be times when we do not eat when hungry, due to lack of financial resources or time. Numerous factors are known to determine or guide eating behavior in an automatic and implicit fashion,[9] which include nutritional and nonnutritional cues. For instance, eating may be initiated or prolonged by the presence of others, i.e., influenced by social factors.[10] Food choices and consumption are also strongly influenced by environmental factors, e.g., advertising, packaging, portion sizes, lighting, and many more.[11,12] Therefore, constant monitoring and self-regulation of eating is necessary in order to eat healthily, i.e., to provide the body both qualitatively and quantitatively with nutrients for optimal health. At the same time, eating healthily also means being able to enjoy the rewarding aspects of food without falling prey to a loss of control over eating. In most cases, obesity is the result of poor dietary habits over a period of time, rather than extreme compulsive eating binges—which contribute to a modest average daily excess of energy intake (EI) over energy expenditure.[13]

We learn about food as we transition through weaning from baby to child to adult,[14] and it is argued that infants actually begin life with very few innate taste preferences and a strong capacity to learn to like new foods. Birch and Anzman[15] identified that in children, weaning to around 3 years of age is of major importance for learning about food and developing lifelong preferences. Associative learning or conditioning occurs when a positive evaluation of a stimulus arises through its association with a second, already-liked stimulus. This is reinforced by "familiarization, referring to the positive impact of repeated exposure on liking of the exposed stimulus." The terms "observational learning" or "social learning" refer to the natural human inclination to observe and imitate the behaviors of others such as mother and peers. For example, the theory and application of repeated exposure and associative conditioning has been applied to increase vegetable acceptance in children.[16]

Associative learning processes play many important roles in the control of food consumption. Most of our likes and dislikes are learned through classical conditioning. In Fig. 8.1, this is summarized as a simple Pavlovian-style conditioning procedure, where a response is arranged between two events, with respect to the subject's behavior.[17] It has been demonstrated that choices of foods and drinks are achieved by learning the relative preferences/aversions for foods and drinks and appetite/satiety for nutrients, regardless of the source of energy. This is explained by Thibault,[18] where food intake becomes part of a "learned ingestive response." We therefore can learn to like and dislike foods, and with repeated exposure, we can become familiar with the postingestive consequences of eating that food/beverage (which can be pleasant or unpleasant). When sensory cues from foods are paired with prompt nutritional aftereffects of eating (unconditioned stimuli), conditioned responses of food choice and intake can be induced.[19]

A. Restrained Eating Behavior and Disinhibition

Dietary restraint refers to the tendency to restrict food intake in order to control body weight. Investigators commonly use questionnaires such as the Dutch Eating Behavior Questionnaire[21] or the Three-Factor Eating Inventory[22] to classify subjects as restrained eaters. Dietary restraint can also be associated with "disinhibition" and loss of control over eating, resulting in binge eating. Examples from the literature where dietary restraint can influence study results include two studies conducted by Westerterp-Plantenga et al.,[23,24] where restrained women responded to covert manipulations of meals by failing to compensate for dietary inclusion of the fat mimetic (olestra) as an energy deficit, lean women who are not restrained compensated EI by 44%. In addition, the EIs of restrained women were actually (or were self-reported as) lower than those of their unrestrained counterparts.

B. Emotional and External Eating Behavior

The DEBQ and TFEI questionnaires can also identify the extent to which the external environment and internal emotional aspects influence food intake. The *externality theory* of human obesity was developed by Schachter in the 1960s,[25] where he proposed that obese subjects are more reactive to external food-related cues and less sensitive to internal hunger and satiation cues than lean individuals, for example, walking past a baker's shop and buying a nice cake/pastry to eat, with no prior plan to purchase and consume a snack. Inter-individual differences in susceptibility to weight gain may be due, in part, to variability in responsiveness to environmental (external) triggers, particularly in an obesogenic environment. The phenomenon of food craving ("an irresistible urge to consume a specific food"), in particular for high-fat foods,[26] has been

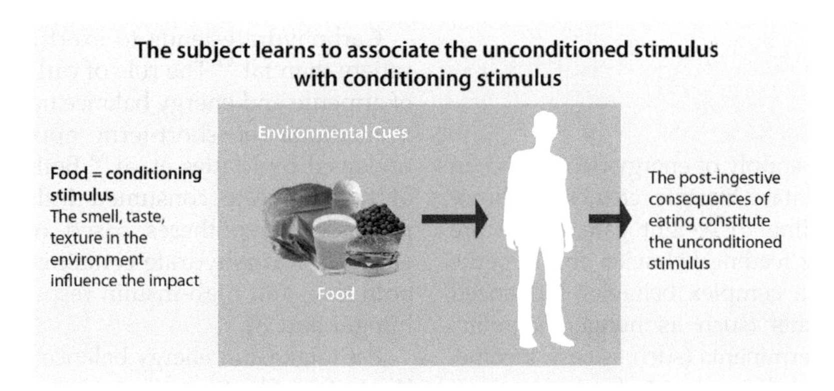

FIGURE 8.1 Eating as a form of learned behavior through associative conditioning.[20]

implicated as an important factor influencing appetite control. Burton et al.[27] identified an association between food craving and external eating scores among a mixed-age sample of both males and females. More specifically, this was in relation to total food cravings and cravings for high-fat foods, with food craving accounting for approximately 8%–20% of the variance in BMI. This area merits further investigation, since the link between eating behavior(s), externality, and food craving as a risk factor for obesity is not well understood.

C. Emotionality Theory

Food intake can have a remarkable effect on mood, and most individuals will have their own food-associated, mood-related habits, e.g., a cup of coffee to get going in the morning or eating sweet foods to reduce anxiety. Emotional states can have major effects on eating behavior and result in either over eating or under eating. There have been several reviews of studies concerning emotional eating in relation to body weight.[28] These studies have almost always dealt with negative emotions such as depression or fear, comparing obese and normal-weight subjects, with results indicating relative over-eating in obese individuals during negative emotional states. Eating by obese individuals in response to negative emotions is a learned behavior to reduce the negative state[29] and has been interpreted as psychosomatic. Geliebter and Aversa[30] conducted a questionnaire study of underweight, normal weight, and obese subjects and also similarly reported that the overweight group ate more than the other weight groups when experiencing negative emotions and situations, whereas underweight individuals reported eating more when experiencing positive emotions and situations. Most striking was the undereating by underweight individuals during negative emotions and situations, which may contribute to their body weight status. The relationship between mood and food will continue to be hotly debated at an individual and population level.

III. NUTRITIONAL INFLUENCES ON FOOD CHOICE

A cheap and plentiful supply of energy-dense food, in combination with a sedentary lifestyle, creates an obesogenic environment, leading to weight gain. There are many factors influencing feeding behavior and appetite control. Food choice is a complex behavior influenced by biological determinants (such as hunger, appetite, and taste); economic determinants (such as cost, income, and availability); physical determinants (such as access, education, skills, and time); social determinants (such as culture, family, peers, and meal patterns); psychological determinants (such as mood, stress, and guilt); and attitudes, beliefs, and knowledge about food. However, individuals do not always initiate eating due to (learned) internal physiological symptoms of hunger. It is recognized that psychological and external (environmental) cues can promote overeating, at least in the short term. Highly palatable food and snacks can contribute to overconsumption of calories, particularly through promotion of hedonic or reward mechanisms. For example, stress or "daily hassle" has been shown to increase snacking behavior, particularly for high-fat and high-sugar foods, which may contribute to our "obesogenic environment."[31]

A. Diet Composition—Not All Calories Are Equal When Influencing Satiety

The dietary macronutrients provide energy as protein, fat, carbohydrate, and alcohol. It is generally accepted that diet composition strongly affects ad libitum EI, under laboratory[32] and free-living conditions,[33] with protein highlighted as the most satiating macronutrient.[34] Even when ingested at the same level of ED, protein is the most satiating macronutrient.[35,36] Under these conditions, differences between carbohydrate and fat are less clear-cut.

Recent findings suggest that an elevated protein intake seems to play a key role in body-weight management, through (i) increased satiety related to increased diet-induced thermogenesis, (ii) its effect on thermogenesis, (iii) body composition, and (iv) decreased energy efficiency.[37] Supported by these mechanisms, a relatively larger WL and stronger body-weight maintenance thereafter have been observed with protein-enriched diets. The safety and efficacy of high-protein diets for WL has been questioned, with Eisenstein et al.[38] summarizing the experimental and epidemiological data. Protein-induced satiety has been shown acutely, within single meals that contain between 25% and 81% of energy from protein, leading to subsequent EI. Protein-induced satiety has been shown with high protein ad libitum diets, lasting up to 14 days[39] and up to 6 months.[40]

Carbohydrate tends to exert a more acute effect on satiety than fat.[41] The role of carbohydrate in regulation of appetite and energy balance has attracted attention as a mediator of short-term appetite[42] and has been reviewed by Mattes et. al.[43] Both the type and amount of carbohydrate consumed influence many ingestive processes. Hypotheses based on the glycemic index value of carbohydrate-containing foods suggest that both low- and high-insulin responses to foods promote hunger and EI.[44]

Fat intake and energy balance have been reviewed by Westerterp-Plantenga.[45] A paradox becomes apparent when considering fat intake and satiety.[46] Although the body appears to generate potent physiological responses that are triggered by fat ingestion, many studies have demonstrated that people who consume high-fat foods (either through personal choice or in experimental situations) tend to overconsume energy, termed passive overconsumption. Rodent studies suggest that fat delivered to the intestine (duodenum or jejunum) generates potent satiety signals. On the other hand, exposure to high-fat foods leads to a form of passive overconsumption that suggests that fat has a weak effect on satiety (poor fullness feedback). When human subjects are given a range of high-fat foods, they increase their EI and gain weight compared with subjects eating a medium- or low-fat diet.[47] This may be explained as fat consumed orally takes some time to reach the intestine, and its negative feedback action is likely to be diluted by other nutrients. Fat produces potent oral stimulation (positive feedback) that facilitates intake; high-fat foods normally have a high ED, which means that a large amount of fat as energy can be consumed before fat-induced satiety signals become operative. The signals are apparently too delayed to prevent the intake of large amounts of this food.[48]

B. Energy Density—The Amount of Energy Per Gram of Food

ED is the amount of energy in a particular weight of food (kJ/g). Dietary ED tends to act as a constraint on feeding behavior[49] influencing satiety or the feeling of fullness after eating. It is influenced by the moisture content of food (adding weight with no calories), fiber content (adding volume with limited calories), and macronutrient composition, mainly from fat content, because of its high energy content per gram. One classic experiment on how ED affects satiety and food intake is the provision of a soup-based preload before eating, which reduces EI at the next meal[50]; interestingly, provision of a glass of water does not have the same effect on satiety as incorporating it into food to lower ED,[51] which also suggests a role for viscosity on gut responsiveness.

A diet that is low in ED will induce an energy deficit, determined by the rate (volume over time) at which low ED foods can be digested and absorbed. This might be a useful strategy to achieve WL. One dietary strategy to decrease ED is to increase the intake of water-rich foods such as fruit and vegetables, allowing a satisfying portion size while decreasing EI. Data from clinical trials suggest that substantial WL can be achieved with this approach.[52] Conversely, if a diet is too high in ED, overconsumption will tend to occur because the amount of food people eat tends to be conditioned and there is relatively weak defense against excess EI.[53] Consumption of foods with a high ED may increase the risk of passive overconsumption and weight gain. As a general rule then, decreasing the fat content either of individual foods or the diet as a whole should decrease the ED of the diet. Studies performed in subjects who were fed a diet where the ED was varied while maintaining the macronutrient composition found that subjects ate a similar weight of food regardless of macronutrient composition, thus promoting energy overconsumption on diets with a high ED.[54,55] Conversely, several studies have shown that if the amount of fat in the diet was varied while keeping the ED constant, subjects consumed a similar weight of food and hence EI remains unchanged.[56,57] These studies, however, involved diets that were highly constructed in terms of macronutrient composition and ED in order to create dissociations and hence do not reflect typical population diets. What these studies suggest is that the overall ED of the diet is strongly influenced by fat content and is probably a major contributor to total EI.

While many previous studies have focused on the link between ED and foods, beverages can also make a significant contribution to the total EI of an individual. In Australia, beverages contribute to 16.3% of the total daily EI for all persons.[58] In the United States, soft drink consumption has increased by more than 60% between 1977 and 1998.[59]

IV. NON NUTRITIONAL INFLUENCES ON FOOD CHOICE

Research into the effect of nonnutritional influences on eating behavior has tended to focus on what we eat (food choice), whereas the physiological or metabolic aspects focus on how much we eat (calorie or weight of food intake). The sensory (odor, texture, taste, appearance) aspects of a food or meal can significantly alter our choice, at least in the short term. These sensory or hedonic parameters influence the reward aspects of eating behavior, and much research focuses on assessing responses to changing single parameters.

A. Palatability—Sensory Capacity to Increase Food Consumption

The palatability of a food can be thought of as its sensory capacity to stimulate ingestion of that food.[60] This definition takes account of the fact that the palatability of the food is jointly determined by the nature of the food (odor, taste, texture, and state), the sensory capabilities and metabolic state of the subject, and the environment in which the food and subject interacts. Palatability is therefore not stable. Satiety is said to be sensory specific in relation to foods because the palatability of a food declines as its ingestion proceeds, while unsampled foods do not change in perceived pleasantness.[61] This has been called sensory-specific satiety.[62,63] This in turn should promote subsequent selection of those other foods and so maintain a variety of foods ingested in a meal. In this context, it is important to ascertain exactly why the pleasantness of a specific food declines as its ingestion proceeds. The texture of foods can influence palatability and calorie intake. Both people and rodents can consume more ad libitum from liquid foods than they can consume in solid foods. This is related to rate of eating, which is higher for liquids when compared to semisolids. For example, eating 500 g of apples takes about 17 min, whereas drinking the equivalent amount of apple juice can be done in 1.5 min.[64] A recent US study[65] has highlighted that limiting the intake of ultraprocessed foods could be an effective strategy for obesity prevention and treatment, since eliminating ultraprocessed foods from the diet decreases EI and results in WL in healthy adults. However, commercially available foods are largely designed to maximize both the sensory and dietary parameters, which in turn make foods appealing to enhance consumer demand and repeat sales. This new research highlights that such foods are likely to promote weight gain. Further knowledge about the importance of palatability and food intake in the long term and how to alter food processing to maximize palatability of food during WL is likely to be a future research area.

B. Sensory Variety—We Are Offered More We Eat More

In summary, short-term studies (within-day) have indicated that increasing sensory variety leads to an increase in food intake.[63] It has been shown that increased variety of foods made available either sequentially or simultaneously increases very short-term food intake (i.e., within a meal).[63,66–68] Spiegel and Stellar[67] have shown this to be the case in both lean and overweight women. They also found that simultaneous increases in the variety of foods offered elevates intake as compared to sequential increases in the variety of foods offered in a single meal. Rolls has reported that the greater the dissimilarity between different foods, the greater the variety-stimulating effect on the short-term intake of foods.[68] This is explained by the phenomenon, "sensory-specific satiety." Sensory specific satiation refers to the decline in reward value during consumption of a food because of repeated exposure to a particular sensory signal. This can be simply described as increased boredom with the taste of a particular product.

It has also been shown by Blundell's group that combinations of sensory attributes associated with mixtures of fat and sugar can have a large effect on EI at a specific feeding episode.[69] This suggests that increases in EI will be promoted by the combination of sensory attributes of foods. More food is often consumed in the presence of other people, a phenomenon known as "social facilitation of energy intake,"[70] a feature of social eating.

One long-term study conducted over a week[71] assessed increasing the variety of nutritionally very similar but sensorially distinct foods available ad libitum in lean and overweight men. Offering 5, 10, or 15 food items per day led to a significant increase in food and EI in the lean men. These data indicate that increasing the variety of sensorially distinct but nutritionally similar foods increased food intake. This had a potent effect on EI and energy balance because subjects actively increased the amount of food they ingested in response to the variety offered. It is not clear if this effect would be maintained over a more prolonged period of time (weeks or months).

C. Portion Size—Plate Size or Meal Size to Influence How Much We Eat

Since the 1970s, the portion size of commercially available foods and beverages has increased, a trend observed in a variety of settings including restaurants, supermarkets, and also in the home environment.[53] Laboratory-based studies examining single-meal eating episodes have suggested that increased portion size promotes increased EI. There is a clear relationship between amount served and amount consumed, even when participants serve themselves. The "bottomless soup bowl experiment," where subjects received tomato soup with a hidden self-filling tube, consumed 73% more soup (113 kcal), compared to when refilled by a server.[72] Other studies suggest this effect persists for up to 4 days,[73] but this would have to be sustained over an extended period of time to contribute to weight gain. Studies in a more natural environment, such as a cafeteria-style restaurant or workplace, have also indicated that increasing the size of a meal portion by 50% increases intake with no apparent compensatory reduction in intake, even when studied for a month.[74] Self-reports of food intake also suggest poor regulation with increased portion size.[75] One study reports men and women eating 19.4 MJ extra (a 16% increase in EI) over an 11-day period when provided with larger portions, which would equate to a 0.5 kg weight gain.[76] This feature of modern eating behavior has, in particular, been the focus of media attention with "supersize" portions being blamed for the rise in obesity in children and adults. Roughly, 41% of Americans report consuming three or more commercially prepared meals a week in 1999–2000.[77] The ready availability and low cost of large portions of energy-dense foods can contribute to a positive energy balance over a prolonged period. However, the data do not prove that portion size plays a role in etiology of obesity, and there is little evidence that decreasing portion size is acceptable or effective for weight control. Smaller-portion controlled foods or marketing of foods for "dieting" is not straightforward, since consumers equate large portions with good value and small portions with feeling deprived. Improving consumer awareness about nutritional information at point-of-sale and incentives for the food industry to offer a variety of portions is likely to be future incentives considered by policy makers to control food provision within the "obesogenic" eating environment.

D. Stress—Do You Eat More or Less When Stressed?

There is evidence to suggest that the majority of people tend to change their eating behavior when they believe themselves to be stressed, with an estimated 80% of people altering their caloric intake either by increasing or decreasing their consumption.[78] The direction of change of calorie intake is highly dependent on eating behavior profile and personality phenotype. For example, it is well documented that individuals who are "restrained" in their eating behavior are more susceptible to stress-induced eating and have been shown to be more susceptible to the deleterious effects of stress on eating behavior (overeating). Dietary restraint can also be associated with 'disinhibition" and loss of control over eating resulting in binge eating. Zellner et al.[79] reported that 71% of those woman who reported increasing their food intake when stressed were categorized as restrained eaters, compared to only 35% of those who did not alter their eating behavior, or reduced their food intake, in response to stress. Zellner's study was based on a self-report questionnaire of eating behavior when stressed, and, as such, it is not possible to conclude what manner of stressor people were considering when responding. Wallis and Hetherington[80] also found evidence that highly restrained individuals increased their snacking after ego-threatening stressors compared to unrestrained individuals.

E. Food Addiction—Does This Phenomenon Exist?

We hear a lot about "food addiction" in the popular media, and we use the word "addiction" very casually to describe our relationships with a wide range of everyday activities. Are people really addicted to chocolate, sugar, or mobile phone use in the same way that they can become physically addicted to nicotine or heroin? Furthermore, since weight gain, body fat accumulation, and obesity are driven by the over consumption of calories relative to energy expenditure, if food addiction does exist, is it responsible for, or a major contributor to, the current obesity epidemic?

There are a number of different definitions of addiction. Until recently, the medically established diagnosis of addiction was limited to substance-related disorders only, with the disorder defined as a chronic relapsing brain disease. The phenomena of "food craving" and "food addiction" are not well researched, and indeed many researchers would question their existence.[81] Food craving is "an irresistible urge to consume a specific food," in particular linked to high-sugar and high-fat foods. Humans who overeat do not generally target specific nutrients, but rather a range of palatable foods. Consequently, food addiction cannot be diagnosed according to any set of criteria that have general medical or psychological recognition. Based on current knowledge, the term food addiction appears inappropriate. By contrast, disorders of eating behavior can resemble the addictive, behavioral patterns observed in substance dependency. Currently, the greatest clinical similarity between an abnormal food consumption behavior and drug addiction exists in binge-eating disorder, an eating disorder characterized by binge eating without subsequent purging episodes and which is prevalent within the obese, human population. Food ingestion is satisfying if we are hungry and palatable food is appealing to us and rewarding because it activates specific parts of the brain, naturally triggering signals in the opioid and dopamine systems. No single food substance or specific neurobiological mechanism can account for the fact that many people overeat and develop obesity. As in many aspects of everyday life, our relationships with food fall along a continuum, with eating disorders at extreme ends. In contrast, it is the gradual accumulation of excess body weight over prolonged periods of time, years, or decades that characterizes the development of overweight and obesity. It is almost certainly inappropriate to invoke food addiction or eating addiction in this context.

This area merits further investigation, since the link between eating behavior(s) and food craving or addiction as a risk factor for obesity is not well known or recognized. The neuropsychology of food reward and food choice and the links between the appetite regulatory network, eating behavior, and food preference are not understood. Future research will likely focus on brain neuroanatomy and interactions with food to challenge whether food is indeed "addictive" and to investigate the pathways involved in the "rewarding" aspects of food and whether this experience can be replicated in healthier food product alternatives, to control body weight.

V. PHYSIOLOGY INFLUENCING FOOD CHOICE

While the influence of psychology in eating behavior is important, it is not the only influence by any means. Physiology also plays an important and influential role in individuals' eating behavior. Food intake is regulated by two complementary drives: the homeostatic and hedonic pathways. The energostatic or homeostatic pathway controls energy balance by increasing the motivation to eat following depletion of energy stores. Feedback is more potent during negative energy balance than during positive energy balance (which is why it is easy to gain weight but difficult to lose weight). In contrast, hedonic or reward-based regulation can override the homeostatic pathway during periods of relative energy abundance by increasing the desire to consume foods that are highly palatable. In summary, we also eat for pleasure, not just to provide energy.

Energostatic pathways—Considered broadly, energy homeostasis consists of the interrelated processes integrated by the brain to maintain energy stores at appropriate levels. When food is ingested, physiological and psychological responses are induced, which depend on its energy and macronutrient content and structure. The macronutrient composition determines the caloric content, digestibility, and the rate of passage of a meal through the gastrointestinal tract (GIT) (the gut) and strongly influences the secretion of peptide hormones from the gut. These hormones, in turn, feedback on brain centers that control eating behavior, metabolism, and energy utilization. During meal processing, the gut secretes a number of newly identified hormones that signal to the brain to suppress future food intake. Physiological changes, such as gut peptide concentrations, are related to appetite ratings or food intake and can be used as biomarkers of appetite. The regulation of appetite is, however, complex, and it is not surprising that multiple control systems exist.[82]

The brain connected to the central nervous system (CNS) is seen as the traditional "control center" for body weight; it has the elaborate task of interpreting continuous information provided to it by neural networks and chemical messengers with respect to the body's energy state. The brain uses this information to initiate an appropriate reaction to maintain homeostasis. These signals vary throughout time, and the responses alter depending on what type of food has been ingested. The gut becomes responsible for generating the majority of inputs communicated to the CNS regarding the content and size of a meal, thus establishing a complex bidirectional communication system, referred to as the gut–brain axis.[83,84]

Hedonic pathways—Eating is essential for survival and is underpinned by the fundamental physiological need to consume energy. However, people often consume in excess of the basic nutrient and energy requirement needed to maintain physiological *homeostasis*, particularly when there is an abundance of readily available food and drink. Eating is more often than not controlled by external cues and stimuli, the time of the day, and social factors, rather the need to replenish energy stores (we eat for pleasure—*hedonic* influence). The modern environment is replete with food-associated cues that encourage eating in the absence of metabolic demands. "Cues" refer to external, environmental cues, such as the sight and smell of particular foods, or locations where certain foods are procured.

It is worthy to note that Blundell and Finlayson have developed understanding and assessment techniques for quantifying "liking" and "wanting" of foods. Liking is the hedonic evaluation (pleasantness, appreciation) of tasting a particular food, whereas wanting refers to the desire to actually ingest a particular food. Wanting has a much more direct effect on food intake than liking.[85] This is incorporated into Fig. 8.2. This figure shows schematic overview of the variety of inputs (biological signals or triggers) linked with hedonic stimulation or satiety. The hedonic signals (activation of dopamine, cannabinoids, or opiods) tend to encourage consumption.[86] There can also be external triggers to the perception of hedonics or the reward factor of the food or beverage, stimulated from the visual or olfactory cues. These cues will also feed into the satiety signals (namely the gut hormones such as cholecystokinin [CCK] or GLP), which in turn can influence the neuropeptide expression (such as NPY, AgPR, MSH). This is not a simple system, rather a highly complex one.

Satiety cascade—Blundell proposed the satiety cascade nearly 30 years ago[87] to provide a conceptual framework for examining the impacts of foods on satiation (processes that bring an eating episode to an end) and satiety (processes that inhibit further eating in the postprandial period). This is shown in Fig. 8.3[87] and has been updated to include emerging evidence on the role of meal timing as an influence on appetite and energy balance. As a general rule, signals arising in the periphery that influence food intake and energy expenditure can be partitioned into two broad categories:

- One comprises the signals generated during meals that cause satiation (i.e., feelings of fullness that contribute to the decision to stop eating)
- And/or satiety (i.e., prolongation of the interval until hunger or a drive to eat reappears).

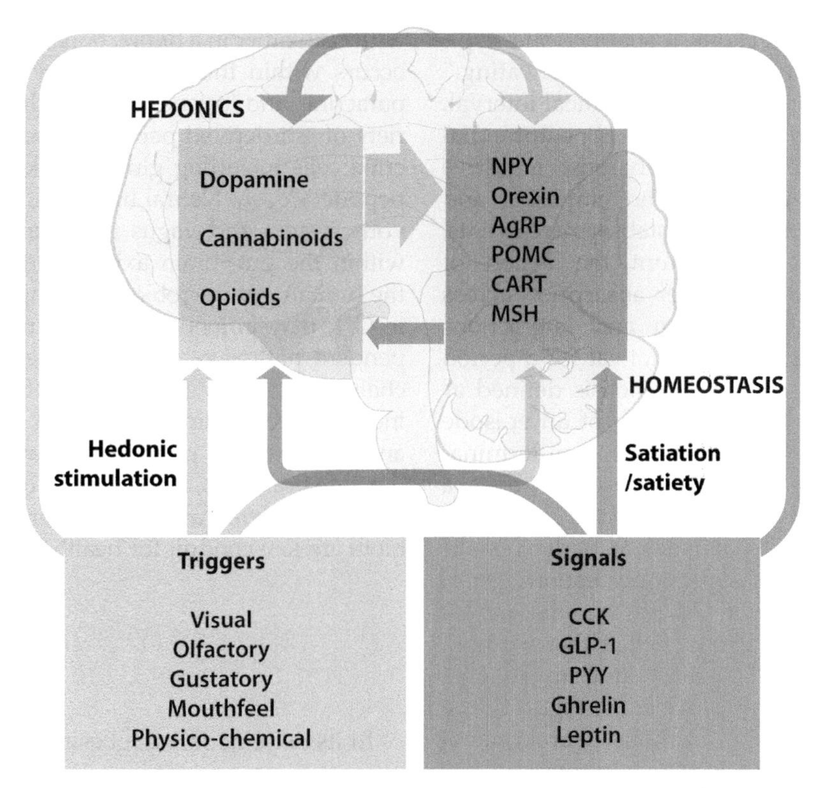

FIGURE 8.2 Energostatic and homeostatic influence on eating, showing the relationship between triggers for consumption and signals for satiety and the interaction between hedonic and homeostatic systems in the brain. CCK is cholecystokinin; GLP-1 is glucagon-like peptide-1; PYY is peptide tyrosine.

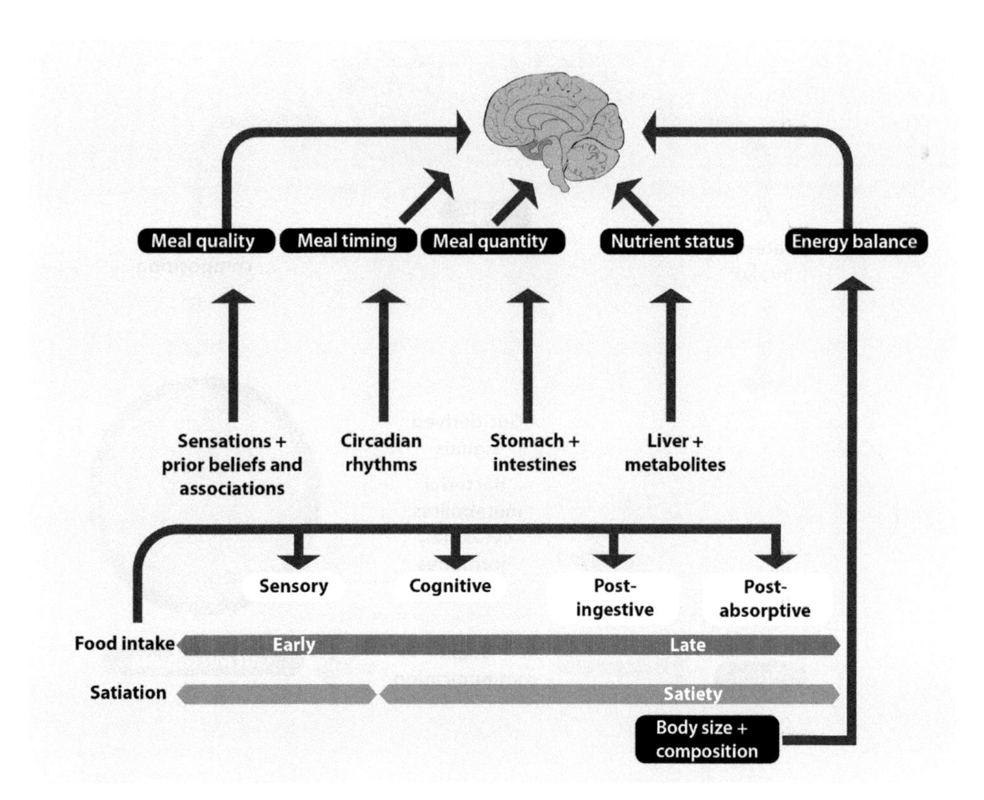

FIGURE 8.3 The satiety cascade describes a series of behavioral and physiological events that occur following food intake and that inhibit further eating until the return of hunger signals. *(Adapted from Blundell et al., 2010).*[20]

Satiety is another motivational construct and typically is used to refer to "a state of inhibition of eating." Simply, this can be considered as the intermeal interval. This is mainly influenced by physiological postprandial and CNS effects. For example, early post ingestive events include gastric distension and emptying and release of hormones followed by postabsorptive events, including mechanisms arising from the action of glucose, fats, and amino acids after absorption across the intestine into the bloodstream and interactions with the CNS. After a meal, we do not eat for a period of time and this reflects satiety. Satiation is defined as "the process leading to the termination of an episode of eating." This describes the process of meal termination or stopping eating and may be expressed as a feeling of fullness. Meal termination is affected by psychological events and behavior, as well as an early cephalic phase response. These are the sensory perceptions generated by smell, taste, temperature, and texture that inhibit eating in the short term. Cognitive beliefs that we hold about food may inhibit eating in the short term.

The food–gut–brain axis is detailed in Fig. 8.4. The gut–brain axis is comprised of various neurohumoral components that allow the gut and brain to communicate with each other in a bidirectional manner. Communication occurs within this axis via may routes including local, paracrine, and/or endocrine mechanisms, involving a variety of gut-derived peptides produced from enteroendocrine cells including glucagon-like peptide 1, CCK, and peptide YY_{3-36}. Neural networks, such as the enteric nervous system and vagus nerve, also convey information within the gut–brain axis. Emerging evidence suggests the human gut microbiota, a complex ecosystem residing in GIT, may influence the brain through several interdependent pathways, including the fermentation of short-chain fatty acids (SCFA), and behavior modifications, including controlling satiety and influencing energy balance. Some recent publications have eloquently described the gut–brain axis, in the context of food intake, where the gut is considered as a "second brain" and the gut microbiota are key conduit for health.[88,89]

VI. BODY COMPOSITION ASSESSMENT OF BODY STORES

In its extreme forms, obesity is easily recognized. Significant excess weight is readily visible, and most adults

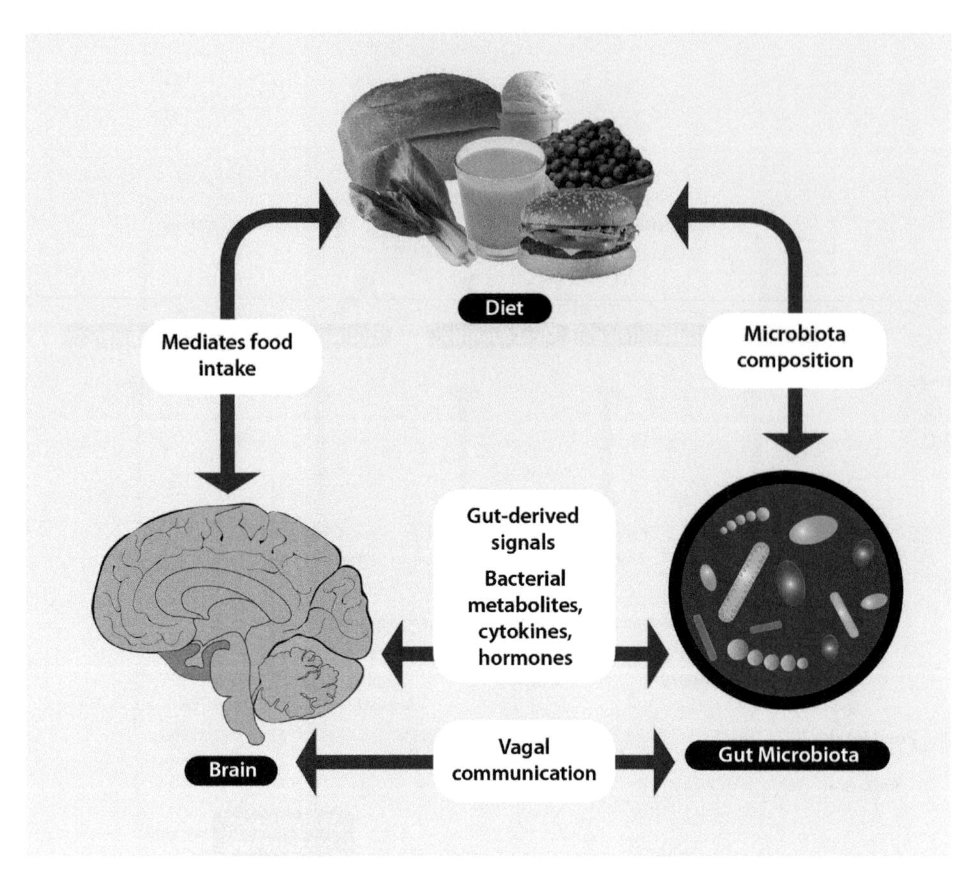

FIGURE 8.4 Food–gut–brain axis shows that food and dietary components interact with the gastrointestinal tract, which in turn signals to the brain in a complex network.

TABLE 8.1 Reference man's body composition with individual components and density (from Snyder et al. 1974).

Component	Density (g/ml)	Reference body %
Water	0.9937	62.4
Protein	1.34	16.4
Mineral (osseous)	3.038	5.9
Mineral (non-osseous)	3.317	4.8
Fat	0.9007	15.3
Fat-free mass	1.100	84.7
Total reference body	1.064	100

can identify the difference between a highly trained and muscular athlete and a person who is obese, where excess weight is dominated by body fat. The specific measurement of body composition requires more sophisticated measures of the body stores. At a minimum, the body is considered to be composed of two compartments, fat mass (FM) and fat-free mass (FFM). FM is relatively homogeneous, but the FFM component includes bone mineral, protein, water, glycogen, and other minor constituents. Analysis of a limited number of cadavers has shown that these principal body constituents exist in relatively constant proportions and, through the measurement of one or more of these components, the composition of the whole body may be inferred (Table 8.1).[90]

Multicompartment models are commonly used for research purposes and have been described in detail elsewhere.[91] In brief, a three-compartment model usually combines measures of total body water with densitometry to estimate water, fat, and dry, fat-free tissue, while a four-compartment model extends this analysis to include bone mineral, usually measured by dual energy X-ray absorptiometry, to give bone, water, fat, and soft, dry, fat-free tissue.[92] Different body composition techniques have their advantages and disadvantages with respect to simplicity, precision, and accuracy.[93] Correct interpretation of the changes in body composition requires understanding of the limitations of the techniques employed. For example, Wells et al.[94] examined the propagation of methodological errors on estimations of fat and FFM and concluded that the four-component model estimates FM and FFM (or protein, as TBW and body mineral mass are already accounted) to within ± 0.54 kg. Elia[95] also suggested, in a review of body composition analysis using various component models, that body fat and protein can be estimated to within 0.5 ± 0.75 kg using the four-component model.

A. Body Composition Assessment of Energy Balance

Excess fat accumulates in response to a prolonged period in which EI exceeds energy expenditure and treating obesity requires this situation to be reversed. There is an ongoing debate as to the relative importance of intake and expenditure in the etiology of obesity. At a population level, it is likely that both are important, while the error in the measurement of intake and expenditure at an individual level precludes specific conclusions in the majority of cases. Nonetheless, an understanding of dietary intake and energy expenditure is important in understanding the etiology of obesity and helps to establish a personalized approach to weight management.

Successful WL strategies aim to optimize fat mass loss and minimize lean tissue loss. Prevention of the excessive loss of lean body mass (LBM) is desirable because this can assist in attenuating the counterproductive decline in resting metabolism associated with WL. Reducing body fat by diet and exercise can improve the health and quality of life of patients, as well as lowering mortality and morbidity risk.[96] Monitoring body weight (mass) reduction alone does not allow changes in body composition (fat, protein, bone, and water) to be assessed and thus the suitability of the regime to be determined. In a research environment, the composition of WL is usually obtained from a two-compartment model, with changes in FFM and FM measured by air displacement plethysmography (Bod Pod) or bioimpedance (BIA). Because FFM consists of water, protein, and mineral, any change in one of these compartments will affect the estimate of FFM. The four-compartment model assumes that body weight is equal to the sum of FM and FFM, where FFM is composed of water, protein, and minerals. Total mineral is the sum of osseous mineral and cell mineral.[92]

Osseous mineral is derived from the measurement of bone mineral ash, and cell mineral is considered as a constant ratio of bone ash. After correcting for water and mineral content at 36°C, data from the DEXA are used to correct for bone content; body density is used to calculate the proportion of FM and FFM. Finally, the TBW data can be used to calculate the proportion of protein in FFM. Water, protein, and mineral are summed to yield FFM. This model has been described in detail.[90]

The density of FM and FFM is assumed as 1.34 kg/l and 0.9 kg/L, respectively.[90] Protein and FM are calculated indirectly from body density calculation. First, the contribution of water and mineral is subtracted from body weight and body volume, and then the residual values are used to estimate the combined density of protein and fat. The model does not consider glycogen separately; this is primarily included in the protein estimation.

B. Energy Cost of Weight Gain and Weight Loss

It has been suggested that the energy content of WL is approximately 3500 kcal or 32.2 MJ/kg per pound of body weight (relative to requirements). Work by Hall et al., 2011, challenges this approach as being too simplistic and leading to an overestimation of WL, based on extreme WL modeling.[97] This value assumes exclusive loss of adipose tissue consisting of 87% fat,[95] which is oversimplified, since there is likely to be loss of LBM during energy deficit (and influenced by degree of obesity, diet composition, physical activity level, rate, and duration of WL). The metabolizable energy densities of body glycogen, protein, and fat are 17.6, 19.7, and 39.5 MJ kg^{-1}, respectively, where loss of body water results in a significant mass change but contributes nothing to the metabolizable energy content. The energy content per kg change of body fat is 39·5 MJ and 7·6 MJ for a kg of lean mass when working with a two-compartment model of body composition (such as air displacement plethysmography).

Hall et al.[97] propose a dynamic mathematical modeling approach whereby calorie deficits can be calculated over a prolonged period of time, and they propose an approximate and alternative rule of thumb that for an average overweight adult, a change in EI of 100 KJ per day could lead to an eventual bodyweight change of about 1 kg (equivalent to 10 kcal/d per 1 lb of weight change), with half of the weight change being achieved in about 1 year and 95% over 3 years.

C. Weight Change in Response to Overfeeding

The classical studies of Bouchard et al.[98] are worthy of mention. These researchers undertook very well-controlled studies to determine whether there are true differences in the responses among individuals to long-term overfeeding and to assess the possibility that genotypes are involved in such differences. In response to 84 days of 1000 kcal day^{-1} of overfeeding, 12 pairs of monozygotic twins gained on average 8.1 kg, but the range was from 4.3 to 13.3 kg. However, the similarity within each twin pair in response to overfeeding was significant with respect to body weight gain, percentage of fat, and total FM with about three times more variance among pairs than within pairs. The Quebec group have more attempted to identify predictors of body composition and body energy changes in response to overfeeding.[99] They highlight that prior to overfeeding FFM, muscle oxidative enzyme activities, VO_2 max, low androgenicity, and high levels of leptin appear to be biomarkers of more favorable body composition changes and less body energy gains in response to a fixed amount of excess calories. The similarity in the adaptation to long-term overfeeding within the pairs of twins clearly indicated that genetic factors are involved in the partitioning between fat and lean mass deposition and in determining the energy expenditure response.

Additional factors affecting the energy cost of tissue deposition was the body composition of the subjects under study. The energy cost of weight gain is higher in the obese than in the lean. It has been observed that, during weight gain, thin individuals gain proportionately more lean tissue; obese individuals gain proportionately more adipose tissue.[100,101] Since the energy required to gain a gram of adipose tissue is about six times greater than for lean tissue, it is actually energetically *costlier* for the obese to gain weight. Under conditions of a positive EB, it is pertinent to consider the patterns of tissue storage and the energetic cost of weight gain, since it is often claimed by the obese that the energy cost of weight gain may be less for the lean compared to the obese; when excess energy is ingested, thin individuals gain proportionately more lean tissue, whereas obese individuals gain proportionately more adipose tissue. Per gram of tissue gained, the energy cost for adipose tissue gain is about six times greater than for lean tissue. Thus *per unit of weight gain*, it is actually energetically more costly for the obese to gain weight (Forbes et al.).[102,103]

To examine this concept more closely, it is necessary to consider the composition of specific tissues. The adipose tissue content of reference man comprises 80% fat (mainly triglyceride), 15% water, and 5% protein as wet tissue.[102,103] The gross energy content of fat (adipose tissue triglyceride) is 39.9 kJ/g and for average meat protein is 23.6 kJ/g[104]. The energy content of adipose tissue should therefore be $[(0.8 \times 39.9) + (0.15 \times 0) + (0.05 \times 23.6)] = 33.1$ kJ/g. For subjects of BMI 20–25, Forbes has estimated the ratio of LBM to FM gained or lost to be 39% LBM and 61% FM.[103,105]

Given the composition of adipose tissue, this would approximate to 25% lean tissue and 75% adipose tissue, for reference man.[90] Therefore, the energy content of weight gain would amount to approximately 29 MJ/kg. When calculating the energy cost of weight gain, consideration has to be given not only to the energy content of weight gain but also to the energy costs associated with assimilating and maintaining that tissue. Forbes, using data from his own and other overfeeding studies in predominantly lean males, performed regression analysis of excess energy ingested against weight gain. He determined that the energy cost of weight gain was 33.7 kJ/g from these analyses. Because obese individuals gain proportionately more fat, this figure is likely to be higher.[101,103]

VII. CONCLUSION

Although consumers search for the "magic bullet" approach for fast and safe WL diet for weight control, these do not exist! This chapter has outlined why we have not solved the obesity epidemic. Namely, the complex systems in the human body, including physiology, psychology, and behavior of humans, identify many pathways to influence food choice and eating behavior. Furthermore, a one-diet approach does not fit all people! We do not have current knowledge to be able to direct nutrition advice for an individual, but this will likely come in the future, whereby a detailed assessment of psychology and physiology will indicate what dietary approaches will work best for which type of people.

RESEARCH GAPS—FUTURE PERSPECTIVES

Research gaps in energy balance

- Gut microbiota influence on energy balance—There is now compelling evidence of a direct bidirectional cross talk between the brain and the gut, pinpointing they have a reciprocal influence on each other's physiology and (dys)function. Diet is a major modulator of gut–microbiota profile and the metabolites they produce, thus dietary modification can impact on health. The role of the gut microbiota to influence EI and energy expenditure and understanding the role of individual dietary components to support precision or personalized nutrition (e.g., effect of dietary fiber to influence SCFA production) will continue to be a hot topic in years to come.
- Functional food to support appetite across the life course—With an aging population, dietary approaches to promote health and independence later in life are needed. In part, this can be achieved by maintaining muscle mass and strength as people age. Functional foods can offer an additional health benefit beyond the nutrition. New evidence suggests that current dietary recommendations for protein intake may be insufficient to achieve this goal and that individuals might benefit by increasing their intake and frequency of consumption of high-quality protein. More research is needed to explore how to build consumer awareness about the importance of sufficient protein intake for healthy aging.
- Sustainable and healthy plant protein to support health—Exploring alternative protein sources and transitioning toward more sustainable, plant-based diets has been a recent research priority. The high proportion of animal protein consumption in developed countries raises both health and environmental concerns. Dietary patterns characterized by a high intake of animal protein have been associated with increased risk of obesity, diabetes, cardiovascular disease mortality, and some cancers. Animal protein consumption requires large areas of dedicated land, water, nitrogen, and fossil energy for production and transportation. It is still unclear whether plant proteins affect appetite in the same way as animal proteins and whether they compromise subsequent EI.
- Chrononutrition (role of circadian rhythms and timing of eating)—It is now becoming apparent that not only what we eat but also when eat can influence body weight and appetite control. This may be due to circadian rhythms or a behavioral response to eating. For example, consuming more calories in the morning (big breakfast) and less in the evening (small dinner) may lead to greater feeling of fullness throughout the day and higher levels of physical activity. Thus, the timing of eating and fasting and the translation of results from preclinical trials into humans will be an exciting development.

VIII. REFERENCES

1. Mela D. Eating behavior, food preferences and dietary intake in relation to obesity and body-weight status. *Proc Nutr Soc*. 1996; 55:803–816.
2. World Health Organization. *Diet, Nutrition and the Prevention of Chronic Disease. Report of the Joint WHO/FAO Expert Consultation. WHO Technical Report Series, No.96*. Geneva, Switzerland: World health Organization; 2003 (TRS 916).
3. The Government Office for Science, UK. *Foresight- Tackling Obesities - Future Choices. Project Report*. 2nd ed. UK: The Government Office for Science; 2007.
4. Timmins KA, Green MA, Radley D, Morris MA, Pearce J. How has big data contributed to obesity research? A review of the literature. *Int J Obes*. 2018;42(12):1951–1962.

5. Innovative UK. Knowledge Transfer Network. (https://ktn-uk.co.uk/news/protein-for-life-a-framework-for-action; Accessed, 1st June 2019).
6. Morris J, Puttick M, Clark J, et al. The timescale of early land plant evolution. *Proc Natl Acad Sci. USA*. 2018:115.
7. Mercer J, Johnstone AM, Halford J. Approaches to influencing food choice across the age groups: from children to the elderly. *Proc Nutr Soc.* 2015;74(2):149–157.
8. Meule A, Vögele C. The psychology of eating. *Front Psychol.* 2013; 4:215. https://doi.org/10.3389/fpsyg.2013.00215.
9. Cohen D, Farley TA. Eating as an automatic behavior. *Prev Chronic Dis.* 2008;5:A23.
10. Herman CP, Polivy J. The self-regulation of eating: theoretical and practical problems. In: Baumeister RF, Vohs KD, eds. *In Handbook of Self-Regulation: Research, Theory, and Applications*. New York: The Guilford Press; 2004:492–508.
11. Stroebele N, De Castro JM. Effect of ambience on food intake and food choice. *Nutrition*. 2004:821–838. https://doi.org/10.1016/j.nut.2004.05.012.
12. Cohen DA, Babey SH. Contextual influences on eating behaviours: heuristic processing and dietary choices. *Obes Rev.* 2012; 13:766–779.
13. Rogers PJ. Obesity – is food addiction to blame? *Addiction*. 2011; 106:1213–1214. https://doi.org/10.1111/j.1360-0443.2011.03371.
14. Paroche M, Caton SJ, Vereijken CMJL, Weenen H, Houston-Price C. How infants and young children learn about food: a systematic review. *Front Psychol.* 2017;25(8):1046.
15. Birch LL, Anzman SL. Learning to eat in an obesogenic environment: a developmental systems perspective on childhood obesity. *Child Dev. Perspect.* 2010:138–143. https://doi.org/10.1111/j.1750-8606.2010.00132.
16. Keller KL. The use of repeated exposure and associative conditioning to increase vegetable acceptance in children: explaining the variability across studies. *J Acad Nutr Diet.* 2014;114(8):1169–1173.
17. Holland PC, Petrovich GD. A neural systems analysis of the potentiation of feeding by conditioned stimuli. *Acad Nutr Diet.* 2014;114(8):1169–1173.
18. Thibault L. *Obesity Prevention; the Role of Brain and Society on Individual Behavior. Chapter 10 - Associative Learning and the Control of Food Intake*. Academic Press; 2010.
19. Le Magnen J. Effects of the duration of a post prandial fast on the acquiaition of appetites in the white rat (first published in French in 1957). *Appetite*. 1999;3:27–29.
20. Blundell J. Making claims. Functional foods for managing appetite and weight. *Nat Rev Endocrinol.* 2010;6:53–56.
21. Strien T, Frijters JER, Bergers GPA, Defares PB. The Dutch Eating Behavior Questionnaire (DEBQ) for assessment of restrained, emotional and external eating behavior. *Int J Eat Disord.* 1986; 5(2):295–315.
22. Stunkard AJ, Messick S. The three-factor eating questionnaire to measure dietary restraint, disinhibition and hunger. *J Psychosom Res.* 1985;22:71–83.
23. Westerterp Plantenga MS, Wijckmans Duijsens NEG, TenHoor F, Weststrate A. Effect of replacement of fat by nonabsorbable fat (sucrose polyester) in meals or snacks as a function of dietary restraint. *Physiol Behav.* 1997;61(No.6):939–947.
24. Westerterp-Plantenga MS, Wijckmans-Duijsens NEG, Verboeket-van de Venne WPG, De Graaf K, Van het Hof KH, Weststrate JA. Energy intake and body weight effects of six months reduced or full fat diets, as a function of dietary restraint. *Int J Obes*. 1998;22:14–22.
25. Schachter S. Some extraordinary facts about obese humans and rats. *Am Psychol.* 1971;26:129–144.
26. Waters A, Hill A, Waller G. Bulimics' responses to food cravings: is binge-eating a product of hunger or emotional state? *Behav Res Ther.* 2001;39:877–886.
27. Burton P, Smit HJ, Lightowler HJ. The influence of restrained and external eating patterns on overeating. *Appetite*. 2007;49:191–197.
28. Allison DB, Heshka S. Emotion and eating in obesity? A critical analysis. *Int J Eat Disord.* 1993;13(3):289–295.
29. Kaplan HI, Kaplan HS. The psychosomatic concept of obesity. *J Nerv Ment Dis.* 1957;125:181–201.
30. Geliebter A. Aversa emotional eating in overweight, normal weight, and underweight individuals. *Eat Behav.* 2003;3: 341–347.
31. O'Connor D, Jones F, Conner M, McMillan B, Ferguson E. Effects of daily hassles and eating style on eating behavior. *Health Psychol : Off J Division Health Psychol, Am Psychol Ass.* 2008;27:S20–S31. https://doi.org/10.1037/0278-6133.27.1.S20.
32. Poppitt SD, Swann D, Black AE, Prentice AM. Assessment of selective under-reporting of food intake by both obese and non-obese women in a metabolic facility. *Int J Obes Relat Metab Disord.* 1998;22:303–311.
33. De Castro JM. Varying levels of food energy self-reporting are associated with between-group, but not within-subject, differences in food intake. *J Nutr.* 2006;136:1382–1388.
34. Halton TL, Hu FB. The effects of high protein diets on thermogenesis, satiety and weight loss: a critical review. *J Am Coll Nutr.* 2004; 23:373–385.
35. Johnstone AM, Stubbs RJ, Harbron CG. Effect of overfeeding macronutrients on day-to-day food intake in man. *Eur J Clin Nutr.* 1996;50(7):418–430.
36. Stubbs RJ, Harbron CG, Prentice AM. Covert manipulation of the dietary fat to carbohydrate ratio of isoenergetically dense diets: effect on food intake in feeding men ad libitum. *Int J Obes Relat Metab Disord.* 1996;20:651–666.
37. Lejeune M, Kovacs E, Westerterp-Plantenga M. Additional protein intake limits weight regain after weight loss in humans. *Br J Nutr.* 2005;93(2):281–289.
38. Eisenstein J, Roberts SB, Dallal G, Saltzman E. High-protein weight-loss diets: are they safe and do they work? A review of the experimental and epidemiologic data. *Nutr Rev.* 2002;60(7):189–200.
39. Johnstone AM, Horgan GW, Murison SD, Bremner DM, Lobley GE. Effects of a high-protein ketogenic diet on hunger, appetite, and weight loss in obese men feeding ad libitum. *Am J Clin Nutr.* 2008;87:44–55.
40. Skov AR, Toubro S, Bulow J, et al. Changes in renal function during weight loss induced by high vs low protein diets in overweight subjects. *Int J Obes.* 1999;23:1170–1177.
41. Raben A, Jensen NJ, Marckmann P, SandstroÈm B, Astrup A. Spontaneous weight loss during 11 weeks' ad libitum intake of a low fat, high fiber diet in young, normal weight subjects. *Int J Obes.* 1995;19:916–923.
42. Stubbs RJ, Mazlan N, Whybrow S. Carbohydrates, appetite and feeding behavior in humans. *J Nutr.* 2001;131(10):277–278.
43. Mattes RD, Hollis J, Hayes D, Stunkard AJ. Appetite measurement and manipulation misgivings. *J Am Diet Assoc.* 2005:87–89.
44. Flint A, Gregersen NT, Gluud LL, et al. Associations between postprandial insulin and blood glucose responses, appetite sensations and energy intake in normal weight and overweight individuals: a meta-analysis of test meal studies. *Br J Nutr.* 2007; 98:17–25.
45. Westerterp-Plantenga MS. Fat intake and energy-balance effects. *Physiol Behav.* 2004;83:579–585.
46. Blundell JE, Lawton CL, Halford J, Serotonin C. Eating Behavior, and fat intake. *Obesity.* 1995;3:471S–476S.
47. Blundell JE, Stubbs RJ. High and low carbohydrate and fat intakes: limits imposed by appetite and palatability and their implications for energy balance. *Eur J Clin Nutr.* 1999;53:S148–S165.
48. Blundell J, Lawton C, Cotton J, Macdiarmid J. Control of human appetite: implications for the intake of dietary fat. *Annu. Rev. Nutr.* 1996;16:285–319.

49. Rolls BJ. The relationship between dietary energy density and energy intake. *Physiol Behav.* 2009;97:609–615.
50. Himaya A, Louis-Sylvestre J. The effect of soup on satiation. *Appetite.* 1998;30:199–210.
51. Rolls BJ, Bell EA, Castellanos VH, Chow M, Pelkman CL, Thorwart ML. Energy density but not fat content of foods affected energy intake in lean and obese women. *Am J Clin Nutr.* 1999;69: 863–871.
52. Yao M, Roberts SB. Dietary energy density and weight regulation. *Nutr Rev.* 2001;59:247–258.
53. Rolls BJ, Roe LS, Meengs JS. Portion size can be used strategically to increase vegetable consumption in adults. Experiment 1 *Am J Clin Nutr.* 2010;91(4):913–922.
54. Stubbs RJ, Johnstone AM, Harbron CG, et al. Covert manipulation of energy density of high carbohydrate diets in in 'pseudo free-living' humans. *Int J Obes Relat Metab Disord.* 1998a;22: 885–892.
55. Stubbs RJ, Johnstone AM, O'Reillly LM, et al. The effect of covertly manipulating the energy density of mixed diets on ad libitum food intake in 'pseudo free-living' humans. *Int J Obes.* 1998b;22:980–987.
56. Stubbs RJ, Ritz P, Coward WA, Prentice AM. Covert manipulation of the ratio of dietary fat to carbohydrate and energy density: effect on food intake and energy balance in free-living men eating ad libitum. *Am J Clin Nutr.* 1995;62(2):330–337.
57. Bell EA, Castellanos VH, Pelkman CL, Thorwart ML, Rolls BJ. Energy density of foods affects energy intake in normal weight women. *Am J Clin Nutr.* 1998;67:412–420.
58. McLennan W, Podger A. *National Nutrition Survey: User's Guide.* Canberra (AUST): AGPS; 1998.
59. Economics Research Service. Food Consumption, Prices, and Expenditures, 1970-97. Judith Jones Putnam and Jane E. Allshouse. Food and Rural Economics Division, U.S. Department of Agriculture. Statistical Bulletin No. 965.
60. Mela DJ, Rogers PJ. Hunger, palatability and satiation: physiological and learned influences on eating. In: *Food, Eating and Obesity.* Boston, MA: Springer; 1998.
61. O'Doherty J, et al. Sensory-specific satiety-related olfactory activation of the human orbitofrontal cortex. *Neuroreport.* 2000;11:893–897.
62. Le Magnen J. Advances in studies on the physiological control and regulation of food intake. *Prog Physiol Psychol.* 1971;4:203–261.
63. Rolls BJ, Rolls ET, Rowe EA, Sweeney K. Sensory-specific satiety in man. *Physiol Behav.* 1981;27:137–142.
64. Flood-Obbagy JE, Rolls BJ. The effect of fruit in different forms on energy intake and satiety at a meal. *Appetite.* 2009;52(2):416–422.
65. Hall KD, et al. Ultra-processed diets cause excess calorie intake and weight gain: an Inpatient randomized randomized controlled trial of ad libitum food intake. *Cell Metabol.* 2019. https://doi.org/10.1016/j.cmet.2019.05.008 ([Epub ahead of print]).
66. Bellisle, Le Magnen J. The structure of meals in humans: eating and drinking patterns in lean and obese subjects. *Physiol Behav.* 1981;27(4):649–658.
67. Spiegel TA, Stellar E. Effects of variety on food intake of underweight, normal-weight and overweight women. *Appetite.* 1990; 15:47–61.
68. Rolls B. Experimental analyses of the effects of variety in a meal on human feeding. *Am J Clin Nutr.* 1985;42:932–939.
69. Green S, Blundell J. Effect of fat-and sucrose-containing foods on the size of eating episodes and energy intake in lean dietary restrained and unrestrained females: potential for causing overconsumption. *Eur J Clin Nutr.* 1996;50(9):625–635.
70. De Castro J. Socio-cultural determinants of meal size and frequency. *Br J Nutr.* 1997:S39–S55. https://doi.org/10.1079/BJN19970103.
71. Stubbs RJ, Johnstone AM, Mazlan N, et al. Effect of altering the variety of sensorially distinct foods, of the same macronutrient content, on food intake and body weight in men. *Eur J Clin Nutr.* 2001;55:19–28.
72. Wansink B, Painter J, North J. Bottomless bowls: why visual cues of portion size may influence intake. *Obes. Res.* 2005;13: 93–100.
73. Kelly MT, Wallace JM, Robson PJ, Rennie KL, Welch RW, Hannon-Fletcher MP, Brennan S, Fletcher A, Livingstone MB. Increased portion size leads to a sustained increase in energy intake over 4 d in normal-weight and overweight men and women. *British Journal Nutrition.* 2009;102(3):470–477.
74. Diliberti N. Increased portion size leads to increased energy intake in a restaurant meal source. *Obes Res.* 2004;123:562–568.
75. Bray GA, Nielsen SJ, Popkin BM. Consumption of high-fructose corn syrup in beverages may play a role in the epidemic of obesity. *Am J Clin Nutr.* 2004;79(4):537–543. https://doi.org/10.1093/ajcn/79.4.537.
76. Rolls BJ, Roe LS, et al. The effect of large portion sizes on energy intake is sustained for 11 days. *Obesity.* 2007;15:1535–1543.
77. Kant AK, Graubard BI. Predictors of reported consumption of low-nutrient density foods in a 24-h recall by 8-16 year old U.S. children and adolescents. *Appetite.* 2003;41:175–180.
78. Scott C, Johnstone AM. Stress and eating behavior: implications for obesity. *Obes. Facts.* 2012;5(2):277–287.
79. Zellner DA, Loaiza S, Gonzalez JP, et al. Food selection changes under stress. *Physiol Behav.* 2006;87:789–793.
80. Wallis DJ, Hetherington MM. Stress and eating: the effects of ego-threat and cognitive demand on food intake in restrained and emotional eaters. *Appetite.* 2004;43(1):39–46.
81. Hebebrand OJ, Albayrak RA, Antel J, Dieguez C,J, et al. "Eating addiction", rather than "food addiction", better captures addictive-like eating behavior. *Neurosci Biobehav Rev.* 2014;47: 295–306. https://doi.org/10.1016/j.neubiorev.2014.08.016.
82. Friedman M. An energy sensor for control of energy intake. *Proc Nutr Soc.* 1997;56(1A):41–50. https://doi.org/10.1079/PNS19970008.
83. Bauer KC, Huus KE, Finlay BB. Microbes and the mind: emerging hallmarks of the gut microbiota-brain axis. *Cell Microbiol.* 2016;18: 632–644.
84. Gribble FM, Reimann F. Enteroendocrine cells: chemosensors in the intestinal epithelium. *Annu Rev Physiol.* 2016;78:277–299. https://doi.org/10.1146/annurev-physiol-021115-105439.
85. Finlayson G, King N, Blundell JE. Is it possible to dissociate 'liking' and 'wanting' for foods in humans? A novel experimental procedure. *Physiol Behav.* 2007;90:36–42.
86. Blundell J. Pharmacological approaches to appetite suppression. *Trends Pharmacol Sci.* 1991;12:147–157.
87. Blundell JE, Lawton CL, Hill AJ. Mechanisms of appetite control and their abnormalities in obese patients. *Horm Res.* 1993;39(Suppl 3):72–76.
88. Oriach CS, Robertson RC, Catherine S, Cryan JF, Dinan TG. Food for thought: the role of nutrition in the microbiota-gut–brain axis. *Clin Nutr Experi.* 2016;6:25–38.
89. Cryan, et al. The microbiota-gut-brian Axis. *Physiol Rev.* 2019; 99(4):1877–2013.
90. Snyder WS, Cook MJ, Nasset ES. *Report of the Task Group on Reference Man.* Oxford, UK: Pergamon Press; 1974.
91. Heymsfield SB, Wang ZM, Withers R. Multicomponent molecular level models of body composition analysis. In: Roche A, Heymsfield SB, Lohman TG, eds. *Human Body Composition.* Champaign, IL: Human Kinetics; 1996:129–147.
92. Coward WA, Parkinson SA, Murgatroyd PR. Body composition measurements for nutrition research. *Nutr Res Rev.* 1988;1:115–124.
93. Fuller NJ, Jebb SA, Laskey MA, Coward WA, Elia M. Four compartment model for the assessment of body composition in human. Comparison with alternative methods; and evaluation of the density and hydration of fat free mass. *Clin Sci.* 1992;82:687–693.

94. Wells JCK, Fuller NJ, Dewit O, Fewtrell MS, Elia M, Cole TJ. Four-compartment model of body composition in children: density and hydration of fat-free mass and comparison with simpler models. *Am J Clin Nutr.* 1999;69:904–912.
95. Elia M. Organ and tissue contribution to metabolic rate. In: Kinney JM, Tucker HN, eds. *Energy Metabolism: Tissue Determinants and Cellular Corollaries.* New York: Raven Press; 1992:61–80.
96. World Health Organization. *Obesity: Preventing and Managing the Global Epidemic. Technical Report Series 894.* Geneva: WHO; 2000.
97. Hall KD, Sacks G, Chandramohan D, et al. Quantification of the effect of energy imbalance on bodyweight. *Lancet.* 2011;378: 826–837. https://doi.org/10.1016/S0140-6736(11)60812-X.
98. Bouchard C, Tremblay A, Despres JP, et al. The response to long-term overfeeding in identical twins. *N Engl J Med.* 1990;322: 1477–1482.
99. Bouchard C, Tchernof A, Tremblay A. Predictors of body composition and body energy changes in response to chronic overfeeding. *Int J Obes.* 2014;38:236–242.
100. Forbes GB. *Human Body Composition: Growth, Aging, Nutrition and Activity.* New York: Springer-Verlag; 1987a.
101. Forbes GB, Welle SL. Lean body mass in obesity. Int J Obes. 1983; 7(2):99–107.
102. Forbes GB, Kreipe ER, Lipinski BA. Body composition and the energy cost of weight gain. *Hum Nutr Clin Nutr.* 1982;36: 485–487.
103. Forbes GB, Brown MR, Welle SL, Lipinski BA. Deliberate overfeeding in women and men: energy cost and composition of the weight gain. *Br J Nutr.* 1986;56:1–9.
104. Elia M, Livesey G. Energy expenditure and fuel selection in biological systems: the theory and practice of calculations based on indirect calorimetry and tracer methods. *World Rev Nutr Diet.* 1992;70:68–131.
105. Forbes G. Do obese individuals gain weight more easily than non-obese individuals? *Am J Clin Nutr.* 1990;52:224–227. https://doi.org/10.1093/ajcn/52.2.224.

CHAPTER

9

EATING BEHAVIORS AND STRATEGIES TO PROMOTE WEIGHT LOSS AND MAINTENANCE

Donna H. Ryan[1], *MD*
Stephen Anton[2], *PhD*

[1]Pennington Biomedical Research Center, Baton Rouge, LA, United States
[2]University of Florida, Gainesville, FL, United States

SUMMARY

It may at times seem like we are searching for a cure for obesity with a magic diet, evidenced by past fad diets and the current attraction to low-carbohydrate diets and ketogenic diets. This chapter discusses the biologic basis of our eating behaviors and the biologic basis of health improvement with weight loss. With this understanding, we discuss the behavioral change approaches that can be used to navigate the modern food environment and lose enough weight to improve health. First, we review the evidence base for lifestyle intervention with a purpose of understanding the push by all professional societies to implement intensive behavioral therapy for obesity. The chapter discusses calorie targets and calorie deficits, episodic fasting, mindfulness, and the emergence of electronic self-monitoring tools. All of these approaches are based on our understanding of the biology of food intake. But weight loss is only the beginning; the hard part of losing weight for most patients with obesity is weight loss maintenance, and we discuss the important shift in focus to maintain lost weight, along with promising methods to achieve this goal.

Keywords: Adaptive thermogenesis; Calorie deficits; Calorie targets; Eating behavior; Episodic fasting; Food intake biology; Intensive behavioral therapy for obesity; Lifestyle intervention; Metabolic adaptation; Mindfulness; Self-monitoring; Weight loss maintenance.

I. INTRODUCTION AND BACKGROUND

Malnutrition comes in the form of undernutrition and obesity. Since the United States first documented the rise in rates of obesity and overweight in the late 1980s,[1] the prevalence of obesity in adults has steadily climbed. This rising prevalence has been noted across the world as the leading nutritional problem in high-income countries.[2] More recently, obesity has become a significant public health burden in low- and middle-income countries.[2] The most recent (2016–17) US obesity rates determined by measurement of height and weight of a representative sample of United States adults showed that 39.8% of adults have a BMI >30 kg/m^2.[2,3] This represents an increase from 14.5% in the measurements taken in 1976–80,[3] meaning that the prevalence of obesity has nearly tripled in 35 years.[1,3] This epidemic has spawned enormous interest by public health authorities, health care providers, and from people affected by overweight and obesity.

The approach to losing weight has been largely a self-help enterprise; in a survey, 82% of 3008 US adults with obesity reported that they felt "completely responsible" for their weight loss.[4] This survey also asked those persons with obesity and 606 health care providers in the United States whether they endorsed different weight

Present Knowledge in Nutrition, Volume 2
https://doi.org/10.1016/B978-0-12-818460-8.00009-5

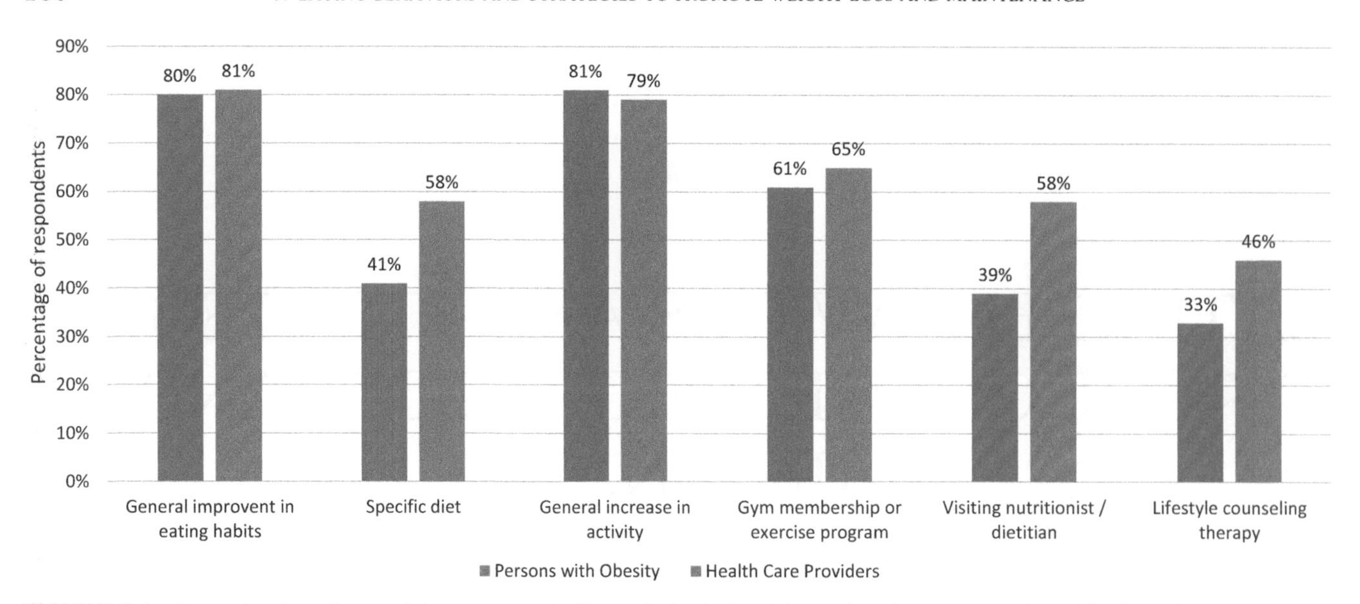

FIGURE 9.1 Overvaluation of general improvement in diet and physical activity and undervaluation of specific therapies: proportion of persons with obesity and health care providers who reported treatment is "completely effective."[4] *Adapted from Kaplan LM, Golden A, Jinnett K et al. Perceptions of barriers to effective obesity care: results from the national ACTION study.* Obesity. *2018;26, 61–69.*

loss treatment approaches as "completely effective" and the results are shown in Fig. 9.1.[4]

While health care providers generally rated efficacy higher, a minority (39%) of persons with obesity endorsed visits to a dietitian or nutritionist as efficacious and even fewer (33%) endorsed lifestyle counseling for efficacy.[4] It should be noted that patients and providers were even more skeptical of efficacy of medical interventions.[4] As is also shown in Fig. 9.1, persons with obesity and health care providers value the efficacy of "Healthy Eating" over a specific diet and also endorse the efficacy of generally being more active over a specific exercise program.[4] While self-monitoring is a key element of behavioral approaches to weight loss, the minority of people with obesity value tracking of food and physical activity and only a bare majority of health care providers value these proven tools.[4] This survey demonstrates that persons with obesity and many health care providers do not have realistic views of weight loss and are uniformed about evidence-based weight loss principles.

> Patients and providers are overvaluing a generalized approach to healthy eating and physical activity, while at the same time undervaluing behavioral intervention for weight management.

The vast majority of US adults with obesity report a desire to weigh less.[5] The commercial weight loss industry in the United States is estimated to be $70.3 billion annually (https://blog.marketresearch.com/2018-outlook-strong-for-the-u.s.-weight-loss-market).

It is obvious that individuals with overweight and obesity are struggling to lose weight and to sustain weight loss. All too often, weight loss is sought through Internet searches yielding supplement advertisements and fad approaches for which there is no evidence of weight loss efficacy and safety. Further, even though there are some commercial weight loss program that provide evidence of successful weight loss and weight loss maintenance,[6] these programs are challenged by high attrition rates and lack of long-term efficacy.

Given this background, there is a need to understand why effective weight loss approaches have been so challenging for persons with overweight and obesity, and to identify strategies that have proven efficacy. In this chapter, we will begin by reviewing the biology of eating behaviors and body weight regulation, discuss the current state of the art in achieving and sustaining effective weight loss, discuss the biologic-based approaches to supporting changes in eating behaviors, and then review emerging effective strategies to maintaining lost weight.

A. Biology of Eating Behaviors and Body Weight Regulation

The traditional way that energy balance has been conceptualized is as a simple equation whereby if more energy is consumed than is expended, then the excess energy will be stored as body fat. This simplistic paradigm, while true, implies that one can reduce food intake with "willpower" and belies the biologic basis of food intake and the complexity of body weight regulation.

We provide a brief discussion below and refer our readers to excellent recent reviews in this area.[7,8]

Food intake is biologically regulated. The homeostatic system of food intake regulation is driven by neural and hormonal signals in a "gut–brain axis" informing the brain of hunger to initiate food intake; other signals, both hormonal and neural, that occur after food is ingested or nutrients are absorbed signal the brain that food intake has occurred and the process of satiety and cessation of food intake begins. Another food intake regulatory system, the reward system, occurs when we see or smell food cues that we recognize as having high hedonic value. The rewarding aspects of food can override the homeostatic system and we can eat foods of high hedonic value, even when we have satiated our hunger. In addition, habit and lack of mindfulness may contribute to increase in food intake.

B. Homeostatic System of Food Intake Regulation

The chief "hunger hormone" is ghrelin,[9] which is produced by the stomach. High ghrelin levels occur before food intake and ghrelin falls after feeding. After ingestion of food, stretch receptors in the stomach signal fullness through the vagus nerve.[10] When nutrients enter the small intestine, a series of hormones are released including GLP-1, PYY, and oxyntomodulin; these hormones signal satiety.[8,10] When nutrients are absorbed, amylin, insulin, and pancreatic polypeptide are released from the pancreas, which signal the brain to reduce food intake. This gut–brain axis regulates the homeostatic intake of foods and generally occurs in three cycles (breakfast, lunch, and dinner) throughout the day. The chief areas of the brain involved in homeostatic regulation are the hypothalamus, corticolimbic system, and hindbrain.[8,10] It has been proposed that genetic and epigenetic alterations of gut signaling mechanisms contribute to obesity via alterations in homeostatic regulation.[8]

C. Reward System of Hedonic Food Intake Regulation

The reward system consists of brain circuitry including cortical and subcortical brain areas that receive external cues and recall rewarding aspects of food, and involving cognition, and executive functions. Hedonic controls interact with homeostatic controls to regulate body weight.[8,10] In the modern environment, increased exposure to energy-dense foods of high hedonic value and increased exposure to food cues may contribute to increased food intake[8,10] Further, stress-induced overeating can be seen as a disorder of the reward system.[11]

D. Habit-Driven Food Intake

In modern life, most eating episodes have become disconnected from the procurement and preparation of food. This mindless and habit-driven food intake poses a challenge to the homeostatic control of food intake. Watching television or movies, text messaging, and playing computer games result in impaired cognition and memory of a meal and increases snacking later. This suggests that mindful experience of a meal may be needed to produce adequate satiation.[10]

E. Leptin and Regulation of Energy Stores

Leptin is a hormone produced by body fat; leptin levels correspond to body fat; and individuals with obesity have high leptin levels. When leptin levels fall, energy is conserved by reduction in resting energy expenditure and increase in food intake. Thus, leptin serves as a modulator of chronic food intake and energy expenditure status.[12] The leptin regulatory system seems to be more sensitive to reductions in leptin to produce increased food intake and reduced resting energy expenditure.[8,10,12]

It is crucial to understand the role of leptin in the metabolic adaptation (reduction in energy expenditure greater than would be predicted for loss of active metabolic mass) that follows weight loss if one is to understand the challenges of long-term weight loss maintenance. With weight loss, there is a reduction in resting energy expenditure that is disproportionate to the amount of reduction in lean body mass.[13] The metabolic adaptation is thought to be closely related to the degree of leptin reduction.[14] This is subject to individual variation with some individuals displaying greater or lesser reduction in energy expenditure with a given amount of weight loss. However, this is also a "spring-loaded model."[15] The greater the weight loss, the greater the metabolic adaptation and therefore the greater the reduction in resting energy expenditure.[16] Thus, it may be easier for individuals to maintain lesser reductions in body weight than larger reductions in body weight.[17]

F. Biologic and Metabolic Adaptations to Weight Loss

Body fat is defended by normal physiology. Both sides of the energy balance equation are affected by weight reduction.

Body weight reduction induces hormonal changes that occur when body weight is reduced, which drives increased hunger, decreased satiety, and reduction in resting energy expenditure.

A seminal study describing the effect of weight loss on gut hormone responses (which drive hunger and satiety) and on leptin changes was conducted by Sumithran et al.[18] The results of this study are summarized in Fig. 9.2. There were 50 subjects with overweight and obesity who entered a metabolic unit and received a very–low-energy diet for 10 weeks. The mean weight loss was 14%. The subjects were allowed to be free-living but were counseled to support weight loss maintenance. At week 62 (1 year out of the unit), weight regain was 5% on average and individuals were reduced by 8% from baseline. Weight loss at 10 weeks resulted in statistically significant hormonal changes in response to a test meal—reductions in leptin, PYY, CCK, insulin, and amylin and to statistically significant increases in levels of ghrelin. Subjective appetite was also measured by visual analog scales. In response to the test meal, there were significant increases in subjective appetite and desire to eat. Even at 62 weeks, there were significant differences from baseline including leptin, PYY, CCK, insulin, and ghrelin as well as hunger ratings. The reductions in leptin levels were disproportionate to the amount of weight loss. At 14% loss, there was a 65% reduction in leptin and at 8% weight loss, leptin was still reduced 35% from baseline. These changes indicate that patients who successfully lose weight through low-calorie diets experience many biologic changes including increased hunger, reduced satiety, and reduction in resting energy expenditure. Thus, reduced patients have a "double whammy"; they have changes in appetite regulation and energy expenditure that favor weight regain.

G. Biology of Weight Loss Benefits

It is not necessary for patients to achieve an ideal body weight or even a body mass index (BMI) 30 kg/m^2 to achieve health benefits.

Weight loss beginning at just 3% can produce improvements in glycemia and triglycerides.[19] Modest weight loss (5%–10%) improves glycemia, blood pressure, lipids, need for medications, mobility, and quality of life.[20] Of course, larger weight loss produces greater benefits. Further, more substantial weight loss is needed to improve some weight-related complications, such as obstructive sleep apnea and nonalcoholic steatotic hepatitis.[20] Additionally, organs respond differently to different amounts of weight loss.[20]

Weight loss of just 5% has been shown to maximize liver and adipose tissue insulin sensitivity, accounting for the power of modest weight loss to impact diabetes prevention in patients with prediabetes.[21] The message to weight counselors is that our weight loss goals should be aligned with the amount of weight loss needed to produce health improvement. For patients

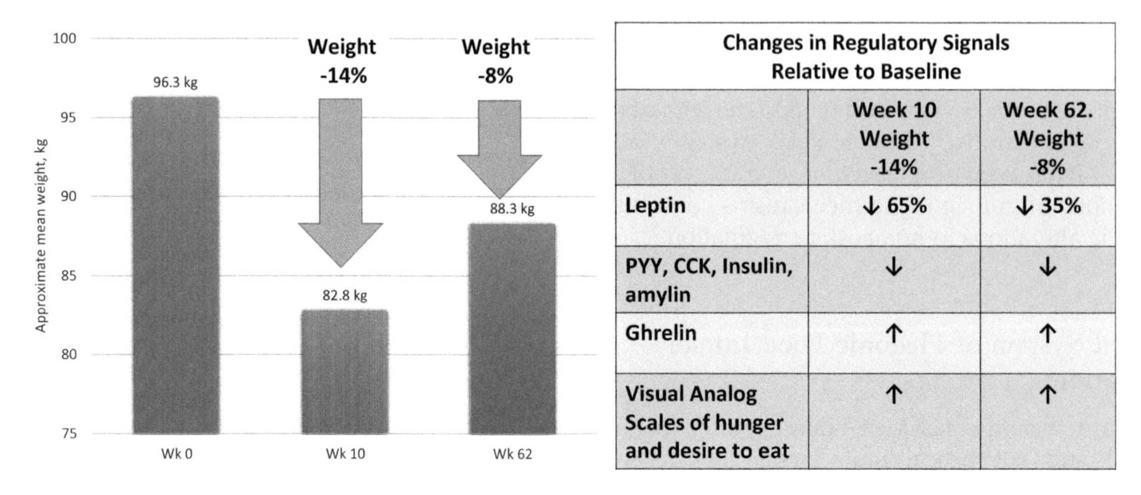

Changes in Regulatory Signals Relative to Baseline		
	Week 10 Weight -14%	Week 62. Weight -8%
Leptin	↓ 65%	↓ 35%
PYY, CCK, Insulin, amylin	↓	↓
Ghrelin	↑	↑
Visual Analog Scales of hunger and desire to eat	↑	↑

FIGURE 9.2 Weight reduction produces changes in regulatory hormones and measurable changes in appetite. Patients were reduced in a metabolic unit over 10 weeks by, on average, −14%. Allowed to be free-living for a year, but with continued counseling, they regained to −8% below baseline. At week 10, leptin was reduced by 65% and at week 62 by 35%. In response to a test meal, there were measurable decreases in satiety hormones (decreased) and ghrelin (increased) at week 10 and at week 62. Visual analog scale measurements of appetite showed increased hunger and desire for food at both 10 and 62 weeks. *Adapted from Sumithran P et al.* N Engl J Med. *2011;365:1597–1604.*

with early metabolic complications of obesity, modest weight losses may produce dramatic risk reduction, especially in terms of diabetes progression. Remembering that metabolic adaptation is a spring-loaded model, more moderate amounts of weight loss will be easier to maintain over the long term as they will not be challenged by the extreme metabolic adaptation that occurs with extreme weight loss.

Furthermore, diet is not only about weight. Diet quality needs to be kept in mind. All Americans have been recommended to consume a dietary pattern that emphasizes intake of vegetables, fruits, and whole grains; includes low-fat dairy products, poultry, fish, legumes, nontropical vegetable oils, and nuts; and limits intake of sodium, sweets, sugar-sweetened beverages, and red meats.[22] Additionally, the only randomized clinical trial evaluating cardiovascular events as outcomes favored a Mediterranean diet approach.[23]

> A dietary approach that focuses on eating behaviors to limit caloric intake and favors high diet quality would seem to be ideal for producing both short- and long-term weight loss.

II. CURRENT STATE OF THE ART AND BEST PRACTICES IN ACHIEVING AND SUSTAINING WEIGHT LOSS THROUGH LIFESTYLE MODIFICATION

The current US Preventive Services Task Force (USPSTF) recommendations[24] for weight management provide a strong endorsement for weight management for persons with BMI >30 kg/m^2 and, in particular, for primary health care providers to use intensive behavioral therapy approaches to achieve and sustain weight loss. In these recommendations, intensive behavioral therapy is intended to be comprehensive, that is addressing behaviors around both food intake and PA. Further, the recommendations prescribe that the behavioral therapy be delivered in 14–16 sessions over the first 6 months and that therapy should be continued for at least 1 year.[25] These endorsements rest primarily on several large, long-term studies of lifestyle intervention for weight loss, primarily Diabetes Prevention Program (DPP),[26–28] Look AHEAD,[29,30] and Weight Loss Maintenance (WLM).[31] In Table 9.1, we describe the food intake and PA behaviors that were utilized in the three studies, along with the weight loss outcomes.

A. Learnings From Large Randomized Clinical Trials Demonstrating Weight Reduction Over The Long Term

Lifestyle interventions, such as those described above (DPP, Look AHEAD, and WLM) in which participants are taught to reduce their caloric intake and increase PA levels to achieve a negative energy balance, typically produce average weight losses of 5–10 kg in obese adults.[32] Weight losses of this magnitude generally results in significant improvements in a number of cardiovascular risk factors including hypertension,[33] glucose intolerance,[34] and hyperlipidemia,[35] as well as psychological well-being.[36] Programs that advocate greater calorie restriction and more intense strategies for behavior change have yielded better compliance and greater weight loss,[37] and the amount of weight lost is generally associated with greater satisfaction by participants.[38] Similarly, lifestyle interventions have been shown to delay or prevent diabetes in individuals with screen detected prediabetes in several landmark diabetes prevention trials,[39] including DPP illustrated above. Most randomized controlled trials have found that lifestyle interventions slow the progression from impaired glucose tolerance to diabetes by 30%–60% across a broad range of racial groups.[39] A good example of this long-term intensive approach for lifestyle behavior modification is the DPP,[26–28] which is now offered at a low cost in YMCAs across the country.[40]

B. Long-Term Weight Loss Maintenance and The National Weight Control Registry

The large-scale studies described above suggest that some individuals who lose 10% or more of their body weight are able to keep it off for several years. For example, the Look AHEAD (Action in Health for Diabetes) study, a clinical trial testing the effects of a lifestyle intervention in more than 5,000 adults with type 2 diabetes, found that 42% of the 887 participants who lost at least 10% of their body weight at Year 1 maintained a 10% or greater weight loss over 4 years.[41]

As discussed earlier, a multitude of factors appear to increase the difficulty of achieving long-term weight loss. A number of compensatory mechanisms occur following calorie restriction and weight loss, including reductions in metabolic rate combined with neuroendocrine signals to increase food intake and decrease energy expenditure, to promote weight regain until the defended body weight is reached.[13–15] Moreover, a complex interaction of physiological, environmental, and psychological factors makes the maintenance of lost weight difficult to achieve. Many internal and external

TABLE 9.1 Food intake and physical activity behavioral approaches in three influential lifestyle intervention trials.

	DPP[26–28]	Look AHEAD[29,30]	WLM[31]
Baseline description of lifestyle intervention participants	1079 participants with impaired glucose tolerance; mean age 50.6 years; mean BMI 33.6 kg/m^2	2570 participants with type 2 diabetes; mean age 58.6 years; mean BMI 36.3 kg/m^2 (women) and 35.3 kg/m^2 (men)	1685 participants, aged $\geq$ 25, overweight or obese (BMI = 25–45 kg/m^2) and on medications for hypertension and or dyslipidemia
Goal	7% weight loss	10% weight loss	Weight loss $\geq$ 4 kg
Weight loss achieved	Year 1 weight loss 7.2% Year 2 weight loss 5.8% Year 3 weight loss 4.5%	Year 1 weight loss 8.6% Year 4 weight loss 6.15%	69% of all participants who started the program lost $\geq$ 4 kg by the end of Phase 1
Diet quality	Reduce total dietary fat to <25% of calories; if weight loss was not achieved by lowering fat, calorie goals were introduced	$\leq$30% total calories from fat (with $\leq$10% total calories from saturated fat) and $\geq$15% total calories from protein Liquid meal replacements (provided free of charge) and frozen food entrees and structured meal plans (conventional foods) for those who declined the meal replacements	Encourage to follow DASH eating pattern (high-fiber and low-fat diet) during Phase 1; participants provided with caloric intake goals based on personal need during Phase 2
Physical activity	Engage in and maintain moderate-intensity activity, such as brisk walking, for at least 150 min per week	Home-based exercise with gradual progression to goal of 175 min of moderate-intensity physical activity per week	180 min per week of moderate physical activity during Phase 1; increased moderate-intensity physical activity an average of at least 45 min per day $\geq$ 5 times each week (i.e., > 225 min per week) during Phase 2
Curriculum	16-Lessons in 6 months, covering diet, exercise, and behavior modification; taught individually, face-to-face; then monthly individual and group sessions; toolbox approach	Based on DPP; 24 sessions in 6 months; taught in 3 group and 1 individual sessions per month; after 6 months, 2 group and 1 individual sessions for 1 year; toolbox approach from DPP	Phase 1: 20 weekly group sessions, designed to be participant centered and interactive, approximately one and a half to 2 hours with 18–25 participants per group
Behavioral techniques	Self-monitoring of weight, dietary intake, and physical activity; Regular meal pattern; Eating slowly; Stimulus control; Label reading; Contingency planning.	Self-monitoring of weight, dietary intake, and physical activity; Regular meal pattern; Eating slowly; Stimulus control; Label reading; Contingency planning Orlistat optional after 6 months	Self-monitoring of behavior, skill development, individual specific behavior change plans, goal setting
Health benefits associated with the intervention	Diabetes prevention: 58% reduction in progression from impaired glucose tolerance to type 2 diabetes after about 3 years.	After 9.5 years no difference in cardiovascular event rate; improved biomarkers of glucose and lipid control, less sleep apnea, lower liver fat, less depression, improved insulin sensitivity, less urinary incontinence, less kidney disease, reduced need of diabetes medications, maintenance of physical mobility, improved quality of life, and lower costs.[189]	After 30 months of the personal contact maintenance intervention, continuation for another 30 months provided no additional benefit. However, across the entire study, weight loss was slightly greater in those originally assigned to personal contact intervention as compared to self-directed control participants.[190]

cues (in addition to hunger) may prompt an orientation toward certain foods and an increased desire to eat.[42] Moreover, compared to lean individuals, overweight individuals have been reported to have a stronger preference for energy-dense foods.[42]

As a consequence of this unfriendly combination of factors, most individuals experience some regain of weight during the postdieting period. This weight regain typically occurs during a time when there are fewer reinforcements to maintain adherence to lifestyle changes initiated during treatment. Thus, the individual may perceive there to be greater behavioral "cost" to continued dietary restriction and/or PA and less "benefits" in terms of weight loss.

There are, however, some individuals who have been successful in maintaining large weight losses (>30 lbs) over 10 years. These individuals are part of the National Weight Control Registry (NWCR), which was founded in 1993 to identify successful weight loss maintainers and describe strategies they use to achieve and maintain weight loss.[43,44] Thomas and colleagues (2014) reported long-term weight losses in this highly select group of individuals.[45]

Although some weight regain occurred over time, these individuals were able to maintain 74% of their initial weight loss at 10 years, and 88% of them had maintained a 10% weight loss at Year 10. Noteworthy, the individuals who had larger initial weight losses at entry into the NWCR maintained larger weight losses throughout the entire follow-up period.

Given that individuals in the NWCR represent only a minority of Americans, an important question to ask is what behaviors these individuals engage in to achieve such impressive long-term weight losses.

> In most studies, the members of the NWCR reported high levels of physical activity (PA) (approximately 2000 kcal expended per week), low calorie and fat intake, high levels of dietary restraint, and low levels of disinhibition.[45–47] In addition, most participants reported weighing themselves several times a week.[46]

A noteworthy limitation is that the behavioral factors were examined only at the 1 year follow-up, rather than annually, which would have provided more information on the connection between behavioral changes and weight trajectories. Nevertheless, such findings indicate that long-term weight loss maintenance is possible but requires sustained behavior change.[45] As noted above, sustaining these behaviors is difficult for the vast majority of individuals in the current obesogenic environment.

C. National Recommendations and Guidelines

The impact of the US prevalence of overweight and obesity on disease burden and health care costs demands that public health policy address prevention and remediation of excess body weight. The demonstration of health benefits with 3%–10% weight loss described above has been an incentive for the USPSTF to endorse behavioral intervention for weight management.[24] The Center for Medicare and Medicaid Services (CMMS) has endorsed reimbursement for "intensive behavioral therapy for obesity."[25]

The current evidence-based Obesity Guidelines[19] endorse advising individuals "who would benefit from weight loss to participate for >6 months in a comprehensive lifestyle program that assists participants in adhering to a lower calorie diet and in increasing physical activity through the use of behavioral strategies" with preference given to "on site, high intensity (i.e., >14 sessions in 6 months) comprehensive weight loss interventions provided in individual or group sessions by a trained interventionist." Further, these guidelines recommend that providers "advise overweight and obese individuals who have lost weight to participate long-term (at least 1 year) in a comprehensive weight loss maintenance program." These recommendations are "Grade A (strong)" and are echoed by the USPSTF[24] and the CMMS.[25]

III. EATING BEHAVIORS TO PRODUCE WEIGHT LOSS

A. Calorie Targets, Deficits, Points, and Exchanges

Lifestyle interventions for weight loss represent the first line of intervention in the treatment of obesity.[48] The behavioral component of most interventions typically includes group sessions and some individual counseling. During these sessions, the interventionist will provide specific and individualized dietary information to help the participant adhere to the low-calorie regimen and meet his/her calorie target. Prior to lifestyle interventions, estimated energy needs may be calculated either through indirect calorimetry to determine resting metabolic rate (RMR) or through established equations. For example, Kevin Hall's energy balance models[49] have been incorporated into the NIDDK Body Weight Planner[49] to determine participants' individual baseline energy requirements, their energy intake targets, and the expected rate of weight loss. Specifically, the NIDDK Body Weight Planner provides a graph (Fig. 9.3) and data output that depicts individual participant's expected rate of weight loss. This model considers that interindividual

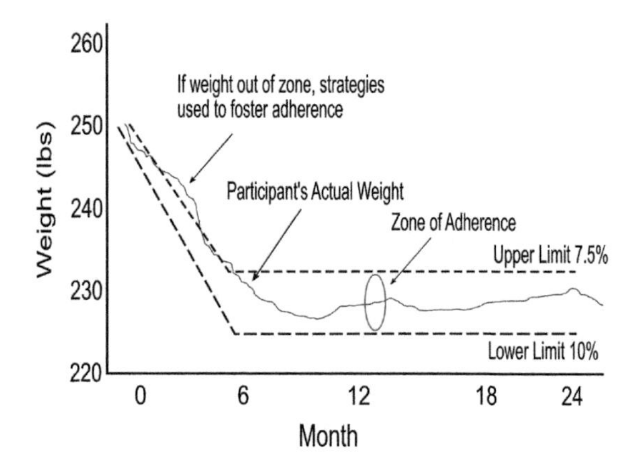

FIGURE 9.3 NIDDK weight graph with zone of adherence.

variability in weight loss from the same intervention can be due to differences in initial body composition as well as uncertainly in baseline energy expenditure.[49]

Weight loss typically occurs during the first 6 months of treatment, although participants are usually encouraged to lose weight for as long as possible. The targeted goals typically entail a low-calorie eating pattern (i.e., a calorie deficit of 500–1000 kcal/day below steady state) coupled with increases in moderate-intensity PA (e.g., walking for 30 min/day) to produce a weight loss of approximately 1–2 pounds per week. Dietary intake is frequently adjusted at 3 and 6 months, as deemed appropriate by the lifestyle interventionists, to account for the weight loss, and subsequent reduction in metabolic rate, to keep the calorie deficit constant.

The intervention approach is typically tailored to the needs of the individual participant, with specific nutritional and behavioral strategies selected from an intervention "toolbox." Example dietary strategies include increasing dietary fiber, modifying recipes to decrease energy density, adding novel foods to relieve boredom, strategies to avoid impulse eating, obtaining desired foods through home delivery or take-home meals, and developing strategies to limit caloric intake in public settings such as restaurants, parties, and work. In terms of macronutrient intake, most individuals find it easier to follow nutritionally "balanced" dietary regimens compared to those that are very low with respect to either carbohydrates or fats.[50]

Dietary Exchanges, based on the American Dietetic Association (ADA) Exchange System, are another tools that have been used to help participants adhere to their calorie targets with the corresponding number of ADA exchanges/day adjusted for the specific diet. The exchange system affords the participant the most flexibility in diet planning once the concept is learned. The meal plans can be followed exactly to achieve the targets and enable the participant to reinforce the exchange concept. These types of exchanges and/or points systems have also been successfully used to produce clinically meaningful weight loss in many commercial weight loss programs.[6]

Successful attempts to modify eating behavior to produce weight loss typically utilize empirically supported behavioral skills including self-monitoring (which addresses mindfulness and habit-driven food intake), environmental control (which reduces food cues to reward eating), eating regular meals and contingency management (to avoid excessive hunger from the homeostatic system of food intake regulation) and skills training in slowing eating rate, increasing oral processing and other behaviors such as encouraging low energy density foods (to allow the satiety hormones time to act), use of meal replacements (MRs) (to provide fixed energy, portion-controlled option to facilitate dietary adherence),[51] and increasing social support through skills training or recruitment of participants with friends/family.[52,53]

In Table 9.2, we describe empirically supported behavioral strategies and provide examples of how these strategies could be used in weight loss interventions to enhance adherence levels.

The strategies described above have been shown to enhance both short-term and long-term weight loss. Adherence levels unfortunately decline in most individuals over time, even with strong behavioral skills training and support. Thus, there is a need to explore alternative or complementary approaches that may facilitate adherence and complement traditional lifestyle interventions to make long-term behavior change more sustainable. In the sections below, we describe a few promising complementary and alternative approaches.

B. Episodic Fasting

One alternative dietary approach that may produce similar biological changes as caloric restriction that has received increasing interest from the scientific community is Intermittent Fasting.[54] In contrast to traditional caloric restriction paradigms, food is not consumed during designated fasting time periods but is typically not restricted during designated eating time periods. The length of the fasting time period can also vary but is frequently 12 or more continuous hours. There are many types of intermittent fasting approaches, but the two most popular and well-studies approaches are alternate day fasting (ADF) or alternate day modified fasting (ADMF) and time-restricted feeding (TRF).

Alternate day or ADMF involves consuming no or very little food on fasting days and then alternating with a day of unrestricted food intake or a "feast" day. In a recent review by Anton and colleagues,[55] ADF and/or ADMF produced significant reductions in body weight and fat mass in 10 of the 10 eligible trials. In 9 of the 10 trials, an ADMF approach was used. In 3 of the 10 trials, there was also a significant loss of fat-free

TABLE 9.2 Strategies for increasing adherence to treatment.

Strategy	Description	Examples	Supportive citations
Extended care	Providing long-term contact individually or by group, either in-person, by phone, or via the Internet	Providing biweekly or monthly follow-up sessions	Ross Middleton, Patidar, and Perri[191] Perri et al.[192]
Skills training	Specific training in problem-solving skills or relapse prevention	Training participants how to address barriers that interfere with treatment adherence, such as time constraints	Witkiewitz and Marlatt[193]; Perri et al.[194]; Baum, Clark, and Sandler[195]
Social support	Increasing social support through skills training or recruitment of participants with friends/family	Recruiting participants with their friends and family; conducting group-based interventions rather than individual-based interventions	Wing and Jeffery[53]
Treatment tailoring	Making flexible treatment recommendations that can be tailored to individual preferences and schedule	Allowing individuals to choose their own methods of physical activity and allowing multiple short bouts of physical activity rather than requiring long bouts	Jakicic et al.[196] Perri et al.[197]
Self-monitoring	Having participants keep records of their adherence behaviors	Having participants weight themselves daily to assess weight loss maintenance	Butryn et al.[46]
Multicomponent strategies	Combining multiple strategies to promote long-term adherence	Providing biweekly or monthly follow-up, group-based sessions that focus on skills training and continued self-monitoring	Perri, Sears, and Clark[198]; Perri et al.[199]
Ongoing feedback	Providing feedback to participants on how they are doing or how they could improve	Providing weekly or monthly communication in which feedback is given, along with potential strategies that may help the participant adapt/adjust	Cook[200]; Sherrington et al.[201]
Stimulus control	Stimulus control strategies alter an individual's environment to maximize healthy choices	Having participant's manipulating their environment to adhere to behavior, such as moving unhealthy foods out of the house or setting notes on fridge to exercise	Kelley et al.[202]
Cognitive restructuring	Help participants identify and alter stress-inducing thought/s	Training that allows participant to shift negative thoughts that interfere with treatment to more positive	Foreyt and Poston[203]
Problem solving	Train participants on the process of finding solutions to challenging obstacles	Allow participants to define the problem, identify the causes, and formulate solutions to overcome barriers of adherence	Murawski et al.[204]; Perri et al.[194]
Relapse prevention	Providing training to prevent and manage relapse in participants	Training participants in how to prevent and cope with relapse	Witkiewitz and Marlat[193]; Perri et al.[194] Baum, Clark, and Sandler[195]
Mindful eating	An individual maintaining a neutral (nonjudgmental) awareness of one's physical and emotional sensations while earing or in a food-related environment.	Training participants to be more aware of their bodies cues, satiety, hunger, and also external cues related to the eating environment	Dunn et al.[56] Framson et al.[205]
Slowing of eating rate	Having participants slow down the process of eating by extending the time of mastication (chewing) of food	Having participants increase the number of mastication cycles before swallowing of food	Hollis[206] Hurst and Fukuda[207] Shah et al.[208]

mass (FFM), with the amount of FFM lost being greatest in the only trial that used an ADF approach. TRF interventions, a popular type of intermittent fasting where individuals engage in daily fasts between 14 and 18 h, have also been found to produce significant reductions in body fat without significant loss of lean tissue in middle-age and younger individuals.[55]

C. Mindfulness, Slowing the Rate of Food Intake, and Increasing Oral Processing Time

Another approach that has the potential to enhance long-term weight loss is mindful eating, which refers to "maintaining a non-judgmental awareness of [one's] physical and emotional sensations while eating or in a food-related environment." The approaches used to teach mindful eating through intervention include acceptance-based behavioral therapy, meditation, mindfulness-based stress reduction, and group mindful eating. Participants are typically taught to be more aware of their bodies, hunger, and satiety, as well as recognize external cues to eat and have self-compassion. Participants are also encouraged to exercise and change eating habits to be consistent with a healthy lifestyle.

The finding of a recent review by Dunn and colleagues supports the inclusion of mindful eating as a strategy to promote long-term weight loss.[56] All 12 studies included in this review reported modest weight losses when mindful eating strategies were used. Noteworthy, four of the five studies that conducted follow-up assessments reported continued weight loss with only one study reporting weight regain. More studies are needed to narrow down the specific strategies, messages, and methodologies that should be included in a mindful eating-centered weight management program.

An approach in line with mindful eating practices is to slow the rate of eating to potentially reduce total food consumption at each meal by increasing satiety levels. Some studies indeed show slow eating, but still at a moderate speed, increases satiety and decreases hunger levels in overweight and obese individuals with type 2 diabetes.[57] This eating approach, however, did not lead to any differences in glucose, insulin, or gastrointestinal hormonal signals. Other studies have found that reducing eating rate results in less food intake compared to a baseline meal for men but not women.[58] Such findings suggest the need to better understand how rate of eating could differentially affect satiety responses in men and women.

D. Meal Replacements (Partial and Total)

Nutrient-rich MR diet plans have been shown to yield significant health benefits in a safe and effective manner. Weight management interventions utilizing MRs or partial MRs typically produce greater weight reduction, sufficient nutrition, higher satisfaction, and better long-term adherence rates compared to those that focus on conventional foods.[51] Findings from a recent metaanalysis indicate that MR products produce statistically greater weight loss of approximately 1.5 kg over 1 year compared to interventions that focus on conventional foods.[51] Two studies reported weight loss outcomes at 4 years with both favoring interventions with MRs over control (self-directed dieting). These findings indicate that use of MR products can enhance long-term weight loss. Importantly, MRs appear to be safe and have not been associated with higher rates of adverse events.[59]

E. Tools to Help Modify Eating Behaviors (Selfmonitoring and Tracking Tools, Oral Device, and Waist Cord)

There is substantial research demonstrating a relationship between self-monitoring and weight loss;[60] however, less is known about the effects of different recording formats on long-term adherence. Traditionally, pen and paper methods have been employed for tracking variables such as calorie intake, daily weights, and minutes of exercise. The use of digital devices, specifically "smartphones," as modalities for recording food intake and exercise behavior, however, has significantly increased over the past decade and appears to have replaced traditional pen and paper methods as the primary modality for recording dietary intake.

Initial studies suggest that apps on mobile phones for self-monitoring may produce higher levels of adherence than either websites or pen and paper. For example, Burke et al. found that participants who used a personal device to self-monitor had much higher rates of adherence (80%) than those who used a pen and paper (55%) to record dietary adherence over a 6 month period.[61] There were small differences in the percentages of individuals who achieved clinically meaningful weight losses (>5% baseline weight) with no significant differences between groups (49% vs. 46%). Carter et al. also found a significantly higher level of adherence among individuals using a smartphone compared to individuals who either used a website or a food diary to self-monitor (92 vs. 35 vs. 29 days over a 6 month period).[62] In this study, the participants in the smartphone group lost a greater amount of body fat than either the website or diary group.

Although initial studies support the superiority of a mobile app over other methods of self-monitoring, adherence levels unfortunately decline over time regardless of the modality used.[63,64] Thus, there is a need to continue to explore strategies to enhance long-term adherence to self-monitoring, regardless of the modality used.

Smartphone applications

One of the major barriers to successfully disseminating interventions to free-living individuals is lack of methodologies that can accurately assess calorie and nutrient intake, as well as provide real-time feedback to individuals about their dietary intake and energy expenditure levels. Smartphone apps can help overcome this barrier by providing real-time feedback to users regarding dietary intake and PA monitoring.[65] Two noteworthy findings of a recent scoping review by Rivera and colleagues[65] on apps for weight management were that (1) a large percentage of weight loss apps (139 out of 393) utilize a self-monitoring feature and (2) most mobile apps for weight loss/management lack important evidence-based features and have not undergone rigorous scientific testing.

One exception to these findings is the "SmartLoss" app. This app incorporates many empirically supported weight management strategies, including remote monitoring, personalized nutritional counseling, and weekly feedback "toolboxes" that contain information on how to improve eating habits. In a 12 week intervention trial, use of this app led to statistically significant weight loss at weeks 4, 8, and 12 (mean weight change of 10% body weight at 12 weeks).[66] Additionally, participants receiving the SmartLoss intervention had significant reductions in waist circumference at weeks 8 and 12 and a significant reduction in systolic and diastolic blood pressure at week 12.[66]

Wearable technology

Wearable technologies, including watches (FitBit, Garmin, and Apple Watches) and bracelets, may also assist with weight loss by providing real-time feedback about an individual's daily activities and total energy expenditure. In a review by Cheatham and colleagues, a total of 25 studies were identified, which investigated the use of wearable technology on changes in body weight and PA levels in overweight and obese populations.[67] 19 of the 25 identified trials reported positive effects of wearable technology on body weight and PA, as assessed by step count, accelerometer monitored PA, and exercise energy expenditure. The findings of this review indicate that activity trackers can enhance the effects of standard weight loss programs, specifically in middle-age and older adults. Notably, the studies included in this review focused on short-term (<6 months) weight loss. There is currently a dearth of evidence on the effects of wearable technology on long-term weight loss.

eHealth interventions

In contrast to smartphone apps, there have been a considerable number of trials that have tested the effectiveness of ehealth interventions for weight loss. The most common modalities for delivering these interventions include email, text messages, monitoring devices, mobile applications, computer programs, and personal digital assistants. A systematic review and metaanalysis by Hutchesson and colleagues[68] examined the efficacy of eHealth interventions to aid in the prevention and treatment of obesity and overweight in adults. A total of 84 clinical trials were identified with 61 having the primary aim of weight loss, 10 weight loss maintenance, 8 weight gain prevention, and 5 weight loss and maintenance. Using metaanalytic techniques, they found that eHealth interventions produced significantly greater weight loss compared to control groups (mean difference = 2.7 kg). Additionally, interventions with evidence-based behavioral skills training, such as self-monitoring and personalized feedback, produced significantly greater weight loss.

> Although the findings of this review of eHealth interventions as a treatment option support weight loss efficacy, the findings were much less positive for weight loss maintenance. Seven trials were identified, which compared eHealth interventions to a control condition for long-term weight loss, with no difference observed between groups in any of these trials.[68]

Thus, the evidence to date does not support the effectiveness of eHealth interventions for weight loss maintenance.

Devices/strategies to modify eating behavior

Taking smaller bites of food leads to more oral processing and slower rate of food intake, potentially increasing satiety, and decreasing the risk of overeating.[69–72] For this reason, there has been an increased interest in the potential of oral devices to be used as a simple intervention to promote weight loss by reducing food intake. Oral devices can modify eating behaviors by decreasing the size of the oral cavity, forcing the user to take smaller bites or less frequent bites. These devices, which are made of soft material that is contoured to an individual's palate shape, are typically worn during mealtimes and can be easily removed during all other activities besides eating. Oral devices can also have a monitor that tracks the amount of food and bites an individual takes during a meal.[72]

To date, four studies have examined the effects of different types of oral devices to restrict the size of the oral cavity to determine if decreased oral cavity size could impact food consumed, and subsequently short- and long-term weight loss. These studies found that use of oral devices produced a reduction in body weight ranging from 3% to 11%, with an average weight loss of 4.9 kg ± 0.9 kg.[69–72] All four of these studies showed the experimental group lost a statistically significant amount of weight over the course of both weeks and months, and three studies found use of the oral device produced a clinically significant weight loss (>5% total body loss).

An important question is whether or not these devices would need to used indefinitely. As a first step toward answering this question, Von Seck et al. implemented a two-phase intervention: phase one involving the issue of the oral device while eating, and in phase two, the participants removed the oral device while eating to determine if the oral device would have long-term effects on weight loss.[72] Noteworthy, the participants continued to lose a statistically significant amount of weight in phase two, despite not using the oral device. This strongly suggests that the participants continued to eat less food even when they stopped using the device.

IV. WEIGHT LOSS MAINTENANCE CHALLENGES

> Following traditional lifestyle interventions, many compensatory mechanisms occur to both the metabolic and neuroendocrine systems that signal the body to decrease energy expenditure and increase food intake, which combine to promote weight regain.

As noted earlier, the body has several compensatory mechanisms that occur following calorie restriction and weight loss to increase food intake and decrease energy expenditure.[14–16]

These mechanisms, such as decreased leptin response after meals (a protein hormone that signals satiety) and an increased ghrelin response (a gut peptide associated with the sensation of hunger), tend to promote weight regain following weight loss, and these physical changes appear to remain present until an individual has returned to their baseline weight.[15,16,18,73] As a result, individuals desiring to maintain a reduced body weight would have to consume fewer calories than suggested through the signals received from the brain and periphery.[74] Unfortunately, these strong neuroendocrine signals to increase food intake and decrease energy expenditure following weight reduction do not appear to decrease over time and thus remain present until the defended weight is reached (i.e., the lost weight is regained).[75]

As a consequence of these behavioral, environmental, and physiological factors, most individuals experience some weight regain following weight loss.[76] This weight gain often occurs after the end of initial treatment, a time when there is the least amount of contact with treatment providers. After the end of intervention, most individuals no longer have contact with providers and/or group members for social reinforcement, which may be needed as steady weight loss tends to slow after completion of treatment. As a result, the behavioral "costs" of continued dietary control can seem too high in comparison to the diminished "benefit" in terms of weight loss, decreasing motivation to maintain behavioral changes. This may lead individuals to perceive the costs of weight management efforts to exceed the benefits, which could ultimately lead to an abandonment of weight management efforts.[77]

With the current physical and social environment supporting unhealthy dietary practices and sedentary behavior, it is not surprising that initial success in lifestyle programs is commonly followed by a return to pretreatment patterns of eating and PA.[24,76] Indeed, the potency of environmental challenges often initiates a behavioral "cascade" wherein initial lapses in the maintenance of behavioral changes undermine the individual's confidence in their self-management skills and thereby lead to poor long-term adherence and the eventual abandonment of the entire behavior change effort for many individuals.[77,78]

We know, however, that there is a population that has been succeeding in maintaining substantial weight losses over the long term. Thus, it is important to carefully study the behaviors in which these individuals consistently engage.

V. RECOMMENDATIONS BASED ON EATING AND ACTIVITY BEHAVIORS IN NWCR

A. Eating Behavior

Successful weight loss maintainers in the NWCR report many of the same habits, including: eating a low-fat, high-carbohydrate diet, regular self-monitoring of body weight, with 36% reporting weighing once daily and 79% reported weighing once weekly, and high levels of PA averaging 2827 kcal/week in energy expenditure.[46,79,80] Approximately 75% of these individuals reported expending >1000 kcal/week (or walking > 10 miles/week), 54% expending >2000 kcal/week, and 35% expending >3000 kcal/week through various forms of PA. Individuals who reported more PA also reported consuming diets lower in fat and higher cognitive restraint.[79] Walking was the most popular form of PA reported, with resistance training being the second most common.

Successful weight loss maintainers continue to limit and monitor their calorie intake as well as engage in high levels of PA.

In addition to the key behaviors mentioned above, Wyatt et al. determined that consistently eating breakfast was also a common characteristic found in successful weight loss maintainers, with approximately 78% of successful weight loss maintainers reporting eating regular breakfast whereas ≤5% reported never eating breakfast.[80] Individuals with greater weight loss also demonstrated better eating habits, such as higher cognitive restraint, flexible and rigid control, lower intake of fat, more restrained eating, fewer fast food meals per week, and frequently eating breakfast.[79] A noteworthy limitation of these conclusions is that these psychological and behavioral factors were only assessed at the 1 year follow-up, rather than at all annual visits, which would have provided more information on the connection between behavioral changes and weight trajectories. Nevertheless, such findings indicate that long-term weight loss maintenance is possible but requires sustained behavior change in eating and exercise habits.[45] As noted above, sustaining these behaviors is difficult for the vast majority of individuals in the current obesogenic environment.

B. Physical Activity Levels

The variability in reported PA among members of the NWCR presents a challenge to create a single PA recommendation for weight loss and weight loss maintenance.[81] Fortunately, findings from RCTs can help inform the optimal amount and type of exercise for weight loss maintenance.

In 2001, the American College of Sports Medicine published a Position Statement that recommended adults obtain 150 min per week of moderate-intensity aerobic PA (PA) for health benefits, but 200–300 min per week, or 60 min of walking per day for weight loss maintenance.[82] In 2009, the evidence was reexamined based on studies conducted since 1999, and the following conclusions were reached: (1) Evidence supports moderate-intensity PA between 150 and 250 min (−1) to be effective to prevent weight gain. (2) Moderate-intensity PA between 150 and 250 min per week (−1) will provide only modest weight loss. (3) Greater amounts of PA (>250 min/week [−1]) are associated with clinically significant weight loss.[83] These conclusions suggest that PA levels of as little as 150 min per week may be effective in preventing weight gain.

Higher amounts of PA, however, appear to be particularly effective for promoting long-term weight loss. For example, the Studies of a Targeted Risk Reduction Intervention through Defined Exercise followed previously obese women for 12 months. This study determined that an average of 80 min/day (or 1.3 h/day) of moderate or 35 min/day (0.6 h/day) of vigorous activity added to a sedentary lifestyle resulted in the least weight regain.[84] Activity levels were assessed by doubly labeled water, and women in the "highly active" group (who engaged in the aforementioned PA duration) regained only 2.5 kg at the 1 year follow-up assessment. The moderate activity level group regained 9.9 kg, and the sedentary group regained 7 kg at the 1 year follow-up.[84]

Most studies to date have looked at the effects of aerobic exercise for weight loss maintenance. Fewer studies have examined the potential of resistance training to enhance long-term weight loss. Resistance training has the potential to enhance long-term weight loss by stimulating increased levels of fat oxidation both during and acutely following the exercise session.[85,86] Additionally, resistance training may have a positive effect on weight loss maintenance by preserving or increasing FFM and thereby enhancing metabolic rate.[87]

A growing body of evidence supports the potential of resistance training to be a weight loss maintenance tool. For example, Hunter and colleagues determined that resistance training (3 days/week) enhanced weight loss maintenance among African American and European women following a very–low-calorie diet (800 kcal/day).[88] The proposed mechanism through which resistance training enhanced weight loss maintenance was by preserving FFM, which helped to avert the decline in resting energy expenditure typically seen following calorie restricted weigh loss.[88]

A study by Borg et al (2002) investigated the effects of resistance training versus walking on weight loss maintenance in 90 middle-aged obese men and found it produced favorable changes in body composition but did not lead to greater weight loss maintenance.[89] Following an 8 week very–low-calorie diet, participants were randomized to one of three groups: control, walking, and resistance training. Both of the exercise groups (walking and resistance training) engaged in 45 minute sessions, three times weekly. Target walking intensity was 60%–70% VO_2 max, as assessed by a treadmill test, and had an estimated energy expenditure of 1.7 MJ (400 kcal). Resistance training comprised eight repetitions of each exercise for three sets, at an intensity of 60%–80% of the subject's 1 rep maximum, and the estimated energy expenditure was 1.2 MJ (300 kcal) for each session. All three groups regaining an average of 9.6 kg over the 23 month unsupervised follow-up. However, the resistance training group has the smallest regain in the waist-to-hip ratio and kept off more fat mass than the other groups.[89]

> Resistance training has the potential to enhance weight loss maintenance by maintaining or potentially enhancing FFM and thereby averting the decline in RMR that typically occurs following weight loss interventions.

VI. OBESITY ACROSS THE LIFE SPAN AND IMPORTANCE OF PREVENTING DRIVERS OF GAIN

A. Obesity and Aging

Of significant concern, the number and proportion of obese, older women has increased dramatically over the past two decades.[90] Recent estimates indicate that 35% of older Caucasian women are obese and another 33% are overweight, placing them at risk for obesity.[90] Even more alarming, approximately 50% of African American women age 60 and over are currently obese, with an additional 30% classified as overweight.[90] In line with the high prevalence of obesity, older, postmenopausal African American also have higher rates of obesity-related illnesses, including diabetes and hypertension,[90,91] as well as functional limitations due to obesity than other populations.[91,92]

Both women and men show an increase in central adiposity and subcutaneous abdominal tissue with increasing age, which has been shown to negatively affect skeletal muscle metabolism[93] and increase the risk of cardiometabolic abnormalities.[94–96] The decline in estrogen following menopause can disrupt energy metabolism and predispose women to gain adipose tissue, as well as increase risk of obesity-related disease conditions.[97] Moreover, postmenopausal status also leads to deleterious changes in fat distribution, especially with abdominal adiposity increased and an increase in lipid profile that points to the higher risk of chronic disease conditions.[98]

Similar to obesity, diabetes is highly prevalent among older adults. Diabetes currently afflicts more than one in five adults age 65 years and older.[99] Additionally, the prevalence of diabetes among older adults is rising and projected to reach 30% in the next three decades.[100]

Although obesity is a significant contributor to diabetes-related disability,[101,102] there appears to be a distinct effect of diabetes on risk for disability independent of BMI.[101–103] For example, investigators from the Women's Health and Aging Study reported that adjusting for obesity minimally reduced the association between diabetes and objective measures of physical function.[104] In addition, Park and colleagues (2006) found a linear relationship between duration of diabetes and poor glycemic control with changes in muscle quality.[103]

The causes of these age-related biological changes are multifactorial and include environmental, social, and behavioral factors. Among the behavioral factors, low levels of PA combined with excessive and unhealthy calorie intake appear to strongly contribute to functional decline among older adults.[105] For example, sedentary time has been associated with the development of both metabolic syndrome[106] and major mobility disability (defined as inability to walk one block)[107] in a large sample of generally healthy older adults with moderate mobility limitations. In line with these findings, a recent review of trends in US health by the US Burden of Disease Collaborators found that high BMI, smoking, and high fasting plasma glucose are the three most important risk factors for disease and disability in the United States.[108] Among these, only smoking is decreasing, while BMI and fasting plasma glucose levels are steadily increasing.

B. Drivers of Weight Gain Across The Life Span

Stress

Stress can be defined as "the generalized, non-specific response of the body to any factor that overwhelms, or threatens to overwhelm, the body's compensatory abilities to maintain homeostasis can be either acute or chronic, with the type of stress having specific consequences." While acute stress activates the "flight or fight" response and suppresses appetite, chronic stress has generally been associated with a greater preference for energy dense foods, particularly those high in fat and sugar.[109] Findings from longitudinal studies suggest that chronic life stress is linked to weight gain, with the effects being greater in men than women.[109] Perceived stress may also promote weight gain through its effects on PA levels with most studies finding that higher levels of perceived stress lead to reductions in PA levels.[110]

In addition to the behavioral changes noted above, there are a few physiological mechanisms through which chronic stress can lead to weight gain. First, chronic stress can dysregulate the HPA axis and induce secretion of glucocorticoids, which target the hypothalamus that can alter glucose metabolism, promote insulin resistance, and influence multiple appetite-related hormones and hypothalamic neuropeptides.[111,112] Chronic stress can also lead to overactivation of the hypothalamic–pituitary–adrenal axis and sympathetic adrenal medullary system, as well as the release of circulating hormones that could promote fat storage.[112] The hormones ghrelin and cortisol in particular have been associated with weight gain following elevated levels of perceived stress.[113] For example, Chao et al. found that higher fasting levels of ghrelin predicted future (6 months) food cravings for starchy, carbohydrate heavy foods.[114]

To our knowledge, no study has examined the potential of stress management interventions to enhance weight loss maintenance, and only two studies have examined the potential of stress management interventions to enhance the effects of weight loss interventions in overweight adults. In both of these studies, the addition of a stress management program, which incorporated diaphragmatic breathing, progressive muscle relaxation, and guided visualization, to a dietary intervention was found to produce larger reductions in BMI and weight compared to a control group (diet only).[115,116] Additionally, participants receiving the stress management intervention reported greater reductions in anxiety and depression and higher levels of dietary restraint comparted to participants in the control group.[115,116]

Sleep

Self-reported mean sleep time has decreased 10–15 min from 1985 to 2010, with adults self-reporting less than 6 h of sleep per night increasing from 22.3% to 29.2%.[117] This is of concern as short sleep time can increase risk for obesity.[118] In a 16 year longitudinal study of 68,183 women, a clear relationship between self-reported sleep duration and weight gain was observed.[118] Women who reported sleeping between 7 and 8 h per night had the lowest risk for major weight gain. Risk of developing obesity began to increase for women who slept less than 7 h per night, with the risk progressively increasing for women who reported sleeping less than 6 and 5 h per night (6% and 15% increase, respectively).[118] In the MedWeight Study, a registry of individuals who lost at least 10% of their body weight in the past and either maintained the loss or regained it, short sleep duration and poor sleep quality were also directly linked to poor weight loss maintenance.[119] Although the exact mechanism linking sleep to weight gain is not known, there are a number of potential mechanisms through which short sleep duration could affect body weight including reduction in PA, increased ghrelin levels, and decreased leptin sensitivity.[120] To our knowledge, no studies have tested the effects of a sleep intervention on weight loss or weight loss maintenance.

Medications for obesity

Current medications for obesity are indicated to be used as adjuncts to a reduced-calorie diet and increased PA for chronic weight management in adults with a BMI $\geq$30 kg/m^2 or those with a BMI $\geq$27 kg/m^2 who have at least one weight-related comorbid condition, such as diabetes mellitus, hypertension, hyperlipidemia, or sleep apnea.[121] At present, there are five major FDA approved antiobesity medications: phentermine, orlistat, phentermine/topiramate extended release, naltrexone sustained release (SR)/bupropion SR, and liraglutide (the only injectable formulation). Four of these five medications work by activating CNS pathways that reduces appetite or enhances satiety, and the other medication (i.e., Orlistat) works by reducing the absorption of dietary fat.[121]

Obesity medications have an efficacy of 3%–7% (estimated net weight loss) compared to placebo.[121] Several classes of FDA-approved medications, along with off-label medications, have also been found effective in enhancing weight loss maintenance.[122,123] When used as an adjunct to lifestyle intervention, obesity medications have been found to produce greater mean weight loss and an increased likelihood of achieving clinically meaningful 1 year weight loss relative to placebo.[122,123] Thus, obesity medications appear to be a useful adjunct to lifestyle interventions to maintain weight loss and prevent weight regain.

Although medications can enhance weight loss and weight loss maintenance, limitations to long-term use of obesity medications exist. First, it is necessary to carefully evaluate their safety, efficacy, contraindications, and drug interactions before prolonged use.[122,123] This is especially important in regards to cardiovascular safety, as increased rates of adverse cardiac events have been reported with previously approved medications.[122,123] Additionally, there is a high variability of responses to these medications, reluctance of some patients and providers to initiate pharmacotherapy, high attrition rates, and a risk of regaining weight despite treatment. Finally, there are currently no recommendations for which type or class of patients the particular medications will be best suited. This decision is often left to providers who do not have the requisite expertise or experience to recognize the specific phenotypes that would differentially responds to certain medications.

> Medications hold promise to enhance weight loss maintenance, but more research is needed to determine the types of medications that would be most appropriate for specific patient populations.

VII. OBESITY ACROSS THE LIFE SPAN AND BODY COMPOSITION CHANGES WITH AGING, MENOPAUSE

A. Role of Dietary Macronutrient Composition in Long-Term Weight Loss

Although calorie restriction produces short-term weight loss, intense debate remains about the importance of macronutrient composition in the treatment of obesity.

There are currently strong advocates of diets that emphasize protein, those that emphasize carbohydrates, or those that emphasize fat.[124–126] Yet findings to date from studies in which macronutrient composition was manipulated have been mixed. In a number of studies, low-carbohydrate, high-protein diets have been found to produce superior short-term (i.e., 6 month) weight loss as compared to conventional, low-fat diets.[127–132] In contrast, other researchers found that a very–high-carbohydrate, very–low-fat vegetarian diet was superior to a conventional high-carbohydrate, low-fat diet in improving cardiovascular disease risk factors.[133,134] Other studies, however, have not reported that macronutrient composition can influence weight loss outcomes.

Relatively few studies that have examined the role of dietary composition in weight loss outcomes have followed participants for 1 year or longer, and among these studies, the findings have been mixed. For example, one study found an ad lib low-fat diet was superior to a diet with fixed energy intakes,[135] while other studies found a moderate-fat, Mediterranean-style diet and a low-carbohydrate diet produced greater long-term weight loss than a low-fat diet.[136,137] In contrast, other studies have found no differences between high-protein and low-protein diets in long-term weight loss.[128] Until recently, most trials involved relatively small samples comprised of mostly women and did not adequately report on adherence to the assigned diets. Thus, the most important question is whether overweight people have a better response in the long-term to diets that emphasize a specific macronutrient composition.

The Pounds Lost trial was conducted in an effort to answer this question. In this large-scale, 2 year intervention trial, conducted at two different sites, a total of 811 participants were randomly assigned to one of four diets that emphasized different contents of carbohydrates, fats, and proteins.[138] Specifically, participants were assigned to follow one of the following four diets: 20% fat, 15% protein, and 65% carbohydrates (low-fat, average-protein); 20% fat, 25% protein, and 55% carbohydrates (low-fat, high-protein); 40% fat, 15% protein, and 45% carbohydrates (high-fat, average-protein); and 40% fat, 25% protein, and 35% carbohydrates (high-fat, high-protein). Participants in all four dietary conditions were provided with a state-of-the-art behavioral intervention throughout the entire 2 year intervention. The key findings of this trial were that all four diets produced clinically meaningful weight loss and that there were no differences in weight loss or maintenance of weight loss between the diets over the course of 2 years.[138] Other noteworthy findings were that many participants had difficulty achieving the macronutrient goals for their assigned group and that adherence steadily declined regardless of which dietary macronutrient condition the participant was assigned.[63,139] Overall, these findings with respect to adherence to macronutrient goals suggest that participants in weight loss programs revert to their customary macronutrient intakes over time but may nonetheless be able to maintain some weight loss.

The findings of the Pounds Lost trial would suggest that there is not an ideal macronutrient composition for weight loss maintenance. Although it was a well-conducted, large-scale, long-term trial, it was only one trial. Another approach to look at the potential effects of macronutrient composition on weight loss outcomes is to examine the effects of popular diets on weight loss.

Based in part on such trends in weight gain, the creators of many popular diets (e.g., Atkins, Zone) have suggested that diets in which carbohydrate intake is significantly higher than other macronutrients are not an optimal approach for weight loss and may even contribute to weight gain. Most of these diets were published and promoted by one or more health and wellness "expert" who attests to the health and weight loss benefits observed when following their recommended diet.

Two reviews have evaluated the effects of popular diets on both short- and long-term weight loss outcomes. The first was a metaanalysis by Johnston et al. in 2014, which attempted to answer the question of whether any popular diets were effective in producing weight loss over the short term (6 months or less) and/or long term (12 months).[140] The primary findings of this metaanalysis were that reductions in calorie intake were the primary driver of weight loss and that differences between diets differing in macronutrient composition were relatively small. A noteworthy limitation of this metaanalysis, however, was that it included studies in which calorie restriction was a component of some of the popular diets tested.

As a follow-up to the Johnston et al. review, Anton and colleagues conducted a review of the effects of popular diets that did not include specific calorie targets on both short-term ($\leq$6 months) and long-term ($\geq$1 year) weight loss outcomes.[141] The diets selected for this review were based on the popular diets listed in the 2016 US News and World Report. A noteworthy finding of this review was that only 7 of the 20 eligible popular diets in the US News & World Report had been tested in a clinical trial and that there was a large disparity in the evidence base for these 7 diets (without calorie targets). In contrast to the Johnston et al. review, Anton and colleagues found that the Atkins diet had substantially more support from clinical trials than any other popular diet. Specifically, six of seven clinical trials supported the efficacy of the Atkins diet to produce clinically meaningful short-term weight loss, with findings from four of five trials supporting the ability of this diet to produce long-term weight loss. In contrast to the Atkins diet, there were few clinical trials published on the other six empirically tested diets (i.e., the DASH diet, the glycemic index diet, the Mediterranean diet, the Ornish diet, the Paleolithic diet, the low-fat vegan diet, and the zone diet).

Noteworthy, current recommendations of the Dietary Guidelines Advisory Committee, which state that diets with less than 45% of calories as carbohydrates are not successful for long-term weight loss (1months), are not in line with low-carbohydrate diets such as Atkins.[22] In support of current dietary guidelines, a metaanalyses by Hall and Guo of 32 controlled feeding studies found that isocaloric substitution of dietary carbohydrate for fat produced greater energy expenditure (26 kcal/d) and fat loss (16 g/d).[142] Thus, the low-fat diet, rather than low-carbohydrate diet, produced more favorable changes in energy expenditure and fat loss in this metaanalytic review of isocaloric diets. Given the mixed findings reported in the literature and different conclusions reached by recent reviews and metaanalyses, it is not surprising that the role of diet composition in weight loss and weight loss maintenance remains a topic of significant debate.

> Despite extensive research, there is not a clear answer to what the optimal diet is to promote weight loss and/or weight loss maintenance. The best diet is therefore likely to be the diet that an individual will follow over the long term.

B. Metabolic Dysregulation and Aging

With aging, there are changes in body composition that can contribute to unhealthy metabolic states, further increasing risk for unhealthy weight gain, and ultimately chronic disease conditions. First, there is often a loss of FFM, which seems to parallel the reduction in metabolic rate, particularly after the age of 50.[143] Due to the combination of aging and corresponding reduction in activity levels, loss of muscle mass progresses faster with increasing age.[144,145] This age-related muscle loss (sarcopenia) can diminish both the metabolic and mechanical functions of the skeletal muscle,[146,147] which is of concern as skeletal muscle has the greatest contribution to an individual's metabolic rate.[148]

In addition to loss of total muscle mass, the quality of muscle declines with age due to increased fat infiltration within the muscle, which can result in a loss of muscle strength[149] and power.[150] Noteworthy, these age-related changes in muscle composition appear to be even more pronounced in older adults with obesity[151,152] and can lead to a reduction in energy expenditure and increased risk of weight gain.[143] Over time, the progressive reduction of the structural and mechanical function of skeletal muscle during aging can ultimately lead to impairments in the functional capacity[153] and contribute to metabolic disease conditions (e.g., metabolic syndrome).[154]

At a cellular level, a decrease in skeletal muscle oxidative capacity and mitochondrial function is typically observed with aging, resulting in impaired oxidative capacity for fat utilization.[155] Over time, this can lead to an imbalance between fatty acid uptake and fatty acid oxidation and utilization and lead to lipotoxicity, a condition in which the body is unable to convert excess lipid into lipid droplets to be utilized for fatty acid oxidation.[156] Lipotoxicity also results from lipids being synthesized from excess glucose in both adipose and nonadipose tissue.[157] During aging, these physiological changes can contribute to body weight gain and a redistribution of body fat to the abdominal area, visceral organs, and even the bone. Notable metabolic changes that are related to lipotoxicity include a decline of insulin sensitivity, alteration in substrate utilization, and reduction in mitochondrial function and number.[158]

Chronic overnutrition is a key contributor to the development of lipotoxicity, as frequently consumption of calories results in an increase of carbohydrate utilization and decrease of fatty acid oxidation. Over time, this can contribute to the accumulation of toxic fatty acids, as the skeletal muscle is less able to switch between metabolizing lipids and carbohydrates. Lipotoxicity appears to be an important factor contributing to muscle loss with age and associated decline in physical functioning.[159–161] Moreover, the combination of muscle loss and fat gain may act synergistically to increase risk of physical disability in the elderly.[143,162,163]

The complexity of the physiological changes with aging and the development of metabolic dysfunction, which predisposes individuals to further weight gain, warrants further investigation.

> Metabolic changes occur during aging that can promote adiposity and loss of lean mass. Therefore, it is particularly important that middle-age and older adults continue to engage in lifestyle behaviors that can promote metabolic health.

C. Treatment Targets—Fat Versus Weight Loss and Muscle Retention

The metabolic changes described above can put the weight reduced older adult in a bit of a precarious situation. On the one hand, they need to reduce their calorie consumption to match the reduction in their metabolic rate, due to loss of skeletal muscle. On the other hand, there appears to be an increased need for protein to maintain levels of FFM.[164] Additionally, with the reduction in metabolic rate comes an increased susceptibility to gain weight, specifically body fat.

Due to the body composition and metabolic changes that occur with aging, there remains significant debate regarding how to best treat obesity in older adults.[165] This controversy primarily revolves around concerns that weight loss may accelerate the rate of muscle and bone loss that normally occurs with aging and thereby adversely affect physical function.[166,167] Indeed, a relatively large proportion of FFM (25%) is typically lost following traditional lifestyle interventions (caloric restriction and aerobic exercise).[168]

On the other hand, lifestyle interventions represent potential treatment methods that could delay or even prevent the most common and disabling conditions experienced by obese, older adults.[169,170] For example, a large-scale clinical trial found that intentional weight loss was associated with reduced mortality risk in obese adults 60 years and older,[171] and another recent trial found weight loss reduces arterial stiffness in obese, older adults,[172] suggesting that weight loss should be recommended for this population. Recent clinical trials also suggest that the addition of resistance training to a diet plus aerobic exercise program can attenuate the loss of skeletal muscle during weight loss in adults age 65 and over.[169] Diet plus supervised resistance and aerobic exercise regimens have also been found to substantially improve mobility (i.e., walking speed) and function in obese, older adults.[170,173]

Although some risk may be associated with weight loss in older adults, obesity and sedentary lifestyle, without intervention, are known to predict the development of disability in otherwise well-functioning older adults.[174,175] Confidence in use of these interventions on a broad scale will require a study to demonstrate that the benefits of these interventions outweigh potential risks. Thus, enhancing and/or maintaining FFM represents a very important focus of treatment, as high-quality muscle is the primary driver of metabolic rate. A very important secondary focus should be on the effects of treatment on mobility and physical function, as walking speed is an excellent proxy of overall health status in older adults.[176,177]

Another important secondary focus should be on enhancing metabolic flexibility, so that the individual is able to utilize and switch between glucose and fat-derived ketones as sources of energy.[55] For many sedentary, overweight older adults, this switch rarely occurs and thus their body remains in fat storage mode for the majority of time. In contrast, the activation of the metabolic switch appears to be a useful strategy to prevent lipotoxicity, as it causes a shift from fat storage to utilization of body fat as an energy source. To induce this metabolic switch, it is critical to focus on lifestyle habits, such as intermittent fasting and resistance training that can increase resting energy metabolism, total energy expenditure, and fat oxidation.

D. Promising Approaches to Enhance Long-Term Weight/Fat Loss

Although the optimal intervention strategy for improving health and metabolic function in overweight adults is not currently known, there are several promising approaches worthy of investigation to enhance long-term weight/fat loss. Standard lifestyle approaches (i.e., diet plus aerobic exercise) have demonstrated efficacy for weight loss and have also been found to improve self-reported physical function.[178] Additionally, calorie-restricted diets have been shown to reduce intrahepatic fat and improve insulin sensitivity in obese, older adults.[179] These effects are observed with or without the addition of aerobic exercise, though aerobic exercise does appear to enhance the beneficial metabolic changes produced by calorie restriction.[179]

As positive as these findings are in regards to weight loss and metabolic improvements, standard lifestyle interventions have not been successful to date in producing long-term weight loss for the majority of individuals. Thus, the long-term weight loss maintenance remains the Achilles heel of obesity treatment. Below, we review promising approaches that could be used as an alternative or integrated with standard lifestyle treatments to produce better long-term weight/fat loss.

Resistance training

One promising approach to enhance the effects of standard lifestyle interventions is to add a resistance training component to the exercise intervention. The addition of resistance training to a hypocaloric diet has been found to attenuate the loss of lean mass during weight loss in older adults.[169] Other trials have found that calorie restricted diets combined with comprehensive exercise programs involving resistance training improve physical function and ameliorate frailty in older adults with obesity.[170] Additionally, the combination of moderate-intensity resistance training plus diet was recently found to be more effective than diet alone in producing fat loss and reducing intermuscular adipose tissue following a 10 week weight loss intervention in overweight, older adults.[180] Noteworthy, the improvements in functional capacity appear to be directly related to enhanced muscle quality due to the reduction in fat infiltration into muscle bundles.[181] A growing body of evidence indicates resistance training may have the potential to enhance weight loss maintenance, though findings of initial

Activation of the metabolic switch in fuel metabolism from glucose to ketones through lifestyle habits can encourage both fat loss and muscle retention. Unfortunately, this switch rarely occurs in most sedentary, overweight adults.

studies are mixed.[88,89] The proposed mechanism through which resistance training enhanced long-term weight loss was by preserving FFM, which helped to avert the decline in resting energy expenditure typically seen following calorie restricted weigh loss.[88]

High-protein diets

Increasing dietary protein intake has been shown to increase muscle protein synthesis in older adults and stimulate postprandial muscle accretion in older men.[182,183] Therefore, higher protein diets could be an intervention to preserve FFM in older populations, particularly when combined with resistance training.[182,183] In line with this, the combination of a high dietary protein diet plus resistance exercise training was recently shown to significantly increase FFM during weight loss in overweight and obese older adults.[184] Noteworthy, the high-protein diet, independent of the resistance exercise, did not significantly affect changes in FFM during weight loss. The participants who received the combined intervention of high-protein diet plus resistance exercise, however, had a significant increase in their FFM. In line with the findings of this trial, a recent review by Anton and colleagues found that dietary interventions involving protein supplementation improved functional and strength outcomes in older adults with sarcopenia.[164] Such findings suggest that the combination of high-protein, calorie-restricted diets, particularly when combined with resistance training, can help maintain or even increase FFM during weight loss and thus may be a promising approach for enhancing weight loss maintenance, particularly in older adults.

Portion control plates

Increased portion sizes appear to be directly related to increased energy intake,[185] and thus portion size is likely an important factor contributing to the current obesity epidemic. This suggests that reducing portion size through portion control plates may have an attractive strategy to promote weight loss and weight loss maintenance. In a recent study by Hughes and colleagues, students who used a portion control plate served themselves significantly less food in comparison to when they used a regular dinner plate.[69] In another 6 month clinical trial of type 2 diabetic patients with obesity, a dietary intervention utilizing portion control plates produced significantly greater weight loss than dietary teaching alone.[70] Noteworthy, this weight loss resulted in a larger percentage of patients in the control group going off of their diabetes medications compared to the usual care group.[70] Such findings suggest that portion control plates could be a promising method for enhancing long-term weight loss.

Intermittent fasting

Recent reviews have highlighted the potential of less traditional dietary approaches, specifically intermittent fasting,[54,55] to produce substantial weight and fat loss and thereby potentially improve unhealthy age-related changes in body composition. The two types of intermittent fasting that have the most supportive evidence for producing clinically meaningful weight loss are ADF and TRF.[55] Noteworthy, TRF approaches seemed to be particularly effective for maintaining FFM during weight loss. To date, only one study has tested the effects of ADF on weight loss maintenance over 1 year and found it was not superior to calorie restriction,[186] and no studies, to our knowledge, have tested the effects of TRF on long-term weight loss. Thus, future trials are needed to evaluate the potential that this eating pattern may have for enhancing weight loss maintenance.

VIII. CONCLUSION

Although obesity is an intractable problem for most, there remains a small percentage (but large number) of individuals who have successfully lost substantial amounts of weight (>30 lbs) and maintained this loss for several years. This indicates two things: (1) successful long-term weight loss with the current treatment paradigm is possible and (2) the current treatment paradigm does not work well for most individuals.

Despite strong evidence indicating that lifestyle intervention programs involving diet, exercise, and behavior modification can reduce risk factors for many chronic diseases and improve physical function, long-term adherence to lifestyle interventions to date is notoriously low.[187] Consequently, the "adherence problem" represents an important challenge to weight loss interventions.[187] As we discussed in this chapter, this is not due to a failure of willpower or other character flaw, but rather because the body defends against weight loss through a number of different biological mechanisms, which makes sustained weight loss extremely difficult to achieve. This is particularly true for older adults because of the decline in FFM, the primary driver of metabolism (or metabolic rate), that occurs with aging. For most people, the degree of willpower required to maintain a calorie-restricted diet and high levels of PA in the current obesogenic environment is simply too difficult.

Ultimately, weight gain and weight regain is an energy balance problem. Much focus to date has been on the energy intake side for both weight loss and weight loss maintenance, but the energy expenditure side may deserve more attention for preventing weight regain and enhancing weight loss maintenance. We say this because there is an inevitable reduction in resting and total energy expenditure with the current treatment paradigm of caloric restriction and subsequent loss of FFM. This puts the weight-reduced person in a precarious position because the moment they deviate too far from their target calorie intake, either body fat will accumulate or lean mass will be lost, both of which lead to unhealthy metabolic changes. As noted above, this approach will work but only a small percentage of the population on a long-term basis. Thus, it is very important to carefully evaluate what types of behavioral changes the majority of adults are likely to adhere to over the long term.

For the reasons mentioned above, we believe a potentially more efficacious approach to enhancing long-term weight loss would be to focus on strategies to enhance energy expenditure, rather than reducing energy intake, following weight loss. A few notable ways in which this could be accomplished include (1) increasing or maintaining high-quality, FFM through increased protein intake and resistance training, (2) increasing PA (all types) levels and reducing sedentary behavior, (3) temporarily increasing metabolic rate and fat oxidation through acute exercise sessions, and (4) activating brown fat by flipping the metabolic switch through intermittent fasting. By enhancing both resting and total energy expenditure through these methods, the target calorie intake to maintain a reduced body weight would increase to a potentially more sustainable level.

Fortunately, there is evidence that the defended body weight can be changed by influencing hormonal, metabolic, and neural functions that regulate food intake and energy expenditure in response to weight loss.[74] The success of bariatric surgery, which is the only treatment to date scientifically demonstrated to produce long-term, sustainable weight loss, attests to the potential benefits of this type of treatment approach.[188] While there a number of promising treatments that have the potential to enhance long-term weight loss, ultimately the best approach for a given individual is likely to be the one that they can adhere to over time.

Our hopes for the future are that greater understanding of the biology of body weight regulation will yield new approaches. It should be a high-profile area of research investment. Similarly, understanding how bariatric surgery seems to be successful should be a priority for research because it will drive new approaches. And finally, we will need research in understanding how weight loss differs from weight maintenance because two different approaches may be needed for long-term success.

RESEARCH GAPS

- Better phenotyping and genotyping of individuals to direct recommendations for behaviors around food intake, so as to maximize weight loss.
- Understanding the biology of food intake and energy balance regulation and development of tools to produce weight loss in persons whose health would benefit from weight loss.
- Understanding the biology of reactive thermogenesis (metabolic adaptation) and the biologic alterations in hunger and satiety signals to develop tools to sustain weight loss in the reduced weight state.
- Strategies to enhance energy expenditure, both resting and total, following weight loss to promote weight loss maintenance.
- Role of intermittent fasting and/or other lifestyle behaviors in shifting metabolism from lipogenesis (fat storage) to fat mobilization for energy through fatty acid oxidation.

IX. REFERENCES

1. Flegal KM, Carroll MD, Kuczmarski RJ, Johnson CL. Overweight and obesity in the United States: prevalence and trends, 1960–1994. *Int J Obes Relat Metab Disord*. 1998;22:39–47.
2. Trends in adult body-mass index in 200 countries from 1975 to 2014: a pooled analysis of 1698 population-based measurement studies with 19.2 million participants. *Lancet*. 2016;387:1377–1396.
3. Hales CM, Carroll MD, Fryar CD, Ogden CL. Prevalence of obesity among adults and youth: United States, 2015–2016. *NCHS Data Brief*. 2017:1–8.
4. Kaplan LM, Golden A, Jinnett K, et al. Perceptions of barriers to effective obesity care: results from the national ACTION study. *Obesity*. 2018;26:61–69.
5. Martin CB, Herrick KA, Sarafrazi N, Ogden CL. Attempts to lose weight Among adults in the United States, 2013–2016. *NCHS Data Brief*. 2018:1–8.
6. Gudzune KA, Doshi RS, Mehta AK, et al. Efficacy of commercial weight-loss programs: an updated systematic review. *Ann Intern Med*. 2015;162:501–512.
7. Berthoud HR, Munzberg H, Morrison CD. Blaming the brain for obesity: integration of hedonic and homeostatic mechanisms. *Gastroenterology*. 2017;152:1728–1738.

8. MacLean PS, Blundell JE, Mennella JA, Batterham RL. Biological control of appetite: a daunting complexity. *Obesity.* 2017;25(Suppl 1):S8–S16.
9. Muller TD, Nogueiras R, Andermann ML, et al. Ghrelin. *Mol Metab.* 2015;4:437–460.
10. Schwartz GJ. The role of gastrointestinal vagal afferents in the control of food intake: current prospects. *Nutrition.* 2000;16: 866–873.
11. Hemmingsson E. A new model of the role of psychological and emotional distress in promoting obesity: conceptual review with implications for treatment and prevention. *Obes Rev.* 2014;15: 769–779.
12. Munzberg H, Morrison CD. Structure, production and signaling of leptin. *Metabolism.* 2015;64:13–23.
13. Astrup A, Gotzsche PC, van de Werken K, et al. Meta-analysis of resting metabolic rate in formerly obese subjects. *Am J Clin Nutr.* 1999;69:1117–1122.
14. Knuth ND, Johannsen DL, Tamboli RA, et al. Metabolic adaptation following massive weight loss is related to the degree of energy imbalance and changes in circulating leptin. *Obesity.* 2014;22:2563–2569.
15. Rosenbaum M, Leibel RL. Models of energy homeostasis in response to maintenance of reduced body weight. *Obesity.* 2016; 24:1620–1629.
16. Fothergill E, Guo J, Howard L, et al. Persistent metabolic adaptation 6 years after "The Biggest Loser" competition. *Obesity.* 2016;24: 1612–1619.
17. Ravussin E, Ryan DH. Energy expenditure and weight control: is the biggest loser the best loser? *Obesity.* 2016;24:1607–1608.
18. Sumithran P, Prendergast LA, Delbridge E, et al. Long-term persistence of hormonal adaptations to weight loss. *N Engl J Med.* 2011;365:1597–1604.
19. Jensen MD, Ryan DH, Apovian CM, et al. 2013 AHA/ACC/TOS guideline for the management of overweight and obesity in adults: a report of the American College of Cardiology/American Heart Association Task Force on Practice Guidelines and The Obesity Society. *Circulation.* 2014;129:S102–S138.
20. Ryan DH, Yockey SR. Weight loss and improvement in comorbidity: differences at 5%, 10%, 15%, and over. *Curr Obes Rep.* 2017;6: 187–194.
21. Magkos F, Fraterrigo G, Yoshino J, et al. Effects of moderate and subsequent progressive weight loss on metabolic function and adipose tissue biology in humans with obesity. *Cell Metabol.* 2016;23:591–601.
22. U.S.Department of Health and Human Services, U.S.Department of Agriculture. *2015–2020 Dietary Guidelines for Americans.* 8th ed. 2015 (Ref Type: Report).
23. Estruch R, Ros E, Salas-Salvado J, et al. Primary prevention of cardiovascular disease with a Mediterranean diet. *N Engl J Med.* 2013;368:1279–1290.
24. LeBlanc ES, Patnode CD, Webber EM, Redmond N, Rushkin M, O'Connor EA. Behavioral and pharmacotherapy weight loss interventions to prevent obesity-related morbidity and mortality in adults: updated evidence report and systematic review for the US preventive services task force. *JAMA.* 2018;320(11):1172–1191.
25. U.S.Centers for Medicare, Medicaid Services. *Medicare Coverage Database.* 2019 (Ref Type: Report).
26. The Diabetes Prevention Program. Design and methods for a clinical trial in the prevention of type 2 diabetes. *Diabetes Care.* 1999;22:623–634.
27. The Diabetes Prevention Program (DPP): description of lifestyle intervention. *Diabetes Care.* 2002;25:2165–2171.
28. Knowler WC, Barrett-Connor E, Fowler SE, et al. Reduction in the incidence of type 2 diabetes with lifestyle intervention or metformin. *N Engl J Med.* 2002;346:393–403.
29. Pi-Sunyer X, Blackburn G, Brancati FL, et al. Reduction in weight and cardiovascular disease risk factors in individuals with type 2 diabetes: one-year results of the look AHEAD trial. *Diabetes Care.* 2007;30:1374–1383.
30. Ryan DH, Espeland MA, Foster GD, et al. Look AHEAD (Action for Health in Diabetes): design and methods for a clinical trial of weight loss for the prevention of cardiovascular disease in type 2 diabetes. *Contr Clin Trials.* 2003;24:610–628.
31. Svetkey LP, Stevens VJ, Brantley PJ, et al. Comparison of strategies for sustaining weight loss: the weight loss maintenance randomized controlled trial. *J Am Med Assoc.* 2008;299:1139–1148.
32. Perri MG, Nezu AM, Patti ET, McCann KL. Effect of length of treatment on weight loss. *J Consult Clin Psychol.* 1989;57:450–452.
33. Whelton PK, Appel LJ, Espeland MA, et al. Sodium reduction and weight loss in the treatment of hypertension in older persons: a randomized controlled trial of nonpharmacologic interventions in the elderly (TONE). TONE Collaborative Research Group. *J Am Med Assoc.* 1998;279:839–846.
34. Wing RR, Koeske R, Epstein LH, Nowalk MP, Gooding W, Becker D. Long-term effects of modest weight loss in type II diabetic patients. *Arch Intern Med.* 1987;147:1749–1753.
35. Dattilo AM, Kris-Etherton PM. Effects of weight reduction on blood lipids and lipoproteins: a meta-analysis. *Am J Clin Nutr.* 1992;56:320–328.
36. Wing RR, Epstein LH, Marcus MD, Kupfer DJ. Mood changes in behavioral weight loss programs. *J Psychosom Res.* 1984;28: 189–196.
37. Jeffery RW, Drewnowski A, Epstein LH, et al. Long-term maintenance of weight loss: current status. *Health Psychol.* 2000;19: 5–16.
38. Karlsson J, Sjostrom L, Sullivan M. Swedish obese subjects (SOS)–an intervention study of obesity. Two-year follow-up of health-related quality of life (HRQL) and eating behavior after gastric surgery for severe obesity. *Int J Obes Relat Metab Disord.* 1998;22: 113–126.
39. Crandall JP, Knowler WC, Kahn SE, et al. The prevention of type 2 diabetes. *Nat Clin Pract Endocrinol Metabol.* 2008;4:382–393.
40. Ackermann RT. Working with the YMCA to implement the diabetes prevention program. *Am J Prev Med.* 2013;44:S352–S356.
41. Wadden TA, Neiberg RH, Wing RR, et al. Four-year weight losses in the Look AHEAD study: factors associated with long-term success. *Obesity.* 2011;19:1987–1998.
42. Mela DJ. Determinants of food choice: relationships with obesity and weight control. *Obes Res.* 2001;9(Suppl 4):249S–255S.
43. Klem ML, Wing RR, McGuire MT, Seagle HM, Hill JO. A descriptive study of individuals successful at long-term maintenance of substantial weight loss. *Am J Clin Nutr.* 1997;66: 239–246.
44. McGuire MT, Wing RR, Klem ML, Seagle HM, Hill JO. Long-term maintenance of weight loss: do people who lose weight through various weight loss methods use different behaviors to maintain their weight? *Int J Obes Relat Metab Disord.* 1998;22:572–577.
45. Thomas JG, Bond DS, Phelan S, Hill JO, Wing RR. Weight-loss maintenance for 10 years in the national weight control registry. *Am J Prev Med.* 2014;46:17–23.
46. Butryn ML, Phelan S, Hill JO, Wing RR. Consistent self-monitoring of weight: a key component of successful weight loss maintenance. *Obesity.* 2007;15:3091–3096.
47. Phelan S, Wyatt HR, Hill JO, Wing RR. Are the eating and exercise habits of successful weight losers changing? *Obesity.* 2006;14: 710–716.
48. Cefalu WT, Bray GA, Home PD, et al. Advances in the science, treatment, and prevention of the disease of obesity: reflections from a diabetes care editors' expert forum. *Diabetes Care.* 2015; 38:1567–1582.

49. Hall KD, Sacks G, Chandramohan D, et al. Quantification of the effect of energy imbalance on bodyweight. *Lancet*. 2011;378: 826–837.
50. Dansinger ML, Gleason JA, Griffith JL, Selker HP, Schaefer EJ. Comparison of the Atkins, Ornish, Weight Watchers, and Zone diets for weight loss and heart disease risk reduction: a randomized trial. *J Am Med Assoc*. 2005;293:43–53.
51. Astbury NM, Piernas C, Hartmann-Boyce J, Lapworth S, Aveyard P, Jebb SA. A systematic review and meta-analysis of the effectiveness of meal replacements for weight loss. *Obes Rev.* 2019;20:569–587.
52. Dimatteo MR. Social support and patient adherence to medical treatment: a meta-analysis. *Health Psychol*. 2004;23:207–218.
53. Wing RR, Jeffery RW. Benefits of recruiting participants with friends and increasing social support for weight loss and maintenance. *J Consult Clin Psychol*. 1999;67:132–138.
54. Anton S, Leeuwenburgh C. Fasting or caloric restriction for healthy aging. *Exp Gerontol*. 2013;48:1003–1005.
55. Anton SD, Moehl K, Donahoo WT, et al. Flipping the metabolic switch: understanding and applying the health benefits of fasting. *Obesity.* 2018;26:254–268.
56. Dunn C, Haubenreiser M, Johnson M, et al. Mindfulness approaches and weight loss, weight maintenance, and weight regain. *Curr Obes Rep*. 2018;7:37–49.
57. Angelopoulos T, Kokkinos A, Liaskos C, et al. The effect of slow spaced eating on hunger and satiety in overweight and obese patients with type 2 diabetes mellitus. *BMJ Open Diabetes Res Care*. 2014;2. e000013.
58. Martin CK, Anton SD, Walden H, Arnett C, Greenway FL, Williamson DA. Slower eating rate reduces the food intake of men, but not women: implications for behavioral weight control. *Behav Res Ther.* 2007;45:2349–2359.
59. Flechtner-Mors M, Ditschuneit HH, Johnson TD, Suchard MA, Adler G. Metabolic and weight loss effects of long-term dietary intervention in obese patients: four-year results. *Obes Res.* 2000;8:399–402.
60. Burke LE, Wang J, Sevick MA. Self-monitoring in weight loss: a systematic review of the literature. *J Am Diet Assoc.* 2011;111:92–102.
61. Burke LE, Conroy MB, Sereika SM, et al. The effect of electronic self-monitoring on weight loss and dietary intake: a randomized behavioral weight loss trial. *Obesity.* 2011;19:338–344.
62. Carter MC, Burley VJ, Nykjaer C, Cade JE. Adherence to a smartphone application for weight loss compared to website and paper diary: pilot randomized controlled trial. *J Med Internet Res*. 2013; 15:e32.
63. Anton SD, LeBlanc E, Allen HR, et al. Use of a computerized tracking system to monitor and provide feedback on dietary goals for calorie-restricted diets: the POUNDS LOST study. *J Diabetes Sci Technol*. 2012;6:1216–1225.
64. Turner-McGrievy GM, Beets MW, Moore JB, Kaczynski AT, Barr-Anderson DJ, Tate DF. Comparison of traditional versus mobile app self-monitoring of physical activity and dietary intake among overweight adults participating in an mHealth weight loss program. *J Am Med Inf Assoc*. 2013;20:513–518.
65. Rivera J, McPherson A, Hamilton J, et al. Mobile apps for weight management: a scoping review. *JMIR Mhealth Uhealth*. 2016;4:e87.
66. Martin CK, Gilmore LA, Apolzan JW, Myers CA, Thomas DM, Redman LM. Smartloss: a personalized mobile health intervention for weight management and health promotion. *JMIR Mhealth Uhealth*. 2016;4:e18.
67. Cheatham SW, Stull KR, Fantigrassi M, Motel I. The efficacy of wearable activity tracking technology as part of a weight loss program: a systematic review. *J Sports Med Phys Fit*. 2018;58:534–548.
68. Hutchesson MJ, Rollo ME, Krukowski R, et al. eHealth interventions for the prevention and treatment of overweight and obesity in adults: a systematic review with meta-analysis. *Obes Rev.* 2015;16:376–392.
69. Hughes JW, Goldstein CM, Logan C, et al. Controlled testing of novel portion control plate produces smaller self-selected portion sizes compared to regular dinner plate. *BMC Obes*. 2017;4:30.
70. Pedersen SD, Kang J, Kline GA. Portion control plate for weight loss in obese patients with type 2 diabetes mellitus: a controlled clinical trial. *Arch Intern Med*. 2007;167:1277–1283.
71. Ryan DH, Parkin CG, Longley W, Dixon J, Apovian C, Bode B. Efficacy and safety of an oral device to reduce food intake and promote weight loss. *Obes Sci Pract*. 2018;4:52–61.
72. von SP, Sander FM, Lanzendorf L, et al. Persistent weight loss with a non-invasive novel medical device to change eating behaviour in obese individuals with high-risk cardiovascular risk profile. *PLoS One*. 2017;12. e0174528.
73. Ravussin E. Metabolic differences and the development of obesity. *Metabolism*. 1995;44:12–14.
74. Levin BE. The drive to regain is mainly in the brain. *Am J Physiol Regul Integr Comp Physiol*. 2004;287:R1297–R1300.
75. MacLean PS, Higgins JA, Jackman MR, et al. Peripheral metabolic responses to prolonged weight reduction that promote rapid, efficient regain in obesity-prone rats. *Am J Physiol Regul Integr Comp Physiol*. 2006;290:R1577–R1588.
76. McEvedy SM, Sullivan-Mort G, McLean SA, Pascoe MC, Paxton SJ. Ineffectiveness of commercial weight-loss programs for achieving modest but meaningful weight loss: systematic review and meta-analysis. *J Health Psychol*. 2017;22:1614–1627.
77. Elfhag K, Rossner S. Who succeeds in maintaining weight loss? A conceptual review of factors associated with weight loss maintenance and weight regain. *Obes Rev.* 2005;6:67–85.
78. Jeffery RW, French SA, Schmid TL. Attributions for dietary failures: problems reported by participants in the Hypertension Prevention Trial. *Health Psychol*. 1990;9:315–329.
79. Catenacci VA, Odgen L, Phelan S, et al. Dietary habits and weight maintenance success in high versus low exercisers in the National Weight Control Registry. *J Phys Activ Health*. 2014;11: 1540–1548.
80. Wyatt HR, Grunwald GK, Mosca CL, Klem ML, Wing RR, Hill JO. Long-term weight loss and breakfast in subjects in the National Weight Control Registry. *Obes Res*. 2002;10:78–82.
81. Catenacci VA, Ogden LG, Stuht J, et al. Physical activity patterns in the National Weight Control Registry. *Obesity.* 2008;16:153–161.
82. Jakicic JM, Clark K, Coleman E, et al. American College of Sports Medicine position stand. Appropriate intervention strategies for weight loss and prevention of weight regain for adults. *Med Sci Sports Exerc*. 2001;33:2145–2156.
83. Donnelly JE, Blair SN, Jakicic JM, Manore MM, Rankin JW, Smith BK. American College of Sports Medicine Position Stand. Appropriate physical activity intervention strategies for weight loss and prevention of weight regain for adults. *Med Sci Sports Exerc*. 2009;41:459–471.
84. Schoeller DA, Shay K, Kushner RF. How much physical activity is needed to minimize weight gain in previously obese women? *Am J Clin Nutr.* 1997;66:551–556.
85. Burt DG, Lamb K, Nicholas C, Twist C. Effects of exercise-induced muscle damage on resting metabolic rate, sub-maximal running and post-exercise oxygen consumption. *Eur J Sport Sci*. 2014;14: 337–344.
86. Moghetti P, Bacchi E, Brangani C, Dona S, Negri C. Metabolic effects of exercise. *Front Horm Res*. 2016;47:44–57.
87. Petridou A, Siopi A, Mougios V. Exercise in the management of obesity. *Metabolism*. 2019;92:163–169.
88. Hunter GR, Byrne NM, Sirikul B, et al. Resistance training conserves fat-free mass and resting energy expenditure following weight loss. *Obesity.* 2008;16:1045–1051.
89. Borg P, Kukkonen-Harjula K, Fogelholm M, Pasanen M. Effects of walking or resistance training on weight loss maintenance in

obese, middle-aged men: a randomized trial. *Int J Obes Relat Metab Disord*. 2002;26:676–683.
90. Flegal KM, Carroll MD, Ogden CL, Curtin LR. Prevalence and trends in obesity among US adults, 1999–2008. *J Am Med Assoc*. 2010;303:235–241.
91. Ford ES, Giles WH, Dietz WH. Prevalence of the metabolic syndrome among US adults: findings from the third National Health and Nutrition Examination Survey. *J Am Med Assoc*. 2002;287: 356–359.
92. Sundquist J, Winkleby MA, Pudaric S. Cardiovascular disease risk factors among older black, Mexican-American, and white women and men: an analysis of NHANES III, 1988–1994. Third National Health and Nutrition Examination Survey. *J Am Geriatr Soc*. 2001; 49:109–116.
93. Calvani R, Joseph AM, Adhihetty PJ, et al. Mitochondrial pathways in sarcopenia of aging and disuse muscle atrophy. *Biol Chem*. 2013;394:393–414.
94. Lee JJ, Pedley A, Hoffmann U, Massaro JM, Fox CS. Association of Changes in Abdominal Fat Quantity and Quality With Incident Cardiovascular Disease Risk Factors. *J Am Coll Cardiol*. 2016;68: 1509–1521.
95. Lovejoy JC, Champagne CM, de JL, Xie H, Smith SR. Increased visceral fat and decreased energy expenditure during the menopausal transition. *Int J Obes*. 2008;32:949–958.
96. Wajchenberg BL. Subcutaneous and visceral adipose tissue: their relation to the metabolic syndrome. *Endocr Rev*. 2000;21:697–738.
97. Chen H, Guo X. Obesity and functional disability in elderly Americans. *J Am Geriatr Soc*. 2008;56:689–694.
98. Reddy KS, Chandala SR. A comparative study of lipid profile and oestradiol in pre- and post-menopausal women. *J Clin Diagn Res*. 2013;7:1596–1598.
99. Caspersen CJ, Thomas GD, Boseman LA, Beckles GL, Albright AL. Aging, diabetes, and the public health system in the United States. *Am J Publ Health*. 2012;102:1482–1497.
100. Boyle JP, Thompson TJ, Gregg EW, Barker LE, Williamson DF. Projection of the year 2050 burden of diabetes in the US adult population: dynamic modeling of incidence, mortality, and prediabetes prevalence. *Popul Health Metrics*. 2010;8:29.
101. de R N, Volpato S. Physical function and disability in older adults with diabetes. *Clin Geriatr Med*. 2015;31:51–65. viii.
102. Gregg EW, Beckles GL, Williamson DF, et al. Diabetes and physical disability among older U.S. adults. *Diabetes Care*. 2000;23:1272–1277.
103. Park SW, Goodpaster BH, Strotmeyer ES, et al. Decreased muscle strength and quality in older adults with type 2 diabetes: the health, aging, and body composition study. *Diabetes*. 2006;55: 1813–1818.
104. Volpato S, Blaum C, Resnick H, Ferrucci L, Fried LP, Guralnik JM. Comorbidities and impairments explaining the association between diabetes and lower extremity disability: the Women's Health and Aging Study. *Diabetes Care*. 2002;25:678–683.
105. Goisser S, Kemmler W, Porzel S, et al. Sarcopenic obesity and complex interventions with nutrition and exercise in community-dwelling older persons–a narrative review. *Clin Interv Aging*. 2015;10:1267–1282.
106. Mankowski RT, Aubertin-Leheudre M, Beavers DP, et al. Sedentary time is associated with the metabolic syndrome in older adults with mobility limitations–The LIFE Study. *Exp Gerontol*. 2015;70:32–36.
107. Mankowski RT, Anton SD, Axtell R, et al. Device-measured physical activity as a predictor of disability in mobility-limited older adults. *J Am Geriatr Soc*. 2017;65:2251–2256.
108. Mokdad AH, Ballestros K, Echko M, et al. The state of US health, 1990–2016: burden of diseases, injuries, and risk factors among US states. *J Am Med Assoc*. 2018;319:1444–1472.
109. Torres SJ, Nowson CA. Relationship between stress, eating behavior, and obesity. *Nutr*. 2007;23:887–894.
110. Stults-Kolehmainen MA, Sinha R. The effects of stress on physical activity and exercise. *Sports Med*. 2014;44:81–121.
111. Sominsky L, Spencer SJ. Eating behavior and stress: a pathway to obesity. *Front Psychol*. 2014;5:434.
112. Yau YH, Potenza MN. Stress and eating behaviors. *Minerva Endocrinol*. 2013;38:255–267.
113. Richardson AS, Arsenault JE, Cates SC, Muth MK. Perceived stress, unhealthy eating behaviors, and severe obesity in low-income women. *Nutr J*. 2015;14:122.
114. Chao AM, Jastreboff AM, White MA, Grilo CM, Sinha R. Stress, cortisol, and other appetite-related hormones: prospective prediction of 6-month changes in food cravings and weight. *Obesity*. 2017;25:713–720.
115. Christaki E, Kokkinos A, Costarelli V, Alexopoulos EC, Chrousos GP, Darviri C. Stress management can facilitate weight loss in Greek overweight and obese women: a pilot study. *J Hum Nutr Diet*. 2013;26(Suppl 1):132–139.
116. Xenaki N, Bacopoulou F, Kokkinos A, Nicolaides NC, Chrousos GP, Darviri C. Impact of a stress management program on weight loss, mental health and lifestyle in adults with obesity: a randomized controlled trial. *J Mol Biochem*. 2018;7:78–84.
117. Ogilvie RP, Patel SR. The epidemiology of sleep and obesity. *Sleep Health*. 2017;3:383–388.
118. Patel SR, Hu FB. Short sleep duration and weight gain: a systematic review. *Obesity*. 2008;16:643–653.
119. Yannakoulia M, Anastasiou CA, Karfopoulou E, Pehlivanidis A, Panagiotakos DB, Vgontzas A. Sleep quality is associated with weight loss maintenance status: the MedWeight study. *Sleep Med*. 2017;34:242–245.
120. Taheri S. The link between short sleep duration and obesity: we should recommend more sleep to prevent obesity. *Arch Dis Child*. 2006;91:881–884.
121. Srivastava G, Apovian CM. Current pharmacotherapy for obesity. *Nat Rev Endocrinol*. 2018;14:12–24.
122. Van GL, Dirinck E. Pharmacological approaches in the treatment and maintenance of weight loss. *Diabetes Care*. 2016;39(Suppl 2): S260–S267.
123. Yanovski SZ, Yanovski JA. Long-term drug treatment for obesity: a systematic and clinical review. *J Am Med Assoc*. 2014;311:74–86.
124. Freedman MR, King J, Kennedy E. Popular diets: a scientific review. *Obes Res*. 2001;9(Suppl 1):1S–40S.
125. Jequier E, Bray GA. Low-fat diets are preferred. *Am J Med*. 2002; 113(Suppl 9B):41S–46S.
126. Willett WC, Leibel RL. Dietary fat is not a major determinant of body fat. *Am J Med*. 2002;113(Suppl 9B):47S–59S.
127. Brehm BJ, Seeley RJ, Daniels SR, D'Alessio DA. A randomized trial comparing a very low carbohydrate diet and a calorie-restricted low fat diet on body weight and cardiovascular risk factors in healthy women. *J Clin Endocrinol Metab*. 2003;88:1617–1623.
128. Due A, Toubro S, Skov AR, Astrup A. Effect of normal-fat diets, either medium or high in protein, on body weight in overweight subjects: a randomised 1-year trial. *Int J Obes Relat Metab Disord*. 2004;28:1283–1290.
129. Foster GD, Wyatt HR, Hill JO, et al. A randomized trial of a low-carbohydrate diet for obesity. *N Engl J Med*. 2003;348:2082–2090.
130. Gardner CD, Kiazand A, Alhassan S, et al. Comparison of the Atkins, Zone, Ornish, and LEARN diets for change in weight and related risk factors among overweight premenopausal women: the A TO Z Weight Loss Study: a randomized trial. *J Am Med Assoc*. 2007;297:969–977.
131. Skov AR, Toubro S, Ronn B, Holm L, Astrup A. Randomized trial on protein vs carbohydrate in ad libitum fat reduced diet for the treatment of obesity. *Int J Obes Relat Metab Disord*. 1999;23:528–536.
132. Yancy Jr WS, Olsen MK, Guyton JR, Bakst RP, Westman EC. A low-carbohydrate, ketogenic diet versus a low-fat diet to treat

obesity and hyperlipidemia: a randomized, controlled trial. *Ann Intern Med*. 2004;140:769–777.

133. Barnard ND, Cohen J, Jenkins DJ, et al. A low-fat vegan diet improves glycemic control and cardiovascular risk factors in a randomized clinical trial in individuals with type 2 diabetes. *Diabetes Care*. 2006;29:1777–1783.
134. Ornish D, Scherwitz LW, Billings JH, et al. Intensive lifestyle changes for reversal of coronary heart disease. *J Am Med Assoc*. 1998;280:2001–2007.
135. Toubro S, Astrup A. Randomised comparison of diets for maintaining obese subjects' weight after major weight loss: ad lib, low fat, high carbohydrate diet v fixed energy intake. *BMJ*. 1997;314:29–34.
136. McManus K, Antinoro L, Sacks F. A randomized controlled trial of a moderate-fat, low-energy diet compared with a low fat, low-energy diet for weight loss in overweight adults. *Int J Obes Relat Metab Disord*. 2001;25:1503–1511.
137. Shai I, Schwarzfuchs D, Henkin Y, et al. Weight loss with a low-carbohydrate, Mediterranean, or low-fat diet. *N Engl J Med*. 2008;359:229–241.
138. Sacks FM, Bray GA, Carey VJ, et al. Comparison of weight-loss diets with different compositions of fat, protein, and carbohydrates. *N Engl J Med*. 2009;360:859–873.
139. Williamson DA, Anton SD, Han H, et al. Adherence is a multi-dimensional construct in the POUNDS LOST trial. *J Behav Med*. 2010;33:35–46.
140. Johnston BC, Kanters S, Bandayrel K, et al. Comparison of weight loss among named diet programs in overweight and obese adults: a meta-analysis. *J Am Med Assoc*. 2014;312:923–933.
141. Anton SD, Hida A, Heekin K, et al. Effects of popular diets without specific calorie targets on weight loss outcomes: systematic review of findings from clinical trials. *Nutrients*. 2017;9.
142. Hall KD, Guo J. Obesity energetics: body weight regulation and the effects of diet composition. *Gastroenterology*. 2017;152:1718–1727.
143. Baumgartner RN. Body composition in healthy aging. *Ann N Y Acad Sci*. 2000;904:437–448.
144. Jurca R, Lamonte MJ, Church TS, et al. Associations of muscle strength and fitness with metabolic syndrome in men. *Med Sci Sports Exerc*. 2004;36:1301–1307.
145. Stephen WC, Janssen I. Sarcopenic-obesity and cardiovascular disease risk in the elderly. *J Nutr Health Aging*. 2009;13:460–466.
146. Bouchard DR, Heroux M, Janssen I. Association between muscle mass, leg strength, and fat mass with physical function in older adults: influence of age and sex. *J Aging Health*. 2011;23: 313–328.
147. Sayer AA, Dennison EM, Syddall HE, Gilbody HJ, Phillips DI, Cooper C. Type 2 diabetes, muscle strength, and impaired physical function: the tip of the iceberg? *Diabetes Care*. 2005;28: 2541–2542.
148. Blondin DP, Labbe SM, Phoenix S, et al. Contributions of white and brown adipose tissues and skeletal muscles to acute cold-induced metabolic responses in healthy men. *J Physiol*. 2015;593: 701–714.
149. Delmonico MJ, Harris TB, Visser M, et al. Longitudinal study of muscle strength, quality, and adipose tissue infiltration. *Am J Clin Nutr*. 2009;90:1579–1585.
150. Tuttle LJ, Sinacore DR, Mueller MJ. Intermuscular adipose tissue is muscle specific and associated with poor functional performance. *J Aging Res*. 2012;2012, 172957.
151. Barbat-Artigas S, Pion CH, Leduc-Gaudet JP, Rolland Y, Aubertin-Leheudre M. Exploring the role of muscle mass, obesity, and age in the relationship between muscle quality and physical function. *J Am Med Dir Assoc*. 2014;15:303–320.
152. Koster A, Ding J, Stenholm S, et al. Does the amount of fat mass predict age-related loss of lean mass, muscle strength, and muscle quality in older adults? *J Gerontol A Biol Sci Med Sci*. 2011;66: 888–895.
153. Barbat-Artigas S, Dupontgand S, Pion CH, Feiter-Murphy Y, Aubertin-Leheudre M. Identifying recreational physical activities associated with muscle quality in men and women aged 50 years and over. *J Cachexia Sarcopenia Muscle*. 2014;5:221–228.
154. Vieira DC, Tibana RA, Tajra V, et al. Decreased functional capacity and muscle strength in elderly women with metabolic syndrome. *Clin Interv Aging*. 2013;8:1377–1386.
155. Newgard CB, Pessin JE. Recent progress in metabolic signaling pathways regulating aging and life span. *J Gerontol A Biol Sci Med Sci*. 2014;69(Suppl 1):S21–S27.
156. Engin AB. What is lipotoxicity? *Adv Exp Med Biol*. 2017;960: 197–220.
157. Slawik M, Vidal-Puig AJ. Lipotoxicity, overnutrition and energy metabolism in aging. *Ageing Res Rev*. 2006;5:144–164.
158. Finkel T. The metabolic regulation of aging. *Nat Med*. 2015;21: 1416–1423.
159. Harridge SDR, Young A. *Skeletal Muscle 3. Principles and Practices of Geriatric Medicine*. London: Wiley; 1998:898–905.
160. Baumgartner RN, Stauber PM, McHugh D, Koehler KM, Garry PJ. Cross-sectional age differences in body composition in persons 60+ years of age. *J Gerontol A Biol Sci Med Sci*. 1995;50: M307–M316.
161. Forbes GB. Longitudinal changes in adult fat-free mass: influence of body weight. *Am J Clin Nutr*. 1999;70:1025–1031.
162. Blaum CS, Xue QL, Michelon E, Semba RD, Fried LP. The association between obesity and the frailty syndrome in older women: the Women's Health and Aging Studies. *J Am Geriatr Soc*. 2005;53: 927–934.
163. Cesari M, Kritchevsky SB, Baumgartner RN, et al. Sarcopenia, obesity, and inflammation–results from the trial of Angiotensin converting enzyme inhibition and novel cardiovascular risk factors study. *Am J Clin Nutr*. 2005;82:428–434.
164. Anton SD, Hida A, Mankowski R, et al. Nutrition and exercise in sarcopenia. *Curr Protein Pept Sci*. 2018;19:649–667.
165. Waters DL, Ward AL, Villareal DT. Weight loss in obese adults 65 years and older: a review of the controversy. *Exp Gerontol*. 2013;48: 1054–1061.
166. Houston DK, Nicklas BJ, Zizza CA. Weighty concerns: the growing prevalence of obesity among older adults. *J Am Diet Assoc*. 2009;109:1886–1895.
167. Miller SL, Wolfe RR. The danger of weight loss in the elderly. *J Nutr Health Aging*. 2008;12:487–491.
168. Stiegler P, Cunliffe A. The role of diet and exercise for the maintenance of fat-free mass and resting metabolic rate during weight loss. *Sports Med*. 2006;36:239–262.
169. Frimel TN, Sinacore DR, Villareal DT. Exercise attenuates the weight-loss-induced reduction in muscle mass in frail obese older adults. *Med Sci Sports Exerc*. 2008;40:1213–1219.
170. Villareal DT, Banks M, Sinacore DR, Siener C, Klein S. Effect of weight loss and exercise on frailty in obese older adults. *Arch Intern Med*. 2006;166:860–866.
171. Shea MK, Houston DK, Nicklas BJ, et al. The effect of randomization to weight loss on total mortality in older overweight and obese adults: the ADAPT Study. *J Gerontol A Biol Sci Med Sci*. 2010;65:519–525.
172. Dengo AL, Dennis EA, Orr JS, et al. Arterial destiffening with weight loss in overweight and obese middle-aged and older adults. *Hypertension*. 2010;55:855–861.
173. Chomentowski P, Dube JJ, Amati F, et al. Moderate exercise attenuates the loss of skeletal muscle mass that occurs with intentional caloric restriction-induced weight loss in older, overweight to obese adults. *J Gerontol A Biol Sci Med Sci*. 2009; 64:575–580.

174. Vincent HK, Vincent KR, Lamb KM. Obesity and mobility disability in the older adult. *Obes Rev.* 2010;11:568–579.
175. Landi F, Onder G, Carpenter I, Cesari M, Soldato M, Bernabei R. Physical activity prevented functional decline among frail community-living elderly subjects in an international observational study. *J Clin Epidemiol.* 2007;60:518–524.
176. Hardy SE, Perera S, Roumani YF, Chandler JM, Studenski SA. Improvement in usual gait speed predicts better survival in older adults. *J Am Geriatr Soc.* 2007;55:1727–1734.
177. Purser JL, Weinberger M, Cohen HJ, et al. Walking speed predicts health status and hospital costs for frail elderly male veterans. *J Rehabil Res Dev.* 2005;42:535–546.
178. Morey MC, Snyder DC, Sloane R, et al. Effects of home-based diet and exercise on functional outcomes among older, overweight long-term cancer survivors: RENEW: a randomized controlled trial. *J Am Med Assoc.* 2009;301:1883–1891.
179. Shah K, Stufflebam A, Hilton TN, Sinacore DR, Klein S, Villareal DT. Diet and exercise interventions reduce intrahepatic fat content and improve insulin sensitivity in obese older adults. *Obesity.* 2009;17:2162–2168.
180. Avila JJ, Gutierres JA, Sheehy ME, Lofgren IE, Delmonico MJ. Effect of moderate intensity resistance training during weight loss on body composition and physical performance in overweight older adults. *Eur J Appl Physiol.* 2010;109:517–525.
181. Manini TM, Buford TW, Lott DJ, et al. Effect of dietary restriction and exercise on lower extremity tissue compartments in obese, older women: a pilot study. *J Gerontol A Biol Sci Med Sci.* 2014; 69:101–108.
182. Gorissen SH, Horstman AM, Franssen R, et al. Ingestion of wheat protein increases in vivo muscle protein synthesis rates in healthy older men in a randomized trial. *J Nutr.* 2016;146:1651–1659.
183. Paddon-Jones D, Leidy H. Dietary protein and muscle in older persons. *Curr Opin Clin Nutr Metab Care.* 2014;17:5–11.
184. Verreijen AM, Engberink MF, Memelink RG, van der Plas SE, Visser M, Weijs PJ. Effect of a high protein diet and/or resistance exercise on the preservation of fat free mass during weight loss in overweight and obese older adults: a randomized controlled trial. *Nutr J.* 2017;16:10.
185. Hollands GJ, Shemilt I, Marteau TM, et al. Portion, package or tableware size for changing selection and consumption of food, alcohol and tobacco. *Cochrane Database Syst Rev.* 2015. CD011045.
186. Trepanowski JF, Kroeger CM, Barnosky A, et al. Effect of alternate-day fasting on weight loss, weight maintenance, and cardioprotection among metabolically healthy obese adults: a randomized clinical trial. *JAMA Intern Med.* 2017;177:930–938.
187. Middleton KR, Anton SD, Perri MG. Long-term adherence to health behavior change. *Am J Lifestyle Med.* 2013;7:395–404.
188. Golzarand M, Toolabi K, Farid R. The bariatric surgery and weight losing: a meta-analysis in the long- and very long-term effects of laparoscopic adjustable gastric banding, laparoscopic Roux-en-Y gastric bypass and laparoscopic sleeve gastrectomy on weight loss in adults. *Surg Endosc.* 2017;31:4331–4345.
189. Pi-Sunyer X. The look AHEAD trial: a review and discussion of its outcomes. *Curr Nutr Rep.* 2014;3:387–391.
190. Coughlin JW, Brantley PJ, Champagne CM, et al. The impact of continued intervention on weight: five-year results from the weight loss maintenance trial. *Obesity.* 2016;24:1046–1053.
191. Middleton KM, Patidar SM, Perri MG. The impact of extended care on the long-term maintenance of weight loss: a systematic review and meta-analysis. *Obes Rev.* 2012;13:509–517.
192. Perri MG, Limacher MC, Durning PE, et al. Extended-care programs for weight management in rural communities: the treatment of obesity in underserved rural settings (TOURS) randomized trial. *Arch Intern Med.* 2008;168:2347–2354.
193. Witkiewitz K, Marlatt GA. Emphasis on interpersonal factors in a dynamic model of relapse. *Am Psychol.* 2005;60:341–342.
194. Perri MG, Nezu AM, McKelvey WF, Shermer RL, Renjilian DA, Viegener BJ. Relapse prevention training and problem-solving therapy in the long-term management of obesity. *J Consult Clin Psychol.* 2001;69:722–726.
195. Baum JG, Clark HB, Sandler J. Preventing relapse in obesity through posttreatment maintenance systems: comparing the relative efficacy of two levels of therapist support. *J Behav Med.* 1991; 14:287–302.
196. Jakicic JM, Winters C, Lang W, Wing RR. Effects of intermittent exercise and use of home exercise equipment on adherence, weight loss, and fitness in overweight women: a randomized trial. *J Am Med Assoc.* 1999;282:1554–1560.
197. Perri MG, Martin AD, Leermakers EA, Sears SF, Notelovitz M. Effects of group- versus home-based exercise in the treatment of obesity. *J Consult Clin Psychol.* 1997;65:278–285.
198. Perri MG, Sears Jr SF, Clark JE. Strategies for improving maintenance of weight loss. Toward a continuous care model of obesity management. *Diabetes Care.* 1993;16:200–209.
199. Perri MG, McAllister DA, Gange JJ, Jordan RC, McAdoo G, Nezu AM. Effects of four maintenance programs on the long-term management of obesity. *J Consult Clin Psychol.* 1988;56: 529–534.
200. Cook W. The effect of personalised weight feedback on weight loss and health behaviours: evidence from a regression discontinuity design. *Health Econ.* 2019;28:161–172.
201. Sherrington A, Newham JJ, Bell R, Adamson A, McColl E, Araujo-Soares V. Systematic review and meta-analysis of internet-delivered interventions providing personalized feedback for weight loss in overweight and obese adults. *Obes Rev.* 2016;17:541–551.
202. Kelley CP, Sbrocco G, Sbrocco T. Behavioral modification for the management of obesity. *Prim Care.* 2016;43:159–175. x.
203. Foreyt JP, Poston WS. What is the role of cognitive-behavior therapy in patient management? *Obes Res.* 1998;6(Suppl 1):18S–22S.
204. Murawski ME, Milsom VA, Ross KM, et al. Problem solving, treatment adherence, and weight-loss outcome among women participating in lifestyle treatment for obesity. *Eat Behav.* 2009;10: 146–151.
205. Framson C, Kristal AR, Schenk JM, Littman AJ, Zeliadt S, Benitez D. Development and validation of the mindful eating questionnaire. *J Am Diet Assoc.* 2009;109:1439–1444.
206. Hollis JH. The effect of mastication on food intake, satiety and body weight. *Physiol Behav.* 2018;193:242–245.
207. Hurst Y, Fukuda H. Effects of changes in eating speed on obesity in patients with diabetes: a secondary analysis of longitudinal health check-up data. *BMJ Open.* 2018;8. e019589.
208. Shah M, Copeland J, Dart L, Adams-Huet B, James A, Rhea D. Slower eating speed lowers energy intake in normal-weight but not overweight/obese subjects. *J Acad Nutr Diet.* 2014;114: 393–402.

CHAPTER

10

TASTE, COST, CONVENIENCE, AND FOOD CHOICES

Adam Drewnowski[1], *PhD*
Pablo Monsivais[2], *PhD, MPH*

[1]**Center for Public Health Nutrition, University of Washington, Seattle, WA, United States**
[2]**Department of Nutrition and Exercise Physiology, Elson S. Floyd College of Medicine, Washington State University, Spokane, WA, United States**

SUMMARY

Food choices are complex decisions that are largely guided not only by perceptions of taste, cost, and convenience but also by consumer concerns about health, safety, and increasingly, the environment. The concept of taste refers to taste, aroma, texture, and the pleasure response to foods. The cost component covers food prices and the relative affordability of alternative food patterns. Convenience refers to ease of physical access to food sources and to the time spent buying and preparing food. The healthfulness of foods has been measured using nutrient density metrics. The environmental cost of food production is increasingly cited as a potential driver of future food choices and a predictor of future diets. While taste is an important driver of food choices, it is not the only one. The current emphasis in public health nutrition is on sustainable food systems and on the adequacy, quality, and, above all, affordability of the global food supply. All too often, good-tasting empty calories are cheap, whereas nutrient-rich foods are more expensive. Public health programs to improve nutrient density of population diets ought to consider taste, cost, and convenience among the key drivers of food choice and food consumption patterns.

Keywords: Affordability; Convenience; Cost; Food choice decisions; Food patterns; Food systems; Health; Nutrient density; Nutrient profiling; Taste; Variety.

I. OVERVIEW

The principal drivers of consumer food choice are taste, cost, and convenience. Each of these domains has its own interdisciplinary research tools, metrics, and measures. Sensory aspects of food and its reward value are covered by the psychology of taste and smell and the neurobiology of the brain processes of reward. The relations between food prices, diet quality, and diet cost are covered by consumer economics. Affordability is given by food costs in relation to household incomes. Convenience has been defined as the ease of interactions between the consumer and the food environment. Though physical aspects of the food environment such as food deserts were once given research priority, the food environment has even more important economic and policy components. The relation between energy intakes, diet quality, and health outcomes across populations has been the topic of multiple studies in nutritional epidemiology. The study of food patterns and their variety draws on studies in ethnography, sociology, and anthropology. Finally, measuring the environmental impact of alternative food patterns requires additional input from geography, agricultural modeling, and studies on climate change. Nutrition has become much more interdisciplinary in recent years. Effectively, present knowledge in nutrition is being transformed into present interdisciplinary knowledge in food systems, nutrition, and health.

Present Knowledge in Nutrition, Volume 2
https://doi.org/10.1016/B978-0-12-818460-8.00010-1

II. INTRODUCTION

The current goal of public health nutrition is to promote the consumption of healthy diet from sustainable food systems. Consumers are advised to seek out foods that are healthy, affordable, appealing, and environmentally friendly.[1–3] The four principal domains of sustainable diets, as defined by the Food and Agriculture Organization of the United Nations,[2] were health, economics, society, and the environment. Reports now define sustainable food systems as those that produce nutrient-rich foods that are affordable, socially and culturally acceptable, and sparing of both natural and human resources.[4] Yet, taste, cost, and convenience remain the primary drivers of food choices and therefore have implications for the sustainability of food systems.

There are few foods (and few diets) that are simultaneously nutrient rich, affordable, acceptable, and planet friendly. Paradoxes abound. In general, energy-dense processed foods based on refined grains, sugars, and fats are highly palatable,[5] yet excessive consumption of these foods of minimal nutritional value is at the root of the global obesity epidemic.[6–8] However, these processed foods also tend to be affordable[9–11] and widely accessible,[12,13] and their production is associated with relatively low production of climate-changing greenhouse gasses.[14] Conversely, many nutrient-rich foods have larger climate impacts,[14] including sources of high-quality protein, an essential nutrient for development and growth, cost more per calorie,[15,16] and can have lower palatability[17] and lower reward value.[18]

Herein lies the paradox: foods that are good-tasting, inexpensive, and convenient have been associated with adverse health outcomes. Conversely, foods that are healthier and more nutrient-rich may not offer the same reward value, can be more expensive, and are not always available in neighborhoods with limited purchasing power. Taste, cost, and convenience are closely tied to the quality of food patterns and the likely health outcomes.

Proposed nutrition interventions in public health uniformly stress the need to improve the quality of the population diet. Yet many of the interventions to reduce sugar intakes, promote the consumption of fresh produce, limit access to fast foods, or put taxes on snacks or ultraprocessed foods tend to ignore the importance of taste, cost, and convenience in shaping food choices. By contrast, consumers often cite these three factors ahead of nutrition as the most important influences on their food choices.[19]

A. Background

Taste refers to the physiologic sensations of taste, aroma, and texture[1] and to the sensory pleasure response to foods.[5,20] Although sweet taste responsiveness (or lack of it) has been linked to obesity risk in past studies, the reality is that taste responses are highly variable and not necessarily closely tied to body weight. Furthermore, sweet taste responsiveness is only one of the several factors driving food choice, alongside myriad other economic, social, and cultural variables. The underlying assumption that food-seeking behaviors and therefore energy intakes were driven by individual taste alone was never tenable: other factors need to be taken into account.

There are multiple steps between a person's taste responses, their food choices,[5,20] and the risk of diet-related noncommunicable disease (NCD). First, very few studies have examined taste responses, food preferences, and nutrient intakes in the same subject population. No direct association between taste function and health outcomes can be made, and in the absence of longitudinal data, no causal pathways can be drawn. Second, population eating habits are influenced by age, gender, and energy needs, as well as by demographic and socioeconomic factors, making it difficult to link taste-related variables with particular health outcomes.

B. Key Issues

The factors that influence taste responses and food preferences operate at multiple levels. The conventional position taken by researchers in physiology and pharmacology is that dietary sugars and fats unleash pleasure, lead to drastic changes in food intake, and are comparable in every way to drugs of abuse.[18] The position taken by economic determinism is that sugar and fat influence food intake primarily through their widespread availability and very low cost. There can be little doubt that the global obesity epidemic owes much to the palatability, convenience, and low cost of energy-dense foods.[5,9,21,22] Examining the physiological, economic, and social determinants of food choices in relation to potential health outcomes is the topic of this review.

III. TASTE, PALATABILITY, AND SATIETY

A. Measuring Human Taste

The five primary tastes are sweet, sour, salty, bitter, and umami. Typical tastants are sucrose (sweet), hydrochloric acid (sour), sodium chloride (salty), caffeine or quinine (bitter), and monosodium glutamate (MSG) (umami). When dissolved in water, these substances stimulate the taste response, which can be measured through taste acuity, taste perception, or taste preference.

Taste acuity is measured using detection and recognition thresholds for the lowest detectable amounts. Taste perception is based on the scaling of perceived intensity of more concentrated (i.e., suprathreshold) taste stimuli.[23,24] Studies on taste and food choice also examined intensity scaling of suprathreshold solutions. Among the methods used for intensity scaling have been 9-point category scales, visual analog scales, the labeled magnitude estimation scale, magnitude estimation, and other ratio scales.[25,26] Intensity ratings often have used a logarithmic scale, since taste, like other sensory systems, has sensitivity to stimulus concentrations that span several orders of magnitude. Early studies on the genetics of bitter taste involved stimuli based on the thiourea-containing compounds propylthiocarbamide and 6-n-propylthiouracil (PROP), which taste extremely bitter to some people but not to others.[27,28]

Most behavioral research on the impact of taste on food choices has been on the detection and perception of sweet, sour, salty, bitter, and umami. However, when it came to food choices, neither taste acuity nor taste scaling predicted individual likes or dislikes for the tasted substance. In general, humans like sweet and dislike sour, salty, and bitter tastes; however, a great deal of individual variability has been observed.[29,30] Sensory preferences for sweet, sour, salty, or bitter solutions (or foods) have typically used a 9-point hedonic preference scale that ranged from dislike extremely to like extremely with a neutral point at 5 (neither like nor dislike). However, hedonic preferences for a given taste had limited predictive value. Preferences for sugar solutions in water were linked to preferences for sugar sweetened beverages, but not necessarily for other sweet foods.[31,32]

B. Sweet, Bitter, Sour, Salty, and Umami

Taste responses are critical for survival. Sweetness signals food energy, and at least for naturally sweet foods such as ripe fruits, it also signals the presence of nutrients. Children equate palatability with sweetness and selectively consume the sweetest and the most energy-dense foods.[33] For children, sweetness is one of the most salient attributes of a food or beverage. Indeed young children categorized foods according to whether they were familiar or sweet.[33] Sweet foods and beverages are universally liked across all cultures and by all age groups.[5,20] By contrast, bitterness signals dietary danger,[34] which is why bitter-tasting vegetables and fruits are often rejected by children and by pregnant women. The savory umami taste, elicited by glutamate salts, may signal the protein content of foods. The underlying taste receptor mechanisms have been broadly grouped into those that function as ion channels (salty and sour) and those that function via G-protein–coupled pathways (sweet, bitter, and umami).

Hedonic responses to sweetness depend on age. While children aged 3–5 years typically show a monotonic rise in hedonic ratings with increasing sweetness, taste preferences for intense sweetness decline during adolescence, coinciding with maturation and the cessation of growth.[35,36] For most adults, 7%–10% of sugar in water is the ideal sweetness level or "breakpoint," corresponding precisely to the amount of sugar in most sugar-sweetened beverages.[37,38]

The notion that food choices of persons with obesity are driven by abnormal sensory or hedonic preferences for sweet has been most persistent. Numerous studies tried to show that persons with obesity either fail to perceive sweetness or are extremely sensitive to sweet taste.[39–43] However, studies using sucrose solutions, sweetened soft drinks, or chocolate milkshakes found no connection between preferences for sweetness and body weight.[44–46]

Sweet taste can be modulated by hormones and other signaling molecules. The activation of CB-1 cannabinoid receptors by anandamide, an endocannabinoid, has been shown to increase the physiological response to sweetness.[47] Sweet taste acuity was reportedly lowered by serotonin.[48] Countering this effect, the responsiveness of sweet taste receptors was reduced by leptin, a circulating peptide hormone produced by adipocytes.[49]

From birth, humans dislike and reject bitter tastes,[32–34] a universal signal for potential dietary danger. The sensitivity to bitter taste is highest in infants, young children, and pregnant women who would be the groups most vulnerable to bitter-tasting dietary toxins, and more intensely tasting bitter stimuli are most likely to be rejected.[34] Recent studies show that the newborn infant's rejection of sour and bitter solutions has changed to partial acceptance after the first year of life.[50] Even so, young children dislike bitter chocolate preferring instead white chocolate, a substance from which all bitter-tasting compounds have been removed. Adults learn to tolerate bitter taste later in life, especially when the bitter taste is accompanied by fat (chocolate), caffeine (coffee), or alcohol (beer).[34,51]

While plant-based diets, rich in cruciferous and other vegetables, may be protective against cancer, active phytochemicals are almost always bitter, acrid, or astringent.[51,52] Chemopreventive phenols, tannins, lignans, flavonoids, isoflavones, and glucosinolates impart a perceptible bitter taste to many vegetables and fruit.[52] Drewnowski and Rock[53] first suggested that genetic taste markers might have an influence on the ability of cancer patients' compliance with therapeutic diets that were phytonutrient-rich, namely bitter-tasting vegetables and fruit. Based on previous research,[54,55] bitter brassica vegetables, such as Brussels sprouts, cabbage, spinach, and kale, are often disliked the most.[52]

Interest in the genetic basis of bitter taste sensitivity has been systematically explored using two bitter compounds: phenylthiocarbamide and PROP. Individual taste sensitivity to these compounds is an inherited trait with an identified genetic basis.[56] The ability to taste phenylthiocarbamide/PROP has been associated with higher sensitivity to selected bitter compounds and with aversions to some bitter foods.[57] While studies have been able to link PROP taster status to taste responses to some bitter foods and some food preferences, associations with food consumption patterns and diet quality have been less consistent[27] with greater PROP sensitivity associated with both lower[58] and higher[59] dietary quality compared to people with less sensitivity to PROP. The argument that "supertasters" of PROP were at lower risk for heart disease because of their alleged dislike of the texture of dairy fat[60] has not been supported by studies of fat consumption in controlled feeding studies.[61] In a sample of women, PROP tasters did not consume less fat but did consume fewer calories overall at a buffet meal, compared to nontasters.[61] However, another study of dietary patterns, biomarkers, and BMI of over 350 women found no link between PROP taster status and nutrition and health outcomes.[62] The lack of consistent associations between PROP sensitivity and dietary habits suggests that many moderating and mediating factors are interposed between the taste acuity measures and food-seeking behavior.[27] Moreover, being highly sensitive to PROP might also reflect heightened sensitivity to other taste and texture stimuli.[63,64]

Sour stimuli and sour-tasting foods are instinctively aversive.[65] Sourness in foods is associated with acid content, which can be higher in foods that have spoiled. However, fresh fruit can also be sour. Studies have linked greater sour preference in children to the consumption of fresh fruit,[66] suggesting the potential value of increasing sour taste preferences among children. While repeated exposure over a period of 8 days was not effective,[67] adding sugar to sour solutions did work.[68] Other research indicates that, at least for children, a liking for very sour tastes may be part of a broader acceptance toward novel and intense stimuli.[69]

The taste for salty foods is partially a reflection of homeostatic requirements for sodium, which is continuously excreted into the environment. Taste responses to sodium chloride can be modified when dietary sodium intake is restricted through medication or diet, with liking for salty stimuli rising to salt levels that would be aversive under normal, nondepleted conditions.[70] Depletion induced by drugs or exercise can also induce liking for salty foods[71] and can induce conditioned preferences for flavors paired with the saltier tastes.[72] The liking for salty taste thus appears to be dynamic, responding to physiological demands.

A person's sensitivity and liking for salty taste may have implications for health. For instance, in some studies, higher sodium recognition thresholds were associated with hypertension and history of type-2 diabetes.[73,74] However, sodium recognition thresholds are not consistently associated with either liking for salty taste or with the amounts of sodium consumed.[75] Shifts in liking for salty taste can occur without changes in detection or recognition thresholds.[75–77] Other studies have failed to link liking for salty state with a higher risk of hypertension.[77]

Observations that the liking for salty taste could be modified by the levels of dietary sodium has led the 2010 Dietary Guidelines to suggest that the best population-based approach to lowering sodium intake[78] would be a systematic and gradual reduction to the sodium content of processed foods.[79] That approach was largely based on one study showing that limiting dietary sodium to 1600 mg/day led to heightened preferences for unsalted foods and lower hedonic ratings for salty soups.[76] The same study, based on participants undergoing treatment with diuretics, showed that participants added lower amounts of table salt to unsalted soups. The current Dietary Guidelines call for reducing sodium intakes to less than 2300 mg per person per day. Reducing dietary sodium gradually over time can allow consumers to adjust taste preferences to the lower level of sodium in their habitually consumed foods.[80,81]

Together with salt taste, umami contributes to the savoriness of foods. For over 100 years, glutamate salts including MSG have been used to evoke the umami taste, enhancing the sensory quality of certain savory foods.[82] The identification of a G-protein−coupled receptor[83] established umami as a distinct taste pathway. Laboratory-based sensory studies have shown that MSG can potentiate the perceived savoriness of foods and improve hedonic response overall.[84−89]

The umami taste may be important for signaling nutritional characteristics of foods. Glutamate salts are related to glutamic acid, an amino acid integral to food proteins.[90,91] Protein hydrolysis that occurs during fermentation and aging can release free glutamate.[92] For example, free glutamate is found in abundance in soy sauces, aged cheeses, and even some fresh foods such as tomatoes and shellfish. Foods that are higher in protein or higher in free glutamate may be favored by persons with greater sensitivity to MSG.[93]

The flavor-enhancing effects of MSG and other glutamate salts could promote food consumption, but evidence that MSG is associated with excess energy intake is mixed. In short-term experimental studies, no significant differences in hunger ratings or differences in subsequent energy intake were observed following MSG supplemetation.[94] In other studies, adding MSG to foods led a selective increase in the consumption of those foods but did not increase the total food energy consumed.[95] In still other studies, the addition of MSG led to higher energy intakes at the next meal[96] or had no effect.[97,98] While some have found a negative relation between MSG consumption and body weight,[99−101] others have pointed to a link between MSG consumption and weight gain.[102−104]

C. Sensory Response to Fats

Fats endow foods with their characteristic taste and texture and contribute to the overall palatability of the diet. The first sensory response to fat involves perception through the nose or mouth of fat-soluble volatile flavor molecules. Oral perception of fat content has been described as sensitivity to food texture as sensed by the oral cavity during chewing or swallowing.[105] This form of fat perception is akin to somatosensation, mediated by nerve endings responsive to pressure or pain.[106] Other mechanisms of chemosensation have been implicated, involving G-protein–coupled receptors, lipid transporters, and potassium channels inhibited by free polyunsaturated fatty acids.[107–109]

The orosensory experience evoked by fat depends on the food product. In dairy products, fat takes the form of emulsified globules that are perceived as smooth and creamy. Water-binding qualities of fat account for the tenderness and juiciness of steaks and the moistness of cakes and other baked goods. Heat transfer at high temperature gives rise to food textures that are crispy, crunchy, and brittle. Among textural qualities that depend on the fat content of foods are hard, soft, juicy, chewy, greasy, viscous, smooth, creamy, crunchy, crisp, and brittle. Generally, high-fat content of foods has been a desirable sensory feature and one that is often linked with higher product quality by the consumer. Sensory preferences and consumption patterns are often linked. People seem to like the foods they already consume. As with salt preferences, self-reported preferences for fat in foods may be influenced to some extent by the amount of fat in the habitual diet.[110]

Fat potentiates the hedonic response to sweetness. A 1983 behavioral study found evidence for hedonic synergy by using 20 different mixtures of dairy products of different fat content and sweetened with different amounts of sugar.[38] Peak hedonic ratings were obtained for stimuli containing 20% fat and 8% sucrose by weight, corresponding to whipping cream with sugar.[38] These studies made early use of response surface methodology and three-dimensional projections of the hedonic response surface. These findings of a hedonic synergy for sugar and fat mixtures were later extended to sweetened cream cheese, the French creamy white cheese fromage blanc, cake frostings, and ice cream.

More recently, a 2019 study using repeated measures functional magnetic resonance found that the neural response to palatable fat—sugar mixtures was associated with weight gain.[111] Weight -gainers exhibited greater decreases in activation in the anterior insula and lateral orbitofrontal cortex in response to a high-fat/high-sugar compared with low-fat/low-sugar milkshake than those who remained weight stable. Exposure to low-fat/high-sugar as compared with a low-fat/low-sugar milkshake did not distinguish between the two groups. The study concluded that blunted brain responsiveness of regions associated with the taste and reward value of high-fat and high-fat/high-sugar foods was the cause of weight gain. The notion that obesity is caused by a taste (and more recently) brain dysfunction is as popular as ever.

D. Palatability and Satiety

Satiety is one among many mechanisms regulating energy balance.[112] Palatability and satiety have opposite effects on food intakes. While palatability increases appetite and therefore food consumption, satiety limits consumption by reducing meal size or by delaying the onset of the next meal.[22] As such, both palatability and satiety help to adjust energy intakes to energy needs. However, in experimental studies, both palatability and satiety tend to be measured in terms of the amounts of food consumed. As a result, the foods that are overeaten are by definition the most palatable and the least satiating.[5]

Standard measures of palatability include the perceived pleasantness of a given food, intent to eat, or the amount of food consumed. Among standard measures of satiety are reduced hunger, fullness, reduced intent to consume a meal or a snack, or the amount of food consumed. Some investigators have made a distinction between satiety and satiation.[26] While satiation is responsible for the termination of a given meal and reduced meal size, satiety, defined as a state of internal repletion, delays the onset or reduces the size of the next meal.

Increased satiety has also been measured in terms of reduced palatability. Sensory-specific satiety was specifically defined as reduced palatability of the just-consumed food relative to other foods.[5] In other words, given the reciprocal nature of palatability and satiety measures, the most palatable foods are by definition the least satiating and vice versa.

The low satiating power of energy-dense sweet and fat-rich foods has been singled out for special scrutiny.[113,114] Some researchers have argued that the palatability of sugar overrides normal satiety signals, leading to overeating and overweight.[115] Others have noted that fat had low satiating power, judging by the "passive overeating" of fat-rich foods.[116] One question is whether palatable fat-rich foods are overeaten because of their high energy density or because of their fat content.[116] If satiety is macronutrient driven, fat may be overeaten because it affects satiety less than a corresponding amount (in kcal) of carbohydrate or protein. The creation of palatable and yet highly satiating foods, the avowed goal of the weight loss industry,[5] may represent a contradiction in terms.

E. Hedonic Responses and Food Liking

Intensity and hedonic ratings for the same taste stimuli follow different psychophysical curves. Laboratory studies have generally tested hedonic ratings for sugar solutions, sweetened lemonade, salted soups or tomato juice, or mixtures of milk, cream, and sugar. However, studies have shown that taste preferences for sweet and salty tastes in aqueous solution were not a good predictor of self-reported liking for sweet or salty foods.[26]

Industry studies on the taste acceptability of more complex foods, conducted in commercial sensory evaluation labs, generally asked respondents to rate the acceptability of flavor, color, and texture, as well as the overall acceptability of the food product.[117] The key measure of liking has been the 9-point hedonic scale, commonly known and the hedonic preference scale.[20]

Food preferences are said to predict food consumption. However, people may have positive attitudes toward the foods they already eat so that food preferences may merely be a reflection of existing eating habits. For instance, a study of school children found that higher liking for vegetables and fruit was associated with higher consumption.[118] Given cross-sectional nature of study designs, it may be that higher consumption led to the reports of higher liking.[119] Another key limitation of the research is how preferences were assessed. Many studies of food likes and dislikes employed not actual foods but printed lists of food names. Such tools merely capture respondents' attitudes toward a verbal concept of a given food, since the food itself was never presented.

Taste preferences and food choices differ over the life course and in relation to our physical conditions.[33,72,120] Preferences and aversions are modifiable by growth, maturation, and hormonal status.[121–123] Both taste preferences and food choices are further shaped by prior experience and associative learning. Preferences for aversive tastes including bitter (caffeine), alcohol, and hot spices are all said to be the result of associating the often unpleasant taste with the desirable postingestive consequences.[124] A previously neutral or even unpleasant taste can become preferred, provided it is linked with a suitable mechanism of reward.

IV. TIME, MONEY, AND HEALTH

A. Food Prices and Dietary Costs

Consumer food choices are economic decisions made in response to taste, reward value prices, incomes, time constraints, and the perceived nutritional value of foods. Taste response or the liking for foods alone does not always predict purchase intent or actual consumer behavior. Consumption patterns are also influenced by price, convenience, safety, and nutritional concerns.[124,125] Other demographic, cultural, and socioeconomic factors also modulate the connection between taste responsiveness and food choice.

Food cost is a dominant factor guiding food selection. Disparities in food prices and the costs of diets contribute to the observed disparities in health outcomes by socioeconomic status.[126] Several economic studies have made the association between the declining monetary and time cost of food and rising obesity rates.[127,128] Those studies pointed to the widespread availability of palatable energy-dense fast foods, the entry of women into the labor force, and lower physical activity associated with work.[128,129]

Even though expenditures on foods as a proportion of household budgets have steadily declined over the last 50 years,[130] not all foods have become equally affordable. There is a growing price disparity between the low-cost, energy-dense foods based on refined grains, added sugars, and added fats and the more nutrient-dense foods including lean meats, dairy products, whole grains, and fresh vegetables and fruit that are generally more expensive.[11,131,132] Providing adequate empty calories has become cheaper than providing more nutrient-rich foods.

Further, healthier foods are not always available in economically disadvantaged areas with reduced food budgets and lower purchasing power.[12,133] Unequal access to affordable healthy foods is another barrier to the adoption of healthier diets by low-income groups. Disparities in food access, together with decreasing time devoted to food preparation and consumption by working households, may help explain some of the observed disparities in health.[134,135] Identifying food patterns that are nutrient rich, affordable, and appealing should be a priority to fight social inequalities in nutrition and health.

The nature of the relation between diet quality and diet cost has important implications for the study of diets and disease risk as well as for food security and public health.[9,136–139] If diets that can help prevent disease are more costly than unhealthy diets, then diet-related socioeconomic inequities in obesity and health may be challenging to overcome with information and encouragement alone. That inequities in diet at least partly explain inequities in health is not new,[140,141] but the notion that the higher cost of healthier diets may present a structural barrier to the adoption of healthier diets by populations with fewer resources is newer.[142,143]

Studies have found that diets that are higher in nutrients of public health concern, such as potassium, fiber, and calcium, were associated with higher consumer food costs.[144,145] Similarly, diets that met food- and nutrient-based targets in the United Kingdom were systematically more costly than diets that failed to meet these targets.[146–148] For example, U.S. diets that were more costly, in terms of dollars per 2000 kcal, were more closely aligned to the Dietary Guidelines for Americans, as measured by the Healthy Eating Index (HEI) compared to cheaper diets (Fig. 10.1).[149,150] Diets that were more accordant with the Dietary Approaches to Stop Hypertension were more costly than diets that were inconsistent with this healthy dietary pattern.[151,152] More diverse diets, which were associated with lower risk of type-2 diabetes, were substantially more costly than more homogenous diets, which were associated with higher diabetes risk.[153] Yet, following

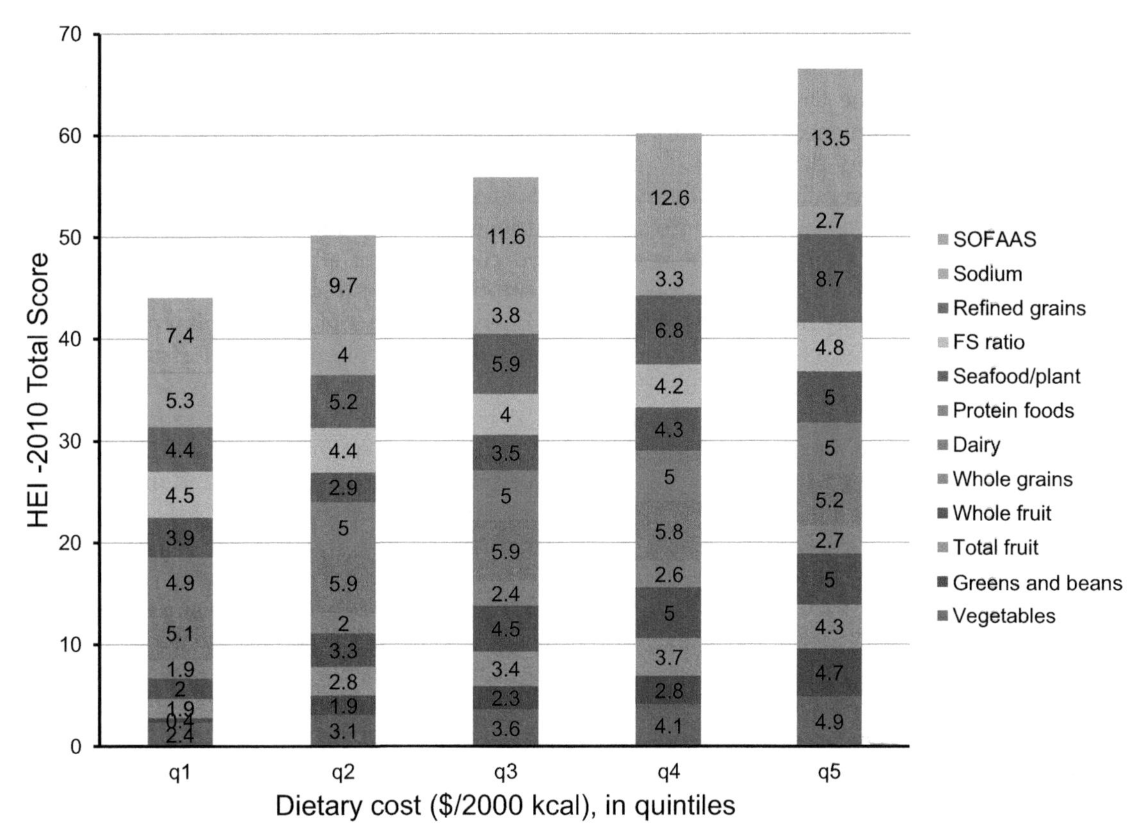

FIGURE 10.1 Dietary quality in relation to dietary cost, expressed as US dollars per 2000 kcal of dietary energy. Dietary cost categorized into quintiles. Dietary quality indexed by the Healthy Eating Index (HEI) 2010. Plot shows contribution of different HEI-2010 subcomponents for each group. Empty calories represent SoFAAS, solid fat, alcohol, and added sugars. *Data from 11,181 adults from the 2007–10 National Health and Nutrition Examination Survey. Figure adapted from Rehm et al.*[150]

other evidence-based dietary patterns may not necessarily be more costly for consumers. For example, some studies have found that diets that adhered to the Mediterranean diet pattern were more costly,[154] while others have found that cost was not associated with following this pattern.[155,156]

While spending more money does not guarantee a healthier diet, reducing food costs below a certain limit virtually guarantees that the resulting diet will be nutrient-poor.[157] One key question is whether palatable, low-cost, energy-dense diets are associated with higher energy consumption overall? In other words, can BMI values be linked directly to food prices and to diet costs, after adjusting for covariates? Although some preliminary data on diet quality and diet cost are available,[158,159] the answers to all these questions are far from clear.

B. Time and Convenience

The pursuit of nutritious food and healthy eating by consumers may conflict with time constraints and the need for convenience. In the United States, social and economic trends have coincided with less time allocated to food preparation and a greater demand for convenience, with time spent in home food preparation declining by more than one-third between 1965 and 2008.[160] Although there are signs of a slight increase in time allocated to cooking in recent years,[161] Americans now spend an estimated 37 min per day engaging in all aspects of cooking and food preparation, including cooking, serving, and cleaning up afterward.[162]

Although home-cooked, family meals are widely deemed to be integral to healthy diets, time scarcity may undermine these habits. Cooking freshly prepared meals at home requires a time commitment that many cannot afford, given time poverty and competing demands.[163,164] For example, working parents earing low wages considered family meals important but often served their families foods that were fast and easy to prepare,[165] including hot dogs, pizza, and macaroni and cheese.[166] Research on low- and middle-income working parents showed that they coped with time pressures by relying more on take-out and restaurant meals and basing family meals on prepared entrees and other quick options.[167]

The need for convenience may also be at odds with recommended meal plans that are optimized for nutrition and affordability. Economic analyses of the USDA's Thrifty Food Plan have found that these nutritious, low-cost meal plans were time-intensive to prepare and much more costly when time was explicitly included in analysis.[134,135,168]

Attitudes toward and convenience have been shown to affect diet quality.[126,169–174] For example, in the US Continuing Survey of Food Intake by Individuals (CSFII 1994–96), prioritizing convenience over nutrition in foods was associated with lower quality diets and higher consumption of fats, added sugars, and sodium.[126,169] Similarly, studies from Finland and the United States found that adults who prioritized convenience consumed fewer fruits and vegetables, more energy-dense foods,[175] and more fast food[176] and had lower overall dietary quality.[177] Having the skills, time, and other resources to forgo convenience and prepare food at home may hold the key to affordable, yet nutritious diets. For example, a study of US adults found that those who more frequently engaged in food preparation at home spent less money on food overall, yet had healthier diets, as indicated by the HEI-2010.[178] Fig. 10.2 shows how HEI-2010 scores and components varied with frequency of cooking at home for this sample of adults.

C. Nutrient Density and Health

Ideally, the food supply should offer foods that are nutrient-rich, healthful, affordable, culturally appropriate, and appealing.[2,4,179] Balancing innate human preferences for sweet and energy-rich foods with population health goals has been a challenge.[180] It has become a matter of public health concern that low-income consumers in high-income countries are over -supplied with low-cost calories while falling short of some key nutrients.[181] Many populations suffer from chronic deficiencies in high-quality protein, vitamin A, calcium, iron, and zinc.

Here we review the concepts of nutrient density and the nutrients-to-energy ratio, as they apply to public health nutrition. Ways to improve the nutrient density of individual foods and the total diet include product (re)formulation, fortification, and reshaping of food industry product portfolios. The manipulation of the nutrients-to-energy ratio, without substantially increasing food cost, is more effectively achieved with processed as opposed to fresh foods.

Energy density of foods is defined in terms of kcal per unit weight or volume.[21,182] The range of energy densities runs from 0 kcal/100 g (water) to 900 kcal/100 g (oil). For the most part, energy-dense foods that are dry are foods. Water in foods provided weight and bulk but no dietary energy and no nutrients. While sugar and fat can contribute to energy density, it is largely an inverse function of the foods water content. Dietary energy density is defined as calories per total weight of all foods and caloric beverages consumed. In general, water and noncaloric beverages are excluded from dietary energy density calculations.

In many studies, excess consumption of energy-dense foods of low nutritional value has been linked to an increased risk of obesity[183] and related NCDs.[184–186] Economics may hold part of the key for solving the dilemma. "Empty" calories that are nutrient-poor calories cost less, while naturally nutrient-rich foods can cost more.[16,131,132] Obesity and poverty may be linked by the low-cost, high reward value and easy access to

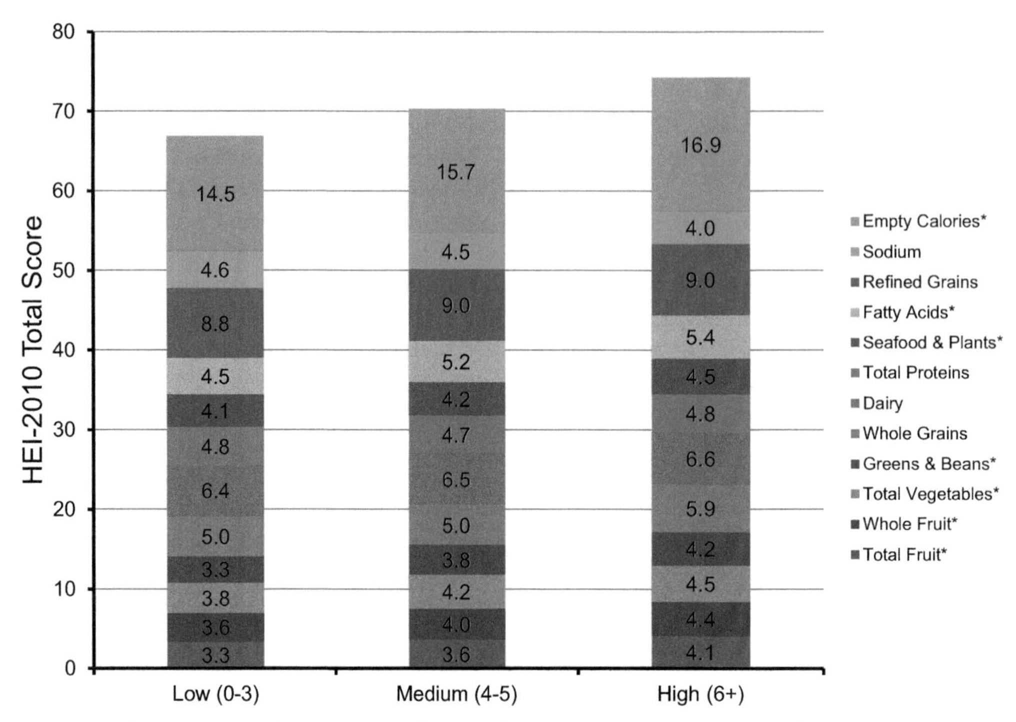

FIGURE 10.2 Dietary quality in relation to frequency of cooking at home. Dietary quality indexed by the HEI-2010. Plot shows contribution of different HEI-2010 subcomponents for each group. Empty calories represent SoFAAS, solid fat, alcohol, and added sugars. Asterisks indicate where subcomponents are significantly different across quintiles at $P < .05$. *Data from a stratified random sample of 437 King County, Washington adults. Figure adapted from Tiwari et al.*[178]

energy-dense foods.[9] Supplying sufficient dietary energy while avoiding caloric excess and improving nutrient-to-calories ratios for key nutrients are twin priority areas for the food industry and for public health.

Nutrient profiles of foods have been used as a basis for targeting fiscal or informational interventions. For example, some countries have imposed taxes on snacks with energy density in excess of 275 kcal/100 g.[187] Others have placed warning labels on foods where energy exceeded 200 kcal per serving.[188] Energy density may not have been the main point, since low–energy density sugar-sweetened beverages have also been the target of taxes, though these measures are usually predicated on the low nutrient density of these beverages.[188–190] Foods containing added sugars and fats have been under scrutiny as possible candidates for regulation and taxation.[189,191,192] Nutrition and health claims and regulation of marketing and advertising to children have emphasized a food's nutrient density and a favorable nutrient profile.[193]

Nutrient density is usually defined as the ratio of nutrients to calories. It is measured in terms of amounts of selected key nutrients per reference amount of food, where the latter is 100 kcal, 100 g, or a serving. While the US Food and Drug Administration has defined servings as Reference Amounts Customarily Consumed, no government-mandated serving sizes exist in the European Union at this time.[194] Generally, energy density and nutrient density are inversely linked.[15,132]

Nutrient profiling (NP) of foods is the technique used to assess nutrient density by scoring the content of foods against health objectives such as dietary recommendations.[195] Several NP models and scoring systems have been developed by researchers, regulatory agencies, and by the food industry. Some of these tools have focused on nutrients to limit: usually saturated fat, sugar (added or total), and salt, which are often consumed to excess in comparison to recommendations. Other NP models have emphasized shortfall nutrients, those consumed in inadequate amounts. Some models have balanced the beneficial nutrients to encourage with nutrients to limit. In these NP classifications, each food was assigned a single score that best reflected its nutritional quality overall.[196] Science-driven scores and indices may be helpful for consumers in making better food choices and may also assist the food industry in designing and promoting healthier food items. With few exceptions, existing NP models have focused on scoring individual foods without considering different meals, menus, or the whole diet.[193,197,198]

Two approaches to validating NP models have been suggested. For example, construct validity of the Nutrient Rich Foods (NRF) index was established with reference to an independent measure of a healthy diet.[199] An alternative approach was to validate a different NP model (SAIN,LIM) against dietary guidelines using linear programming.[200] The NRF system also benefited from a predictive validity test: higher NRF scores were linked to

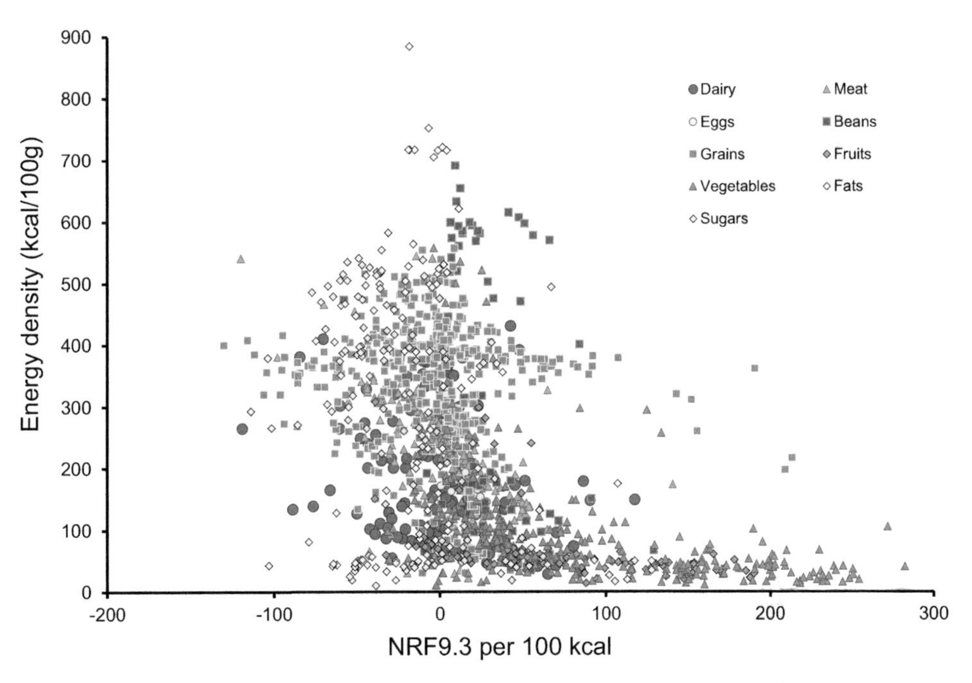

FIGURE 10.3 Nutrient density of foods in relation to energy density. Nutrient density based on the Nutrient Rich Food (NRF) Score, 9.3,[132] computed per 100 kcal of food; energy density calculated as kcal/100 g edible portion. *Data for 1603 foods and beverages from the Food and Nutrient Database for Dietary Studies.*

reduced mortality in the Rotterdam Cohort Study.[201] Nutrient density typically varies inversely with energy density. Fig. 10.3 illustrates the interrelation between nutrient density, based on the NRF score, and energy density for 1603 foods consumed in the United States.

Nutrient profile models are often tailored to specific public health goals. For example, NP models have become the basis for regulating health and nutrition claims, front-of-pack labels, marketing and advertising to children, and for taxation of selected foods and food groups,[193,202,203] as well as measuring and monitoring nutritional quality in food banks.[204] The food industry has used nutrient profiles to (re)evaluate and (re)formulate their product portfolios.[198,205,206]

Improving the nutrient-to-energy ratio of processed foods would be a major step forward toward better public health.[207] Here, the food industry has improved the product nutrient density by reducing energy from added sugars and saturated fats. Fortified foods also improve nutrient-to-energy ratios. However, if the concept of nutrient density is to be translated into effective dietary guidance, it is necessary to ensure that the more nutrient-rich foods do not cost more.

V. CONCLUSION

The last 20 years of nutrition research have seen a shift from biological determinism of dietary behavior to a wider appreciation of multilevel determinants of food choices and diet quality. Academic research is now playing catch-up with the food industry, which has long understood that consumer food choices are largely motivated by pleasure, cost, and convenience. Only by understanding these drivers of dietary behaviors can nutrition professionals hope to develop effective interventions, programs, and policies that might lead to healthier eating habits. With consumers also increasingly concern about the environmental implications of food choices, nutrition professionals, including researchers and dietitians, will need to appreciate how some food choices that may be good for health may not necessarily be environmentally sustainable. Collaboration and coordination of research and policy across the food system will be necessary to identify and promote foods and dietary patterns that are appealing and affordable to consumers and still are nutritious and sustainable.

RESEARCH GAPS

Current research and knowledge in nutrition increasingly draw on studies in social, environmental, and climate sciences to complement biology, physiology, and behavior. The concepts of personal, population, and planetary health, introduced in the Giessen Declaration,[208] have opened the door to multidisciplinary research on the relation between food systems and health.

First, the research focus has shifted from the relation between individual nutrients and disease outcomes to territorial food patterns and food-based dietary guidelines. However, while nutrients can be obtained from different cost sources, the inclusion of specific foods in healthy dietary patterns is likely to be associated with a corresponding higher cost. While empty calories are relatively inexpensive, the more nutrient-rich foods and food patterns are likely to cost more.[6] Attitudes toward food have also changed. Although taste, cost, and convenience still drive food choices, there are growing concerns with social values, with cultural and ethical norms, and about sustainability and animal welfare. Mixed methods studies should combine epidemiologic research on dietary intakes with social and ethnographic studies on motivations, ambitions, and desires.

There is also a need to explore diet quality in relation to food prices, diet costs, and household incomes. The evolution of the food supply over the past 100 years was shaped in part by rapid urbanization and the entry of women into the labor force.[128,129,209] The food chain had lengthened as urban dwellers have become more remote from the food supply,[210–212] relying increasingly on processed foods and foods eaten away from home. Policies and actions aimed at improving one aspect of the food system may have broad-ranging and unintended side effects. Product reformulation may not only improve nutrient content but also affect palatability and price. Healthier, more sustainable diets may be less affordable and may be economically out of reach for low-income populations.[213] Taxes on low-cost foods can represent regressive taxation. In crafting interventions, it is important to consider potential impacts on the entire food supply chain including, but not limited to, nutritional and health considerations.[214,215]

These research gaps can only be filled by interdisciplinary studies on food systems, nutrition, and health. Public health interventions to improve diet quality and nutritional status will need to account for the multilevel determinants of dietary behavior, including the social and environmental factors that are known determinants of obesity and health.[216]

VI. REFERENCES

1. *Agriculture USD of H and HS and USD of. 2015 – 2020 Dietary Guidelines for Americans.* 8th ed. 2015. https://doi.org/10.1097/NT.0b013e31826c50af.
2. Food and Agricultural Organization to the United Nations (FAO). *Sustainable Diets and Biodiversity.* 2010. https://doi.org/10.1017/S002081830000607X.
3. Willett W, Rockström J, Loken B, et al. Food in the Anthropocene: the EAT–Lancet Commission on healthy diets from sustainable food systems. *Lancet.* 2019;393(10170):447–492.
4. Macdiarmid JI, Kyle J, Horgan GW, et al. Sustainable diets for the future: can we contribute to reducing greenhouse gas emissions by eating a healthy diet? *Am J Clin Nutr.* 2012;96(3):632–639. https://doi.org/10.3945/ajcn.112.038729.
5. Drewnowski A. Energy density, palatability, and satiety: implications for weight control. *Nutr Rev.* 1998;56(12):347–353.
6. Butland B, Jebb S, Kopelman P, et al. Foresight tackling obesities: future choices – project report. *Gov Off Sci;* 2007:1–161. https://www.gov.uk/government/uploads/system/uploads/attachment_data/file/287937/07-1184x-tackling-obesities-future-choices-report.pdf.
7. Crino M, Sacks G, Vandevijvere S, Swinburn B, Neal B. The influence on population weight gain and obesity of the macronutrient composition and energy density of the food supply. *Curr Obes Rep.* 2015;4(1):1–10.
8. Rolls BJ, Ello-Martin JA, Tohill BC. What can intervention studies tell us about the relationship between fruit and vegetable consumption and weight management? *Nutr Rev.* 2004;62(1):1–17. https://doi.org/10.1301/nr.2004.jan.1.
9. Drewnowski A, Specter SE. Poverty and obesity: the role of energy density and energy costs. *Am J Clin Nutr.* 2004;79(1):6–16.
10. Powell LM, Chaloupka FJ. Food prices and obesity: evidence and policy implications for taxes and subsidies. *Milbank Q.* 2009. https://doi.org/10.1111/j.1468-0009.2009.00554.x.
11. Jones NRV, Conklin AI, Suhrcke M, Monsivais P. The growing price gap between more and less healthy foods: analysis of a novel longitudinal UK dataset. *PLoS One.* 2014;9(10). https://doi.org/10.1371/journal.pone.0109343.
12. Larson NI, Story MT, Nelson MC. Neighborhood environments: disparities in access to healthy foods in the U.S. *Am J Prev Med.* 2009;36(1):74–81.
13. Farley TA, Baker ET, Futrell L, Rice JC. The ubiquity of energy-dense snack foods: a national multicity study. *Am J Public Health.* 2010;100(2):306–311.
14. Drewnowski A, Rehm CD, Martin A, Verger EO, Voinnesson M, Imbert P. Energy and nutrient density of foods in relation to their carbon footprint. *Am J Clin Nutr.* 2014;101(1):184–191.
15. Maillot M, Darmon N, Darmon M, Lafay L, Drewnowski A. Nutrient-dense food groups have high energy costs: an econometric approach to nutrient profiling. *J Nutr.* 2007;137(7):1815–1820.
16. Jones NRV, Monsivais P. Comparing prices for food and diet research: the metric matters. *J Hunger Environ Nutr.* 2016;11(3). https://doi.org/10.1080/19320248.2015.1095144.
17. Liem DG, Russell CG. The influence of taste liking on the consumption of nutrient rich and nutrient poor foods. *Front Nutr.* 2019;6:174.
18. de Macedo IC, de Freitas JS, da Silva Torres IL. The influence of palatable diets in reward system activation: a mini review. *Adv Pharmacol Sci.* 2016;2016.
19. Aggarwal A, Rehm CD, Monsivais P, Drewnowski A. Importance of taste, nutrition, cost and convenience in relation to diet quality: evidence of nutrition resilience among US adults using National Health and Nutrition Examination Survey (NHANES) 2007–2010. *Prev Med.* 2016;90. https://doi.org/10.1016/j.ypmed.2016.06.030.
20. Drewnowski A. Taste preferences and food intake. *Annu Rev Nutr.* 1997;17(1):237–253.
21. Prentice AM, Jebb SA. Fast foods, energy density and obesity: a possible mechanistic link. *Obes Rev.* 2003;4(4):187–194. https://doi.org/10.1046/j.1467-789X.2003.00117.x.
22. Rolls BJ. The role of portion size, energy density, and variety in obesity and weight management. *Handb Obes Treat.* 2018;93.
23. Drewnowski A. Genetics of human taste perception. *Neurol Dis Ther.* 2003;57:847–860.
24. Beauchamp GK. Sensory and receptor responses to umami: an overview of pioneering work. *Am J Clin Nutr.* 2009;90(3):723S–727S.
25. Bartoshuk LM. The biological basis of food perception and acceptance. *Food Qual Prefer.* 1993;4(1–2):21–32.
26. Mattes RD, Hollis J, Hayes D, Stunkard AJ. Appetite: measurement and manipulation misgivings. *J Am Diet Assoc.* 2005;105(5):87–97.
27. Tepper BJ, White EA, Koelliker Y, Lanzara C, d'Adamo P, Gasparini P. Genetic variation in taste sensitivity to 6-n-propylthiouracil and its relationship to taste perception and food selection. *Ann N Y Acad Sci.* 2009;1170:126–139. https://doi.org/10.1111/j.1749-6632.2009.03916.x.
28. Keller KL, Adise S. Variation in the ability to taste bitter thiourea compounds: implications for food acceptance, dietary intake, and obesity risk in children. *Annu Rev Nutr.* 2016;36:157–182.
29. Keskitalo K, Tuorila H, Spector TD, et al. Same genetic components underlie different measures of sweet taste preference. *Am J Clin Nutr.* 2007;86(6):1663–1669.
30. Wise PM, Hansen JL, Reed DR, Breslin PAS. Twin study of the heritability of recognition thresholds for sour and salty taste. *Chem Senses.* 2007;32(8):749–754.
31. Mattes RD. Gustation as a determinant of ingestion: methodological issues. *Am J Clin Nutr.* 1985;41(4):672–683.
32. Drewnowski A, Brunzell JD, Sande K, Iverius PH, Greenwood MR. Sweet tooth reconsidered: taste responsiveness in human obesity. *Physiol Behav.* 1985;35(4):617–622. http://www.ncbi.nlm.nih.gov/entrez/query.fcgi?cmd=Retrieve&db=PubMed&dopt=Citation&list_uids=4070436.
33. Birch LL. Development of food preferences. *Annu Rev Nutr.* 1999;19(1):41–62.
34. Drewnowski A. The science and complexity of bitter taste. *Nutr Rev.* 2001;59(6):163–169. http://www.ncbi.nlm.nih.gov/entrez/query.fcgi?cmd=Retrieve&db=PubMed&dopt=Citation&list_uids=11444592.
35. Enns MP, Van Itallie TB, Grinker JA. Contributions of age, sex and degree of fatness on preferences and magnitude estimations for sucrose in humans. *Physiol Behav.* 1979;22(5):999–1003.
36. Barragán R, Coltell O, Portolés O, et al. Bitter, sweet, salty, sour and umami taste perception decreases with age: sex-specific analysis, modulation by genetic variants and taste-preference associations in 18 to 80 year-old subjects. *Nutrients.* 2018;10(10):1539.
37. Moskowitz HR, Kluter RA, Westerling J, Jacobs HL. Sugar sweetness and pleasantness: evidence for different psychological laws. *Science.* 1974;184(4136):583–585.
38. Drewnowski A, Greenwood MR. Cream and sugar: human preferences for high-fat foods. *Physiol Behav.* 1983;30(4):629–633. http://www.ncbi.nlm.nih.gov/entrez/query.fcgi?cmd=Retrieve&db=PubMed&dopt=Citation&list_uids=6878464.
39. Bartoshuk LM, Duffy VB, Hayes JE, Moskowitz HR, Snyder DJ. Psychophysics of sweet and fat perception in obesity: problems, solutions and new perspectives. *Philos Trans R Soc B Biol Sci.* 2006;361(1471):1137–1148.
40. Grinker J. Obesity and sweet taste. *Am J Clin Nutr.* 1978;31(6):1078–1087.
41. Thompson DA, Moskowitz HR, Campbell RG. Taste and olfaction in human obesity. *Physiol Behav.* 1977;19(2):335–337.

42. Rodin J, Moskowitz HR, Bray GA. Relationship between obesity, weight loss, and taste responsiveness. *Physiol Behav.* 1976;17(4): 591–597.
43. Hardikar S, Höchenberger R, Villringer A, Ohla K. Higher sensitivity to sweet and salty taste in obese compared to lean individuals. *Appetite.* 2017;111:158–165.
44. Malcolm R, O'Neil PM, Hirsch AA, Currey HS, Moskowitz G. Taste hedonics and thresholds in obesity. *Int J Obes.* 1980;4(3): 203–212.
45. Thompson DA, Moskowitz HR, Campbell RG. Effects of body-weight and food-intake on pleasantness ratings for a sweet stimulus. *J Appl Physiol.* 1976;41(1):77–83.
46. Bobowski N, Mennella JA. Personal variation in preference for sweetness: effects of age and obesity. *Child Obes.* 2017;13(5): 369–376.
47. Yoshida R, Ohkuri T, Jyotaki M, et al. Endocannabinoids selectively enhance sweet taste. *Proc Natl Acad Sci USA.* 2010;107(2): 935–939. http://www.pnas.org/content/107/2/935.abstract.
48. Heath TP, Melichar JK, Nutt DJ, Donaldson LF. Human taste thresholds are modulated by serotonin and noradrenaline. *J Neurosci.* 2006;26(49):12664–12671. https://doi.org/10.1523/JNEUROSCI.3459-06.2006.
49. Jyotaki M, Shigemura N, Ninomiya Y. Modulation of sweet taste sensitivity by orexigenic and anorexigenic factors. *Endocr J.* 2010; 57(6):467–475.
50. Schwartz C, Issanchou S, Nicklaus S. Developmental changes in the acceptance of the five basic tastes in the first year of life. *Br J Nutr.* 2009;102(9):1375–1385. https://doi.org/10.1017/S0007114509990286.
51. Barratt-Fornell A, Drewnowski A. The taste of health: nature's bitter gifts. *Nutr Today.* 2002;37(4):144–150. http://www.ncbi.nlm.nih.gov/entrez/query.fcgi?cmd=Retrieve&db=PubMed&dopt=Citation&list_uids=12352830.
52. Drewnowski A, Gomez-Carneros C. Bitter taste, phytonutrients, and the consumer: a review. *Am J Clin Nutr.* 2000;72(6): 1424–1435. http://www.ncbi.nlm.nih.gov/entrez/query.fcgi?cmd=Retrieve&db=PubMed&dopt=Citation&list_uids=11101467.
53. Drewnowski A, Rock CL. The influence of genetic taste markers on food acceptance. *Am J Clin Nutr.* 1995;62(3):506–511. http://www.ncbi.nlm.nih.gov/entrez/query.fcgi?cmd=Retrieve&db=PubMed&dopt=Citation&list_uids=7661111.
54. Fischer R, Griffin F, Kaplan AR. Taste thresholds, cigarette smoking, and food dislikes. *Med Exp Int J Exp Med.* 1963;9:151–167. http://www.ncbi.nlm.nih.gov/entrez/query.fcgi?cmd=Retrieve&db=PubMed&dopt=Citation&list_uids=14083335.
55. Glanville EV, Kaplan AR. Food preference and sensitivity of taste for bitter compounds. *Nature.* 1965;205(4974):851–853. https://doi.org/10.1038/205851a0.
56. Kim UK, Jorgenson E, Coon H, Leppert M, Risch N, Drayna D. Positional cloning of the human quantitative trait locus underlying taste sensitivity to phenylthiocarbamide. *Science.* 2003;299(5610): 1221–1225. https://doi.org/10.1126/science.1080190299/5610/1221.
57. Tepper BJ. Nutritional implications of genetic taste variation: the role of PROP sensitivity and other taste phenotypes. *Annu Rev Nutr.* 2008; 28:367–388. https://doi.org/10.1146/annurev.nutr.28.061807.155458.
58. Stevenson RJ, Boakes RA, Oaten MJ, Yeomans MR, Mahmut M, Francis HM. Chemosensory abilities in consumers of a western-style diet. *Chem Senses.* 2016. https://doi.org/10.1093/chemse/bjw053.
59. Sharafi M, Rawal S, Fernandez ML, Huedo-Medina TB, Duffy VB. Taste phenotype associates with cardiovascular disease risk factors via diet quality in multivariate modeling. *Physiol Behav.* 2018. https://doi.org/10.1016/j.physbeh.2018.05.005.
60. Duffy VB. Associations between oral sensation, dietary behaviors and risk of cardiovascular disease (CVD). *Appetite.* 2004;43(1):5–9. https://doi.org/10.1016/J.Appet.2004.02.007.
61. Tepper BJ, Neilland M, Ullrich NV, Koelliker Y, Belzer LM. Greater energy intake from a buffet meal in lean, young women is associated with the 6-n-propylthiouracil (PROP) non-taster phenotype. *Appetite.* 2011;56(1):104–110. https://doi.org/10.1016/j.appet.2010.11.144.
62. Drewnowski A, Henderson SA, Cockroft JE. Genetic sensitivity to 6-n-propylthiouracil has no influence on dietary patterns, body mass indexes, or plasma lipid profiles of women. *J Am Diet Assoc.* 2007;107(8):1340–1348. https://doi.org/10.1016/J.Jada.2007.05.013.
63. Lim J, Urban L, Green BG. Measures of individual differences in taste and creaminess perception. *Chem Senses.* 2008;33(6): 493–501. https://doi.org/10.1093/chemse/bjn016.
64. Reed DR. Birth of a new breed of supertaster. *Chem Senses.* 2008; 33(6):489–491. https://doi.org/10.1093/chemse/bjn031.
65. Desor JA, Maller O, Andrews K. Ingestive responses of human newborns to salty, sour, and bitter stimuli. *J Comp Physiol Psychol.* 1975;89(8):966–970. http://www.ncbi.nlm.nih.gov/entrez/query.fcgi?cmd=Retrieve&db=PubMed&dopt=Citation&list_uids=1184802.
66. Liem DG, Bogers RP, Dagnelie PC, de Graaf C. Fruit consumption of boys (8—11 years) is related to preferences for sour taste. *Appetite.* 2006;46(1):93–96. https://doi.org/10.1016/j.appet.2005.11.002.
67. Liem DG, de Graaf C. Sweet and sour preferences in young children and adults: role of repeated exposure. *Physiol Behav.* 2004;83(3):421–429. https://doi.org/10.1016/j.physbeh.2004.08.028.
68. Capaldi ED, Privitera GJ. Decreasing dislike for sour and bitter in children and adults. *Appetite.* 2008;50(1):139–145. https://doi.org/10.1016/j.appet.2007.06.008.
69. Liem DG, Westerbeek A, Wolterink S, Kok FJ, de Graaf C. Sour taste preferences of children relate to preference for novel and intense stimuli. *Chem Senses.* 2004;29(8):713–720. https://doi.org/10.1093/chemse/bjh077.
70. Johnson AK. The sensory psychobiology of thirst and salt appetite. *Med Sci Sport Exerc.* 2007;39(8):1388–1400. https://doi.org/10.1249/mss.0b013e3180686de800005768-200708000-00023.
71. Beauchamp GK, Bertino M, Burke D, Engelman K. Experimental sodium depletion and salt taste in normal human volunteers. *Am J Clin Nutr.* 1990;51(5):881–889. http://www.ncbi.nlm.nih.gov/entrez/query.fcgi?cmd=Retrieve&db=PubMed&dopt=Citation&list_uids=2185626.
72. Wald N, Leshem M. Salt conditions a flavor preference or aversion after exercise depending on NaCl dose and sweat loss. *Appetite.* 2003;40(3):277–284. doi:S0195666303000138.
73. Michikawa T, Nishiwaki Y, Okamura T, Asakura K, Nakano M, Takebayashi T. The taste of salt measured by a simple test and blood pressure in Japanese women and men. *Hypertens Res.* 2009;32(5):399–403. https://doi.org/10.1038/hr.2009.31.
74. Isezuo SA, Saidu Y, Anas S, Tambuwal BU, Bilbis LS. Salt taste perception and relationship with blood pressure in type 2 diabetics. *J Hum Hypertens.* 2008;22(6):432–434. https://doi.org/10.1038/jhh.2008.1.
75. Lucas L, Riddell L, Liem G, Whitelock S, Keast R. The influence of sodium on liking and consumption of salty food. *J Food Sci.* 2011;76(1):S72–S76. https://doi.org/10.1111/j.1750-3841.2010.01939.x.
76. Blais CA, Pangborn RM, Borhani NO, Ferrell MF, Prineas RJ, Laing B. Effect of dietary sodium restriction on taste responses to sodium chloride: a longitudinal study. *Am J Clin Nutr.* 1986;44(2):232–243. http://www.ncbi.nlm.nih.gov/

entrez/query.fcgi?cmd=Retrieve&db=PubMed&dopt=Citation&list_uids=3728360.
77. Mattes RD. The taste for salt in humans. *Am J Clin Nutr.* 1997;65(2 suppl):692S–697S. http://www.ncbi.nlm.nih.gov/entrez/query.fcgi?cmd=Retrieve&db=PubMed&dopt=Citation&list_uids=9022567.
78. Dotsch M, Busch J, Batenburg M, et al. Strategies to reduce sodium consumption: a food industry perspective. *Crit Rev Food Sci Nutr.* 2009;49(10):841–851. https://doi.org/10.1080/10408390903044297.
79. Cook NR, Cutler JA, Obarzanek E, et al. Long term effects of dietary sodium reduction on cardiovascular disease outcomes: observational follow-up of the trials of hypertension prevention (TOHP). *BMJ.* 2007;334(7599):885. https://doi.org/10.1136/bmj.39147.604896.55.
80. Wyness LA, Butriss JL, Stanner SA. Reducing the population's sodium intake: the UK Food Standards Agency's salt reduction programme. *Public Health Nutr.* 2012;15(2):254–261.
81. He FJ, Brinsden HC, MacGregor GA. Salt reduction in the United Kingdom: a successful experiment in public health. *J Hum Hypertens.* 2014;28(6):345.
82. Bellisle F. Glutamate and the UMAMI taste: sensory, metabolic, nutritional and behavioural considerations. A review of the literature published in the last 10 years. *Neurosci Biobehav Rev.* 1999;23(3):423–438. doi:S0149-7634(98)00043-8.
83. Nelson G, Chandrashekar J, Hoon MA, et al. An amino-acid taste receptor. *Nature.* 2002;416(6877):199–202. https://doi.org/10.1038/nature726nature726.
84. Bellisle F, Monneuse MO, Chabert M, Larue-Achagiotis C, Lanteaume MT, Louis-Sylvestre J. Monosodium glutamate as a palatability enhancer in the European diet. *Physiol Behav.* 1991;49(5):869–873. doi:0031-9384(91)90196-U.
85. Roininen K, Lahteenmaki L, Tuorila H. Effect of umami taste on pleasantness of low-salt soups during repeated testing. *Physiol Behav.* 1996;60(3):953–958. S0031938496000984.
86. Okiyama A, Beauchamp GK. Taste dimensions of monosodium glutamate (MSG) in a food system: role of glutamate in young American subjects. *Physiol Behav.* 1998;65(1):177–181. S0031-9384(98)00160-7.
87. Schiffman SS. Intensification of sensory properties of foods for the elderly. *J Nutr.* 2000;130(4S suppl l), 927S-30S http://www.ncbi.nlm.nih.gov/entrez/query.fcgi?cmd=Retrieve&db=PubMed&dopt=Citation&list_uids=10736354.
88. Ball P, Woodward D, Beard T, Shoobridge A, Ferrier M. Calcium diglutamate improves taste characteristics of lower-salt soup. *Eur J Clin Nutr.* 2002;56(6):519–523. https://doi.org/10.1038/sj.ejcn.1601343.
89. Carter BE, Monsivais P, Drewnowski A. The sensory optimum of chicken broths supplemented with calcium di-glutamate: a possibility for reducing sodium while maintaining taste. *Food Qual Prefer.* 2011;22(7). https://doi.org/10.1016/j.foodqual.2011.05.003.
90. Beyreuther K, Biesalski HK, Fernstrom JD, et al. Consensus meeting: monosodium glutamate—an update. *Eur J Clin Nutr.* 2007;61(3):304.
91. Jinap S, Hajeb P. Glutamate. Its applications in food and contribution to health. *Appetite.* 2010;55(1):1–10.
92. Kurihara K. Glutamate: from discovery as a food flavor to role as a basic taste (umami). *Am J Clin Nutr.* 2009;90(3):719S–722S.
93. Luscombe-Marsh ND, Smeets AJ, Westerterp-Plantenga MS. Taste sensitivity for monosodium glutamate and an increased liking of dietary protein. *Br J Nutr.* 2008;99(4):904–908. https://doi.org/10.1017/S000711450788295X.
94. Rogers PJ, Blundell JE. Umami and appetite: effects of monosodium glutamate on hunger and food intake in human subjects. *Physiol Behav.* 1990;48(6):801–804. http://www.ncbi.nlm.nih.gov/entrez/query.fcgi?cmd=Retrieve&db=PubMed&dopt=Citation&list_uids=2087510.
95. Bellisle F. Experimental studies of food choices and palatability responses in European subjects exposed to the Umami taste. *Asia Pac J Clin Nutr.* 2008;17(suppl 1):376–379. http://www.ncbi.nlm.nih.gov/entrez/query.fcgi?cmd=Retrieve&db=PubMed&dopt=Citation&list_uids=18296383.
96. Luscombe-Marsh ND, Smeets AJ, Westerterp-Plantenga MS. The addition of monosodium glutamate and inosine monophosphate-5 to high-protein meals: effects on satiety, and energy and macronutrient intakes. *Br J Nutr.* 2009:1–9. https://doi.org/10.1017/S0007114509297212.
97. Carter Monsivais P, Perrigue MP, Drewnowski ABE. Supplementing chicken broth with monosodium glutamate reduces hunger and desire to snack but does not affect energy intake in women. *Br J Nutr.* 2011. https://doi.org/10.1017/S0007114511001759.
98. Anderson GH, Fabek H, Akilen R, Chatterjee D, Kubant R. Acute effects of monosodium glutamate addition to whey protein on appetite, food intake, blood glucose, insulin and gut hormones in healthy young men. *Appetite.* 2018;120:92–99.
99. Shi Z, Luscombe-Marsh ND, Wittert GA, et al. Monosodium glutamate is not associated with obesity or a greater prevalence of weight gain over 5 years: findings from the Jiangsu Nutrition Study of Chinese adults. *Br J Nutr.* 2010;104(3):457–463. https://doi.org/10.1017/S0007114510000760.
100. Essed NH, van Staveren WA, Kok FJ, de Graaf C. No effect of 16 weeks flavor enhancement on dietary intake and nutritional status of nursing home elderly. *Appetite.* 2007;48(1):29–36. https://doi.org/10.1016/j.appet.2006.06.002.
101. Kondoh T, Torii K. MSG intake suppresses weight gain, fat deposition, and plasma leptin levels in male Sprague-Dawley rats. *Physiol Behav.* 2008;95(1–2):135–144. https://doi.org/10.1016/j.physbeh.2008.05.010.
102. Hermanussen M, Garcia AP, Sunder M, Voigt M, Salazar V, Tresguerres JA. Obesity, voracity, and short stature: the impact of glutamate on the regulation of appetite. *Eur J Clin Nutr.* 2006;60(1):25–31. https://doi.org/10.1038/sj.ejcn.1602263.
103. Hirata AE, Andrade IS, Vaskevicius P, Dolnikoff MS. Monosodium glutamate (MSG)-obese rats develop glucose intolerance and insulin resistance to peripheral glucose uptake. *Braz J Med Biol Res.* 1997;30(5):671–674. http://www.ncbi.nlm.nih.gov/entrez/query.fcgi?cmd=Retrieve&db=PubMed&dopt=Citation&list_uids=9283637.
104. He K, Zhao L, Daviglus ML, et al. Association of monosodium glutamate intake with overweight in Chinese adults: the INTERMAP Study. *Obes (Silver Spring).* 2008;16(8):1875–1880. https://doi.org/10.1038/oby.2008.274.
105. Schiffman SS, Graham BG, Sattely-Miller EA, Warwick ZS. Orosensory perception of dietary fat. *Curr Dir Psychol Sci.* 1998;7(5):137–143.
106. Mattes RD. Is there a fatty acid taste? *Annu Rev Nutr.* 2009;29(1):305–327. https://doi.org/10.1146/annurev-nutr-080508-141108.
107. Gilbertson TA, Liu L, Kim I, Burks CA, Hansen DR. Fatty acid responses in taste cells from obesity-prone and -resistant rats. *Physiol Behav.* 2005;86(5):681–690. https://doi.org/10.1016/j.physbeh.2005.08.057.
108. Khan NA, Besnard P. Oro-sensory perception of dietary lipids: new insights into the fat taste transduction. *Biochim Biophys Acta Mol Cell Biol Lipids.* 2009;1791(3):149–155. http://www.sciencedirect.com/science/article/B6VNN-4VCNPBV-2/2/50aa6372c4186aaa86bf7fff09551127.
109. Besnard P, Passilly-Degrace P, Khan NA. Taste of fat: a sixth taste modality? *Physiol Rev.* 2015;96(1):151–176.
110. Cooling J, Blundell J. Are high-fat and low-fat consumers distinct phenotypes? Differences in the subjective and behavioural response to energy and nutrient challenges. *Eur J Clin Nutr.* 1998;52(3):193–201. http://www.ncbi.nlm.nih.gov/entrez/query.fcgi?cmd=Retrieve&db=PubMed&dopt=Citation&list_uids=9537305.

111. Yokum S, Stice E. Weight gain is associated with changes in neural response to palatable food tastes varying in sugar and fat and palatable food images: a repeated-measures fMRI study. *Am J Clin Nutr.* 2019;110(6):1275–1286.
112. Romieu I, Dossus L, Barquera S, et al. Energy balance and obesity: what are the main drivers? *Cancer Causes Control.* 2017;28(3): 247–258.
113. Holt SH, Miller JC, Petocz P, Farmakalidis E. A satiety index of common foods. *Eur J Clin Nutr.* 1995;49(9):675–690. http://www.ncbi.nlm.nih.gov/entrez/query.fcgi?cmd=Retrieve&db=PubMed&dopt=Citation&list_uids=7498104.
114. Erlanson-Albertsson C. How palatable food disrupts appetite regulation. *Basic Clin Pharmacol Toxicol.* 2005;97(2):61–73.
115. Green SM, Burley VJ, Blundell JE. Effect of fat- and sucrose-containing foods on the size of eating episodes and energy intake in lean males: potential for causing overconsumption. *Eur J Clin Nutr.* 1994;48(8):547–555. http://www.ncbi.nlm.nih.gov/entrez/query.fcgi?cmd=Retrieve&db=PubMed&dopt=Citation&list_uids=7956999.
116. Blundell JE, Burley VJ, Cotton JR, Lawton CL. Dietary fat and the control of energy intake: evaluating the effects of fat on meal size and postmeal satiety. *Am J Clin Nutr.* 1993;57(5 Suppl):772S–777S. Discussion 777S–778S http://www.ncbi.nlm.nih.gov/entrez/query.fcgi?cmd=Retrieve&db=PubMed&dopt=Citation&list_uids=8475895.
117. Clydesdale FM. Color as a factor in food choice. *Crit Rev Food Sci Nutr.* 1993;33(1):83–101.
118. Brug J, Tak NI, te Velde SJ, Bere E, de Bourdeaudhuij I. Taste preferences, liking and other factors related to fruit and vegetable intakes among schoolchildren: results from observational studies. *Br J Nutr.* 2008;99(suppl 1):S7–S14. https://doi.org/10.1017/S0007114508892458.
119. Aldridge V, Dovey TM, Halford JCG. The role of familiarity in dietary development. *Dev Rev.* 2009;29(1):32–44. http://www.sciencedirect.com/science/article/B6WDH-4V5NT2K-1/2/3f1aaafc39dbf16175cdf83facfc3c73.
120. Leshem M, Abutbul A, Eilon R. Exercise increases the preference for salt in humans. *Appetite.* 1999;32(2):251–260.
121. Berthoud H-R, Zheng H. Modulation of taste responsiveness and food preference by obesity and weight loss. *Physiol Behav.* 2012; 107(4):527–532.
122. Faas MM, Melgert BN, de Vos P. A brief review on how pregnancy and sex hormones interfere with taste and food intake. *Chemosens Percept.* 2010;3(1):51–56.
123. Miras AD, le Roux CW. Bariatric surgery and taste: novel mechanisms of weight loss. *Curr Opin Gastroenterol.* 2010;26(2):140–145.
124. Logue AW. *The Psychology of Eating and Drinking.* New York: Brunner-Routledge; 2004.
125. Glanz K, Basil M, Maibach E, Goldberg J, Snyder D. Why Americans eat what they do: taste, nutrition, cost, convenience, and weight control concerns as influences on food consumption. *J Am Diet Assoc.* 1998;98(10):1118–1126. https://doi.org/10.1016/S0002-8223(98)00260-0.
126. Beydoun MA, Wang Y. How do socio-economic status, perceived economic barriers and nutritional benefits affect quality of dietary intake among US adults? *Eur J Clin Nutr.* 2008;62(3):303–313. https://doi.org/10.1038/sj.ejcn.1602700.
127. Lakdawalla D, Philipson T. The growth of obesity and technological change. *Econ Hum Biol.* 2009;v7(n3):283–293.
128. Philipson T. The world-wide growth in obesity: an economic research agenda. *Health Econ.* 2001;10(1):1–7.
129. Cutler DM, Glaeser EL, Shapiro JM. Why have Americans become more obese? *J Econ Perspect.* 2003;17(3), 93(118) http://find.galegroup.com/itx/infomark.do?&contentSet=IAC-Documents&type=retrieve&tabID=T002&prodId=EAIM&docId=A121241855&source=gale&srcprod=EAIM&userGroupName=wash_main&version=1.0.
130. *Americans' Budget Share for Total Food Has Changed Little during the Last 20 Years.* USA: Kansas City; 2019. https://www.ers.usda.gov/data-products/chart-gallery/gallery/chart-detail/?chartId=76967. Accessed December 2, 2019.
131. Monsivais P, Drewnowski A. The rising cost of low-energy-density foods. *J Am Diet Assoc.* 2007;107(12). https://doi.org/10.1016/j.jada.2007.09.009.
132. Monsivais P, Mclain J, Drewnowski A. The rising disparity in the price of healthful foods: 2004–2008. *Food Policy.* 2010;35(6). https://doi.org/10.1016/j.foodpol.2010.06.004.
133. Jetter KM, Cassady DL. The availability and cost of healthier food alternatives. *Am J Prev Med.* 2006;30(1):38–44.
134. Rose D. Food stamps, the Thrifty Food Plan, and meal preparation: the importance of the time dimension for US Nutrition Policy. *J Nutr Educ Behav.* 2007;39(4):226–232. https://doi.org/10.1016/j.jneb.2007.04.180.
135. Davis GC, You W. The Thrifty Food Plan is not thrifty when labor cost is considered. *J Nutr.* 2010;140(4):854–857. https://doi.org/10.3945/jn.109.119594.
136. Chan M. *Statement at the High-Level Conference on World Food Security.* Italy: World Heal Organ Rome; 2008.
137. De Schutter O. The right to an adequate diet: The agriculture-food-health nexus. In: *Rep Present 19th Sess United Nations Hum Rights Counc Geneva, Switz.* 2011.
138. Monsivais P, Perrigue MM, Adams SL, Drewnowski A. Measuring diet cost at the individual level: a comparison of three methods. *Eur J Clin Nutr.* 2013;67(11). https://doi.org/10.1038/ejcn.2013.176.
139. Aaron GJ, Keim NL, Drewnowski A, Townsend MS. Estimating dietary costs of low-income women in California: a comparison of 2 approaches. *Am J Clin Nutr.* 2013;97(4):835–841.
140. Orr JB. *Food Health and Income: Report on a Survey of Adequacy of Diet in Relation to Income.* London: Macmillan and Company Limited; 1937.
141. James WP, Nelson M, Ralph A, Leather S. Socioeconomic determinants of health. The contribution of nutrition to inequalities in health. *BMJ.* 1997. https://doi.org/10.1136/bmj.314.7093.1545.
142. Monsivais P, Aggarwal A, Drewnowski A. Are socio-economic disparities in diet quality explained by diet cost? *J Epidemiol Community Health.* 2012;66(6). https://doi.org/10.1136/jech.2010.122333.
143. Aggarwal A, Monsivais P, Cook AJ, Drewnowski A. Does diet cost mediate the relation between socioeconomic position and diet quality? *Eur J Clin Nutr.* 2011;65(9). https://doi.org/10.1038/ejcn.2011.72.
144. Monsivais P, Aggarwal A, Drewnowski A. Following federal guidelines to increase nutrient consumption may lead to higher food costs for consumers. *Health Aff.* 2011;30(8). https://doi.org/10.1377/hlthaff.2010.1273.
145. Aggarwal A, Monsivais P, Drewnowski A. Nutrient intakes linked to better health outcomes are associated with higher diet costs in the US. *PLoS One.* 2012;7(5). https://doi.org/10.1371/journal.pone.0037533.
146. Timmins KA, Hulme C, Cade JE. The monetary value of diets consumed by British adults: an exploration into sociodemographic differences in individual-level diet costs. *Public Health Nutr.* 2015;18(1):151–159.
147. Morris MA, Hulme C, Clarke GP, Edwards KL, Cade JE. What is the cost of a healthy diet? Using diet data from the UK Women's Cohort Study. *J Epidemiol Community Health.* 2014;68(11): 1043–1049.
148. Jones NR, Tong TY, Monsivais P. Meeting UK dietary recommendations is associated with higher estimated consumer food costs: an analysis using the National Diet and Nutrition Survey and consumer expenditure data, 2008–2012. *Public Health Nutr.* 2017. https://doi.org/10.1017/S1368980017003275.

149. Rehm CD, Monsivais P, Drewnowski A. The quality and monetary value of diets consumed by adults in the United States. *Am J Clin Nutr.* 2011;94(5). https://doi.org/10.3945/ajcn.111.015560.
150. Rehm CD, Monsivais P, Drewnowski A. Relation between diet cost and healthy eating index 2010 scores among adults in the United States 2007–2010. *Prev Med.* 2015;73. https://doi.org/10.1016/j.ypmed.2015.01.019.
151. Monsivais P, Rehm CD, Drewnowski A. The DASH diet and diet costs among ethnic and racial groups in the United States. *JAMA Intern Med.* 2013;173(20). https://doi.org/10.1001/jamainternmed.2013.9479.
152. Monsivais P, Scarborough P, Lloyd T, et al. Greater accordance with the dietary approaches to stop hypertension dietary pattern is associated with lower diet-related greenhouse gas production but higher dietary costs in the United Kingdom. *Am J Clin Nutr.* 2015;102(1). https://doi.org/10.3945/ajcn.114.090639.
153. Conklin AI, Monsivais P, Khaw K-T, Wareham NJ, Forouhi NG. Dietary diversity, diet cost, and incidence of type 2 diabetes in the United Kingdom: a prospective cohort study. *PLoS Med.* 2016;13(7). https://doi.org/10.1371/journal.pmed.1002085.
154. Lopez CN, Martinez-Gonzalez MA, Sanchez-Villegas A, Alonso A, Pimenta AM, Bes-Rastrollo M. Costs of Mediterranean and western dietary patterns in a Spanish cohort and their relationship with prospective weight change. *J Epidemiol Community Health.* 2009;63(11):920–927.
155. Goulet J, Lamarche B, Lemieux S. A nutritional intervention promoting a Mediterranean food pattern does not affect total daily dietary cost in North American women in free-living conditions. *J Nutr.* 2008;138(1):54–59.
156. Tong TYN, Imamura F, Monsivais P, et al. Dietary cost associated with adherence to the Mediterranean diet, and its variation by socio-economic factors in the UK Fenland Study. *Br J Nutr.* 2018; 119(6). https://doi.org/10.1017/S0007114517003993.
157. Darmon N, Ferguson EL, Briend A. A cost constraint alone has adverse effects on food selection and nutrient density: an analysis of human diets by linear programming. *J Nutr.* 2002;132(12): 3764–3771. http://www.ncbi.nlm.nih.gov/entrez/query.fcgi?cmd=Retrieve&db=PubMed&dopt=Citation&list_uids=12468621.
158. Andrieu E, Darmon N, Drewnowski A. Low-cost diets: more energy, fewer nutrients. *Eur J Clin Nutr.* 2006;60(3):434–436. https://doi.org/10.1038/Sj.Ejcn.1602331.
159. Drewnowski A, Monsivais P, Maillot M, Darmon N. Low-energy-density diets are associated with higher diet quality and higher diet costs in French adults. *J Am Diet Assoc.* 2007;107(6). https://doi.org/10.1016/j.jada.2007.03.013.
160. Hamrick KS, Andrews M, Guthrie J, Hopkins D, McClelland K. How much time do Americans spend on food?. In: *Americans and Food Choices: Select Research on Time and Diet.* 2012.
161. Anekwe TD, Zeballos E. *Food-Related Time Use: Changes and Demographic Differences.* 2019.
162. Hamrick K. *Americans Spend an Average of 37 Minutes a Day Preparing and Serving Food and Cleaning Up.* 2016.
163. Gustat J, Lee Y-S, O'Malley K, et al. Personal characteristics, cooking at home and shopping frequency influence consumption. *Prev Med Rep.* 2017;6:104–110.
164. Mills S, White M, Brown H, et al. Health and social determinants and outcomes of home cooking: a systematic review of observational studies. *Appetite.* 2017;111:116–134.
165. Jabs J, Devine CM, Bisogni CA, Farrell TJ, Jastran M, Wethington E. Trying to find the quickest way: employed mothers' constructions of time for food. *J Nutr Educ Behav.* 2007; 39(1):18–25. https://doi.org/10.1016/j.jneb.2006.08.011.
166. Devine CM, Jastran M, Jabs J, Wethington E, Farell TJ, Bisogni CA. "A lot of sacrifices:" work-family spillover and the food choice coping strategies of low-wage employed parents. *Soc Sci Med.* 2006;63(10):2591–2603. https://doi.org/10.1016/j.socscimed.2006.06.029.
167. Devine CM, Farrell TJ, Blake CE, Jastran M, Wethington E, Bisogni CA. Work conditions and the food choice coping strategies of employed parents. *J Nutr Educ Behav.* 2009;41(5):365–370. https://doi.org/10.1016/j.jneb.2009.01.007.
168. Davis GC, You W. Not enough money or not enough time to satisfy the Thrifty Food Plan? A cost difference approach for estimating a money, Äìtime threshold. *Food Policy.* 2011;36(2):101–107.
169. Beydoun MA, Wang Y. Do nutrition knowledge and beliefs modify the association of socio-economic factors and diet quality among US adults? *Prev Med.* 2008. https://doi.org/10.1016/j.ypmed.2007.06.016.
170. Lê J, Dallongeville J, Wagner A, et al. Attitudes toward healthy eating: a mediator of the educational level–diet relationship. *Eur J Clin Nutr.* 2013;67(8):808.
171. Acheampong I, Haldeman L. Are nutrition knowledge, attitudes, and beliefs associated with obesity among low-income Hispanic and African American women caretakers? *J Obes.* 2013;2013.
172. Traill WB, Chambers SA, Butler L. Attitudinal and demographic determinants of diet quality and implications for policy targeting. *J Hum Nutr Diet.* 2012;25(1):87–94.
173. Turrell G, Kavanagh AM. Socio-economic pathways to diet: modelling the association between socio-economic position and food purchasing behaviour. *Public Health Nutr.* 2006;9(3): 375–383.
174. Gittelsohn J, Anliker JA, Sharma S, Vastine AE, Caballero B, Ethelbah B. Psychosocial determinants of food purchasing and preparation in American Indian households. *J Nutr Educ Behav.* 2006;38(3):163–168.
175. Konttinen H, Sarlio-Lähteenkorva S, Silventoinen K, Männistö S, Haukkala A. Socio-economic disparities in the consumption of vegetables, fruit and energy-dense foods: the role of motive priorities. *Public Health Nutr.* 2013;16(5):873–882.
176. Monsivais P, Aggarwal A, Drewnowski A. Time spent on home food preparation and indicators of healthy eating. *Am J Prev Med.* 2014;47(6). https://doi.org/10.1016/j.amepre.2014.07.033.
177. Aggarwal A, Monsivais P, Cook AJ, Drewnowski A. Positive attitude toward healthy eating predicts higher diet quality at all cost levels of supermarkets. *J Acad Nutr Diet.* 2014;114(2). https://doi.org/10.1016/j.jand.2013.06.006.
178. Tiwari A, Aggarwal A, Tang W, Drewnowski A. Cooking at home: a strategy to comply with U.S. Dietary guidelines at no extra cost. *Am J Prev Med.* 2017;52(5):616–624.
179. Nelson ME, Hamm MW, Hu FB, Abrams SA, Griffin TS. Alignment of healthy dietary patterns and environmental sustainability: a systematic review. *Adv Nutr.* 2016;7(6):1005–1025.
180. Morris MJ, Beilharz JE, Maniam J, Reichelt AC, Westbrook RF. Why is obesity such a problem in the 21st century? The intersection of palatable food, cues and reward pathways, stress, and cognition. *Neurosci Biobehav Rev.* 2015;58:36–45.
181. Swinburn BA, Sacks G, Hall KD, et al. The global obesity pandemic: shaped by global drivers and local environments. *Lancet.* 2011;378(9793):804–814.
182. Rolls BJ. The role of energy density in the overconsumption of fat. *J Nutr.* 2000;130(2):268S–271S.
183. Mendoza JA, Drewnowski A, Christakis DA. Dietary energy density is associated with obesity and the metabolic syndrome in US adults. *Diabetes Care.* 2007;30(4):974–979.
184. Wang J, Luben R, Khaw K-T, Bingham S, Wareham NJ, Forouhi NG. Dietary energy density predicts the risk of incident

type 2 diabetes: the European Prospective Investigation of Cancer (EPIC)-Norfolk Study. *Diabetes Care*. 2008;31(11):2120–2125.
185. Hartman TJ, Gapstur SM, Gaudet MM, et al. Dietary energy density and postmenopausal breast cancer incidence in the cancer prevention study II nutrition cohort. *J Nutr*. 2016;146(10):2045–2050.
186. Johns DJ, Lindroos A, Jebb SA, Sjöström L, Carlsson LMS, Ambrosini GL. Dietary patterns, cardiometabolic risk factors, and the incidence of cardiovascular disease in severe obesity. *Obesity*. 2015;23(5):1063–1070.
187. Batis C, Rivera JA, Popkin BM, Taillie LS. First-year evaluation of Mexico's tax on nonessential energy-dense foods: an observational study. *PLoS Med*. 2016;13(7):e1002057.
188. Caro JC, Ng SW, Taillie LS, Popkin BM. Designing a tax to discourage unhealthy food and beverage purchases: the case of Chile. *Food Policy*. 2017;71:86–100.
189. Novak NL, Brownell KD. Taxation as prevention and as a treatment for obesity: the case of sugar-sweetened beverages. *Curr Pharmaceut Des*. 2011;17(12):1218–1222.
190. Backholer K, Blake M, Vandevijvere S. Sugar-sweetened beverage taxation: an update on the year that was 2017. *Public Health Nutr*. 2017;20(18):3219–3224.
191. Powell LM, Chriqui JF. *Food Taxes and Subsidies: Evidence and Policies for Obesity Prevention*. New York: Oxford Handb Soc Sci obesity Oxford Univ Press; 2011:639–664.
192. Franck C, Grandi SM, Eisenberg MJ. Taxing junk food to counter obesity. *Am J Public Health*. 2013;103(11):1949–1953.
193. Rayner M. Nutrient profiling for regulatory purposes. *Proc Nutr Soc*. 2017;76(3):230–236.
194. Guidance for Industry: Reference Amounts Customarily Consumed: List of Products for Each Product Category. Rockville, MD. https://www.fda.gov/regulatory-information/search-fda-guidance-documents/guidance-industry-reference-amounts-customarily-consumed-list-products-each-product-category.
195. Drewnowski A, Fulgoni III V. Nutrient profiling of foods: creating a nutrient-rich food index. *Nutr Rev*. 2008;66(1):23–39.
196. Drewnowski A. Defining nutrient density: development and validation of the nutrient rich foods index. *J Am Coll Nutr*. 2009;28(4):421S–426S.
197. Drewnowski A. Uses of nutrient profiling to address public health needs: from regulation to reformulation. *Proc Nutr Soc*. 2017. https://doi.org/10.1017/S0029665117000416.
198. Lehmann U, Charles VR, Vlassopoulos A, Masset G, Spieldenner J. Nutrient profiling for product reformulation: public health impact and benefits for the consumer. *Proc Nutr Soc*. 2017;76(3):255–264.
199. Fulgoni III VL, Keast DR, Drewnowski A. Development and validation of the nutrient-rich foods index: a tool to measure nutritional quality of foods. *J Nutr*. 2009;139(8):1549–1554.
200. Darmon N, Vieux F, Maillot M, Volatier J-L, Martin A. Nutrient profiles discriminate between foods according to their contribution to nutritionally adequate diets: a validation study using linear programming and the SAIN, LIM system. *Am J Clin Nutr*. 2009;89(4):1227–1236.
201. Streppel MT, Sluik D, Van Yperen JF, et al. Nutrient-rich foods, cardiovascular diseases and all-cause mortality: the Rotterdam study. *Eur J Clin Nutr*. 2014;68(6):741.
202. Ni Mhurchu C, Mackenzie T, Vandevijvere S. *Protecting New Zealand Children from Exposure to the Marketing of Unhealthy Foods and Drinks: A Comparison of Three Nutrient Profiling Systems to Classify Foods*. 2016.
203. Rayner M, Scarborough P, Kaur A. Nutrient profiling and the regulation of marketing to children. Possibilities and pitfalls. *Appetite*. 2013;62:232–235.
204. Seidel M, Laquatra I, Woods M, Sharrard J. Applying a nutrient-rich foods index algorithm to address nutrient content of food bank food. *J Acad Nutr Diet*. 2015;115(5):695–700.
205. Vlassopoulos A, Masset G, Charles VR, et al. A nutrient profiling system for the (re) formulation of a global food and beverage portfolio. *Eur J Nutr*. 2017;56(3):1105–1122.
206. INDEX G. *Access to Nutrition Index*. 2018.
207. Drewnowski A. Nutrient density: addressing the challenge of obesity. *Br J Nutr*. 2018;120(s1):S8–S14.
208. Beauman C, Cannon G, Elmadfa I, et al. The principles, definition and dimensions of the new nutrition science. *Public Health Nutr*. 2005;8(6a):695–698.
209. Sturm R, An R. Obesity and economic environments. *CA Cancer J Clin*. 2014. https://doi.org/10.3322/caac.21237.
210. Kearney J. Food consumption trends and drivers. *Philos Trans R Soc B Biol Sci*. 2010;365(1554):2793–2807.
211. Steel C. *Hungry City: How Food Shapes Our Lives*. Random House; 2013.
212. Weaver LJ, Meek D, Hadley C. Exploring the role of culture in the link between mental health and food insecurity: a case study from Brazil. *Ann Anthropol Pract*. 2014;38(2):250–268.
213. Hirvonen K, Bai Y, Headey D, Masters WA. Affordability of the EAT–Lancet reference diet: a global analysis. *Lancet Glob Heal*. 2020;8(1):e59–e66.
214. Rutter H, Bes-Rastrollo M, De Henauw S, et al. Balancing upstream and downstream measures to tackle the obesity epidemic: a position statement from the European Association for the Study of Obesity. *Obes Facts*. 2017;10(1):61–63.
215. Egan M, Penney T, Anderson de Cuevas R, et al. *NIHR SPHR Guidance on Systems Approaches to Local Public Health Evaluation. Part 2: What to Consider when Planning a Systems Evaluation*. 2019.
216. Savona N, Rutter H, Cummins S. *Tackling Obesities: 10 Years on*. 2017.

SECTION B

Nutrition Monitoring, Measurement, and Regulation

CHAPTER

11

PRESENT KNOWLEDGE IN NUTRITION—NUTRIENT DATABASES

David B. Haytowitz[1], *MSc*
Pamela R. Pehrsson[2], *PhD*

[1]USDA-ARS-Beltsville Human Nutrition Research Center, Nutrient Data Laboratory (Retired), Silver Spring, MD, United States
[2]USDA-ARS-Beltsville Human Nutrition Research Center, Methods and Application of Food Composition Laboratory, Beltsville, MD, United States

SUMMARY

Nutrient or Food Composition Databases (FCDB) are developed to provide a source of reference for the many constituents found in the foods consumed by humans. Among the many use of these databases are assessing dietary intake of populations, nutrition research, development of health policy, and nutrition education. In addition, the food industry provides and uses data from these databases for nutrition labeling programs and product development. Data are the result of chemical analysis, calculations, or estimations/imputations. The steps needed to develop a program for the analysis of foods are described in detail. Other sources of analytical data include the scientific literature and work performed at other institutions, i.e., government agencies, trade associations, and food companies. Procedures for evaluating data from other sources are also described. FoodData Central—a resource for FCDB developed and maintained by United States Department of Agriculture and released in 2019—is also described. The chapter concludes with a discussion of future directions for FCDB.

Keywords: Food composition databases; Nutrient analysis; Nutrient databases.

I. INTRODUCTION

Nutrient databases or Food Composition Databases (FCDB) have a long history and were developed to establish representative values for use in dietary assessment and providing dietary guidance to large population groups. They are not suitable for providing a precise estimate of dietary intake by an individual, for example, for use in a clinical study or for giving dietary advice in medical situations. However, they can provide useful estimates in these cases, particularly for planning purposes. Each analysis is a snapshot in time of the composition of a particular food sample. So, if one acquires a sample of the same food several weeks or months later, it may be the same food, but it is not the same sample, and its composition can be very different. Therefore, one cannot rely on a single sampling of a food, but must collect a statistically suitable number of samples, to ensure that one can generate estimates of variability to go along with the mean value. The number of samples required will depend on both the variability of the food and the nutrients within the food. For example, a highly processed food like a ready-to-eat breakfast cereal will require fewer samples than a fresh piece of fruit.

In the future, personalized nutrition would allow one to point a handheld scanner at a food sample and have the complete nutrient profile of the food displayed and stored, and dietary recommendations made based on synchronized personal medical information. Of course, such scanners must be programmed to not include

Present Knowledge in Nutrition, Volume 2
https://doi.org/10.1016/B978-0-12-818460-8.00011-3

inedible components, such as bones, rinds, seeds, etc., which depend on the food or preferences of the person consuming the food. Some seeds are consumed, while others are not. Some people will eat the peel on certain fruits, while others will not. A scanning device will need to look at the entire edible portion of the food, as composition can vary within a food. If the food is scanned in the market, the scanner has to omit any packaging in its measurement. Once such a scanner is built and the sampling problems solved, we may not need nutrient databases. Until then, nutrient databases must be accurate, comprehensive, and representative of foods in the United States (US) food supply, so that scientists, government policy makers, educators, health professionals, and the general public have the required food composition data to make sound decisions in order to meet their diverse needs. New FCDB, with connections to data on specific agricultural information, will also become available, enabling further research.

The production and processing of agricultural commodities constitutes major portions of our global economy as well as human well-being. Nutrient and FCDB are intricately woven into these areas and used for a variety of purposes relating to nutrition and dietetics including nutrition monitoring, research, nutrition and health policy, and education. (Fig. 11.1). Dietitians and researchers use FCDB to provide dietary advice to clients, assessing dietary intake of populations, and designing meal plans for patients as part of a healthcare environment. In addition, the food industry provides and uses data for and from these databases for nutrition labeling programs and product development. Government agencies use these data to determine nationwide estimates of nutrient intake[1,2] and to develop dietary guidelines.[3] These databases contain many compounds found in foods beyond those classically defined as nutrients, such as carotenoids, tocopherols and tocotrienols, menaquinones, flavonoids, and choline metabolites as well as information related to the food samples—or metadata. While some forms of these compounds act as vitamins and are theorized to have potential health benefits, the metabolic roles for others are yet to be determined

In the early 2000s, the World Health Organization (WHO)[5] reported that up to 90% of diabetes, 80% of CHD, and one-third of all cancers could be prevented through physical activity and dietary behaviors. An update issued in 2015 suggested that noncommunicable diseases (NCDs)—cardiovascular diseases, cancers, respiratory diseases, and diabetes—still accounted for 82% of deaths worldwide.[5] While the distribution of diseases may vary globally, it is clear that improving personal nutrition, which depends upon knowing the composition of foods in the diet, along with increases in physical activity, is important in the monitoring and reduction of NCDs.

Agriculture, food production, monitoring, and research in nutrition/health outcomes include the processes behind

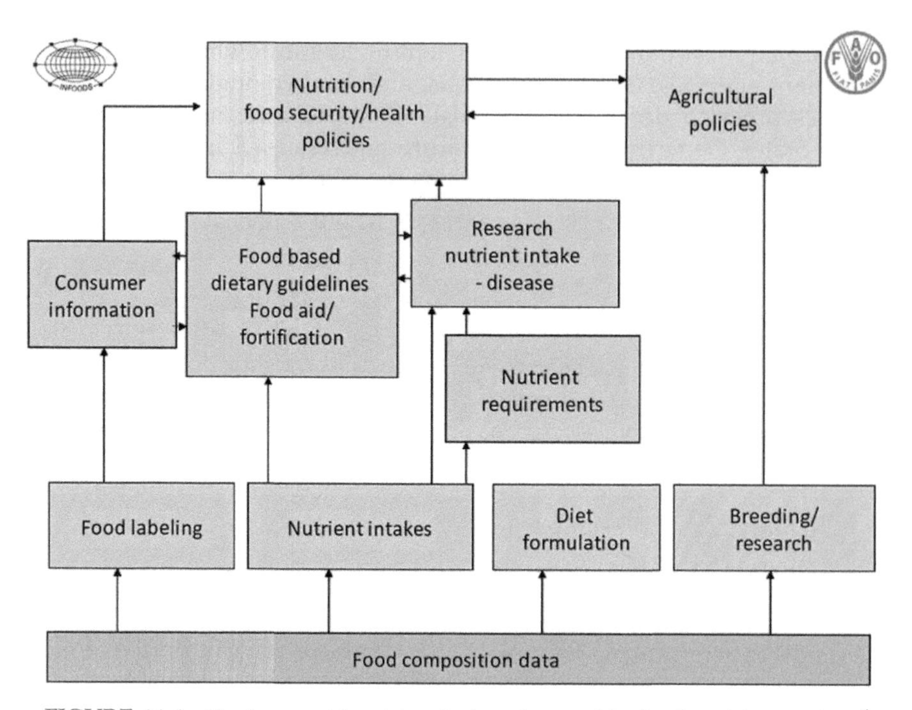

FIGURE 11.1 Food composition data—the base for a multitude of nutrition activities.[4]

the raw materials and processing and food science that connects raw commodities to the wide spectrum of different foods available in the food supply.[6] These processes impact the chemical composition of foods and the determination of the amounts of individual components included in FCDB or tables. The United States Department of Agriculture (USDA) databases are the foundation for other databases, both nationally and abroad; they are used in research, nutrition education, and nutrition monitoring and policies. Food composition database uses are multidimensional, serving not only the above but also as a tool to serve a wide consumer base. FCDB are important in national and world trade, especially considering the diversity of foods now available globally. In addition, commodity-level foods are sold based on specific components and, in some cases, components that may yield information about contamination or adulteration. In many countries, use of dietary supplements has increased significantly, and, since this contributes to nutrient intake, they become an important complement to FCDB. Many standards for acceptance of foods into national and international food supplies have been established, e.g., the USDA School Lunch Program foods (https://www.fns.usda.gov/nslp/national-school-lunch-program-nslp) and many from Codex Alimentarius (http://www.fao.org/fao-who-codexalimentarius/en/), a set of international food standards, guidelines, and codes of practice for globally traded foods.

It is important to consider the limitations present in FCDB, so they may be used appropriately and remain a valuable tool for these applications. Most FCDB are published electronically, though abbreviated versions are often available in hard copy for nonprofessional uses. The development of accurate and comprehensive FCDB is a complex and demanding task requiring knowledgeable scientists and a well-thought-out analytical program, which insures that key research questions are addressed.

II. BACKGROUND

A. Food Composition Tables

With the development of analytical methods to determine the nutrient content of foods during the 1800s, tables of food composition were assembled to meet the needs of the burgeoning science of nutrition and related fields. These early tables included only the proximate components (protein, fat, moisture, and ash)—carbohydrate was determined by difference. Also included was what we now know as crude fiber, which was defined as the nondigestible component of carbohydrates. In 1892, Atwater and Woods[7] published the first table of composition data in the US for 178 food items. 1n 1950, USDA published "Composition of Food—Raw, Processed and Prepared," also referred to as Agriculture Handbook No. 8 (AH-8). This publication was revised and expanded in 1963. Starting in 1976, a complete overhaul of AH-8 began, resulting in 21 sections by food group plus 4 supplements to update and expand previously released tables.

As the files were getting too large for floppy disks or keypunch cards and magnetic tapes were also infrequently used, these were phased out as users moved to personal computers. First available on floppy disks, and more recently CD-ROMs, FCDB are now available for downloading on the Internet.

As each section of AH-8 was released in hard copy, a corresponding release of the USDA National Nutrient Database for Standard Reference (SR) was made available. After 1992 with the last of AH-8 supplements, hard copy updates ceased and all updates to the database occurred with annual updates to SR. These continued through SR28 (2016). Periodically, additional food components were added to the database with subsequent release of the database. Some were made due to changes in the DRI's published by the National Academies, such as different forms of folate. Others, such as choline, were added to meet expanded research interests. The final release of SR was made in 2018 and is known as SR Legacy. A large number of nutrient databases have been developed globally, and, given the complexity of these databases and the resources needed to create them, source databases are most often developed by national organizations affiliated with government agencies. In the US, this activity is hosted at the Beltsville Human Nutrition Research Center, part of USDA's Agricultural Research Service (ARS).

One compilation of food composition database is the *International Nutrient Databank Directory*, developed by the National Nutrient Database Conference.[8] This Directory lists most US databases, as well as a number of international ones, and consists of voluntary submissions from database developers. There is a host of commercial composition databases that use USDA FCDB as their foundations. Another useful international compilation of FCDB developed in other countries is maintained by FAO/INFOODS.[9] Behind each FCDB are database management systems of varying complexity. These are used to generate electronic files that can be downloaded by interested users, who can then query the database to find the information they need. The databases can also be used to create printed reports, though a complete report of a large database may contain thousands of pages and as a result be difficult to use. In these cases, abridged versions of the large databases are available in printed forms that are easier to use.

B. Food Components

The nutrients covered by the various food composition tables and databases have changed over the years. The first tables contained only proximates. Various minerals and vitamins were added as their role in nutrition was identified, and analytical methodology was developed to determine their amounts in various food stuffs. The multivolume version of AH-8 also included data on amino acids and fatty acids. The number of nutrients increased over the years (Table 11.1) as research and public health interest emphasized the need for data on the content of these nutrients in food composition tables and databases.

The definition of fiber also changed over the years, starting out as crude fiber. In 1989, neutral detergent fiber was reported through 1992. Starting in 1990, total dietary fiber by the enzymatic-gravimetric method was reported (AOAC 985.29, 991.43).[10] Nutrient Databases have changed over the years to reflect these shifting definitions and as analytical methods have been developed to accurately determine the amount of dietary fiber in foods as defined.

Sugars are a large category of chemical compounds. For food purposes, the 6-carbon mono- and disaccharides are the most common. Monosaccharides or simple sugars are comprised of glucose, fructose, and galactose. The disaccharides—sucrose, lactose, and maltose,—are made of two of the monosaccharides. Sucrose is made of a molecule of glucose and fructose; lactose is made of a molecule of glucose and galactose; while maltose is composed of two molecules of glucose. For labeling purposes,[11] total sugars are defined as the sum of these mono- and disaccharides.

Folate is a B vitamin found in several forms with differing biological activities. According to the National Academies,[12] naturally present food folate is equivalent to 1 ug dietary folate equivalents (DFE), while added folic acid is equivalent to 0.6 ug DFE. Accordingly, it is necessary to perform these calculations to properly

TABLE 11.1 Nutrients in Food Composition Databases (FCDBs).

Customary nutrients	Less common nutrients/compounds often found in separate databases or publications
Proximates:	Individual amino acids
Moisture (water)	Individual fatty acids
Protein	Individual sugars
Total lipids	
Total saturated fatty acids	
Total monounsaturated fatty acids	
Total polyunsaturated fatty acids	
Carbohydrates	
Starch	
Sugar	
Dietary fiber	
Ash	
Minerals:	
Calcium, iron, magnesium, phosphorus, potassium, sodium, zinc, copper, manganese	Selenium, iodine, aluminum, chloride
Vitamins:	
Thiamin, riboflavin, niacin, pantothenic acid, vitamin, B_6, vitamin B_{12}, folate, vitamin E (α-tocopherol), vitamin K, (phylloquinone)	Folate vitamers, choline and their metabolites, biotin, tocopherols and tocotrienols, dihydrophylloquinone and menaquinones
	Bioactive compounds:
	Flavonoids
	Flavones
	Flavonols
	Flavan-3-ols
	Flavonones
	Anthocynadins
	Isoflavones
	Proanthocyanidins
	Sulphorophanes
	Glucosinolates

report DFE's in the FCDB. In 1996, the US Food and Drug Administration (FDA) published rules requiring the fortification of breads, rolls, noodles, and pasta in order to prevent neural tube defects in newborn infants. In these cases, the added folic acid greatly outweighs the naturally present food folate. However, to generate an accurate value, each amount of each form must be determined and the above calculations performed. The analytical methodology for determining the folate content of foods is complex as it is necessary to extract the folate from the food matrix without destroying it. Various enzymes are used to perform this extraction. The folate is then quantified by a microbiological technique. It is also possible to quantify total folate by an HPLC technique that measures several forms of tetrahydrofolate: 5-methyltetrahydrofolate, 10-formyl folic acid, and 5-formyltetrahydrofolic acid, but outside of government and university research laboratories, this technique is not frequently utilized.

Vitamin K is found naturally in two different forms: (1) phylloquinone in plants and (2) menaquinones in animal products and fermented foods. Phylloquinones are also found as dihydrophylloquinones. Menaquinones have from 4 to 15 additional units in a side chain. Typically, FCDB contain only vitamin K and do not differentiate between the various forms. Furthermore, few labs are experienced in analyzing these forms.

The active form of vitamin E is α-tocopherol,[13] although previously other tocopherols were thought to have vitamin E activity and a value for α-tocopherol equivalents was determined using different factors for each of the tocopherols. Values for the individual tocopherols and tocotrienols are provided in USDA tables, as they have antioxidant activity and other biological roles.

Interest in the choline content of foods arose due to the establishment of a DRI for it in 1998[12] and its role in trimethylaminuria or fish malodor syndrome. This syndrome results from the lack of an enzyme to metabolize choline and results in a strong fish in individuals suffering from this condition. Choline also may have a role in lowering the risk of dementia.[14] There are six choline metabolites: betaine, glycerophosphocholine, phosphocholine, phosphatidylcholine, sphingomyelin, and total choline found in foods.

Starting in the 1990s, research into various chronic diseases focused on the role of oxidizing compounds on cellular health. Concomitantly, interest grew in a class of compounds in foods known collectively as antioxidants. One of the biological roles of a few of the customary nutrients is to act as antioxidants. These include vitamin C, carotenoids—some which contribute to vitamin A, tocopherols, and tocopherols—of which only α-tocopherol contributes to vitamin E activity. Another class of antioxidants are the flavonoids.

While over 5000 types of flavonoids are found in plants, only about 30 are commonly found in food plants. They are:

- Flavonols: quercetin, kaempferol, myricetin, isorhamnetin
- Flavones: luteolin, apigenin
- Flavanones: hesperetin, naringenin, eriodictyol
- Flavan-3-ols: (+)-catechin, (+)-gallocatechin, (−)-epicatechin, (−)-epigallocatechin, (−)-epicatechin 3-gallate, (−)-epigallocatechin 3-gallate, theaflavin, theaflavin 3-gallate, theaflavin 3′-gallate, theaflavin 3,3′ digallate, thearubigins
- Anthocyanidins: cyanidin, delphinidin, malvidin, pelargonidin, peonidin, petunidin
- Isoflavones: daidzein, genistein, glycitein, and total isoflavones
- Proanthocyanidin: dimers, trimers, 4–6 mers (tetramers, pentamers, and hexamers), 7–10 mers (heptamers, octamers, nonamers, and decamers), and polymers (dp > 10)

USDA has published three different Special Interest Databases starting in the 1990s,[15–17] which have focused on these compounds.

C. Available Databases

New technology in database management is crucial to streamline data flow, analysis, and dissemination in production of timely and accurate databases for researchers and other users. At USDA, this resulted in the development of a completely new system, FoodData Central (FDC),[1] which was launched in April 2019 (Fig. 11.2).

FoodData Central puts five different FCDB maintained at the Beltsville Human Nutrition Research Center under one integrated web site; two of these databases have been hosted at BHNRC for many years: SR Legacy and the Food and Nutrient Database for Dietary Studies (FNDDS).[18] SR has been hosted at USDA for over 30 years and has covered many foods, including key foods, in the US food supply—up to 150 components and analytical, calculated, imputed data, with the latter based on linear programming tools and label information and similar foods. FNDDS is the dietary component ("What We Eat in America") of the National Health and Nutrition Examination Survey (NHANES). For this database, among other sources and recipes, nutrient data from SR for foods and beverages in WWEIA, NHANES

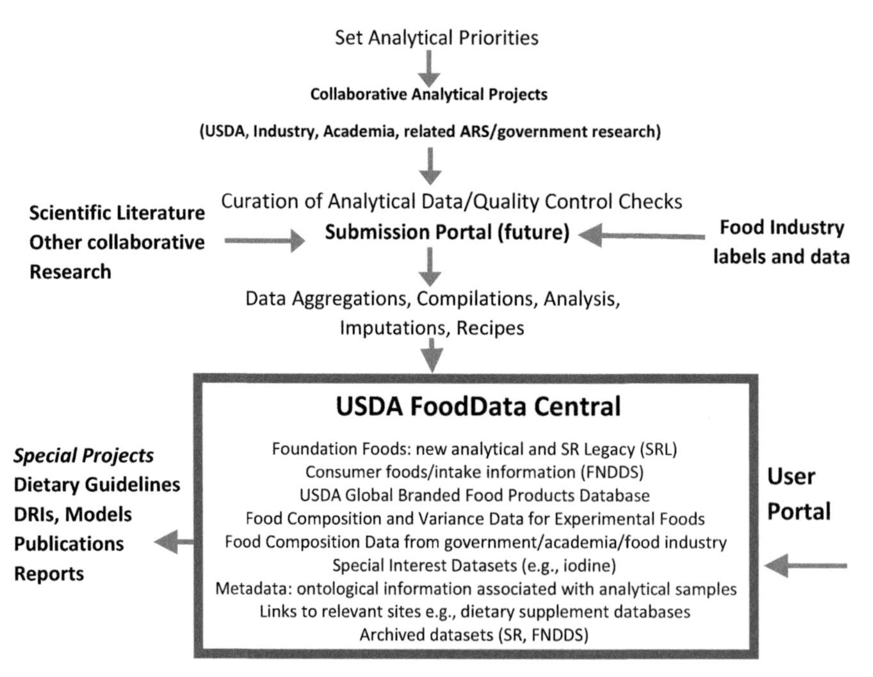

FIGURE 11.2 USDA FoodData central: data and information flow.

are converted into gram amounts and their nutrient values determined. FNDDS is updated and released every 2 years prior to release of WWEIA, NHANES, and it includes food/beverage descriptions, mainly generic, for ~9000 items, food/beverage portions and weight—40,000+ portions in grams; food energy; and 64 nutrients. The USDA Global Branded Food Products Database (BFPDB) is a more recent addition, launched in 2016 as the result of a public–private partnership and is detailed below. Each of these data types is unique and was developed to meet specific needs. For example, the data in the FNDDS make it possible for researchers to conduct enhanced analyses of dietary intakes reported in the NHANES. FoodData Central adds two new types of data that are grouped under the categories: (1) "Foundation Foods" provides expanded nutrient information and extensive underlying metadata that will help users understand the variability in the nutrient values of foods and (2) "Experimental Foods" links to data about foods produced by agricultural researchers that will allow users to see for themselves how factors such as climate, soils, and agricultural practices can affect a food's nutritional profile. The latter foods, grown under experimental conditions, are not necessarily available to consumers.

In order to provide a complete assessment of nutrient intakes, one must include dietary supplements. USDA has worked with the Office of Dietary Supplements (ODS) and National Institutes of Health (NIH)—who host these databases—to develop the Dietary Supplement Ingredient Database (DSID) (https://dsid.usda.nih.gov/), which is based on the analyses of various dietary supplements. A companion database is the Dietary Supplement Label Database (DSLD) (http://dsld.nlm.nih.gov/dsld/index.jsp), which is a compilation of data taken from the supplements fact panels on each package. The DSID was developed by USDA in collaboration with the ODS and other federal agencies and provides estimated levels of ingredients in dietary supplement product categories commonly sold in the US. These statistically predicted estimates may differ from labeled amounts and are based on chemical analysis of nationally representative products. The DSLD contains information from the labels of approximately 76,000 dietary supplement products available in the US marketplace. In addition to a list of the contents and other added ingredients (such as fillers, binders, and flavorings), the DSLD includes information such as directions for use, health-related claims, and cautions.

III. SOURCES OF DATA AND DATA TYPES

The sources of food composition data are varied and include sponsored contracts, data from the food industry, scientific literature, other government agencies, and data generated by calculations (e.g., standard factors [energy calculations, nitrogen-to-protein conversion, and calculations of missing values], and recipes and formulations). Early food composition tables were often based on the efforts of a single scientist or organization that performed all the analyses in their own laboratories. This may still occur in the case of emerging nutrients where a limited number of scientists have the knowledge and resources to properly analyze the compound in question.

As interest in a compound grows, other scientists use and often modify the methodology developed by the first scientist and publish additional manuscripts. The resulting manuscripts can then be assembled into a more comprehensive table and/or database.

While some national databases may be comprised from data solely from analyses conducted in one lab or in conjunction with affiliated labs, most do not have the resources to analyze all foods in their database for all nutrients on a regular schedule. Therefore, most use a hybrid approach combining data from their own or affiliated labs, contracts with commercial labs, data from the scientific literature, and reports generated by government agencies, food companies, and trade associations.

A. Contracts

If an organization developing and maintaining an FCDBB does not have analytical laboratories of their own or wants to analyze a food compound, for which they do not have the necessary expertise or equipment, contracts can be utilized to perform the analyses at either commercial laboratories or by agreements with university scientists. Starting in the 1970s, USDA, in addition to published data from the scientific literature, began to obtain data for its food composition tables from contracts.

In order to design an analytical program to support the development of an FCDB, the following set of steps should be followed:

1) Identify foods and critical nutrients for sampling and analysis;
2) Evaluate existing data for scientific quality;
3) Devise and implement a probability-based national sampling plan or food-specific sampling plan (e.g., crop growing areas);
4) Analyze sampled foods in-house or under supervised laboratory contracts; and
5) Compile newly generated data to update FCDB.

In 1997, USDA's Nutrient Data Laboratory (NDL) used these steps to develop a comprehensive food analysis program, known as the National Food and Nutrient Analysis Program (NFNAP) with support from a number of Institutes within the NIH, and later the FDA and the Centers for Disease Control and Prevention.

Identify foods and critical nutrients for sampling and analysis

Existing food composition and food consumption data can be used to identify and prioritize foods and nutrients for analysis.[19,20] For example, the USDA Key Foods are those foods, which in aggregate, that contri bute 75% of the nutrient intake for selected nutrients of public health importance from the diet.

The latest Key Foods list was generated using weighted two-day food consumption data from the NHANES 2013–14 Data Files[18] and food composition data from SR26 (2013). The Key Foods approach allows an organization to concentrate analytical resources on those foods that contribute significant amounts of nutrients of public health interest to the diet.

Evaluate existing data for scientific quality

At the initiation of NFNAP in 1997, the food composition values in SR were reviewed for scientific quality by NDL staff. Data for many of the foods in the database at that time were found to be more than 10 year old and based on a limited number of values, lacked complete and accurate documentation, and included some samples of uncertain origin. To assess the quality of existing data and to improve the level of documentation, NDL scientists developed an expert system for evaluating data quality.[21,22] See Section V for more details. Many of the food profiles in the database were found to be missing all or some of the information that would permit expert system evaluation of the data. For these reasons, and to establish a core set of data of known sampling, analytical methodology, and quality control (QC), it was determined that a comprehensive update of the food items on the Key Foods list would be needed.

Devise and implement a probability-based sampling survey of US foods

A probability-proportional-to-size food sampling plan was developed by NDL staff in collaboration with statisticians from the USDA National Agricultural Statistics Service based on a stratified three-stage design using 2010 Census Bureau projected state population sizes and census regions.[23] Forty-eight geographically dispersed counties were selected at the first stage, pickup locations at the second stage, and specific food products at the third stage. Subsets of these locations can be selected according to the requirements of the specific food item and nutrients. For example, nutrients with greater variability, such as fluoride, would be sampled in more locations. Another consideration in designing the sampling strategy was that fewer samples would be analyzed for lower consumption foods as identified during the Key Foods process or for nutrients found at lower concentrations. Details of the sampling design are discussed in Perry et al. [24] Pickup locations will depend on the nature of the food sample. Agricultural commodities can be procured at the farm or processing facility, which could be packing plant or slaughterhouse. Retail products can be purchased at a supermarket or restaurant.

Once food items are identified using the Key Foods approach, it was necessary to further refine the specific food items to be sampled and analyzed. For brand name products, a sampling approach utilizing market share information was used. For example, after examining the Key Foods list, it was determined that pizza was a major contributor of many nutrients. However, the SR Link file in the FNDDS did not differentiate between pizzas purchased from a fast food pizza restaurant versus those purchased frozen and heated and served at home. Consequently, both types were sampled and analyzed. Several different types (e.g., cheese, pepperoni, pepperoni and sausage, and meat/vegetable combinations) and brands (e.g., major national brands and store brands) were purchased in supermarkets as described above. Later, several different types (e.g., cheese, pepperoni, and deluxe) of fast food restaurant pizza from major national chains were purchased from individual restaurants.

For commodity foods, samples can be picked up at retail outlets in the locations described above. However, to better link samples and analytical results to agricultural practices, a different sampling approach is needed. This would identify specific cultivars and major growing areas. This way such information as weather, soil conditions, and other agricultural practices such as fertilization and irrigation can also be collected. For meats, information on breed and feeding regimes can be collected. As a result, to better capture the variability inherent in these foods, a greater breadth of sampling is required than those that would be adequate for a retail product manufactured in one or two processing plants.

The sampling plan can be modified to meet the requirements of specific studies, e.g., the sampling of drinking water in homes to analyze fluoride. It can also be used for special population groups who may be located in geographically distinct areas (e.g., American Indians and Alaska Natives on reservations, and Hispanic Americans).[24]

Foods were purchased under contract by a USDA-directed professional product pickup company using tested selection protocols in retail outlets.[25] Commodities such as fresh fruits and vegetables, along with various meats and seafood, can be purchased at retail outlets or obtained at the point-of-harvest, catch, or slaughter. At this point, specific information on the food sampled, such as the postal or GPS coordinates of the sampling location, along with specific cultivar and breed, part of the plant or animal, for commodity foods is collected. The foods were shipped to the Food Analysis Laboratory Control Center (FALCC) at Virginia Polytechnic Institute and State University in Blacksburg, Virginia, for sample preparation. For brand name products, food labels are also retained, and the complete descriptive information, such as full name, ingredients, nutrition facts, and UPC codes, can be entered into a database for eventual matching with the analytical results. Procedures were developed for sample unit receipt, preparation, and storage, which can be modified as needed for new food samples. FALCC continuously develops protocols for homogenizing and compositing samples based on instructions from NDL, collects relevant weights and dissection information for edible and nonedible portions as required, and documents processing and preparation procedures. Processed samples are shipped to qualified, analytical laboratories for analysis as directed by NDL. Reserve and archive samples of each food are maintained at FALCC.

Analyze sampled foods under USDA-supervised laboratory contracts

Most analytical values in nutrient databases were determined by the Official Methods of Analysis of AOAC International[10] or equivalent. AOAC utilizes the contributions of the worldwide scientific community to develop standards and methods and conduct a systematic evaluation and review of methods. As many analysts may make slight modifications to these methods and commercial laboratories establish their own Standard Operating Procedures, it is vital to make sure the modification does not appreciably change the results from the published method. Commercial laboratories must also validate the method for use within their facility and ensure that employees are properly trained in the performance of particular method and that they follow good laboratory practices.

While robust methods exist for proximate components, mineral and vitamins, there are exceptions. For example, as described above, a definition and method for determining dietary fiber has been sought for decades. While it appears that the scientific community has settled on a definition, finding a precise, easy-to-use analytical method remains elusive. For emerging nutrients, such as various bioactive compounds (flavonoids, phenolics, isothiocyanates, and glucokinases), methods have been developed by various researchers and may not have gone through the procedures to be accepted as an AOAC method. To develop a database of these compounds, one must make sure that the analyst is acquainted with the methodology and knows how to modify it for different foods. First, one needs to extract it from the food matrix without destroying the compound being determined. Then one needs to remove any similar compounds that might be extracted at the same time. Finally, the amount in the food is determined.

To ensure that it contracts with laboratories that follow these procedures, NDL employs a two-step process for awarding contracts for the analysis of foods.[26]

Aliquots of each composite are sent to the laboratories by FALCC for analysis according to work plans developed by NDL. Along with the samples, a QC sample is included to be analyzed at the same time as the food samples. For a QC sample, an organization can use certified reference materials (CRMs) such as those developed at the National Institute of Standards and Technology. However, these materials are expensive and may not be available in sufficient quantiles to support a large food analysis program, so the organization should develop their own in-house control composite. While many commercial analytical laboratories have their own in-house samples, it is important for an organization to have an independent set of samples for the comparison of results. The use of both CRMs and in-house materials is an important factor to consider when selecting a laboratory to perform the analyses. The results, including both those for the analytical samples and the QC samples from the laboratories, are then reviewed by a QC committee comprised of experts within an organization as well as those from an outside group. The QC data for CRMs are compared to the certificate values for the material, and the results for control composites are compared to a database of all results obtained for the particular control composites. Any questions about the results are referred to the laboratories for clarification, and, if necessary, the analyses are repeated.

Compile newly generated data to update the composition database

Data from the analytical laboratories are then combined with the descriptive information collected on the sample units and are migrated to USDA food composition database. Previously, data were disseminated in annual releases of the SR database. New data are disseminated through FoodData Central under the rubric of "Foundation Foods." Users can download files for all of the data types hosted at FoodData Central, either individually or as one large file, for use on their own computers. Since many research efforts are connected to FCDB, it is important to capture the metadata attached to analytical samples, the scientific names, the date of harvest or procurement, the date of analysis, sample storage/shipping/handling protocols, preparation/cooking methods, analytical methods by compound studied, etc. Only then can data be accurately tracked in the event of formulation changes, new data, analytical method changes, or replacements and used for data analyses over time. Without precise sample descriptions, as has been a problem in past data, data cannot be connected.

B. Food Industry

Prior to the launch of the USDA BFPDB in 2016, data were also obtained from food companies willing to share data on their food products, which they were having analyzed as part of their nutrition labeling programs, which was required by regulation starting in the early 1970s and updated with the passage of the Nutrition Labeling and Education Act in 1990.[27] FDA then promulgated regulations to implement the Act.[28] However, these data are limited to the approximately 14 nutrients required by the legislation. Many nutrition researchers are interested in vitamins, minerals, and various bioactive compounds not included in the legislation and regulations developed by FDA. These regulations were then modified in 2016[11] and were initially effective in July 2018 for large companies and July 2019 for small companies. The effective dates were then extended to January 2020 and 2021, respectively.

USDA also collaborates with the food industry; trade associations either contract with various companies to sample, prepare, and analyze the food samples or they fund USDA to contract for analyses. Sampling, analysis, and QC protocols must be approved by the USDA or whoever is conducting the study, prior to initiation. Results are then sent to USDA, which evaluates the data and identifies any concerns, and if necessary, repeats the analyses. Once reviewed for QC, nutrient profiles are released in updates to the FCDB.

In 2016, USDA, as part of a public–private partnership with ARS, USDA, International Life Sciences Institute ILSI North America, GS1 US, 1WorldSync, Label Insight, University of Maryland, and Joint Institute for Food Safety and Applied Nutrition released the BFPDB. Initially released in September 2016 at the Global Open Data for Agriculture and Nutrition Summit with over 75,000 food items. At the launch of FoodData Central in April 2019, the BFPDB contained around 280,000 food items at the writing of this chapter. The BFPDB largely supplants data submitted directly by the food industry to be included in SR. Now it stands alone, and similar label databases have been or are being produced in other countries.

Information in the BFPDB is received from food industry data providers and is primarily based on nutrition label declarations. This database also includes ingredient lists for each of the foods; this functionality allows parsing of ingredients into researchable categories, another dimension of the US food supply. In addition, nutrient information is presented on a per serving basis for consumers and a 100-gram basis for researchers and some consumers. Data per serving are presented as both per serving and as % Daily Value. These data are used in consumer education, research studies, and food label regulatory efforts.

C. Literature

A wide variety of manuscripts on the composition of foods are published each year in the scientific literature. Many of these focus on emerging compounds of scientific interest. These include various bioactive compounds, such as flavonoids, glucosinolates, phenolic acids, and lignans. Fewer articles on proximates, minerals, and vitamins are published in developed nations, though many articles on these compounds are published in developing countries on indigenous foods. Manuscripts on emerging nutrients, such as certain trace minerals, e.g., iodine and certain vitamins, particularly lesser known forms, e.g., folate vitamers, choline metabolites, and menaquinones, are also found. Most of these manuscripts are written with a specific research goal in mind and may not necessarily be designed for inclusion in a nutrient database. Consequently, they may be missing certain information that is critical for use in a nutrient database.

One of the most important pieces of information is a complete and accurate food description for each food item in the journal article. Foods that are vaguely named or that have inconsistent or ambiguous descriptive terms will cause confusion for the user and may lead to improper use of the data. Indicating the form of the food, such as raw or cooked; whether ingredients been added such as breading in fried chicken; whether certain parts, that some may consider inedible, but others may not, have been removed will affect the nutrient content of the food, as well as the weight of the portion. Guidelines and methods for describing foods have been developed, and issues related to food descriptions and to the development of descriptive terms have been discussed.[29] It is also critical to properly identify the units of measure, e.g., grams, milligrams, and micrograms as well as the portion size, e.g., cups and pieces including the size and form. A cup of finely diced potatoes will weigh more than a cup of 1″ cubes. Similarly, when describing certain foods, it is necessary to give the dimensions—to properly know the nutrient content of a large apple one needs to know the dimensions applicable to are large apple, compared to a small apple, in order to make proper nutrient assessments.

D. Calculations

A number of calculations are integral to the development of nutrient databases; however, these have limitations. These include (1) protein from nitrogen by the use of factors; (2) calculation of energy from proximate components (protein, fat, carbohydrate, and, when present, alcohol) by the use of factors; (3) carbohydrate by difference; (4) total sugars by the summation of individual sugars; (5) vitamin A in RAE from provitamin A carotenoids; and (6) total saturated fatty acids, total monounsaturated fatty acids, and total polyunsaturated fatty acids by summing the individual fatty acids in each class.

Nitrogen-to-protein conversion factors

These factors were first developed in the 1880s along with the Kjeldahl method, which actually measures nitrogen. At that time, protein was assumed to be 16% nitrogen, which results in factor of 6.25. Jones[30] expanded the factors by looking at the amino acid profile of isolated proteins. However, this approach depended on the degree of purification and the representativeness of that protein to the all proteins found in the food. He proposed different nitrogen-to-protein for some foods, i.e., soybeans, and based on the foods he studied, specific factors were assigned to broad categories of foods. Also, 6.25 was used if a specific factor for a food did not exist. This process did not consider nonprotein nitrogenous compounds (nucleic acids, amines, urea, nitrates/nitrites, nitrogenous glycosides, etc.). Furthermore, specific proteins and amino acids can vary by cultivar and growing conditions. These reasons can result in overestimating protein content. In 2002, an FAO/WHO expert consultation recommended summing amino acids to determine protein content.[31] While summing amino acids to determine protein content could be more precise, protein analysis is much cheaper than amino acid analysis, and this could be an issue in developing countries, where protein malnutrition is more prevalent. Conversion factors, most commonly 6.25, are built into regulations for nutrition labeling in the US and many other countries. The price in trade for many products is based on protein content calculated by these factors; hence, there are many barriers to moving away from the use of the nitrogen-to-protein conversion factors. Including amino acids profiles in nutrient databases will also facilitate the calculation of various measures of protein quality, such as protein digestibility-corrected amino acid score.

Energy factors

The energy content of food is calculated and not measured directly. While bomb calorimetry provides a method for determining the gross energy in a food item, it does not consider that not all the compounds that can be burned in a food can be metabolized. Therefore, to determine metabolizable energy, one must also determine the energy in feces and urine and subtract both from gross energy. This is complicated and time-consuming. Therefore, the data are limited (small sample sizes, short feeding periods, limited foods). It is not possible to use this method to determine the energy content of a single food, as one cannot have human subject consume a diet a just one food, so the factors were derived for mixed diets. The first factors were developed by Atwater in 1896.[7] When specific factors were not available, the generic factors of 4-9-4 for protein, fat, and carbohydrates, respectively, are used. Based on this approach, Merrill and Watt[32] developed energy factors for a wide group of foods, but like nitrogen-to-protein conversion factors, sometimes these factors are fairly specific and other times they cover a large group of foods, such as mature dry beans, cowpeas, peas, other legumes, and nuts or other vegetables (not potatoes and starch roots, other underground crops and mushrooms). These factors, whether the specific Atwater factors or the generic 4-9-4 are also built into nutrition labeling regulations, so like the nitrogen-to-protein conversion factors, there are barriers to changing the approach to calculating food energy.

Total sugars

Total sugars are calculated by summing up individual sugars (sucrose, glucose, fructose, lactose, maltose, and galactose). These are the mono- and disaccharides defined as the constituents comprising total sugar for the purpose of nutrition labeling, yet chemically many other compounds are identified as sugars. To eliminate confusion, USDA has, with the release of FoodData Central in April 2019, renamed this nutrient to "Sugars, Total NLEA." Starting in January 2020, companies will be required to display the amount of added sugars in the food item as part of an overhaul of the Nutrition Facts Panel (FDA, 2016). However, there is no analytical method for determining the quantity of added sugars in a food item. Therefore, food companies will calculate this value based on their formulation for the food item.

Carbohydrate by difference

As there is no direct analytical method for determining total carbohydrates in a food, it is calculated by subtracting the sum of the moisture, protein, fat, ash, and alcohol (if present) from 100. A better method, though more costly, is to calculate carbohydrate by summing analytical values for sugars, starch, and dietary fiber and other carbohydrate fractions. However, there are problems associated with methodology for these constituents. As described above, total sugars only include six mono- and disaccharides. Over the years, the definition of dietary fiber has changed, and multiple analytical methods are accepted for labeling products in the US. While the scientific community has defined dietary fiber as "nondigestible carbohydrates and lignin that are intrinsic and intact in plants," analytical methodology has struggled to keep up. The best current method is the modified enzymatic-gravimetric ("McCleary") method (AOAC 2009.01, 2011.25), but it is complex, time-consuming, and more expensive[33] than the original enzymatic-gravimetric method (AOAC 985.29, 991.43). Both the original and modified enzymatic-gravimetric methods measure a series of extracts and precipitates, which do not identify specific dietary fiber constituents, e.g., cellulose, nondigestible oligosaccharides, beta-glucans, pectin, chitin, inulin, and resistant starch. Knowing the quantity of each of these specific dietary fiber constituents would enable researchers to better identify their role in the maintenance of the microbiome and general health.

Other calculations to fill-in missing values

With the large variety of foods available, it is not possible to properly analyze every food for every nutrient. Therefore, over the years, a number of procedures have been developed to estimate the quantity of a particular nutrient in a food item. While the results from these procedures may not be as accurate as those obtained by direct analysis of samples obtained through a statistically based sampling plan, they can provide estimates appropriate in certain applications, such as large-scale dietary assessment and guidance. The precision of the estimate is dependent on the food item and the nutrient. They would not be appropriate in clinical studies and for individualized dietary advice, particular in medical situations. Some of the approaches used are discussed below.

Assumed zero

This approach is used when a given nutrient is not found in a particular food, such as cholesterol in apples or dietary fiber in beef steak. This occurs when there is no metabolic pathway that would produce the specific nutrient, and it is not added in preparation. For example, while chicken naturally does not contain dietary fiber, if breading is added in preparing fried chicken, the finished product would contain some fiber. Other nutrients such as certain minerals and some vitamins may be found in such low levels that, when measured analytically, they are below the level of detection, and for certain purposes could be assumed to be zero. Of course, with better analytical methods, this nutrient may be detectable and actual result reported.

Another form of the same food

This approach can be used to fill in missing values for one food where you have values for a similar food. For example, missing nutrients for cooked kale could be calculated from raw kale by adjusting for changes in total solids and applying the appropriate nutrient retention factors. Another example would be calculating missing values for butterhead lettuce from leafy green lettuce, again adjusting for differences in the total solids. Since both food items are raw, no retention factors are needed.

Recipes

Complete nutrient profiles or specific missing nutrients for more complex foods can be calculated by using a recipe program. Such programs incorporate many ingredients as well as using yield factors to adjust for changes in total solids and total fat. If a nutrient profile for a prepared ingredient is not available, the recipe program can incorporate both retention and yield factors. For the recipe-based nutrient profile to be calculated properly, full nutrient profiles are required for all ingredients.

Formulations

For many processed foods in order to calculate missing values, one needs to know the ingredients and the quantity used. While the ingredients are listed on the package from highest to lowest amount used, the exact quantities used are proprietary and not available. It is possible to estimate the proportions using linear programming techniques. The program will use the known nutrients in the target food and the nutrients in the nutrient database for each ingredient. Values for the target food can be (1) analytical data; (2) claim on label/serving; or (3) data supplied by the manufacturer. Values taken from nutrition labels may be rounded or otherwise adjusted to reach certain public health goals, such as encouraging people to avoid low-sodium foods or to consume higher amounts of foods with beneficial minerals and vitamins. Therefore, the ingredient proportions calculated by the formulation program may be less reliable. The ingredients listed on the package label may not contain enough specificity to accurately match them with comparable items in the source database. For example, the ingredient list may state "soy flour" but does not indicate if it is full fat, partially defatted, or defatted. The developer could try each one and see which comes up with the best estimate for the known nutrients in the target foods and then use those calculated values for the missing ones.

IV. DATA QUALITY EVALUATION SYSTEM

When using data from diverse sources, a method for ascertaining the quality of the data from each source is needed. USDA developed just such a system[20] that looks at five parameters: (1) sampling plan; (2) number of samples; (3) sample handling; (4) analytical method; and (5) analytical QC. Within this scheme, points are assigned to each parameter based on specific criteria and all are summed to develop a rating score for each food component within a food item. Therefore, authors of scientific papers should include this information in their manuscript. Of course, as mentioned earlier, an accurate and complete food description is critical.

A. Sampling Plan

The sampling plan should be statistically based and incorporate information on food type, cultivar, brand name geographic distribution, and market share. It should also consider the demographics of the population consuming the food in question. The geographic area studied needs to be defined and can be national, regional, or local depending on the food being studied or the sample design must be structured accordingly. Historically, many reported studies relied on a convenience sample obtained from the institution's own experimental or local farms or a nearby retail outlet. This is often inadequate for the purpose of developing a national database. However, if many studies are available within a country or region, the data from each can be aggregated to develop national estimates. It may be useful for many researchers to make the individual estimates available.

B. Number of Samples

Cleary having more individual samples from each location within the sampling plan is preferable. However, funding limitations can restrict the number of samples that can be collected and analyzed. Sometimes compositing samples from many pickup sites within a sampling location or within a region is an alternative, but at the cost of losing variability information on the foods. Again, nutrient data on multiple samples of a food item can be aggregated and univariate statistics generated. Depending on the nature of the food item, these data can be weighted using productions or market share information.

C. Sample Handling

Steps must be taken to insure nutrient stability of the food items between the time they are acquired either in the field or retail outlet and when they are analyzed. Some foods must be prepared by removing inedible parts, or in the case where a cooked food is being analyzed, appropriate procedures must be followed. Additional steps to prepare the sample for analysis, such as drying and homogenization, must be followed and scored.

D. Analytical Methodology

Each food component and food has an optimum method for determining the amount of the specific component in the food. Each analytical method contains processing (extraction, digestion, etc.), identification (detection, limits of detection, percent recoveries), and quantitation steps (limits of quantitation, calibration cures, calculations, etc.), and each must be meticulously performed. Furthermore, the lab conducting the analysis must validate the method within their facility, and each analyst performing the analysis must be trained and demonstrate competence. When using data from many published sources, older methods not currently used may be encountered. While many of these methods can provide accurate methods, it is important to make sure the method yields the specificity required to properly measure the amount of the food component in the food sample.

E. Analytical Quality Control

As day-to-day performance of the analyses can vary, it is essential to include QC materials of known composition along with the test samples. These materials can be developed in-house or purchased from various agencies such as the National Institutes for Standards and Technology in the US (https://www.nist.gov/srm) or the Joint Research Center of the European Commission (https://ec.europa.eu/jrc/en/reference-materials/catalogue). As foods are complex, it is important to select an appropriate QC material that has a similar matrix to the food being analyzed. The rating for this criterion is based on the suitability of the QC material and its frequency of use.

Although not part of the expert system, a compete food description is critical. After all, you can have the best analytical data, but if you do not know the details about the food, it is useless. For example, if you have data on "beef," what cut does it represent, how was it prepared, how was the fat trimmed before cooking, and were any seasonings or other ingredients added during cooking? Another example applies to fruits and vegetables—is it raw, cooked, frozen, or canned? If raw, what was the portion consumed? If cooked, how was it cooked; was anything added during cooking? If canned, was the can drained and only the drained solids analyzed or were the total can contents analyzed. Was it packed in brine, heavy syrup, light syrup, or juice? All of these processing and preparation procedures affect the nutrient content, so it is essential to know what form of the food is contained in your database, so the user can select the item that matches their needs.

V. CONCLUSION

Globally, most food supplies have expanded, diversified, and are far more complex than at any point in human history. In order for a better understanding of the interrelationship between food composition, dietary patterns, genetics, environments, and health, food composition tables must be readily, easily, and affordably accessible and transparent. At the USDA, food composition research and additions to and changes in FCDB reflect the need for more relevant information to connect agricultural practices, commercial and home processing and preparation, food composition, dietary patterns, and health outcomes. In a complicated food supply, which, in recent decades, includes a surge of imported international foods from diverse cultures, organic to genetically engineered crops and crops grown under the impact of climate change, new technologies and agricultural practices, fish farming and changes in animal husbandry, and a complex commercially processed sector of the food industry, the need to discern how nutrient variability is measured is as important as the mean or median amount. Metadata describes the farm to fork information about foods at the agricultural commodity level. For examples, for crop products, genetics of the plant, soil composition, growth and harvest information and dates, fertilizers, organic versus conventional, location (GPS coordinates), shipping and storage information, and any other factors in the supply chain and processing flow. For animal products, this may include breed, feed, age of the animal, animal husbandry practices, etc., which may impact the nutrient profiles of the meat, dairy, or egg products. Tracking this information is essential to analyses of composition as it relates to dietary patterns and ultimately, health outcomes. With new existing software, interconnected information can be joined with other databases, regionally, nationally, and globally to research diet and health.

RESEARCH GAPS

- Keeping up with an ever-changing and complicated food supply
- Improved sampling for commonly consumed foods and ingredients
- Metadata describing the farm-to-fork information about foods at the agricultural commodity level
- Need for more relevant information to connect agricultural practices, commercial and home processing and preparation, food composition, dietary patterns, and health outcomes
- Comprehensive data on emerging food components of public health interest

VI. REFERENCES

1. *U.S. Department of Agriculture, Agricultural Research Service*. FoodData Central; 2019. fdc.nal.usda.gov.
2. National Center for Health Statistics, CDC. *NHANES, National Health and Nutrition Examination Survey*; 2017. https://www.cdc.gov/nchs/nhanes/about_nhanes.htm.
3. U.S. Department of Health and Human Services, U.S. Department of Agriculture. *2015 – 2020 Dietary Guidelines for Americans*. 8th ed.; 2015. December 2015. Available at: https://health.gov/dietaryguidelines/2015/guidelines/.
4. *International Network of Food Data Systems (INFOODS)*; 2017. http://www.fao.org/infoods/infoods/food-composition-challenges/en/.
5. World Health Organization (WHO), Food and Agricultural Organization (FAO). report*Noncommunicable Diseases Fact Sheet*. Updated June 2017. Report of the joint WHO/FAO expert consultation on diet, nutrition and the prevention of chronic diseases. http://www.who.int/mediacentre/factsheets/fs355/en/. Accessed October 27, 2017.
6. Pehrsson PR, Haytowitz DB. *Food Composition Databases in: The Encyclopedia of Food and Health*. Vol. 3. 2016:16–21. https://doi.org/10.1016/B978-0-12-384947-2.00308-1.
7. Atwater WO, Woods CD. *The Chemical Composition of American Food Materials*. Bulletin No. 28. U.S. Department of Agriculture; 1896. Online: https://www.ars.usda.gov/ARSUserFiles/80400525/Data/Classics/es028.pdf.
8. National Nutrient Databank Conference (NNDB). *International Nutrient Databank Directory*; 2018. version 3.10 http://www.nutrientdataconf.org/indd/.
9. International Network of Food Data Systems (INFOODS). *International Food Composition Tables Directory*; 2017. http://www.fao.org/infoods/infoods/tables-and-databases/en/.
10. AOAC International. *Official Methods of Analysis of AOAC International*. 21st ed. 2019 (Rockville, Maryland).
11. U.S. Food and Drug Administration. *Changes to the Nutrition Facts Label*; 2016. https://www.fda.gov/Food/GuidanceRegulation/GuidanceDocumentsRegulatoryInformation/LabelingNutrition/ucm385663.htm.
12. The National Academies of Science, Engineering and Medicine. *Dietary Reference Intakes for Thiamin, Riboflavin, Niacin, Vitamin B6, Folate, Vitamin B12, Pantothenic Acid, Biotin, and Choline*. National Academy Press; 1998. https://www.nap.edu/catalog/6015/dietary-reference-intakes-for-thiamin-riboflavin-niacin-vitamin-b6-folate-vitamin-b12-pantothenic-acid-biotin-and-choline.
13. The National Academies of Science, Engineering and Medicine. *Dietary Reference Intakes for Vitamin C, Vitamin E, Selenium, and Carotenoids*. National Academy Press; 2000. https://www.nap.edu/catalog/9810/dietary-reference-intakes-for-vitamin-c-vitamin-e-selenium-and-carotenoids.
14. Ylilauri MPT, Voutilainen S, Lönnroos E, et al. Associations of dietary choline intake with risk of incident dementia and with cognitive performance: the Kuopio Ischaemic Heart Disease Risk Factor Study. *Am J Clin Nutr*. 2019. https://doi.org/10.1093/ajcn/nqz148.
15. Haytowitz DB, Wu X, Bhagwat S. *USDA Database for the Flavonoid Content of Selected Foods, Release 3.3*. U.S. Department of Agriculture, Agricultural Research Service; 2018. Nutrient Data Laboratory Home Page: https://www.ars.usda.gov/ARSUserFiles/80400535/Data/Flav/Flav3.3.pdf.
16. Haytowitz D, Wu X, Bhagwat S. *USDA's Database for the Proanthocyanidin Content of Selected Foods, Release 2.1*. U.S. Department of Agriculture, Agricultural Service; 2018. Nutrient Data Laboratory Home Page: https://www.ars.usda.gov/ARSUserFiles/80400535/Data/PA/PA02-1.pdf.
17. Bhagwat SA, Haytowitz DB. *USDA Database on the Isoflavone Content of Selected Foods, Release 2.1*; 2015. https://www.ars.usda.gov/ARSUserFiles/80400525/Data/isoflav/Isoflav_R2-1.pdf.
18. U.S. Department of Agriculture, Agricultural Research Service. *USDA Food and Nutrient Database for Dietary Studies 2015–2016*. Food Surveys Research Group Home Page; 2018. http://www.ars.usda.gov/nea/bhnrc/fsrg.
19. Haytowitz DB, Pehrsson PR, Holden JM. Setting Priorities for nutrient analysis in diverse populations. *J Food Compos Anal*. 2000;13:425–433.
20. Haytowitz DB, Pehrsson PR, Holden JM. The identification of key foods for food composition research. *J Food Compos Anal*. 2002;15:183–194.
21. Holden JM, Bhagwat SA, Patterson KY. Development of a multi-nutrient data quality evaluation system. *J Food Compos Anal*. 2002;15:339–348.
22. Holden JM, Bhagwat SA;, Haytowitz D, et al. Development of a database of critically evaluated flavonoid data: application of USDA's data quality evaluation system. *J Food Compos Anal*. 2005;18:829–844.
23. US Census Bureau. *US Census Bureau Population Estimates*; 2001. Version current 2002. Internet: http://www.census.gov/programs-surveys/popest/data/data-sets.2001.html.
24. Perry CR, Pehrsson PR, Holden J. A Revised Sampling Plan for Obtaining Food Products for Nutrient Analysis for the USDA National Nutrient Database. Version current 2003. Internet: http://www.amstat.org/sections/srms/proceedings/y2003f.html (Accessed 03 August 2015).
25. Trainer D, Pehrsson PR, Haytowitz DB, et al. Development of sample handling procedures for foods under USDA's national food and nutrient analysis program. *J Food Compos Anal*. 2008;23(8):843–851.
26. Haytowitz DB, Pehrsson PR. USDA's national food and nutrient analysis program (NFNAP) produces high-quality data for USDA food composition databases: two decades of collaboration. *Food Chem*. 2016;238:134–138. https://doi.org/10.1016/j.foodchem.2016.11.082.
27. U.S. Congress. *Public Law 101–535. Nutrition Labelling and Education Act*. Government Printing Office; 1990. https://www.govinfo.gov/content/pkg/STATUTE-104/pdf/STATUTE-104-Pg2353.pdf.
28. U.S. Food and Drug Administration, Office of Regulatory Affairs. *Guide to Nutrition Labeling and Education Act (NLEA) Requirements*; 1994. https://www.fda.gov/regulatory-information/search-fda-guidance-documents/guidance-industry-food-labeling-guide.
29. Truswell AS, Bateson DJ, Madafiglio KC, Pennington JAT, Rand WM, Klensin JC. INFOODS guidelines for describing foods: a systematic approach to facilitate international exchange of food composition data. *J Food Compos Anal*. 1991;4:18–38.
30. Jones DB. *Factors for Converting Percentages of Nitrogen in Foods and Feeds into Percentages of Protein*. Vol. 83. Circular: US Department of Agriculture; 1941. Slight revision, 1941.
31. World Health Organization of the United Nations. *Joint FAO/WHO/UNU Expert Consultation on Protein and Amino Acid Requirements in Human Nutrition*. Geneva, Switzerland: WHO Technical Report Series 935; 2002.
32. Merrill AL, Watt BK. *Energy Value of Foods: Basis and Derivation, Revised*. US Department of Agriculture, Agriculture Handbook 74; 1976.
33. Phillips KM, Haytowitz DB, Pehrsson PR. Implications of two different methods for analyzing total dietary fiber in foods for food composition databases. *J Food Compos Anal*. 2019. https://doi.org/10.1016/j.jfca.2019.103253.

CHAPTER

12

NUTRITION SURVEILLANCE

Kirsten A. Herrick[1,2], *PhD, MSc*
Cynthia L. Ogden[2], *PhD*
[1]National Institutes of Health, Bethesda, MD, United States
[2]Centers for Disease Control and Prevention, Hyattsville, MD, United States

SUMMARY

Nutrition surveillance includes assessment of physical size and growth (anthropometry), biological samples (e.g., saliva, blood, and urine), and dietary intake. The target group may be individuals, households, schools, communities, or even a nation. Nutrition surveillance serves many purposes: monitoring nutritional status or changes in the food supply, informing changes in policy, and identifying locations or individuals in need of resources. Central to all these functions is collection of timely, relevant, high-quality data and communication of results that lead to action. Common features unite nutrition surveillance; however, implementation can vary widely depending on context. In this chapter, the National Health and Nutrition Examination Survey, a national nutrition and health surveillance system in the United States, is described, as well as examples from five high-income countries—Canada, Japan, South Korea, Australia, and the United Kingdom—three middle- or low-income countries—Mexico, India, and Ethiopia—and two internationally supported household surveys—the Demographic and Health Survey and Multiple Indicator Cluster Survey

Keywords: Australia; Canada; Ethiopia; India; Japan; Mexico; Monitoring; NHANES; South Korea; Surveillance; United Kingdom.

"If you cannot measure it, you cannot improve it." *Lord Kelvin.*

I. INTRODUCTION

Nutrition is critical to health and development. Better nutrition is associated with improved infant, child, and maternal health, better pregnancy outcomes for mothers and babies, increased productivity, and a lower risk of many chronic diseases including diabetes and cardiovascular disease.[1] Despite an extensive evidence base to document these associations, the 2018 Global Nutrition Report showed that progress to reduce malnutrition worldwide has been slow and that some populations face a triple burden from malnutrition (i.e., child stunting, anemia in adult women, and overweight in adult women). Globally, among children under 5 years old, 150.8 million are stunted and 50.5 million are wasted, while at the other end of the spectrum, 38.3 million are overweight.[2] The General Assembly of the United Nations (UN) proclaimed the UN Decade of Action on Nutrition 2016–25 in April at the start of the 10-year period. The announcement marked the beginning of a concerted effort on the part of the Member States to address malnutrition, both under- and overnutrition, globally.[3]

II. DEFINITIONS AND EXPLANATORY RELATIONSHIPS

At the heart of this effort to address malnutrition are data. Data are crucial to identifying the answers to the interrogatory questions that guide action.[4] Data are collected through nutrition surveillance: "the continuous assessment of dietary intake and nutrition status of a population or a selected population subgroup for the purposes of detecting changes and initiating public

https://doi.org/10.1016/B978-0-12-818460-8.00012-5
2020 Published by Elsevier Inc.

BOX 12.1

Objectives of a Surveillance System

- To describe the nutritional status of the population and subgroups within the population.
- To provide information that contributes to the analysis of causes and associated factors and therefore permits a selection of preventive measures.
- To promote decisions by governments concerning priorities and the disposal of resources to meet the needs of both "normal development" and emergencies.
- To enable predictions to be made based on current trends in order to indicate the probable evolution of nutritional problems to assist in the formulation of policy.
- To monitor nutritional programs and to evaluate their effectiveness.

In emergency settings, the objectives specifically focus on:

- Providing a warning system to highlighting an evolving crisis.
- Identifying appropriate response strategies, both food and non-food assistance.
- Triggering a response.
- Targeting areas that are more at risk or in greater need of assistance.
- Identifying malnourished children.

Source: World Health Organization[161]

health action"[5] (see Box 12.1). Nutrition surveillance is multifaceted and interrelated, including assessment of physical size and growth (anthropometry), biological samples (e.g., saliva, blood, and urine), and dietary intake. It can be collected at the individual, institutional, regional, national, and international level. The target group of interest may be an individual, a household, a school, a community, or even a nation. Nutrition surveillance can also be used for a variety of purposes: to monitor nutritional status or changes in the food supply, including contaminants; to inform changes in policy; and to identify locations or individuals in need of resources.

A. Anthropometry

The physical measures used in nutritional surveillance depend on the setting. Because of the high nutritional needs during growth and development, children are often the target of nutritional surveillance, acting as a harbinger of nutritional risks.

Common anthropometric indicators for children birth to 24 months of age include height/length and weight that are used to determine the following: low height-for-age (stunting), low weight-for-age (underweight), and low weight-for-height (wasting), which are routinely used to monitor the burden of nutritional deprivation.[6] In severe situations, such as nutrition emergencies, mid-upper arm circumference may be measured and clinical signs of disease such as kwashiorkor (protein malnutrition), pellagra (niacin deficiency), Bitot's spots (vitamin A deficiency), and scurvy (vitamin C deficiency) may also be used.[7] Often, physical measurements are compared to age and sex-specific distributions from a reference population (usually a growth chart) to assess growth. There are many growth charts available for use. US Centers for Disease Control and Prevention recommends the use of the WHO growth charts for children birth to 24 months of age. In children and adolescents aged 2–19 years, the 2000 CDC growth charts are recommended.[8] For these older children, the 5th and 95th percentiles on the sex-specific CDC body mass index (BMI)–for-age growth charts are used to define underweight and obesity. Among adults, height, weight, BMI, and skin folds are used.

B. Biological Samples

A detailed discussion of biological samples is beyond the focus of this chapter because such assessment is less suitable for large-scale nutrition surveillance. In addition to being invasive and dependent on expensive and elaborate equipment, the interpretation of results is often difficult without additional contextual information.[9] Laboratory assessment can be used to measure both deficiency and excess for a range of macronutrients and micronutrients; however, use is typically limited to high-income countries, and even in this setting, measurement may be periodic and focused only on subgroups of the greatest concern.

C. Dietary Assessment

In general, there are three broad levels that dietary assessment falls into: national, household, and individual. At the national level, assessment tools include food balance sheets, total diet studies, and universal product codes (UPCs) with electronic scanning devices (UPC assessment can be applied at all three levels). Dietary assessment at the household level may include the food account method, household food record, and household 24-hour recall method. Measurement at the individual level may be captured via 24-hour recall, in addition to many other assessment tools, e.g., food frequency questionnaires (FFQs), food records (weighed or estimated), and screeners.[9] National and household level measurements provide per capita estimates.

Dietary assessment at the individual level, rather than national or household, is a critical piece of national nutrition surveillance in many countries. Resources, literacy and numeracy, and final use of the data collected determine which method is best suited to a particular need.[9] For a detailed discussion of dietary assessment instruments to assess individual intake, see the Dietary Assessment Primer[10] or Chapter 14, Assessment of Dietary Intake by Self-reports and Biological Markers.

Below several dietary assessment methods used at the national, household, and individual levels are described:

Tools used for dietary assessment

Food balance sheets; Food balance sheets record a country's food supply over a specified period by considering annual production, changes in stocks, imports and exports, and distribution of food used within the country.[11] Waste arising from farm activities and during distribution and processing is accounted for; however, waste at the household or food service level is not included.[9]

Total diet studies; total diet studies are chemical analyses of food that measure dietary intake of food contaminants, macronutrients, and vitamins by an individual consuming a typical diet.[12] The foods assessed, and methods used to assess them, can be based on market baskets studies, individual food items, and duplicate portions.[9] For example, the US Food and Drug Administration (FDA) monitors over 800 contaminants and nutrients in the diet four times a year by purchasing, preparing, and analyzing about 280 kinds of foods and beverages from four market basket regions in the United States.[12]

UPCs and electronic scanning devices; UPCs and electronic scanning devices capture purchases of canned and packaged foods at retail establishments.[9] This method provides estimates of per capita purchases based on the total population.

The food account method; the food account method is a daily record, typically undertaken by the person responsible for food purchases and preparation in the home. It captures all food coming into the household, whether purchased, received as a gift, or produced, as in a home garden, over a specified time frame. The food account is typically quantified by recording the retail units or household measures of each food item.[9]

The household food record; the household food record can be completed by the individual most knowledgeable about food preparation in the home or recorded by an interviewer. This is an open-ended, self-reported account of all foods and beverages eaten by members of the household. It is typically done concurrently or soon after eating, and the amounts consumed can be either weighed or estimated. Dietary supplements used can also be captured with this method. In addition to measuring food consumed, plate waste can also be collected and subtracted from the amount consumed. The individuals completing the food record are asked to provide detailed information about the methods of preparation used.[9]

Individual food records; individual food records are conducted in a manner like a household food record; however, the individual reports only the foods and beverages they consume rather than the whole household.

The 24-hour; the 24-hour recall is a structured, open-ended interview that captures the type and quantity of food and beverages consumed in the previous 24 h. There is a quick listing of reported foods consumed, followed by probes to elicit details about preparation method and quantity consumed and finally a review with additional probes about commonly forgotten foods. It can be administered by an interviewer, and recently, with advances in technology, can be self-administered via a computer, e.g., the Automated Self-Administered 24-Hour (ASA24) Dietary Assessment Tool.[13] Dietary supplements can also be captured in this tool. It can be administered at both the individual and household level. At the household level, the method relies on the household member responsible for food preparation to remember all foods and beverages consumed in the household in the previous 24-hour period.

The FFQ; the FFQ is a finite list of foods and beverages consumed, which includes response categories to indicate usual pattern of consumption, typically over a month or year. With the inclusion of portion sizes, the tool can be quantitative to indicate the amount in addition to the type of foods consumed. It is typically self-administered and captures information about an individual, rather than a household.

Screeners; screeners are short dietary assessment instruments, which may include questions about dietary behaviors, e.g., "What type of milk do you typically drink?", or it can include questions about a very limited number of foods and beverages. They can be self-administered or interviewer-administered but are generally shorter than an FFQ and ask about a particular aspect of the diet, but not the total diet.

Process of nutrition surveillance

The process of nutrition surveillance is the same irrespective of country context. Data are collected from individuals and then aggregated above the individual level, allowing analysis and interpretation to uncover patterns among groups of individuals. Results are then communicated and disseminated so that public health practitioners can make informed decisions to improve the nutritional status of individuals.[14]

Resources and purpose for conducting nutrition surveillance often differ among high-, middle-, and low-income countries. Nutrition surveillance systems can be complex and expensive, so their implementation can look different depending on the context. Many high-income countries have a dedicated nutrition surveillance system; their primary purpose is to collect data for public health practitioners for monitoring and action. The data collection methods are designed to produce high-quality, valid, nationally representative data. Nutrition surveillance may also capitalize on data collected from administrative sources, such as clinics. In this context, the need for high quality and validity is still present, but the data are not necessarily representative. Thus, a distinction can be made between primary data collection—data collected for the sole purpose of nutrition surveillance—and secondary data collection—data used for surveillance that are initially collected for other purposes, such as administrative (e.g., use of service, distance traveled to find service, etc.).[15]

Primary data for nutrition surveillance may include repeated cross-sectional surveys, data collection at sentinel sites in communities, and data collected about children attending schools. Secondary data may include administrative data from feeding centers or programs, data from health facilities, and data collected in the community in mass screenings.[15]

III. CURRENT STATUS OF FIELD

The National Health and Nutrition Examination Survey (NHANES), a national nutrition and health surveillance system in the Unites States, provides a case study of the many ways that nutritional surveillance data can be used. Drawing on examples from NHANES, the use of nutrition surveillance data is explained. As previously mentioned, nutritional surveillance activities vary widely globally. To highlight this variation, the collection, analysis, dissemination, and use of data collected from a variety of national nutritional surveillance systems are presented. Examples from five high-income countries (Canada, Japan, South Korea, Australia, and the United Kingdom), three middle- or low-income countries (Mexico, India, and Ethiopia), and two internationally supported household surveys (the Demographic and Health Survey [DHS] and Multiple Indicator Cluster Survey [MICS]) are followed by a discussion of current challenges and new directions that are emerging in the field.

A. Nutrition Surveillance in the United States

NHANES is the primary source of nutrition data in the United States; it illustrates both surveillance and action at different levels of the socioecologic framework. An additional resource is from the National Collaborative on Childhood Obesity Research (NCCOR), which maintains a Catalog of Surveillance Systems (https://www.nccor.org/nccor-tools/catalogue/) in the United States. While a detailed description of the many nutrition surveillance systems in the US is beyond the scope of this chapter, the NCCOR catalog provides access to over 100 data sources with information on health behaviors (e.g., diet and physical activity), health outcomes, determinants, policies, and environmental factors.

Nutrition surveillance of early childhood in the United States

Federal dietary guidance efforts at the population level in the United States have been focused at age 2 years and above, primarily due to the lack of high-quality dietary consumption data for infants younger than 2 years.[16] Legislation passed in 2014 mandated that the Dietary Guidelines for Americans 2020–25 include infants younger than 2 years.[17] However, there are considerable research gaps that make meeting this mandate a challenge.

One challenge is a dearth of information about the consumption amount and the composition of human breast milk. For infants fed expressed breast milk, it is possible to capture consumption volume, but for infants fed breast milk at the breast, it can be quite difficult to estimate consumption volume.[18] Additionally, irrespective of feeding mode, data on the nutrient composition of breast milk is lacking.[19] The estimates of nutritional content of human breast milk in the US National Nutrient Database for Standard Reference have been criticized for being outdated and of uncertain data quality.[20] Efforts at the national,[21,22] federal,[19] and international[23] level are underway to help fill the gap surrounding the estimation of the volume and nutrient content of breast milk.

The US National Health and Nutrition Examination Survey

NHANES, conducted by the National Center of Health Statistics, was designed to monitor the nation's health and nutritional status. The precursor to NHANES, the National Health Examination Survey, was conducted in the 1960s and did not include dietary assessment measures. In the early 1970s, dietary assessment and nutrition were added to the survey and the first NHANES was conducted (1971–74). It was a periodic survey until 1999, when NHANES became continuous, releasing data on about 10,000 persons of all ages every 2 years.[24] NHANES is an example of primary data collection (repeated cross-sectional survey) for nutrition surveillance. Of note, NHANES currently collects dietary data, among other measures, on infants younger then 2 years; however, the abovementioned limitations apply, and they hamper the ability of these data to be widely used to inform policy.

NHANES now includes an interview in the home and a subsequent standardized physical exam, including laboratory testing, in a mobile exam center (MEC) (Fig. 12.1). NHANES is designed to be representative of the civilian, noninstitutionalized US population and uses a complex, multistage, probability sampling design to select participants of all ages.[26] Various subgroups may be oversampled in order to obtain reliable and precise estimates of specific concern for these populations.[27,28]

NHANES collects anthropometry (including height, weight, length, and waist circumference, among other measures), dietary intake, and nutritional biochemistries. Dietary assessment in NHANES is conducted with both questionnaires and 24-hour dietary recalls. The questionnaires are not static; between 2-year cycles, questionnaires can be modified to meet research needs, or new questionnaires may be developed and included for a finite time. For example, between 2005 and 2010, NHANES included questions on the use of the Nutrition Facts Label on food products that help inform food buying decisions.[24] NHANES currently also includes a questionnaire on household food security, timing, and introduction of solid foods, food program participation, and a seafood FFQ.

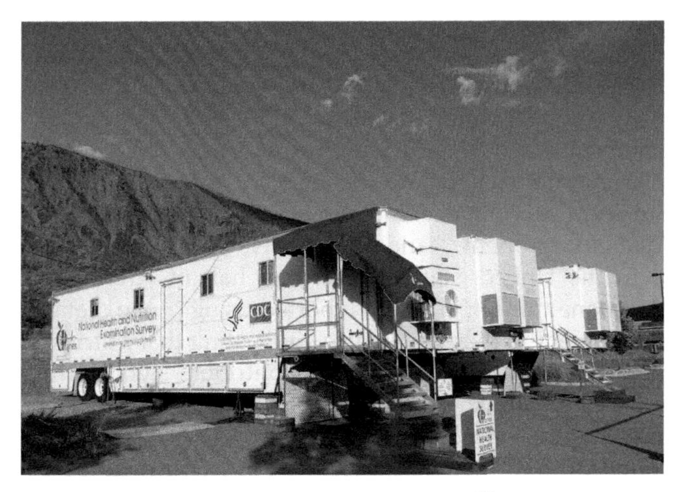

FIGURE 12.1 NHANES Mobile Exam Center.[25] The Mobile Exam Center (MEC) used in NHANES is a mobile, state-of-the-art, medical facility used to measure and collect health data from US participants.

Two 24-hour dietary recalls are collected by trained interviewers, the first during the MEC visit and the second by phone 3–10 days later. Both interviews use US Department of Agriculture's (USDA's) Automated Multiple-Pass Method (AMPM), a computer-assisted dietary interview system with standardized probes[29] that capture the type and quantity of food consumed over the 24 h from midnight to midnight before the interview.

The biological samples collected in NHANES vary over time, depending on funding, research priorities, and feasibility. They include, or have included in the past, blood, urine, hair, and saliva and are used to address research needs relevant to specific age and sex groups.[30–32] Nutritional biochemistries have included iron, sodium, vitamin A, vitamin C, and vitamin D, among others.[33]

Use of NHANES nutrition surveillance data: examples; NHANES plays a prominent role in the development of the periodic Dietary Guidelines for Americans and the assessment of the extent to which different subgroups are following the guidelines.[34] For example, the eighth edition and most recent version, the Dietary Guidelines for Americans 2015–20, included an evaluation of US eating patterns using NHANES data from 2007–2010.[34] Based on the Dietary Guidelines, programs such as MyPlate (Fig. 12.2) have been developed.[35]

NHANES nutrition data help inform national policy development and evaluation. For instance, estimates of sodium intake among infants and toddlers,[37] infants and preschool children,[38] school-aged children,[39] and adults[40,41] in the United States obtained from NHANES have been used in efforts to reduce sodium consumption and the amount of sodium in various food products that children consume.[42,43] Additionally, USDA used NHANES data in updating the standards for the amount of sodium in school meals.[44] NHANES weight, height, and BMI data on children and adolescents were used to create the 2000 CDC pediatric growth charts that are widely used by clinicians and researchers to monitor growth and define obesity.[45]

As a national source of dietary information, NHANES has also been used to assess the impact of food supply changes and of policies on the health of Americans. For example, starting in 1998, federal regulations requiring the fortification of grains in the US food supply with folic acid to reduce the risk of neural tube defects (serious birth defects of the brain, spine, and spinal cord) were implemented.[46] Data from NHANES show an increase in serum folate and red blood cell folate from surveys in 1988 and 1994 (prefortification) compared to values from surveys 1999–2000 through 2005–06 (postfortification).[47] Over a similar time period, data from the US National Vital Statistics System observed a roughly 26% reduction in the portion of neural tube defect–affected pregnancies.[48]

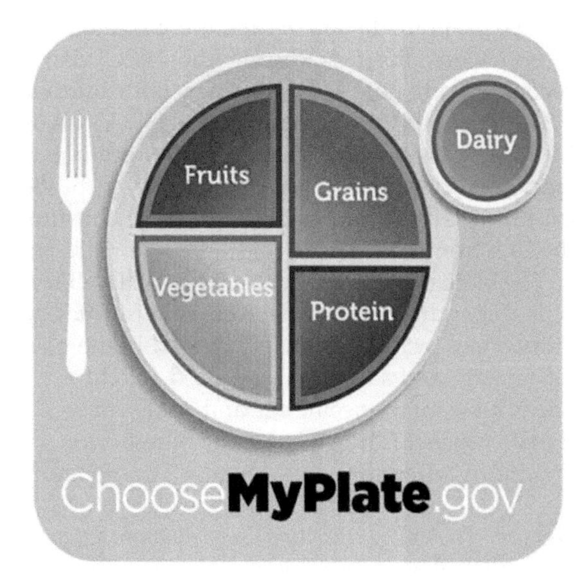

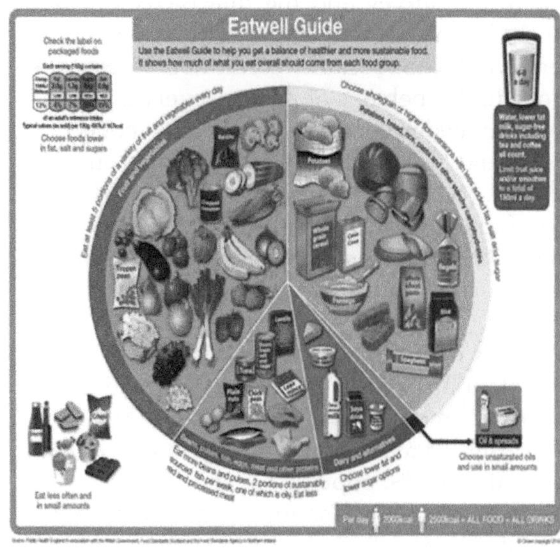

FIGURE 12.2 Food guides derived from nutrition surveillance data: US my Plate[86] and UK Eatwell Guide.[36] Both the United States and the United Kingdom have plate-based food guides to help educate individuals about healthy eating patterns.

In April 2016, the US FDA announced the expansion of fortification to include corn masa flour.[49] NHANES data played an important role in this decision. Analyses of NHANES data were used to determine the additional amount of folic acid that US population and subgroups, such as women of reproductive age, would consume if corn masa flour were also fortified with folic acid[50–52] and to estimate the number of neural tube defect births that could be averted with folic acid fortification of corn masa flour.[53] Corn masa flour is a staple consumed routinely and in appreciable amounts by Mexican American women, a subgroup that experiences higher rates of neural tube defects compared to non-Hispanic white women, in part due to low folate intake as a consequence of low consumption of wheat flour fortified with folic acid.[51]

Databases that support nutrition surveillance in the United States; Underpinning the data collected in NHANES are databases that are fundamental to nutritional surveillance. These databases are needed to translate the foods and beverages people report consuming into the nutrients contained in those foods and beverages. USDA's Agricultural Research Service (ARS) maintains FoodData Central,[54] an integrated data system for nutrient data and agricultural and experimental research.

The NHANES food and beverage data are routinely linked to two databases found on FoodData Central: the Food and Nutrient Database for Dietary Studies that translates foods and beverages into nutrients and the Food Patterns Equivalents Database that disaggregates foods and beverages into their component parts and matches these parts with the food pattern components identified in the US Dietary Guidelines (see also Chapter 11 on nutrient databases).

Nutrient intakes from dietary supplements can also be evaluated using the Dietary Supplement Labels Database (https://ods.od.nih.gov/Research/Dietary_Supplement_Label_Database.aspx) and Dietary Supplements Ingredients Database (https://dietarysupplementdatabase.usda.nih.gov/).

Other databases also available at FoodData Central include Foundation Foods, Experimental Foods, and the USDA Global Branded Food Products. Foundation Foods includes extensive metadata that allow users to see the variability associated with nutrient values, such as the number of samples an estimate is based on, the date and location of collection, the analytical approach used, and potentially, agricultural information such as genotype and production practices. Experimental Foods links to agricultural research data. Information in the USDA Global Branded Food Products database is voluntarily reported by food industry and data presentation is standardized by FoodData Central. The United States also maintains databases to monitor other aspects of nutrition surveillance, including food availability,[55] the food environment,[56] and food safety.[57,58]

In the United States, more than half of adults and about one-third of children reported using $\geq$ one dietary supplement in the past 30 days, indicating that nutrients from dietary supplements may contribute significantly to dietary intake and should be considered when monitoring nutritional status.[59] NHANES has been collecting information on dietary supplement usage in the US population since 1971 and maintains a dietary supplement database.[59,60] The database maintained by

NHANES only captures supplements reported by participants in NHANES. However, two other federal databases exist, which capture all dietary supplements that are currently or have ever been available for purchase in the United States: the Dietary Supplement Label Database[61] and the Dietary Supplement Ingredient Database.[62]

B. Nutrition Surveillance—High-Income Countries

Canada

Similar to the United States, Canada collects nutrition surveillance data through multiple national surveillance activities.[63] The Canadian Community Health Survey (CCHS) includes questionnaires related to food security, fruit and vegetable consumption, and height and weight. On a periodic basis, detailed nutritional information, including a 24-hour recall, suitable to estimate usual nutrient intakes and population intake distributions, has been collected in a special survey, called CCHS—Nutrition.[64]

The most recent detailed nutrition data were collected in 2015, with a prior data collection in 2004. CCHS samples respondents aged 1 and over in the 10 provinces through a stratified, multistage, cross-sectional sampling design.[65] The targeted sample in 2004 was n = 29,000 and n = 24,000 in 2015.

The Canadian Health Measures Survey (CHMS) began data collection in 2007. This continuous survey collects data on approximately 5000 individuals every 2 years and covers the 10 provinces, enrolling participants between the ages of 3 and 79 years through a complex, multistage, cluster sampling design to obtain a nationally representative sample.[66] Like NHANES, CHMS conducts a household interview and collects anthropometric measures and nutritional biomarkers in a mobile clinic. The household interview includes an FFQ to collect information on food group consumption: meat, milk, dairy, grains, salt, dietary fat, fruits, and vegetables. Nutritional biomarkers, collected through blood and urine samples, include vitamin B12, vitamin D, ferritin, iodine, sodium, and potassium.[67]

Two other surveillance systems of note are the Canadian Total Diet Study (TDS) and the National Nutrition Food Basket. The Canadian TDS, referred to as a Market Basket Study in other country contexts, is conducted by the Bureau of Chemical Safety at Health Canada's Food Directorate and monitors contaminants, such as lead, mercury, arsenic, cadmium, PCBs, dioxins, and pesticides in the food supply.[68] It has been a continuous survey since 1969. Sampling takes place in a different major city each year with the goal of sampling cities spread across Canada. Approximately 210 individual food items are sampled from 3-4 supermarkets and sent to a centralized laboratory for testing.[68]

The National Nutrition Food Basket was first conducted in 1974. It describes the quantity and cost of about 60 foods that represent a nutritious diet by specific age and gender groups. The government uses the data to monitor cost and affordability of healthy eating. The last revision of the National Nutrition Food Basket was in 2008. This revision incorporates food choices reflected in the 2004 CCHS Cycle 2.2, Nutrition.[69] The latest revision of Canada's dietary guidelines, Canada's Food Guide, published in January 2019,[70] included evidence from CCHS 2004 Nutrition and the CHMS.[71]

Japan

Japan's National Health and Nutrition Survey (NHNS) started as the National Nutrition Survey (NNS) in 1945 in response to food shortages, concerns about the nutritional status of the civilian population, and the need to solicit food aid after World War II.[72] This makes it the oldest continuing NNS in the world. By 2003, the health and nutritional status of the population had transitioned from concerns about undernutrition to concerns relating to chronic disease, prompting a redesign to include chronic disease surveillance under the current NHNS name.

Since 2003, the survey has been administered as a stratified, two-stage clustered sample of the civilian population ages 1 year and over with a physical examination, lifestyle survey, and dietary intake survey.[72] Dietary intake collection is conducted on a single day, freely chosen by study participants, between October and December, excluding Sundays and public holidays, and includes a four-part, self-administered questionnaire with a household roster that collects information on meal patterns, daily step counts, and dietary records.[72,73] Household representatives responsible for food preparation are instructed by trained interviewers on how to weigh foods and beverages consumed in the household and complete the food records. In addition, food waste is captured. Following completion of the dietary intake and lifestyle surveys, participants attend a designated facility, within walking distance of their home, where the physical examination is performed. Weight, height, abdominal circumference, and blood pressure measurement are taken. In addition, a blood sample is collected and a medical interview performed. Data from NHNS is used to evaluate the national health promotion initiative, Health Japan 21[72]; the survey is the only source of national data on risk factors for chronic disease.

South Korea

The first Korean National Health and Nutrition and Examination Survey (KNHANES) was administered in 1998, after the Korean National Nutrition Survey merged with the National Health and Health Knowledge and Behavior Survey.[74,75] Starting in 2007, KNHANES became an annual survey that evaluates the health and nutritional status of the South Korean people. The survey is conducted by the Korean Centers for Disease Control and Prevention and captures a nationally representative cross-sectional sample of 10,000 people, ages 1 year and over each year. The survey includes a health interview and health examination (e.g., body measurements, blood pressure, laboratory tests [blood and urine], dental exam and lung function), conducted by trained staff in a MEC, and a nutrition survey, conducted by dietitians in the participant's home about 1 week following the physical exam in the MEC. The nutrition survey includes an interview-administered FFQ, 24-hour recall, and dietary behavior questionnaire that asks about meal skipping, eating out, use of dietary supplements, and use of food labeling, among other topics.[76]

Data from KNHANES have been used to establish and evaluate national health and nutrition objectives, develop Korean children and adolescent growth charts, establish Dietary Reference Intakes, monitor the nutritional status of vulnerable groups, and compare health indicators internationally.[75] KNHANES data are also a resource to examine dietary patterns and chronic disease, mental health, and functional outcomes in both adults and children.[76]

Australia

Australia collected nutrition data on adults in 1995 when the National Nutrition Survey was conducted and in 2007 for children ages 2–16 years when the Australian National Children's Nutrition and Physical Activity Survey was conducted.[77] Since then, there has been no regular, national Nutrition Surveillance Program (NSP). In 2011–13, two new components were added to the Australian Health Survey (AHS): the National Nutrition and Physical Activity Survey (NNPAS) and the National Health Measures Survey (NHMS) (Fig. 12.3).[77,78]

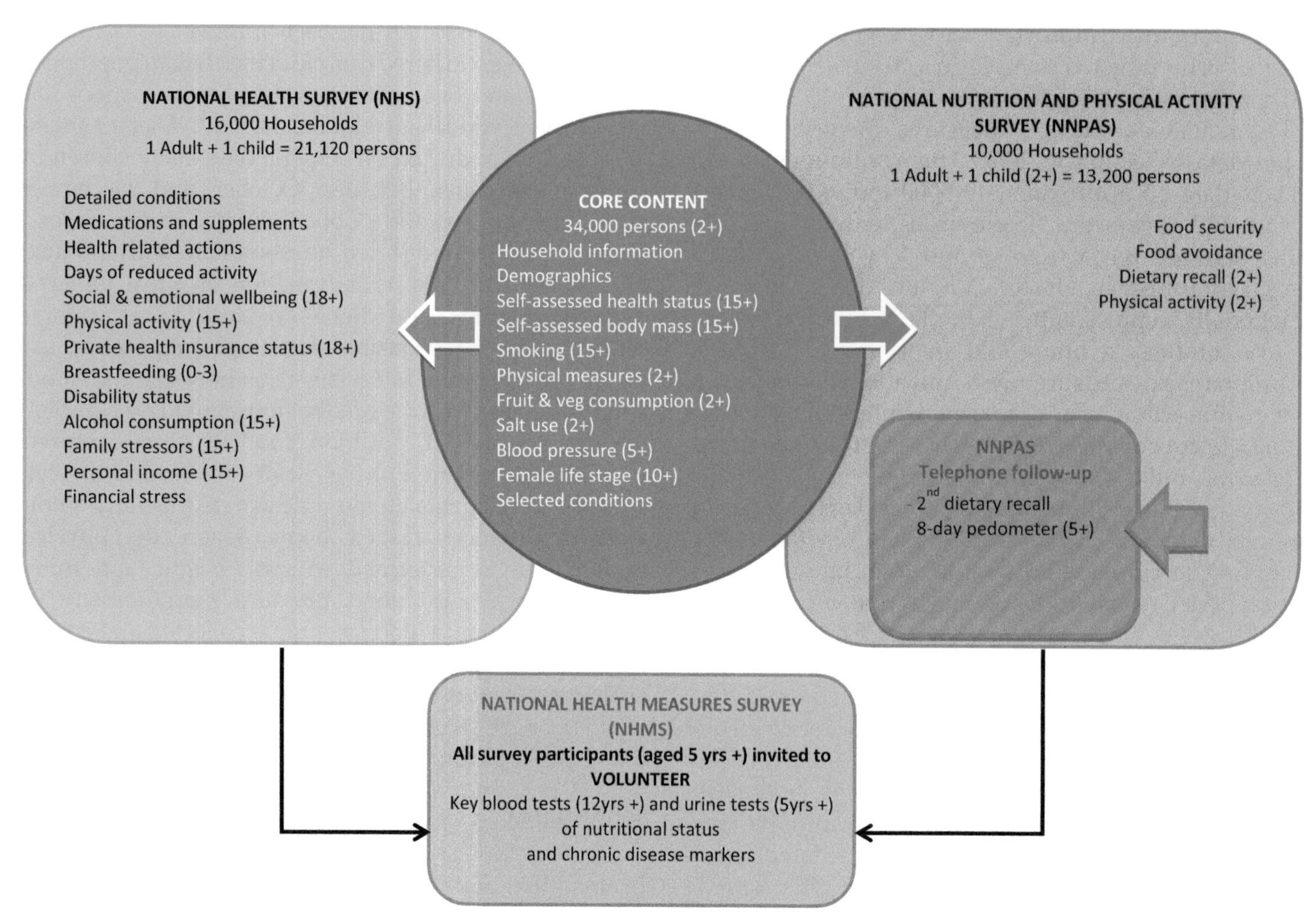

FIGURE 12.3 Structure of the 2011–13 Australian Health Survey.[77] The Australian Health Survey comprises separate surveys with some measures linked to produce a rich data source to examine multiple dimensions of health in the Australian population. *Australian Bureau of Statistics.*

These additions made AHS the largest and most com prehensive health survey ever conducted in Australia. NNPAS was administered in 9500 households and captured a maximum of one adult and one child (aged $\geq$2 years) yielding a sample of 12,000 individuals. Sample selection was designed to ensure that reliable estimates could be produced for each state and territory. Trained interviewers administered questions on food security, food avoidance, select medical conditions, sedentary behavior, and tobacco smoking. Physical measurements (height, weight, waist circumference, and blood pressure) were collected, in addition to a 24-hour dietary recall. Respondents were also asked to wear a pedometer for 8 days and provide a second 24-hour dietary recall by phone. Participants ages 5 and over were invited to participate in the NHMS, where blood and urine samples were collected and assessed for nutritional status and markers of chronic disease.

The usual nutrient intakes based on the Nutrient Reference Values for Australia and New Zealand showed that 73% of females and 51% of males ages 2 and over had inadequate intakes of calcium from food consumption.[79] Similarly, 23% of females and 3% of males had inadequate iron intakes from food and 76% of males and 42% of females exceeded the Upper Level of Intake for sodium.[79]

The next iteration of the NNPAS is planned for data collection in 2020–21, with the goal of establishing a National Food and Nutrition Monitoring Surveillance system, with a commitment to conduct a national nutrition survey every 10 years.[80] Some of the many aims for this nutrition surveillance system are to (1) inform policy and regulation, (2) monitor trends over time in the composition of foods, overall diet, dietary behaviors, and nutritional status of population (or population subgroups), (3) assess dietary and nutrient inadequacies and excesses, (4) identify barriers to healthy eating, (5) assess risk of exposure to substances in food, and (6) assess the use of nutritional supplements and their implications for nutritional intake, nutritional status, and the health of the population.[80]

United Kingdom

The National Diet and Nutrition Survey (NDNS) was initiated in 1992 as a series of periodic, cross-sectional surveys that were administered to different age groups of the UK population.[81,82] The NDNS Rolling Program (NDNS RP) began in 2008 and is funded by Public Health England and the UK Food Standards Agency. It is a continuous cross-sectional survey that assesses the diet, nutrient intake, and nutritional status of UK residents aged 1.5 years and above. Approximately 1000 individuals are sampled each year, half of them adults and half children. This survey includes an interview, a 4-day diet record, physical measurements, and blood and urine samples. The primary goals of the NDNS RP are to monitor food consumption, nutrient intakes, and nutritional status of the UK population and assess exposure to food chemicals.[83] Data from NDNS RP are used to assess the impact of health promotion initiatives aimed at improving diet quality and nutrient intakes.[84]

Data from NDSNS RP were used to develop the UK Eatwell Guide,[85] similar to US national data being used to develop MyPlate in the United States[86] The Eatwell Guide is a model of a plate that illustrates a balanced diet in the United Kingdom[36,85] (see Fig. 12.2). The foods depicted on the plate are derived from the NDNS RP and represent the most commonly consumed foods in the United Kingdom, but the amounts reflect what is needed to achieve dietary recommendations.[87]

Nutrition surveillance with the NDNS program has been used to monitor changes in dietary quality. Comparing data obtained in an early periodic survey with that from the NDNS RP, positive changes have occurred in the diets of younger children, such as lower consumption of soft drinks, crisps (i.e., chips) and savory snacks, and chocolate confectionary among children 4–10 years in 2008–09 compared with 1997. However, the need for nutrition surveillance is illustrated by the proportion of girls aged 11–18 years (46%) and women aged 19–64 years (21%) with mean iron intakes below the UK lower reference nutrient intake.[84]

Other health surveys, such as the Health Survey for England,[88] the Scottish Health Survey,[89] and Health Survey Northern Ireland,[90] objectively collect information on health and health-related behaviors (e.g., measured height, weight, blood pressure, and blood samples). A brief module on fruit and vegetable consumption is typically included and can be used to monitor trends in the percentage of adults who consume five or more portions of fruit and vegetables per day, in line with the 5 A DAY guidelines developed by WHO.[91,92]

C. Nutrition Surveillance—Middle- and Low-Income Countries

Recent reviews of nutrition surveillance in middle- and low-income countries have provided a snapshot of the current situation and highlight the continued need for surveillance.[15,93–95] In these settings, nutrition surveillance is often constrained by a myriad of factors such as hazardous conditions related to safety or a harsh physical environment that limit access to more nutritious foods, in addition to a lack of human and monetary resources.[94]

Many middle- and low-income countries also face a triple burden from malnutrition (child stunting, anemia in adult women, and overweight in adult women).[2] Additionally, undernutrition in these settings can be life-threatening, and thus requires data to inform quick action. For these reasons, nutrition surveillance in middle- and low-income countries can vary significantly from country to country, as there is no "one-size-fits-all" approach.

To meet the timely need for data, nutrition surveillance in middle- and low-income countries often relies on multiple data collections. Repeated nutrition surveys that collect data on anthropometry and food security is one type of data collection. Other data sources include community-based sentinel sites, feeding program admissions, and health clinics.[94] Many middle- and low-income countries rely on anthropometry as a primary indicator and dietary intake as a secondary indicator.[15,93,94] In the context of chronic deprivation, admissions to feeding programs and data from health clinics can inform nutrition surveillance.

Some middle- and low-income countries have national nutrition surveillance programs, while others rely on programs conducted by international organizations, such as the DHS supported by the US Agency for International Development (USAID)[96] and the MICS, supported by the United Nations Children's Fund.[97] DHS began in the mid-1980's and MICS began 10 years later, in the mid-1990's. These surveys are periodic; however, one usually takes place every 3–5 years in a country or region, thus enabling monitoring of trends.

Local interviewers with local knowledge are hired to conduct the survey, but training and supervising a vast force of interviewers is both challenging and expensive. DHS and MICS provide estimates of nutritional status for national and regional assessment, including urban/rural areas about a year after data collection. However, like many high-income countries, finer granularity at the subregional or local level is not possible.

Two additional tools used in many low-income countries include the Standardized Monitoring and Assessment of Relief and Transition (SMART) methodology[98] and software for Emergency Nutrition Assessment (ENA).[99] SMART, launched in 2002, is a broad, interagency collaborative of humanitarian practitioners (donors, policymakers, experts in the field, international and UN agencies, universities, research institutes, and governments). It was initiated in 2002 to address the difficulty in comparing monitoring results across surveys due to the lack of standardization of methodology and measures. SMART therefore provides a framework to compare data collected on two indicators to assess the magnitude and severity of a humanitarian crisis: the nutritional status of children under 5 and the mortality rate in the population.[98]

To further aid this effort, ENA was developed for SMART to make recording and calculating indicators easy and reliable.[99] The latest version of the ENA software is available for download on the SMART website, http://smartmethodology.org.

Another resource to find data on nutrition and health is the Global Health Data Exchange, http://ghdx.healthdata.org/countries. Below, case studies of nutrition surveillance from three middle- and low-income countries are presented.

Mexico

Mexico is considered an upper middle-income country by the World Bank, and a newly industrialized country. The contrast between Mexico and other middle- and low-income countries illustrates why there is no "one-size-fits-all" for nutrition surveillance. The first National Nutrition Survey (NNS-1988) in Mexico was conducted in 1988 by the Ministry of Health and the National Institute of Public Health.[100] Prior surveys in Mexico were not probabilistic, nor did they cover both urban and rural zones, thus they were not nationally or regionally representative. NNS-1988 focused on two groups considered the most nutritionally vulnerable: children <5 years and women of reproductive age (12–49 years). The survey collected measured height and weight, dietary intake (24-hour recall), sociodemographic characteristics, and health and illness indicators.[100]

Ten years later, a follow-up survey, NNS-1999, was conducted to collect updated information on the nutritional status of the country considering the high prevalence of both malnutrition and overweight found in 1988.[101] NNS-1999 showed that the stunting, anemia, and micronutrient deficiencies were the leading problems related to poor nutrition. However, overweight and obesity were also identified as a public health concern.[100]

Beginning in 2006, the cross-sectional survey was renamed the Mexican National Health and Nutrition Survey (ENSANUT 2006) and expanded to cover all individuals ages 1 year and older. The survey collected information on the household, general health, and anthropometry and also included biochemical tests and dietary assessment. Dietary data were collected using a semiquantitative FFQ.[102] ENSANUT 2006 showed that the national prevalence of underweight (3.4%), stunting (15.5%), and wasting (2.0%) in children <5 years were considerably lower than two decades earlier.[100] In contrast, the prevalence of overweight and obesity among adults ages 20 years and over was 70%, and among children and adolescents ages 2–18 years, almost one-quarter had overweight or obesity (24%).[100] In 2012, the survey was repeated using the same methodology and instruments, and data have been used to monitor trends in nutrition status in both children and adults.[103]

ENSANUT MC 2016 is the most recent version of the survey, administered to gather information on the impact of nutritional policies that had been enacted since ENSANUT 2012, in addition to general surveillance activities. Due to concerns about the rising rates of obesity and the widespread consumption of sugar-sweetened beverages (SSBs) in Mexico, a national SSB excise tax of one-peso per liter (a 10% increase) was passed on January 1, 2014.[104]

Data from ENSANUT 2016 have been used to evaluate the impact of an SSB excise tax on the probability of decreased SSB consumption, conditional on multiple sociodemographic factors, such as awareness of the tax, and beliefs about its effectiveness. One study found that adults who were aware of the SSB data were more likely to report a decrease in SSB consumption, compared to those who were not aware.[104] Additional results on anemia[105] and physical activity[106] have been generated from ENSANUT 2016.

India

India has multiple surveys that provide information on nutrition and health, collected at national, state, and vulnerable area levels.[107,108] For example, the Ministry of Agriculture monitors food production. The Indian Government's National Sample Survey conducted by the Ministry of Statistics and Programme Implementation monitors household expenditures. Recent estimates found that Indian households spend nearly half of their income (45%) on food and India's food subsidy program provides for nearly 800 million people, receiving nearly 1% of Gross Domestic Product.[109] The National Sample Survey Office (NSSO) of the Ministry of Statistics and Programme Implementation has collected data on poverty, affordability, and food expenditures since 1975. On an annual basis, NSSO publishes reports that can be used to monitor per capita consumption of bulk food items. However, this information can only be used to monitor what was purchased for consumption at the household level. It does not measure the foods actually consumed and it does not capture foods consumed outside the household.[110]

Of the large-scale, national-level, community-based surveys, only the National Nutrition Monitoring Bureau (NNMB) collects information on actual intakes at the household and individual level using a 24-hour recall. Many of the other surveys collect nutrition and food information at the household or individual level using FFQs (National Sample Survey, National Family Health Survey, District Level Household Survey, India Health and Development Survey, Indian Migration Study, and the Andhra Pradesh Child and Parent Study).[107,108] The NNMB,[111] established in 1972, is part of the National Institute of Nutrition and has administered national nutrition surveys, starting in 1975–79, that have been repeated in the same villages in 1988–89, 1996–97,[108] 2004–05, and 2011–12.[107] In 1993, the Government of India adopted their National Nutrition Policy which called for strengthening of the existing NNMB to allow for comparison of data from all over India to inform policy aimed at eliminating malnutrition for all.[111]

NNMB surveys have been conducted in 10 of the 27 states of India (Andhra Pradesh, Gujarat, Karnataka, Kerala, Madhya Pradesh, Maharashtra, Orissa, Tamil Nadu, Uttar Pradesh, and West Bengal). They collect sociodemographics, measured height, weight, and waist circumference, and one 24-hour recall for respondents ages 1 y and over and are typically repeated every 3 years.[95] A comparison of data from three time points in NNMB (1975–79, 1996–95, and 2011–12) found a significant decline over time in chronic energy deficiency among rural, nonpregnant, nonlactating (NPNL) women aged 18–60 years, from 52% to 46%–34%. Over the same period, the prevalence of overweight/obesity increased from 7% to 13%–24% among NPNL women 18–60 years.[112] NNMB data have also been used to document underweight, stunting, and wasting and associated factors among infants <3 years[113] and children <5 years[114] and the prevalence of overweight/obesity, hypertension, and diabetes among the adult rural population.[115]

Ethiopia

For several decades, recurrent droughts have led to crop and livestock failures in Ethiopia, creating a food insecure situation ripe for malnutrition.[116] The National Surveillance Program (NSP) in Ethiopia, run by Save the Children between 1986 and 2001, provided information to the Ethiopian government's Early Warning System to identify areas of food insecurity.[15] The program was comprised of annual cross-sectional cluster surveys with quarterly longitudinal follow-up of 50 children younger than 5 years in areas prone to famine.[15] A total of 9250 children were followed each year. Data collected included anthropometry and food security questionnaires and were mainly used to inform requests for food aid.[15]

The Ethiopian government did not have the capacity to take over the NSP after a planned 3-year transfer of administration by Save the Children beginning in 1998,[15] and this led to the establishment of the Ethiopian Emergency Nutrition Coordination Unit (ENCU) within the Early Warning Department of the current Disaster Risk Management and Food Security Sector in the Ministry of Agriculture and Rural Development.[116]

With this change, the NSP has become an "as-needed" survey, with more emphasis on rapid nutrition assessment rather than monitoring a deterioration in food security.[15] To ensure comparability across surveys and rapid results, SMART technology is used, with EMA software.[15,94,116] The ENCU approves all nutrition surveys before they are administered to ensure data quality, while the Complex Emergency Database (CE-DAT) team compiles the data on health and nutrition indicators into a publicly available database used to monitor nutritional status.[116,117] Analyses using data from CE-DAT and other publicly available databases found that the estimated pooled prevalence of wasting was 11% between 2000 and 2013 among children ages 6–59 months.[117] In contrast, data from the Ethiopian DHS for 2016 found that 14% of infants 0–24 months had wasting and 8% of older infants 25–59 months were wasted.[118] The Ethiopian DHS was conducted in 2016 by the Central Statistical Agency under the guidance of the Ministry of Health and is the fourth nationally representative survey.

IV. ISSUES SPECIFICALLY RELATED TO NUTRITION SURVEILLANCE

There is a stark contrast between the challenges associated with nutrition surveillance in middle- and low-income countries compared to high-income countries. The metrics used can differ (anthropometry vs. dietary assessment), resources vary widely, and critically, the outcomes monitored (undernutrition vs. overnutrition) have different timelines, consequences, and challenges. Middle- and low-income countries are often faced with the triple burden of nutritional issues as mentioned earlier, a situation that stretches already limited resources.

A. Importance of Data Quality

Data quality, however, is a key necessity in nutrition surveillance, irrespective of context. The need for high data quality applies across country settings, data capture tools, measurement techniques, and nutrient databases. High-quality anthropometric data reflect standardized measurements. Participant-reported values do not provide the same level of accuracy as measured values.[119] Moreover, training ensures that measurements are comparable over time and across settings.[120] Nutrition surveillance in the United States relies on food and nutrient databases, maintained by the Methods and Application of Food Composition Laboratory at the Beltsville Human Nutrition Research Center, ARS of USDA. Nutrient databases translate the detailed information collected about the type and quantity of foods consumed into information about the composition (i.e., protein, fat, vitamin, minerals) of foods and diets. If the database is lacking in current values, any analysis using the database will also be lacking. ARS scientists have developed and maintained the databases to ensure accuracy by using up-to-date laboratory practices, nationally representative analytical samples, establishing protocols for handling missing values and limitations, prioritizing nutrients and foods commonly consumed in the US diet, documenting changes in methodology over time, and performing integrity checks to ensure high data quality.[121,122] In addition to nutrient values, portion sizes, food names, and recipes need to be updated and tracked on a continuous basis.[123] Keeping these databases current requires significant investments in time and money.

High quality in data collection tools is also critically important. The USDA AMPM developed by the Food Surveys Research Group at ARS/USDA was validated through a series of studies to enhance and improve data collection with a 24-hour recall.[124] As previously mentioned, the SMART methodology[98] and ENA system[99] were developed to ensure high data quality in low-income settings and allow for comparability across surveys.

The foil to high data quality is measurement error. Measurement error is the difference between observed (or measured) value and the true value; it is a part of any measurement, not just dietary assessment. Measurement error is not a new concept in the field of nutrition surveillance,[125] and a great deal of progress has been made to describe measurement error and its impact on dietary assessment.[126] In addition, analytic methods have been developed to mitigate the effect of measurement error.[127–129] No single tool is perfect, and a combination of tools draws on the strengths of all tools employed,[130] and innovations in the field of dietary assessment continue, as discussed below.

B. Introduction of New Technologies

Widespread access to the Internet, mobile phones, and mobile phones with integrated cameras has led to an explosion of advances to both improve speed of data collection and analysis, while also addressing limitations associated with measurement error in dietary assessment.[131] Many new technologies are web-based, which allow for both self-administration of questionnaires and use anywhere with Internet connectivity, allowing more flexibility and immediate analysis of the food and nutrients reported as consumed.[132] Wearable technology[133–135] and natural language processing are also areas of active research.[136,137]

The ASA24[138] is a web-based, automatically coded, self-administered dietary assessment tool that can capture 24-hour recalls and/or single or multiple day food records. It was developed by the NIH's National Cancer Institute, under contract with Westat, a social science research firm, and is based on the USDA's AMPM method that is used to collect individual 24-hour recalls in the nationally representative sample of the US population in NHANES.[124] ASA24 can be self-administered, allowing respondents to complete the 24-hour recall at their leisure, so long as they have connection to the Internet. Because ASA24 is autocoded, food and nutrient composition of the reported foods and beverages is available immediately after completing the recall or record, allowing timely feedback for use in both clinical and epidemiological settings.

ASA24 has also been adapted for use in Canada and Australia and is available in English and Spanish (US version) and English and French (Canadian version).[138] Self-administered ASA24 requires basic literacy, numeracy, and computer savvy, limiting its use in some populations (e.g., young children, elderly); however, some of these limitations can be mitigated with interviewer administration. ASA24 use is also limited by the need for continuous Internet connection while completing the 24-hour recall or record.[138] Other web-based dietary assessment tools include myfood24, Intake24, NutriNet-Santé, DietDay[139], and INDDEX24.[140,141]

The Technology Assisted Dietary Assessment or TADA mobile food record application (mFR)[142,143] layers digital images, taken with a cell phone, with a traditional food record. Using a single photo with a fiducial marker (an object that is placed next to the food before the photo is taken to provide context as to the size and color of the food) and mathematical algorithms, the TADA system identifies the food item and estimates the portion size of the foods consumed. This information is paired with the food record to capture the details about the type of foods and beverages consumed. Other mobile dietary assessment systems under development include FoodLog,[144] DietCam,[145] and Im2Calories.[146]

Other technological advances that merit further investigation include wearable technology, such as glasses with cameras to capture real-time eating occasions,[134,147] bite or chew sensors,[148–151] and voice-based nutrition records that utilize natural language processing to convert the spoken word to text.[136] These tools need not be used in isolation; in fact, combining data from multiple instruments may improve precision.[130]

C. Merger of Environmental Data With Nutrition Surveillance Efforts

Novel linkages to established databases or linkages to newly created databases provide opportunities to explore new aspects about food and diet. Increasingly, the impact of diet on both human health and environmental sustainability has garnered attention.[152] Metrics to measure this aspect of diet are still under development, but efforts to link average daily greenhouse gas emissions, in carbon dioxide equivalents, to individual foods reported by participants in the US NHANES data[153] are underway. The result is a database that presents a unique opportunity to investigate the carbon footprint of common dietary patterns in the United States and may shed light on the environmental impact of food choices.

Another facet of diet that has recently been explored is the degree of processing a food item has undergone and the purported impact on diet quality[154,155] and health.[156] The NOVA[157] system of food classification is one of the many systems that has been developed to identify possible effects of ultraprocessed foods on diet quality and the sustainability of food systems.[158] Additional areas of active research include the "omics," such as metabolomics, genomics, proteomics,[159] and the microbiome[160] that seek to characterize and quantify all the molecules in a system (i.e., cell, organ, individual) to provide insight into the function of the system. These fields may one day be included in future surveillance efforts.

RESEARCH GAPS

- Research on human milk composition
- Research on methodologies to obtain quality food/formula consumption data in infants and young children
- Continued technological innovations in dietary assessment to reduce measurement error and respondent burden
- Integration of surveillance system methodology to enhance comparisons between countries and organizations
- Validation that resources put into surveillance result in improved public health programming and serve as the factual basis for public health policies in support of, or in refuting, political agendas

Acknowledgments

This chapter includes material taken from the chapter titled Nutrition Monitoring in the United States by Briefel RR and McDowell MA in Present Knowledge in Nutrition, 10th Edition, edited by Erdman JW, Macdonald IA, and Zeisel SH and published by Wiley-Blackwell. 2012 International Life Sciences Institute. The contributions of previous authors are thereby acknowledged.

V. REFERENCES

1. WHO. *10 Facts on Nutrition*; 2017. https://www.who.int/features/factfiles/nutrition/en/. Accessed May, 2019.
2. Development Initiatives. *2018 Global Nutrition Report: Shining a Light to Spur Action on Nutrition*. Bristol, UK: Development Initiatives; 2018.
3. United Nations System Standing Committee on Nutrition. *The UN Decade of Action on Nutrition 2016–2025*. https://www.unscn.org/en/topics/un-decade-of-action-on-nutrition. Accessed May 2019.
4. Inernational Food Policy Research Institute. *Global Nutrition Report 2014: Actions and Accountability to Accelerate the World's Progress on Nutrition*; 2014. http://www.ifpri.org/publication/global-nutrition-report-2014-actions-and-accountability-accelerate-worlds-progress. Accessed May, 2019.
5. Zwald M, Ogden C. Population surveillance and monitoring. In: Jones-Smith J, ed. *Public Health Nutrition*. Baltimore, MD: Johns Hopkins University Press; (in press).
6. Caulfield LE, Richard SA, Rivera JA, Musgrove P, Black RE. Stunting, wasting, and micronutrient deficiency disorders. In: Jamison DT, Breman JG, et al., eds. *Disease Control Priorities in Developing Countries*. 2006. Washington (DC).

7. World Health Organization. United nations high commissioner for refugees. In: *United Nations Children's Fund, Programme. WF. Food and Nutrition in Emergencies*. 2004.
8. Grummer-Strawn LM, Reinold C, Krebs NF, Centers for Disease C, Prevention. Use of World Health Organization and CDC growth charts for children aged 0-59 months in the United States. *Morb Mortal Wkly Rep*. 2010;59(RR-9):1–15.
9. Gibson RS. *Principles of Nutritional Assessment*. 2nd ed. New York, NY: Oxford University Press; 2005.
10. Dietary Assessment Primer. *Dietary Assessment Instrument Profiles*. National Institutes of Health, National Cancer Institute. https://dietassessmentprimer.cancer.gov/profiles/. Accessed May 2019.
11. Food and Agriculture Organization (FAO). *FAO Food Balance Sheets: A Handbook*. Rome: Food and Agriculture Oranization of hte United Nations; 2001.
12. FDA (U.S. Food & Drug Administration). *Total Diet Study*; 2018. https://www.fda.gov/food/science-research-food/total-diet-study. Accessed May , 2019.
13. Subar AF, Kirkpatrick SI, Mittl B, et al. The Automated Self-Administered 24-hour dietary recall (ASA24): a resource for researchers, clinicians, and educators from the National Cancer Institute. *J Acad Nutr Diet*. 2012;112(8):1134–1137.
14. Tuffrey V, Hall A. Methods of nutrition surveillance in low-income countries. *Emerg Themes Epidemiol*. 2016;13:4.
15. Tuffrey V. *Nutrition Surveillance Systems: Their Use and Value*. London: Save the Children and Transform Nutrition; 2016.
16. Raiten DJ, Raghavan R, Porter A, Obbagy JE, Spahn JM. Executive summary: evaluating the evidence base to support the inclusion of infants and children from birth to 24 mo of age in the Dietary Guidelines for Americans–"the B-24 Project". *Am J Clin Nut*. 2014;99(3):663s–691s.
17. U.S. Congress. *Pub. L. 113–79. The 2014 Farm Bill*. Washington, DC: 113th Congress; 2014.
18. Stam J, Sauer PJ, Boehm G. Can we define an infant's need from the composition of human milk? *Am J Clin Nutr*. 2013;98(2): 521S–528S.
19. Casavale KO, Ahuja JKC, Wu X, et al. NIH workshop on human milk composition: summary and visions. *Am J Clin Nutr*. 2019; 110(3):769–779. https://doi.org/10.1093/ajcn/nqz123.
20. Wu X, Jackson RT, Khan SA, Ahuja J, Pehrsson PR. Human milk nutrient composition in the United States: current knowledge, challenges, and research needs. *Curr Dev Nutr*. 2018;2(7):nzy025.
21. Lackey KA, Williams JE, Meehan CL, et al. What's normal? Microbiomes in human milk and infant feces are related to each other but vary geographically: the INSPIRE study. *Frontiers in nutrition*. 2019;6:45.
22. Moossavi S, Sepehri S, Robertson B, et al. Composition and variation of the human milk microbiota are influenced by maternal and early-life factors. *Cell Host Microbe*. 2019;25(2), 324–335.e324.
23. The International Society for Research in *Human Milk and Lactation (ISRHML)*. https://www.isrhml.com/i4a/pages/index.cfm?pageid=1&pageid=3267. Accessed May 2019.
24. National Center for Health Statistics. *National Health and Nutrition Examination Survey*; 2016. http://www.cdc.gov/nchs/nhanes.htm. Accessed March 3, 2016.
25. NHANES' MEC Collects Health Data. *Inside NCHS: Featured Topics from the National Center for Health Statistics 2013*; 2019. https://blogs.cdc.gov/inside-nchs/2013/04/17/nhanes-mec-collects-health-data/.
26. Zipf G, Chiappa M, Porter KS, Ostchega Y, Lewis BG, Dostal J. National health and nutrition examination survey: plan and operations, 1999–2010. *Vital Health Stat 1*. 2013;(56):1–37.
27. Mirel LB, Mohadjer LK, Dohrmann SM, et al. National health and nutrition examination survey: estimation procedures, 2007–2010. National Center for Health Statistics *Vital Health Stat*. 2013;2(159).
28. Johnson CL, Dohrmann SM, Burt VL, Mohadjer LK. National health and nutrition examination survey: sample design, 2011–2014. National Center for Health Statistics *Vital Health Stat*. 2014;2(162).
29. Blanton CA, Moshfegh AJ, Baer DJ, Kretsch MJ. The USDA Automated Multiple-Pass Method accurately estimates group total energy and nutrient intake. *J Nutr*. 2006;136(10):2594–2599.
30. Curtin LR, Mohadjer LK, Dohrmann SM, et al. National health and nutrition examination survey: sample design, 2007–2010. *Vital Health Stat*. 2013;2(160):1–23.
31. Curtin LR, Mohadjer LK, Dohrmann SM, et al. The national health and nutrition examination survey: sample design, 1999–2006. *Vital Health Stat*. 2012;2(155):1–39.
32. Johnson CL, Dohrmann SM, Burt VL, Mohadjer LK. National health and nutrition examination survey: sample design, 2011–2014. *Vital Health Stat Ser 2 Data Eval Methods Res*. 2014;(162):1–33.
33. National Center for Health Statistics. *National Health and Nutrition Examination Survey 1999-2016 Survey Contents Brochure*; 2016. http://www.cdc.gov/nchs/data/nhanes/survey_content_99_16.pdf. Accessed April 26, 2016.
34. U.S. Department of Health and Human Services and U.S. Department of Agriculture. *2015-2020 Dietary Guidelines for Americans*. December 2015.
35. Tagtow A, Haven J, Maniscalco S, Johnson-Bailey D, Bard S. MyPlate celebrates 4 years. *J Acad Nutr Diet*. 2015;115(7):1039–1040.
36. *Public Health England in association with the Welsh Government Food Standards Scotland and the Food Standards Agency in Northern Ireland. Eatwell Guide*. https://assets.publishing.service.gov.uk/government/uploads/system/uploads/attachment_data/file/528193/Eatwell_guide_colour.pdf. Accessed May 2019.
37. Maalouf J, Cogswell ME, Yuan K, et al. Top sources of dietary sodium from birth to age 24 mo, United States, 2003–2010. *Am J Clin Nutr*. 2015;101(5):1021–1028.
38. Tian N, Zhang Z, Loustalot F, Yang Q, Cogswell ME. Sodium and potassium intakes among US infants and preschool children, 2003–2010. *Am J Clin Nutr*. 2013;98(4):1113–1122.
39. Cogswell ME, Yuan K, Gunn JP, et al. Vital signs: sodium intake among U.S. school-aged children - 2009–2010. *Morb Mortal Wkly Rep*. 2014;63(36):789–797.
40. Cogswell ME, Zhang Z, Carriquiry AL, et al. Sodium and potassium intakes among US adults: NHANES 2003–2008. *Am J Clin Nutr*. 2012;96(3):647–657.
41. Pfeiffer CM, Hughes JP, Cogswell ME, et al. Urine sodium excretion increased slightly among U.S. adults between 1988 and 2010. *J Nutr*. 2014;144(5):698–705.
42. Choi SE, Brandeau ML, Basu S. Expansion of the national salt reduction initiative: a mathematical model of benefits and risks of population-level sodium reduction. *Med Decis Mak*. 2016; 36(1):72–85.
43. New York City Department of Health and Mental Hygiene. *National Salt Reduction Initiative Corporate Commitments*. National Salt Reduction Initiative corporate commitments; 2014. http://www.nyc.gov/html/doh/downloads/pdf/cardio/nsri-corporate-commitments.pdf. Accessed April 26, 2016.
44. Food and Nutrition Service Federal Register. Nutrition standards in the national school lunch and school breakfast programs. *Fed Regist*. 2016;77:4088–4167. Nutrition Standards in the National School Lunch and School Breaskfast Programs https://www.gpo.gov/fdsys/pkg/FR-2012-01-26/pdf/2012-1010.pdf. Accessed March 3, 2016.
45. Kuczmarski RJ, Ogden CL, Guo SS, et al. 2000 CDC Growth Charts for the United States: methods and development. *Vital Health Stat 11*. 2002;(246):1–190. Data from the National Health Survey.
46. Crider KS, Bailey LB, Berry RJ. Folic acid food fortification-its history, effect, concerns, and future directions. *Nutrients*. 2011;3(3): 370–384.

47. McDowell MA, Lacher DA, Pfeiffer CM, et al. Blood folate levels: the latest NHANES results. *NCHS Data Brief.* 2008;(6):1–8.
48. Spina bifida and anencephaly before and after folic acid mandate–United States, 1995-1996 and 1999-2000. *Morb Mortal Wkly Rep.* 2004;53(17):362–365.
49. Food and Drug Administration. *FDA Approves Folic Acid Fortification of Corn Masa Flour;* 2016. http://www.fda.gov/NewsEvents/Newsroom/PressAnnouncements/ucm496104.htm. Accessed April 22, 2016.
50. Hamner HC, Tinker SC, Berry RJ, Mulinare J. Modeling fortification of corn masa flour with folic acid: the potential impact on exceeding the tolerable upper intake level for folic acid, NHANES 2001–2008. *Food Nutr Res.* 2013;57.
51. Hamner HC, Mulinare J, Cogswell ME, et al. Predicted contribution of folic acid fortification of corn masa flour to the usual folic acid intake for the US population: national Health and Nutrition Examination Survey 2001–2004. *Am J Clin Nutr.* 2009;89(1):305–315.
52. Hamner HC, Tinker SC, Flores AL, Mulinare J, Weakland AP, Dowling NF. Modelling fortification of corn masa flour with folic acid and the potential impact on Mexican-American women with lower acculturation. *Public Health Nutrition.* 2013;16(5):912–921.
53. Tinker SC, Devine O, Mai C, et al. Estimate of the potential impact of folic acid fortification of corn masa flour on the prevention of neural tube defects. *Birth Defects Res A Clin Mol Teratol.* 2013; 97(10):649–657.
54. US Department of Agriculture. *FoodData Central.* https://fdc.nal.usda.gov/. Accessed May 2019.
55. U.S. Department of Agriculture Economic Research Service. *Food Availability (Per Capita) Data System (FADS).* https://www.ers.usda.gov/data-products/food-availability-per-capita-data-system/. Accessed May 2019.
56. U.S. Department of Agriculture Economic Research Service. *Food Environment Atlas.* https://www.ers.usda.gov/data-products/food-environment-atlas.aspx. Accessed May 2019.
57. Centers for Disease Control and Prevention. *Foodborne Disease Active Surveillance Network (FoodNet).* https://www.cdc.gov/foodnet/index.html. Accessed May 2019.
58. Centers for Disease Control and Prevention. *National Outbreak Reporting System (NORS).* https://www.cdc.gov/nors/index.html. Accessed May 2019.
59. Gahche JJ, Bailey RL, Potischman N, et al. Federal monitoring of dietary supplement use in the resident, civilian, noninstitutionalized US population, national health and nutrition examination survey. *J Nutr.* 2018;148(Suppl 2):1436s–1444s.
60. National Center for Health Statistics. In: *National Health and Nutrition Examination Survey, 1999-2014 Data Documentation, Codebook, and Frequencies, Dietary Supplement Database, September 2014.* Hyattsville (MD): National Center for Health Statistics; 2016.
61. Dwyer JT, Bailen RA, Saldanha LG, et al. The dietary supplement Label database: recent developments and applications. *J Nutr.* 2018;148(Suppl 2):1428s–1435s.
62. Andrews KW, Gusev PA, McNeal M, et al. Dietary supplement ingredient database (DSID) and the application of analytically based estimates of ingredient amount to intake calculations. *J Nutr.* 2018;148(suppl_2):1413S–1421S.
63. Health Canada. *Food and Nutrition Surveillance.* https://www.canada.ca/en/health-canada/services/food-nutrition/food-nutrition-surveillance.html. Accessed May 2019.
64. Heath Canada Canadian Community Health Survey, Cycle 2.2, Nutrition (2004). *A Guide to Accessing and Interpreting the Data.* Health Canada; 2006. https://www.canada.ca/en/health-canada/services/food-nutrition/food-nutrition-surveillance/health-nutrition-surveys/canadian-community-health-survey-cchs/canadian-community-health-survey-cycle-2-2-nutrition-2004-guide-accessing-interpreting-data-health-canada-2006.html#a1.1.2. Accessed May , 2019.
65. Statistics Canada. Canadian Community Health Survey - Nutrition (CCHS). http://www23.statcan.gc.ca/imdb/p2SV.pl?Function=getSurvey&SDDS=5049. Accessed May 2019.
66. Health Canada. *Canadian Health Measures Survey.* https://www.canada.ca/en/health-canada/services/food-nutrition/food-nutrition-surveillance/health-nutrition-surveys/canadian-health-measures-survey.html. Accessed May 2019.
67. Tremblay M, Wolfson M, Connor Gorber S. Canadian Health Measures Survey: rationale, background and overview. *Health Reports.* 2007;18(Suppl):7–20.
68. Health Canada. *Canadian Total Diet Study.* https://www.canada.ca/en/health-canada/services/food-nutrition/food-nutrition-surveillance/canadian-total-diet-study.html. Accessed May 2019.
69. Health Canada. *National Nutritious Food Basket.* https://www.canada.ca/en/health-canada/services/food-nutrition/food-nutrition-surveillance/national-nutritious-food-basket.html. Accessed May 2019.
70. Health Canada. *Canad's Food Guide.* https://food-guide.canada.ca/en/. Accessed May 2019.
71. Health Canada. *Evidence Review for Dietary Guidance: Summary of Results and Implications for Canada's Food Guide 2015;* 2016. https://www.canada.ca/content/dam/canada/health-canada/migration/publications/eating-nutrition/dietary-guidance-summary-resume-recommandations-alimentaires/alt/pub-eng.pdf.
72. Ikeda N, Takimoto H, Imai S, Miyachi M, Nishi N. Data resource profile: the Japan national health and nutrition survey (NHNS). *Int J Epidemiol.* 2015;44(6):1842–1849.
73. Okada E, Saito A, Takimoto H. Association between the portion sizes of traditional Japanese seasonings-soy sauce and miso-and blood pressure: cross-sectional study using national health and nutrition survey, 2012–2016 data. *Nutrients.* 2018;10(12).
74. Park HA. The Korea national health and nutrition examination survey as a primary data source. *Korean J Fam Med.* 2013;34(2):79.
75. Korean Center for Disease Control & Prevention. *Korean National Health and Nutrition Examination Survey.* https://knhanes.cdc.go.kr/knhanes/eng/index.do. Accessed May 2019.
76. Kweon S, Kim Y, Jang MJ, et al. Data resource profile: the Korea national health and nutrition examination survey (KNHANES). *Int J Epidemiol.* 2014;43(1):69–77.
77. Australian Bureau of Statistics. *Australian Health Survey: Users' Guide, 2011–13: Structure of the Australian Health Survey* https://www.abs.gov.au/ausstats/abs@.nsf/Lookup/74D87E30B3539C53CA257BBB0014BB36?opendocument. Accessed May 2019.
78. Australian Bureau of Statistics. *Australian Health Survey: Biomedical Results for Chronic Diseases, 2011-12; About the National Health Measures Survey.* https://www.abs.gov.au/ausstats/abs@.nsf/Lookup/4364.0.55.005Chapter1102011-12. Accessed May 2019.
79. Australian Bureau of Statistics. *Australian Health Survey: Usual Nutrient Intakes, 2011-12* https://www.abs.gov.au/ausstats/abs@.nsf/Lookup/by%20Subject/4364.0.55.008∼2011-12∼Main%20Features∼Key%20findings∼100. Accessed May 2019.
80. Publich Health Association Australia. *Food and Nutirtion Monitoring and Surveillance in Australia: Policy Position Statement.* https://www.phaa.net.au/documents/item/2866. Accessed May 2019.
81. GOV.UK. *Collection: National Diet and Nutrition Survey.* https://www.gov.uk/government/collections/national-diet-and-nutrition-survey. Accessed May 2019.
82. Food Standards Agency. *NDNS Previous Survey Reports.* https://webarchive.nationalarchives.gov.uk/20101209182513/http://www.food.gov.uk/science/dietarysurveys/ndnsdocuments/ndnspreviousurveyreports/. Accessed May 2019.
83. Ashwell M, Barlow S, Gibson S, Harris C. National diet and nutrition surveys: the British experience. *Public Health Nutr.* 2006;9(4): 523–530.

84. Whitton C, Nicholson SK, Roberts C, et al. National Diet and Nutrition Survey: UK food consumption and nutrient intakes from the first year of the rolling programme and comparisons with previous surveys. *Br J Nutr.* 2011;106(12):1899–1914.
85. Public Health England. *From Plate to Guide: What, why and how for the Eatwell Model* https://assets.publishing.service.gov.uk/government/uploads/system/uploads/attachment_data/file/579388/eatwell_model_guide_report.pdf. Accessed May 2019.
86. U.S. Department of Agriculture Center for Nutrition Policy and Promotion. *Choose My Plate.* https://www.choosemyplate.gov/. Accessed May 2019.
87. Public Health England. *The Eatwell Guide: How Does it Differe to the Eatwell Plate and Why?* https://assets.publishing.service.gov.uk/government/uploads/system/uploads/attachment_data/file/528201/Eatwell_guide_whats_changed_and_why.pdf Accessed May 2019.
88. *National Health Service (NHS) Digital. Health Survey for England;* 2016. https://digital.nhs.uk/data-and-information/publications/statistical/health-survey-for-england/health-survey-for-england-2016#summary. Accessed May, 2019.
89. Scottish Government. *Scottish Health Survey.* https://statistics.gov.scot/data/scottish-health-survey. Accessed May 2019.
90. Health Survey Northern Ireland Department of Health. *Health Survey (NI) First Results 2017/2018.* https://www.health-ni.gov.uk/sites/default/files/publications/health/hsni-first-results-17-18.pdf. Accessed May 2019.
91. Joint WHO/FAO Expert Consultation. *Diet, Nutirtion and the Prevention of Chronic Diseases: A Repot of a Joint FAO/WHO Expert Consultation.* WHO Technical Report Series, No. 916. Geneva: World Health Organization; 2003.
92. World Health Organization. *Healthy Diet;* 2019. https://www.who.int/en/news-room/fact-sheets/detail/healthy-diet. Accessed May, 2019.
93. *Nutrition in the WHO African Region.* Brazzaville: World Health Organization; 2017.
94. Friedman G. *Review of National Nutrition Surveillance Systems.* Washington, D.C: FHI 360/FANTA; 2014.
95. Song S, Song WO. National nutrition surveys in Asian countries: surveillance and monitoring efforts to improve global health. *Asia Pac J Clin Nutr.* 2014;23(4):514–523.
96. U.S. Agency for International Development. *Demographic and Health Surveys.* https://www.dhsprogram.com/What-We-Do/Survey-Types/DHS.cfm. Accessed May 2019.
97. UNICEF. *The Multiple Indicator Cluster Surveys (MICS).* http://mics.unicef.org/faq. Accessed May 2019.
98. Linking Complex Emergency Response and Transition Initiative (CERTI). *Standardized Monitoring and Assessment of Relief and Transitions.* http://www.smartindicators.org/. Accessed May 2019.
99. NutriSurvey ENA for SMART - *Software for Emergency Nutrition Assessment.* http://www.nutrisurvey.de/ena/ena.html. Accessed May 2019.
100. Rivera JA, Irizarry LM, Gonzalez-de Cossio T. Overview of the nutritional status of the Mexican population in the last two decades. *Salud Publica Mex.* 2009;51(Suppl 4):S645–S656.
101. Resano-Perez E, Mendez-Ramirez I, Shamah-Levy T, Rivera JA, Sepulveda-Amor J. Methods of the national nutrition survey 1999. *Salud Publica Mex.* 2003;45(Suppl 4):S558–S564.
102. Rodriguez-Ramirez S, Mundo-Rosas V, Jimenez-Aguilar A, Shamah-Levy T. Methodology for the analysis of dietary data from the Mexican national health and nutrition survey 2006. *Salud Publica Mex.* 2009;51(Suppl 4):S523–S529.
103. Gaona-Pineda EB, Mejia-Rodriguez F, Cuevas-Nasu L, Gomez-Acosta LM, Rangel-Baltazar E, Flores-Aldana ME. Dietary intake and adequacy of energy and nutrients in Mexican adolescents: results from Ensanut 2012. *Salud Publica Mex.* 2018;60(4):404–413.
104. Alvarez-Sanchez C, Contento I, Jimenez-Aguilar A, et al. Does the Mexican sugar-sweetened beverage tax have a signaling effect? ENSANUT 2016. *PLoS One.* 2018;13(8):e0199337.
105. De la Cruz-Gongora V, Villalpando S, Shamah-Levy T. Prevalence of anemia and consumption of iron-rich food groups in Mexican children and adolescents: ensanut MC 2016. *Salud Publica Mex.* 2018;60(3):291–300.
106. Medina C, Jauregui A, Campos-Nonato I, Barquera S. Prevalence and trends of physical activity in children and adolescents: results of the Ensanut 2012 and Ensanut MC 2016. *Salud Publica Mex.* 2018;60(3):263–271.
107. Aleksandrowicz L, Tak M, Green R, Kinra S, Haines A. Comparison of food consumption in Indian adults between national and sub-national dietary data sources. *Br J Nutr.* 2017;117(7):1013–1019.
108. Rathi K, Kamboj P, Bansal PG, Toteja GS. A review of selected nutrition & health surveys in India. *Indian J Med Res.* 2018; 148(5):596–611.
109. Alderman H, Bhattacharya S, Gentilini U, Puri R. *Is India ready for choice-based PDS [Public Distribution System]? 2019;* https://www.hindustantimes.com/india-news/is-india-ready-for-choice-based-pds/story-VGuow7n6cYSl4e79K6BTML.html. Accessed May 2019.
110. National Sample Survey Office. *Key Indicators of Household Expenditure on Service and Durable Goods.* https://www.thehinducentre.com/multimedia/archive/02914/Key_Indicators_of__2914425a.pdf. Accessed May 2019.
111. National Insitute of Nutrition Hyderabad India. *National Nutrition Monitoring Bureau.* http://nnmbindia.org/aboutus.html. Accessed May 2019.
112. Meshram II, Balakrishna N, Sreeramakrishna K, et al. Trends in nutritional status and nutrient intakes and correlates of overweight/obesity among rural adult women (>/=18–60 years) in India: national Nutrition Monitoring Bureau (NNMB) national surveys. *Public Health Nutrition.* 2016;19(5):767–776.
113. Meshram II, Mallikharjun Rao K, Balakrishna N, et al. Infant and young child feeding practices, sociodemographic factors and their association with nutritional status of children aged <3 years in India: findings of the National Nutrition Monitoring Bureau survey, 2011–2012. *Public Health Nutrition.* 2019;22(1):104–114.
114. Joe W, Rajpal S, Kim R, et al. Association between anthropometric-based and food-based nutritional failure among children in India, 2015. *Matern Child Nutr.* 2019:e12830.
115. Meshram II, Vishnu Vardhana Rao M, Sudershan Rao V, Laxmaiah A, Polasa K. Regional variation in the prevalence of overweight/obesity, hypertension and diabetes and their correlates among the adult rural population in India. *Br J Nutr.* 2016; 115(7):1265–1272.
116. Manyama IB, Abate GA, Tamiru M. *The Emergency Nutrition Coordination Unit of Ethipopia roles, reponsibilities and achievements.* https://www.ennonline.net/fex/40/nutrition. Accessed May 2019.
117. Delbiso TD, Rodriguez-Llanes JM, Donneau AF, Speybroeck N, Guha-Sapir D. Drought, conflict and children's undernutrition in Ethiopia 2000–2013: a meta-analysis. *Bull World Health Organ.* 2017;95(2):94–102.
118. Gebreegziabher T, Regassa N. Ethiopia's high childhood undernutrition explained: analysis of the prevalence and key correlates based on recent nationally representative data. *Public Health Nutrition.* 2019;22(11):2099–2109.
119. Akinbami LJ, Ogden CL. Childhood overweight prevalence in the United States: the impact of parent-reported height and weight. *Obesity.* 2009;17(8):1574–1580.
120. World Health Organization and the United Nations Children's Fund (UNICEF). *Recommendations for Data Collection, Analysis and Reporting on Anthropometric Indicators in Children under 5 Years Old;* 2019. https://www.who.int/nutrition/publications/anthropometry-data-quality-report/en/. Accessed May, 2019.

121. Bodner JE, Perloff BP. Databases for analyzing dietary data–the latest word from what We Eat in America. *Subtrop Plant Sci.* 2003;16(3):347–358.
122. Perloff B, Ahuja JK. Development and maintenance of nutrient databases for national dietary surveys. *Public Health Rev.* 1998; 26(1):43–47.
123. Anderson E, Perloff B, Ahuja JKC, Raper N. Tracking nutrient changes for trends analysis in the United States. *Subtrop Plant Sci.* 2001;14(3):287–294.
124. Moshfegh AJ, Rhodes DG, Baer DJ, et al. The US Dpartment of Agriculture Automated Multiple-Pass Method reduces bias in the collection of energy intakes. *Am J Clin Nutr.* 2008;88(2):324–332.
125. Beaton GHBJ, Ritenbaugh C. Errors in the interpretation of dietary assessments. *Am J Clin Nutr.* 1997;65(4:Suppl):1100S–1107S.
126. Subar AF, Freedman LS, Tooze JA, et al. Addressing current criticism regarding the value of self-report dietary data. *J Nutr.* 2015; 145(12):2639–2645.
127. Dodd KW, Guenther PM, Freedman LS, et al. Statistical methods for estimating usual intake of nutrients and foods: a review of the theory. *J Am Diet Assoc.* 2006;106(10):1640–1650.
128. Kipnis V, Midthune D, Buckman DW, et al. Modeling data with excess zeros and measurement error: application to evaluating relationships between episodically consumed foods and health outcomes. *Biometrics.* 2009;65(4):1003–1010.
129. Tooze JA, Midthune D, Dodd KW, et al. A new statistical method for estimating the usual intake of episodically consumed foods with application to their distribution. *J Am Diet Assoc.* 2006; 106(10):1575–1587.
130. Carroll RJ, Midthune D, Subar AF, et al. Taking advantage of the strengths of 2 different dietary assessment instruments to improve intake estimates for nutritional epidemiology. *Am J Epidemiol.* 2012;175(4):340–347.
131. Cade JE. Measuring diet in the 21st century: use of new technologies. *Proc Nutr Soc.* 2017;76(3):276–282.
132. Stumbo PJ. New technology in dietary assessment: a review of digital methods in improving food record accuracy. *Proc Nutr Soc.* 2013;72(1):70–76.
133. Bedri A, Li R, Haynes M, et al. EarBit: using wearable sensors to detect eating episodes in unconstrained environments. *Proc ACM Interact Mob Wearable Ubiquitous Technol.* 2017;1(3).
134. Chung J, Chung J, Oh W, Yoo Y, Lee WG, Bang H. A glasses-type wearable device for monitoring the patterns of food intake and facial activity. *Sci Rep.* 2017;7:41690.
135. Yiru S, Salley J, Muth E, Hoover A. Assessing the accuracy of a wrist motion tracking method for counting bites across demographic and food variables. *IEEE J Biomed Health Inform.* 2017; 21(3):599–606.
136. Hezarjaribi N, Mazrouee S, Ghasemzadeh H. Speech2Health: a mobile framework for monitoring dietary composition from spoken data. *IEEE J Biomed Health Inform.* 2018;22(1):252–264.
137. Mezgec S, Eftimov T, Bucher T, Koroušić Seljak B. Mixed deep learning and natural language processing method for fake-food image recognition and standardization to help automated dietary assessment. *Public Health Nutr.* 2019;22(7):1193–1202.
138. *Automated Self-Administered 24-Hour Dietary Assessment Tool.* https://epi.grants.cancer.gov/asa24/. Accessed May 2019.
139. Conrad J, Nöthlings U. Innovative approaches to estimate individual usual dietary intake in large-scale epidemiological studies. *Proc Nutr Soc.* 2017;76(3):213–219.
140. *International Dietary Data Expansion Project. INDDEX24.* https://inddex.nutrition.tufts.edu/inddex24. Accessed May 2019.
141. Coates JC, Colaiezzi BA, Bell W, Charrondiere UR, Leclercq C. Overcoming dietary assessment challenges in low-income countries: technological solutions proposed by the international dietary data expansion (INDDEX) project. *Nutrients.* 2017;9(3).
142. Zhu F, Bosch M, Woo I, et al. The use of mobile devices in aiding dietary assessment and evaluation. *IEEE J Sel Top Signal Process.* 2010;4(4):756–766.
143. Zhu F, Mariappan A, Boushey CJ, et al. Technology-assisted dietary assessment. *Proc SPIE-Int Soc Opt Eng.* 2008;6814:681411.
144. Aizawa K. FoodLog: multimedia food recording tools for diverse applications. In: Nishida T, ed. *Vertical Impact.* Tokyo: Springer Japan; 2016:77–95. Human-Harmonized Information Technology; Vol. 1.
145. He H, Kong F, Tan J. DietCam: multiview food recognition using a multikernel SVM. *IEEE J Biomed Health Inform.* 2016;20(3): 848–855.
146. Myers A, Johnston N, Rathod V, et al. Im2Calories: towards an automated mobile vision food diary. In: *Paper Presented at: 2015 IEEE International Conference on Computer Vision (ICCV); 7–13 Dec. 2015.* 2015.
147. Zhang R, Amft O. Monitoring chewing and eating in free-living using smart eyeglasses. *IEEE J Biomed Health Inform.* 2018;22(1):23–32.
148. Farooq M, Sazonov E. Automatic measurement of chew count and chewing rate during food intake. *Electronics.* 2016;5(4).
149. Farooq M, Sazonov E. Segmentation and characterization of chewing bouts by monitoring temporalis muscle using smart glasses with piezoelectric sensor. *IEEE J Biomed Health Inform.* 2017;21(6):1495–1503.
150. Fontana JM, Higgins JA, Schuckers SC, et al. Energy intake estimation from counts of chews and swallows. *Appetite.* 2015;85:14–21.
151. Papapanagiotou V, Diou C, Lingchuan Z, van den Boer J, Mars M, Delopoulos A. A novel approach for chewing detection based on a wearable PPG sensor. In: *Conference Proceedings : Annual International Conference of the IEEE Engineering in Medicine and Biology Society IEEE Engineering in Medicine and Biology Society Annual Conference. 2016.* 2016:6485–6488.
152. Willett W, Rockström J, Loken B, et al. Food in the Anthropocene: the EAT–Lancet Commission on healthy diets from sustainable food systems. *The Lancet.* 2019;393(10170):447–492.
153. O'Malley K, Willits-Smith A, Aranda R, Heller M, Rose D. Vegan vs paleo: carbon footprints and diet quality of 5 popular eating patterns as reported by US consumers (P03-007-19). *Curr Dev Nutr.* 2019;3(suppl 1).
154. Martinez Steele E, Popkin BM, Swinburn B, Monteiro CA. The share of ultra-processed foods and the overall nutritional quality of diets in the US: evidence from a nationally representative cross-sectional study. *Popul Health Metrics.* 2017;15(1):6.
155. Moubarac JC, Batal M, Louzada ML, Martinez Steele E, Monteiro CA. Consumption of ultra-processed foods predicts diet quality in Canada. *Appetite.* 2017;108:512–520.
156. Gibney MJ, Forde CG, Mullally D, Gibney ER. Ultra-processed foods in human health: a critical appraisal. *Am J Clin Nutr.* 2017; 106(3):717–724.
157. Monteiro CA, Cannon G, Levy RB, et al. Ultra-processed foods: what they are and how to identify them. *Public Health Nutr.* 2019;22(5):936–941.
158. Moubarac JC, Parra DC, Cannon G, Monteiro CA. Food classification systems based on food processing: significance and implications for policies and actions: a systematic literature review and assessment. *Curr Obesity Rep.* 2014;3(2):256–272.
159. Sebedio JL. Metabolomics, nutrition, and potential biomarkers of food quality, intake, and health status. *Adv Food Nutr Res.* 2017;82: 83–116.
160. Rowland I, Gibson G, Heinken A, et al. Gut microbiota functions: metabolism of nutrients and other food components. *Eur J Nutr.* 2018;57(1):1–24.
161. Regional Office for the Eastern Mediterranean, Al Jawaldeh A, Osman D, Tawfik A. *Food and nutrition surveillance systems: a manual for policy-makers and programme managers.* World Health Organization, Regional Office for the Eastern Mediterranean; 2014. https://apps.who.int/iris/handle/10665/259796[A1].

CHAPTER

13

DIETARY PATTERNS

Sarah A. McNaughton, PhD, APD, FDAA

Institute for Physical Activity and Nutrition (IPAN), School of Exercise and Nutrition Sciences, Deakin University, Geelong, VIC, Australia

SUMMARY

Dietary patterns examine the combinations, types, and amounts of foods consumed in the diet. There is now global consensus that food and nutrition policies should be informed by evidence regarding dietary patterns. Dietary patterns are assessed using two main approaches, namely, data-driven approaches based on multivariate statistical techniques (e.g., principal component analysis, cluster analysis, and reduced rank regression) or investigator-defined patterns commonly based on "a priori" dietary guidelines or recommendations (e.g., diet quality scores). Dietary pattern methods can be used to address a range of nutrition science issues including etiological research using observational and experimental designs, behavioral research, monitoring, and surveillance and in dietary guideline development. Despite large developments in the field of dietary patterns, key research gaps remain such as a lack of primary studies for some health outcomes and populations, an understanding of the role of dietary patterns in diet–gene interactions and individual responses to diet, and methodological issues that impact the synthesis of evidence for use in the development of dietary guidelines.

Keywords: Data-driven methods; Diet quality index; Dietary patterns; Healthy Eating Index; Investigator-defined methods; Principal component analysis; Total diet.

I. INTRODUCTION

The study of dietary patterns is now an established field in nutrition that has evolved over the last 40 years. The first studies on what we now consider dietary patterns were published in the early 1980s.[1–3] These studies used multivariate statistical methods to capture the complexity of food intake. Subsequently, the field grew during the 1990s with the addition of studies capturing dietary patterns using methods to assess diet quality[4,5] and dietary diversity.[6] The study by Slattery et al. on diet and colon cancer[7,8] is considered a seminal publication and a key time in nutritional epidemiology for dietary patterns. Since that time, dietary patterns research has continued to flourish and research studies using these methodologies have grown exponentially.[9,10] These early studies used a variety of definitions; however, over time, there has been increasing consensus in terminology and approaches. This chapter will outline commonly used definitions of dietary patterns, key concepts, and the major methodologies used commonly in the field. It will also summarize the applications and use of dietary patterns evidence and identify research gaps and limitations in the evidence base.

II. DEFINITIONS

Dietary intake is a complex exposure, with multiple layers reflecting a continuum from nutrients to foods to eating occasions to dietary patterns (Fig. 13.1). Each of these layers, and the interplay between them, is important to health and provides a unique perspective to our understanding of contemporary nutrition problems.

Definitions of dietary patterns have evolved over time, and there are a number of different definitions of

Present Knowledge in Nutrition, Volume 2
https://doi.org/10.1016/B978-0-12-818460-8.00013-7

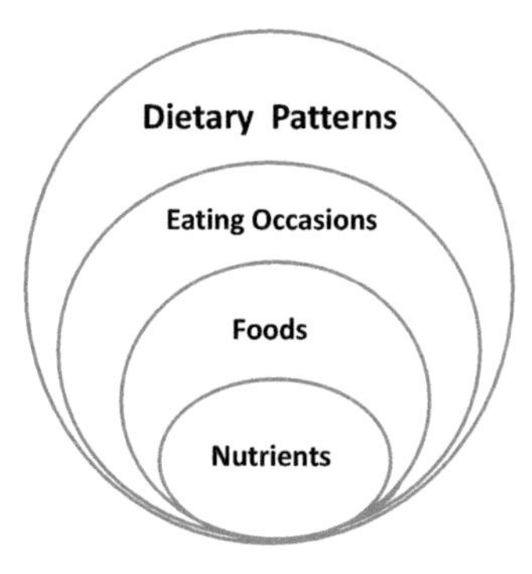

FIGURE 13.1 Dietary intake is a multilevel exposure reflecting a continuum from nutrients to foods to eating occasions to dietary patterns. Each of these layers and the interaction between them are important for health.

dietary patterns in the literature (see Box 13.1). Early research used a variety of terms and definitions, with Slattery et al.[7] using the term "eating patterns" to describe statistically derived patterns from food consumption data. The two most commonly accepted definitions now in use are the United States Department of Agriculture (USDA) Dietary Patterns Systematic Review Project definition[11] and the definition put forward by Hu et al.[12] and acknowledged in the taxonomy of dietary behaviors by Stok et al.[13] The USDA definition describes dietary patterns as the quantities, proportions, variety, or combination of different foods, drinks, and nutrients (when available) in diets and the frequency with which they are habitually consumed. Notably, this 2014 definition has been subsequently modified to describe "food patterns" or "food-based dietary patterns" and removes any reference to nutrients.[14]

Researchers have often defined dietary patterns using an operational definition, that is, according to how dietary patterns are measured or assessed.[15,16] This approach is useful in some contexts, for example, when conducting systematic reviews and meta-analyses as it can provide clear inclusion and exclusion criteria. However, it important to remember that conceptually, the study of dietary patterns aims to capture the multidimensional and complex nature of diet, assessing the total diet rather than intakes of individual nutrients or foods, and restricting the definition to the methodological approaches used may limit the emergence of new approaches and techniques to capture dietary patterns.

III. CURRENT STATUS OF FIELD

A. Why Are Dietary Patterns Important?

Dietary patterns have emerged as an important exposure in nutritional epidemiology. This interest has increased alongside the lack of success of dietary intervention studies focused on single nutrients such as those examining β-carotene[17] and the development of interventions based on the "total diet" such as the Lyon Diet Heart Study and the Dietary Approaches to Stop Hypertension (DASH) trial.[18,19] Additional evidence of the inadequacies of a single-nutrient approach is provided by meta-analyses of the role of saturated fat and cardiovascular disease which demonstrated inconsistencies in the existing literature when examining nutrient-focused research.[20]

There are a number of advantages of using dietary patterns to reflect dietary exposure rather than individual nutrients or even individual foods. Biologically, dietary pattern research has the potential to capture

BOX 13.1

Evolution of different definitions for dietary patterns

1981
Food eating patterns: Foods as they are actually consumed in various characteristic combinations.[2]
2002
Dietary patterns: Specific combination of foods and beverages one eats on a regular basis, which includes a specific mix of nutrients.[12,13]

2014
Dietary patterns: The quantities, proportions, variety, or combination of different foods, drinks, and nutrients (when available) in diets and the frequency with which they are habitually consumed.[11]
2018
Food patterns: The quantities, proportions, variety, or combinations of different food and beverages in diets and the frequency with which they are habitually consumed.[14]

interactions that may occur between a variety of food components and constituents and reflects the potentially important role played by the food matrix. Additionally, there are still components in foods where the biological action is unknown or not well characterized; therefore, food-based approaches to dietary patterns can account for this. Dietary patterns research can capture the concept of dietary balance as it can incorporate multiple aspects or dimensions of diet simultaneously and recognize that a critical factor in disease prevention may be the balance between protective and harmful components of diet. It is also acknowledged that intakes of most nutrients are highly correlated, and statistically, it can be difficult to examine the effects of one nutrient[21]; therefore, dietary patterns can address this issue of multicollinearity. Finally, a dietary patterns approach can address the fact that small changes or differences in individual foods may not demonstrate associations with health outcomes, but there may be cumulative and synergistic health benefits of multiple foods.[22]

B. Assessing Dietary Patterns

A number of key methodologies have emerged over time in the dietary pattern literature (Table 13.1). These are grouped into two major types: (1) data-driven methods (also referred to as empirical methods or "a posteriori" methods) and (2) investigator-defined methods (also referred to as "a priori" methods). Each of these methods provides a composite or summary measure of dietary behaviors; however, it is important to recognize that each of these methods addresses the issue from a different perspective and the particular method of choice will depend on the research question.

Data-driven methods

Data-driven methods utilize a range of multivariate statistical approaches to summarize a large number of dietary variables into integrated measures of diet and are often considered data reduction techniques. Dietary intake variables are known to be highly correlated, and the statistical approaches utilized take advantage of this characteristic. There are three commonly used methods in the literature, namely, principal component analysis, cluster analysis, and reduced rank regression, with principal component analysis currently the most popular method.[9] Data-driven approaches allow the data to determine the dietary patterns and hence describe the patterns of eating that actually exist in the population rather than depending on the researcher's previous knowledge or preconceived ideas of population intakes or diet–disease relationships. They can provide useful insights into existing dietary behaviors.

One of the major criticisms of data-driven approaches is that there a number of decisions that must be made by the researcher during the analysis process, and some of these decisions may be considered subjective. One of the decisions that influence all types of data-driven methods relates to the development of the food groups used as the input variables for the statistical analysis.[23] This is a subjective step, and there are a large range of different food groupings applied in the literature to date.[24,25] Food groupings and categorizations may be based on existing food categorization systems used in national food composition databases, which in turn may apply food commodity approaches and nutrient composition considerations. Dietary patterns research also commonly incorporates other theoretical considerations such as culinary uses of foods and behavioral aspects of how foods are consumed; however, these factors are likely to vary across countries and population groups. Approaches to food categorizations may reflect different goals and research questions. There has been little research on the impact of different food categorizations on the outcomes of dietary patterns research. However, one early study by McCann et al.[26] addressed this issue indirectly. McCann et al.[26] conducted analyses assessing dietary patterns using factor analysis and compared the dietary patterns when using 36 broad food groups versus 168 single food items. The authors found that the number of patterns, and qualitatively the type of patterns identified (in terms of the types of foods associated with each pattern), was not impacted. However, associations between the dietary patterns and the health outcome (cancer) were attenuated when using the broad foods groups. This suggests that important information was lost and that more detailed food information may be beneficial when examining relationships with diet and health.

Factor analysis and principal component analysis; Factor analysis and principal component analysis (which is a type of factor of factor analysis) are the most common data-driven methods used to derive dietary patterns.[9,12,27] These methods employ the correlations between foods consumed in the diet to describe the variations in food intakes that exist in a population. These methods result in latent variables or "factors," which are the dietary patterns. These factors are defined by the foods whose consumption is highly correlated with the factor. Specific criteria are applied when determining the number of dietary patterns to extract including the eigenvalues (usually >1.0), the identification of a break point in the scree plot, and interpretability of the patterns.[28,29] To date, the majority of studies have identified three or fewer patterns.[9] The foods that load "highly" are the major contributors to the dietary

TABLE 13.1 Dietary pattern assessment and methodology.

Method	Description	Examples	Challenges in use or interpretation	Use	Research gaps
Data-driven dietary patterns—*"a posteriori"*	• Use a range of multivariate statistical techniques to reduce a large number of dietary components • Utilize the highly correlated nature of dietary intake variables • Describe patterns that exist in the population • Methods vary according to whether they are outcome independent (e.g., principal component analysis) or outcome	• Factor analysis and principal component analysis • Cluster analysis • Reduced rank regression	• Multiple different methods and some aspects of methods are well defined • Some steps require subjective decisions • Dietary patterns identified do not always reflect current knowledge/guidelines on optimal eating patterns	• Identify relationships between diet and health • Identify groups of people (cluster analysis) • Understand pathways or mechanisms between diet and health (reduced rank regression)	• How many foods groups are optimal? • Reduced rank regression—what are the optimal type and number of intermediate markers? • Can data-driven dietary patterns be used to develop quantitative dietary recommendations?

	dependent (e.g., reduced rank regression)				
Investigator-defined dietary patterns—"*a priori*"	• Describe intakes according to prespecified criteria, guidelines, recommendations, or knowledge • Investigator defines the attributes of the dietary patterns and the criteria and cut points to assess the degree of concordance • Attributes may be nutrient-based, food-based, or both nutrient and food intakes combined • Most commonly calculated as indexes or "diet quality scores" operationalizing national dietary guidelines • May also reflect other selective or predefined diets, e.g., vegetarian diets • Recent approaches may be based on single attributes such as level of processing or level of plant-based foods versus animal-based foods • Large number of existing indices worldwide	• Healthy Eating Index, • Diet Quality Index, • Mediterranean Diet Scores, • Dietary Inflammatory Index, • Dietary variety scores	• Low proportion of participants consuming a diet consistent with the dietary guidelines can lead to lack of variation in the population • Single summary score can be achieved in multiple ways that can make interpretation difficult	• Identify relationships between diet and health • Assessing intervention outcomes • Monitoring and surveillance	• Refining the development of diet quality indices • How do we know which attributes or dietary factors are the most important to include? What are the best indicators or measures of these attributes? What criteria or cutpoints should be used? • What is the minimum set of indicators to include? • What is the impact on small changes in an index or score?

patterns and often the foods used to label or develop a name for the dietary pattern. Considerable variability exists in the literature related to the cut point for factor loadings; however, loadings from 0.20 to 0.40 are most commonly utilized. For each dietary pattern identified, a dietary pattern score is calculated based on the food intake input variable and the factor loading for each food. This score reflects how well a participant's dietary intake reflects the dietary pattern of interest.[30,31]

When using this method, it should be recognized that a person's overall dietary pattern is most adequately represented by the combination of all the dietary patterns identified in the population. For example, if a study identifies two dietary patterns, a participant will have a score describing their intake of the foods for each of these patterns. Often the dietary patterns are investigated separately with the outcome of interest, but it may also be important to investigate the impact of both patterns simultaneously. One of the major analytical advantages of the factor analysis or principal component analysis approaches is that it results in a continuous score. A continuous score is an advantage with respect to interpretation, as it aligns with concepts of other nutrient and food intake variables. From a statistical perspective, it maximizes statistical power to detect diet–disease relationships (compared to cluster analysis and other person-centered approaches).

Cluster analysis and other person-centered approaches; Cluster analysis is a statistical method that aims to describe variations in food intakes and separates individuals into mutually exclusive groups or clusters.[32] People are clustered in groups based on difference and similarities in food intakes. The aim is to generate clusters where people within clusters have as similar food intakes as possible and to maximize the difference in food intake between clusters ensuring the within-cluster variability is small compared to the difference between clusters.[30] Food and beverage intakes (the input variables) are commonly expressed as either frequency of intake or percentage of energy intake[15] and standardized food intakes may be used as cluster analysis is sensitive to outliers. The two most common clustering techniques include the K-means method and Ward's hierarchical clustering.[15]

As with PCA, a number of steps in cluster analysis require subjective decisions, and a key issue in using cluster analysis is determining the number of clusters to report. The K-means method requires that the number of clusters extracted is predefined by the researcher, while the Ward's method does not. These methods are often used together to determine the number of clusters to report from the data.[33] The subjective nature of this analysis can be minimized using empirical stopping rules such as the Calinski–Harabasz index (K-means CA) or the Duda–Hart stopping rule (Ward's hierarchical clustering method), to determine the optimal number of clusters.[34] The number of clusters is often also determined based on size of the cluster where clusters containing less than <10% of the total sample are considered too small for adequate statistical power. Finally, the interpretability of dietary pattern clusters is also examined to confirm the final solution.[34]

More recently, latent class and latent profile analysis has been used as an alternative method for cluster analysis, and there are a growing number of studies applying this methodology.[35] Conceptually, they are similar to cluster analysis in that it attempts to create mutually exclusive groups or classes based on variations in food consumption, maximizing variation between the groups. Latent class and latent profile analysis use different algorithms and assumptions based on maximum likelihood methods. They have a number of advantages over cluster analysis including the ability to use input variables with different scales or units, with no requirement for standardization before analysis. Furthermore, there are formal criteria based on goodness-of-fit tests for selecting the number of dietary patterns to retain reducing the criticism of subjectivity involved with data-driven dietary pattern assessment.

Cluster analysis and other person-centered approaches are intuitive from a public health or clinical perspective as conceptually these approaches identify groups of people and may be useful to identify target groups for intervention. However, cluster analysis has a number of disadvantages in a research context. It can result in limited statistical power, particular in studies with smaller sample sizes or where the groupings result in clusters with small numbers of participants. These analysis methods also can be particularly challenging when conducting longitudinal studies in terms of assessing clusters at different time points and changes over time.[36]

Reduced rank regression; Reduced rank regression is commonly considered a hybrid method in that it is primarily a data-driven approach and also incorporates prior knowledge.[37,38] It is a statistical technique that aims to examine pathways through which food intake impacts health outcomes and the pathway or mechanisms through which diet may act. In reduced rank regression, the researcher identifies the food groups and the health outcome of interest and a set of intermediate variables that are chosen on the basis of previous knowledge. The intermediate variables that have been commonly used are nutrient intakes, biomarkers of nutritional status or other biomarkers of the disease process, or risk factors for the health outcome. The analysis is conducted in two steps. The first step examines the combinations of foods that predict the intermediate variables using regression.

Loadings for each food are derived and used to calculate a dietary patterns score (similar to the approaches used to calculate scores for factor or principal component analysis). Unlike factor or principal component analysis, the maximum number of dietary patterns that can be extracted is fixed and is determined on the number of intermediate variables used in the analysis. This reduces the number of subjective decisions required when developing the dietary patterns. Many studies have only examined the first pattern extracted, which by default explains the greatest variation in intermediat variables. In the second step, the relationship between dietary pattern scores and disease outcome is tested using standard epidemiological designs and methods.

Reduced rank regression methodology has been used to study dietary influences on obesity,[39] CVD,[40,41] diabetes,[42] and all-cause mortality.[43–45] This method is different from other dietary pattern approaches as it identifies foods that explain variation in intermediate markers rather than explaining variation in food intakes.[37] Therefore, it is particularly suited to etiological work and can be used to identify or confirm pathways through which dietary patterns may act, rather than identifying underlying behavioral food intake patterns.

Compared to other methods of dietary pattern assessment, reduced rank regression has been used less frequently. This may be due to the complexity of the method as many decisions are required including identifying suitable intermediate variables. Nutrient variables have commonly been used, perhaps reflecting the lack of appropriate biomarkers of nutritional status available or lack of other markers of the disease processes. More research is required to understand the optimal number and combination of intermediate markers to include and the impact of using different markers. For example, it is likely that some disease outcomes have multiple mechanisms through which diet may act, each with multiple potential markers, and it is unclear whether these should be examined separately in reduced rank regression modeling.

Investigator-defined patterns methods

The second major approach to assessing dietary patterns is the use of investigator-defined methods that are also referred to as "*a priori*" methods. Within this category, there are a number of different ways to construct the dietary patterns. However, the overarching principal is that the dietary patterns are defined by the researcher, and the aim is to describe intakes according to previous knowledge, guidelines, and recommendations using prespecified criteria. The researcher selects the attributes, that is, the food components or items that make up the dietary pattern, the indicators to include, and the criteria and cut points to assess the degree of concordance with those attributes. The attributes may be nutrient-based, food-based, or combine both nutrient and food intakes. The attributes and cut points are commonly selected on the basis on national dietary guidelines, food selection guides, and nutrient reference values. Dietary intakes of individuals are then scored against these prespecified attributes and criteria to determine how well their dietary pattern aligns. Dietary indices or diet quality scores are the most well-known and commonly used form of investigator-defined dietary patterns. Other approaches to investigator-defined patterns are the use of selective dietary patterns, for example, vegetarian diets, or a focus on single attributes such as dietary diversity.[6] More recently, the level of food processing has been suggested as a key attribute for defining dietary patterns.[46]

As noted, dietary scores or indices may be based on nutrients, foods, or both nutrients and food. Food-based dietary indices have theoretical and practical advantages over those that incorporate other dietary constituents such as nutrients.[47] From a theoretical perspective, using a food-based approach is a less reductionist paradigm. It retains the complexity of food intake, including the food matrix and the variety of nutrient and non-nutrient components in food, and these are principles that underpin the study of dietary patterns. Food-based indices and scores are also consistent with international calls for food-based dietary guidelines.[48] Conceptually, food-based scores also are more similar to the other data-driven methods of assessing dietary patterns, which are solely focused on food intakes.[15] Food-based scores also have practical benefits. Food-based scores can be more readily applied to brief dietary assessment tools that assess food intakes rather than those diet quality scores that required detailed assessments of nutrient intake. Therefore, food-based scores may be more suitable for some monitoring and surveillance activities.[49]

Table 13.2 describes a range of commonly used diet quality scores within the literature and the key characteristics of these scores. From this table, it can be seen that scores have been developed to capture a wide range of dietary profiles, and each one contains varying attributes, and have different criteria. Different scores or indices may have different primary aims and may address different research questions. Therefore, when selecting a diet quality tool, it is important to evaluate the underlying objective and its appropriate application in each context. One of the most well-know diet quality scores is the Healthy Eating Index (HEI).[5,50,51] USDA developed this score to assess compliance with the Dietary Guidelines for Americans. The HEI was first released in 1995[5] and has been continually refined and updated to reflect ongoing updates to the Dietary Guidelines.[52,53] It was originally applied to assess the diet quality of individuals, and subsequently, the HEI

TABLE 13.2 Examples of commonly used diet quality scores.

Name	Description of attributes and key concepts
Healthy Eating Index (HEI-2015)[84]	• Developed to reflect Dietary Guidelines for Americans. • 13 items: Wholegrains, refined grains, total vegetables, greens and beans, total fruits, whole fruits, dairy, total protein foods, seafood and plant proteins, fatty acids, sodium, added sugars, and saturated fats.
Recommended Foods Score[85]	• Foods on the dietary questionnaire are identified as "recommended" according to dietary guidelines. • Food consumption classified according to frequency of consumption with foods consumed more than once per week scoring 1. • Total score is the sum of recommended foods consumed regularly.
Mediterranean Diet Score[86,87]	• Large range of different scores in the literature. • Commonly includes indictors of fruit, vegetables, cereals, fish, olive oil, alcohol, meat and meat products, and dairy. • Predominantly scored according to median intakes except for alcohol intake (quantitative intakes scored).
Dietary Inflammatory Index[58]	• 45 components: Macro- and micronutrients (28 components), bioactive compounds/phytochemicals (8 components), foods (2 components), and herbs and spices (7 components). • 36 components are antiinflammatory, 9 components are proinflammatory.
Dietary Approaches to Stop Hypertension (DASH) score[88]	• Based on the DASH diet • 8 components: Fruits, vegetables, whole grains, nuts and legumes, low-fat dairy, red and processed meats, sweetened beverages, and sodium. • Scored according to quintiles of dietary intake.
Alternative Healthy Eating Index (AHEI)-2010[89,90]	• Originally developed in 2002 and subsequently updated. • 12 components: Vegetables, fruit, wholegrains, sugar-sweetened beverages and fruit juice, nuts, legumes, red/processed meat, *trans* fat, long-chain (n-3) fats (EPA + DHA), PUFA, sodium, alcohol. • Quantitative cut points.
Plant-based Diet Index (PDI)[91]	• 18 food groups in three categories: 1. Plant food groups—Healthy (whole grains, fruits, vegetables, nuts, legumes, vegetable oils, tea, and coffee) 2. Plant food groups—Less healthy (fruit juices, refined grains, potatoes, sugar-sweetened beverages, sweets, and desserts) 3. Animal food groups (animal fat, dairy, egg, fish or seafood, meat miscellaneous animal based foods) • Scored according to quintiles of dietary intake, animal foods reverse scored.
EAT-Lancet Score[92]	• 14 components: Whole grains, tubers and starchy vegetables, vegetables, fruits, dairy foods, protein sources (4 items: beef, lamb, pork; chicken, other poultry; eggs; fish), legumes (dry beans, lentils, peas; soy foods; peanuts; or tree nuts), added fats, added sugars. • Quantitative cut-points for each component used as criteria. • Components scored as 0 (not meeting) or 1 (meeting).

has been used to assess diet quality of multiple layers of the food system. The HEI is commonly used in other countries; however, often the cutoffs or criteria for specific components of the dietary index are altered to reflect local guidelines and nutrient reference values.[54–57]

C. Comparability of Dietary Patterns

A significant issue facing dietary pattern research is comparability across studies using different methods and in different populations groups. Some of the reasons for this arise from use of different methodological approaches, the subjective nature of some aspects of methodology (particularly in relation to data-driven approaches), the different food groups and definitions of items included within these food groups, and different treatment of alcohol intake across dietary patterns approaches and studies.[9] Specifically, with respect to reduced rank regression, there has been considerable variability in the intermediate markers (different combinations of nutrients and different combinations of disease biomarkers) that have been used, even when examining the same health outcomes.

Investigator-defined methods are often considered a solution to issues of comparability, given that the attributes, criteria, and scoring are prespecified. Theoretically this is true, and for many diet quality scores, comparability is less of an issue, as they can be applied across populations more systematically. However, this may not be the case across all of the subtypes of dietary scores and indices and there are some situations where comparability is still an issue for investigator-defined approaches. The Mediterranean diet score is one such example.[9] Firstly, there are a number of scores available in the literature, which vary with respect to the food and nutrient attributes and indicators that are included. However, even when the same score is used across populations, it may be difficult to compare across studies. The scoring approaches for the Mediterranean diet scores often utilize a population-based approach, with scoring based on the distribution of intakes of each component in that population (e.g., those participants with an intake above the median intake receive a score of 1 for that component). Therefore, while the foods and nutrients that make up the score may be similar, across different studies, participants who score highly may have different quantitative levels of intake or consumption. Similarly, the dietary inflammatory index is an investigator-defined dietary pattern score based on evidence from 1943 studies examining the effect of dietary components on inflammatory markers.[58] The index contains 45 components; however, when applied across populations, studies have included anywhere between 18 and 37 components due to data availability.[59,60] Issues of comparability are also raised when existing indices such as the US HEI[51,52] are adapted for use in different countries and different criteria or cut-offs are applied.[54–57] Without further evaluation, it can be difficult to assess the impact of these changes and it can be unclear whether an individual's score on the HEI dietary index still reflects the same dietary intake profile.

The Dietary Patterns Method Project was specifically designed to address issues relating to variability in methods and approaches across cohorts and inform updates to the Dietary Guidelines for Americans.[61] The project conducted standardized and parallel analyses and applied four dietary indices (HEI 2010, the Alternate HEI 2010, the alternate Mediterranean Diet score, and the DASH score) to three cohorts. The analyses were standardized in terms of calculating the dietary indices (for example, ensuring the food groups were constructed in a standardized way) and conducting the statistical analyses (for example, utilizing standard covariates and harmonizing the outcomes). The project was able to show good concordance across the scores and cohorts, with significant reductions in all-cause, CVD, and cancer mortality associated with higher dietary quality as measured by the four diet quality scores.[61]

D. Application of Dietary Patterns to Nutrition Science

Dietary pattern methods can be used in a range of study designs and across a range of nutrition science questions and applications, including etiological research using observational and experimental designs, behavioral research, monitoring and surveillance, and in dietary guideline development. Given the diversity of methods described previously, an important consideration is to ensure that the most appropriate method is used to answer a particular research question.

Etiological research (understanding diet and health relationships)

In nutritional epidemiology, research questions relating to understanding diet and health relationships is the primary research question and has been the primary use of dietary pattern research to date.[62] Measures of dietary patterns may be used in epidemiological studies either to investigate associations of overall healthy eating patterns with particular health outcomes or as a confounder when investigating other exposure–disease relationships. Dietary pattern exposures have been used in randomized controlled trials to understand diet and health, for example, through the application of Mediterranean dietary patterns and DASH. Specifically, they have been used to design dietary interventions, and subsequently dietary patterns assessment methods may be used to assess compliance with the dietary interventions.

Behavioral research

Behavioral epidemiology is primarily concerned with the distribution and determinants of behaviors that influence health and focuses on research that aims to identify influences on the behavior and evaluate behavior change interventions.[63] Dietary patterns methods are useful in behavioral research as they capture multiple aspects of the diet that are often interrelated, and changing one behavior may impact other parts of the diet with both positive and negative consequences.[64] In behavioral research, measures of dietary patterns are the outcome of interest and may be used to as an integrated measure of dietary behavior to examine predictors or determinants.[65] They may also be used to investigate interactions with other health behaviors, and finally, they may be the outcome used when evaluating interventions. All dietary patterns methods have been used when examining predictors and determinants of dietary patterns or when examining associations with other health behaviors. When evaluating interventions, the investigator-defined methods may be most appropriate, as the intervention will target specific dietary behaviors, and these approaches allow the investigator to define the dietary elements relevant to their intervention. Diet quality scores may be particularly useful when evaluating tailored interventions where participants select their individual dietary goals as there will be multiple ways to achieve changes in overall diet quality score.

Monitoring and surveillance

Nutrition monitoring and surveillance is important for evaluating and reviewing food and nutrition policy and programs, identifying vulnerable groups, and identifying emerging nutrition issues.[66] Key characteristics of monitoring and surveillance activities are the need for collection and analysis of routine measurements that allow detection of changes over time, progress toward established goals or targets, and therefore involve ongoing or repeat measures over time. While nutrition monitoring and surveillance systems should consider the entire food and nutrition system from food production, supply, distribution, consumption, nutritional status, and metabolism to health outcomes for the population, assessment of food and nutrient consumption patterns is a cornerstone of these activities. Given the need for comparability over time and population groups, investigator-defined approaches to dietary patterns are most suited to monitoring and surveillance objectives. As described above, many diet quality scores have been designed to reflect compliance with national dietary guidelines. They are suited to examining how well people comply with those dietary guidelines, examine changes over time, and monitor trends at the population level.[50] The United States HEI has been applied at multiple levels of the food system, namely, the individual, community, and food environment level.[67] It has been used to examine diet quality of the food supply using food balance data over time[68,69] and to examine other aspects of the food environment such as supermarkets and fast food restaurants[51,67,69,70] demonstrating that it can be used to evaluate multiple components of the food and nutrition system. The HEI can be used to assess other levels of the food system or food environment such as the food supply because the criteria are based on energy density. That is, the required quantities are based on the amounts of food groups per 1000 kcal, which translates the proportion between amounts of groups of food per amounts of energy, reflecting the balance of the diet rather than the quantity of the diet.[51]

Use of dietary pattern research in dietary guideline development

There is now global consensus that dietary guidelines should be informed by evidence regarding dietary patterns given the multifactorial nature of diet-related disease,[10,71] and there has been increasing use of dietary pattern evidence to inform dietary guidelines. Recognizing the importance of dietary patterns, the United States Dietary Guidelines has increasingly incorporated evidence relating to dietary patterns. The 2020 Dietary Guidelines Advisory Committee (DGAC) Dietary Patterns Subcommittee reviewed evidence relating to eight major topics including growth, body composition and obesity, cardiovascular disease, type 2 diabetes, cancer, bone health, sarcopenia, and all-cause mortality.[72] In addition, there were nine topics addressed relating to dietary patterns in pregnancy and lactation, and the guidelines will be informed by data analysis and modeling that includes assessment of dietary patterns. This builds on work by the 2015 DGAC, where the dietary patterns structure was a key underlying concept.[73] The 2015 Committee examined research questions relating to dietary patterns and cardiovascular disease, body weight and obesity, type 2 diabetes, cancer, congenital anomalies, neurological and psychological illnesses, and bone health and utilized evidence from the Nutrition Evidence Library (now known as the Nutrition Evidence Systematic Review) Dietary Patterns Systematic Review Project.[11] This was the first time systematic reviews on dietary patterns had been incorporated into the dietary guidelines process. Given the nature of the evidence in dietary patterns research, the DGAC utilized qualitative descriptions of healthy dietary patterns based on scientific evidence for several health outcomes. Of note, dietary patterns evidence was prioritized such that where strong or moderate evidence related to dietary patterns and health outcomes was available, this evidence was utilized, and the food and nutrient characteristics identified were summarized to guide recommendations. When only limited or insufficient evidence related to dietary patterns and a particular health outcome was available, existing evidence on specific foods and/or nutrients was used. Food modeling also incorporated dietary patterns concepts to develop the USDA Food Patterns (including the Healthy US-style Pattern, the Healthy Mediterranean-style Pattern, and the Healthy Vegetarian Pattern) and provided the basis for quantitative recommendations.

Other agencies worldwide have also moved to using dietary patterns concepts and research to inform guidelines and recommendations. The World Cancer Research Fund has produced Cancer Prevention Recommendations based on expert review of evidence with a major focus on dietary exposures, published in three expert reports in 1997,[74] 2007,[75] and 2018.[76] The First Expert report was published in 1997[74] and did not include any reference to dietary patterns, while the second expert report published in 2007 included a review of dietary pattern exposures.[75] In 2007, the evidence was considered insufficient in that dietary patterns were infrequently studied and the existing evidence was conflicting primarily due to variations in the methods used; therefore, a narrative summary of evidence was provided. For the third expert report in 2018, systematic reviews were conducted focusing on studies examining dietary patterns using dietary indices American Cancer Society Cancer prevention Guidelines Score, HEI 2005, the alternate Mediterranean Diet Score and the WCRF/AICR Score.[76] As the underlying evidence base of primary studies increases, there will be more use of dietary patterns in policy and practice.

IV. CONCLUSION

The field of dietary patterns research emerged almost 40 years ago and has gained significant interest and increased exponentially over the last 20 years. Dietary patterns methods provide an important tool for studying many nutrition questions and can provide important insights into dietary behaviors and associations with health outcomes. A range of methods can be used for dietary patterns analysis, and there is a need to develop greater consensus in the use, application, and reporting of dietary patterns research. It is important to consider the continuum of dietary intake when understanding the role of diet in health rather than focusing solely on nutrients or foods, and it is critical that we integrate dietary pattern approaches when developing nutrition policies and guidelines.

RESEARCH GAPS

Dietary patterns research has developed substantially in the last 15 years, and research shows that dietary patterns are important predictors of chronic disease and all-cause mortality.[14] However, there are still significant knowledge gaps. As with studies of individual foods, there is a lack of primary studies for some health outcomes such as mental and neurological health.[77,78] There is also a lack of evidence for some population groups. For example, the 2015 DGAC acknowledged that where dietary patterns were assessed, the majority of evidence on dietary patterns was restricted to adults,[73] and there were more limited data on children and adolescents. There is also limited data using longitudinal assessment of dietary intake and life-course analyses of dietary patterns and health outcomes. Furthermore, there is a significant lack of published data for low- and middle-income countries.[10,79] This lack of primary data is a major barrier for the development of national level dietary guidelines.

Another significant research gap relates to the assessment of individual variation in responses to dietary intake.[80] This is a critical area for nutritional epidemiology, as failure to consider diet–gene interactions may in part explain the mixed findings in relation to diet and health outcomes across a number of areas. This is fundamental knowledge to underpin interventions of personalized nutrition. While new studies are emerging,[81,82] most existing studies investigating diet–gene interactions have focused on relationships with specific nutrients and have largely ignored dietary patterns, and there are few studies of outcomes other than cardiovascular disease or cancer.

There are also research gaps in relation to aspects of the methodology used to assess dietary patterns. Different methodological approaches may be best suited to particular research questions and may not be interchangeable. However, within a particular analytical approach, there are differences in the application of each method across studies.[9] As described earlier, comparability across studies due to different methodological approaches, particularly the data-driven methodologies, is an important issue.[9] The impact of the variability in application of each of the methods in unclear and requires further evaluation. Also, this diversity of approaches adds significant complexity to the synthesis of dietary patterns research in systematic reviews and meta-analyses.[83] Further research is required to develop consensus in the conduct and reporting of dietary patterns research and agreed upon approaches for synthesizing evidence generated from dietary pattern studies to allow best use of dietary pattern evidence in the development of dietary guidelines.

V. REFERENCES

1. Margetts BM, Campbell NA, Armstrong BK. Summarizing dietary patterns using multivariate analysis. *J Hum Nutr.* 1981;35(4): 281–286.
2. Schwerin HS, Stanton JL, Riley Jr AM, et al. Food eating patterns and health: a reexamination of the Ten-State and HANES I surveys. *Am J Clin Nutr.* 1981;34(4):568–580.
3. Schwerin HS, Stanton JL, Smith JL, Riley Jr AM, Brett BE. Food, eating habits, and health: a further examination of the relationship between food eating patterns and nutritional health. *Am J Clin Nutr.* 1982;35(5 Suppl):1319–1325.
4. Kant AK. Indices of overall diet quality: a review. *J Am Diet Assoc.* 1996;96:785–791.
5. Kennedy ET, Ohls J, Carlson S, Fleming K. The healthy eating index: design and applications. *J Am Diet Assoc.* 1995;95(10): 1103–1108.
6. Kant AK, Block G, Schatzkin A, Ziegler RG, Nestle M. Dietary diversity in the US population, NHANES II, 1976-1980. *J Am Diet Assoc.* 1991;91(12):1526–1531.

7. Slattery ML, Boucher KM, Caan BJ, Potter JD, Ma KN. Eating patterns and risk of colon cancer. *Am J Epidemiol.* 1998;148(1):4–16.
8. Slattery ML, Boucher KM. Factor analysis as a tool for evaluating eating patterns. *Am J Epidemiol.* 1998;148(1):20–21.
9. Borges CA, Rinaldi AE, Conde WL, Mainardi GM, Behar D, Slater B. Dietary patterns: a literature review of the methodological characteristics of the main step of the multivariate analyzes. *Rev Bras Epidemiol.* 2015;18(4):837–857.
10. Kumanyika S, Afshin A, Arimond M, Lawrence M, McNaughton S, Nishida C. Background paper on healthy diets. In: *Sustainable Healthy Diets Guiding Principles.* 2019. International Expert Consultation Healthy and Sustainable Diets. In: Rome: Food and Agriculture Organization of the United Nations and World Health Organization.
11. United States Department of Agriculture. *A Series of Systematic Reviews on the Relationship Between Dietary Patterns and Health Outcomes.* 2014.
12. Hu FB. Dietary pattern analysis: a new direction in nutritional epidemiology. *Curr Opin Lipidol.* 2002;13(1):3–9.
13. Stok FM, Renner B, Allan J, et al. Dietary behavior: an interdisciplinary conceptual analysis and taxonomy. *Front Psychol.* 2018;9: 1689.
14. Schulze MB, Martinez-Gonzalez MA, Fung TT, Lichtenstein AH, Forouhi NG. Food based dietary patterns and chronic disease prevention. *BMJ.* 2018;361:k2396.
15. Newby PK, Tucker KL. Empirically derived eating patterns using factor or cluster analysis: a review. *Nutr Rev.* 2004;62(5):177–203.
16. Wirfalt E, Drake I, Wallstrom P. What do review papers conclude about food and dietary patterns? *Food Nutr Res.* 2013;57.
17. Albanes D. B carotene and lung cancer: a case study. *Am J Clin Nutr.* 1999;69:1345S–1350S.
18. De-Lorgeril M, Salen P, Martin JL, Monjaud I, Delaye J, Mamelle N. Mediterranean diet, traditional risk factors, and the rate of cardiovascular complications after myocardial infarction: final report of the Lyon Diet Heart Study. *Circulation.* 1999;99(6):779–785.
19. Appel LJ, Moore TJ, Obarzanek E, et al. A clinical trial of the effects of dietary patterns on blood pressure. DASH Collaborative Research Group. *N Engl J Med.* 1997;336(16):1117–1124.
20. Siri-Tarino PW, Sun Q, Hu FB, Krauss RM. Meta-analysis of prospective cohort studies evaluating the association of saturated fat with cardiovascular disease. *Am J Clin Nutr.* 2010;91(3): 535–546.
21. Freudenheim JL. Study design and hypothesis testing: issues in the evaluation of evidence from research in nutritional epidemiology. *Am J Clin Nutr.* 1999;69(6):1315s–1321s.
22. McNaughton SA, Mishra GD, Brunner EJ. Food patterns associated with blood lipids are predictive of coronary heart disease: Whitehall II prospective study. *Br J Nutr.* 2009;102(4):619–624.
23. Tapsell LC, Neale EP, Probst Y. Dietary patterns and cardiovascular disease: insights and challenges for considering food groups and nutrient sources. *Curr Atheroscler Rep.* 2019;21(3):9.
24. Moubarac JC, Parra DC, Cannon G, Monteiro CA. Food classification systems based on food processing: significance and implications for policies and actions: a systematic literature review and assessment. *Curr Obes Rep.* 2014;3(2):256–272.
25. Fardet A, Rock E, Bassama J, et al. Current food classifications in epidemiological studies do not enable solid nutritional recommendations for preventing diet-related chronic diseases: the impact of food processing. *Adv Nutr.* 2015;6(6):629–638.
26. McCann SE, Marshall JR, Brasure JR, Graham S, Freudenheim JL. Analysis of patterns of food intake in nutritional epidemiology: food classification in principal components analysis and the subsequent impact on estimates for endometrial cancer. *Public Health Nutr.* 2001;4(5):989–997.
27. Tucker KL. Dietary patterns, approaches, and multicultural perspective. *Appl Physiol Nutr Metabol.* 2010;35(2):211–218.
28. Jannasch F, Riordan F, Andersen LF, Schulze MB. Exploratory dietary patterns: a systematic review of methods applied in pan-European studies and of validation studies. *Br J Nutr.* 2018; 120(6):601–611.
29. Kline P. *An Easy Guide to Factor Analysis.* London: Routledge; 1994.
30. Moeller SM, Reedy J, Millen AE, et al. Dietary patterns: challenges and opportunities in dietary patterns research an Experimental Biology Workshop, April 1, 2006. *J Am Diet Assoc.* 2007;107(7): 1233–1239.
31. Krebs-Smith SM, Subar AF, Reedy J. Examining dietary patterns in relation to chronic disease: matching measures and methods to questions of interest. *Circulation.* 2015;132(9):790–793.
32. Schulze MB, Hoffmann K. Methodological approaches to study dietary patterns in relation to risk of coronary heart disease and stroke. *Br J Nutr.* 2006;95(5):860–869.
33. Leech RM, McNaughton SA, Timperio A. Clustering of children's obesity-related behaviors: associations with sociodemographic indicators. *Eur J Clin Nutr.* 2014;68(5):623–628.
34. Thorpe MG, Milte CM, Crawford D, McNaughton SA. A comparison of the dietary patterns derived by principal component analysis and cluster analysis in older Australians. *Int J Behav Nutr Phys Act.* 2016;13:30.
35. Lobo AS, de Assis MAA, Leal DB, et al. Empirically derived dietary patterns through latent profile analysis among Brazilian children and adolescents from Southern Brazil, 2013–2015. *PLoS One.* 2019;14(1):e0210425.
36. Leech RM, McNaughton SA, Timperio A. Clustering of diet, physical activity and sedentary behavior among Australian children: cross-sectional and longitudinal associations with overweight and obesity. *Int J Obes.* 2015;39(7):1079–1085.
37. Hoffmann K, Schulze MB, Schienkiewitz A, Nothlings U, Boeing H. Application of a new statistical method to derive dietary patterns in nutritional epidemiology. *Am J Epidemiol.* 2004;159(10): 935–944.
38. Weikert C, Schulze MB. Evaluating dietary patterns: the role of reduced rank regression. *Curr Opin Clin Nutr Metab Care.* 2016; 19(5):341–346.
39. Livingstone KM, McNaughton SA. Dietary patterns by reduced rank regression are associated with obesity and hypertension in Australian adults. *Br J Nutr.* 2017;117(2):248–259.
40. Nazari SSH, Mokhayeri Y, Mansournia MA, Khodakarim S, Soori H. Associations between dietary risk factors and ischemic stroke: a comparison of regression methods using data from the Multi-Ethnic Study of Atherosclerosis. *Epidemiol Health.* 2018;40: e2018021.
41. Sauvageot N, Leite S, Alkerwi A, et al. Association of empirically derived dietary patterns with cardiovascular risk factors: a comparison of PCA and RRR methods. *PLoS One.* 2016;11(8):e0161298.
42. Jannasch F, Kroger J, Schulze MB. Dietary patterns and type 2 diabetes: a systematic literature review and meta-analysis of prospective studies. *J Nutr.* 2017;147(6):1174–1182.
43. Heroux M, Janssen I, Lam M, et al. Dietary patterns and the risk of mortality: impact of cardiorespiratory fitness. *Int J Epidemiol.* 2010; 39(1):197–209.
44. Hoffmann K, Boeing H, Boffetta P, et al. Comparison of two statistical approaches to predict all-cause mortality by dietary patterns in German elderly subjects. *Br J Nutr.* 2005;93(5):709–716.
45. Meyer J, Doring A, Herder C, Roden M, Koenig W, Thorand B. Dietary patterns, subclinical inflammation, incident coronary heart disease and mortality in middle-aged men from the MONICA/KORA Augsburg cohort study. *Eur J Clin Nutr.* 2011;65(7): 800–807.
46. Herforth A. *Seeking Indicators of Healthy Diets.* Gallup and Swiss Agency for Development and Cooperation; 2016.
47. Waijers PM, Feskens EJ, Ocke MC. A critical review of predefined diet quality scores. *Br J Nutr.* 2007;97(2):219–231.

48. *World Health Organization and Food and Agriculture Organization of the United Nations, Preparation and Use of Food-Based Dietary Guidelines. Joint FAO/WHO Consultation (WHO Technical Report Series 880)*. World Health Organization; 1998.
49. Rafferty AP, Anderson JV, McGee HB, Miller CE. A healthy diet indicator: quantifying compliance with the dietary guidelines using the BRFSS. *Prev Med*. 2002;35(1):9–15.
50. Kirkpatrick SI, Reedy J, Krebs-Smith SM, et al. Applications of the healthy eating index for surveillance, epidemiology, and intervention research: considerations and caveats. *J Acad Nutr Diet*. 2018; 118(9):1603–1621.
51. Guenther PM, Reedy J, Krebs-Smith SM. Development of the Healthy Eating Index-2005. *J Am Diet Assoc*. 2008;108(11): 1896–1901.
52. Guenther PM, Casavale KO, Reedy J, et al. Update of the Healthy Eating Index: HEI-2010. *J Acad Nutr Diet*. 2013;113(4):569–580.
53. Krebs-Smith SM, Pannucci TE, Subar AF, et al. Update of the Healthy Eating Index: HEI-2015. *J Acad Nutr Diet*. 2018;118(9): 1591–1602.
54. Yuan YQ, Li F, Wu H, et al. Evaluation of the validity and reliability of the Chinese healthy eating index. *Nutrients*. 2018;10(2).
55. Woodruff SJ, Hanning RM. Development and implications of a revised Canadian Healthy Eating Index (HEIC-2009). *Public Health Nutr*. 2010;13(6):820–825.
56. Previdelli AN, Andrade SC, Pires MM, Ferreira SR, Fisberg RM, Marchioni DM. A revised version of the Healthy Eating Index for the Brazilian population. *Rev Saude Publica*. 2011;45(4): 794–798.
57. Taechangam S, Pinitchun U, Pachotikarn C. Development of nutrition education tool: Healthy Eating Index in Thailand. *Asia Pac J Clin Nutr*. 2008;17(Suppl 1):365–367.
58. Shivappa N, Steck SE, Hurley TG, Hussey JR, Hebert JR. Designing and developing a literature-derived, population-based dietary inflammatory index. *Public Health Nutr*. 2014;17(8):1689–1696.
59. Ruiz-Canela M, Bes-Rastrollo M, Martinez-Gonzalez MA. The role of dietary inflammatory index in cardiovascular disease, metabolic syndrome and mortality. *Int J Mol Sci*. 2016;17(8).
60. Shivappa N, Godos J, Hebert JR, et al. Dietary inflammatory index and colorectal cancer risk-a meta-analysis. *Nutrients*. 2017;9(9).
61. Liese AD, Krebs-Smith SM, Subar AF, et al. The Dietary Patterns Methods Project: synthesis of findings across cohorts and relevance to dietary guidance. *J Nutr*. 2015;145(3):393–402.
62. Mozaffarian D, Rosenberg I, Uauy R. History of modern nutrition science-implications for current research, dietary guidelines, and food policy. *BMJ*. 2018;361:k2392.
63. Sallis JF, Owen N, Fotheringham MJ. Behavioral epidemiology: a systematic framework to classify phases of research on health promotion and disease prevention. *Ann Behav Med: Publ Soc Behav Med*. 2000;22(4):294–298.
64. Baranowski T, Cullen KW, Nicklas T, Thompson D, Baranowski J. Are current health behavioral change models helpful in guiding prevention of weight gain efforts? *Obes Res*. 2003;11(Suppl): 23s–43s.
65. McNaughton S. Understanding the eating behaviors of adolescents: application of dietary patterns methodology to behavioral nutrition research. *J Am Diet Assoc*. 2011;111(2):226–229.
66. *Australian Institute of Health and Welfare, Australia's Food & Nutrition. Cat. No. PHE 163*. Canberra: AIHW. Australian Institute of Health and Welfare; 2012.
67. Jahns L, Scheett AJ, Johnson LK, et al. Diet quality of items advertised in supermarket sales circulars compared to diets of the US population, as assessed by the Healthy Eating Index-2010. *J Acad Nutr Diet*. 2016;116(1), 115–122.e111.
68. Reedy J, Krebs-Smith SM, Bosire C. Evaluating the food environment: application of the Healthy Eating Index-2005. *Am J Prev Med*. 2010;38(5):465–471.
69. Krebs-Smith SM, Reedy J, Bosire C. Healthfulness of the U.S. food supply: little improvement despite decades of dietary guidance. *Am J Prev Med*. 2010;38(5):472–477.
70. Kirkpatrick SI, Reedy J, Kahle LL, Harris JL, Ohri-Vachaspati P, Krebs-Smith SM. Fast-food menu offerings vary in dietary quality, but are consistently poor. *Public Health Nutr*. 2014;17(4):924–931.
71. Tapsell LC, Neale EP, Satija A, Hu FB. Foods, nutrients, and dietary patterns: interconnections and implications for dietary guidelines. *Adv Nutr*. 2016;7(3):445–454.
72. 2020 Dietary Guidelines Advisory Committee Dietary Patterns Subcommittee. *Topics and Questions Under Review by the Committee*. https://www.dietaryguidelines.gov/work-under-way/review-science/topics-and-questions-under-review.
73. Dietary Guidelines Advisory Committee. *Scientific Report of the 2015 Dietary Guidelines Advisory Committee: Advisory Report to the Secretary of Health and Human Services and the Secretary of Agriculture*. Washington, DC: U.S. Department of Agriculture, Agricultural Research Service; 2015.
74. *World Cancer Research Fund and American Institute for Cancer Research, Food, Nutrition and the Prevention of Cancer: a Global Perspective*. Washington, DC: American Institute for Cancer Research; 1997.
75. World Cancer Research Fund. *Food, Nutrition, Physical Activity, and the Prevention of Cancer: A Global Perspective* [Second Expert Report]. London: World Cancer Research Fund & American Institute for Cancer Prevention; 2007.
76. World Cancer Research Fund. *Diet, Nutrition, Physical Activity and Cancer: a Global Perspective* [Third Expert Report]. London: World Cancer Research Fund & American Institute for Cancer Prevention; 2018.
77. Fardet A, Boirie Y. Associations between food and beverage groups and major diet-related chronic diseases: an exhaustive review of pooled/meta-analyses and systematic reviews. *Nutr Rev*. 2014; 72(12):741–762.
78. Milte CM, McNaughton SA. Dietary patterns and successful ageing: a systematic review. *Eur J Nutr*. 2016;55(2):423–450.
79. Trijsburg L, Talsma EF, de Vries JHM, Kennedy G, Kuijsten A, Brouwer ID. Diet quality indices for research in low- and middle-income countries: a systematic review. *Nutr Rev*. 2019; 77(8):515–540.
80. Ohlhorst SD, Russell R, Bier D, et al. Nutrition research to affect food and a healthy lifespan. *Adv Nutr*. 2013;4(5):579–584.
81. Laddu D, Hauser M. Addressing the nutritional phenotype through personalized nutrition for chronic disease prevention and management. *Prog Cardiovasc Dis*. 2019;62(1):9–14.
82. Wang T, Heianza Y, Sun D, et al. Improving adherence to healthy dietary patterns, genetic risk, and long term weight gain: gene-diet interaction analysis in two prospective cohort studies. *BMJ*. 2018:360.
83. 2015 Dietary Guidelines Advisory Committee. *Scientific Report of the 2015 Dietary Guidelines Advisory Committee (Advisory Report)*. 2015.
84. Reedy J, Lerman JL, Krebs-Smit SM, et al. Evaluation of the Healthy Eating Index-2015. *J Acad Nutr Diet*. 2018;118(9): 1622–1633.
85. Kant AK, Schatzkin A, Graubard BI, Schairer C. A Prospective study of diet quality and mortality in women. *JAMA*. 2000; 283(16):2109–2115.
86. Bach A, Serra-Majem L, Carrasco JL, et al. The use of indexes evaluating the adherence to the Mediterranean diet in epidemiological studies: a review. *Public Health Nutr*. 2006;9(1a):132–146.
87. D'Alessandro A, De Pergola G. Mediterranean diet and cardiovascular disease: A critical evaluation of A priori dietary indexes. *Nutrients*. 2015;7(9):7863–7888.
88. Fung TT, Chiuve SE, McCullough ML, Rexrode KM, Logroscino G, Hu FB. Adherence to a DASH-style diet and risk of coronary heart

disease and stroke in women. *Arch Intern Med*. 2008;168(7): 713–720.

89. Chiuve SE, Fung TT, Rimm EB, et al. Alternative dietary indices both strongly predict risk of chronic disease. *J Nutr*. 2012;142(6): 1009–1018.
90. McCullough ML, Willett WC. Evaluating adherence to recommended diets in adults: the Alternate Healthy Eating Index. *Public Health Nutr*. 2006;9(1a):152–157.
91. Satija A, Bhupathiraju SN, Rimm EB, et al. Plant-based dietary patterns and incidence of type 2 diabetes in US men and women: Results from three prospective cohort studies. *PLoS Med*. 2016;13(6): e1002039.
92. Knuppel A, Papier K, Key TJ, Travis RC. EAT-Lancet score and major health outcomes: the EPIC-Oxford study. *Lancet (London, England)*. 2019;394(10194):213–214.

CHAPTER

14

ASSESSMENT OF DIETARY INTAKE BY SELF-REPORTS AND BIOLOGICAL MARKERS

Marga C. Ocké[1,2], *PhD*
Jeanne H.M. de Vries[1], *PhD*
Paul J.M. Hulshof[1], *MSc*

[1]Wageningen University & Research, Division of Human Nutrition and Health, Wageningen, the Netherlands
[2]National Institute for Public Health and the Environment, Bilthoven, the Netherlands

SUMMARY

Accurate assessment of dietary intake is crucial in the field of nutrition. In this chapter, different dietary assessment methods and types of biomarkers of dietary intake, their strengths and weaknesses, and the importance of examining the sources of error and variation are described. There is no best method of diet assessment for all purposes; therefore, the investigator has to select the method appropriate for the purpose and target group of the survey. Performing validation studies is essential to further improve dietary assessment methods, for a better interpretation of dietary assessment results, and for the correction of associations with outcomes for measurement errors, so that such associations are not obscured by these errors. Innovations in dietary assessment methods and validated biomarkers of intake will certainly improve assessments, but they are not the solution to all of the inherent problems in applying dietary assessment methods.

Keywords: 24-Hour food recall; Automatic dietary monitoring; Diet history; Dietary assessment; Food frequency questionnaire; Food record; Intake biomarker; Technology.

I. INTRODUCTION

A. Background

Accurate assessment of food consumption is a crucial element of research or clinical care within the field of nutrition. Within this field, the underlying purpose of estimations of dietary intake may vary. For instance, clinical studies are focused on the fate of nutrients in the body, while public health studies monitor the adequacy of the diet and study the relationship between food consumption and health.

The focus of this chapter is on dietary methods to assess the intake of individuals and not on indirect approaches such as food balance sheets or household consumption surveys. Several dietary assessment methods directed at the individual are available. They mainly differ in their concept (e.g., time frame used), their goals (e.g., obtaining information on foods, nutrients, or diet pattern), underlying assumptions, and cognitive approaches. Assessment of dietary intake is not easy and is prone to measurement error. However, errors in dietary assessment have been studied for decades and repeatedly recognized. By

https://doi.org/10.1016/B978-0-12-818460-8.00014-9

understanding, acknowledging, and minimizing measurement error, the performance of assessments can be improved.

B. Key Issues

This chapter describes the main methods to assess dietary exposure. The concept of the traditional methods has changed little, but the application of technology-based methods, including mobile applications and wearable devices, and the use of biomarkers have increased accuracy and convenience for responders and reduced costs. Nevertheless, innovative technologies largely rely on the basic principles of the traditional methods (see Table 14.1 for definitions of methods). Therefore, the present chapter describes the traditional methodologies with a focus on innovative technologies and includes the use of biomarkers to assess dietary exposure.

II. CURRENT STATUS OF THE FIELD

A. Different Purposes of Dietary Assessment

Dietary assessment is needed in many types of dietary studies, such as nutritional epidemiology, national or regional food consumption surveys, experimental or dietary intervention studies, and methodological studies. Interest can be in a group of persons or in the individual. The individual or group may consist of one or various age groups such as infants, toddlers, children, adolescents, adults, or older adults. Also, interest may be focused on specific population groups such as immigrants, persons with disabilities or illnesses, persons with low or high socioeconomic status, or persons in low- and middle-income countries.

The reason to collect dietary data can also vary greatly. There can be interest in intake of individual foods, food groups, nutrients, potentially toxic or

TABLE 14.1 Definitions of relevant terms and their relationships in the context of this chapter.

Term	Description
Dietary assessment	A comprehensive evaluation of a person's food intake
Dietary assessment method	A method/approach for conducting a dietary assessment
Food description	Characterization of a consumed food in dietary assessment
Portion size aid	Tool for quantifying the consumed food in dietary assessment
Self-report	Food intake reported by the participant/consumer (e.g. in a questionnaire/to an interviewer/in a tool)
Biomarkers of intake	A biological characteristic that is objectively measured as an indicator of intake
Reference period	Time window to which the dietary assessment/biomarker pertains
Validity study	Study to identify how well a dietary assessment actually measures the true intake
Relative validity study	Study to identify how a dietary assessment method compares to another dietary assessment method
Repeatability study	Study to identify how repeated administration of a dietary assessment method provides the same results
Test method	Dietary assessment method for which (relative) validity is assessed in a validity study
Reference method	Dietary assessment method to which the test method is compared to in a validity study
Measurement error	Systematic and random misestimations of dietary intake caused by errors in responding, coding, portion sizes, food composition databases, techniques, and biochemical analyses

healthy compounds, or on dietary patterns, meal patterns, environmental impact of diets, overall health profiles, etc. Moreover, the interest may be in the actual intake, in the habitual intake, or intake in a specific period of time. These different purposes are important for determining which dietary assessment method is most appropriate. After describing the main types of dietary assessment methods in the next paragraph, the considerations for choosing an appropriate dietary assessment method will be discussed.

B. Available Methods

Two primary methods to assess dietary intake include self-reports and biomarkers of exposure. In general, methods can be divided into two basic categories: those that reflect data at the time of eating (prospective methods consisting of weighed and estimated records or biomarkers reflecting short-term intake) and those that collect data about diet eaten in the recent past or over a longer period of time (retrospective methods consisting of 24-hour recalls [24 hR], dietary history [DH], food frequency questionnaire [FFQ], or biomarkers reflecting long-term intake).

Prospective self-reports may include several days of recording, sometimes accompanied by collecting duplicate samples for chemical analysis or performed by proxies, e.g., by observation. Retrospective methods may refer to recent diet (24 hR) or habitual diet (DH and FFQ). The three methods differ, but if they are performed as an interview, some practical aspects are similar.

Interviewers should have a thorough knowledge about the purpose of the method, the typical food habits of the target population, foods available in the marketplace, and preparation practices. The location and mode (e.g., written questionnaire, face-to-face or telephone interview, web-based application) of the assessment may affect respondent's willingness and ability to report their diet.

Cognitive aspects should also be taken into account. The success of the report relies on the respondent's ability to remember and adequately describe their diet. It is important to take advantage of what is known about how respondents retrieve, judge, and report their food consumption to the interviewer.

In collaborative research that involves multiple locations with multiple interviewers, interviewers should be trained and checks made to decrease systematic differences among them in data collecting and coding.

The need for biomarkers of intake was proposed by several researchers who addressed poor associations between diet, as determined from subject information and health outcome.[1,2] These poor associations were partly attributed to measurement error in intake (see Section II.F). The dependency on self-reported intake, and the incompleteness of food composition databases,[3] has spurred the search for and utilization of biomarkers as indicators of food and nutrient intake. The application of dietary biomarkers has been boosted further by more and better analytical techniques (including ~ omics techniques) to measure multiple metabolites in response to an altered food intake.[4] The main premise of intake biomarkers is that the errors are considered to be independent of errors related to self-reports.

Self-reports to assess *actual* intake

Food records (FR); In the weighed food record (FR), the subject is taught to weigh and record the food and its weight immediately before eating and to weigh any leftovers. Where weighing would interfere with normal eating habits, for example, in a restaurant, describing the quantity of foods consumed is acceptable. The weighed method differs from the estimated record where subjects do not weigh but keep records of foods eaten and portion sizes. These portion sizes are described in natural units (household measures) by using the utensils commonly found in homes.

The form used to record intake, kept in a record book, may be closed or open.[5] A closed form is a precoded list of all of the commonly eaten foods in units of specified portion size. This list allows for rapid coding but can be unfamiliar to the subjects. A semiopen form may be preconstructed with foods and amount options but includes sufficient space for other foods and/or amounts. Respondents must be trained to record the level of detail needed to describe adequately the foods and amounts consumed. After recording, the record should be checked and coded by a nutritionist.

FR may be completed by someone other than the subject. For example, children <10 years old or fragile older persons will need the help of a caregiver as proxy. Instead of recording, the respondent may be asked to collect a similar portion of all the foods in their diet in a container to be chemically analyzed in the laboratory. This method is preferred if the food composition database does not provide sufficiently accurate values on the component(s) of interest.

The advantage of FRs is that they do not rely on memory. However, they have a high respondent burden, and respondents must be literate and highly cooperative. This requirement may lead to response bias as a result of overrepresentation of more highly educated individuals interested in diet and health. Also, food consumed away from home may be less accurately reported, and the usual eating pattern may be influenced by the recording process. Substantial underreporting is suspected in specific subpopulations because of altered intake or reporting according to social norms.

New technologies reduce the burden of FRs to both respondent and researcher. These technologies include the use of digital images, nutrient databases making coding superfluous, and image analysis to provide automatic determination of food and nutrient intake and estimation of portion sizes. For example, mobile telephones with an integrated camera to record food intake allow real-time data collection and automatic coding of food intake.[6] This may lead to fewer omissions and a higher acceptability in younger or less literate populations. However, using technology does not completely overcome the problems of FRs. Also, development of technologies is associated with high cost and technical problems, may require training of respondents, and may, if a precoded food list is used, provide less detail on the intake of foods.[6,7]

Twenty-four hour food recall; In a 24 hR, an individual recalls actual food and beverage intake, mostly for the immediate past 24 h but sometimes also for 48 h or the preceding day. Food quantities are usually assessed by use of household measures, food models, or photographs.

The 24 hR was traditionally conducted by a personal interview, face-to-face or by telephone, or with open forms or precoded questionnaires, but computer-assisted interviews have become common. More recently, self-administered computerized 24 hRs have been developed.[8] The 24 hR, including computerized versions, is often modeled on the USDA multiple-pass method.[9] In this method, participants start with a quick list of foods consumed and in a following step describe the type and amount of these foods in more detail.

In the case of interviews, training of the interviewers is crucial because improved accuracy of the dietary recall is obtained by asking probing questions. At the end of the interview, a checklist with foods or snacks that might be easily forgotten may be added. For children[10] and elderly people,[11] specific adaptations to their cognitive processes can improve the recall process. Because the 24 hR depends on a subject's ability to remember and adequately describe their diet, this method is not suitable for children younger than 8–10 years and many adults ≥75 years. The 24 hR method is considered appropriate for describing the mean intakes of groups of individuals.[12] Different days of the week must be used to obtain recalls as respondents may eat differently on days of the week they work or go to school versus holidays. It is advised that no prior notification be given to the subjects about the interview to avoid changes in their usual diet.

Diet recalls as open interviews are not culture-specific, administration time can be short, the time period (e.g., past 24 h) is well defined, and, if interviewer administered, literacy is not required. Administration by a dietitian or trained professional requires fewer callbacks. Web-based 24 hRs are considered an important step forward,[8] as the costs are reduced because an interviewer and coding of the consumption data are not required. Also web-based 24 hRs have the advantage that participants can fill in the recall at a time of their own choice. These advantages have made web-based 24 hR feasible for large-scale epidemiological studies.

Weaknesses of 24 hR are that respondent's recall depends on short-term memory. The method is also vulnerable to variability between interviewers and requires substantial staff time; this is not the case for self-administered computerized 24 hR. However, the latter method requires access to computers or the Internet, and participants may have difficulty finding the actual food consumed in the food databases used.

Self-reports to assess usual intake

Dietary history; The DH assesses an individual's total daily food intake and usual meal pattern over varied periods of time, e.g., the past month, 6 months, or 1 year. Originally, Burke[13] developed the DH technique in three parts: (1) an interview about the subject's usual daily pattern of food intake with quantities specified in household measures; (2) a cross-check using a detailed list of foods; and (3) a 3-day FR. Today, the perfor mance of the DH differs between studies, and the 3-day FR is often omitted. The purpose of the study defines how detailed information should be collected, which may substantially influence the duration of the interview. Usual portion sizes are estimated with standard household measures and may be checked by weighing.

Because a DH aims to record a food pattern, it is a more complex interview than the 24 hR. Also, the interview is very liable to evoke socially desirable answers. Therefore, highly trained nutritionists with well-developed social skills are required to conduct the interview. Exceptions may be DHs guided and controlled by a precoded interview form or computer software, especially if they are developed to be completed by the subject.

The DH is also rather demanding for the subject. Respondents are asked to make many judgments about the usual food intake and the amounts of those foods, and the recall period is difficult to conceptualize accurately. Reports covering a longer period may be influenced by present consumption and reveal higher (or lower) estimates[14] than assessed by recalls or records. In order to obtain adequate data, respondents need to follow a regular dietary pattern and have a good memory, which may hamper getting a representative sample of the population. A satisfactory DH is not always obtained from young children, people preoccupied with weight problems, or mentally retarded individuals. Respondent literacy is not required for an interviewer-administered DH.[15]

The data of a DH can be applied to classify categories (e.g., quantiles) of intake and to assess the relative average intakes of groups of people and the distribution of intakes within these groups. A short version of this method with a limited checklist of foods is often used in the clinical setting for diagnosis and as a basis for therapeutic dietary guidelines.[16]

Food frequency questionnaire method; The first FFQs were developed for large epidemiological studies investigating the relationship between diet and health outcomes. The questionnaire used is a preprinted list of foods on which subjects are asked to estimate the frequency and often also the amount of habitual consumption during a specified period. The types of foods vary on each FFQ depending on the interest of the researcher, which may be the intake of a specific nutrient or a more comprehensive assessment.[17]

The list of foods in an FFQ can be developed in several ways.[18] For epidemiological studies, the best way is to select foods found to contribute most to the variance of intake from a recent food consumption database of a population similar to the target population. The nutrient value assigned to each food group item listed is based on weighting each food included in the group item by usage.

The first FFQs did not include quantitative estimates, other than servings or portions per day, week, or month.[17,18] The use of these nonquantitative FFQs is based on the assumption that total intake is more determined by variation in consumption frequency than by variation in portion size and that consumption frequency is unrelated to consumed quantities. Nevertheless, some investigators have built a quantitative aspect into the technique and called their method a semiquantitative FFQ. Not all investigators advocate inclusion of portion sizes because errors made by the estimation may outweigh the variance in intake of most foods.[17,18]

FFQs vary in the foods listed, the reference period, answer categories, procedure for estimating portion size, and mode of administration. The longer the food list, the more detailed the information, but the respondent may become less precise in answering the questions. Nevertheless, a review by Molag et al.[19] showed that more accurate results were obtained with longer FFQ (200 vs. 100 items).

The advantage of an FFQ is that the food list is standardized.[20] For some respondents, it may be cognitively difficult to combine the intake of similar foods or mixed dishes over a longer period of time and to report about them in one question. On the other hand, introducing separate questions may lead to double counting.

It is also important to address the best time frame for the study objective and to take seasonal variation into account. However, it may be questioned whether respondents can accurately report over a period longer than 2 months.[21] A solution may be to repeat the FFQ over time. If the questionnaire is self-administered, the accompanying instructions are important. Web-based questionnaires have the advantage that they can easily give cognitive support and prevent respondents skipping questions.

As mentioned earlier, FFQs are suitable for large-scale epidemiological studies. They estimate the usual food (group) intake of an individual. When portion size questions are included or when portion sizes are assumed, individuals can be ranked according to nutrient intake. A self-administered web-based questionnaire may require little time to complete and to process; the response burden is generally low, and response rates, therefore, are high. The method can be automated easily and is not very costly.

A problem of FFQ is that memory of food use in the past is required and that the respondent's burden is governed by number and complexity of foods listed and the quantification procedure. The listing of foods may be incomplete or missing details. The quantification of portion sizes may be less accurate than in records or recalls. Also, the development and testing of the food list takes significant time, no information on day-to-day variation is provided, and the suitability is questionable for subpopulations who consume culture-specific foods.

Other methods

Several brief dietary assessment methods have also been developed. These instruments may be useful in clinical settings or for health-promoting activities when only information of a part of the diet or qualitative information of the total intake is required. For example, a screener regarding fat consumption might be useful to increase awareness about unhealthy eating habits.[15] In addition, new technologies may allow the so-called snapshot techniques, which collect detailed information on dietary practice at a specific point in time, such as single meals.[22]

Multiple food records (FR) or 24-hour recalls (24hR) and combined methods

In order to assess usual intake by FR or 24 hR, these methods have to be repeated over a representative number of days. The number of days needed depends on the aim of the survey and the expected between- and within-individual variation in intakes of the nutrients of interest.[18] However, in practice, often no more than three or four consecutive days are included because of respondent fatigue. For monitoring and surveillance studies, two or more nonconsecutive repeated 24 hRs in combination with statistical modeling allow estimation of the usual intake distribution of individuals. Several statistical methods for estimating the usual intake distribution from repeated 24 hRs are available.[23] Multiple days of recording may also allow individuals to be classified according to their usual intakes, which is required for epidemiological studies. For infrequently consumed foods, FRs or 24 hRs may be combined with an FFQ or propensity questionnaire.[24] The information from the records or recalls provides details about the type and amount of foods consumed while the FFQ provides information on the propensity of a person to consume the food.

Another example of a combined method is the 24 hR assisted by an FR. This appears to be a valid method for assessing the dietary intake of children and older people.[25] Diaries are used to record their food intake and then are used as a memory prompt during 24 hRs. Combined methods are more time consuming for respondents and fieldworkers, although computers have facilitated the blending of methods.

C. Biomarkers of Intake

Types of biomarkers to assess actual and usual intake

Intake biomarkers can be classified based on their relationship with intake and intended use into four categories: "recovery" markers, "concentration" markers, "predictive" markers, and "replacement" markers.[26]

Recovery markers; recovery markers show a direct quantitative relationship with intake of a substance and can be measured in bodily excretion (typically urine). The assumption is that the body is in equilibrium (homeostasis) and that no accumulation or depletion occurs in the body over a fixed time period. Examples of recovery markers are carbon dioxide fluxes reflecting total energy intake in weight stable subjects, measured by subjects drinking a defined amount of doubly labeled water.[27] Urinary nitrogen, sodium, and potassium are other recovery markers, with which the correlation with intake is generally high. These types of biomarkers have been shown to be very valuable when evaluating dietary assessment methods.[28]

Concentration markers; concentration markers have an indirect relationship with intake and are measured in urine, plasma, and other specimen or tissues. The level of the marker in the biological specimen is dependent on portion size, frequency of consumption, absorption, distribution, metabolism, elimination, and homeostatic control. Concentration markers cannot be translated into absolute levels of intake, but the concentration in the biological specimen will correlate with intake of specific nutrients or foods. However, the strength of the correlation is lower than what is found for recovery markers. Most biomarkers are concentration markers.

Replacement biomarkers; replacement biomarkers are more or less similar to concentration markers with the exception that they specifically refer to components for which information in food composition databases is scarce or unreliable. This category of biomarkers covers mainly bioactive components or nutrients, such as selenium, for which the concentration is very variable and dependent on local soil conditions.[29]

Predictive biomarkers; predictive biomarkers as a separate category was suggested in 2005 based on controlled studies in a metabolic ward.[30] This type of marker shows a dose–response relationship with intake but a low recovery, and the relationship may be more dependent on subject characteristics, resulting in lower correlations with intake. The only predictive marker described so far is urinary fructose and sucrose as markers of sugar intake.

Specific biomarkers of nutrients and foods

To date, more than 25,000 compounds have been identified in food.[31] This includes classical nutrients, nonnutrient components, and bioactive components with putative health effects. Dietary biomarkers are discussed extensively in many reports with detailed examples given of metabolic profiles reflecting specific food intake.[3,18] Table 14.2 gives a brief overview of some selected dietary biomarkers.

Biomarker requirements

The utility of a biomarker of intake for applications in research depends on several factors. There are several minimum requirements for a marker of intake. First of all, the biomarker measured in a biological specimen should be sensitive to intake so that an increase in intake of a specific food or nutrient should be reflected in a measurable change of a nutrient or metabolite in the specimen. Ideally, a broad range of intakes should be reflected accordingly in the level of the biomarker, resulting in a high correlation between intake and biomarker level. The magnitude of the correlation is however dependent on the bioavailability of the nutrient and homeostatic mechanisms. Subject-related factors such as biological variation in nutrient absorption, metabolism, turnover, and excretion; metabolic stress; or colonic microbiota are factors that may influence the sensitivity to intake.[26] Also, lifestyle factors such as smoking, physical activity, or alcohol consumption may result in a differential response to dietary intake. For many nutrients, the relationship between intake and concentration is not linear but plateaus due to homeostatic control. A classic example is plasma vitamin A: at low intakes, there is a linear relationship of intake with plasma levels of vitamin A. At higher intakes, intake is no longer reflected in the level of the biomarker.

TABLE 14.2 Proposed biomarkers and time window of consumption for some selected nutrients and foods.

Nutrient/Food	Biomarker Examples	Medium	Time Window
Energy	Fractional turnover rate of water isotopes[a]	Spot urine, plasma, saliva	Short–medium
Available carbohydrates	Sucrose/fructose[b]	24-h urine	Short
Fatty acids	Essential, trans, and odd-chain fatty acids	Plasma cholesteryl esters, phospholipids	Short–medium
		Erythrocyte membrane, platelets	Medium
		Adipose tissue	Long
Protein	Organic nitrogen[a]	24-h urine	Short
Dietary fiber	Alkylresorcinol; stool weight	24-h urine, plasma; faeces	Short–medium
Na^+/K^+	Na/K[a]	24-h urine	Short
Thiamin	Thiamin	24-h urine	Short
Riboflavin	Riboflavin; erythrocyte glutathione reductase	24-h urine; erythrocytes	Short–long
Folate	Folate	Serum; erythrocytes	Short–medium
Vitamin C	Ascorbic acid, dehydroascorbic acid	Plasma; leukocytes	Short–medium
Alcohol	Ethylglucuronide	Urine	Short
Fruit and vegetables	Carotenoids, vitamin C	Plasma, urine	Short–medium
Citrus fruits	Proline, betaine	Urine	Short
Fish	Eicosapentaenoic acid (EPA), docosahexaenoic acid (DHA), trimethylamine N-oxidase (TMAO)	Plasma, tissue, urine	Short–long
Whole cereals	Alkylresorcinols	Plasma, urine	Short–medium
Meat	1-Methylhistidine	Urine	Short
Olive oil extra vierge	Hydroxytyrosol sulfate	Urine, plasma	Short–medium
Dairy	Odd-chain fatty acids, phytanic acid	Plasma	Short–medium

[a]*Recovery marker.*
[b]*Predictive marker.*

Second, biomarker kinetics must be described adequately to make a good choice of sample type, frequency, and time window for a specific research question. For instance, nutrient exposures relevant to chronic disease are long term. Therefore, a biomarker of intake should ideally reflect the cumulative effect of diet over an extended period of time when studying diet–disease relationships using biomarkers. Thus, information on the time integration of the marker (short-term responses vs. long-term responses to intake) is required. A 24-h urine collection is more likely to be representative of the intake for that day (e.g., of sodium) than a spot urine sample. In general, blood cells are more representative of long-term intake for a number of nutrients than is plasma. Fig. 14.1 shows the time integration of several nutritional biomarker media in relation to two dietary methods.

Another important requirement is that the chosen biomarker of intake should be specific for the nutrient or food consumed. This is often not the case. A dietary biomarker may reflect intake of multiple dietary components or can result from the metabolism of other dietary components.

Strengths and limitations

Biomarkers are useful as reference measurements to assess the validity of dietary assessment methods and for estimating intake of specific nutrients or compounds when there is a lack of detailed and reliable food composition data and/or when large variability within

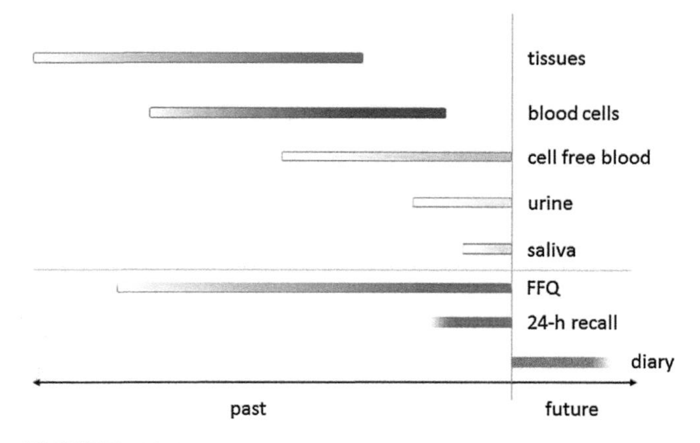

FIGURE 14.1 Time window that represents consumption of several biomarker media and dietary assessment techniques by self-reports.

foods makes it difficult to estimate exposure otherwise. Combining self-reported intake with biomarker information has been shown to increase the power to detect diet–disease associations.[32] One of the main limitations of biomarkers is that only a few good biomarkers of intake currently available have been thoroughly validated: e.g., time–response relationships for acute and repeated intakes under controlled conditions are often lacking.

Most currently available biomarkers are concentration markers, and their correlation with the intake of specific foods appears to be low to moderate,[3] which makes it very difficult to assess intake of food groups. Biomarkers alone will not give data on food intake and/or dietary patterns, and therefore biomarkers are complementary to dietary assessment methods. Another limitation is that many biomarkers have a short half-life, especially when measured in urine. This means that for many biomarker applications, more than one specimen is required to address within-person variability. The access to media from respondents may present another limitation.

Blood is often chosen as the medium because it is easily accessible, but it is not necessarily the best medium reflecting intake, since blood is a transport vehicle for substrates and metabolites and not a target tissue for storage or metabolism. Also, in some cultural settings, and for children, it may be difficult to get access to blood because of resistance to venepuncture.

D. Assessment of Diet Quality

Diet quality (DQ) metrics are increasingly used. These indices or indicators aim to evaluate the overall diet and categorize individuals according to the extent to which they conform to a defined healthy diet based on current nutritional knowledge.[33,34] They are used for nutritional epidemiology to assess dietary risk factors for noncommunicable diseases or to monitor the quality of an individual's diet and give feed-back to improve their DQ. Indicators of DQ may assess to what extent an individual adheres to national food-based dietary guidelines or nutrient recommendations, or they may address the variety of the individual's entire diet. Several healthy diet indices and diversity scores are available to evaluate DQ[35] or to study the association between food components and health outcomes in different target populations. A higher score usually means a higher DQ. DQ of an individual's diet based on the food components or nutrients included can be evaluated based on moderation, adequacy, an optimum range of intake, or as a ratio.[36] For this, self-reports such as 24 hR, FR, or FFQ are used. Also, brief FFQ or screeners specifically developed to ask questions about intake can be directly scored for evaluating the different components of DQ.[37]

DQ measures have some methodological limitations. For example, they do not always capture the complete daily or usual intake, the development of the components and the scores are often designed for specific purposes not always restricted to nutritional disciplines (e.g., including physical activity), and they evolve over time. However, they may give a more complete picture of a diet pattern and consistently show inverse associations with adverse health outcomes and mortality.[35] If they are assessed with a technology-based FFQ screener, they are easy to apply.[37]

Assessing dietary supplements and fortified foods

To have a complete picture of the intake of nutrients, it is important to assess the intake of dietary supplements, such as vitamin supplements, and fortified foods, i.e., foods enriched with micronutrients. Collection of valid data on (components of) supplement use and fortified foods is difficult,[38] especially if their use is substantial, as it is in Northern American and Western European populations. Still, research is needed about the best methodology for assessing intake of dietary supplements combined with other dietary information and related measurement error.[39] Dietary supplements can contribute >50% of micronutrient intake for an individual.[39] Failure to include such important sources of nutrient intake can result in poor estimates of intake. Supplement users may take supplements irregularly. Therefore, to take a measure of supplement use on one or a few days as a proxy for long-term intake incorporates measurement error. Depending on the food supply, the same will probably hold for fortified foods with high concentrations of a specific micronutrient.

In large-scale studies focusing on diet–disease relationships, the frequency and number of supplements taken seem to be much more important than accuracy about content. Within each of these types of supplements (e.g., a vitamin C supplement), the exact brand name or exact content does not seem to be necessary.[39]

For assessment of actual intake—in contrast to usual intake—and for quantitative assessment of the distribution of nutrient intakes for a population, brand name and dose information are relevant.

An approach similar to that used for dietary supplements will probably work for foods marketed in a fortified version as well as the ordinary version. However, for many other types of fortified foods, information at the brand name level and subtype will be required. This may be the case because the consumer is unaware of consuming a fortified product, the consumer does not know the specific content of the product, or the amounts of added components in some products vary enormously.

Technology-based tools and automatic dietary monitoring

Several aspects of the application of dietary assessment methodology may be facilitated by technology to help standardization of interviewers and to reduce costs of data collection and processing. A number of dietary assessment methods now available utilize technology.[40] Many of these tools are based on traditional methods and may have similar problems regarding misreporting due to errors in response, coding, food composition databases, and portion size estimations, but they also have many advantages for research and consumers. An important attribute is that such tools meet general quality standards; this can be achieved by publishing information on tool development and tool characteristics, including food identification and quantification, food composition databases used, and validity testing.[40]

During the last 20 years, novel technology under development can automatically identify dietary intake and collect data for diet coaching. Automatic dietary monitoring (ADM) tracks dietary activities such as preparation, ingestion, processing, and swallowing immediate to food intake.[41] Examples of this technology include smart eyeglasses and chewing sensors. This research field is still in an early stage, especially with respect to application and validation in free-living populations. Some problems in ADM are a lack in functional performance, comfort of the eyeglasses or sensors, ease of use, social acceptance, and privacy protection.[41] They may also have high costs and interfere with daily activities. Although it will be hard to develop ADM systems that are fully suitable for dietary monitoring, these systems may be valuable because of adding objective measurements to other methods of dietary assessment.

Quantification of portions

It is well-known that considerable error is made in quantifying food portions. The consumed amounts of foods need to be quantified into gram portions in most dietary assessment methods that rely on self-reporting. Particularly in the case of shared plate eating, quantifying the consumed amount is an even larger challenge.[42] The quantities consumed can be assessed in various ways although not all approaches are suitable for all purposes. Different types of portion size estimation aids seem more or less effective for different types of foods.[15]

Description (without equipment); Portion sizes for foods can be expressed in household measures, natural or commercial units, or typical serving sizes.[15] Examples are the amount of coffee expressed as the number of cups of coffee and the quantity of egg as the number of eggs. Information on the weight of reported units is then required for portions to be converted into weights. It is important to check whether standard portion sizes apply. The approach of using such standard measures is cognitively easier and preferable overestimation of consumed amounts in weights but may be less accurate for some foods such as vegetables and meats.

Scales; The most accurate method for obtaining the quantity of a food is the use of calibrated kitchen scales in food or table service. However, the weighed quantity may not represent the quantity that would have been eaten if the weighing process was not necessary.[43] When scales are used, they should be robust, be accurate to at least 5 g, and weigh amounts up to 1.5 kg so that a normal plate can be used when weighing the food to be eaten.

Food models; food replicas are three-dimensional models representing specific foods and amounts. They are lifelike in size and color and are often made of plastic. Portion size models are more abstract than food replicas and represent sizes of portions (mounds, cubes, balls, etc.) rather than specific foods. Drawings are alternative ways to help estimating amounts of foods.

Food photographs; food photographs are increasingly being used for estimating portion sizes. In most cases, a series of photographs representing different quantities of the same food are offered to the subject, who is asked to identify the photograph that most resembles the quantity consumed. Sometimes, only one photograph is available for each food and the quantity is indicated as a fraction or multiple of the amount shown. This latter approach gives rise to larger systematic error than does a series of food photographs.[15] Several studies have examined the validity of this type of portion size estimation or the added value of food photographs versus standard amounts. The angle at which the photographs are taken as well as the number and range of depicted quantities are important for the perception of the shown quantities.[44]

With innovative image-assisted and image-based methods, participants can take images of consumed foods and leftovers, or images are automatically taken by wearable cameras for subsequent portion size estimation via estimation of the food volume or through comparison with standard portions.[45] These technologies have the potential to improve the estimation of portion size in dietary assessment, though need some further development.

E. Choice of a Method to Estimate Intake

It is important to carefully select the method for estimating intake based on the objective and design of the study, the target population, and the dietary component(s) of interest. Also, the choice of method may be decided by that of a previous study to allow comparison of results between the studies. Some researchers may choose the most convenient or cheapest method, even though the method is not the best choice to answer the study question. This might explain why the FFQ is often the method of choice.

There are several dietary assessment toolkits available to assist researchers in selecting the best approach in assessment of diet.[46] It is advisable to take into account several considerations for choosing a method from most to least important.

When selecting a method to answer a study question, the following considerations should be addressed:

1. What is the main objective of the study? Is it the assessment of foods or nutrients, other food or intake components, or dietary patterns?
2. What type of information is needed for the data analyses and what analytical approach will be used?
3. What is the desired reference period or time frame for the assessment?
4. What characteristics of the study population may influence the performance of the methods?
5. Should the results be comparable to other studies?
6. What resources (budget and expertise) are available?

Objective of the study

When choosing a method, first consider in what type of study the dietary assessment method will be applied and decide whether the main interest is to determine intake of foods, nutrients, other components, or a diet pattern. For example, in experimental or clinical studies, a biomarker of exposure may be appropriate if the interest is a nutrient for which a biomarker is available, whereas in an epidemiological study to investigate the association between a food group such as plant proteins and a health outcome, only a self-report can provide the answer. Also, for assessing dietary patterns, self-reports are indispensable.

Both self-reports, especially an FFQ, and biomarkers can be used to assess dietary exposure in order to be able to rank subjects according to intake and then to relate intake to a health outcome. A biomarker is often used in (nested) case–control studies or cohort studies complementary to the use of self-reports.[18,47] Open methods such as 24 hRs and FRs and, if available, dietary biomarkers are also frequently used to assess compliance in human intervention trials. An example of the latter are measurements of α-linolenic acid, EPA, and DHA in plasma as compliance markers for the intake of margarines supplemented with these fatty acids in patients who have had a myocardial infarction.[48] An important application of dietary biomarkers is their use as reference measurements to assess the validity of self-reports. They provide an estimate of absolute (recovery markers) or relative intake (concentration markers) and can be used to calibrate self-reports.[49]

Analytical approach and type of information

Related to the objective, the approach used for data analysis is essential in selecting the method. It is important to know whether data analysis will be aimed at the population or the individual level. In surveillance or monitoring studies, the interest is to assess the proportion of the population with inadequate or excessive intakes.[50] For this interest, it is sufficient to assess the intake distribution on the population level. In epidemiological studies, often correlation or regression analysis is performed to assess relationships between intake and health outcomes. For this type of research question, the method must be able to rank or classify individuals according to the intake of interest.[50] Thus, for surveillance studies, 2 one-day assessments per individual may be sufficient, whereas for epidemiological studies at least 2 days would be necessary. The number of days needed depends on the number of participants and the within-person variation or day-to-day variation of the nutrient.[18]

The most difficult aim is to assess the absolute level of individual intake. This detail of information, for example, may be needed to calculate a nutrient balance such as of fat or protein. However, this is mostly only done under clinical or experimental conditions in small populations. Most self-reports are not accurate enough to generate such data, so recovery biomarkers of exposure are essential.

Reference period

For some studies, the interest regarding intake may be the actual or short-term intake, whereas for other research questions, it may be the long-term usual intake. For example, in experiments, the objective of knowing intake may be short-term (while the experiment is underway), while the adherence to the intervention diet is evaluated. In clinical practice, an estimate of actual intake is needed to relate to symptoms of patients suspected of having a food allergy. On the other hand, in epidemiological studies, when investigating the relationship of diets with chronic disease, for example, the focus is on long-term and usual intake.

In case–control studies, the reference period of intake is not always the recent past but may be also the distant past, depending on the start of the disease. It is, of course, questionable whether respondents are capable of providing such retrospective reports, especially because their reports may be influenced by current intake or current culturally acceptable practices. Some methods are more suitable to assess actual intake, such as 24 h recalls and FRs, whereas other methods such as food frequency and diet history methods are characterized by their ability to assess usual intake (see Section II.B).

The study population

Methods may perform differently in diverse age groups, in males versus females, or in individuals with disabilities, so the method should be chosen in light of the characteristics of the target population. Even within similar populations, methods may have to be adapted because of heterogeneity of subgroups.

For example, respondents above 65 years of age include healthy older individuals for whom all methods may be appropriate but also fragile older people for whom methods must be adapted because of their inability to report intake. Thus, competence of older adults to participate in dietary assessment studies requires careful consideration. Adapted recording methods and diet histories have resulted in valid reports for older adults. A picture-sort technique including a cognitive processing approach helps elderly people to remember what they usually eat.[11] With regard to 24 hR and FFQ, the possibility of cognitive decline needs to be borne in mind. It may also be helpful to combine different techniques, for example, an FR combined with 24 hR.[51]

When respondents are unable to answer, surrogate responders may be used. Individuals who are closest to the subject (e.g., caregivers) are assumed to be the best proxy responders, not only because they know the most about a subject's lifestyle but also because their commitment is greater.[52] In institutionalized persons, e.g., care-dependent elderly, proxies or interviewers may use an observation method, although it is typically not possible to apply such an intensive method to large numbers of residents.[51]

Within the age group of children from 0 to 18 years, methods may also perform differently as was shown by Livingstone,[53] who evaluated different self-reports against doubly labeled water as a reference method. Self-reported intake with children is more prone to errors due to a child's limited food knowledge, memory, and concept of time.[54] Young children up to the age of 6 years have insufficient ability to cooperate in dietary assessment procedures.[54] For very young children, in-nursery or in-school meal composition can be observed or intake recorded by a caregiver or teacher and the information combined with parental reports at home. Parents are reliable reporters of food intake at home but not of consumption outside the home.[18] In children of 6 years and older, more accurate information can be obtained by interviewing the child and parent together. From the age of 8 years onwards, there is a rapid increase in the ability to self-report food intake.[53]

Of key importance in designing appropriate methods is to understand how food-related information is memorized and subsequently recalled. The most usual retrieval mechanisms utilized with children are images (the color and shape of foods); usual practice (familiarity of the food); behavior chaining (linking foods to other foods or meal practices); and food preference.[53] By adolescence, cognitive abilities should be fully developed; limiting problems in that age are usually issues of motivation and body image. Web-based technologies may be of added value in this age group.

In one study, the 24 hR method conducted over no less than 3 days which included parents was found to be the most valid method to estimate total energy intake in children aged 4–11 years.[55] Using this approach, timing of the interview appears to be a very important factor. Reporting accuracy was found to be greater with a shorter recalling period interval covering the 24 h directly preceding the time of the interview. Using photographs and technology, children could estimate food portion size with an accuracy approaching that of adults. Using innovative technologies may improve reports as well because they may increase motivation, cooperation, and recognition of types of foods and portion sizes.[10]

Most methods have been developed and validated for Western populations but often not for populations in non-Western low-income countries. In these countries, the 24 hR is mostly used for population assessment because it is culturally sensitive and cognitively easy.[56] However, procedures of 24 hR may need to be adapted, for example, with respect to interviewing and cultural practices, as well as seasonal fluctuations.

Another important characteristic of all populations that may influence the choice of a method is the presence of overweight or obesity. A higher body mass index is an important determinant of underreporting and should therefore always be considered.[57]

Comparability with other studies

If dietary intake has been assessed with different methods in different studies, it is difficult and probably not possible to compare or combine their results.

Therefore, a prerequisite for such comparison is that the chosen methods are similar. An alternative may be to perform a calibration study to identify the differences in performance between the methods. An FFQ is culturally based and developed for a certain target population. The application of this method, therefore, limits the comparability of many epidemiological studies.

In general, researchers can use information from validation studies to allow comparison between methods. In the Netherlands, a national FFQ has been developed for application in Dutch cohort studies.[58] To facilitate the development of new high-quality FFQs and validate existing FFQs, the National Dietary Assessment Reference Database study developed a reference database with detailed information about the level and variation in dietary intake of the general Dutch population.[59] Comparability may be increased by such use of standardized and transparent procedures.

Costs, feasibility, and expertise

When different methods are suitable to answer the study question, the choice can be narrowed to choosing the method with the lowest cost and burden or requiring the least expertise. For example, a precoded or web-based method that can be self-administered requires fewer resources than an open method asking for a skilled interviewer and coding. Particularly in the case of use of biomarkers, feasibility aspects are important. In some cultural settings, it may be difficult to get access to blood because of the resistance to venepuncture. Similarly, in many situations, it may be difficult to collect 24-h urines because of the expense as well as the high respondent burden.

If a relatively cheap instrument cannot meet the objective of the planned dietary assessment, it should not be applied because of scientific and ethical reasons. When it is difficult to select a single method that meets all the requirements, it may be best to concurrently administer different self-reports or to combine self-reports with the collection of dietary biomarkers to overcome possible sources of error.

F. Measurement Error

Since measurement error cannot be avoided, it is essential to know how type and size of measurement error can be assessed. With adequate insight into measurement error, a dietary assessment method can be improved, an appropriate dietary assessment method chosen, proper power calculations performed, results of a dietary study interpreted, and study results corrected for the observed measurement error.

Sources of variation

At the level of the individual, dietary intake is characterized by daily variation superimposed on an underlying consistent pattern.[18] There are two types of daily intake variation: systematic, where factors such as day of the week or season contribute to variation in a systematic way, and random, which cannot be attributable. Dietary data collected on multiple days incorporate these types of variation. In FFQ and DH, participants are asked to provide information about their usual intake, which requires that they filter out their underlying consistent dietary pattern themselves. This becomes more difficult in the absence of a regular dietary pattern. Urine and blood specimens are the most frequently collected media for dietary biomarkers and represent a short-to-medium term time window of dietary intake (see Fig. 14.1).

The degree of random and systematic variation in dietary data differs across nutrients. For example, total energy and macronutrient intake have relatively little random variation, whereas intake of some nutrients such as retinol or marine fatty acids is characterized by large random variation resulting from large variation in their daily intakes because they are found in few foods.[18]

Types of error

From a methodological point of view, four types of measurement error exist: random within-person error, systematic within-person error, random between-person error, and systematic between-person error.[18] Systematic error is also called bias. The types and size of error vary with the particular dietary assessment method and probably also with the population to which it is applied. Table 14.3 provides an overview of the main sources of error related to the four main types of self-report dietary assessment methods.[18]

Random within-person error; Random within-person error may be due to day-to-day variation in an individual's daily intake when habitual intake is estimated. Thus, error in this methodological sense is not a mistake in the data collection but rather a mismatch in time frame. Random within-person error also includes errors in the measurement of intake on any occasions that are not systematic. Examples of this type of error are the result of foods omitted or included falsely in FRs or 24 hRs, of portion sizes estimated inaccurately, and of coding mistakes. When random within-person error is the only type of error present, the precision of the estimated mean value for an individual depends on the within-subject variation and the number of replicate measurements. Similarly, the number of days required to estimate mean intake for an individual given the size of the random variation and the precision that is needed can be estimated.[50]

Systematic within-person error; systematic within-person error, or person-specific bias, may be caused when a

TABLE 14.3 Sources of error in assessing dietary intake in four types of self-report dietary assessment methods.[18]

Sources of error:	Weighed record	24-hour recall	Diet history	Food frequency
Variation in intake with time	+	+	−	−
Response errors				
Omitting foods	+	+	+	+
Including foods	−	+	+	+
Estimation of weight of foods	−	+	+	+
Estimation of frequency of foods consumed	n.a.	n.a.	+	+
Changes in real diet due to burden of method	+	+/−	−	−
Errors in conversion into nutrients				
Food composition database	+	+	+	+
Coding/choosing correct food	+	+	+	−

+, error is likely.
−, error is unlikely.
n.a., not applicable.

person consciously or unconsciously underestimates or exaggerates food intake. An important food for an individual who is not included in a questionnaire, or a question that is systematically misunderstood by an individual, will also lead to systematic within-person error. If the dietary assessment method is repeatedly administered, the error will occur again, thus leading to person-specific bias. Consequently, the estimation of mean intake for an individual is not improved by repeated measurements and remains biased. Increasing evidence suggests that most self-reported intakes are likely to be flawed with person-specific biases.[28]

Random between-person error; random between-person error or person-specific error may be due to random and systematic within-person error if they are distributed randomly across individuals; an overestimation by some individuals is counterbalanced by an underestimation by others (see Table 14.4). The estimated mean intake is consequently not biased but the precision is affected, and the distribution of measured intake is artificially widened.[23] Estimates of the percentage of subjects below or above a certain cut-off level (e.g., Estimated Average Requirement) are therefore not accurate. Also, the validity of measures of associations with health parameters is hampered and for univariate association is attenuated.[28] The precision of the estimate of the mean group intake where random between-person error exists can be improved by increasing the number of subjects or the number of replicate measurements.[50]

Systematic between-person error; systematic between-person error is caused by systematic within-person error that is not randomly distributed across individuals. Questionnaires that fail to include important foods for a population, use incorrect standard portion sizes, and obtain socially desirable answers (untrue) by groups of people and 24 hRs or FRs that do not include weekend days will all result in systematic between-person error.[18] As a result, the mean intake is not estimated correctly nor is the percentage of persons above or below a certain cut-off level.

Testing whether an association with a health parameter exists is not affected by systematic between-person error that applies equally to all subjects. However, this error may be associated with a variable for which the relation with dietary intake is the topic of study, and a misleading conclusion may be drawn. An example is body mass index: subjects with a higher body mass index underreport their energy intake more than those with lower body mass index.[60]

TABLE 14.4 The effects of random and systematic between-person error in dietary intake on parameters to be estimated.

	Type of between-person error	
Parameter to be estimated	**random**	**systematic**
Mean intake	Precision ↓	Validity ↓
Variation of intake	Validity ↓	No effect
Percent of subjects below EAR	Validity ↓	Validity ↓
Association with health outcome	Validity ↓	No effect

Prepared by Jan Burema.

The effects of random and systematic between-person measurement error on various parameters to be estimated are summarized in Table 14.4.

Biomarker errors; although biomarkers of intake are considered objective (and thus not subject to subject bias) and can be measured in a wide array of specimens, they are also prone to error. Errors in biomarker concentrations are related to specimen collection, processing, and storage (preanalytical errors), laboratory errors, and errors related to within-person variation over time.[61] In order to reduce the uncertainty in the concentration of a biomarker, these issues need to be addressed by standardizing the preanalytical stage as much as possible, by validating and standardizing measurements in the laboratory to reduce bias and assay variation, and by increasing the number of samples obtained to take into account biological variation.

With respect to blood samples, the easiest way is to collect finger-prick blood, but the volume that can be obtained is usually low and is unsuitable to aliquot into smaller portions for storage. Dividing the specimen into different aliquots is in general advisable to prevent losses due to repeated freeze-thawing cycles when multiple components are of interest and only one aliquot is available.[61]

Concentrations of biomarkers in blood are dependent on the procedure followed, e.g., fasting state, previous exercise, posture of the subject (supine or sitting), and skills of the phlebotomist. In addition, for some nutrients such as folate or vitamin C, stabilization may be required after collection. The preanalytical stage contributes most to the "turnaround time" of a specimen, and therefore fast processing of a sample after collection is necessary to avoid unwanted changes in the sample.[62] Storage at very low temperature (liquid nitrogen, −80°c freezer) is required, especially when long-term storage is necessary for a biomarker study. Ideally, stability studies should be included. Losses of biomarker content can occur due to inadequate storage, which may lead to attenuated effect estimates.[63]

Urine, either spot or 24-h urine, is available in larger quantities. Urine sampling represents short-term exposure to diet and, especially with 24-h urine sample collection, e.g., for assessing protein or sodium intake, requires perceptive and cooperative subjects. One of the main challenges is assuring completeness of a 24-hour urine collection. This is often monitored by the subjects taking PABA tablets, and then excretion of PABA in the collected urine is measured to monitor compliance. Specific preservation techniques during collection may be necessary depending on the analyte of interest, ambient temperature of the sample collected, and collection period.

Evaluation of measurement error; Information on the size of random measurement error can be obtained from dietary repeatability and validity studies. In repeatability studies, the dietary assessment method is readministered. Such studies only give information on part of the total error, i.e., not that based on systematic within-person error.[18] In theory, validity studies supply information on the total error. However, in practice, this is limited by the lack of a true gold standard, that is, dietary assessment methods without errors or with completely independent errors. In the absence of a true gold standard, it is important that the test method for which the validity is being assessed is compared to a reference method with independent types of measurement error. The OPEN study is an example of a study that gives insight in the error matrix for 24 hRs and FFQs.[28]

An often-used check for misestimation of energy intake is the ratio of energy intake to estimated basal metabolic rate. If this ratio is below the confidence limit of the expected value of PAL for the individual, energy intake is very likely underreported. These checks can be done at the study population level as well as the level of the individual; confidence limits of PAL differ for these situations.[27]

Removing measurement error

Formulas and statistical models that correct for the effects of random measurement error are available for many outcome measures, such as the distribution of intakes and measures of associations with other variables such as correlation coefficients, regression coefficients, and relative risks.[18,64] Techniques for adjustments are not well developed for systematic measurement error associated with parameters of interest.

III. DEVELOPMENT AND APPLICATION OF METHODS

A. Self-Reports

Recent developments in dietary assessment methods by self-reports focus mainly on applying new technology tools. Accessibility of the new technology to participants needs to be considered, as well as how food is identified and how consumed foods are quantified. Customization to the population group of interest should be carefully considered, and it is essential that the data output, data flow, and linkage to other data like food composition databases are developed well. New tools need to be pretested in the population group for later implementation. Usability tests and focus group discussions can be appropriate approaches for such pretests. Usually, many iterations are required. After the tool is developed, performing a validity study is of utmost importance. In case the new tool will replace another existing tool, a comparison or calibration study is important.[40]

B. Discovery and Validation of Biomarkers

Several approaches have been used in the past to identify markers of intake: either well-controlled dietary intervention studies have been used or correlation studies of self-reported intake of specific foods or food groups with urinary profiles or blood concentrations.[4] Most biomarkers of food intake were identified using compound-specific analytical procedures. In this hypo thesis-driven or targeted-approach candidate, biomarkers are selected based on knowledge of their presence in foods or food groups and by information on their metabolism or excretion. Subsequently, the suitability of the candidate biomarkers is further confirmed in dietary intervention studies.

C. Metabolomics

The emergence of metabolomics techniques allows the measurement of multiple components simultaneously, often by a nontargeted or discovery-driven approach, and this has been increasingly used during the last decade to explore the food metabolome. The food metabolome is the change in metabolite concentrations due to the digestion, absorption, and biotransformation of foods in the body or by microbiota.[31] Proline betaine as biomarker of citrus fruits intake was one of the first biomarkers discovered using this approach in an intervention study.[65] Correlation studies using nontargeted approaches and self-reported intakes has revealed many candidate biomarkers as well.[31,66] Metabolomics uses high throughput techniques based on NMR, GC-MS, or LC-MS, and these techniques offer a promising opportunity to discover novel biomarkers of intake at very low concentrations.[4] However, a challenge is to process and statistically analyze a huge amount of raw data by multivariate techniques. The identification and quantification can also be challenging due to poor availability of standards and the need for interlaboratory biomarker validation (reproducibility) studies.

Ideally, the validity of any biomarker should be established in well-controlled studies. The number of thoroughly validated dietary biomarkers however is limited, and the lack of a systematic approach, or well-defined validation criteria, has been brought up recently by some researchers.[67] The aim of the Food Biomarkers Alliance (FoodBAll) project is "to develop clear strategies for food intake biomarker discovery and validation, and to identify and validate biomarkers for a range of foods consumed across Europe."[47]

D. Validation of Biomarkers

Validation criteria to critically assess candidate biomarkers have been suggested to address the following attributes of the biomarker: (1) sensitivity and specificity of analytical method; (2) specificity of the marker for its food/food group; (3) dose–response relationship; (4) time–response relationship for acute intakes; (5) time–response relationship for repeated intakes; (6) robustness after intake of complex meals; (7) validation against other markers for same food (group); and (8) verification of sensitivity and specificity shown in a validation study.[67] For most biomarkers, only a few of these attributes have been evaluated thoroughly.

RESEARCH GAPS

Future directions for dietary assessment and biomarkers of intake include further development of

- Innovative technologies for dietary assessment including food identification and portion size estimations and their evaluation;
- Validation in specific population groups, especially non-Western populations;
- Assessment of intake of dietary supplements combined with intake from foods, and related measurement error;
- Biomarkers of intake using controlled feeding studies.

Acknowledgments

This chapter is an update of the chapter titled Estimation of Dietary Intake by van Staveren WA, Ock MC, and de Vries JHM in *Present Knowledge in Nutrition*, 10th Edition, edited by Erdman JW, Macdonald IA, and Zeisel SH and published by Wiley-Blackwell. © 2012 International Life Sciences Institute. Portions of this update are from the previously published chapter, and the contributions of previous authors are acknowledged.

IV. REFERENCES

1. Bingham SA. Biomarkers in nutritional epidemiology. *Public Health Nutr.* 2002;5(6a):821–827.
2. Favé G, Beckmann ME, Draper JH, Mathers JC. Measurement of dietary exposure: a challenging problem which may be overcome thanks to metabolomics? *Genes Nutr.* 2009;4(2):135–141.
3. Scalbert A, Huybrechts I, Gunter MJ. The food exposome. In: Dagnino S, Macherone A, eds. *Unraveling the Exposome: A Practical View.* Cham: Springer International Publishing; 2019:217–245.
4. O'Gorman A, Brennan L. The role of metabolomics in determination of new dietary biomarkers. *Proc Nutr Soc.* 2017;76(3):295–302.
5. Nydahl M, Gustafsson IB, Mohsen R, Becker W. Comparison between optical readable and open-ended weighed food records. *Food Nutr Res.* 2009;53. https://doi.org/10.3402/fnr.v53i0.1889.
6. Boushey CJ, Spoden M, Zhu FM, Delp EJ, Kerr DA. New mobile methods for dietary assessment: review of image-assisted and image-based dietary assessment methods. *Proc Nutr Soc.* 2017; 76(3):283–294.
7. Ortega RM, Perez-Rodrigo C, Lopez-Sobaler AM. Dietary assessment methods: dietary records. *Nutr Hosp.* 2015;31(Suppl 3):38–45.
8. Timon CM, van den Barg R, Blain RJ, et al. A review of the design and validation of web- and computer-based 24-h dietary recall tools. *Nutr Res Rev.* 2016;29(2):268–280.
9. Conway JM, Ingwersen LA, Moshfegh AJ. Accuracy of dietary recall using the USDA five-step multiple-pass method in men: an observational validation study. *J Am Diet Assoc.* 2004;104(4):595–603.
10. Baxter SD. Cognitive processes in children's dietary recalls: insight from methodological studies. *Eur J Clin Nutr.* 2009;63(Suppl 1): S19–S32.
11. Kumanyika SK, Tell GS, Shemanski L, Martel J, Chinchilli VM. Dietary assessment using a picture-sort approach. *Am J Clin Nutr.* 1997;65(4 Suppl):1123s–1129s.
12. De Keyzer W, Bracke T, McNaughton SA, et al. Cross-continental comparison of national food consumption survey methods—a narrative review. *Nutrients.* 2015;7(5):3587–3620.
13. Burke B. The dietary history as a tool in research. *J Am Diet Assoc.* 1947;23:1041–1046.
14. Strassburg A, Eisinger-Watzl M, Krems C, Roth A, Hoffmann I. Comparison of food consumption and nutrient intake assessed with three dietary assessment methods: results of the German National Nutrition Survey II. *Eur J Nutr.* 2019;58(1):193–210.
15. Thompson FE, Subar AF. Dietary assessment methodology. In: Coulston A, Boushey C, eds. *Nutrition in the Prevention and Treatment of Disease.* 4th ed. Amsterdam: Elsevier; 2017:5–48.
16. Moran Fagundez LJ, Rivera Torres A, Gonzalez Sanchez ME, de Torres Aured ML, Perez Rodrigo C, Irles Rocamora JA. Diet history: method and applications. *Nutr Hosp.* 2015;31(Suppl 3): 57–61.
17. Cade J, Thompson R, Burley V. Warm D. Development, validation and utilisation of food-frequency questionnaires – a review. *Public Health Nutr.* 2002;5(4):567–587.
18. Willett WC. *Nutritional Epidemiology.* 3rd ed. New York: Oxford University Press; 2013.
19. Molag ML, de Vries JH, Ocke MC, et al. Design characteristics of food frequency questionnaires in relation to their validity. *Am J Epidemiol.* 2007;166(12):1468–1478.
20. Perez Rodrigo C, Aranceta J, Salvador G, Varela-Moreiras G. Food frequency questionnaires. *Nutr Hosp.* 2015;31(Suppl 3):49–56.
21. Smith AF, Jobe JB, Mingay DJ. Retrieval from memory of dietary information. *Appl Cognit Psychol.* 1991;5(3):269–296.
22. Illner AK, Freisling H, Boeing H, Huybrechts I, Crispim SP, Slimani N. Review and evaluation of innovative technologies for measuring diet in nutritional epidemiology. *Int J Epidemiol.* 2012; 41(4):1187–1203.
23. Souverein OW, Dekkers AL, Geelen A, et al. Comparing four methods to estimate usual intake distributions. *Eur J Clin Nutr.* 2011;65(Suppl 1):S92–S101.
24. Conrad J, Nothlings U. Innovative approaches to estimate individual usual dietary intake in large-scale epidemiological studies. *Proc Nutr Soc.* 2017;76(3):213–219.
25. Trolle E, Amiano P, Ege M, et al. Evaluation of 2 × 24-h dietary recalls combined with a food-recording booklet, against a 7-day food-record method among schoolchildren. *Eur J Clin Nutr.* 2011; 65(Suppl 1):S77–S83.
26. Jenab M, Slimani N, Bictash M, Ferrari P, Bingham SA. Biomarkers in nutritional epidemiology: applications, needs and new horizons. *Hum Genet.* 2009;125(5):507–525.
27. Livingstone MBE, Black AE. Markers of the validity of reported energy intake. *J Nutr.* 2003;133(3):895S–920S.
28. Kipnis V, Subar AF, Midthune D, et al. Structure of dietary measurement error: results of the OPEN biomarker study. *Am J Epidemiol.* 2003;158(1):14–21. discussion 22-16.
29. Longnecker MP, Taylor PR, Levander OA, et al. Selenium in diet, blood, and toenails in relation to human health in a seleniferous area. *Am J Clin Nutr.* 1991;53(5):1288–1294.
30. Tasevska N, Runswick SA, McTaggart A, Bingham SA. Urinary sucrose and fructose as biomarkers for sugar consumption. *Cancer Epidemiol Biomark Prev.* 2005;14:1287–1294.
31. Scalbert A, Brennan L, Manach C, et al. The food metabolome: a window over dietary exposure. *Am J Clin Nutr.* 2014;99(6): 1286–1308.
32. Freedman LS, Tasevska N, Kipnis V, et al. Gains in statistical power from using a dietary biomarker in combination with self-reported intake to strengthen the analysis of a diet-disease association: an example from CAREDS. *Am J Epidemiol.* 2010;172(7):836–842.
33. Trijsburg L, Talsma EF, de Vries JHM, Kennedy G, Kuijsten A, Brouwer ID. Diet quality indices for research in low- and middle-income countries: a systematic review. *Journal.* 2019. https://doi.org/10.1093/nutrit/nuz017.
34. Gil A, Martinez de Victoria E, Olza J. Indicators for the evaluation of diet quality. *Nutr Hosp.* 2015;31(Suppl 3):128–144.
35. Wirt A, Collins CE. Diet quality—what is it and does it matter? *Public Health Nutr.* 2009;12(12):2473–2492.
36. Looman M, Feskens EJ, de Rijk M, et al. Development and evaluation of the Dutch healthy diet index 2015. *Public Health Nutr.* 2017; 20(13):2289–2299.
37. van Lee L, Feskens EJ, Meijboom S, et al. Evaluation of a screener to assess diet quality in the Netherlands. *Br J Nutr.* 2016;115(3):517–526.
38. Yetley EA. Multivitamin and multimineral dietary supplements: definitions, characterization, bioavailability, and drug interactions. *Am J Clin Nutr.* 2007;85(1):269s–276s.
39. Bailey RL, Dodd KW, Gahche JJ, et al. Best practices for dietary supplement assessment and estimation of total usual nutrient intakes in population-level research and monitoring. *J Nutr.* 2019; 149(2):181–197.
40. Eldridge AL, Piernas C, Illner AK, et al. Evaluation of new technology-based tools for dietary intake assessment-an ILSI Europe dietary intake and exposure task force evaluation. *Nutrients.* 2018;11(1).
41. Schiboni G, Amft O. Automatic dietary monitoring using wearable accessories. In: Tamura T, Chen W, eds. *Seamless Healthcare Monitoring: Advancements in Wearable, Attachable, and Invisible Devices.* Cham: Springer; 2018:369–412.
42. Burrows T, Collins C, Adam M, Duncanson K, Rollo M. Dietary assessment of shared plate eating: a missing link. *Journal.* 2019; 11(4). https://doi.org/10.3390/nu11040789.
43. Goris AH, Westerterp KR. Underreporting of habitual food intake is explained by undereating in highly motivated lean women. *J Nutr.* 1999;129(4):878–882.

44. Turconi G, Guarcello M, Berzolari FG, Carolei A, Bazzano R, Roggi C. An evaluation of a colour food photography atlas as a tool for quantifying food portion size in epidemiological dietary surveys. *Eur J Clin Nutr.* 2005;59(8):923–931.
45. Gemming L, Utter J, Ni Mhurchu C, et al. Image-assisted dietary assessment: a systematic review of the evidence. Measuring food intake with digital photography. *J Acad Nutr Diet.* 2015;115(1):64–77.
46. Dao MC, Subar AF, Warthon-Medina M, et al. Dietary assessment toolkits: an overview. *Public Health Nutr.* 2019;22(3):404–418.
47. Brouwer-Brolsma EM, Brennan L, Drevon CA, et al. Combining traditional dietary assessment methods with novel metabolomics techniques: present efforts by the Food Biomarker Alliance. *Proc Nutr Soc.* 2017;76(4):619–627.
48. Kromhout D, Giltay EJ, Geleijnse JM. n−3 fatty acids and cardiovascular events after myocardial infarction. *N Engl J Med.* 2010; 363(21):2015–2026.
49. Kaaks RJ. Biochemical markers as additional measurements in studies of the accuracy of dietary questionnaire measurements: conceptual issues. *Am J Clin Nutr.* 1997;65(4):1232S–1239S.
50. Beaton GH, Milner J, Corey P, et al. Sources of variance in 24-hour dietary recall data: implications for nutrition study design and interpretation. *Am J Clin Nutr.* 1979;32(12):2546–2559.
51. de Vries JH, de Groot LC, van Staveren WA. Dietary assessment in elderly people: experiences gained from studies in the Netherlands. *Eur J Clin Nutr.* 2009;63(Suppl 1):S69–S74.
52. Emmett P. Workshop 2: the use of surrogate reporters in the assessment of dietary intake. *Eur J Clin Nutr.* 2009;63(Suppl 1):S78–S79.
53. Livingstone MB, Robson PJ, Wallace JM. Issues in dietary intake assessment of children and adolescents. *Br J Nutr.* 2004;92(Suppl 2):S213–S222.
54. Foster E, Bradley J. Methodological considerations and future insights for 24-hour dietary recall assessment in children. *Nutr Res.* 2018;51:1–11.
55. Burrows TL, Martin RJ, Collins CE. A systematic review of the validity of dietary assessment methods in children when compared with the method of doubly labeled water. *J Am Diet Assoc.* 2010; 110(10):1501–1510.
56. Gibson RS, Charrondiere UR, Bell W. Measurement errors in dietary assessment using self-reported 24-hour recalls in low-income countries and strategies for their prevention. *Adv Nutr.* 2017;8(6):980–991.
57. Trijsburg L, Geelen A, Hollman PC, et al. BMI was found to be a consistent determinant related to misreporting of energy, protein and potassium intake using self-report and duplicate portion methods. *Public Health Nutr.* 2017;20(4):598–607.
58. Eussen SJ, van Dongen MC, Wijckmans NE, et al. A national FFQ for the Netherlands (the FFQ-NL1.0): development and compatibility with existing Dutch FFQs. *Public Health Nutr.* 2018;21(12): 2221–2229.
59. Brouwer-Brolsma EM, Streppel MT, van Lee L, et al. A national dietary assessment reference database (NDARD) for the Dutch population: rationale behind the design. *Nutrients.* 2017;9(10). https://doi.org/10.3390/nu9101136.
60. Pietilainen KH, Korkeila M, Bogl LH, et al. Inaccuracies in food and physical activity diaries of obese subjects: complementary evidence from doubly labeled water and co-twin assessments. *Int J Obes.* 2010;34(3):437–445.
61. Tworoger SS, Hankinson SE. Use of biomarkers in epidemiologic studies: minimizing the influence of measurement error in the study design and analysis. *Cancer Causes Control.* 2006;17(7): 889–899.
62. Guder WG, Narayanan S, Wisser H, Zawta B. *Samples: From the Patient to the Laboratory: the Impact of Preanalytical Variables on the Quality of Laboratory Results.* Weinheim: Wiley-VCH Verlag GmbH & Co. KGaA; 2007.
63. Ocké MC, Schrijver J, Obermann-De Boer GL, Bloemberg BPM, Haenen GRMM, Kromhout D. Stability of blood (pro)vitamins during four years of storage at −20 °C: consequences for epidemiologic research. *J Clin Epidemiol.* 1995;48(8):1077–1085.
64. Freedman LS, Midthune D, Dodd KW, Carroll RJ, Kipnis V. A statistical model for measurement error that incorporates variation over time in the target measure, with application to nutritional epidemiology. *Stat Med.* 2015;34(27):3590–3605.
65. Heinzmann SS, Brown IJ, Chan Q, et al. Metabolic profiling strategy for discovery of nutritional biomarkers: proline betaine as a marker of citrus consumption. *Am J Clin Nutr.* 2010;92(2):436–443.
66. Zamora-Ros R, Achaintre D, Rothwell JA, et al. Urinary excretions of 34 dietary polyphenols and their associations with lifestyle factors in the EPIC cohort study. *Sci Rep.* 2016;6:26905.
67. Dragsted LO, Gao Q, Scalbert A, et al. Validation of biomarkers of food intake-critical assessment of candidate biomarkers. *Genes & nutrition.* 2018;13:14.

CHAPTER

15

ESTABLISHING NUTRIENT INTAKE VALUES

Janine L. Lewis[1], *BSc, Grad Dip Nut & Diet, Grad Dip Public Health*
Johanna T. Dwyer[2,3], *DSc, RD*

[1]Food Standards Australia New Zealand, Canberra, ACT, Australia
[2]Tufts University Medical School, Boston, MA, United States
[3]Office of Dietary Supplements, National Institutes of Health, Bethesda, MD, United States

SUMMARY

Nutrient intake values (NIVs) are recommendations for nutrient intakes throughout the life cycle that meet human nutrient requirements. These values are necessary for nutrition science and policy making, including assessing the adequacy of food supplies and diets to support health. They also serve as a basis for reference values used in nutrition labeling. NIVs may apply internationally or to national or regional populations. They are established by international, regional, or national government agencies or professional scientific societies. Because of this diversity, NIVs often differ from country to country, not only for relevant scientific reasons but also because of local choice of terminology and derivation. The reasons for the similarities and differences across countries are described for major sets of NIVs that are published in English. Efforts over the past decade to harmonize terminology and methodological approaches have been made by the international agencies, but progress is slow.

Keywords: Dietary reference intakes; Dietary reference value; Harmonization; Nutrient reference value; Terminology.

I. INTRODUCTION

A. Background

A set of reference values for nutrient intake to sustain health throughout the life cycle is an essential nutrition policy tool. Various sets of such reference values have been developed, expanded, and updated over the years for international, regional, or national use. Their development is resource intensive, time consuming and expensive and requires a wide range of scientific expertise. Therefore, this work has been carried out primarily by United Nations agencies, governments, or professional/scientific nutrition societies. Some countries do not establish their own nutrient intake recommendations. Instead, they adopt or modify those from other sources appropriate to their situation or use those that are available internationally. The terminology used in these recommendations differs widely among the various sources although each suite of terms relates to similar concepts. This chapter has adopted the internationally proposed collective term for nutrient intake recommendations called *nutrient intake values* (NIVs).[1] NIVs are numeric, evidence-based values that describe and quantify the amounts of nutrients from the diet needed to meet human requirements. Regardless of whether a set of NIVs applies to a national, regional, or international population, these values are derived for age-sex groups and certain life stages (such as pregnancy or lactation) throughout the life cycle.

In an increasingly global nutrition world, scientists and policy makers need to understand the basis for NIVs, their derivation, proper interpretation, and use. Now that the

https://doi.org/10.1016/B978-0-12-818460-8.00015-0

range of national, regional, and international publications of NIVs is highly accessible on the Internet, it is important to understand how these reference sets vary. The following sections describe the similarities and differences of sets of NIVs available in English, their uses, terminology, methodological approaches employed, and efforts over the last decade to improve global harmonization.

II. DEFINITIONS AND EXPLANATORY RELATIONSHIPS

A. Uses

NIVs are used for many purposes, including assessment of individual intakes and in the examination and interpretation of nutrition surveys to provide an estimate of probable nutrient intake adequacy of populations. They are also used for planning of individual diets, food labeling, formulating criteria for food programs, institutional feeding, and other nutritional interventions (Fig. 15.1). When NIVs are used appropriately, they help to harmonize nutrient-based dietary assessment and planning, both within and between countries.

B. Terminology

In 2010, the Food and Agriculture Organization (FAO) and the World Health Organization (WHO) were requested to survey reference sources of NIVs for vitamins and minerals from around the world. The report[2] surveyed 55 national, regional, and international sets of NIVs published between 1998 and 2010. In so doing, it importantly observed that a lack of common naming terminology among countries made it difficult to compare and classify the basis for the numeric values. Different terms were used for the same concept, and the same term was used for different concepts depending on the country or organization.

Table 15.1 presents a summary of the various terms applied to NIVs by expert bodies in various countries including the Institute of Medicine (IOM) for the United States and Canada; the European Food Safety Authority (EFSA) for countries in the European Union (EU); and the FAO of the United Nations and the WHO for use internationally. In 2007, a consortium of international experts convened by the United Nations University (UNU), with help from FAO and WHO, also proposed new terminology for NIVs in recognition of the lack of global uniformity in this field.[6] The most notable new term, the INL_X, was built on an existing concept to indicate that any percentile in the statistical distribution of requirements could be adopted as the recommended intake level. Generally, the new terminology refers to similar concepts and uses a similar framework to others, but, so far, it has not been widely adopted.

In Table 15.1, the term "intake" in the Description column respectively takes the general meaning of a

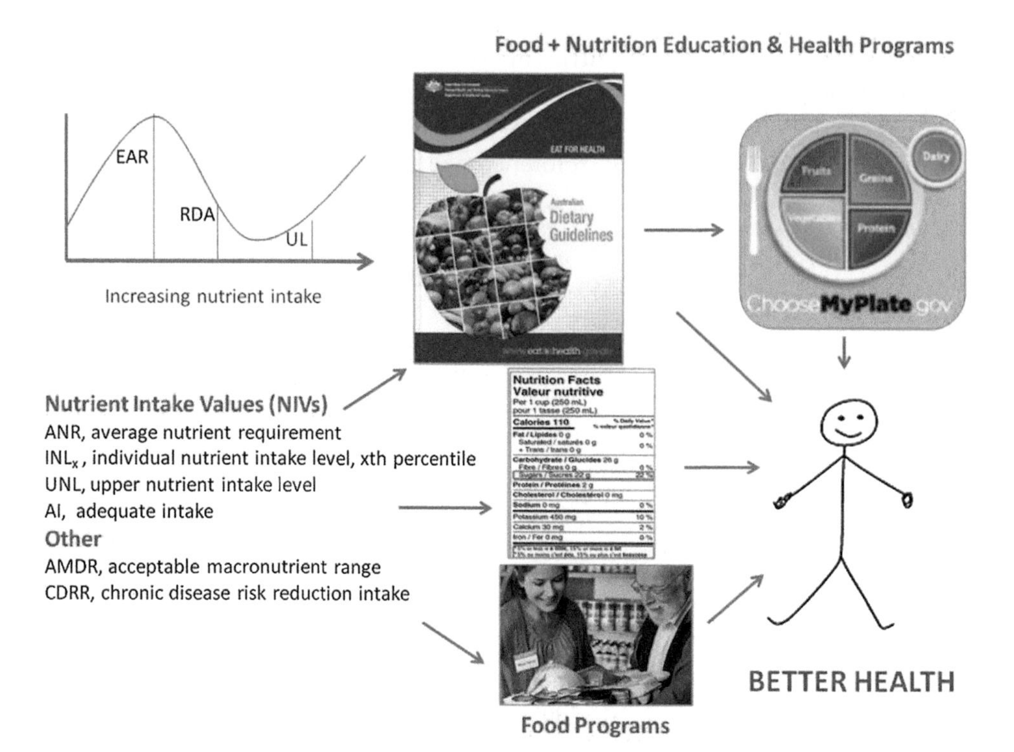

FIGURE 15.1 Relationship between dietary standards, dietary guidelines, and associated interventions and better health.

TABLE 15.1 Glossary of terms used for describing NIVs by various expert bodies.

Term	Abbreviation	General description	Term used by
Acceptable macronutrient distribution range	AMDR	Range of intakes for carbohydrate, fat, and protein associated with reduced risk of chronic disease while providing adequate intake of essential nutrients	IOM[3] for the United States and Canada; NHMRC/MOH[4] for Australia and New Zealand
Adequate Intake	AI	An observed or experimentally determined intake by a population that is assumed to be adequate	IOM[3]; EFSA[5] for the european union; NHMRC/MOH[4]
Average nutrient requirement	ANR	The average requirement estimated from a statistical distribution of requirements for a population	Proposed by UNU/FAO/WHO[6]
Average requirement	AR	Intake that is adequate for half the population, given a normal distribution of requirement	EFSA[5]; Nordic council of ministers for nordic Countries[a,7]
Chronic disease risk reduction intake	CDRR	Intake above which an intake reduction is expected to reduce chronic disease risk	NASEM[8]
Dietary Reference Intake	DRI	Set of reference nutrient intake values: EAR, RDA, AI, AMDR, CDRR, UL	IOM[3]
Dietary Reference Value	DRV	Set of reference nutrient intake values: EAR, RNI, LRNI, SI	Committee on medical Aspects of Food and Nutrition Policy (COMA)[b,9] for the United Kingdom (UK)
		Set of reference nutrient intake values: AR, PRI, LTI, AI, RI, safe and adequate intake, UL	EFSA[5]
		Nordic Nutrient Recommendations: AR, RI, LI, UL	Nordic Council[7]
Estimated Average Requirement	EAR	Intake estimated to meet the requirement of half the population	IOM[3]; NHMRC/MOH[4]; COMA[b,9]; FAO/WHO[10]
Guideline recommendation	WHO guideline	See Box 15.1	WHO[11–13]
Individual nutrient level, x = percentile chosen	INL x	Intake at the chosen percentile of the normal distribution of requirement	Proposed by UNU/WHO/FAO[6]; Adopted by codex alimentarius[14]

Continued

TABLE 15.1 Glossary of terms used for describing NIVs by various expert bodies.—cont'd

Term	Abbreviation	General description	Term used by
Lower intake level	LI	A cutoff intake below which could lead to clinical deficiency symptoms in most individuals	Nordic Council[7]
Lower reference nutrient intake	LRNI	Intake enough for only a small group in a population who have low requirements (2.5%)	COMA[b,9]
Lower threshold intake	LTI	Intake below which almost all are unable to maintain "metabolic integrity," according to a chosen criterion	EFSA[5]
Nutrient intake values	NIV	Set of reference nutrient intake values: ANR, INL_x, UNL	Proposed by UNU/WHO/FAO[6]
Nutrient Reference Values	NRV	Set of reference nutrient intake values: EAR, RDI, AI, AMDR, UL	NHMRC/MOH[4]
Population Reference Intake	PRI	Intake that is adequate for virtually all in a population	EFSA[5]
Recommended Dietary Allowance	RDA	Intake sufficient to meet the requirements of nearly all in a population	IOM[3]
Recommended Dietary Intake	RDI	Intake sufficient to meet the requirements of nearly all in a population	NHMRC/MOH[4]
Recommended Intake	RI	Intake that meets the requirements and maintains good nutritional status among practically all in a population	Nordic Council[7]
Recommended Nutrient Intake	RNI	Intake that meets the requirements of almost all in a population	FAO/WHO[10]
Reference intake range of macronutrients	RI	The intake range for macronutrients, expressed as % energy intake that are adequate for maintaining health and associated with a low risk of selected chronic diseases	EFSA[5]
Reference Nutrient Intake	RNI	Intake that is enough or more than enough for about 97% of a population	COMA[b,9]

TABLE 15.1 Glossary of terms used for describing NIVs by various expert bodies.—cont'd

Term	Abbreviation	General description	Term used by
Safe and adequate intake	Not established	Intake that does not give rise to concerns about adverse health effects, in instances when a UL could not be established and assumed to be sufficient based on observations from a population	EFSA[c,15]
Safe intake	SI	Intake enough for almost everyone, but below a level that could have undesirable effects	COMA[b,9]
Tolerable Upper Intake Level	UL	Highest average intake likely to pose no risk of adverse health effects to almost all in a population	IOM[3]
		Maximum chronic intake unlikely to pose a risk of adverse health effects	EFSA[16]
Upper Intake Level	UL	Maximum chronic intakes unlikely to pose a risk of adverse health effects	Nordic Council[7]
Upper level of intake	UL	Highest average intake likely to pose no adverse health effects to almost all in the population	NHMRC/MOH[4]
		Maximum habitual intake likely to lead to adverse health effects	WHO[17]
Upper nutrient level	UNL	Highest average intake likely to pose no risk of adverse health effects to almost all in a population	Proposed by UNU/FAO/WHO[6]

[a]*Nordic countries comprise Denmark, Finland, Norway, Sweden, Iceland, the Faroe Islands, Greenland, and Åland.*
[b]*COMA was disbanded and replaced by the Scientific Advisory Committee on Nutrition (SACN) that updated selected DRVs from 2011.*
[c]*This term applies only to sodium and chloride.*

(average) daily nutrient intake level; the term "population" is assumed to be a group of apparently healthy individuals of a particular age, sex, and life stage.

Table 15.2 provides selected abbreviations from Table 15.1 arranged by concept and expert body to indicate the level of similarity and difference in terminology for NIVs.

C. Methodological Approaches Employed

Similarities

Today, nomenclature and methods for ascertaining nutrient requirements are becoming more widely accepted and harmonized between expert groups and countries, with the result that recommendations for

TABLE 15.2 Comparison of terminology used by selected expert bodies for describing NIVs.

	UNU/FAO/WHO[6]	IOM[3]	EFSA[5,16]	FAO/WHO[10,17]
Terms used	NIV	DRI	DRV	
Average requirement	ANR	EAR	AR	
Recommended intake for almost all in a population	INL_x, where x = 97.5	RDA	PRI	RNI
Adequate intake		AI	AI	
Macronutrient distribution range		AMDR	RI	Guideline recommendation[11–13]
Upper level	UNL	UL	UL	UL

AI, Adequate Intake; *AMDR*, acceptable macronutrient distribution range; *ANR*, Average Nutrient Requirement; *AR*, Average Requirement; *DRI*, Dietary Reference Intake; *DRV*, Dietary Reference Value; *EAR*, Estimated Average Requirement; INL_x, individual nutrient level, where x = percentile chosen; *NIV*, Nutrient Intake Value; *PRI*, Population Reference Intake; *RDA*, Recommended Dietary Allowance; *RIs*, reference intake range for macronutrients; *RNI*, Recommended Nutrient Intake; *UL*, Tolerable Upper Intake Level/upper intake level; *UNL*, upper nutrient level.

nutrient intakes are converging more than ever before. The data on which NIVs are based are generally similar when reviewed by expert groups and then adopted by one country or another. They include relevant human clinical and experimental data (such as depletion–repletion studies, dose–response studies, and balance studies), epidemiological studies, and relevant animal studies. The methods used in formulating NIVs generally involve a review of the literature and recommendations by expert scientists on the nutrient in question.

Most expert bodies setting NIVs now provide values for protein, vitamins, and minerals and newer sections on dietary components that are relevant to the reduction in risk of diet-related diseases.[18,19] For example, the recent revisions of the US/Canadian Dietary Reference Intakes (DRIs) for sodium and potassium provide additional focus on such outcomes with a new chronic disease risk reduction (CDRR) intake value.[8] Developing CDRR values such as acceptable macronutrient distribution ranges (AMDRs) and CDRRs are challenging since the causes of the diseases are multifactorial, including, but not limited to, one or more dietary components. When experimental studies are possible for studying chronic diseases, they are usually of short duration with high doses and surrogate markers from which lower intakes over many years and chronic disease endpoints are inferred. Risk reduction values are therefore not usually determined experimentally; rather, they are based largely on observational epidemiology, with all the difficulties this method creates for establishing causal inference.

There is variability in nutrient requirements even among individuals who are similar in age and sex or life stage, and therefore statistical concepts are essential in the derivation and interpretation of NIVs.[20] The use of probability models and statistical techniques is vital in the formulation of human nutrient requirements since such requirements all have a probability distribution that must be dealt with by a probability approach.[21] For individuals, the values are stated in probabilistic terms since an individual's nutrient requirements are never known with certainty.

Virtually all expert bodies setting NIVs now use similar statistical approaches for determining the midpoint of the distribution of requirements for a given function for each nutrient, and for deriving an estimate of the standard deviation (SD) of the requirements. These bodies also use probability theory to state a level that ensures nutritional adequacy for most individuals at some point above the mean requirement, such as 2 SDs. Although data are often lacking at present, a second set of distributions of risk of excessive intakes is used when it is available as the basis for establishing the upper nutrient levels (UNL).

Most expert bodies setting NIVs base them on criteria that reflect a meaningful biomarker of a nutrient-related function.[22] This is critical since the choice of indicator or function will determine the amount of the nutrient that is needed. Desirable criteria exhibit a dose–response function, are responsive to inadequacy or excess of a single nutrient, resist rapid day-to-day changes in response to inadequate, adequate, or excessive intakes, are easily measurable or assessable with noninvasive methods, and are unresponsive to environmental changes other than nutrient intakes.[1] Although functional criteria that reflect chronic disease endpoints are often the most relevant, the data for using them are often not available.[23]

Methods for using NIVs in dietary assessment and planning are also becoming increasingly popular and uniform. One such use is for nutrition labeling, which is discussed later in the chapter.

Differences

In spite of the similarities noted above, there are still many differences between the processes used by expert bodies to set NIVs and in their estimates of nutrient requirements.

Terminology and nomenclature are still not harmonized even though NIVs are defined in similar ways by most expert bodies. Inconsistencies in the conceptual frameworks used may lead the unwary to assume that differences in expert reports are much greater than they actually are. The reasons for the differences in estimates of NIVs include the relative emphasis given to different types of evidence (human epidemiological or experimental studies and studies from other species) and the functional criteria chosen, whereas the literature available when the reviews were conducted also contributes to differences in conclusions. Differences also exist as a result of variations in dietary composition (which affect nutrient absorption and bioavailability), the anthropometric reference standards used (e.g., height, weight, or growth rates of reference individuals), definitions of reference groups or groups at risk (e.g., premature infants), and assumptions about the climate, altitude, and temperature. NIVs also vary according to underlying assumptions about nutrient bioavailability and how these values are extrapolated if evidence is unavailable for certain age-sex or life stage groups. Where there is insufficient biological data, NIVs may also be established based on food consumption surveys of usual intakes of healthy people. This explains to some extent the variability in Adequate Intake (AI) values that reflect diverse dietary patterns.

D. How NIVs Are Developed by Various Expert Groups

Governmental or quasigovernmental bodies are responsible for setting NIVs in some countries (the United States/Canada, EU, Australia/New Zealand) whereas it is professional societies (Korean Nutrition Society) in some others. In addition to the preceding expert groups, other joint collaborations of governments or professional societies set NIVs, such as the Nordic Council of Ministers for Nordic Countries and the nutrition societies of Germany, Austria, and Switzerland (known as D-A-CH—constructed from the initial letters of the country identifications for Germany [D], Austria [A] and Switzerland [CH]). The expert groups also differ in the extent to which the NIV development process is transparent, reproducible, and objective. Some expert groups use systematic evidence-based reviews to support the development of their NIVs in order to promote a transparent and rigorous process for reviewing the relevant data and to facilitate the update of these values as new evidence becomes available.[24,25] However, some modifications to the systematic review process are required for this purpose.[26]

Scientific and technical challenges in applying systematic reviews to the development of NIVs include defining and prioritizing the key research questions, the quality of available studies, and finding biomarkers or intermediate (surrogate) outcomes that can be used when there is a dearth of studies directly linking nutrient intakes to clinical or functional outcomes. There are also logistic challenges in procuring sufficient staffing, time, and economic resources to conduct such systematic reviews on each of the key research questions. Nevertheless, using vitamin A as an example, a modified systematic review process was judged to promise a greater degree of transparency and objectivity in setting NIVs than not using it.[27]

The most recent IOM review of vitamin D and calcium incorporated a systematic evidence-based review in the process of updating these DRIs.[28] An independent panel of technical experts helped informatics experts prioritize and select key questions and outcomes of interest; methods for using existing systematic reviews were refined for determining requirement-related questions; and quality assessment tools and methods for translating results from studies not designed to address the issues of interest were developed and applied.[29] A similar process of defining in advance questions to be addressed by systematic reviews prior to a panel of experts reviewing the results was also used in developing more recent recommendations updating dietary intakes for sodium and potassium.[8]

Methods for using NIVs in assessing nutrient intakes and for planning vary from one expert group to another. Since there is considerable variability in the nutrient intakes of similar individuals under similar circumstances that must be taken into account in dietary assessment and in planning, these procedures also require the application of statistics to adjust food consumption surveys to estimate usual intakes. These methods are briefly described[30] and more extensively in volumes from the IOM devoted to dietary assessment[20] and planning.[31] The methods have been applied to setting intakes to decrease chronic disease risk, make recommendations for meals in child care programs, and devise guidance for developing food packages for pregnant and lactating mothers, infants, and children in several recent reports.[19,32,33]

III. CURRENT STATUS OF THE FIELD

A. Dietary Reference Intakes Developed for the United States and Canada

The DRIs used in the United States and Canada are published in several volumes[3,34–39] and are described in detail elsewhere. Various types of DRIs have been established for energy, 8 macronutrients and their key components, 11 vitamins, and 17 minerals, of which 2 have Tolerable Upper Intake Levels (UL) only. The key types of DRIs are described as follows.

Estimated Average Requirement

The Estimated Average Requirement (EAR) is the amount of a nutrient that meets the requirement for a specific criterion of adequacy for half of the individuals in a population of a given age and sex or life stage. This is an average or median value since the amount of the nutrient needed to achieve adequacy varies from one individual to the next. Because nutrient requirements are usually distributed normally or can be transformed mathematically to achieve a normal distribution, this is a useful summary number. EARs have been established for protein, carbohydrate, and several vitamins and minerals.

For most of these nutrients, there are many different functional criteria that might be chosen for setting the requirement, and therefore it is important to justify the choice of a given criterion. For example, the criteria for vitamin A that could be used as a basis to evaluate adequacy included the presence of xerophthalmia, night blindness, or an amount above a cutoff for plasma retinol–binding protein levels. Because the EAR is a median requirement for a group, and because the variation around the median is considerable, the EAR is not useful for estimating the nutrient adequacy of an *individual*'s intake. At the EAR level of intake, half of the individuals in a group are expected to be below their requirement and half are above it. An individual whose usual intake is below the EAR has a risk of inadequacy between 50% and 100%.

In contrast, by using the EAR, it is possible to assess the prevalence of inadequacy in population groups with a statistical technique known as the probability approach, a derivation of which is commonly referred to as the EAR cutpoint method.[20] Simply stated, the cutpoint method provides an indication of the prevalence of inadequate intakes in a population by the proportion of the population with nutrient intakes below the EAR. Dietary advice to the general public should attempt to promote distributions of intakes by individuals in which as many individuals as possible have usual intakes that are above the EAR and below the UL. For this reason, the Recommended Dietary Allowance (RDA) level of intake is used for most recommendations to the public.

Recommended Dietary Allowance

The RDA is the average daily dietary intake level that is expected to meet the nutrient requirements of nearly all (e.g., 97%–98%) healthy persons of a specific age and sex or life stage. In order to calculate the RDA from the EAR, it is assumed that the requirement distribution is normal or can be transformed to normalcy, and that the amount of the nutrient needed to cover virtually everyone in the population is defined statistically for 97%–98% coverage as 2 SDs above the EAR. When no SD is available, the coefficient of variation is used. It is usually assumed to be 10% (or 1.2 times the EAR) or, on occasion, as 15% (1.3 times the EAR) on the basis of existing nutrient requirement data. If an individual has an intake that is less than the RDA but more than the EAR, his risk of inadequacy would be between 2% and 3% and 50%. As intakes fall further below the RDA, the risk rises but not the certainty of inadequacy. Thus, the RDA is the nutrient intake goal for *planning* the diets of individuals. However, it is not appropriate for *assessing* the diet of an individual since there are many whose intakes are below the RDA but who may still be getting enough of the nutrient to be above their own nutrient requirement level. Because the RDA is set at a level that exceeds the actual needs of all but about 2%–3% of a population group, it is also overly generous as a standard for evaluating adequacy of group intakes and should not be used for that purpose. The EAR is the appropriate nutrient value to determine the adequacy of the average intake of the group. For example, a recent US publication compared subgroup intakes to the EAR.[40]

Adequate Intake

When the EAR for a nutrient is not known for the particular functional criterion that is most relevant, it is not possible to apply statistical theory and derive an RDA. However, often there is enough information to make some quantitative recommendations about adequate and healthful nutrient intake levels. Under such circumstances, an AI is set as a tentative goal or target for the nutrient intake of individuals until more information is available. Since knowledge is limited, and depending on the data used to establish the AI, it is unknown whether the estimate is generous, sufficient, or possibly even inadequate. The definitions and derivation of an AI vary somewhat, but it is often the average or median intake of a group of healthy people, all of whom are assumed to be meeting their nutrient needs. Therefore, falling short of an AI does not signify inadequacy since it is not based directly on a functional requirement. The most common use of AI is for young infants where it is based on estimates of human milk nutrient content and the mean intakes of groups of healthy infants. However, recommendations for water intake from food and beverages are also provided as AIs, based on maintaining serum osmolality and what is known about nutrient needs for water.[38] The DRIs also include an AI for dietary fiber, based on decreasing risk of cardiovascular disease,[3] along with a definition of dietary fiber.

TABLE 15.3 Selected NIVs for adults as a percent of energy (%E) unless otherwise stated.

Nutrient or dietary factor	FAO/WHO[13,41]	EFSA[15]	IOM[3]
Total fat	15%–30%	20%–35%	20%–35%
Saturated fatty acids	<10%	As low as possible	As low as possible
n-6 PUFAS	5%–8%	4% linoleic acid	5%–10% linoleic acid[a]
n-3 PUFAs	1%–2%	0.5% α-linolenic; 250 mg/day EPA + DHA	0.6%–1.2% α-linolenic acid[a]
Trans fatty acids	<1%	As low as possible	As low as possible
Carbohydrate	55%–75%	45%–60%	45%–65%
Dietary sugars	<10% free sugars	Under review	<25% added sugars
Protein	10%–15%	Not given as %E	10%–35%
Cholesterol	<300 mg/day	Not established	As low as possible

DHA, docosahexaenoic acid; *EPA*, eicosapentaenoic acid; *PUFAs*, polyunsaturated fatty acids.
[a]*Approximately 10% of this range can come from long-chain PUFAs.*

Estimated Energy Requirement

Small excesses in energy intake can, over time, result in weight gain. Also enough is known about energy output to enable exact calculations of energy output and intakes. The EAR and RDA do not apply to energy. Instead, energy needs are stated as average requirements for similar individuals. The Estimated Energy Requirement (EER) is calculated from equations derived from experimental data on the energy needs of individuals of normal weight with a healthy body mass index of between 18.5 and 25 for adults of a given age and sex, height, weight, and physical activity level (PAL).[3] The data are derived from a large international set of doubly labeled water data.

In determining an individual's EER, the person's PAL increases the basal energy requirement needed to maintain current body weight. The activity factors needed to estimate physical activity range from 1.2 for Sedentary (little to no exercise + work a desk job), to 1.375 Lightly Active (light exercise 1–3 days/week), to 1.55 Moderately Active (moderate exercise 3–5 days/week), and 1.725 Very Active (heavy exercise 6–7 days/week). Separate equations to maintain body weight were also developed for overweight and obese individuals.[3]

Acceptable Macronutrient Distribution Range

The AMDR is a range of acceptable macronutrient distributions for individuals, usually presented as a percent of total energy intake. Ranges are provided for protein, fat (and n-3 and n-6 fatty acids), and carbohydrates.[3] The AMDR is not experimentally derived but based largely on epidemiological data. The values are estimates that are thought to minimize the potential for chronic disease such as diabetes and cardiovascular disease over the long term, while also allowing for adequate levels of essential nutrients and energy to be consumed. See Table 15.3 for the IOM AMDRs for adults for protein, total carbohydrate, and total fat.[3] Protein also has a separate EAR and RDA based on nitrogen balance studies, as well as an amino acid scoring pattern to evaluate protein quality.[3]

For dietary cholesterol, *trans* fatty acids (TFAs), and saturated fatty acids, intakes as low as possible while consuming a nutritionally adequate diet are recommended.[3] Although not a UL, the recommendation for added sugars was to limit them to no more than 25% of energy intake in order to ensure sufficient intake of some essential vitamins and minerals.[3] However, since the data originally used to model that limit are now over two decades old, it is likely to be appropriate only for very active individuals. For most Americans who are much more sedentary, their energy needs are so low that, after following dietary patterns recommended by the latest edition of the Dietary Guidelines for Americans 2015–20,[42] the percent of kilocalories from added sugars would have to be far lower than 25% to stay in energy balance. The American Heart Association has urged stricter upper limits based on their reviews of the evidence associating dietary sugars and cardiovascular health and suggested a limit closer to 13% of energy intake from added sugars.[43] Values for selected adult AMDRs are shown in Table 15.3.

Chronic Disease Risk Reduction Intake

The recent evaluation by NASEM of DRIs (NIVs) for sodium and potassium concluded that a new NIV, the CDRR intake, was also necessary.[8] The sodium CDRR was defined as the lowest level of intake for which there was sufficient strength of evidence to characterize a CDRR. For adults, the CDRR recommendation is to reduce sodium intakes above 2300 mg/day. The AI for sodium, which was established for nonchronic disease relationships, continues to be 1500 mg/day for adults.[38] For potassium, values for adults were not established for a CDRR, but AIs for adult women and men are 2400 mg/day and 2500 mg/day, respectively,[8] a decrease from the AI of 4700 mg/day established in 2004 based on chronic disease relationships.[38] If population recommendations are to be made for NIVs for CDRR more generally, methods for establishing the levels of nutrient intakes to recommend for populations will also need to be developed and refined.

Tolerable Upper Intake Level

Intakes far in excess of the RDA may also give rise to health problems. A relatively recent innovation in Dietary Reference Values (DRVs) is the tolerable or safe upper intake level (UL) for a nutrient. The UL is the highest level of chronic nutrient intake that is likely to pose no risk of adverse effects on health to almost everyone in the population. As chronic intake levels rise above the UL, adverse effects may increase.[44] The functional criterion or adverse effect used as a basis for setting the UL is observed at a level usually at least a magnitude or greater than the RDA or AI.

A risk assessment model is applied to available data of the intake levels at which the adverse effect occurred or at lower levels at which no adverse effect was noted.[44] Unfortunately, so few data reporting adverse effects are available at present that ULs cannot be set for a number of nutrients. However, lack of a UL does not mean that the risk of adverse effects does not exist from higher intakes. Although the magnitude of the uncertainty factor applied to the available data takes into account the seriousness of the adverse effect when setting the UL, the severity or seriousness of the adverse events associated with exceeding the UL may vary from one nutrient to another. Finally, from a technical standpoint, unlike the EAR, the UL cannot be manipulated statistically and thus is limited to serving as a reference value when providing guidance for consumers.

An online interactive tool that provides current DRIs for Canada and the United States is available at http://ods.od.nih.gov/health_information/dietary_reference_intakes.aspx.

B. Dietary Reference Values Developed for the European Union

Until recently, several countries in the EU had set their own NIVs, which made assessments of dietary adequacy and planning between European countries confusing and difficult. EFSA is now responsible for setting NIVs, referred to as DRVs. In 2005, the European Commission requested EFSA to review and update the previous 1993 DRVs for nutrient and energy intakes established by EFSA's predecessor—the Scientific Committee on Food (SCF). In 2006, EFSA published a report describing the adverse health effects of high vitamin and mineral intakes and establishing UL for seven vitamins and nine minerals. This report also contained ULs previously determined by SCF.[16]

In 2010, EFSA published its opinion on the principles for deriving and applying the DRVs.[5] The agency subsequently published individual scientific opinions on energy, protein, carbohydrates, dietary fiber, fat and its components, and water (2009–12); on 14 vitamins and 13 minerals (2013–17); and on sodium and chloride (2019). This process also updated the ULs for a few nutrients and population groups.[15]

The European DRVs are derived using a similar range of concepts as the DRIs for the United States and Canada as shown in Tables 15.1 and 15.2. The major difference is the use of the Population Reference Intake (PRI) in place of RDA and the reference intake range for macronutrients (RI) instead of the AMDR. Since nutrient requirements vary among individuals, the distribution of nutrient intakes to meet these requirements is given for half the people in a population group as the AR and for nearly all (97.5%) in a population group as the PRI. When individual requirements can be assumed to be normally distributed in a population, the PRI is calculated as the AR plus twice its SD. However since the SD for a particular nutrient is rarely known, a default is then used. In the absence of sufficient scientific evidence and data to determine an AR for a nutrient, an AI similar to its DRI counterpart or an RI may be established as appropriate.

EFSA's scientific opinions for each nutrient are published online and brought together in a virtual issue of the EFSA journal.[15] EFSA completed its development and review work in 2019 with final publications of opinions on sodium and chloride for which a composite term was adopted—safe and adequate intake.

An online interactive tool is available at https://www.efsa.europa.eu/en/topics/topic/dietary-reference-values.

Given the current interest in dietary sugars, EFSA agreed in 2017 to a request from five member states to update its previous 2010 scientific opinion on DRVs for carbohydrates and dietary fiber.[15] EFSA had previously found insufficient data on which to establish a UL for total or added sugars. In its new work, EFSA will consider whether a UL can be established for total or added or free sugars as defined below:

- Total sugars: the monosaccharides glucose, fructose, and galactose and the disaccharides sucrose, lactose, maltose, and trehalose present in foods;
- Added sugars: sugars used as ingredients in processed and prepared foods and sugars eaten separately or added to foods at the table; and

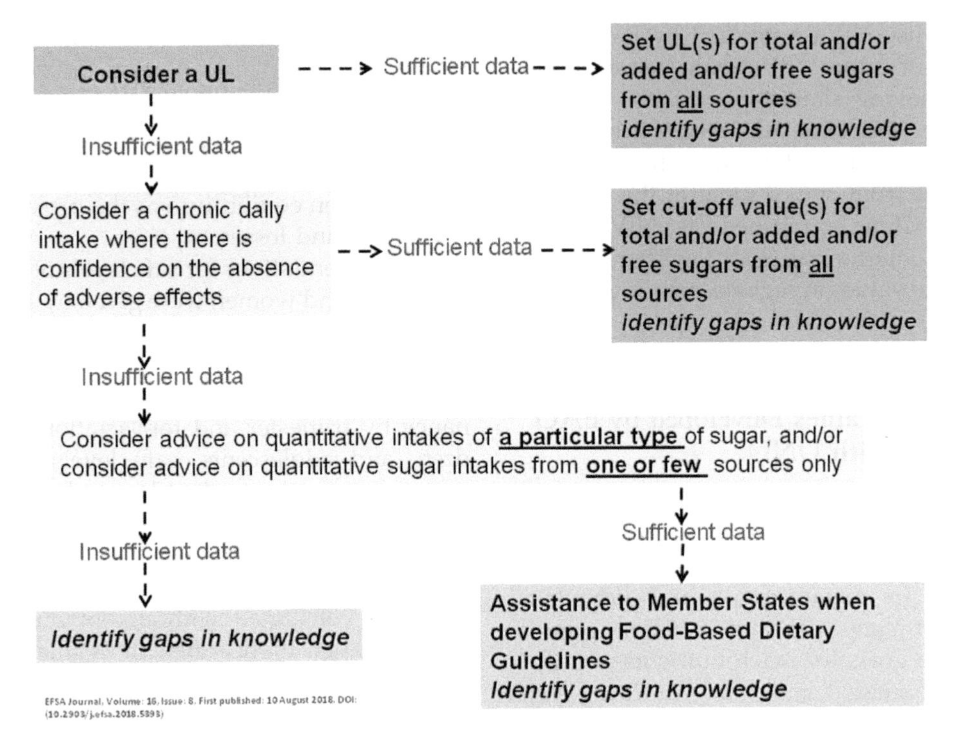

FIGURE 15.2 Stepwise process to provide scientific advice on total/added/free sugars. *From Protocol for the scientific opinion on the Tolerable Upper Intake Level of dietary sugars [Ref. 45]. [© 2018 European Food Safety Authority.* EFSA Journal *published by John Wiley and Sons Ltd on behalf of European Food Safety Authority. This is an open access article under the terms of the Creative Commons Attribution-NoDerivs License, which permits use and distribution in any medium, provided the original work is properly cited and no modifications or adaptations are made.].*

- Free sugars: added sugars plus sugars naturally present in honey, syrups, fruit juices, and fruit juice concentrates.

The protocol to guide the sugars assessment was published in 2018[45] and the updated scientific opinion is planned for completion in 2021. Fig. 15.2 shows the stepwise process intended to be followed.

C. Nutrient Reference Values Developed for Australia and New Zealand

Australia and New Zealand jointly publish NIVs called Nutrient Reference Values (NRVs), which are derived in a manner similar to that given for the United States. and Canada.[4] As a result, many NRVs given as EARs and RDIs (instead of RDA above) have the same or similar values as for the United States and Canada. However, this is not the case for most AIs that are based on population nutrient intake. An interesting and helpful feature of the Australia and New Zealand NRVs is the presentation of a summary of recommendations to reduce chronic disease risk based on expert reviews of the evidence. Suggested dietary targets (SDT) for those aged 14 years and over, based mostly on 90th percentile nutrient intakes in Australia and New Zealand, are provided for vitamins A, C, E, folate, sodium, potassium, dietary fiber, and long-chain n-3 fatty acids. AMDRs designed to reduce chronic disease risk while also ensuring adequate nutrient intakes are given for protein, carbohydrate, fat, linoleic acid, and α-linolenic acid.

In 2017, the recommendation SDT for sodium to reduce chronic disease risk was reviewed in the light of the convincing relationship between sodium intake and blood pressure.[46] The new SDT recommendation was revised from 1600 mg/day[4] to 2000 mg/day based on a new methodological review framework. The highest average intake likely to pose no risk to the general population, i.e., the UL, was also revised from 2300 mg/day[4] to "not determined" because increased sodium intake was associated with increased blood pressure at all measured levels of intake within the analyzed range from 1200 to 3300 mg/day. The AI for sodium remains at 460–920 mg/day for adults to meet basic requirements and allow for AIs of other nutrients, but these levels may not apply to individuals who are highly active on a daily basis to cover sweat and insensible sodium losses.

D. Nutrient Intake Values Developed for Other Countries

The Scandinavian countries have published Nordic Nutrition Recommendations jointly for many years, most recently in 2012.[7] Many countries in the developing world use NIVs published by FAO/WHO (see next section) or adopt NIVs from nearby neighboring countries having similar populations and circumstances. Some countries have established their own NIVs, based in part on data from their countries and in part on data from one or more of the countries discussed above. China published its NIVs, called DRIs, in 2013, but only for national use. There are also efforts to harmonize values in regions such as Southeast Asia.[47]

E. Nutrient Intake Values Developed by FAO and WHO and With UNU

This section describes various jointly prepared or single monographs issued by United Nations agencies for international use. WHO/FAO expert consultations reviewed evidence for dietary intake and diet-related chronic disease over many years and in 2003 set population nutrient intake goals for macronutrients and their components (as % energy) and salt.[41] In 2012, WHO subsequently applied a new approach called WHO Guidelines (see next section) to the development of dietary intake recommendations to reduce the risk of diet-related chronic disease. WHO's previous arrangement of joint expert consultations with FAO and other international collaborators for such dietary recommendations then drew to a close.

Energy requirements (WHO-FAO-UNU)

Humans need energy for basal metabolism (resting energy expenditure), for the metabolic response to food, for varying levels of physical activity and growth, for pregnancy and lactation, and also for special circumstances such as energy expended with fever and shivering thermogenesis accompanying exposure to extreme cold.

A report from an expert consultation[48] Recommended Energy Requirements based on improved data for Total Energy Expenditure, defined as the energy spent on average in a 24-hour period by an individual or group. The report recommended that energy requirements for populations with lifestyles involving different levels of habitual physical activity should diverge from 6 years of age and be expressed as multiples of basal metabolism. PALs should be based on the degree of habitual activity consistent with long-term good health, the reduced risk of diseases associated with sedentary lifestyles, and the maintenance of a healthy body weight.

Protein and amino acids requirements (WHO-FAO-UNU)

A report from an expert consultation on protein requirements was released in 2007.[49] The determination of dietary requirements for protein and amino acids used nitrogen equilibrium as the proxy measure of protein intake and losses.

Recommendations for safe levels of protein intake for adult men and women were given by 10 kg body weight increments. Adult amino acid requirements were given in units of mg/kg body weight/day and mg/g protein. Safe levels of protein intake were also provided for pregnancy by trimester and for lactation. For infants, children, and adolescents, safe levels of protein intake were given both per kg/day and per reference body weight/day. A Tolerable Upper Limit (TUL) was not identified for protein, although the report concluded that, since intakes of three to four times the safe intake could be consumed without obvious harm, the TUL may be much higher than the value of twice the safe intake assumed in previous reports.

The 2007 report also revised the amino acid scoring pattern for adult maintenance and devised scoring patterns for infant and child age groups from the adult maintenance pattern and the amino acid pattern of tissue protein.

Dietary protein quality evaluation (FAO)

An important aspect in developing countries is protein quality. An expert consultation on protein quality evaluation in 2013[50] reviewed the previously recommended Protein Digestibility Corrected Amino Acid Score (PDCAAS) method for evaluating protein quality and recommended that PDCAAS be replaced with a new protein quality measure—Digestible Indispensable Amino Acid Score (DIAAS). The report also recommended that different reference protein amino acid scoring patterns be used in calculating DIAAS applicable to protein intended for different age groups; that amino acids be treated as individual nutrients in dietary protein evaluation; and, wherever possible, that data for digestible amino acids be given in food tables on an individual basis.

Two scoring patterns were recommended for regulatory purposes: the amino acid composition of human milk for infant formulas and a pattern for young children (6 months to 3 years) for all other foods and population groups. Recognizing that available data are insufficient to support the application of the new method in practice, the report called for more data on the true ileal amino acid digestibility of human foods.

Carbohydrates (FAO and WHO)

A scientific update of some of the key issues in the FAO 1998 report on carbohydrates in human nutrition[51] was released in 2007.[52] It provided an improved definition of dietary fiber, recommending that it be based on well-established health benefits and the ability to fulfill regulatory requirements. The experts went further and proposed that dietary fiber be defined as intrinsic plant cell wall polysaccharides and thus the methods of analysis should be such as to accommodate this definition. The scientific update also endorsed a previous recommendation[41] concerning the restriction of beverages high in free sugars and the limitation of total intake of free sugars to reduce the risk of overweight and obesity.

Fats and fatty acids (FAO)

The report of a 2008 joint FAO/WHO expert consultation on lipids[53] emphasized the role of certain fatty acid categories in maintenance of health. One example related to the convincing role of long-chain polyunsaturated fatty acids in neonatal and infant mental development as well as a beneficial role in the maintenance of long-term health and prevention of some chronic diseases. A high intake of saturated fatty acids and to an even greater extent TFAs was found to contribute substantially to adverse blood lipid changes and the development of the cardiovascular diseases that are now a main cause of adult death in developed and developing countries. The WHO Scientific Update on TFAs 54 contributed substantially to this finding of the report. The report also found no conclusive evidence supporting an association of TFAs from ruminant sources with coronary heart disease risk due to the amounts usually consumed.

Vitamins and minerals (FAO and WHO)

The last report of a joint FAO/WHO expert consultation on vitamin and mineral requirements held in 1998 was published in two editions.[10,55] The report contained NIVs for 13 vitamins and 6 minerals including multiple NIVs for iron and zinc based on differing levels of bioavailability according to different local dietary patterns. These NIVs were based on the available scientific evidence and provided values for RNIs (similar to RDAs), although difficulties in data interpretation resulted in some issues remaining unresolved. Average requirements were discussed only in the text, and some values based on dietary intakes were classified as RNIs. Subsequently, a framework for establishing upper levels of intake of nutrients and related substances[17] using an internationally applicable approach (or "model") for a scientifically sound process of nutrient risk assessment was developed.

F. WHO Guidelines

WHO has developed Guidelines on nutrient intake recommendations since 2012 in accordance with the WHO Handbook for Guideline Development.[56] WHO defines its Guidelines as "any document containing recommendations about health interventions whether they are clinical, public health or policy recommendations." WHO adopted the Grading of Recommendations Assessment, Development and Evaluation (GRADE) 57 approach to assess the quality of the evidence base and to develop and report recommendations. This approach aims to ensure that the Guidelines are free from bias, meet a public health need, and are consistent with established principles. The steps in the Guideline procedure are shown in Box 15.1.

BOX 15.1

WHO Guidelines Development[56]

The steps in the Guidelines procedure are

- identification of priority questions and outcomes
- retrieval of evidence
- assessment and synthesis of the evidence
- formulation of recommendations
- identification of research gaps
- planning for dissemination, implementation, impact evaluation, and updating of the guideline.

Recommendations are classified either as strong or conditional. A *strong* recommendation indicates confidence that the desirable effects of adherence outweigh the undesirable consequences and means that it can be adopted as policy in most situations. A *conditional* recommendation indicates less certainty about the balance of benefits and harms or disadvantages so that policy debate and stakeholder consultation should first be undertaken.

WHO Guidelines for sodium intakes for adults and children

Guidelines for sodium and potassium were both based on a review of the evidence related to the health effects of several described changes in sodium or potassium intake, including intakes below or above certain thresholds.[11,12] The Guidelines concluded that reducing sodium intake significantly reduced systolic and diastolic blood pressure in adults and children. An increase in potassium intake was found to result in the same outcomes. WHO thus made a *strong* recommendation to reduce blood pressure to decrease the risk of cardiovascular disease, stroke, and coronary heart disease in adults by reducing sodium intake to less than 5g salt (2g sodium)/day. WHO similarly *strongly* recommended increasing potassium intake from food to at least 90 mmol/day (3510 mg/day) to achieve the same health outcomes. Another *strong* recommendation was made to prevent adverse changes in blood pressure in children by adjusting the adult sodium Guideline amount downwards based on relative energy requirements. However, for potassium, only a *conditional* recommendation was made for children to increase intake for the same reasons and in the same manner.

WHO Guidelines for sugar intake for adults and children

The sugars Guideline[13] reviewed the evidence relating to the health effects, including dental caries and changes in body weight, of several described changes in intake of free sugars, both qualitative directional changes and intakes below two thresholds. The Guidelines made a *strong* recommendation to reduce free sugars intake throughout the life course to less than 10% of total energy intake based on moderate quality evidence from observational studies of a relationship between free sugars and dental caries. A second *conditional* recommendation was made to further reduce free sugars intake to less than 5% of total energy for all groups to minimize the lifelong risk of dental caries based on very low evidence from ecological studies.

G. Examples of International Variation

Tables 15.3 and 15.4 present examples of the numeric variation in NIVs from current international, regional, and binational sources. Some of this variation may reflect the needs of different populations or dietary patterns or other local factors. Other aspects of the variation may be due to maturity of the evidence base at the time the recommendations were made.

Another practical difference among sets of NIVs is the age range classifications. For example, in its most recent publications, WHO set adult age ranges of 19–65 years for males and 19–50 and 51–65 years for females, whereas IOM set an adult age range for each sex of 19–30, 31–50, and 51–70 years, and EFSA set ≥18 years for most nutrient with the balance of nutrients in two age groups 18–24 and ≥ 25 years or other divisions as appropriate for males and females.

TABLE 15.4 Selected NIVs representing protein, vitamin, and mineral requirements of nearly all 19 years old males.

Nutrient	FAO/WHO (RNI)[10]	EFSA (PRI)[15]	IOM (RDA)[3,33–36,38]
Vitamin A	600 μg (RE)	750 μg (RE)	900 μg (RAE)
Vitamin C	45 mg	110 mg	90 mg
Vitamin E	10 mg α-TE	13 mg α-toc	15 mg α-toc
Folate	400 μg (DFE)	330 μg (DFE)	400 μg (DFE)
Calcium	1000 mg	1000 mg	1000 mg
Iron	9.1–27.4[a] mg	11 mg	8 mg
Magnesium	260 mg	350 mg	400 mg
Selenium	34 μg	70 μg	55 μg
Zinc	4.2–14[b] mg	9.4 mg	11 mg

DFEs, dietary folate equivalents; *RAEs*, retinol activity equivalents; *RE*, retinol equivalents.; *α-TE*, alpha-tocopherol equivalents; *α-Toc*, alpha-tocopherol.
[a]*Range includes values for four bioavailabilities.*
[b]*Range includes values for three bioavailabilities.*

H. Food Labeling: Use of Nutrient Reference Values and Daily Values

Many countries and the Codex Alimentarius[14] have derived NRVs for food labeling purposes from either their own or various sets of NIVs. NRVs are listed in food standards to enable food manufacturers to declare the nutrient content of their food as a percent of the relevant NRVs. This label information then allows consumers to interpret the nutrient content of a food portion in terms of its contribution to a healthy nutrient intake.

Because foods are generally available to the population at large and food labels have limited space, and since there are multiple NIVs for a single nutrient according to age and sex, a process is used to derive one NRV that represents the requirements of most of the population. A common approach is to use NIVs for adults—either males only or the average of males and females. If NIVs are given for narrow age ranges within adulthood, the NRV may be a composite of more than one age range. Adult NIVs are usually selected to represent the population at large since NIVs for children aged over 4 years are usually within 80% of the adult value.

Codex Alimentarius, an international foods standards-setting body under the auspices of FAO and WHO, has established guidelines on nutrition labeling for use internationally.[14] These guidelines provide for nutrient amounts declared on food labels to be expressed in metric units such as milligrams and/or as a percent of the NRV. Codex has recently reviewed and extended the list of NRVs in its nutrition labeling guidelines. In so doing, Codex established two types of NRVs—NRV-R (requirement) for protein, 13 vitamins, and 10 minerals and NRV-NCD (noncommunicable diseases) for saturated fat, sodium, and potassium. Codex derived relevant NRVs-R from the $INL_{97.5}$ rather than the average requirement; NRVs were also derived from AIs when $INL_{97.5}$ values were unavailable or unsuitable. The three NRVs-NCD[58,59] were respectively based on recommendations for saturated fat from WHO[41] and FAO[53] based on an energy intake of 2000 kcal (~8.4 MJ) and the WHO guidelines on sodium[11] and on potassium.[12]

The many years of work by the Codex Committee on Nutrition and Foods for Special Dietary Uses to update the Codex NRVs-R for the general population was documented by FAO and WHO in a report about Codex's role in nutrition labeling that included a detailed record of the most recent update of the NRVs-R.[60] Codex is now developing NRVs-R for older infants and for young children for use on foods for the special dietary use of those two age groups.

In the United States and Canada, DRIs have been the basis for the Daily Value (DV), a percent of which is displayed on food labels. Since newer DRIs are now available, they have been used to update the DVs on food labels.[61] Prior to the update, many DVs were based on the 1968 RDAs of the United States, while in Canada, the label values were based on the Canadian RNIs. In the United States, there was debate about whether the RDA or the EAR should be used in food labeling,[62,63] with the adult RDA or AI chosen as the basis of the 2016 revision of the DVs for the United States.

IV. ISSUES SPECIFICALLY RELATED TO NUTRIENT INTAKE VALUES

A. Need for Further Harmonization of NIVs

Evidence-based NIVs are very expensive to develop and therefore there is good reason to harmonize the process globally whenever possible.

Terminology

In the 10 years since the 2007 proposal to internationally harmonize terminology and approaches,[1] advances have been made to adopt the recommended terminology in Codex nutrition labeling guidelines[14] but not at the national or regional level. In 2017, international agencies and the US government[64,65] explored the evidence for achieving global harmonization of methodological approaches to establishing NIVs which built on the prior work. The reasons identified for a lack of further harmonization include those set out in Box 15.2.

In looking forward to the concept of a possible global consultative group on NIVs, a recent meeting concluded that FAO/WHO could convene a reference group to serve as a resource for countries.[64] Special data needs of particular regions or countries were recognized in setting their own NIVs that related to food composition, dietary surveys, bioavailability, and health status. All participants agreed there was still a clear need to fill knowledge gaps and improve the science on which to derive NIVs.[64]

BOX 15.2

Reasons for Lack of Further Harmonization[64,65]

The reasons include

- reluctance to accept global harmonization or lack of access to information on harmonization
- confusing terminology
- lack of resources—not just funding but also scientific interest and political acceptability (e.g., because of trade implications)
- lack of data in some countries or populations
- lack of openness, or sharing, of data, technology, and results because of legal or political constraints
- lack of clarification around uncertainties of recommended values
- difficult decisions about inclusion versus exclusion of evidence when setting recommendations
- different endpoints or criteria chosen among countries and regions
- differences in the updating of recommendations
- difficulties in bringing existing methodologies together from different regions or countries.

A major challenge today is that the ANR (EAR) and UNLs (UL) for some nutrients are not comparable between countries. The variations reflect different studies reviewed, criteria for inclusion and exclusion, differences in interpretation of the evidence, rationales for selecting specific studies to support recommendations, and subjective judgments. NIVs such as the ANR are designed to describe human nutrient requirements and, with adjustments for factors as body size and environmental circumstances, they should be useful globally.[64] The UNLs (UL) also should be broadly applicable.

In order to encourage global harmonization, terminology should also be standardized. It is also important to refine the terminology and use of NIVs expressed as percent of energy, usually related to CDRR. These NIVs for a population are not the same as goals set for individuals because the target for the population depends on the distribution of intakes within the population. For example, if an NIV is set at <5% energy such as the WHO conditional guideline for sugars, the recommendation should state the proportion of the population to which the NIV applies, most likely either as a mean intake value or applicable to nearly all individuals. This fact is widely misunderstood in formulating guidelines and targets and needs to be addressed. NIVs should be used transparently when determining countries' food-based dietary recommendations.[33]

Processes and procedures for setting NIVs

Global harmonization should also involve the standardization of core processes and methods for determining many of the NIVs.[64] Procedures needing refinement for setting NIVs include the choice of data, the transparency of decisions, and scientific evaluation methods employed. Developing values for children include all of these issues as well coping with lack of data and its own unique set of problems.[65]

Use of systematic reviews and expert committees; This is exemplified by the process currently used by the IOM for the United States and Canada to set DRIs. Critical questions are posed, which are then addressed by systematic evidence-based reviews of the literature. The reviews are done by informatics experts who ensure the completeness of the search and who are assisted by content experts. The systematic reviews are then provided to an expert committee that reviews the data and other evidence and sets the final values. The process relies heavily on funders (usually the United States Government and Health Canada). Systematic reviews are expensive and time consuming, and yet, to improve the quality of the derivation of NIVs and guidelines, they must be funded by the public sector. Currently private funding is not considered to be acceptable. Further refinements needed in the DRI process have been summarized.[66]

Predefined analytical networks; predefined analytical frameworks are useful in clarifying systematic review questions. Fig. 15.3 illustrates one framework for considering them.

Dealing with values not amenable to harmonization

Some NIVs are less amenable to global harmonization than others. Factors involving culture, food composition, bioavailability, health status or economics, or other issues have a much greater influence on establishing values such as the AI, which is based more often on usual intakes rather than on a specific biological need, and the AMDR, which is based on epidemiological data gathered in specific countries.[67] Adoption of these values would likely not be appropriate outside of the country or region in which they were derived unless similar conditions applied elsewhere. Countries or regions may also have special needs related to the above factors that would affect the estimation and use of values such as the AI and AMDR in designing food assistance programs and other applications.

It is also important to clarify the influence on some nutrient requirements of diet and host-related factors that vary among countries. For example, habitual diets differ greatly from one country to another and affect the bioavailability of many micronutrients, including protein, calcium, magnesium, iron, zinc, folate, vitamin A, and carotenoids. Host-related factors may also vary from one country to another and affect bioavailability and thus nutrient requirements. They comprise intestinal factors (e.g., secretion of hydrochloric acid, gastric acid, or intrinsic factor; other alterations in the permeability of the intestinal mucosa) and systemic factors (host, age, sex, ethnicity, genotype, and life stages such as pregnancy and lactation, as well as chronic and acute infections). Such factors all may influence estimates of dietary requirements and may necessitate country-specific recommendations that take them into account.[68]

Recent developments toward international harmonization

Following recent publications[64,65] on global harmonization of methodological approaches for NIVs, researchers in the United States developed 26 ANRs (H-AR) for protein, vitamins, and minerals and 19 UNLs (H-ULs) for vitamins and minerals for all age-sex groups and life stages.[69] These values were compiled, as an interim measure, from either US/Canadian DRIs or European DRVs, with priority given to more recent values. Where both sources established only AIs for the

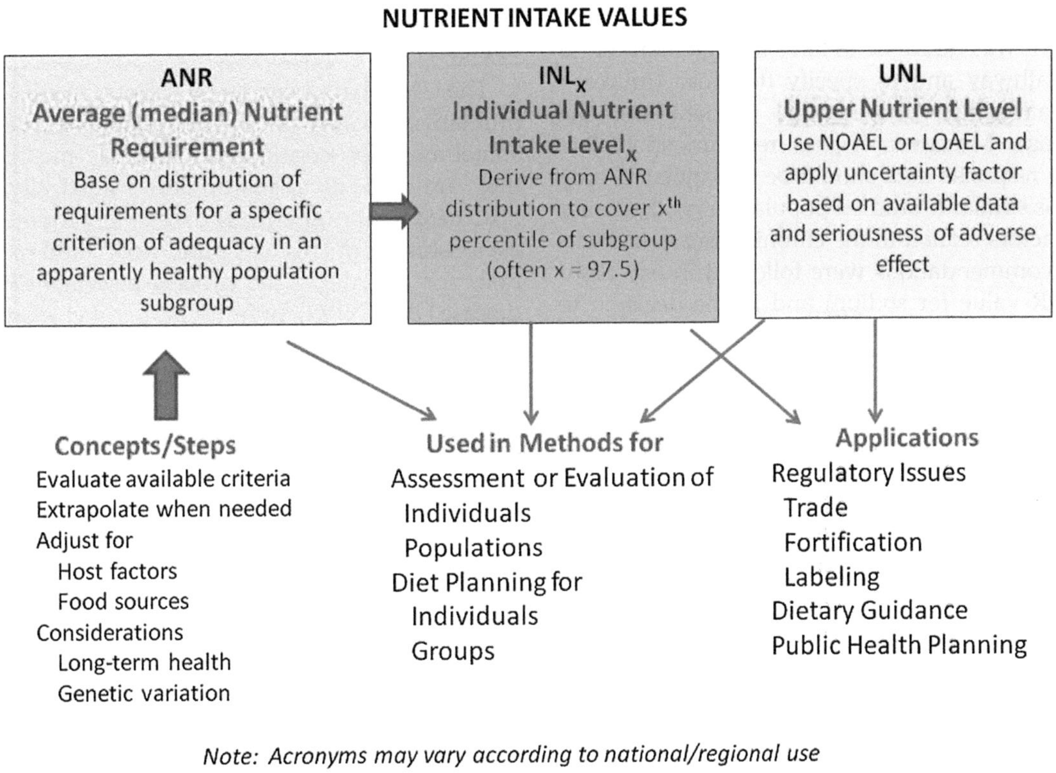

NUTRIENT INTAKE VALUES

ANR
Average (median) Nutrient Requirement
Base on distribution of requirements for a specific criterion of adequacy in an apparently healthy population subgroup

INL_x
Individual Nutrient Intake $Level_x$
Derive from ANR distribution to cover x^{th} percentile of subgroup (often x = 97.5)

UNL
Upper Nutrient Level
Use NOAEL or LOAEL and apply uncertainty factor based on available data and seriousness of adverse effect

Concepts/Steps
Evaluate available criteria
Extrapolate when needed
Adjust for
Host factors
Food sources
Considerations
Long-term health
Genetic variation

Used in Methods for
Assessment or Evaluation of
Individuals
Populations
Diet Planning for
Individuals
Groups

Applications
Regulatory Issues
Trade
Fortification
Labeling
Dietary Guidance
Public Health Planning

Note: Acronyms may vary according to national/regional use

FIGURE 15.3 Concepts, methods of using NIVs, and applications of ANRs, INL_x, and UNL. *Adapted from King and Garza, Food and Nutrition Bulletin, 28:S1-12, 2007.*

same nutrient, H-ARs were calculated assuming a CV of 12.5%. i.e., H-AR = AI/1.25. The authors indicated the lower certainty of these values by italicizing the results and noted the prevalence of inadequacy may be overestimated when such values are used. The harmonized NIVs are particularly intended for international or regional agencies undertaking population nutrient intake assessments in global or regional contexts.

B. NIVs for Chronic Disease Risk Reduction

NIVs for chronic disease are not warranted unless sufficient evidence exists. There is great interest in using chronic disease endpoints as functional criteria for setting such NIVs, but there are so many data gaps that it has not proven possible to do so for any micronutrients, including calcium.[23] The US/Canada AMDRs were set using chronic disease endpoints derived from epidemiological data; they were not based on experimentally determined data. Thus, the standards of evidence for setting the AMDRs were far less rigorous than those used for estimating micronutrient needs.

Causal inference is more difficult with chronic disease endpoints for several reasons. First, most of the data comes from observational studies rather than randomized clinical trials. Second, chronic diseases are multifactorial in their causation. Third, not everyone in the population is at risk for some chronic diseases, while all humans have requirements for the same nutrients. Also, it is unlikely that a threshold exists at which there is zero risk for chronic disease, and intake (dose)–response relationships may be different from those characterizing nutrient requirements. For example, the issues of overlapping recommendations are complex, where optimal intake levels for minimizing risk of one chronic disease may differ from those for another disease or where optimal intake levels that are beneficial for one population subgroup may be harmful for other subpopulations (see Ref. 19, Chapter 7 and Ref. 64 for in-depth discussions of these issues).

The 2017 NASEM report[19] also recommended that analytically validated surrogate markers could be considered instead of outcomes if they were on the causal pathway for disease pathogenesis, were significantly associated with the chronic disease of interest in the target population, and were changed by a nutritional intervention in which a substantial proportion of the change was attributed to that intervention. If all these criteria were met, then findings from surrogate markers could be used as supporting information for results based on the chronic disease in question. A GRADE score of at least moderate certainty would constitute an acceptable level of confidence that the nutrient–disease relationship was causal.[57] It was desirable to have a single marker on the causal pathway and to specify the dose (intake)–response relationships between the nutrient and the chronic disease. Moreover, it was recommended that dose (intake) response data should be extrapolated only to populations similar to studied populations with similar underlying factors related to the chronic disease of interest. These recommendations were followed in establishing the CDRR value for sodium and in the decision to not establish a CDRR value for potassium.[8]

C. NIV Data Gaps

Available data at all life stages

Gaps in requirement data are quite large for some ages and life stages, especially for very young infants, older infants, young children, and the very old, and these must be filled for use in program plans and policy development. When data are lacking, extrapolation and interpolation must be used, introducing uncertainty. Although the needs for further research are usually mentioned in committee recommendations, once reports are issued, the research agenda tends to be neglected. When the time comes to update recommendations, the relevant research may still not be available. Dose–response data rarely exist for these and other age and sex or life stage groups. There is little coordination between countries in developing a research plan to fill the gaps in data that exist. Efforts now being made to synthesize research needs in a systematic way, and to call the attention of researchers to them, should help to move the process forward in the future.[70]

Reference values for special subgroups

Some subgroups within the population such as those with certain diseases or single or multiple gene defects causing inborn errors of nutrient metabolism have special nutrient needs. A framework for developing nutrient recommendations for them is also needed.[71]

Recommendations for nonnutrient bioactive food components

There are many constituents in food that are typically not classified as nutrients but may have beneficial biological effects. Aside from dietary fiber, consumption recommendations for them are lacking. There is a need to develop standards for evaluating safe levels of consumption and potential efficacy. A conceptual framework for developing recommendations for dietary bioactive components in food such as polyphenolics is needed.

Risk assessment methods to support UNL reference values

The UNLs have been set by various groups on the basis of relatively scanty data, with functional criteria that are sometimes not considered clinically meaningful, and they are difficult to manipulate statistically. A WHO/FAO model for nutrient risk assessment for more rigorous establishment of ULs was published,[17] and recommendations for improving the process of establishing chronic disease DRIs (NIVs) for nutrients or other food substances (NOFSs) have been made.[19] Based on the NASEM 2017 report that recommended that ULs be only established based on nonchronic disease endpoints,[19] no ULs were established for either sodium or potassium.[8]

Updates of NIVs

Meaningful triggers for revising and updating NIVs should be adopted to determine when a new review should be conducted. Until recently, countries have usually updated their set of NIVs in one review. This is expensive, time consuming, and means that only a few experts can be engaged to deal with each nutrient. Recently, selective updating has become popular. It is triggered when indicators show that a substantial amount of new data regarding requirements exists, which may lead to improved values. Selective updating also permits greater focus on nutrients of public health significance at a given time. Focusing on only a few nutrients makes it possible to have more expertise on targeted nutrients on scientific advisory committees and may permit the preparation of systematic evidence-based reviews that would be too costly to do for many nutrients simultaneously. Given the costs involved, transparent processes for selecting the nutrients to be evaluated are needed.

Linking personalized nutrition and functional criteria using new genetic findings

The idea of establishing nutrient recommendations based on an individual's nutrient needs as generated by profiling the different single-nucleotide polymorphisms (SNPs) involved in nutrient metabolism has been proposed for minimizing DNA damage and to maximize genomic and ultimately human health, and guidelines have been proposed to evaluate their validity.[72] Also of interest is whether SNPs that create metabolic inefficiencies are distributed by race and ethnicity so that certain large populations are differentially affected. If so, needs for certain nutrients and NIVs for specific population groups might be quite different. While it may be possible to know if this is the case in the future, at present there is little consensus on the nutrient needs and chronic disease–related implications of various SNPs.

D. Appropriateness of Applications in Dietary Assessment and Planning

Over the past decade, techniques for estimating usual intakes and using NIVs for assessment and planning have become available.[73] They have been put to use in many studies of dietary adequacy in the United States, Canada, and elsewhere. Because the methods are relatively new, those who apply them need to be wary of pitfalls that can occur in assessing individuals and groups.[30,74,75] It is important that editorial boards of scientific journals refine their publication standards to insist that appropriate statistical analytic methods be used for dietary assessment and planning. The quality of surveys used for assessing nutrient adequacy varies, which may affect the results obtained.[76] One problem is in determining whether the NIV is flawed in its criterion of adequacy or if a true deficiency exists in a portion of the population. For example, in the United States, the diets of most adults (72% of men and 85% of women > 18 years of age) were inadequate in vitamin E according to 2013–16 intake data from the *What We Eat in America, National Health and Nutrition Examination Survey*[40] and yet no known adverse clinical or functional effect seems to be present. Such findings should trigger additional study of the data used to develop reference standards to determine whether or not adjustments need to be made.

E. Risk–Benefit Assessments

The assessment of the public health burden of nutritional recommendations may include a risk–benefit assessment to determine the risk of inadequacy of low intakes using the ANR and the risks of adverse effects at high intakes using the UNL for the same nutrient. This is particularly important for regulators when assessing the potential impact of food fortification on the extent to which nutrient inadequacy may be improved while also not increasing excess nutrient intakes for the different population age-sex groups.

F. Status of Efforts to Improve NIVs

In conclusion, progress in harmonizing NIVs worldwide has been considerable over the past few decades, and it needs to continue. In the future, it will be helpful to encourage more consultation and collaboration internationally among the various relevant bodies. The goal should be to improve objectivity and transparency and address the many variations in NIVs that are not grounded in real biological differences, but in differences in interpretation, methodology, and terminology. One first step is to synthesize research needs on NIVs and to address them collaboratively, as recommended in an IOM workshop on DRI research needs.[70]

RESEARCH GAPS

- Gaps in data for requirements of young and older infants, young children, and the very old
- Gaps in data on dose–response for NIVs for most sex/age/life stage groups
- Clinically meaningful functional criteria for setting ULs and better statistical methods for establishing the ULs
- Functional criteria for chronic disease NIVs
- Framework for NIVs for specific population groups and subgroups with certain diseases or gene defects causing special nutrient needs including derived from SNP information
- NIVs for bioactive food constituents other than nutrients
- Improved risk–benefit assessments

V. REFERENCES

1. King JC, Garza C. Harmonization of nutrient intake values. *Food Nutr Bull*. 2007;28(28):3S–12S.
2. Food and Agriculture Organization and World Health Organization. *Review of Existing Daily Vitamin and Mineral Intake Reference Values*. Paper CX/NFSDU 11/33/4. Germany: Codex Committee on Nutrition and Foods for Special Dietary Uses; 2011.
3. Institute of Medicine. *Dietary Reference Intakes for Energy, Carbohydrate, Fiber, Fat, Fatty Acids, Cholesterol, Proteins and Amino Acids*. Washington, DC: The National Academies Press; 2002/2005. Available from: http://www.nationalacademies.org/hmd/Reports/2002/Dietary-Reference-Intakes-for-Energy-Carbohydrate-Fiber-Fat-Fatty-Acids-Cholesterol-Protein-and-Amino-Acids.aspx. Accessed October 8, 2019.
4. National Health and Medical Research Council and New Zealand Ministry of Health. *Nutrient Reference Values for Australia and New Zealand Including Recommended Dietary Intakes*; 2006. Available from: https://www.nrv.gov.au/home. Accessed July 14, 2019.
5. European Food Safety Authority. *Scientific Opinion on Principles for Deriving and Applying Dietary Reference Values*. 2010. doi:10.2903/j.efsa.2010.1458. Accessed 8 October 2019.
6. King JC, Vorster HH, Tome DG. Nutrient intake values (NIVs): a recommended terminology and framework for the derivation of values. *Food Nutr Bull*. 2007;28:16S–26S.
7. Nordic Council of Ministers. *Nordic Nutrition Recommendations 2012*; 2012. Available from: https://www.norden.org/en/publication/nordic-nutrition-recommendations-2012. Accessed July 14, 2019.

8. National Academies of Sciences, Engineering, and Medicine. *Dietary Reference Intakes for Sodium and Potassium*. Washington, DC: The National Academies Press; 2019. https://doi.org/10.17226/25353. Accessed October 8, 2019.
9. Committee on Medical Aspects of Food Policy. *Dietary Reference Values for Food Energy and Nutrients for the United Kingdom*; 1991. Available from: https://assets.publishing.service.gov.uk/government/uploads/system/uploads/attachment_data/file/743786/Dietary_Reference_Values_for_Food_Energy_and_Nutrients_for_the_United_Kingdom__1991_.pdf. Accessed October 8, 2019.
10. World Health Organization. *Human Vitamin and Mineral Requirements: Report of a Joint FAO/WHO Expert Consultation*. 2nd ed.; 2004. Available from: https://apps.who.int/iris/bitstream/handle/10665/42716/9241546123.pdf;jsessionid=F67D91E97880DCD6F4D89A8BAF448BC5?sequence=1. Accessed July 14, 2019.
11. World Health Organization. *Guideline: Sodium Intake for Adults and Children*; 2012. Available from: https://www.who.int/nutrition/publications/guidelines/sodium_intake/en/. Accessed July 14, 2019.
12. World Health Organization. *Guideline: Potassium Intake for Adults and Children*; 2012. Available from: https://www.who.int/nutrition/publications/guidelines/potassium_intake/en/. Accessed July 14, 2019.
13. World Health Organization. *Guideline: Sugars Intake for Adults and Children*; 2015. Available from: https://www.who.int/nutrition/publications/guidelines/sugars_intake/en/. Accessed October 8, 2019.
14. Codex Alimentarius Commission. *Guidelines on Nutrition Labelling*; 2017. CAC/GL 2-1985. Revised 2017. Available from: http://www.fao.org/fao-who-codexalimentarius/sh-proxy/en/?lnk=1&url=https%253A%252F%252Fworkspace.fao.org%252Fsites%252Fcodex%252FStandards%252FCXG%2B2-1985%252FCXG_002e.pdf. Accessed July 14, 2019.
15. European Food Safety Authority. *Dietary Reference Values for Nutrients*; 2017. Available from: https://efsa.onlinelibrary.wiley.com/doi/toc/10.1002/(ISSN)1831-4732.021217. Accessed October 8, 2019.
16. European Food Safety Authority. *Tolerable Upper Intake Levels for Vitamins and Minerals*; 2006. Available from: https://www.efsa.europa.eu/sites/default/files/efsa_rep/blobserver_assets/ndatolerableuil.pdf. Accessed October 8, 2019.
17. World Health Organization. *A Model for Establishing Upper Levels of Intake for Nutrients and Related Substances: Report of a Joint FAO/WHO Technical Workshop on Food Nutrient Risk Assessment*; 2006. Available from: https://www.who.int/ipcs/highlights/full_report.pdf. Accessed July 14, 2019.
18. Yetley EA, MacFarlane AJ, Greene-Firestone LS, et al. Options for basing Dietary Reference Intakes (DRIs) on chronic disease endpoints: report from a joint US/Canadian sponsored working group. *Am J Clin Nutr*. 2017;105(1):249S–285S.
19. National Academies of Sciences, Engineering, and Medicine. *Guiding Principles for Developing Dietary Reference Intakes Based on Chronic Disease*. Washington, DC: The National Academies Press; 2017. doi: 10.17226/24828. Accessed 8 October 2019.
20. Institute of Medicine. *Dietary Reference Intakes: Applications in Dietary Assessment*. Washington, DC: National Academy Press; 2000. Available from: http://nationalacademies.org/hmd/Reports/2000/Dietary-Reference-Intakes-Applications-in-Dietary-Assessment.aspx. Accessed October 8, 2019.
21. Rand WM. The probability approach to nutrient requirements. *Food Nutr Bull*. 1990;12:1–8.
22. Yates AA. Using criteria to establish nutrient intake values (NIVs). *Food Nutr Bull*. 2007;28:38S–50S.
23. Trumbo PR. Challenges with using chronic disease endpoints in setting dietary reference intakes. *Nutr Rev*. 2008;66:459–464.
24. Russell RM. Current framework for DRI development: what are the pros and cons? *Nutr Rev*. 2008;66:455–458.
25. Thuraisingam S, Riddell L, Cook K, et al. The politics of developing reference standards for nutrient intakes: the case of Australia and New Zealand. *Publ Health Nutr*. 2009;12:1531–1539.
26. Lichtenstein AH, Yetley EA, Lau J. Application of systematic review methodology to the field of nutrition. *J Nutr*. 2008;138:2297–2306.
27. Russell R, Chung M, Balk EM, et al. Opportunities and challenges in conducting systematic reviews to support the development of nutrient reference values: vitamin A as an example. *Am J Clin Nutr*. 2009;89:728–733.
28. Chung M, Balk EM, Brendel MEA, et al. *Vitamin D and Calcium: A Systematic Review of Health Outcomes*. Evidence Report No. 183, AHRQ publication no. 09-E105; 2009. Available from: https://www.ahrq.gov/downloads/pub/evidence/pdf/vitadcal/vitadcal.pdf. Accessed July 14, 2019.
29. Chung M, Balk EM, Ip S, et al. Systematic review to support the development of nutrient reference intake values: challenges and solutions. *Am J Clin Nutr*. 2010;92:273–276.
30. Murphy SP, Vorster HH. Methods for using nutrient intake values (NIVs) to assess or plan nutrient intakes. *Food Nutr Bull*. 2007;28:51S–60S.
31. Institute of Medicine. *Dietary Reference Intakes: Applications in Dietary Planning*. Washington, DC: The National Academies Press; 2003. Available from: http://www.nationalacademies.org/hmd/Reports/2003/Dietary-Reference-Intakes-Applications-in-Dietary-Planning.aspx. Accessed October 8, 2019.
32. Institute of Medicine. Research methods to assess dietary intake and program participation in child day care. In: *Applications to the Child and Adult Care Food Programs: Workshop Summary*. Washington, DC: The National Academies Press; 2012. https://doi.org/10.17226/13411. Accessed October 8, 2019.
33. National Academies of Sciences, Engineering, and Medicine. *Review of WIC Food Packages: Improving Balance and Choice: Final Report*. Washington, DC: The National Academies Press; 2017. https://doi.org/10.17226/23655. Accessed October 8, 2019.
34. Institute of Medicine. *Dietary Reference Intakes for Calcium, Phosphorous, Magnesium, Vitamin D, and Fluoride*. Washington, DC: National Academy Press; 1997. Available from: http://nationalacademies.org/hmd/reports/1997/dietary-reference-intakes-for-calcium-phosphorus-magnesium-vitamin-d-and-fluoride.aspx. Accessed October 8, 2019.
35. Institute of Medicine. *Dietary Reference Intakes for Thiamin, Riboflavin, Niacin, Vitamin-B6, Folate, Vitamin-B12, Pantothenic Acid, Biotin, and Choline*. Washington, DC: National Academy Press; 1998. Available from: http://nationalacademies.org/hmd/Reports/2000/Dietary-Reference-Intakes-for-Thiamin-Riboflavin-Niacin-Vitamin-B6-Folate-Vitamin-B12-Pantothenic-Acid-Biotin-and-Choline.aspx. Accessed October 8, 2019.
36. Institute of Medicine. *Dietary Reference Intakes for Vitamin C, Vitamin E, Selenium, and Carotenoids*. Washington, DC: National Academy Press; 2000. Available from: http://nationalacademies.org/hmd/Reports/2000/Dietary-Reference-Intakes-for-Vitamin-C-Vitamin-E-Selenium-and-Carotenoids.aspx. Accessed October 8, 2019.
37. Institute of Medicine. *Dietary Reference Intakes for Vitamin A, Vitamin K, Arsenic, Boron, Chromium, Copper, Iodine, Iron, Manganese, Molybdenum, Nickel, Silicon, Vanadium, and Zinc*. Washington, DC: National Academy Press; 2001. Available from: http://nationalacademies.org/hmd/Reports/2001/Dietary-Reference-Intakes-for-Vitamin-A-Vitamin-K-Arsenic-Boron-Chromium-Copper-Iodine-Iron-Manganese-Molybdenum-Nickel-Silicon-Vanadium-and-Zinc.aspx. Accessed October 8, 2019.
38. Institute of Medicine. *Dietary Reference Intakes for Water, Potassium, Sodium, Chloride, And-Sulfate*. Washington, DC: The National Academies Press; 2005. Available from: http://nationalacademies.org/

hmd/Reports/2004/Dietary-Reference-Intakes-Water-Potassium-Sodium-Chloride-and-Sulfate.aspx. Accessed October 8, 2019.
39. Institute of Medicine. *Dietary Reference Intakes for Calcium and Vitamin D*. Washington, DC: The National Academies Press; 2011. Available from: http://nationalacademies.org/hmd/Reports/2010/Dietary-Reference-Intakes-for-Calcium-and-Vitamin-D.aspx. Accessed October 8, 2019.
40. USDA, Agricultural Research Service. *Usual Nutrient Intake from Food and Beverages, by Gender and Age, What We Eat in America*; 2019. NHANES 2013–2016. Available from: https://www.ars.usda.gov/northeast-area/beltsville-md-bhnrc/beltsville-human-nutrition-research-center/food-surveys-research-group/docs/wweia-usual-intake-data-tables/. Accessed October 8, 2019.
41. World Health Organization. *Diet, Nutrition and the Prevention of Chronic Diseases: Report of a Joint WHO/FAO Expert Consultation*. WHO Technical Report Series No. 916; 2003. Available from: https://www.who.int/dietphysicalactivity/publications/trs916/en/. Accessed October 8, 2019.
42. U.S. Department of Health and Human Services and U.S. Department of Agriculture. *2015 – 2020 Dietary Guidelines for Americans*. 8th ed.; 2015. Available from: https://health.gov/dietaryguidelines/2015/guidelines/. Accessed July 20, 2019.
43. Johnson RK, Appel LJ, Brands M, et al. Dietary sugars intake and cardiovascular health: a scientific statement from the American Heart Association. *Circulation*. 2009;120:1011–1020.
44. Institute of Medicine. *Dietary Reference Intakes: A Risk Assessment Model for Establishing Upper Intake Levels for Nutrients*. Washington, DC: National Academy Press; 1998. Available from: http://www.nationalacademies.org/hmd/Reports/1998/Dietary-Reference-Intakes-A-Risk-Assessment-Model-for-Establishing-Upper-Intake-Levels-for-Nutrients.aspx. Accessed October 8, 2019.
45. European Food Safety Authority. *Protocol for the scientific opinion on the Tolerable Upper Intake Level of dietary sugars*; 2018. Available from: https://efsa.onlinelibrary.wiley.com/doi/10.2903/j.efsa.2018.5393. Accessed October 8, 2019.
46. National Health and Medical Research Council and New Zealand Ministry of Health. *Nutrient Reference Values for Australia and New Zealand: Sodium*; 2017. Available from: https://www.nrv.gov.au/nutrients/sodium. Accessed July 14, 2019.
47. Barba CV, Cabrera MI. Recommended dietary allowances harmonization in Southeast Asia. *Asia Pac J Clin Nutr*. 2008;17(Suppl 2): 405–408.
48. Food and Agriculture Organization. *Human Energy Requirements: Report of a Joint FAO/WHO/UNU Expert Consultation*; 2004. FAO Food and Nutrition Technical Report Series No. 1. Available from: https://www.who.int/nutrition/publications/nutrientrequirements/9251052123/en/. Accessed October 8, 2019.
49. World Health Organization. *Protein and Amino Acid Requirements in Human Nutrition: Report of a Joint FAO/WHO/UNU Expert Consultation*; 2007. WHO Technical Report Series No. 935. Available from: https://www.who.int/nutrition/publications/nutrientrequirements/WHO_TRS_935/en/. Accessed October 8, 2019.
50. Food and Agriculture Organization. *Dietary Protein Quality Evaluation in Human Nutrition. Report of an FAO Expert Consultation*; 2013. FAO Food and Nutrition Paper 92. Available from: http://www.fao.org/publications/card/en/c/ab5c9fca-dd15-58e0-93a8-d71e028c8282. Accessed October 8, 2019.
51. Food and Agriculture Organization. *Carbohydrates in Human Nutrition: Report of a Joint FAO/WHO Expert Consultation*. Rome: Food and Agriculture Organization; 1998. FAO Food and Nutrition Paper 66. Available from: http://www.fao.org/docrep/W8079E/W8079E00.htm. Accessed October 8, 2019.
52. Nishida C, Martinez Nocito F, Mann J. Joint FAO/WHO scientific update on carbohydrates in human nutrition. *Eur J Clin Nutr*. 2007; 61(Suppl 1):1S–137S.
53. Food and Agriculture Organization. *Fats and Fatty Acids in Human Nutrition: Report of a Joint FAO/WHO Expert Consultation*; 2010. FAO Food and Nutrition Paper 91. Available from: http://www.fao.org/publications/card/en/c/8c1967eb-69a8-5e62-9371-9c18214e6fce. Accessed October 8, 2019.
54. Nishida C, Uauy R. WHO scientific update on trans fatty acids (TFA). *Eur J Clin Nutr*. 2009;63(Suppl 2):1S–75S.
55. Food and Agriculture Organization. *Human Vitamin and Mineral Requirements: Report of a Joint FAO/WHO Expert Consultation*; 2002. Available from: http://www.fao.org/publications/card/en/c/ceec621b-1396-57bb-8b35-48a60d7faaed. Accessed October 8, 2019.
56. World Health Organization. *WHO Handbook for Guideline Development*. 2nd ed.; 2014. Available from: https://apps.who.int/iris/handle/10665/145714. Accessed July 14, 2019.
57. Welcome to the GRADE Working Group. *From Evidence to Recommendations – Transparent and Sensible*. Available from: http://www.gradeworkinggroup.org/. Accessed 8 October 2019.
58. Codex Committee on Nutrition and Foods for Special Dietary Uses (CCNFSDU). 2012. Report of the 34th Session, REP 13/NFSDU, Paragraph 65.
59. Codex Committee on Nutrition and Foods for Special Dietary Uses (CCNFSDU). 2014. Report of the 36th Session, REP 15/NFSDU, Paragraph 116.
60. Lewis J. *Codex Nutrient Reference Values*; 2019. Available from: http://www.fao.org/documents/card/en/c/ca6969en. Accessed December 18, 2019.
61. Food and Drug Administration. Food Labeling: Revision of the Nutrition and Supplement Facts Labels, May 27, 2016; RIN:0910-AF22; CFR:21 CFR Part 101 Federal Register Number:2016-11867; FDA Docket-2012-N-1210.
62. Institute of Medicine. *Dietary Reference Intakes: Guiding Principles for Nutrition Labeling and Fortification*. Washington, DC: The National Academies Press; 2003. Available from: http://nationalacademies.org/hmd/Reports/2003/Dietary-Reference-Intakes-Guiding-Principles-for-Nutrition-Labeling-and-Fortification.aspx. Accessed October 8, 2019.
63. Murphy SP, Barr SI, Yates AA. The Recommended Dietary Allowance (RDA) should not be abandoned: an individual is both an individual and a member of a group. *Nutr Rev*. 2006;64:313–315. Discussion 315–318.
64. National Academies of Sciences, Engineering, and Medicine. Global harmonization of methodological approaches to nutrient intake recommendations. In: *Proceedings of a Workshop*. Washington, DC: The National Academies Press; 2018. https://doi.org/10.17226/25023. Accessed October 8, 2019.
65. National Academies of Sciences, Engineering, and Medicine. *Harmonization of Approaches to Nutrient Reference Values: Applications to Young Children and Women of Reproductive Age*. Washington, DC: The National Academies Press; 2018. https://doi.org/10.17226/25148. Accessed October 8, 2019.
66. Institute of Medicine. *The Development of DRIs 1994–2004: Lessons Learned and New Challenges – Workshop Summary*. Washington, DC: The National Academies Press; 2008. https://doi.org/10.17226/12086. Accessed October 8, 2019.
67. National Research Council. *Improving Data to Analyze Food and Nutrition Policies*. Washington, DC: The National Academies Press; 2005. https://doi.org/10.17226/11428. Accessed October 8, 2019.
68. Gibson R. The role of diet- and host-related factors in nutrient bioavailability and thus in nutrient-based dietary requirement estimates. *Food Nutr Bull*. 2007;28:77S–100S.
69. Allen LH, Carriquiry AL, Murphy SP. Perspective: proposed harmonized nutrient reference values for populations. *Adv Nutr*. 2019. https://doi.org/10.1093/advances/nmz096, 00:1–15.
70. Suitor C, Meyers L. *Dietary Reference Intakes Research Synthesis, Workshop Summary*. Washington, DC: The National Academies

Press; 2007. https://doi.org/10.17226/11767. Accessed October 8, 2019.

71. National Academies of Sciences, Engineering, and Medicine. *Examining Special Nutritional Requirements in Disease States: Proceedings of a Workshop*. Washington, DC: The National Academies Press; 2018. https://doi.org/10.17226/25164. Accessed October 8, 2019.
72. Grimaldi KA, van Ommen B, Ordovas JM, et al. Proposed guidelines to evaluate scientific validity and evidence for genotype-based dietary advice. *Genes Nutr.* 2017;12:35. https://doi.org/10.1186/s12263-017-0584-0. Accessed October 8, 2019.
73. Barr SI. Applications of dietary reference intakes in dietary assessment and planning. *Appl Physiol Nutr Metabol.* 2006;31:66–73.
74. Murphy SP. Using DRIs for dietary assessment. *Asia Pac J Clin Nutr.* 2008;17(Suppl 1):299S–301S.
75. Murphy SP, Guenther PM, Kretsch MJ. Using the dietary reference intakes to assess intakes of groups: pitfalls to avoid. *J Am Diet Assoc.* 2006;106:1550–1553.
76. Garcia-Alvarez A, Blanquer M, Ribas-Barba L, et al. How does the quality of surveys for nutrient intake adequacy assessment compare across Europe? A scoring system to rate the quality of data in such surveys. *Br J Nutr.* 2009;101(Suppl 2):51S–63S.

CHAPTER

16

NUTRITION IN LABELING

Elizabeth J. Campbell[1], *BSc*
James E. Hoadley[1], *PhD*
Robert C. Post[2], *PhD, MEd, MSc*
[1]EAS Consulting Group, Alexandria, VA, United States
[2]FoodTrition Solutions, LLC, Hackettstown, NJ, United States

SUMMARY

This chapter primarily addresses nutrition-related labeling policies in the United States of America (USA) and provides a limited overview of international policies. The policies covered in this chapter include mandatory and optional nutrition label information in specified formats and optional nutrition-related label claims. Nutrition labeling is required in the USA for most food products, and most of the policy detail provided in the chapter is for conventional foods in the USA. Dietary supplements are discussed in Volume I, Chapter 35. Since in the USA they are a regulatory subset of foods, this chapter also briefly addresses US nutrition labeling requirements for dietary supplements.

Keywords: Dietary guidelines; DRVs; DV; FDS; FSIS; Nutrition; Nutrition facts label; Nutrition-related claims; RDIs.

I. REQUIREMENTS FOR NUTRITION LABELING IN THE USA

A. Introduction

Both the Food and Drug Administration (FDA), in the Department of Health and Human Services (HHS), and the US Department of Agriculture's (USDA) Food Safety and Inspection Service (FSIS) are public health regulatory agencies that assure that foods under their respective jurisdictions are safe, wholesome, and accurately labeled. FDA-regulated products, which include cereal/grain, fruit, vegetable, dairy, seafood, and other food categories, and products made of these, account for about 20 cents of every dollar spent by US consumers and about 75% of the US food supply.[1] FSIS has jurisdiction over about 25% of the food supply, primarily meat, poultry, and processed egg products, and products made from these, and the inspection of catfish.

As part of their missions, both the FDA and FSIS regulate food labeling, including nutrition labeling, and more or less have identical requirements for declaring nutrition information. In some cases, such as with health claims and structure function claims, FSIS defers through policy to FDA regulations. Where there are minor differences between the two agencies' policies, FSIS generally accepts nutrition labeling that is consistent with FDA requirements. This chapter's focus is on requirements and provisions that apply to food products regulated by both agencies.

B. Basis for Nutrients Declared in Labeling

Dietary Guidelines for Americans recommendations

The *Dietary Guidelines for Americans* (DGA) is a Federal policy that guides policy makers, health professionals, and educators on recommendations to help all individuals ages 2 years and older consume a healthy, nutritionally adequate diet.[2] The DGA is updated and revised on a 5-year cycle. The information in the DGA is used in developing Federal food, nutrition, and health policies and programs and is the basis for nutrition education resources designed for the public and components of the HHS and USDA food programs. The goal of the DGA is that, if followed (along with

https://doi.org/10.1016/B978-0-12-818460-8.00016-2

physical activity), the recommendations will contribute to promoting health and helping to reduce risk of chronic illnesses related to diet. Thus, among the areas of scientific evidence that are evaluated to form the recommendations and the healthy eating patterns that embody the recommendations is the latest research on nutritionally adequate intakes of nutrients to promote health.

FDA and FSIS nutrition labeling regulatory requirements

The Nutrition Facts label, which is required on most packaged foods under both FDA and FSIS jurisdiction that are sold at retail, is a primary vehicle for implementing the Dietary Guidelines. The *Dietary Guidelines* consider, apply, and reinforce the Dietary Reference Intakes (DRIs). DRI is the general term for a set of nutrient-based reference values that are quantitative estimates of nutrient intakes to be used for planning and assessing diets for healthy people. DRIs expand on the periodic reports called Recommended Dietary Allowances (RDAs), which were first published by the Institute of Medicine in 1941 (now the National Academy of Medicine [NAM]). By assessing the latest eating habits and patterns among Americans, each edition of the Dietary Guidelines reprioritizes the current nutrients of concern. FDA's latest update to the Nutrition Facts label regulations, which FDA finalized in May 2016, considered the NAM's DRIs used to form the 2015–20 DGA nutrient intake recommendations and nutrients of concern in setting nutrition labeling requirements.[3]

Nutrients of concern are nutrients that are overconsumed or underconsumed in current US dietary patterns and are potentially a substantial public health concern, according to the Dietary Guidelines policy.[2] Data on nutrient intake, corroborated with biochemical markers of nutritional status where available, and association with health outcomes are all used to establish a nutrient as a nutrient of concern. Underconsumed nutrients, or "shortfall nutrients," are those with a high prevalence of inadequate intake either across the US population or in specific groups or segments of the population, relative to NAM-based standards, such as the Estimated Average Requirements or the Adequate Intake. Overconsumed nutrients are those with a high prevalence of excess intake either across the general population or in specific groups or segments, related to NAM-based standards such as the Tolerable Upper Intake Level or other expert group standards. The nutrients declared in Nutrition Facts on food labels and in food labeling are those identified in the Dietary Guidelines as nutrients of concern. Thus, food label Nutrition Facts is an important tool to help consumers make informed food and beverage choices that reflect the recommendations to consume more of the beneficial and less of the negative nutrients of concern.

In addition to the mandatory nutrients declared in the Nutrition Facts label that relate to nutrients of public health concern, other nutrients may be voluntarily declared on labels and in labeling, provided they adhere to FDA and USDA regulatory requirements.

Mandatory and voluntary (optional) nutrients in labeling

In May 2016, FDA published two final rules to update nutrition labeling requirements. "Food Labeling: Revision of the Nutrition and Supplement Facts Labels," established updated rules regarding the mandatory and voluntary declaration of nutrients. The second rule updated Reference Amounts Customarily Consumed (RACCs) and addressed other issues related to determining serving sizes for use in nutrition labeling. All labels applied to foods after January 1, 2021 must comply with these revised requirements.[3]

The FDA final rules amended various aspects of FDA labeling regulations for conventional foods (and dietary supplements) to provide updated nutrition information on the food label to assist consumers in maintaining healthy dietary practices, consistent with current DGA recommendations.[4,1] The updated information is consistent with current data on the associations between nutrients and chronic diseases, health-related conditions, physiological endpoints, and/or maintaining a healthy dietary pattern that impacts current diet-related public health conditions in the United States and corresponds to new information on consumer understanding and consumption patterns. Among several things, the final rules update the list of nutrients that are required or permitted to be declared and provide updated Daily Reference Values and Reference Daily Intake values that are based on current dietary recommendations from consensus reports.

The FDA final rules on the Nutrition Facts label stated that nutrition labeling information is to help consumers make more informed choices to consume a healthy diet and not intended for the clinical management of an

[1] US Federal regulations are compiled in the Code of Federal Regulations (CFR). The CFR is organized by numbered Titles; all FDA regulations are in Title 21 (i.e., 21 CFR). Each CFR Title is subdivided into numbered parts; the FDA regulations relevant to food labels are in "Part 101—Food Labeling" of Title 21 (i.e., 21 CFR 101). Each Part is divided into sections. Regulations pertaining to nutrition information on food labels are in Section 9 of Part 101 (i.e., 21 CFR 101.9).

existing disease. However, FDA said that it considered the large proportion of the US population that is at risk for chronic disease to be the primary target of the Nutrition Facts label's content and format. Simultaneously, FDA recognized in updating the rules on declaring nutrients that there is not room on the label for all information that may be related to maintaining healthy dietary practices and that space constraints on the label of most foods make it impractical to declare all essential nutrients. FDA noted that having a large amount of information on the label could interfere with consumers' abilities to use the information that has the greatest public health significance and that, given the amount and format of information that is required on the label, limits to the voluntary information on the label are necessary so that voluntary information does not clutter the label, does not mislead, confuse, or overwhelm the consumer, and does not take away prominence of and emphasis on the required, mandatory information.

Mandatory nutrients; The Nutrition Facts label—the standard vertical format display with mandatory nutrients—is shown in Fig. 16.1.[5] Mandatory macro and micronutrients are required on labels for the purpose described previously—to help consumers with informed decisions about the nutritional components of foods to achieve better and healthy eating patterns that are consistent with dietary advice. Mandatory macronutrients include total fat, saturated fat, *trans* fat, cholesterol, total carbohydrate, dietary fiber, total sugars/added sugars, and protein. Mandatory micronutrients include sodium, vitamin D, calcium, iron, and potassium.

Nutrition Facts

8 servings per container

Serving size	**2/3 cup (55g)**
Amount per serving	
Calories	**230**
	% Daily Value*
Total Fat 8g	**10%**
Saturated Fat 1g	**5%**
Trans Fat 0g	
Cholesterol 0mg	**0%**
Sodium 160mg	**7%**
Total Carbohydrate 37g	**13%**
Dietary Fiber 4g	**14%**
Total Sugars 12g	
Includes 10g Added Sugars	**20%**
Protein 3g	
Vit. D 2mcg 10% •	Calcium 260mg 20%
Iron 8mg 45% •	Potas. 240mg 6%

* The % Daily Value (DV) tells you how much a nutrient in a serving of food contributes to a daily diet. 2,000 calories a day is used for general nutrition advice.

FIGURE 16.1 Vertical display with micronutrients listed side-by-side.

Voluntary/optional nutrients; US regulations allow voluntary declaration of additional micronutrients within certain regulatory provisions. A Nutrition Facts standard vertical format display with voluntary nutrients is shown in Fig. 16.2.[6]

C. The Basis for Declaring Nutrients—Reference Values for Nutrient Intake Needs: Daily Reference Values and Reference Daily Intakes and the Consumer Friendly "Daily Values"

Daily Reference Values and Reference Daily Intakes

DRVs and RDIs relate to the nutrient needs of the general population 4 years old and above, with applications to certain nutrients and population segments. Both reference values are developed by the NAM, in consensus reports, as noted earlier. These values assist consumers in interpreting information about the amount of a nutrient that is present in a food and in comparing nutritional values of food products. The general population DRVs and RDIs are established for adults and children 4 or more years of age, and subpopulation reference values are established for infants through 12 months, children 1 through 3 years of age, and pregnant women and lactating women. DRVs are provided for total fat, saturated fat, cholesterol, total carbohydrate, dietary fiber, added sugar, sodium, and protein, and RDIs are for dietary essential vitamins and minerals. RDIs, nomenclature, and units of measure for nutrients established for the mandatory and voluntary vitamins and minerals that are essential in human nutrition are shown in Table 16.1[7]

DRVs, nomenclature, and units of measure are established for the food components shown in Table 16.2.[8]

Daily Value

The declaration of nutrient amounts in the Nutrition Facts—both mandatory and voluntary nutrients—must be expressed in the units of measurement shown in Tables 16.1 and 16.2 in the quantitative amount in a labeled serving of the food or beverage, as well as the percent of the Daily Value (DV) contributed.

FDA and FSIS nutrition labeling regulations have a goal of making Nutrition Facts easy for consumers to understand and use. To limit consumer confusion and avoid having to list both "%DRV" and "%RDI" on

Nutrition Facts	
17 servings per container	
Serving size	**3/4 cup (28g)**
Amount per serving	
Calories	**140**
	% Daily Value*
Total Fat 1.5g	**2%**
Saturated Fat 0g	**0%**
Trans Fat 0g	
Polyunsaturated Fat 0.5g	
Monounsaturated Fat 0.5g	
Cholesterol 0mg	**0%**
Sodium 160mg	**7%**
Fluoride 0mg	
Total Carbohydrate 22g	**8%**
Dietary Fiber 2g	**7%**
Soluble Fiber <1g	
Insoluble Fiber 1g	
Total Sugars 9g	
Includes 8g Added Sugars	**16%**
Protein 9g	**18%**
Vitamin D 2mcg (80 IU)	10%
Calcium 130mg	10%
Iron 4.5mg	25%
Potassium 110mg	2%
Vitamin A 90mcg	10%
Vitamin C 9mg	10%
Thiamin 0.3mg	25%
Riboflavin 0.3mg	25%
Niacin 4mg	25%
Vitamin B_6 0.4mg	25%
Folate 200mcg DFE (120mcg folic acid)	50%
Vitamin B_{12} 0.6mcg	25%
Phosphorus 100mg	8%
Magnesium 25mg	6%
Zinc 3mg	25%
Choline 60mg	10%
* The % Daily Value (DV) tells you how much a nutrient in a serving of food contributes to a daily diet. 2,000 calories a day is used for general nutrition advice.	
Calories per gram: Fat 9 • Carbohydrate 4 • Protein 4	

FIGURE 16.2 Vertical display including some voluntary nutrients.

food labels, the regulations use a single term, i.e., DV, for all nutrients. The "%DV" reflects the percentage of a particular nutrient in one serving of a product, based on the daily reference intake level (either DRV or RDI) for that specific nutrient. The %DV helps consumers understand how the amount of a nutrient that is present in a serving of a food fits into their total daily diet. Together with the actual amount of nutrients in a labeled serving, the %DV allows them to compare the nutritional value of food products to build healthy eating patterns consistent with the recommendations of the DGA.

D. Food Package Label Nutrition Information

A goal in devising the Nutrition Facts format was to strike a balance between including as much nutrition information on the label as possible and overwhelming consumers with too much information. Another goal was to ensure that there is uniformity of nutrition information among food labels in order to facilitate comparisons among different foods. To achieve these goals, FDA has compulsory regulations for the Nutrition Facts format that dictate a uniform appearance, content, size, and placement on the food label. Only material prescribed by the nutrition labeling regulations is permitted within the Nutrition Facts panel. The Nutrition Facts regulations are in 21 CFR 101.9.[9] Some of the major Nutrition Facts revisions in the 2016 update were

- Increase the prominence of calories
- Define dietary fiber for nutrition labeling purposes
- Include added sugars as a declared nutrient
- Revise which vitamins and minerals must be declared
- Revise DVs to reflect current recommended dietary levels
- Revise RACCs to reflect current consumption patterns

Nutrition Facts vertical format components

The standard appearance of the Nutrition Facts is as a vertical rectangular box, with the box enclosed in a hairline border. There are alternatives to the *vertical format* that can be used to accommodate a unique package shape or small size (e.g., *tabular* format and *linear* format) or to accommodate a food of minimal nutrient content (e.g., *simplified* format). The Nutrition Facts panel must be placed to the immediate right of the front of a food package (known as the principle display panel), when the package size allows. The information within the box is of a single dark color set on a white, or other neutral color, uniform background. Letters are to be of a single sans serif type style, with lower and upper case, and with bolding and type size as specified by regulation. There are five sections of the vertical format Nutrition Facts, each separated from the next by horizontal lines that are specified as a heavy bar (7-point rule), a medium bar (3-point rule), or hairline (1/4-point rule). The six sections are Heading, Serving size information, Caloric information, Macronutrients content, Vitamin and mineral content, and Footnotes.

TABLE 16.1 Mandatory and optional vitamins and minerals.

Nutrient	Unit of measure	RDI			
		Adults and children ≥4 years	Infants[a] through 12 months	Children 1 through 3 years	Pregnant women and lactating women
Vitamin A	Micrograms RAE[b] (mcg)	900	500	300	1,300
Vitamin C	Milligrams (mg)	90	50	15	120
Calcium	Milligrams (mg)	1,300	260	700	1,300
Iron	Milligrams (mg)	18	11	7	27
Vitamin D	Micrograms (mcg)[c]	20	10	15	15
Vitamin E	Milligrams (mg)[d]	15	5	6	19
Vitamin K	Micrograms (mcg)	120	2.5	30	90
Thiamin	Milligrams (mg)	1.2	0.3	0.5	1.4
Riboflavin	Milligrams (mg)	1.3	0.4	0.5	1.6
Niacin	Milligrams NE[e] (mg)	16	4	6	18
Vitamin B_6	Milligrams (mg)	1.7	0.3	0.5	2.0
Folate[f]	Micrograms DFE[g] (mcg)	400	80	150	600
Vitamin B_{12}	Micrograms (mcg)	2.4	0.5	0.9	2.8
Biotin	Micrograms (mcg)	30	6	8	35
Pantothenic acid	Milligrams (mg)	5	1.8	2	7
Phosphorus	Milligrams (mg)	1,250	275	460	1,250
Iodine	Micrograms (mcg)	150	130	90	290
Magnesium	Milligrams (mg)	420	75	80	400
Zinc	Milligrams (mg)	11	3	3	13
Selenium	Micrograms (mcg)	55	20	20	70

Continued

TABLE 16.1 Mandatory and optional vitamins and minerals.—cont'd

Nutrient	Unit of measure	RDI			
		Adults and children ≥4 years	Infants[a] through 12 months	Children 1 through 3 years	Pregnant women and lactating women
Copper	Milligrams (mg)	0.9	0.2	0.3	1.3
Manganese	Milligrams (mg)	2.3	0.6	1.2	2.6
Chromium	Micrograms (mcg)	35	5.5	11	45
Molybdenum	Micrograms (mcg)	45	3	17	50
Chloride	Milligrams (mg)	2,300	570	1,500	2,300
Potassium	Milligrams (mg)	4,700	700	3,000	5,100
Choline	Milligrams (mg)	550	150	200	550
Protein	Grams (g)	N/A	11	N/A	71[h]

[a]*RDIs are based on dietary reference intake recommendations for infants through 12 months of age.*
[b]*RAE = Retinol activity equivalents: 1 microgram RAE = 1 microgram retinol, 2 microgram supplemental β-carotene, 12 micrograms β -carotene, or 24 micrograms α-carotene or 24 micrograms β-cryptoxanthin.*
[c]*The amount of vitamin D may, but is not required to, be expressed in international units (IU), in addition to the mandatory declaration in mcg. Any declaration of the amount of vitamin D in IU must appear in parentheses after the declaration of the amount of vitamin D in mcg.*
[d]*1 mg α-tocopherol (label claim) = 1 mg α-tocopherol = 1 mg RRR-α-tocopherol = 2 mg* all rac-*α-tocopherol.*
[e]*NE = Niacin equivalents. 1 mg NE = 1 mg niacin = 60 milligrams tryptophan.*
[f]*"Folate" and "folic acid" must be used for purposes of declaration in the labeling of conventional foods and dietary supplements. The declaration for folate must be in mcg DFE (when expressed as a quantitative amount by weight in a conventional food or a dietary supplement) and percent DV based on folate in mcg DFE. Folate may be expressed as a percent DV in conventional foods. When folic acid is added or when a claim is made about the nutrient, folic acid must be declared in parentheses, as mcg of folic acid.*
[g]*DFE = Dietary folate equivalents; 1 DFE = 1 mcg naturally occurring folate = 0.6 mcg folic acid.*
[h]*Based on the reference caloric intake of 2000 calories for adults and children aged 4 years and older and for pregnant women and lactating women.*

TABLE 16.2 Mandatory nutrients.

		DRVs - Food Components			
Food Component	**Unit of measure**	**Adults and Children ≥ 4 years**	**Infants through 12 months**	**Children 1 through 3 years**	**Pregnant women and lactating women**
Fat	Grams (g)	78[a]	30	39[b]	78[a]
Saturated fat	Grams (g)	20[a]	N/A	10[b]	20[a]
Cholesterol	Milligrams (mg)	300	N/A	300	300
Total carbohydrates	Grams (g)	275[a]	95	150[b]	275[a]
Sodium	Milligrams (mg)	2,300	N/A	1,500	2,300
Dietary fiber	Grams (g)	28[a]	N/A	14[b]	28[a]
Protein	Grams (g)	50[a]	N/A	13[b]	N/A[c]
Added sugars	Grams (g)	50[a]	N/A	25[b]	50

[a] *Based on the reference caloric intake of 2000 calories for adults and children aged 4 years and older and for pregnant women and lactating women.*
[b] *Based on the reference caloric intake of 1000 calories for children 1 through 3 years of age.*
[c] *Protein DVs for these groups are in Table 16.1*

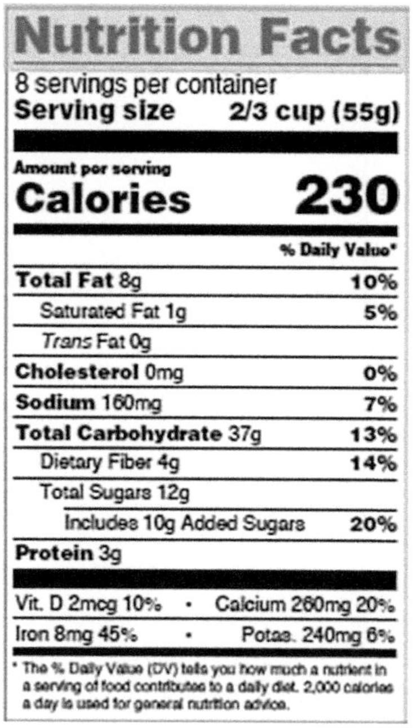

Nutrition Facts

8 servings per container
Serving size **2/3 cup (55g)**

Amount per serving
Calories **230**

	% Daily Value*
Total Fat 8g	**10%**
Saturated Fat 1g	**5%**
Trans Fat 0g	
Cholesterol 0mg	**0%**
Sodium 160mg	**7%**
Total Carbohydrate 37g	**13%**
Dietary Fiber 4g	**14%**
Total Sugars 12g	
Includes 10g Added Sugars	**20%**
Protein 3g	

Vit. D 2mcg 10% • Calcium 260mg 20%
Iron 8mg 45% • Potas. 240mg 6%

* The % Daily Value (DV) tells you how much a nutrient in a serving of food contributes to a daily diet. 2,000 calories a day is used for general nutrition advice.

FIGURE 16.3 Nutrition Facts—heading.

Nutrition Facts

8 servings per container
Serving size **2/3 cup (55g)**

Amount per serving
Calories **230**

	% Daily Value*
Total Fat 8g	**10%**
Saturated Fat 1g	**5%**
Trans Fat 0g	
Cholesterol 0mg	**0%**
Sodium 160mg	**7%**
Total Carbohydrate 37g	**13%**
Dietary Fiber 4g	**14%**
Total Sugars 12g	
Includes 10g Added Sugars	**20%**
Protein 3g	
Vitamin D 2mcg	10%
Calcium 260mg	20%
Iron 8mg	45%
Potassium 240mg	6%

* The % Daily Value (DV) tells you how much a nutrient in a serving of food contributes to a daily diet. 2,000 calories a day is used for general nutrition advice.

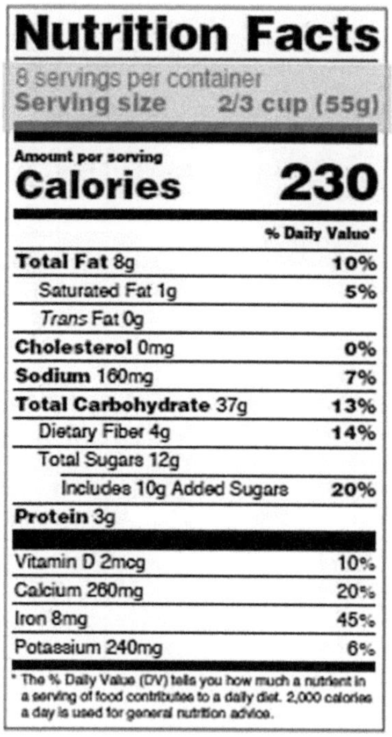

FIGURE 16.4 Nutrition Facts—serving information.

Heading; The Nutrition Facts heading is the top line within in the box as shown in Fig. 16.3.[5] The heading is bolded and set in a sufficiently large type size (at least 16-point) to extend the entire width of the box, where practical; it is the largest type size within the box. A horizontal hairline is placed below the heading. The "Heading" section is followed by the "Servings information" section.

Servings information; As shown in Fig. 16.4, the first line of the "Servings information" section states "__ servings per container" with nonbolded 10-point type.[8] The number of servings per container is to be rounded to a whole number; when rounded, it is preceded with "about." The second line states "serving size" and information describing the serving size with bold 10-point type. The "serving size" heading is left justified; the size information is right justified. The serving size is expressed as a "common household measure" (e.g., teaspoon, cup, slice, piece) followed parenthetically by the metric weight or volume of the serving. Metric values are expressed as whole values; except values less than 5 g (or mL) are rounded to the nearest 0.5 g (or mL), and values less than 2 are rounded to the nearest 0.1 g (or mL). Serving sizes are based on "reference amounts customarily consumed per eating occasion" (RACC or reference amount) that have been compiled by FDA in 21 CFR 101.12.[10] The purpose of the RACC-based serving sizes is to make serving sizes relatively uniform for similar foods across brands, which facilitates comparisons of nutrient content. A horizontal heavy bar is placed below the serving size information.

The number of "servings per container" is declared to the nearest whole number; when the number of servings falls between 2 and 5, it is declared to the nearest 0.5 serving. Rounding is indicated by the term "about" (i.e., about 4 servings per container). The number of "servings per container" for random weight foods (such as cheese) can be declared as "varied." The number of "servings per container" for a package container less than 200% of the applicable reference amount is declared as 1. The servings information is followed by the "Caloric information" section.

Caloric information; The "Caloric information" section begins with the subheading "Amount per serving" in bold 8-point type. Below this subheading is the word "Calories" in bold 16-point type. On the same line, and right justified, is placed the number of calories per serving in bold 22-point type. A horizontal "medium bar" is placed below the "Caloric information" section.

Caloric content per serving can be determined in a couple of ways; one way is use of actual caloric data; another way is to calculate caloric value with the general Atwater caloric factors of 4 calories/g of total carbohydrate and protein and 9 calories/g of fat. FDA also provides for adjusting carbohydrate-derived calories for carbohydrate substances known to have biologically available caloric content lower than 4 calories/g (see Table 16.3).[11] A caloric content of less than 5 calories/g is declared as 0; caloric content between 5 and 50 calories/g is rounded to the nearest 5 calorie increment; and caloric content above 50 calories/g is rounded to the nearest 10

TABLE 16.3 Carbohydrate-derived calories.

Available calories for specific carbohydrate substances
Isomalt 2.0 calories/g
Lactitol 2.0 calories/g
Xylitol 2.4 calories/g
Maltitol 2.1 calories/g
Sorbitol 2.6 calories/g
Hydrogenated starch hydrolyzates 3.0 calories/g
Mannitol 1.6 calories/g
Erythritol 0 calories/g
Soluble dietary fiber 2.0 calories/g
Insoluble dietary fiber 0 calories/g

Source: 21 CFR 101.9(c)(1)(i)(F).

calorie increment (See examples in Figs. 16.5–16.8). The "Caloric information" section is followed by the "Macronutrient content" section.[8]

Macronutrient content; The first line in the "Macronutrient content" section is a right justified "% Daily Value" subheading set in bold 8-point type.[8] Each line in the "Macronutrient content" section is separated from the next by a hairline. There are 10 macronutrients that are declared in this section of the Nutrition Facts (see Table 16.4).[12] The prescribed order for listing these 10 nutrients is the order in which they are listed in the table. These nutrients are declared with 8-point type. Five of these nutrients are the "core" nutrients (total fat, cholesterol, sodium, total carbohydrate, and protein). The core nutrients are differentiated from the other nutrients declared in the

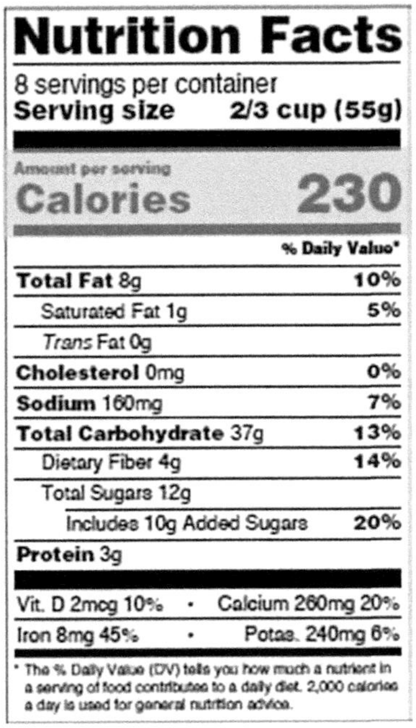

Nutrition Facts
8 servings per container
Serving size 2/3 cup (55g)
Amount per serving
Calories 230
% Daily Value*
Total Fat 8g 10%
Saturated Fat 1g 5%
Trans Fat 0g
Cholesterol 0mg 0%
Sodium 160mg 7%
Total Carbohydrate 37g 13%
Dietary Fiber 4g 14%
Total Sugars 12g
Includes 10g Added Sugars 20%
Protein 3g
Vit. D 2mcg 10% • Calcium 260mg 20%
Iron 8mg 45% • Potas. 240mg 6%
* The % Daily Value (DV) tells you how much a nutrient in a serving of food contributes to a daily diet. 2,000 calories a day is used for general nutrition advice.

FIGURE 16.5 Nutrition Facts—caloric information.

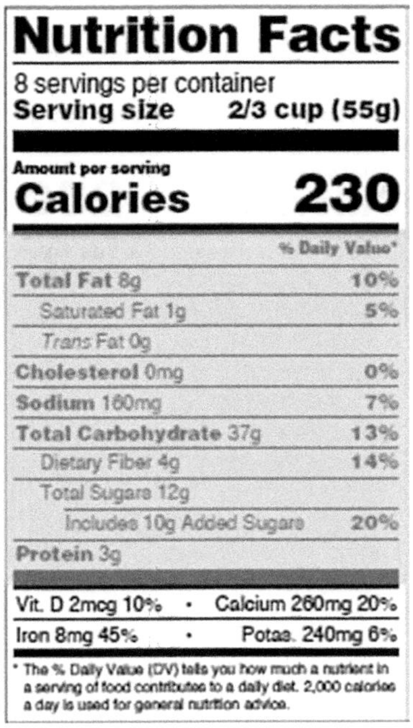

Nutrition Facts
8 servings per container
Serving size 2/3 cup (55g)
Amount per serving
Calories 230
% Daily Value*
Total Fat 8g 10%
Saturated Fat 1g 5%
Trans Fat 0g
Cholesterol 0mg 0%
Sodium 160mg 7%
Total Carbohydrate 37g 13%
Dietary Fiber 4g 14%
Total Sugars 12g
Includes 10g Added Sugars 20%
Protein 3g
Vit. D 2mcg 10% • Calcium 260mg 20%
Iron 8mg 45% • Potas. 240mg 6%
* The % Daily Value (DV) tells you how much a nutrient in a serving of food contributes to a daily diet. 2,000 calories a day is used for general nutrition advice.

FIGURE 16.6 Nutrition Facts—macronutrient content.

Nutrition Facts
8 servings per container
Serving size 2/3 cup (55g)
Amount per serving
Calories 230
% Daily Value*
Total Fat 8g 10%
Saturated Fat 1g 5%
Trans Fat 0g
Cholesterol 0mg 0%
Sodium 160mg 7%
Total Carbohydrate 37g 13%
Dietary Fiber 4g 14%
Total Sugars 12g
Includes 10g Added Sugars 20%
Protein 3g
Vit. D 2mcg 10% • Calcium 260mg 20%
Iron 8mg 45% • Potas. 240mg 6%
* The % Daily Value (DV) tells you how much a nutrient in a serving of food contributes to a daily diet. 2,000 calories a day is used for general nutrition advice.

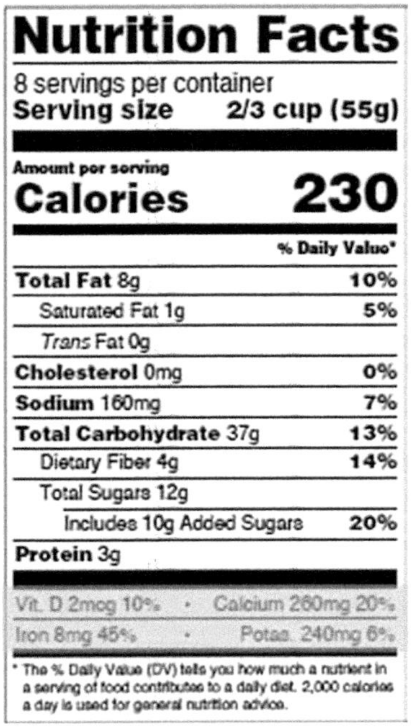

FIGURE 16.7 Nutrition Facts—vitamin and mineral content.

Nutrition Facts by being set in bold type and left justified. The macronutrients other than core nutrients are indented relative to the core nutrients. The weight (grams or milligrams) per serving amount is declared to the right of the nutrient name. The declared weight values are to be rounded using rounding rules for each nutrient as specified in 21 CFR 101.9(c).[9] The percentages of DV per serving are declared in a right

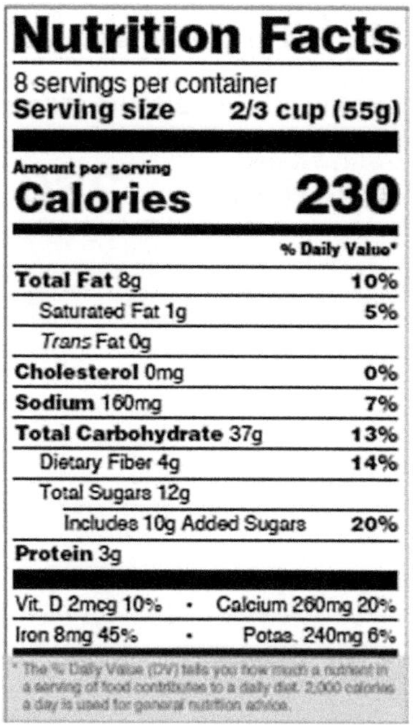

Nutrition Facts

8 servings per container
Serving size 2/3 cup (55g)

Amount per serving
Calories 230

	% Daily Value*
Total Fat 8g	**10%**
Saturated Fat 1g	**5%**
Trans Fat 0g	
Cholesterol 0mg	**0%**
Sodium 160mg	**7%**
Total Carbohydrate 37g	**13%**
Dietary Fiber 4g	**14%**
Total Sugars 12g	
Includes 10g Added Sugars	**20%**
Protein 3g	

Vit. D 2mcg 10% • Calcium 260mg 20%
Iron 8mg 45% • Potas. 240mg 6%

* The % Daily Value (DV) tells you how much a nutrient in a serving of food contributes to a daily diet. 2,000 calories a day is used for general nutrition advice.

FIGURE 16.8 Nutrition Facts—footnote.

TABLE 16.4 Mandatory declared macronutrients and their Daily Values (DVs) (adults and children >4).

Mandatory declared macronutrients and their DVs (adults and children > 4 years)
Total Fat 78 g
Saturated fat 20 g
Trans fat no DV
Cholesterol 300 mg
Sodium 2300 mg
Total carbohydrate 275 g
Dietary fiber 28 g
Total sugars no DV
Added sugars 50 g
Protein 50 g

Source: 21 CFR 101.9(c).

justified column beneath the "% Daily Value" subheading that is at the top of this section. %DV values for the macronutrients are rounded to the nearest whole percent. The %DV is left blank for the two nutrients that have no DV (*trans* fat and total sugars) and for protein. A protein %DV must be declared when there is any information about protein appearing on the label outside the Nutrition Facts. The protein %DV, when it is declared, is calculated using an amount per serving of protein that has been adjusted for both the digestibility and the amino acid completeness of the protein source. The protein adjustment method is called the protein digestibility corrected amino acid score. A horizontal heavy bar is placed below the "Macronutrient content" section. The "Vitamin and mineral content" section follows the "Macronutrient content" section.

Vitamin and mineral content; There are four mandatory vitamins and minerals that must be declared in the Nutrition Facts (vitamin D, calcium, iron, and potassium). They are declared in nonbolded 8-point type. The nutrient name is followed by the weight per serving, and the %DV per serving is aligned in a right justified column.[8] The nutrient weight amounts are declared with a level of significance consistent with the DV. For example, for a DV between 10 and 100, the weight per serving would be expressed to the nearest 1 unit; for a DV between 100 and 1,000, the weight per serving would be expressed to the nearest 10 units. %DV values for vitamins and minerals are declared as 0 for values less than 2%, declared to the nearest 2% for values between 2% and 10%, declared to the nearest 5% for values between 10% and 50%, and declared to the nearest 10% for values above 50%. The vitamins and minerals may either be declared on separate lines, or they may be placed two per line. In addition to the four mandatory vitamin and minerals that must be declared, there are another 23 vitamins and minerals with established DVs that may voluntarily be declared. No vitamin or mineral without a DV may be declared within the Nutrition Facts. The vitamins and minerals with established DVs are listed in Table 16.5. The order of listing vitamins and minerals in Table 16.5 must be observed when any of these nutrients are voluntarily declared in the Nutrition Facts.[13] A horizontal medium bar is placed below the "Vitamin and mineral content" section. The "Footnote" section follows the "Vitamin and mineral content" section.

Footnote; The last section of the Nutrition Facts is for "Footnotes." Footnotes are presented in 6-point type, rather than the 8-point type used elsewhere in the Nutrition Facts. The standard footnote is preceded by an asterisk that refers to the asterisk that follows the "%DV" subheading in the body of the Nutrition Facts.[8] The standard footnote is

> *The % Daily Value (DV) tells you how much a nutrient in a serving of food contributes to a daily diet. 2000 calories a day is used for general nutrition advice.

The complete standard footnote is not always required. Foods that qualify as "calorie free" may either omit the footnote altogether or omit just the second sentence of the footnote. Packages with under 40 square inches available for labeling may replace the standard footnote with "%DV = % Daily Value."

TABLE 16.5 Vitamins and minerals that may be declared in the nutrition facts and their daily values (adults and children > 4 years).

Vitamins and minerals that may be declared in the nutrition facts and their daily values (adults and children > 4 years)

Mandatory

Vitamin D 20 mcg (the International Units (IU) amount may be added in parentheses following the mcg weight amount)
Calcium 1300 mg
Iron 18 mg
Potassium 4700 mg

Voluntary

Vitamin A 900 mcg RAE (retinoic acid equivalents)
Vitamin C 90 mg
Vitamin E 15 mg
Vitamin K 120 mcg
Thiamin 1.2 mg (vitamin B1 may be added in parentheses following the name)
Riboflavin 1.3 mg (vitamin B2 may be added in parentheses following the name)
Niacin 16 mg NE (niacin equivalents)
Vitamin B6 1.7 mg
Folate 400 mcg DFE (dietary folate equivalents)
Vitamin B12 2.4 mcg
Biotin 30 mcg
Pantothenic acid 5 mg
Phosphorus 1250 mg
Iodine 150 mcg
Magnesium 420 mg
Zinc 11 mg
Selenium 55 mcg
Copper 0.9 mg
Manganese 2.3 mg
Chromium 35 mcg
Molybdenum 45 mcg
Chloride 2300 mg
Choline 550 mg

Nutrition Facts

2 servings per container
Serving size **1 cup (255g)**

	Per serving		Per container	
Calories	**220**		**440**	
		% DV*		**% DV***
Total Fat	5g	**6%**	10g	**13%**
Saturated Fat	2g	**10%**	4g	**20%**
Trans Fat	0g		0g	
Cholesterol	15mg	**5%**	30mg	**10%**
Sodium	240mg	**10%**	480mg	**21%**
Total Carb.	35g	**13%**	70g	**25%**
Dietary Fiber	6g	**21%**	12g	**43%**
Total Sugars	7g		14g	
Incl. Added Sugars	4g	**8%**	8g	**16%**
Protein	9g		18g	
Vitamin D	5mcg	25%	10mcg	50%
Calcium	200mg	15%	400mg	30%
Iron	1mg	6%	2mg	10%
Potassium	470mg	10%	940mg	20%

* The % Daily Value (DV) tells you how much a nutrient in a serving of food contributes to a daily diet. 2,000 calories a day is used for general nutrition advice.

FIGURE 16.9 Nutrition Facts—dual columns.

Dual columns; Packages whose contents are between 200% and 300% of the applicable reference amount must have two columns of nutrient content information in their Nutrition Facts (i.e., "dual column format"); the first column declares the quantitative amounts and percent DVs per serving, and the second column is based on the contents of the entire package, as shown in Fig. 16.9.[14] Packages that contain between 150% and 200% of the applicable reference amount must declare the serving size as "1 container," but there is an option to voluntarily use the dual column format with the first column declaring nutrient content information on a "per reference amount" basis and the second column declaring nutrient content information on a "per package" basis.

In addition to the required dual column format for packages containing between 200% and 300% of the applicable reference amount, there is an optional provision for dual columns of nutrient content information for packaged food to which the consumer typically adds additional ingredients prior to consuming (e.g., adding milk to breakfast cereal). In this situation, the first column of nutrient content amounts as "as packaged" and the second column has the "as prepared" amounts.

Alternative formats; There is a SHORTENED format for the Nutrition Facts that provides for moving some of the mandatory declared nutrients to a footnote. Any of the mandatory declared nutrients, other than calories, total fat, sodium, total carbohydrate, and protein, that are present at a level that can be rounded to zero may be omitted from the tabular portion of the Nutrition Facts and instead declared in the footnote portion of the Nutrition Facts.[2] This footnote begins as "Not a significant source of...." The "zero level" nutrients being declared in this footnote are listed in the same order as they normally appear in the tabular portion of the Nutrition Facts. This SHORTENED format Nutrition Facts will declare within the tabular portion of the Nutrition

[2] The mandatory Nutrition Facts nutrients that may be moved from the main body of the Nutrition Facts box to a "Not a significant source of ..." footnote, when present in an amount that is rounded to zero, are saturated fat, *trans* fat, cholesterol, dietary fiber, total sugars, added sugar, protein, vitamin D, calcium, iron, and potassium.

Nutrition Facts	
64 servings per container	
Serving size	**1 tbsp (14g)**
Amount per serving	
Calories	**130**
	% DV*
Total Fat 14g	**18%**
Saturated Fat 2g	**10%**
Trans Fat 2g	
Polyunsaturated Fat 4g	
Monounsaturated Fat 6g	
Sodium 0mg	**0%**
Total Carbohydrate 0g	**0%**
Protein 0g	
Not a significant source of cholesterol, dietary fiber, total sugars, added sugars, vitamin D, calcium, iron, and potassium	
* %DV = %Daily Value	

FIGURE 16.10 Simplified nutrition facts format for foods in which most nutrients are at levels that can be declared as zero.

Facts: (1) calories, (2) four of the five core nutrients (total fat, sodium, total carbohydrate, and protein), regardless of amount, (3) any other mandatory nutrient present at greater than a zero level, (4) nutrients that are required to be declared because there is a claim about them on the label (e.g., total sugars and added sugars must be declared when there is a "Sugar Free" claim on the label), and (5) any voluntarily declared nutrient that the manufacturer may wish to include.

There is a SIMPLIFIED format for the Nutrition Facts that may be used when eight or more of the 15 mandatory declared nutrients are present at zero levels (Fig. 16.10). The SIMPLIFIED Nutrition Facts format includes only calories, four of the five core nutrients (total fat, sodium, total carbohydrate, and protein), and any of the other mandatory nutrients present at more than "zero." The "Not a significant source of..." footnote used in the SHORTENED format is not required with the simplified format unless there are any nutrients declared other than the mandatory nutrients or any nutrition claims are made on the label. The "The % Daily Value (DV) tells you..." footnote is omitted from the SIMPLIFIED format.

The SIMPLIFIED format example shown in Fig. 16.10 is for a hypothetical vegetable oil label that makes a claim about omega-3 fatty acid content, which triggers the requirement to declare polyunsaturated and monounsaturated fat content.[15] The declaration of nutrients other than the core required nutrients, in turn, requires inclusion of a "Not a significant source of..." footnote.

There is a TABULAR format available for packages whose height is insufficient to accommodate the VERTICAL format (Fig. 16.11).[16] The SHORTENED and SIMPLIFIED format options can be combined with the TABULAR format when appropriate. Labels on packages with a surface area 40 square inches or less may omit the "The % Daily Value (DV) tells you..." footnote from a TABULAR format. The TABULAR format is to be used only when the VERTICAL format will not fit on a package label.

There is a LINEAR format available for packages with a surface area less than 12 square inches (Fig. 16.12).[17] The LINEAR format is to be used only when it is impossible to fit the TABULAR format on the label. Minimum allowable type size in the LINEAR format is 6-point. The footnote is omitted from the LINEAR format.

Exemptions; Foods that contain all mandatory declaration nutrients only in amounts defined as zero and bear no nutrition information on the label or in labeling are exempt from placing a Nutrition Facts on their label. A few foods, notably coffee, that have long been exempt from the Nutrition Facts requirement on the basis of having no nutrients to declare will no longer be exempt under the revised Nutrition Facts regulations that have made changes in mandatory declaration nutrients, their DVs, and reference amounts. For example, coffee falls into this situation because potassium is now a mandatory declaration nutrient, and coffee's potassium content per RACC (the new coffee reference amount is 12 fL oz) is greater than 2% of the potassium DV.

Nutrition Facts	**Amount/serving**	**% Daily Value***	**Amount/serving**	**% Daily Value***	*The % Daily Value (DV) tells you how much a nutrient in a serving of food contributes to a daily diet. 2,000 calories a day is used for general nutrition advice.
10 servings per container	**Total Fat** 1.5g	**2%**	**Total Carbohydrate** 36g	**13%**	
Serving size	Saturated Fat 0.5g	**3%**	Dietary Fiber 2g	**7%**	
2 slices (56g)	*Trans* Fat 0.5g		Total Sugars 1g		
	Cholesterol 0mg	**0%**	Includes 1g Added Sugars	**2%**	
	Sodium 280mg	**12%**	**Protein** 4g		
Calories per serving 170	Vitamin D 0mcg 0% • Calcium 80mg 6% • Iron 1mg 6% • Potassium 470mg 10% Thiamin 15% • Riboflavin 8% • Niacin 10%				

FIGURE 16.11 Tabular format nutrition facts for packages less than 3-inches high.

Nutrition Facts Servings: 12, **Serv. size: 1 mint (2g),**
Amount per serving: **Calories 5, Total Fat** 0g (0% DV), Sat. Fat 0g (0% DV), *Trans* Fat 0g, **Cholest.** 0mg (0% DV), **Sodium** 0mg (0% DV), **Total Carb.** 2g (1% DV), Fiber 0g (0% DV), Total Sugars 2g (Incl. 2g Added Sugars, 4% DV), **Protein** 0g, Vit. D (0% DV), Calcium (0% DV), Iron (0% DV), Potas. (6% DV).

FIGURE 16.12 Linear format nutrition facts for packages with surface area less than 12 square inches.

E. Label Requirements for Specific Products

Dietary supplements are a regulatory subcategory of foods. Dietary supplement regulations for labeling, ingredient safety standards, and good manufacturing practice are separate from the corresponding conventional food regulations. Dietary supplements are products intended for oral consumption whose purpose is to supplement the diet, are formulated for consumption in small amounts (e.g., capsules, tablets, spoonful of liquids, etc.), and are not represented as a conventional food. The term "conventional food" is not a defined regulatory term, but FDA uses the term when wishing to make clear where regulatory requirements differ between conventional food and dietary supplements. Nutrition information is presented on dietary supplement labels as Supplement Facts, rather than as Nutrition Facts. The Supplement Facts panel is modeled on the Nutrition Facts, and many of the requirements are the same. A Supplement Facts example for a vitamin and mineral supplement is shown in Fig. 16.13.[18]

Infant formula is another separate food category for which there are nutrition labeling requirements separate from the Nutrition Facts nutrition labeling rules that apply to other foods. Infant formula is defined as a food represented for special dietary use solely as a food for infants by reason of its simulation of human milk or it's suitability as a complete or partial substitute for human milk. There are separate regulations that prescribe what nutrient information is to be presented on infant formula labels.[19]

Supplement Facts

Serving Size 1 Gelcap
Servings Per Container 100

	Amount Per Serving	% Daily Value
Vitamin A (as retinyl acetate and 50% as beta-carotene)	900 mcg	100%
Vitamin C (as ascorbic acid)	90 mg	100%
Vitamin D (as cholecalciferol)	20 mcg (800 IU)	100%
Vitamin E (as dl-alpha tocopheryl acetate)	15 mg	100%
Thiamin (as thiamin mononitrate)	1.2 mg	100%
Riboflavin	1.3 mg	100%
Niacin (as niacinamide)	16 mg	100%
Vitamin B_6 (as pyridoxine hydrochloride)	1.7 mg	100%
Folate	400 mcg DFE (240 mcg folic acid)	100%
Vitamin B_{12} (as cyanocobalamin)	2.4 mcg	100%
Biotin	3 mcg	10%
Pantothenic Acid (as calcium pantothenate)	5 mg	100%

FIGURE 16.13 Supplement facts for a vitamin and mineral dietary supplement.

Medical foods is another food category that is exempt from the Nutrition Facts nutrition labeling rules, although medical foods is not clearly a distinct regulatory category. The 1990 Nutrition Labeling and Education Act included "medical foods" among the list of categories that were to be exempt from the Nutrition Facts nutrition labeling rules.[20] As such, medical food labels can present information about the nutrient content of the medical food in a manner of the manufacturer's choosing. For purposes of defining the character of a food that would be exempt from Nutrition Facts labeling as being a medical food, "medical food" is defined as

> A medical food is a food which is formulated to be consumed or administered enterally under the supervision of a physician and which is intended for the specific dietary management of a disease or condition for which distinctive nutritional requirements, based on recognized scientific principles, are established by medical evaluation.

FDA requires a "medical food" product to meet all the following criteria to qualify for the exemption from Nutrition Facts nutrition labeling:

1. It is a specially formulated and processed product (as opposed to a naturally occurring foodstuff used in its natural state) for the partial or exclusive feeding of a patient by means of oral intake or enteral feeding by tube;
2. It is intended for the dietary management of a patient who, because of therapeutic or chronic medical needs, has limited or impaired capacity to ingest, digest, absorb, or metabolize ordinary foodstuffs or certain nutrients or who has other special medically determined nutrient requirements, the dietary management of which cannot be achieved by the modification of the normal diet alone;
3. It provides nutritional support specifically modified for the management of the unique nutrient needs that result from the specific disease or condition, as determined by medical evaluation;
4. It is intended to be used under medical supervision; and

5. It is intended only for a patient receiving active and ongoing medical supervision wherein the patient requires medical care on a recurring basis for, among other things, instructions on the use of the medical food.

F. 2016 Nutrition Facts Revision—Complex Issues

Several of the changes FDA wanted to make to the Nutrition Facts in the 2016 revisions turned out to be quite complex to implement. Due to the complexities, several of the revised Nutrition Facts components are a source of confusion, particularly so for added sugars, dietary fibers, and folate.

Nutrition Facts revisions—added sugars

FDA established requirements for declaration of added sugars on the Nutrition Facts label because the information would assist consumers in maintaining healthy dietary practices. The declaration would provide them with information necessary to meet the key recommendations of the DGA to construct diets containing nutrient-dense foods and reduce calorie intake from sugars by reducing consumption of added sugars.

The amount per serving of added sugars is declared on a separate line below the "Total Sugars" line and is indented relative to "Total Sugars." The added sugars declaration is "includes __ g Added Sugars." The DV for added sugars is 50 g.

Added sugar includes sugars that are added to foods during processing and also foods that are sugar (e.g., the Nutrition Facts for a bag of sugar will declare 8g per serving total sugar and 8 g per serving added sugar). Ingredients that are considered to be "added sugars" include

- All mono- and disaccharide sugars
- Sugar content of honey
- Sugar content of syrups
- Sugar content of concentrated juices that are in excess of what would be expected from the same volume of 100% juice of the same type
- D-tagatose, isomaltulose, and psicose

A provision included in the 2018 Farm Bill bars FDA from requiring the words "includes X g Added Sugars" in the Nutrition Facts for any single ingredient sugar, honey, agave, or syrup, including maple syrup food product.[21] The FDA interpretation of this legislation is that although the Nutrition Facts for these single ingredient "added sugars" foods need not use the words "includes X g Added Sugars," or declare the grams per serving of added sugars, they still need to declare the %DV for added sugars. FDA does not object to manufacturers of the single ingredient "added sugar" foods named in the 2018 Farm Bill to place a † symbol following the added sugars %DV that references to a truthful and not misleading statement within a footnote at the bottom of the Nutrition Facts that includes a description of the gram amount of sugar added to the diet by one serving of the product and its contribution to the percent DV for added sugars in the diet. FDA also does not object to including a statement such as "All these sugars are naturally occurring in honey" in the footnote.[22]

FDA also has made some concessions in the declaration of added sugars for sweetened cranberry food products. Dried cranberry and cranberry juice beverages sweetened with added sugars that contain total sugars at levels no greater than comparable foods with inherent sugars, but no added sugars, may place a † symbol following the added sugars %DV that references a statement about sugars outside of the Nutrition Facts. Such statement would explain that sweetened dried cranberries and cranberry beverages have amounts of total sugars comparable to comparable noncranberry products. A statement placed outside the Nutrition Facts can provide truthful and not misleading information regarding common practices of adding sugars to increase the palatability of tart cranberries and that sweetened cranberry products contain equivalent amounts of total sugars as comparable fruit products that are inherently sweet and do not declare added sugars on their labels.

Because there is no quantitative analytical method available to distinguish between added sugars and endogenous sugars in a food, manufacturers of foods that contain both added sugars and endogenous sugars must keep records, and make those records available to FDA upon request, that substantiate the amounts of total sugars and added sugars declared in the food's Nutrition Facts.

Nutrition Facts revisions—dietary fiber

FDA's original Nutrition Facts regulations did not define what constituted *dietary fiber,* instead any digestion-resistant carbohydrate substance that could be measured with a validated "dietary fiber" quantitative analytical method would be counted as a dietary fiber. Many new food ingredients that qualified as dietary fiber have been developed subsequent to the 1993 introduction of the Nutrition Facts label. FDA had concerns that not all of the novel dietary fiber ingredients actually had any of the beneficial physiological effects attributable to dietary fiber. Based on the rationale that declaring dietary fiber content solely on the basis of a quantitative analytical measure without knowing whether any dietary fiber attributable benefit is associated with that fiber content, FDA has now defined *dietary fiber* for nutrition labeling purposes as

> ... non-digestible soluble and insoluble carbohydrates (with 3 or more monomeric units), and lignin that are intrinsic and intact in plants; isolated or synthetic non-digestible carbohydrates (with 3 or more monomeric units) determined by FDA to have physiological effects that are beneficial to human health.

This dietary fiber definition entails two categories of dietary fiber: (1) intrinsic and intact and (2) isolated or synthetic. FDA considers the "intact" characteristic as meaning no relevant component present in the edible plant source has been removed or destroyed from the ingredient. FDA considers the "intrinsic" characteristic as meaning the substance is a naturally occurring component of the edible plant food matrix. FDA has illustrated this concept by noting that bran fiber, obtained by grinding of grain outer layers, is the anatomical outer layers of the grain consisting of intact cells and substantial amounts of other plant matrix nutrients (e.g., starch, protein and other nutrients) and is an "intact and intrinsic" dietary fiber source. FDA also includes as "intrinsic and intact" dietary fiber the nondigestible carbohydrates that are created during normal food processing (e.g., cooking, rolling, or milling) such as the digestion-resistant starch in flaked corn meal. However, an ingredient consisting of resistant starch that has been extracted and isolated from flaked corn meal, such that it is no longer part of the food matrix, would be considered an isolated nondigestible carbohydrate.

An "intrinsic and intact" source of dietary fiber automatically qualifies as dietary fiber for nutrition labeling purposes; however, "isolated or synthetic" sources of dietary fiber must be preapproved by FDA before they can be counted toward the dietary fiber content of a food. FDA will approve as dietary fiber a nondigestible carbohydrate substance that has been demonstrated, to FDA's satisfaction, as having beneficial physiological effects for human health. The beneficial physiologic effects of dietary fiber recognized by FDA are (1) lowering of blood total and LDL-cholesterol levels, (2) lowering of blood postprandial glucose levels, (3) reducing gut transit time and improving laxation (as increased fecal bulk), (4) reducing blood pressure, and (5) increasing satiety associated with reduced energy intake and with possible outcomes on body weight. FDA initially recognized 7 "isolated or synthetic" dietary fiber sources in the revised Nutrition Facts regulations and said that additional sources would be added through the Citizen Petition process when interested parties submit a request for an additional isolated or synthetic dietary fiber source, substantiated by evidence establishing a beneficial physiologic effect in humans of the dietary fiber substance. FDA has approved as dietary fiber an additional eight isolated or synthetic nondigestible carbohydrate substances, but the Nutrition Facts regulation has not yet been amended to include any of the additional FDA-approved isolated or synthetic dietary fiber sources. The list of approved isolated fiber sources is on the FDA website in "Guidance for Industry: The Declaration of Certain Isolated or Synthetic Non-Digestible Carbohydrates as Dietary Fiber on Nutrition and Supplement Facts Labels."[23] The FDA-approved isolated or synthetic dietary fiber sources are listed in Table 16.6.[24]

TABLE 16.6 Isolated or synthetic dietary fiber sources.

Isolated or synthetic dietary fiber sources
Beta-glucan fiber
Psyllium seed husk
Cellulose
Guar gum
Pectin
Locust bean gum
Hydroxypropyl methylcellulose
Arabinoxylan
Alginate
Inulin and inulin-type fructans
High amylose starch (resistant starch 2)
Galactooligosaccharides
Polydextrose
Resistant maltodextrin/dextrin
Mixed plant cell wall fibers (ingredients containing 2 or more of cellulose, pectin, lignin, beta-glucan, and arabinoxylan)

Nutrition Facts revisions—folate

The current RDA for folate is expressed as micrograms (mcg) Dietary Folate Equivalents (DFE). The DFE measure accounts for the greater bioavailability of synthetic folic acid added to foods than the bioavailability of folate that occurs naturally in food. 1 mcg food folate is equal to 1 mcg DFE; whereas 1 mcg folic acid is equal to 1.7 mcg DFE. Declaring folate content in the Nutrition Facts is voluntary, however, if any folate information is placed on a label outside the Nutrition Facts, or if folic acid is an added ingredient of the food, then folate content must be declared in the Nutrition Facts.

When folate content is declared in the Nutrition Facts, the nutrient term *folate* is used. The folate content, declared as mcg DFE, includes the total folate content from natural folates, synthetic forms of folate such as L-5-methyltetrahydrofolate, and folic acid. The folate %DV is calculated on the mcg DFE per serving. When a food contains only naturally occurring folate (and no added folic acid), a manufacturer may voluntarily declare "folate" and the folate %DV, without declaring the mcg DFE content. When folic acid is an added ingredient in a food, then the total mcg DFE, the folic acid content, and the folate %DV all be must be declared. The folic acid content is declared within parentheses following the folate mcg DFE content; such as

Folate xx mcg yy__% DV (for food with naturally occurring food folate)

Folate _xx mcg DFE (yy mcg folic acid) zz % DV (for food containing added folic acid)

When the folate content is declared in the Nutrition Facts, and the food contains both naturally occurring food folates and added folic acid, the manufacturer must keep records to verify the amounts of folates and folic acid that are being declared.

II. INTERNATIONAL NUTRITION LABELING: USA, EU, CODEX

The FAO/WHO Codex Alimentarius (Codex) International Food Standards program has developed guidelines for the nutrition labeling of packaged foods. The Codex nutrition labeling guidelines were revised in 1993 and again in 2011. Rules for declaring nutrition information on food labels were introduced in both the USA and the European Union (EU) in the early 1990s. About 25 years later, the nutrition labeling rules have been updated in both the USA and EU. The revised EU nutrition labeling rules went into effect at the end of 2016, and the USA revised nutrition labeling rules are set to go into effect at the beginning of 2020. The EU adopted Regulation (EU) No 1169/2011 in 2011 to modify existing food labeling provisions to provide to consumers updated food information.[25] The nutrition information portion of this regulation went into effect at the end of 2016. With this regulation nutrition labeling of packaged foods became mandatory in the EU. The US FDA issued regulations in 2016 revising the existing mandatory nutrition information food labeling regulation.[9] The nutrition labeling regulation revisions reflect changes in knowledge of nutrient requirements and the link between diet, chronic diseases, and public health. Table 16.7 is a comparison of major features of nutrition labeling requirements in the USA and EU regulations and in the Codex guidelines.[26]

III. NUTRITION AND HEALTH BENEFIT CLAIMS

Manufacturers may choose to make claims on their food labels about their products' attributes or benefits. Unlike in some other countries, in the USA, the term "health claim" applies to only one type of claim. Health claims state or imply a relationship between a substance and reduced risk of a disease. Other types of nutrition or health benefit claims include "nutrient content claims," "structure function claims," and "dietary guidance statements."

A product's intended use will determine whether it is subject to regulation as a food, dietary supplement, or drug. Claims that are made for a product are key to determining its intended use. For example, a claim that a product treats or prevents a disease or abnormal health condition subjects it to regulation as a drug. Because most drugs cannot be marketed until they have received premarket approval, food companies must avoid making claims that would subject their products to regulation as new drugs.[27]

A. Nutrient Content Claims

A nutrient content claim describes the level of a nutrient in a food using terms such as "free," "high," and "low" or compares the level of a nutrient in a food to that of another food, using terms such as "more," "reduced," and "lite." Nutrient content claims cannot be made unless they are authorized by FDA. They can be expressed or implied, and, generally, there must be an established DV for the nutrient that is the subject of the claim. An accurate quantitative statement (e.g., 200 mg of sodium) that does not otherwise "characterize" the nutrient level may be used to describe the amount of a nutrient present. A statement such as "only 200 mg of sodium" characterizes the level of sodium by implying that it is low. Therefore, the food would have to meet the nutritional criteria for a "low" nutrient content claim or carry a disclosure statement that it does not qualify for the claim (e.g., "not a low sodium food").[28] Additional label statements are required for specific nutrient content claims on certain foods.[29]

Special labeling also is required for products that exceed designated "disclosure levels" for fat, saturated fat, cholesterol, and sodium, using a statement such as "See nutrition information for fat content," for a food where the level of fat exceeds the disclosure level and a nutrient content claim is made.

B. Health Claims

A health claim describes the relationship between a substance (food or food component) and a disease or health-related condition.[30] Health claims are limited to statements about reducing disease risk and cannot be claims about the cure, mitigation, treatment, or prevention of disease. Health claims must be authorized by FDA. They must be supported by significant scientific agreement to be established by regulation. Foods are

TABLE 16.7 Comparison of USA and EU nutrition label requirements.

Nutrition information
•Mandatory information

USA	European Union	Codex Alimentarius
Per serving Energy (calories) Macronutrients •Total fat •Saturated fat •Trans fat •Cholesterol •Sodium •Total carbohydrate •Dietary fiber •Total sugars •Added sugars •Protein Micronutrients •Vitamin D •Calcium •Iron •Potassium 21 CFR 101.9	Per 100 g or 100 mL (per serving voluntary) Energy (kcal and kJ) Macronutrients •Fat •Saturates •Carbohydrate •Sugars •Protein •Salt Micronutrients • Added vitamins and minerals Regulation (EU) No 1169/2011, Section 3 (Nutrition declaration), Article 29	Per 100 g or per 100 mL or per serving on single-portion package Energy value Macronutrients • Fat • Saturated fat • Sodium • Available carbohydrates (excluding dietary fiber) • Total sugars Micronutrients • None Any other nutrient for which a nutrition or health claim is made Codex Guidelines on Nutrition Labelling; Sec. 3 Nutrient Declaration [CAC/GL 2-1985 (Rev. 2011)]

Nutrition information
• Voluntary information

USA	European Union	Codex Alimentarius
Macronutrients • Polyunsaturated fat • Monounsaturated fat • Soluble fiber • Insoluble fiber • Sugar alcohol Micronutrients • Fluoride • Vitamins and minerals listed in 21 CFR 101.9(c)(8)(iv)	Macronutrients • Monounsaturates • Polyunsaturates • Polyols • Starch • Fiber Micronutrients • Vitamins and minerals if (1) listed in point 1 of Part A of Annex VIII and (2) present in significant amount (≥ 15% NRV/100 g or mL, for most foods)	Micronutrients • Vitamins and minerals for which recommended intakes have been established and are present at more than 5% of the Nutrient Reference Value per 100 g or 100 mL Codex Guidelines on Nutrition Labelling; Sec. 3 Nutrient Declaration [CAC/GL 2-1985 (Rev. 2011]

Nutrition information
• Nutrient Reference Values

USA	European Union	Codex Alimentarius
Daily Value (DV) Fat 78 g Saturated fat 20 g Cholesterol 300 mg Total carbohydrate 275 g Sodium 2,300 mg Fiber 28 g Total sugars none Added sugar 50 g Protein 50 g Vitamin D 20 mcg Calcium 1,300 mg	Nutrient Reference Value (NRV) Fat 70 g Saturated fat 20 g Cholesterol none Total carbohydrate 260 g Salt 6 g Fiber none Total sugars 90 g Added sugar none Protein Vitamin D 5 mcg Calcium 800 mg Iron 14 mg	Nutrient Reference Value (NRY) Fat none Saturated fat 20 g Cholesterol none Total Carbohydrate Sodium 2,000 mg Fiber none Total sugars Added sugar none Protein 50 g Vitamin D 5 mcg Calcium 1,000 mg

Continued

TABLE 16.7 Comparison of USA and EU nutrition label requirements.—cont'd

Iron 18 mg Potassium 4,700 mg	Potassium 2,000 mg Annex VIII of Regulation 1169/2011/EU	Iron 14 mg Potassium 3,500 mg
Nutrition information • Macronutrient energy values		
USA	**European Union**	**Codex Alimentarius**
Carbohydrate 4 kcal/g Protein 4 kcal/g Fat 9 kcal/g Soluble dietary fiber 2 kcal/g Insoluble dietary fiber 0 kcal/g Polyols (specific individual values 0–3 kcal/g)	Carbohydrate 4 kcal/g (17 kJ) Protein 4 kcal/g (17 kJ) Fat 9 kcal/g (37 kJ) Alcohol 7 kcal/g (29 kJ) Organic acids 3 kcal/g (13 kJ) Polyols 2.4 kcal/g (10 kj) Fiber 2 kcal/f (8 kJ) Erythritol 0 kcal/g (0 kJ) Salatrims 6 kcal/g (25 kJ) Annex XIV of Regulation 1169/2011/EU	Carbohydrate 4 kcal/g (17 kJ) Protein 4 kcal/g (17 kJ) Fat 9 kcal/g (37 kj) Alcohol 7 kcal/g (29 kj) Organic acids 4 kcal/g (17 kj) Codex Guidelines on Nutrition Labelling; 3.3.1 Calculation of Energy [CAC/GL 2-1985 (Rev. 2011)]
Nutrition information • Fiber definitions		
USA	**European Union**	**Codex Alimentarius**
Nondigestible soluble and insoluble carbohydrates (with 3 or more monomeric units), and lignin that are (A) intrinsic and intact in plants or (B) isolated or synthetic nondigestible carbohydrates (with 3 or more monomeric units) determined by FDA to have physiological effects that are beneficial to human health. FDA has determined about 14 isolated or synthetic non-digestible carbohydrate substances qualify as dietary fiber. 21 CFR 101.9(c)(i)	Carbohydrate polymers with three or more monomeric units, which are neither digested nor absorbed in the human small intestine and belong to the following categories: • edible carbohydrate polymers naturally occurring in the food as consumed; • edible carbohydrate polymers that have been obtained from food raw material by physical, enzymatic, or chemical means and that have a beneficial physiological effect demonstrated by generally accepted scientific evidence; • edible synthetic carbohydrate polymers that have a beneficial physiological effect demonstrated by generally accepted scientific evidence. Annex I of Regulation 1169/2011/EU	Carbohydrate polymers with 10 or more monomeric units, which are not hydrolyzed by endogenous enzymes of the small intestine of humans, and belong to the following categories: • edible carbohydrate polymers naturally occurring in the food as consumed; • carbohydrate polymers, which have been obtained from food raw material by physical, enzymatic, or chemical means and which have been shown to have a physiological effect of benefit to health as demonstrated by generally accepted scientific evidence to competent authorities; • synthetic carbohydrate polymers that have been shown to have a physiological effect of benefit to health as demonstrated by generally accepted scientific evidence to competent authorities. Codex Guidelines on Nutrition Labeling [CAC/GL 2-1985 (Rev. 2011)]

ineligible for health claims if they exceed disqualifying levels of total fat, saturated fat, cholesterol, or sodium. Health claims authorized by regulation are listed in FDA's regulations at 21 CFR 101.72–101.83.[31] Health claims can also be authorized by specific decision letters posted on the FDA website.

C. Qualified Health Claims

For a proposed health claim for which there is not significant scientific agreement that the claim is supported, if FDA agrees that the scientific evidence supports a qualified health claim, the agency will provide claim language for which it will exercise enforcement discretion (i.e., generally not take enforcement action). The claim language is tailored to accurately convey the level and quality of the science supporting the claim. Decisions on Qualified Health Claims are in letters posted on the FDA website.[32]

Although FDA's letters are issued to the petitioner requesting the qualified health claim, the qualified claims are available for use on any food or dietary supplement product meeting the conditions specified in the letter.

D. FDAMA Nutrient Content and Health Claims

The Food and Drug Administration Modernization Act of 1997 (FDAMA) allows nutrient content and health claims to be made on the basis of statements issued by certain authoritative federal bodies other than FDA, such as the National Institutes of Health and the National Academies of Sciences, Engineering, and Medicine.[33] The claim is authorized based on a notification by the manufacturer who wishes to use the claim. If FDA does not object to the FDAMA notification, the decision is posted on the FDA website.

E. Structure/Function Claims

Structure/function claims describe the role of substances intended to affect the normal structure or function of the body. Such claims address effects in healthy individuals, for example, "Calcium helps maintain strong bones." In addition, they may characterize the means by which a nutrient acts to maintain such structure or function, for example, "fiber maintains bowel regularity" or "antioxidants maintain cell integrity." Structure/function claims for conventional foods focus on effects derived from nutritive value, while structure/function claims for dietary supplements may focus on nonnutritive as well as nutritive effects.

FDA authorization is not required prior to use of structure/function claims, but structure/function claims may not link the claimed effect to a disease or health-related condition. For example, it is permissible to make the claim that a substance supports memory but not to make the claim the substance reduces memory loss. The one exception to this rule is that claims are permitted to describe a benefit related to a nutrient deficiency disease (e.g., vitamin C and scurvy) as long as the statement also provides information about how widespread such a disease is in the USA.

F. Dietary Guidance

By definition, a "health claim" has two essential components: (1) a substance (includes a food or food component) and (2) a disease or health-related condition. A statement lacking either one of these components does not meet the FDA definition of a health claim. For example, statements that address a role of dietary patterns or of general categories of foods (e.g., fruits and vegetables) in maintaining good health are considered dietary guidance rather than health claims. Dietary guidance statements used on food labels must be truthful and nonmisleading. Unlike health claims, dietary guidance statements are not subject to premarket review and authorization by FDA.

IV. CONCLUSION

The authors of this chapter have presented information on the updated nutrition labeling requirements in the USA that will allow the reader to gain a basic understanding of which information is required and why. For those who need more detail, the authors have listed the three primary resource documents (Refs. 2 and 3). While the FDA has not yet revised the rules for nutrition-related claims to include the updated nutrient and intake data, the agency has committed to making appropriate changes.

RESEARCH GAPS

- Associations between nutrients and chronic diseases and health-related conditions
- Relevant physiological endpoints
- Information on consumer understanding
- Food consumption patterns
- Analytical methodology for determination of nutrient content of foods

V. REFERENCES

1. Food and Drug Administration (FDA). *Fact sheet: FDA at a glance*; 2018. https://www.fda.gov/about-fda/fda-basics/fact-sheet-fda-glance. Accessed September 23, 2019.
2. US Department of Agriculture (USDA). *US Department of Health and Human Services (HHS). Dietary Guidelines for Americans 2015–2020*. 8th ed.; 2015. https://health.gov/dietaryguidelines/2015/guidelines/. Accessed September 23, 2019.
3. Food and Drug Administration. Food Labeling: Revision of the Nutrition and Supplement Facts Labels. *Fed Regist*; May 27, 2016. https://www.federalregister.gov/documents/2016/05/27/2016-11867/food-labeling-revision-of-the-nutrition-and-supplement-facts-labels. Accessed November 16, 2019. https://www.regulations.gov/document?D=FDA-2012-N-1210-1303.
4. Food and Drug Administration. *Electronic Code of Federal Regulations: Title 21 Food and Drugs Part 101 Food Labeling*; 2016. https://www.ecfr.gov/cgi-bin/retrieveECFR?%20gp=&SID=bad23c28ebd662323b3ace1e3f5ee94f&mc=true&n=pt.21.2.101&r=PART&ty=HTML#s%20e21.2.101_154. Accessed September 23, 2019.
5. Food and Drug Administration. *Electronic Code of Federal Regulations: Title 21 Food and Drugs Part 101.9(d)(12) Food Labeling. Derived from Vertical Display with Micronutrients Listed Side-by-Side*; 2016. Adapted 2019 https://www.ecfr.gov/cgi-bin/retrieveECFR?%20gp=&SID=bad23c28ebd662323b3ace1e3f5ee94f&mc=true&n=pt.21.2.101&r=PART&ty=HTML#s%20e21.2.101_154. Accessed September 23, 2019.

6. Food and Drug Administration. *Electronic Code of Federal Regulations: Title 21 Food and Drugs Part 101.9(d)(12) Food Labeling. Vertical Display Including Some Voluntary Nutrients*; 2016. https://www.ecfr.gov/cgi-bin/retrieveECFR?%20gp=&SID=bad23c28ebd662323b3ace1e3f5ee94f&mc=true&n=pt.21.2.101&r=PART&ty=HTML#s%20e21.2.101_154. Accessed September 23, 2019.
7. Food and Drug Administration. *Electronic Code of Federal Regulations: Title 21 Food and Drugs Part 101.9(c)(8)(iv) Food Labeling. RDI – Food Components*; 2016. https://www.ecfr.gov/cgi-bin/retrieveECFR?%20gp=&SID=bad23c28ebd662323b3ace1e3f5ee94f&mc=true&n=pt.21.2.101&r=PART&ty=HTML#s%20e21.2.101_154. Accessed September 23, 2019.
8. Food and Drug Administration. *Electronic Code of Federal Regulations: Title 21 Food and Drugs Part 101.9(c)(8)(iv) Food Labeling*; 2016. https://www.ecfr.gov/cgi-bin/retrieveECFR?%20gp=&SID=bad23c28ebd662323b3ace1e3f5ee94f&mc=true&n=pt.21.2.101&r=PART&ty=HTML#s%20e21.2.101_154. Accessed September 23, 2019.
9. Food and Drug Administration. *Electronic Code of Federal Regulations: Title 21 Food and Drugs Part 101.9 Food Labeling*; 2016. https://www.ecfr.gov/cgi-bin/retrieveECFR?%20gp=&SID=bad23c28ebd662323b3ace1e3f5ee94f&mc=true&n=pt.21.2.101&r=PART&ty=HTML#s%20e21.2.101_154. Accessed September 23, 2019.
10. Food and Drug Administration. *Electronic Code of Federal Regulations: Title 21 Food and Drugs Part 101.12 Food Labeling*; 2016. https://www.ecfr.gov/cgi-bin/retrieveECFR?%20gp=&SID=bad23c28ebd662323b3ace1e3f5ee94f&mc=true&n=pt.21.2.101&r=PART&ty=HTML#s%20e21.2.101_154. Accessed September 23, 2019.
11. Food and Drug Administration. *Electronic Code of Federal Regulations: Title 21 Food and Drugs Part 101.9(c)(1)(i)(F) Food Labeling*; 2016. Available Calories for Specific Carbohydrate Substances https://www.ecfr.gov/cgi-bin/retrieveECFR?%20gp=&SID=bad23c28ebd662323b3ace1e3f5ee94f&mc=true&n=pt.21.2.101&r=PART&ty=HTML#s%20e21.2.101_154. Accessed September 23, 2019.
12. Food and Drug Administration. *Electronic Code of Federal Regulations: Title 21 Food and Drugs Part 101.9(c) Food Labeling. Mandatory Declared Macronutrients and Their Daily Values (Adults and Children >4)*; 2016. https://www.ecfr.gov/cgi-bin/retrieveECFR?%20gp=&SID=bad23c28ebd662323b3ace1e3f5ee94f&mc=true&n=pt.21.2.101&r=PART&ty=HTML#s%20e21.2.101_154. Accessed September 23, 2019.
13. Food and Drug Administration. *Electronic Code of Federal Regulations: Title 21 Food and Drugs Part 101.9(c) Food Labeling. Vitamins & Minerals that May Be Declared in The Nutrition Facts and Their Daily Values (Adults and Children >4)*; 2016. https://www.ecfr.gov/cgi-bin/retrieveECFR?%20gp=&SID=bad23c28ebd662323b3ace1e3f5ee94f&mc=true&n=pt.21.2.101&r=PART&ty=HTML#s%20e21.2.101_154. Accessed September 23, 2019.
14. Food and Drug Administration. *Electronic Code of Federal Regulations: Title 21 Food and Drugs Part 101.9(e)(6)(i) Food Labeling. Dual Column Display, Per Serving and Per Container*; 2016. https://www.ecfr.gov/cgi-bin/retrieveECFR?%20gp=&SID=bad23c28ebd662323b3ace1e3f5ee94f&mc=true&n=pt.21.2.101&r=PART&ty=HTML#s%20e21.2.101_154. Accessed September 23, 2019.
15. Food and Drug Administration. *Electronic Code of Federal Regulations: Title 21 Food and Drugs Part 101.9(f) Food Labeling. Simple Display*; 2016. https://www.ecfr.gov/cgi-bin/retrieveECFR?%20gp=&SID=bad23c28ebd662323b3ace1e3f5ee94f&mc=true&n=-pt.21.2.101&r=PART&ty=HTML#s%20e21.2.101_154. Accessed September 23, 2019.
16. Food and Drug Administration. *Electronic Code of Federal Regulations: Title 21 Food and Drugs Part 101.9(d)(11)(iii) Food Labeling. Tabular Format*; 2016. https://www.ecfr.gov/cgi-bin/retrieveECFR?%20gp=&SID=bad23c28ebd662323b3ace1e3f5ee94f&mc=true&n=pt.21.2.101&r=PART&ty=HTML#s%20e21.2.101_154. Accessed September 23, 2019.
17. Food and Drug Administration. *Electronic Code of Federal Regulations: Title 21 Food and Drugs Part 101.9 (j)(13)(ii)(A)(2) Food Labeling. Linear Display for Small or Intermediate-Sized Packages*; 2016. https://www.ecfr.gov/cgi-bin/retrieveECFR?%20gp=&SID=bad23c28ebd662323b3ace1e3f5ee94f&mc=true&n=pt.21.2.101&r=PART&ty=HTML#s%20e21.2.101_154. Accessed September 23, 2019.
18. Food and Drug Administration. *Electronic Code of Federal Regulations: Title 21 Food and Drugs Part 101.36(e) (11)(ii) Food Labeling. Multiple Vitamins (Includes voluntary listing of vitamin D in IUs)*; 2016. https://www.ecfr.gov/cgi-bin/retrieveECFR?%20gp=&SID=bad23c28ebd662323b3ace1e3f5ee94f&mc=true&n=pt.21.2.101&r=PART&ty=HTML#s%20e21.2.101_154. Accessed September 23, 2019.
19. Food and Drug Administration. *Electronic Code of Federal Regulations: Title 21 Food and Drugs Part 107 Infant Formula*; 2016. https://ecfr.io/Title-21/cfr107_main. Accessed September 23, 2019.
20. 101st Cong (1989-1990). *Nutrition Labeling and Education Act of 1990. H.R. 3562*; 1990. https://www.congress.gov/bill/101st-congress/house-bill/3562. Accessed September 23, 2019.
21. 115th Cong (2017–2018). *Agriculture Improvement Act of 2018. H.R.2*; 2018. https://www.congress.gov/bill/115th-congress/house-bill/2. Accessed September 23, 2019.
22. Food and Drug Administration, U.S, Department of Health and Human Services. *Nutrition and Supplement Facts Labels: Questions and Answers Related to the Compliance Date, Added Sugars, and Declaration of Quantitative Amounts of Vitamins and Minerals: Guidance for Industry*; November 2018. https://www.fda.gov/media/117402/download. Accessed November 16, 2019.
23. Food and Drug Administration, U.S, Department of Health and Human Services. *The Declaration of Certain Isolated or Synthetic Non-digestible Carbohydrates as Dietary Fiber on Nutrition and Supplement Facts Labels; Guidance for Industry*; 2018. Availability https://www.federalregister.gov/documents/2018/06/15/2018-12867/the-declaration-of-certain-isolated-or-synthetic-non-digestible-carbohydrates-as-dietary-fiber-on. Accessed September 23, 2019.
24. Food and Drug Administration. *Electronic Code of Federal Regulations: Title 21 Food and Drugs Part 101.9(c) Food Labeling. Isolated or Synthetic Dietary Fiber Sources*; 2016. https://www.ecfr.gov/cgi-bin/retrieveECFR?%20gp=&SID=bad23c28ebd662323b3ace1e3f5ee94f&mc=true&n=pt.21.2.101&r=PART&ty=HTML#s%20e21.2.101_154. Accessed September 23, 2019.
25. European Commission. *Regulation (EU) No 1169/2011 of the European Parliament and of the Council of 25 October 2011 on the Provision of Food Information to Consumers, Amending Regulations (EC) No 1924/2006 and (EC) No 1925/2006 of the European Parliament and of the Council, and Repealing Commission Directive 87/250/EEC, Council Directive 90/496/EEC, Commission Directive 1999/10/EC, Directive 2000/13/EC of the European Parliament and of the Council, Commission Directives 2002/67/EC and 2008/5/EC and Commission Regulation (EC) No 608/2004 Text With EEA Relevance*; October 25, 2019. http://data.europa.eu/eli/reg/2011/1169/oj. Accessed September 23, 2019.
26. Food and Drug Administration. *Electronic Code of Federal Regulations: Title 21 Food and Drugs Part 101.9(c) Food Labeling. Nutrition Information*; 2016. https://www.ecfr.gov/cgi-bin/retrieveECFR?%20gp=&SID=bad23c28ebd662323b3ace1e3f5ee94f&mc=true&n=-pt.21.2.101&r=PART&ty=HTML#s%20e21.2.101_154. Accessed September 23, 2019.
27. Food and Drug Administration. *Label Claims for Conventional Foods and Dietary Supplements*; 2018. https://www.fda.gov/food/food-labeling-nutrition/label-claims-conventional-foods-and-dietary-supplements. Accessed September 23, 2019.
28. Food and Drug Administration. *Electronic Code of Federal Regulations: Title 21 Food and Drugs Part 101.13 Food Labeling*; 2016. https://www.ecfr.gov/cgi-bin/retrieveECFR?%20gp=&SID=bad23c28ebd662323b3ace1e3f5ee94f&mc=true&n=pt.21.2.101&r=PART&ty=HTML#s%20e21.2.101_154. Accessed September 23, 2019.
29. Food and Drug Administration. *Electronic Code of Federal Regulations: Title 21 Food and Drugs Part 101.54-101.67 Food Labeling*; 2016.

https://www.ecfr.gov/cgi-bin/retrieveECFR?%20gp=&SID=bad23c28ebd662323b3ace1e3f5ee94f&mc=true&n=pt.21.2.101&r=PART&ty=HTML#s%20e21.2.101_154. Accessed September 23, 2019.

30. Food and Drug Administration. *Electronic Code of Federal Regulations: Title 21 Food and Drugs Part 101.14 Food Labeling*; 2016. https://www.ecfr.gov/cgi-bin/retrieveECFR?%20gp=&SID=bad23c28ebd662323b3ace1e3f5ee94f&mc=true&n=pt.21.2.101&r=PART&ty=HTML#s%20e21.2.101_154. Accessed September 23, 2019.
31. Food and Drug Administration. *Electronic Code of Federal Regulations: Title 21 Food and Drugs Part 101.72-101.83 Food Labeling*; 2016. https://www.ecfr.gov/cgi-bin/retrieveECFR?%20gp=&SID=bad23c28ebd662323b3ace1e3f5ee94f&mc=true&n=pt.21.2.101&r=PART&ty=HTML#s%20e21.2.101_154. Accessed September 23, 2019.
32. Food and Drug Administration. *Qualified Health Claims*; 2019. https://www.fda.gov/food/food-labeling-nutrition/qualified-health-claims. Accessed September 23, 2019.
33. Food and Drug Administration. *Food and Drug Administration Modernization Act (FDAMA) of 1997*; 2018. https://www.fda.gov/regulatory-information/selected-amendments-fdc-act/food-and-drug-administration-modernization-act-fdama-1997. Accessed September 23, 2019.

CHAPTER

17

FOOD INSECURITY, HUNGER, AND MALNUTRITION

Katherine Alaimo[1], *PhD*
Mariana Chilton[2], *PhD, MPH*
Sonya J. Jones[3], *PhD*

[1]Food Science and Human Nutrition, Michigan State University, East Lansing, MI, United States
[2]Health Management and Policy, Dornsife School of Public Health, Drexel University, Philadelphia, PA, United States
[3]Arnold School of Public Health, University of South Carolina, Columbia, SC, United States

SUMMARY

Food insecurity and malnutrition in all its forms are responsible for more ill health than any other cause. Maternal and child undernutrition contributes to more than 10% of the world's disease burden. Undernutrition contributes up to 45% of preventable deaths among children under 5 years of age, mainly in low- and middle-income countries. The health consequences of overweight and obesity contribute to an estimated 4 million deaths (7.1% of all deaths) and 120 million healthy years of life lost. The global prevalence of severe food insecurity was 10.2% in 2017, affecting 770 million people. Food insecurity and malnutrition are caused by unequal and unjust distribution of nourishing food due to deficiencies in social, economic, political, and ecological systems. Organizations, politicians, and community leaders are demanding and promising transformative approaches to deep poverty and the climate and nature crises that cause malnutrition and hunger. Policies that protect basic human rights and rights of nature can create well-nourished resilient societies.

Keywords: Food insecurity; Food security; Food sovereignty; Human rights; Hunger; Malnutrition; Neoliberalism; Poverty; Rights of nature; Undernutrition.

I. INTRODUCTION

A. Background

Preventing and alleviating hunger and undernutrition and achieving food security are concerns for all societies. Since the first World Food Conference organized by the United Nations (UN) in 1974, a consensus has emerged that "every man, woman and child has the inalienable right to be free from hunger and malnutrition in order to develop their physical and mental faculties."[1] Today, the international community strives for **Food Security**, defined by the UN as a situation that exists when "all people, at all times, have access to sufficient, safe and nutritious food that meets their dietary needs and food preferences for an active and healthy life."[2] The UN declared the years 2016–25 the Decade of Action on Nutrition with the aim "to eradicate hunger, and malnutrition in all its forms (undernutrition, micronutrient deficiencies, overweight or obesity) and reduce the burden of diet-related noncommunicable diseases (NCDs) in all age groups."[3] The Decade of Action on Nutrition provides an opportunity for consolidation and alignment of programs, initiatives, and policy and invites all member states to make specific nutrition commitments and policy measures.

Present Knowledge in Nutrition, Volume 2
https://doi.org/10.1016/B978-0-12-818460-8.00017-4

A recent Lancet Commission Report declared that we are facing a "global syndemic of obesity, undernutrition and climate change," in other words, a synergy of epidemics that "co-occur in time and place, interact with each other to produce complex sequelae, and share common underlying societal drivers"[4] (p.791). In 2015, the UN adopted the 2030 Agenda for Sustainable Development, which included 17 Sustainable Development Goals (SDGs), an "urgent call for action by all countries" encompassing "a shared blueprint for peace and prosperity for people and the planet, now and into the future".[5] The multinational conventions that wrote the SDGs recognized that achieving food security and ending poverty, malnutrition, and other deprivations are fundamental to all the other sustainable development strategies, such as those that seek to improve health and education, reduce inequality, mitigate the climate crisis, and preserve the natural environment.

Each of these policy initiatives underscores the recognition that all people have a basic right to well-being that encompasses a basic right not only to food but also to economic prosperity, human health, social equity, and healthy ecosystems.

B. Key Issues

Increasing international consensus underscores the necessity of systemic changes to values, philosophies, and principles to achieve food security, health, and well-being, and resilience to social, economic, and climate and other ecological shocks.[4,6] This chapter will outline (1) definitions, measurement, and scope of food insecurity, hunger, and malnutrition; (2) an overall conceptual framework for food insecurity including causes, components, and consequences of food insecurity; and (3) underlying principles and actions needed to address food insecurity and malnutrition.

II. DEFINITIONS, EXPLANATORY RELATIONSHIPS, AND SCOPE

This section provides a brief overview of definitions in the context of evaluating progress in meeting international goals defined in UN SDGs for 2030 of ending hunger and all forms of malnutrition.[7–9] Definitions used here are described in the most recently available international consensus documents.[10,2,11]

A. Food Insecurity and Hunger

The second SDGs commits countries to "End hunger, achieve food security and improve nutrition and promote sustainable agriculture."[12] The Food and Agriculture Organization of the UN (FAO) describes **food security** as multidimensional encompassing: (1) availability of food, (2) access to food, (3) ability to utilize food, and (4) stability of food with regard to climatic, economic, social, and political factors. Food security is a continuum, with food security and food insecurity positioned at opposite ends.[13] Instability can be short-term, leading to acute food insecurity, or medium-to long-term, leading to chronic food insecurity.[2]

Food insecurity is a multifaceted phenomenon, as described in Fig. 17.1. Definitions have evolved as deeper understanding and new sources of data have expanded.[12,13] The most common definitions focus on the household level and include four components: (1) **lack of stability** of food supply resulting in a preoccupation, worry, or uncertainty; (2) Consumption of **poor quality food** that may be unsuitable, not culturally appropriate, unsafe, nonnutritious, or monotonous; (3) **food shortage** for one or more family members, or unequal distribution of enough food within a household; and (4) **lack of control over food situation** resulting in either restricted choice, socially unacceptable food sources, or both.[12,14] Food insecurity can be assessed at multiple levels—individual, household, regions of a country, country, and regions of the globe.

Food insecurity is, at its core, an experience of human suffering. Qualitative studies that have sought to understand people's lived experience of food insecurity in a diverse range of cultures have helped to delineate four common interconnected outcomes of food insecurity. FAO defines **hunger** as "an uncomfortable or painful physical sensation caused by insufficient consumption of dietary energy."[2] Food insecurity may or may not lead to individuals experiencing **hunger of the body**, the pain, discomfort, and poor appetite that can accompany food restriction.[15] Food insecurity can result in diminished nutritional quality of food eaten by both adults and children in households, leading to **poor nutrition**—lower than necessary intakes of essential nutrients such as protein, vitamins, and minerals and higher than needed intake of high-energy, low–nutrient-dense foods.[16] Because the food supply is not adequate or stable, food insecure individuals may report **distorted eating patterns** where people do not eat as frequently or reduce quantity. While food insecure parents consistently report restricting their own food consumption to save food for children, if there simply is not enough, inadequate child or infant feeding and distorted household dynamics regarding food can result.[17–19] **Hunger of the mind** describes the psychological and emotional anguish related to the stresses of food insecurity intertwined with poverty, ill health, and exposure to violence. Respondents to qualitative studies report loss of dignity, shame, embarrassment,

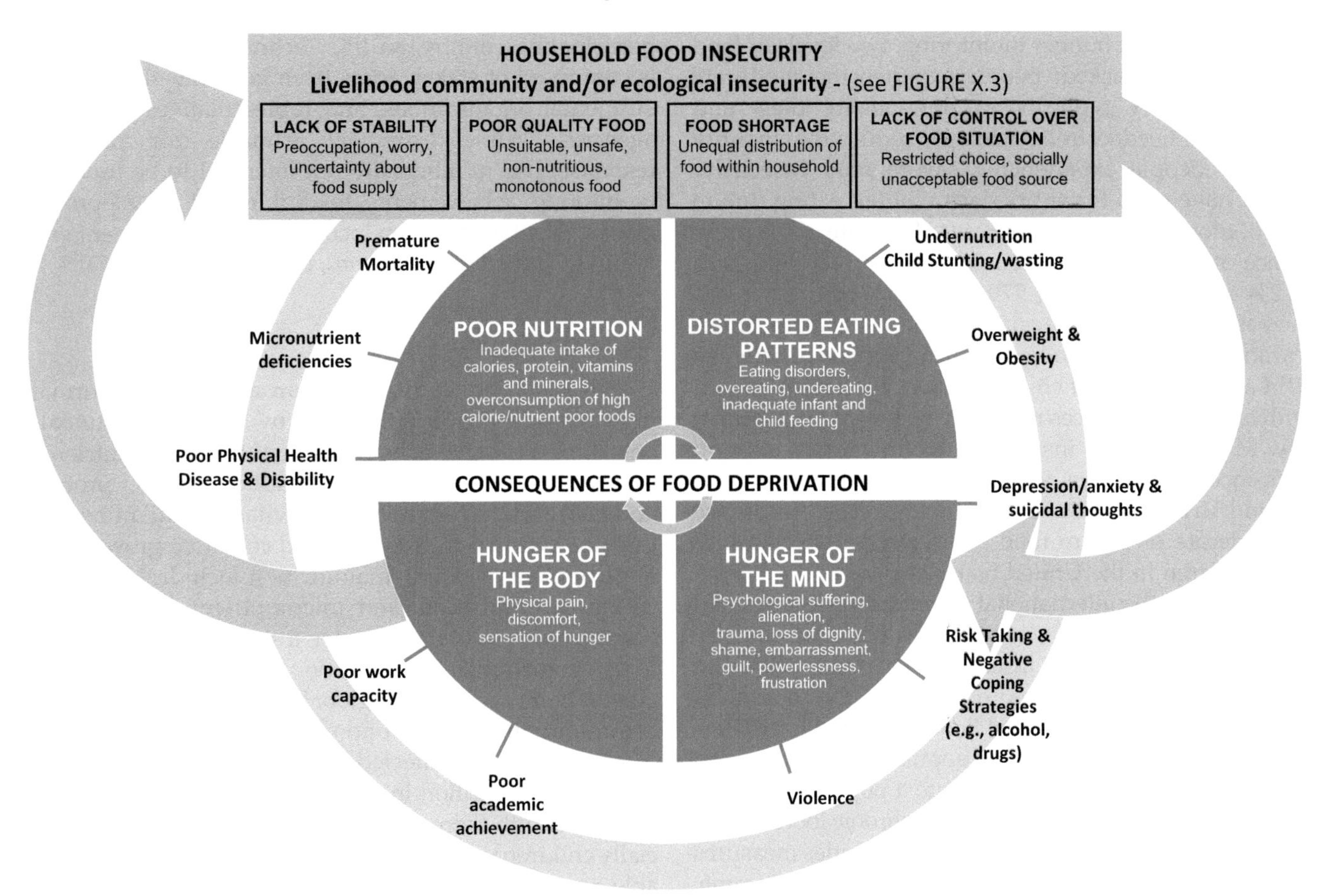

FIGURE 17.1 Components and consequences of household food insecurity.

guilt, powerlessness, stress, fear, alienation, and trauma.[15,20] These experiences of suffering create both individual and collective trauma that have cultural, political, and social implications.[21]

Two measures are used internationally for monitoring and surveillance: Prevalence of Undernutrition and Prevalence of Severe Food Insecurity. For estimating hunger at national and regional levels, the FAO has traditionally used the indicator **prevalence of undernourishment (PoU)**. PoU is an estimate of the proportion of the population whose habitual food consumption is insufficient to provide the dietary energy levels that are required to maintain an active, healthy life. PoU is a percentage based on the cumulative probability that daily habitual dietary energy intakes are below minimum dietary energy requirements.[22] Habitual dietary energy intake levels are computed differently for each country based on available data. Data sources include nationally representative household surveys, and estimates of per capita supply of calories, which are derived from FAO **Food Balance Sheets** for most countries. Food balance sheets estimate the total amount of food available for consumption in a country. Food imported and produced is documented, as are factors that reduce availability such as exports, livestock feed, seed, nonfood uses, and storage and transportation losses.[2,22,23] The global PoU was 10.9% in 2017 affecting 821 million people.[2] Some progress had been made, but the prevalence has been increasing over the past 3 years, reverting to levels seen over a decade ago.[2]

The FAO recently expanded the PoU and adopted a survey instrument based on people's actual food experiences. The **Food Insecurity Experience Scale**, based on the groundwork conducted to develop the 18-item Food Insecurity and Hunger Scale utilized in the United States and other countries, is composed of eight simple yes/no questions that elicit responses along a continuum of severity.[12] The continuum describes experiences beginning with worrying about running out of food, then to compromising on the quality and variety of food, to reducing quantities, and, lastly, to skipping meals and going without eating for days.[24] The questions provide a universal, reliable, and valid metric of the severity of the food insecurity situation of respondents in different cultural, linguistic, and development contexts.[12]

Based on answers to the eight questions, an individual's degree of food insecurity is identified. For the purpose of global hunger monitoring, two levels of food insecurity are tracked: people experiencing **moderate food insecurity** typically eat low-quality diets and might have needed to occasionally reduce the quantity of food. People experiencing **severe food insecurity** would have gone for entire days without eating due to lack of money or other resources.[25] Estimate of the prevalence of severe food insecurity based on the FIES was 10.2% in 2017, affecting 770 million people.[2,12] It has increased since 2014 in every region except North America and Europe.[2] Among countries surveyed between 2014 and 2015, 41% of children under age 15 years lived with an adult who faces moderate or severe food insecurity. Moderate food insecurity ranges greatly even in high-income countries with Japan at the lowest rate at 1% and Uruguay at the highest at 28%. The prevalence of moderate or severe food insecurity among families with children in the United States is 20%.[26]

Since 2004, the international community has benefited from a common global scale for classifying the severity and magnitude of food insecurity and malnutrition to identify populations in need of urgent action to address food insecurity, the **Integrated Food Security Phase Classification (IPC)**.[11,27] For a given population, IPC uses data as recent as 2–3 months to evaluate a population group on three levels: acute food insecurity, chronic food insecurity, and acute malnutrition. Each level includes measures of severity—from non/minimal to catastrophic/famine. The IPC utilizes multiple information sources in the public domain, including direct communication or measurement of individuals at the household level (such as availability of food, patterns of food consumption, ability to purchase food, patterns of livelihood, and degree of stunting in children), and other factors such as drought, tsunami, below-normal food production, rising food prices, conflict, and destruction of means of livelihood. Mitigating factors such as the availability of humanitarian aid are also considered.

To interpret the urgency from various sources of complex information, a consensus process is used. In each participating country, an IPC Technical Working Group is composed of stakeholders from government, nongovernmental organizations, and representatives from UN agencies. While extremely valuable for strategic response, IPC numbers are not intended to be used for monitoring achievements toward global development goals.[27] The IPC has been incorporated into a larger *Early Warning Early Action Initiative*, coordinated by FAO.[28]

B. Malnutrition

The FAO defines **malnutrition** as an "an abnormal physiological condition caused by inadequate, unbalanced, or excessive consumption of the macronutrients that provide dietary energy (carbohydrates, protein and fats) and the micronutrients (vitamins and minerals) that are essential for physical and cognitive growth and development."[29] Thus, malnutrition includes undernutrition, overnutrition, and micronutrient deficiencies.[2] For the purpose of this chapter, a small subset of indicators of malnutrition will be described, which are currently measured on a global basis. The international community has agreed upon these indicators.[7,8]

Every country is affected by malnutrition; food insecurity and malnutrition in all its forms are responsible for more ill health than any other cause.[10,30] Children, especially children under 5 years of age, are extremely vulnerable to malnutrition (see Box 17.1). Even if children survive and recover from early malnutrition, their cognitive ability can be irrevocably damaged, physical development impaired, and risk of obesity and chronic diseases later in life elevated.[31] Monitoring for childhood malnutrition focuses, first, on undernutrition, which contributes to 45% of deaths of children under 5 years of age.[32,33] Maternal and child undernutrition contributes to more than 10% of the world's disease burden.[34] **Undernutrition** is the result of insufficient or poor quality food intake but can also result from an unsanitary environment that exposes children to repeated infections leading to poor absorption or utilization of the nutrients

BOX 17.1

Global Prevalence of Malnutrition in Children Under 5 Years of Age as of 2017–18

- **Wasting** (7.3%)—49 million affected, of whom 17 million are severely wasted.[31]
- **Stunting** (21.9%)—149 million affected.[31]
- **Stunting + wasting** (3.62%)—almost 16 million affected.[35]
- **Overweight** (5.9%)—40 million affected.[31]
- **Trend**: Malnutrition in all its forms remains unacceptably high across all regions of the world. Some reductions have been seen in the prevalence of stunting, but not in wasting. The number of overweight children has increased steadily since 2000.[31]

consumed. The interactions between infection and nutrition create a cycle whereby poor diets compromise immune function making children more susceptible to infections; at the same time, infections can decrease nutrient absorption, worsening nutritional status.[36]

Wasting in children under age 5 (acute malnutrition)

A child who suffers from wasting has a weight that is much lower than expected for her or his height. Wasting is generally the result of weight loss or failure to gain weight associated with a recent period of inadequate calorie intake and/or disease. Children suffering from wasting have weakened immunity, are susceptible to long-term developmental delays, and face increased risk of death, particularly when wasting is severe (12-fold increase in risk).[31,37] Wasting is defined as weight-for-height less than 2 standard deviations below the WHO Child Growth Standard median. Wasting is classified as severe at less than 3 standard deviations below the WHO Child Growth Standard median.[2,31,38]

Stunting in children under age 5 (chronic malnutrition)

A child who is stunted has a height much lower than expected for her or his age and is defined as height or length-for-age less than 2 standard deviations below the WHO Child Growth Standards median.[2,38] Stunting is the devastating result of long-term nutritional deprivation since conception caused by recurrent infections, lack of water, and/or sanitation infrastructures. Children suffering from stunting may never attain their full possible height and their brains may never develop to their full cognitive potential.[31] Stunted children have a higher risk of obesity and chronic disease later in life. Children with severe stunting have a fivefold risk of dying.[37]

Wasting and stunting are interrelated. A child experiencing wasting is more likely to become stunted, and a stunted child is more likely to become wasted.[39] Children who are concurrently wasted and stunted may have even greater mortality risk than those with either wasting or stunting.[35,37,39]

Overweight in children under 5

An overweight child is too heavy for his or her height. For international monitoring, children under 5 are classified as overweight if their weight-for-height is more than 2 standard deviations above median.[38] This form of malnutrition results when a child's energy intakes from food and beverages exceed the child's energy requirements. Overweight in children is a concern because it increases risk for some chronic diseases later in life.[10] However, overweight and malnutrition are not mutually exclusive. Consumption of foods of low-nutrient quality can result in micronutrient deficiencies. Although the precise mechanism is not fully understood, 1.8% of under 5 years of age globally (8.23 million children) experience both stunting and overweight.[40,41]

Micronutrient deficiency and anemia in women of childbearing age

Micronutrient deficiencies are defined as suboptimal nutritional status caused by a lack of intake, absorption, or use of one or more vitamins or minerals. For the purpose of international malnutrition monitoring, the prevalence of anemia, a sign of micronutrient deficiency, in women of childbearing age is monitored in most countries. anemia is prevalent globally, disproportionately affecting children and women of reproductive age. Iron deficiency is one of the most common causes of anemia[42]; it can also be caused by deficiencies of folic acid and/or vitamin B12 or by nonnutritional causes such as cancer and sickle cell anemia.[10,2,43] Whatever its specific cause, anemia negatively affects cognitive and motor development. Among pregnant women, iron deficiency anemia is associated with adverse reproductive outcomes, including preterm delivery and low birth weight among infants.[44] It is estimated that 1.5 billion people in the world are affected by one or more forms of micronutrient deficiency.[30,2] In 2016, 32.8% (632.6 million) of childbearing age women were anemic, 35.3 million of which were pregnant.[43] Prevalence has risen incrementally each year since 2012. No progress has been made toward 2030 goal of a 50% reduction.

Underweight in women of childbearing years

Because of the importance of nutritional status for women of childbearing age, which can profoundly affect the health and survival potential of her children and their families, prepregnancy underweight is measured as a risk for preterm and low birth weight babies.[10] **Moderate underweight** in adults is defined by a body mass index (BMI) less than 18.5, while **severe thinness or underweight** in adult populations is defined as a BMI less than 17.0.[10] Although not currently monitored for the SDGs, moderate underweight increases illness, and severe underweight is associated with dramatic increases in mortality.[10]

Overweight and obesity in adults

Overweight and obesity in adults refers to body weight above normal for height as a result of an excessive accumulation of fat. In adults, overweight is defined as a BMI of more than 25 kg/m^2 but less than 30 kg/m^2 and obesity as a BMI of 30 kg/m^2 or more.[2] (Note: Though a rough estimate, BMI provides a population-level measure of overweight and obesity for both sexes and for all ages of adults.)[45] High BMI (including overweight/obesity) and high waist-to-height ratio are risk factors for chronic diseases such as cardiovascular disease, type 2 diabetes, chronic kidney disease, cancer, and musculoskeletal disorders.[46,47] Prevalence of obesity has nearly tripled since 1975. 38.9% of adults (1.9 billion) are overweight, of whom 13.1% are obese (650 million).

C. Global Nutrition Transition and Triple Burden of Malnutrition

As countries undergo economic globalization, the food supply transitions from subsistence agricultural production to imported food markets of energy-dense, nutrient-poor foods.[36] Twelve commodity plant crops, primarily wheat, corn, and sugar, have in many cases replaced diverse diets of native foods; this nutrition transition that shifts the way the people eat and drink, as well as reduced levels of physical activity, is seen in both urban and rural areas of the world.[36,48–52] Worldwide, most places have dietary patterns that include higher intakes of animal foods, sugars, highly processed foods, and lower intakes of fiber-rich plant foods. This transition gradually leads to increased energy intake leading to increasing rates of noncommunicable chronic diseases, such as obesity and diabetes, while at the same time resulting in micronutrient deficiencies. The coexistence of food insecurity, undernutrition, and overweight and obesity is now referred to as the "triple burden" of malnutrition.[36,53]

D. Mechanisms of Physical and Psychological Consequences of Food Insecurity and Malnutrition

Food insecurity, hunger, and malnutrition create consequences through nutritional and nonnutritional pathways. Food is a fundamental need, but only one of the needs that people have for survival and to participate in society. Other deprivation can be related to war, oppression or conflict, or important societal systems such as health care, education, housing, and ecosystems. These systems are determined by the fundamental causes described in the next section and can intersect with food deprivation to ameliorate or exacerbate consequences. Fig. 17.1 illustrates the interrelationships between the components of food insecurity, malnutrition, and consequences including undernutrition, overweight and obesity, micronutrient deficiencies, premature mortality, poor physical health, depression anxiety and suicidal thoughts, poor work capacity, poor academic achievement, risk taking, and negative coping strategies and violence.

The most direct way to understand the health effects of food insecurity is through how food insecurity affects the quality of food people can buy or grow, which in turn is associated with poor diet quality, nutrient inadequacies, and chronic health conditions such as diabetes, poor self-rated health, and depression.[54,55] Additionally, adults report making "trade-offs" between paying for health care and medications or food, and this makes it difficult to adhere to recommended treatment of chronic diseases such as HIV/AIDS, diabetes, and cancer.[56–59]

Food insecurity and malnutrition affect physical, mental, and emotional health and cognitive well-being across the life span.[60] Food insecurity during pregnancy affects the intrauterine environment, which has an impact on birth outcomes.[61] When young children are food insecure, their social, cognitive, and emotional development falters, diminishing their ability to start school well-prepared. The health effects of food insecurity and malnutrition are most pronounced among young children during the first 3–5 years of life when significant growth and development are taking place. Inadequate or interrupted food intake, even for a short time, can cause long-lasting health problems such as iron-deficient anemia,[62] increased symptoms of respiratory illness, and other types of infections that are associated with increased hospitalizations and overall poor health status.[63,64] Compared to young children living in food secure households, children living in food insecure households have limited cognitive, emotional, and social development.[65] Not only does developmental risk affect their quality of life but also negatively affects school readiness and subsequent success later in life.[66] Food insecurity has similar impacts on school-age children and adolescents.[67] When compared to similar school-aged children in food-secure households, children in food-insecure households were more likely to repeat a grade, have lower reading and math scores, to report challenges in their social relationships,[68,69] and were more likely to exhibit both internalizing and externalizing behavioral problems.[70] The negative consequences can proceed from there, through the school years, to adolescence, and can then translate into greater risk-taking behaviors, such as having many sexual partners, drug and alcohol abuse, greater exposure to violence, and high-risk pregnancy, affecting the next generation in turn.[71] Like the youngest children, adolescents are in a critically important developmental window, and if they are in food-insecure homes, they can struggle with poor mental health and suicidal ideation.[72–74] While household food insecurity affects the children, poor child health can in turn decrease household income by affecting their caregivers' ability to maintain steady employment.[75,76]

Though many believe that parents shield their children from experiencing food insecurity,[77–79] research among children showed that despite their parents' attempts to protect them, school-aged children are aware of food insecurity, find ways to manage household food, and can feel helpless and angry when they have to go without food.[18] Among adults, food insecurity is associated with adverse mental health outcomes.[80] Food insecurity is associated with depressive symptoms, major depression, and anxiety among mothers, which may negatively affect child health outcomes.[81] Mothers who report depressive symptoms experience more employment difficulties.[82,83]

These serious health consequences of food insecurity and malnutrition cannot be considered without addressing the underlying dynamics in family systems, as well as in their economic, social, and political contexts. A significant consideration of family dynamics of food insecurity, poor health, and depression is exposure to violence and trauma. In studies of current and recent exposure to violence, intimate partner violence was found to be associated with increased odds of food insecurity among women,[83,84] and depressive symptoms may mediate this association.[84] Exposure to abuse, neglect, or household instability in childhood is also linked with food insecurity in adulthood. In several studies, women exposed to childhood abuse and/or violence throughout their lives were more likely to report food insecurity compared with those who had not.[85,86] Women who report experiencing posttraumatic stress disorder or associated symptoms are more likely to report household food insecurity.[70,84,87] Such exposure to violence indicates that gender discrimination can reverberate throughout the family through violence, trauma, and food insecurity. Gender discrimination is also at play when considering women's wages compared men's, as well as the disparities in wages between women of color and those who are white. Hence, exposure to violence in the families that are associated with food insecurity is also directly related to gender and racial/ethnic discrimination in society.[88–91]

III. CURRENT STATUS OF FIELD (DOMESTICALLY AND INTERNATIONALLY)

A. Causes of Food Insecurity, Hunger, and Malnutrition

Resilience-based framing and the stress adaption process

Most food security research literature views households through a deficit-based lens, characterizing the seemingly immutable causes of food insecurity, related to issues such as lack of education, limited social networks, depression, household structure such as single-parent homes, unemployment, and low wages.[81,92,93] For example, children in the United States are more likely to be food insecure if they live in certain household structures, including households headed by a single mother, classified as black or Hispanic, in large metropolitan areas, in the South, with older children and with incomes below 185% of the poverty level.[92] A worldwide study examined the global determinants of food insecurity and found that education, social networks, and social capital were the strongest determinants.[26] These studies focused on the deficits in individuals, households, communities, and states, creating an almost overwhelming list of correlates of food insecurity. There is a connective tissue underneath all of these correlates. As shown in Fig. 17.2, we offer an organizing framework for these findings that points to deeper determinants of food insecurity.

Jean Drèze and Amartya Sen suggest that hunger is about "who has control over what."[94] The fact that a society can have plenty of food yet still have people reporting that they are food insecure suggests that hunger is not only about lack of food per se but is rather about but people's lack of power to access food either through equitable access to land and water or the money to secure food. It follows that if people had more control over their own lives, they would be able to secure the necessary food for themselves. People's ability to be resilient in the face of adversity should point to new ways of fostering potential solutions to food insecurity.

All of the factors described through the deficit-based lens can be better framed through resiliency. **Resilience** is defined as the "ability of any system—household, community, ecosystem—to withstand shocks and positively adapt."[95] In the psychology literature, theories such as family adjustment and adaptation response model describe how households balance their demands and capabilities in the face of stressful life events to achieve positive outcomes. A resilience frame can fundamentally alter the focus of food insecurity by recognizing food insecure families as challenged or overwhelmed by disruptive or traumatic events, rather than deficient or dysfunctional.[95]

Many of the correlates of household food security, when framed through resiliency, would be considered as part of a **stress adaptation process**. For instance, the number of stressful life events experienced in the past year and the types and severity of stressful life events are all associated with food security. Experiencing life events laden with **economic stress** (e.g., losing a job, reduction in hours, changing jobs) resulted in a 54% increased odds of food insecurity in one study.[96] Likewise, family or personal stressful life events (e.g., a parent's death) increased the odds of household food insecurity by 22%. In the same study, households with higher incomes, higher Special Supplemental Nutrition Program (SNAP) benefit levels, and greater social support were able to avoid child hunger in the face of stressful life events.[95] Other studies also have found that food insecurity is associated with stressful life events.[97] Temple found in a nationally representative study of Australians that food insecurity was associated with life events laden with **social stress**, such as witnessing violence or being a victim of discrimination or a violent crime, or the stress associated with, or as a result of, having a mental illness, a serious disability, or serious illness, or having an accident.[98] Social stress can also

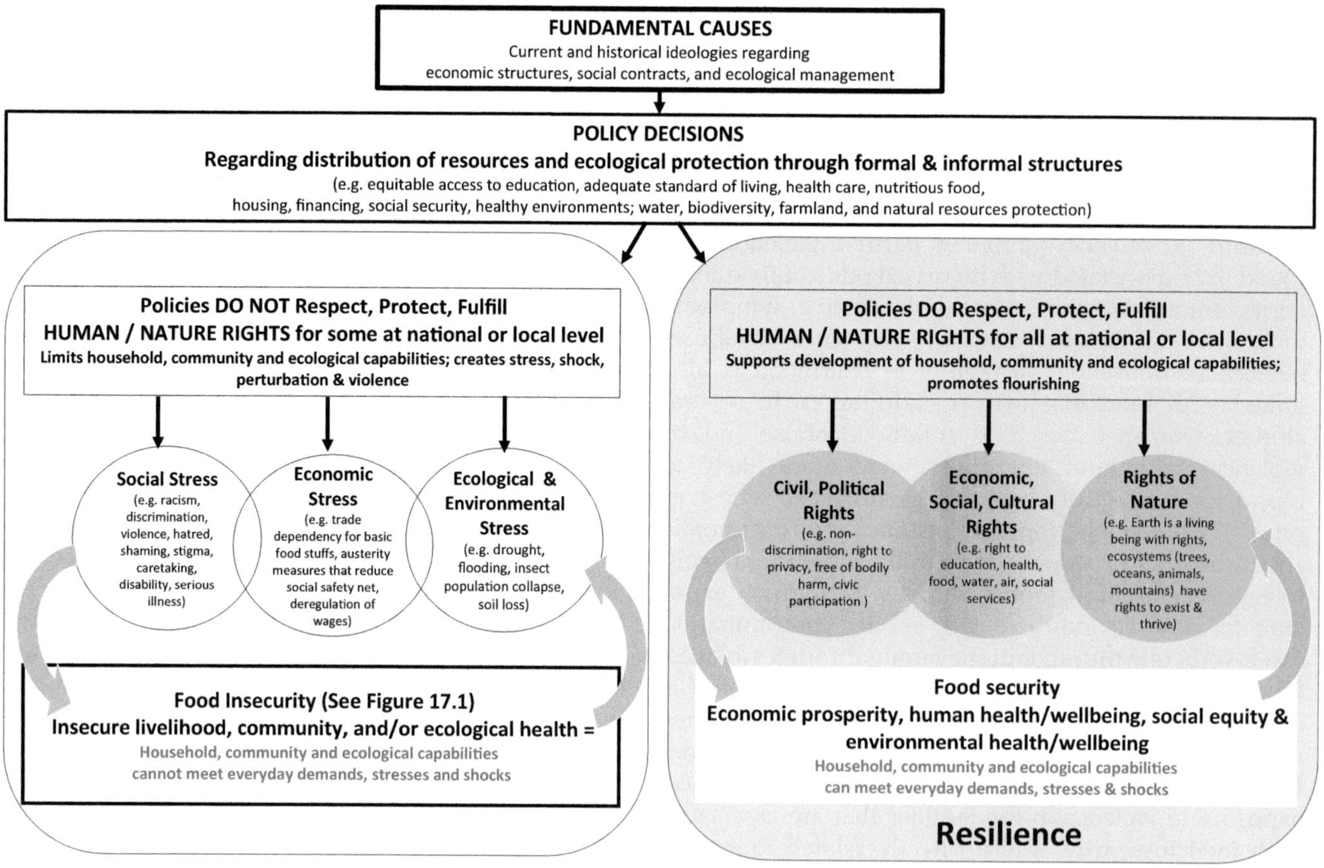

FUNDAMENTAL CAUSES
Current and historical ideologies regarding economic structures, social contracts, and ecological management

POLICY DECISIONS
Regarding distribution of resources and ecological protection through formal & informal structures
(e.g. equitable access to education, adequate standard of living, health care, nutritious food, housing, financing, social security, healthy environments; water, biodiversity, farmland, and natural resources protection)

Policies DO NOT Respect, Protect, Fulfill
HUMAN / NATURE RIGHTS for some at national or local level
Limits household, community and ecological capabilities; creates stress, shock, perturbation & violence

Social Stress (e.g. racism, discrimination, violence, hatred, shaming, stigma, caretaking, disability, serious illness)

Economic Stress (e.g. trade dependency for basic food stuffs, austerity measures that reduce social safety net, deregulation of wages)

Ecological & Environmental Stress (e.g. drought, flooding, insect population collapse, soil loss)

Food Insecurity (See Figure 17.1)
Insecure livelihood, community, and/or ecological health =
Household, community and ecological capabilities cannot meet everyday demands, stresses and shocks

Policies DO Respect, Protect, Fulfill
HUMAN / NATURE RIGHTS for all at national or local level
Supports development of household, community and ecological capabilities; promotes flourishing

Civil, Political Rights (e.g. non-discrimination, right to privacy, free of bodily harm, civic participation)

Economic, Social, Cultural Rights (e.g. right to education, health, food, water, air, social services)

Rights of Nature (e.g. Earth is a living being with rights, ecosystems (trees, oceans, animals, mountains) have rights to exist & thrive)

Food security
Economic prosperity, human health/wellbeing, social equity & environmental health/wellbeing
Household, community and ecological capabilities can meet everyday demands, stresses & shocks

Resilience

FIGURE 17.2 Rights - based approach to understanding food insecurity.

include historical or current colonialism, racism, and discrimination.

Such stressors have been analyzed in the political economic context of the growing hegemony of global neoliberalism. Neoliberalism is a resurgence of laissez faire liberalism and free market capitalism ideas popular in the 19th century. In this type of political economy, the emphasis is on a variety of approaches to economic liberalization including: privatization, austerity, deregulation, trade liberalization, free trade, and extractivism resulting in ecological degradation.

Privatization takes activities done in the interests of the public, such as food distribution, and allows private interests to pursue profits in that activity and shift payment for such activity to individual citizens. For example, since 1996 in the United States, states can spend Temporary Assistance for Needy Families public dollars to purchase private contractor services rather than only in direct assistance to poor families.[99] Of the estimated $233,610 2015 dollars needed to raise a child (similar in both the United States and Sweden), public expenditures are heavily privatized in the United States, so that only 0.7% of US GDP is spent on public family benefits while 3.6% of Swedish GDP is spent on public support for parental leave, daycare, preschool, public school, afterschool activities, summer camps, colleges, and other supports.[100] As a result, children are more vulnerable to income shocks in the US.[101,102]

Austerity policies are designed to reduce government services presumably to keep the tax burden on private entities low and often are implemented when government's debt burdens can no longer be serviced. For instance, European Union countries—Ireland, Italy, Spain, and Greece—all agreed to massive cuts in public spending on their social safety nets as part of their debt restructuring agreements with the International Monetary Fund and the EU Central Bank. After these measures were imposed, the proportion of people who were found to be food insecure (using a proxy measure) across Europe increased from 8.7% to 10.9%, an increase of 13.5 million people.[103]

Deregulation of industries refers to a wide variety of rules that governments usually manage to ensure the public good. Many of them might affect food insecurity, but one of the most significant examples is the de facto deregulation of a federal minimum wage in the United States, which has not increased in 27 years. An economic analysis by the Century Foundation suggests that if instead of deregulating minimum wages, a policy that gradually increased wages in the United States to $15 per hour by 2025 would reduce food insecurity by 6.5%.[104] In this analysis, variations between federal and state minimum wage laws were used to model a gradual increase in wages over 8 years and the numbers of people predicted to become food secure with each increase, based on state estimates of the prevalence of food security.

Trade liberalization policies have been unevenly enacted globally, with the United States, Europe, and Japan endorsing strong protectionism for their own agriculture sector while encouraging trade liberalization in other countries. Trade liberalization has been the primary focus of the World Bank, the FAO, and the UN as a strategy to reduce global hunger. Otero and colleagues have found that trade liberalization policies effectively create relationships of dependency in which economically dominant countries, such as the United States, import "luxury foods," such as fruits and vegetables, while protecting grain and meat markets. Trade partners, such as Mexico, Turkey, and Brazil, on the other hand have shifted their diet toward more imported grains and meats and produce less of the food that their citizens eat. Stable and resilient economic growth are considered important factors in ensuring food security, but 78% of malnourished children live in countries with food surpluses.[105] As more and more economies adopt neoliberalism ideologies, farmers shift from subsistence production and managing commons to privately held land and commodity production. Simply put, neoliberal policies encourage people to sell crops and/or labor to buy food instead of promoting self-sufficiency.

Free trade policies are those that emphasize little government role in how goods are exchanged across counties.[106] Suweis, Carr, Maritan et al. (2015) argue that international trade coupled with growing populations destabilizes local food systems making food insecurity more likely. Free trade agreements are internationally enforceable laws that can limit citizens' abilities to respond to food security crises. Free trade policies that opened up rice markets in Asia, for instance, led to increased hunger and poverty in Indonesia, Ghana, and Honduras.[107] Free trade agreements often include the so-called investor-state dispute settlement agreements that allow investors to sue states if they pass laws that discriminate against a business. When Mexico sought to ensure nutritional security by reducing sweetened beverage consumption through a soda tax, they were sued by Corn Producers International, Cargill, and Archer Daniels Midland and paid millions in fines for discrimination against high-fructose corn syrup.[108]

The type of economic development that accompanies the neoliberal political economic development is focused on the extraction of natural resources from an environment. **Extractionism** has multiple implications for food security, as land and forests that were natural food sources for local populations become sources of minerals, timber, or energy that are traded on free markets and phosphorous and nitrogen are extracted to create chemical fertilizers. Extractionism also impacts our ability to produce food locally as the mining and by-products of extractionism cause **ecological and environmental degradation** of water, fisheries, land cover, soil, and air.[109] Food insecurity currently is an issue of poorly distributed resources, but in the ecology literature, food security is defined as "maintaining production of sufficient and nutritious food in the face of chronic and acute environmental perturbations."[110] The climate and loss of nature crises facing the earth, resulting in more frequent and intense weather events, and loss of important food resources such as topsoil and ocean life have already become significant drivers of hunger and undernutrition.[6,111,112] Countries whose agriculture systems exhibit greater sensitivity to rainfall and temperature variability and those more dependent on fishing and subsistence agriculture are at increased susceptibility.[4]

Many scholars also point to the looming ecological challenges of human-generated inputs to food production, such as fertilizing crops with mined phosphorous and irrigating with redirected rivers. Ensuring a sustainable food supply therefore requires a variety of so-called ecosystems services. Bommarco and colleagues describe the ecosystem services required to support food security as soil formation and nutrient cycling, biological pest controls, and crop pollination. Specifically, they identified the well-documented declines in the organic matter, which are a consequence of fertilization and irrigation. Organic matter feeds microbial communities in soils. These microbial communities increase the nutrient content, and water-holding capacity reduces erosion and ultimately supports higher productivity and efficiency of crops. Weeds and animal pests cause about 30% of maize and 14%–35% of wheat losses worldwide.[113] Chemical controls have not reduced these losses, and ecological management techniques that maintain beneficial checks and balances on pest populations are important ecosystem services for food security. Lastly, about 75% of all food crops require a pollinator to produce foods. Honeybees currently provide most pollination services for crops, and their population declines along with other wild pollinators are a cause of crop yield declines in some areas.

B. Moving Toward Food Security

As described in the previous section, food insecurity is not solely due to a lack of food production or availability but rather to the unequal and unjust distribution of people's entitlements to social, economic, and agroecological support.[114] Food insecurity is a symptom of multiple crises in social, economic, political, and ecological systems. These crises have out-paced conventional approaches to food insecurity worldwide. In order to address food insecurity, governments, community leaders, scientists, and civil society must address the underlying causes that take into account the dynamics of neoliberalism. These societal and political forces cause greater vulnerability that make and/or keep people marginalized, poor, and that test the resilience of individuals and communities to resist, adapt, and thrive.

Governments can implement policies and programs to improve food security worldwide, which are either "nutrition specific" or "nutrition sensitive" as described in Box 17.3. In the global North, many countries such as Sweden, Norway, the Netherlands, and Germany have robust social systems that support families and prevent deep poverty. In the United States, there are examples of nutrition assistance programming that help treat and limit food insecurity but do not eradicate it. Each in their own right, the US SNAP, the Special Supplemental Nutrition Program for Women, Infants, and Children, and school meals programs have helped to reduce food insecurity and improve health.[16] However, these nutrition support programs have not and will not fully protect households against food insecurity without a comprehensive, nationwide strategy to ensure equitable reach and coverage, especially for indigenous, immigrant, and otherwise marginalized communities who are struggling with low wages and lack of steady, predictable, and well-paying employment.[115] Similarly, in the United Kingdom, recent austerity measures and government sanctions have been poorly administered.[116,117] Widespread inadequate supports for families have spurred the institutionalization of emergency food provision against the will of large sectors of society. Australia is experiencing similar dynamics.[118] In the global North, support systems for families are becoming more and more frayed. Simultaneously, trade agreements around the world help to facilitate the march of multinational corporations, which claim to address hunger through donations to emergency efforts, promotion of fortified and genetically altered, patented seeds, and the use of antibiotics, growth hormones, and pesticides. However, these efforts are causing more ecological devastation and further diminish the power and agency of people who are poor.

Organizations, politicians, and community leaders are demanding and promising transformative approaches to deep poverty and hunger. These approaches adopt a human rights framework and link human rights to environmental sustainability, as can be seen in the SDGs (see Box 17.2). Currently, there are growing appeals to the rights of nature to ensure that humans and all other species may survive and thrive with enough food, water, soil, and clean air to sustain life on the planet. Policy protections provided through the intersection of human rights and the rights of nature can create resilient societies (Fig. 17.3).

C. Basic Human Rights, Rights of Nature, and Food Sovereignty

A human rights approach to address malnutrition has captured international attention since the international community agreed on the 1945 Universal Declaration of Human Rights (UDHR). Over the following decades,

BOX 17.2

International Resources for Nutrition Planning

- **Sustainable Development Goals** https://sustainabledevelopment.un.org
- **WHO OneHealth Tool** https://www.who.int/choice/onehealthtool/en/
- **e-Library of Evidence for Nutrition Actions (eLENA)** https://www.who.int/elena/en
- **WHO guidelines for providing nutrition in emergencies** https://www.who.int/nutrition/topics/emergencies/en/
- **Nutrition in health response in emergencies: WHO perspectives and developments** https://www.ennonline.net/fex/56/nutritionhealthresponsewho
- **Core Humanitarian Standard on Quality and Accountability** https://corehumanitarianstandard.org/
- **Voluntary Guidelines to Support the Progressive Realization of the Right to Adequate Food in the Context of National Food Security,** Adopted by the 127th Session of the FAO Council in November 2004 http://www.fao.org/3/a-y7937e.pdf

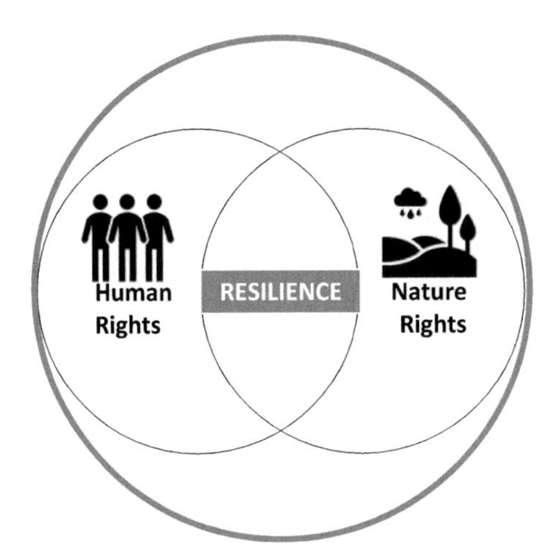

FIGURE 17.3 Resilience is achieved through protection of human and nature rights.

the UDHR bifurcated into two international covenants that have been ratified by most UN member states: the International Covenant of **Civil and Political Rights**, and the 1966 International Covenant on **Economic, Social, and Cultural Rights**. A human rights approach to food, according to the UN Economic and Social Council, aims to ensure that every person, alone or in community with others, has physical and economic access at all times to adequate food or means for its procurement. The right to food does not necessarily require governments to provide food directly. Rather, it obligates governments to respect the right (not prevent people from obtaining food), protect the right (ensure others do not prevent people from obtaining food), and fulfill the right (provide what is necessary for people to nourish themselves).[119,120]

Viewing food security as a human rights issue means that ensuring good nutrition should not be left to benevolence or charity but instead should be viewed as a duty and obligation of a country to its people.[121,122] Central to the human rights approach is ensuring that, at the level of states and or nations, there is a national plan to respect, protect, and fulfill the right to food, and a comprehensive approach to ensure participation of many stakeholders (especially those who are most affected by food insecurity), in the development of solutions, as well as for redress and repair when the right to food is violated. This demands national measurement mechanisms for monitoring and accountability. Some countries (including the United States) have mechanisms for monitoring but still lack a national plan.

Nation state structures are not the only platform through which to protect, respect, and fulfill the right to food. There is a growing surge of grassroots groups that are connecting in spirit and in action to advance the rights of nature in order to protect their lands and rivers, and thereby their food and water. Further consideration that recognizes peoples' right to participate in food systems decision-making and the necessity of caretaking and sustaining the natural resources needed for food production is encompassed in the growing international **Food Sovereignty** movement. Food sovereignty is defined by movement leaders as the "right of peoples to health and culturally appropriate food produced through ecologically sound and sustainable methods, and their right to define their own food and agricultural systems."[123]

The **Rights of Nature** is a burgeoning area of earth law that promotes the concept of the rights of ecosystems to exist, persist, and flourish.[124] Rights of nature arise from indigenous and traditional understandings of human food systems and have been written into laws in countries, such as Bolivia, Ecuador, and New Zealand.[125–127] When the rights of a natural ecosystem,

BOX 17.3

Nutrition-Specific and Nutrition-Sensitive Investments

The 2018 Global Nutrition Report describes nutrition-specific and nutrition-sensitive investments:

> "**Nutrition-specific investments** are considered high impact nutrition interventions that address the immediate determinants of malnutrition. The 2013 *The Lancet* Series on Maternal and Child Nutrition recommends 10 direct interventions such as micronutrient supplementation or fortification, acute malnutrition treatment and exclusive breastfeeding and complementary feeding of young children.
>
> **Nutrition-sensitive investments** address the underlying causes of undernutrition. They include actions from a range of sectors including: health, agriculture and food systems, water, sanitation and hygiene promotion (WASH), education and social protection. Such examples of investments might include improving the purchasing power of women, improving access to food, diversifying agriculture, advancing biofortification, promoting healthy diets, supporting breastfeeding and improving access to WASH."[1](p.98)

such as a forest or river, are recognized, then advocates and regular citizens have legal recourse to protect the ecosystem against degradation and extractivism.[128] The rights of nature bring forth a sense of a global planetary citizenship that transcends state boundaries and is increasingly being incorporated into the food sovereignty movement.[129] As the neoliberal enterprise shifts control of food security away from households, communities, and states toward multinational corporations and global organizations, some countries and communities are responding to this lack of control by asserting their food sovereignty. La Via Campesina, an organization that brings together peasants, farmers, landless people, rural women and youth, indigenous people, migrants, and agricultural workers, and the governments of Ecuador and Bolivia have resisted neoliberal food regimes in their communities and countries by advancing the rights of nature and food sovereignty.[126,130] The Global Alliance for the Rights of Nature was formed in 2010, and at the UN, the Rights to Harmony with Nature were officially recognized. Within these efforts against the conventional and powerful geopolitical tides, ecological and human concerns become central to human well-being and geopolitics, instead of profits, capital, or accumulated wealth. Examples of cases won against government and multinational organizations through the utilization of the rights of nature in national and international courts are growing around the world.

A human rights approach is harmonious with the broader framework of the Rights of Nature and can be fundamental to advancing the opportunity for healthy nutrition and freedom from hunger in the decades to come (see Fig. 17.2). In order for these mechanisms to assist in efforts to address food insecurity, different values are starting to prevail—these are values of solidarity, cooperation, humility, and the decentering of human beings in order to ensure our own safety and security.[91,131]

D. Civic Engagement

Civic engagement can help to mobilize ordinary citizens, experts, and policymakers alike to create meaningful policy solutions that can reduce and ultimately put an end to food insecurity.[120] Such civic engagement can range from taking action to support people in our own surroundings in accessing food, to engaging with local food policy boards, engaging in advocacy around labor, nutrition, housing, and other supports, and demanding better, more accountable programming at all levels of government. But we must go beyond these ad hoc and conventional approaches to poverty and basic needs to an approach to human health and nutrition that is contained within planetary health and boundaries.

These new values may take many years to take hold as it is still quite challenging to encourage people to adopt a human rights approach, especially in the high-income countries most responsible for degradation of the planet and for hoarding wealth. But there is hope. The advancement of the Paris Agreement of 2015, the movement of young people to demand action on climate change, and the coming together of disparate communities—including indigenous people who have long known the struggle against centuries of domination, violence and exploitation, youth, climate scientists, public health professionals, and citizens concerned with everyday safety—point to new levels of civic engagement that might be enough to sway current cultural assumptions of the dominant elite around the globe. Efforts such as the Participation and the Practice of Rights in Northern Ireland, the Detroit Black Community Food Security Network, the Southern Rural Black Women's Initiative for Economic and Social Justice and other organizations of the US Human Rights Network, the international campaign, La Via Campesina, which advocates for food sovereignty, and the Right to Food Coalition in Australia are just a few of many examples where economic social and cultural rights are being advanced by civil society despite cultural, social, and political domination by neoliberal leaders and corporate CEOs. Ways of working with people to help advance this consciousness is through social media, and other types of media, but there is also strength and meaning created through in-person democracy schools—or informal educational sessions designed to improve the critical consciousness of everyday citizens.[132]

IV. CONCLUSION

The high health, social, and economic costs associated with food insecurity have motivated many actors to commit to ending hunger. Hunger is caused by a lack of access to money to purchase food, clean land and water to grow food, and geopolitical stability. The primary driver for these global conditions is a neoliberal model of economic activity. Transforming human relationships to ensure the right to food will involve ensuring the rights of people and nature, honoring the resilience and wisdom of food insecure people and engaging their leadership, and a commitment to build every community's food sovereignty.

RESEARCH GAPS

Transformative political and social change is needed to address food insecurity, malnutrition, and hunger, and we need new ways of carrying out research that take a resilience, strength-based approach, and recognize the importance of many societal processes that cause and exacerbate food insecurity.[4,91,133] In addition, research strategies should be inclusive of perspectives of those who have experienced food insecurity first hand who provide invaluable expert insight into dynamics and solutions. Collaboration between experts with lived experience and professionals from a variety of disciplines—including politics, history, anthropology, economics, systems thinking, psychology, agroecology, war, and others—will enhance our knowledge and engender new solutions to hunger.

Research topics should include special attention to system thinking and interventions that build resilience and prevent food insecurity and go beyond measuring calories, food trade, and specific micronutrients to consider food security and well-being on a broad scale. Some of these may include ensuring that women have greater opportunities to express their wisdom and power in identifying solutions or ensuring that people who have been marginalized, especially those who also have expertise of knowledge about restorative ecology, sustainable agriculture, and in improving water conditions, can be leading investigations. Finally, with the understanding that neoliberal systems are at the root of household food insecurity, looking to other forms of social organization and economics should be paramount. This includes carrying out research on the effectiveness of the sharing economies (such as mutual aid societies) and solidarity economies (such as farm cooperatives) on improving food security, resilience, and well-being.

Acknowledgments

This chapter is a revision of and companion to the chapters titled "Food Insecurity, Hunger, and Undernutrition" by David L. Pelletier, Christine M. Olson, and Edward A Frongillo, and "Public Nutrition in Humanitarian Crises" by Helen Young, Kate Sadler, and Annalies Borrel in *Present Knowledge in Nutrition, 10th Edition*, edited by Erdman JW, Macdonald IA, and Zeisel SH and published by Wiley-Blackwell. © 2012 International Life Sciences Institute. Portions of this chapter are from the previously published chapters and the contributions of previous authors are acknowledged.

V. REFERENCES

1. United Nations. *Key Conference Outcomes in Food*. https://www.un.org/en/development/devagenda/food.shtml. Accessed 15 July 2019.
2. Food and Agriculture Organization of the United Nations. *The State of Food Security and Nutrition in the World: Building Climate Resilience for Food Security and Nutrition*; 2018. www.fao.org/3/i9553en/i9553en.pdf. Accessed July 15, 2019.
3. *United Nations Decade of Action on Nutrition: About*. https://www.un.org/nutrition/about. Accessed 15 July 2019.
4. Swinburn BA, Kraak VI, Allender S, et al. The global syndemic of obesity, undernutrition, and climate change: the Lancet commission report. *Lancet Lond Engl*. 2019;393(10173):791–846. https://doi.org/10.1016/S0140-6736(18)32822-8.
5. *Sustainable Development Goals: Sustainable Development Knowledge Platform*. https://sustainabledevelopment.un.org/?menu=1300. Accessed 17 July 2019.
6. Cullerton K, Donnet T, Lee A, Gallegos D. Effective advocacy strategies for influencing government nutrition policy: a conceptual model. *Int J Behav Nutr Phys Act*. 2018;15. https://doi.org/10.1186/s12966-018-0716-y.
7. *Transforming our World: The 2030 Agenda for Sustainable Development*. https://resources/transforming-our-world-2030-agenda-sustainable-development. Accessed 15 July 2019.
8. *WHO | Comprehensive Implementation Plan on Maternal, Infant and Young Child Nutrition*. WHO. http://www.who.int/nutrition/publications/CIP_document/en/. Accessed 15 July 2019.
9. Angood C. *Extension of 2025 Maternal, Infant and Young Child Nutrition Targets to 2030*. UN Standing Comm Nutr News; 2015:41. www.ennonline.net/newsroom/extensionof2025targetsscnnewspaper. Accessed July 15, 2019.
10. Development Initiatives. *Global Nutrition Report*; 2018. Published 09:58:49.202407+00:00 https://globalnutritionreport.org/reports/global-nutrition-report-2018/. Accessed July 15, 2019.
11. *IPC Global Platform*. http://www.ipcinfo.org/. Accessed 15 July 2019.
12. Cafiero C, Viviani S, Nord M. Food security measurement in a global context: the food insecurity experience scale. *Measurement*. 2018;116:146–152. https://linkinghub.elsevier.com/retrieve/pii/S0263224117307005.
13. Jones AD, Ngure FM, Pelto G, Young SL. What are we assessing when we measure food security? A compendium and review of current metrics. *Adv Nutr Bethesda Md*. 2013;4(5):481–505. https://doi.org/10.3945/an.113.004119.
14. Alaimo K. Food insecurity in the United States: an overview. *Top Clin Nutr*. 2005;20(4):281.
15. Chilton M, Booth S. Hunger of the body and hunger of the mind: African American women's perceptions of food insecurity, health and violence. *J Nutr Educ Behav*. 2007;39(3):116–125. https://doi.org/10.1016/j.jneb.2006.11.005.
16. Holben D. Position of the American Dietetic Association: food insecurity in the United States. *J Am Diet Assoc*. 2010;110(9):1368–1377. http://www.sciencedirect.com/science/article/pii/S0002822310011946.
17. Ralston K. *Children's Food Security and USDA Child Nutrition Programs*:33.
18. Fram MS, Frongillo EA, Jones SJ, et al. Children are aware of food insecurity and take responsibility for managing food resources. *J Nutr*. 2011. https://doi.org/10.3945/jn.110.135988.
19. Fram MS, Ritchie LD, Rosen N, Frongillo EA. Child experience of food insecurity is associated with child diet and physical activity. *J Nutr*. 2015;145(3):499–504. https://doi.org/10.3945/jn.114.194365.

20. Hamelin A-M, Beaudry M, Habicht J-P. Characterization of household food insecurity in Québec: food and feelings. *Soc Sci Med.* 2002;54(1):119–132.
21. Ó Gráda C. Famine, trauma and memory. *Béaloideas.* 2001;69: 121–143. https://doi.org/10.2307/20520760.
22. Loganaden, N. FAO methodology for estimating the prevalence of undernourishment. *Presented at the: 2003; International Scientific Symposium: Measurement and Assessment of Food Deprivation and Undernutrition;* Rome, Italy. http://www.fao.org/3/Y4249E/y4249e06.htm. Accessed 15 July 2019.
23. ESS Website. *Ess: Food Balance Sheets.* http://www.fao.org/economic/ess/fbs. Accessed 15 July 2019.
24. Bickel G, Nord M, Cristofer P, Hamilton W, Cook J. *Measuring Food Security in the United States: Guide to Measuring Household Food Security, Revised 2000.* Alexandria VA: U.S. Department of Agriculture, Food and Nutrition Service; 2000. https://fns-prod.azureedge.net/sites/default/files/FSGuide.pdf. Accessed July 30, 2019.
25. *Voices of the Hungry | Food and Agriculture Organization of the United Nations.* http://www.fao.org/in-action/voices-of-the-hungry. Accessed 15 July 2019.
26. Smith MD, Rabbitt MP, Coleman- Jensen A. Who are the world's food insecure? New Evidence from the Food and Agriculture Organization's food insecurity experience scale. *World Dev.* 2017;93: 402–412. https://doi.org/10.1016/j.worlddev.2017.01.006.
27. IPC Global Partners. *Integrated Food Security Phase Classification Technical Manual Version 3.0. Evidence and Standards for Better Food Security and Nutrition Decisions.* 2019. Rome.
28. Food and Agriculture Organization of the United Nations. *Early Warning Early Action Report on Food Security and Agriculture January – March 2019: FAO in Emergencies;* 2019. http://www.fao.org/emergencies/resources/documents/resources-detail/en/c/1177087/. Accessed July 17, 2019.
29. Food, Agriculture Organization of the United Nations.. *The State of Food and Agriculture 2013;* 2013. http://www.fao.org/3/i3300e/i3300e00.htm.
30. GBD Risk Factors Collaborators. Global, regional, and national comparative risk assessment of 79 behavioral, environmental and occupational, and metabolic risks or clusters of risks, 1990–2015: a systematic analysis for the Global Burden of Disease Study 2015. *Lancet Lond Engl.* 2016;388(10053):1659–1724.
31. *Data and Analytics Section of the Division of Data, Research and Policy, UNICEF, New York Together with the Department of Nutrition for Health and Development, WHO Geneva and the Development Data, United Nations Children's Fund (UNICEF), World Health Organization, International Bank for, Reconstruction and Development/The World Bank, UNICEF/WHO/World Bank Group, Joint Child Malnutrition Estimates. Levels and Trends in Child Malnutrition: Key Findings of the 2019 Edition of the Joint Child Malnutrition Estimates.* Geneva: World Health Organization; 2019. https://www.who.int/nutgrowthdb/jme-2019-key-findings.pdf?ua=1. Accessed July 15, 2019.
32. *The Cost of Malnutrition: Why Policy Action is Urgent | Food Security Portal.* http://www.foodsecurityportal.org/cost-malnutrition-why-policy-action-urgent. Accessed 15 July 2019.
33. *Children: Reducing Mortality.* https://www.who.int/news-room/fact-sheets/detail/children-reducing-mortality. Accessed 15 July 2019.
34. World Health Organization. *Nutrition Challenges.* WHO. https://www.who.int/nutrition/challenges/en/. Accessed 15 July 2019.
35. Khara T, Mwangome M, Ngari M, Dolan C. Children concurrently wasted and stunted: a meta-analysis of prevalence data of children 6–59 months from 84 countries. *Matern Child Nutr.* 2018; 14(2):e12516. https://doi.org/10.1111/mcn.12516.
36. Ghattas H. *Food Security and Nutrition in the Context of the Global Nutrition Transition.* Rome: Food and Agriculture Organization of the United Nations; 2014:21.
37. Olofin I, McDonald CM, Ezzati M, et al. Associations of suboptimal growth with all-cause and cause-specific mortality in children under five years: a pooled analysis of ten prospective studies. *PLoS One.* 2013;8(5):e64636. https://doi.org/10.1371/journal.pone.0064636.
38. *WHO | The WHO Child Growth Standards.* WHO. http://www.who.int/childgrowth/en/. Accessed 15 July 2019.
39. Richard SA, Black RE, Gilman RH, et al. Wasting is associated with stunting in early childhood. *J Nutr.* 2012;142(7):1291–1296. https://doi.org/10.3945/jn.111.154922.
40. Popkin BM, Richards MK, Montiero CA. Stunting is associated with overweight in children of four nations that are undergoing the nutrition transition. *J Nutr.* 1996;126(12):3009–3016. https://doi.org/10.1093/jn/126.12.3009.
41. United Nations Children's Fund D of DR, Policy. *Global UNICEF Global Databases: Overlapping Stunting, Wasting and Overweight.* 2018.
42. Petry N, Olofin I, Hurrell RF, et al. The proportion of anemia associated with iron deficiency in low, medium, and high human development index countries: a systematic analysis of national surveys. *Nutrients.* 2016;8(11). https://doi.org/10.3390/nu8110693.
43. *WHO | Global Health Observatory (GHO) Data.* WHO. http://www.who.int/gho/en/. Accessed 15 July 2019.
44. Xiong X, Buekens P, Alexander S, Demianczuk N, Wollast E. Anemia during pregnancy and birth outcome: a meta-analysis. *Am J Perinatol.* 2000;17(3):137–146. https://doi.org/10.1055/s-2000-9508.
45. *Obesity and Overweight.* https://www.who.int/news-room/fact-sheets/detail/obesity-and-overweight. Accessed 15 July 2019.
46. Afshin A, Forouzanfar MH, Reitsma MB, et al. Health effects of overweight and obesity in 195 countries over 25 yearsGBD 2015 Obesity Collaborators, ed. *N Engl J Med.* 2017;377(1):13–27. https://doi.org/10.1056/NEJMoa1614362.
47. Ashwell M, Gunn P, Gibson S. Waist-to-height ratio is a better screening tool than waist circumference and BMI for adult cardiometabolic risk factors: systematic review and meta-analysis. *Obes Rev.* 2012;13(3):275–286. https://doi.org/10.1111/j.1467-789X.2011.00952.x.
48. N. C. D. Risk Factor Collaboration. Rising rural body-mass index is the main driver of the global obesity epidemic in adults. *Nature.* 2019;569(7755):260–264.
49. Lockie S, Carpenter D. *Agriculture, Biodiversity and Markets: Livelihoods and Agroecology in Comparative Perspective.* London, UK: Earthscan Publications; 2010. http://www.routledge.com/books/details/9780415507356/. Accessed July 17, 2019.
50. Kohl HW, Craig CL, Lambert EV, et al. The pandemic of physical inactivity: global action for public health. *Lancet Lond Engl.* 2012; 380(9838):294–305. https://doi.org/10.1016/S0140-6736(12)60898-8.
51. Thrupp LA. Linking agricultural biodiversity and food security: the valuable role of agrobiodiversity for sustainable agriculture. *Int Aff.* 2000;76(2):265–281.
52. Popkin BM, Adair LS, Ng SW. Global nutrition transition and the pandemic of obesity in developing countries. *Nutr Rev.* 2012;70(1): 3–21. https://doi.org/10.1111/j.1753-4887.2011.00456.x.
53. *Overcoming the Triple Burden of Malnutrition in the MENA Region IFPRI.* http://www.ifpri.org/blog/overcoming-triple-burden-malnutrition-mena-region%E2%80%A8. Accessed 17 July 2019.
54. Leung CW, Epel ES, Ritchie LD, Crawford PB, Laraia BA. Food insecurity is inversely associated with diet quality of lower-income adults. *J Acad Nutr Diet.* 2014;114(12), 1943–1953. e2.
55. Seligman HK, Bindman AB, Vittinghoff E, Kanaya AM, Kushel MB. Food insecurity is associated with diabetes mellitus: results from the National Health Examination and Nutrition Examination Survey (NHANES) 1999–2002. *J Gen Intern Med.* 2007;22(7):1018–1023.

56. Seligman HK, Laraia BA, Kushel MB. Food insecurity is associated with chronic disease among low-income NHANES participants. *J Nutr.* 2010;140(2):304–310.
57. Anema A, Vogenthaler N, Frongillo EA, Kadiyala S, Weiser SD. Food insecurity and HIV/AIDS: current knowledge, gaps, and research priorities. *Curr HIV AIDS Rep.* 2009;6(4):224–231.
58. Seligman HK, Davis TC, Schillinger D, Wolf MS. Food insecurity is associated with hypoglycemia and poor diabetes self-management in a low-income sample with diabetes. *J Health Care Poor Underserved.* 2010;21(4):1227–1233. https://doi.org/10.1353/hpu.2010.0921.
59. Simmons LA, Modesitt SC, Brody AC, Leggin AB. Food insecurity among cancer patients in Kentucky: a pilot study. *J Oncol Pract.* 2006;2(6):274–279.
60. Braveman P, Barclay C. Health disparities beginning in childhood: a life-course perspective. *Pediatrics.* 2009;124(suppl 3).
61. Olson CM, Strawderman MS. The relationship between food insecurity and obesity in rural childbearing women. *J Rural Health.* 2008;24(1):60–66.
62. Skalicky A, Meyers AF, Adams WG, Yang Z, Cook JT, Frank DA. Child food insecurity and iron-deficiency anemia in low-income infants and toddlers in the United States. *Matern Child Health J.* 2006;10(2):177–185.
63. Cook JT, Frank DA, Berkowitz C, et al. Food insecurity is associated with adverse health outcomes among human infants and toddlers. *J Nutr.* 2004;134(6):1432–1438.
64. Casey PH, Szeto KL, Robbins JM, et al. Child health-related quality of life and household food security. *Arch Pediatr Adolesc Med.* 2005;159(1):51–56.
65. Rose-Jacobs R, Black MM, Casey PH, et al. Household food insecurity: associations with at-risk infant and toddler development. *Pediatrics.* 2008;121(1):65–72. https://doi.org/10.1542/peds.2006-3717.
66. Heckman JJ. Skill formation and the economics of investing in disadvantaged children. *Science.* 2006;312(5782):1900–1902.
67. Shankar P, Chung R, Frank DA. Association of food insecurity with children's behavioral, emotional, and academic outcomes: a systematic review. *J Dev Behav Pediatr.* 2017;38(2):135–150.
68. Alaimo K, Olson CM, Frongillo EA. Food insufficiency and American school-aged children's cognitive, academic, and psychosocial development. *Pediatrics.* 2001;108(1):44–53.
69. Jyoti DF, Frongillo EA, Jones SJ. Food insecurity affects school children's academic performance, weight gain, and social skills. *J Nutr.* 2005;135(12):2831–2839.
70. Melchior M, Caspi A, Howard LM, et al. Mental health context of food insecurity: a representative cohort of families with young children. *Pediatrics.* 2009;124(4):e564–e572. https://doi.org/10.1542/peds.2009-0583.
71. Shonkoff JP, Boyce WT, McEwen BS. Neuroscience, molecular biology, and the childhood roots of health disparities: building a new framework for health promotion and disease prevention. *J Am Med Assoc.* 2009;301(21):2252–2259. https://doi.org/10.1001/jama.2009.754.
72. Gundersen C, Kreider B. Bounding the effects of food insecurity on children's health outcomes. *J Health Econ.* 2009;28(5):971–983. https://doi.org/10.1016/j.jhealeco.2009.06.012.
73. Alaimo K, Olson CM, Frongillo EA, Briefel RR. Food insufficiency, family income, and health in U.S. preschool and school-age children. *Am J Public Health.* 2001;91:781–786.
74. Alaimo K, Olson CM, Frongillo EA. Family food insufficiency is associated with dysthymia and suicidal symptoms in adolescents: results from NHANES III. *J Nutr.* 2002;132:719–725.
75. Chavkin W, Wise PH. The data are in: health matters in welfare policy. *Am J Public Health.* 2002;92(9):1392–1395.
76. Romero D, Chavkin W, Wise P, Hess C, Van Landeghem K. State welfare reform policies and maternal and child health services: a national study. *Matern Child Health J.* 2001;5(3):199–206.
77. Hamelin AM, Habicht JP, Beaudry M. Food insecurity: consequences for the household and broader social implications. *J Nutr.* 1999;129(2S Suppl):525S–528S.
78. Rose D, Oliveira V. Nutrient intakes of individuals from food-insufficient households in the United States. *Am J Public Health.* 1997;87(12):1956–1961.
79. Radimer KL, Olson CM, Green JC, Campbell CC, Habicht JP. Understanding hunger and developing indicators to assess it in women and children. *J Nutr Educ.* 1992;24:36S–44S.
80. Jessiman-Perreault G, McIntyre L. Household food insecurity narrows the sex gap in five adverse mental health outcomes among Canadian adults. *Int J Environ Res Public Health.* 2019;16(3):319. https://doi.org/10.3390/ijerph16030319.
81. Whitaker RC, Phillips SM, Orzol SM. Food insecurity and the risks of depression and anxiety in mothers and behavior problems in their preschool-aged children. *Pediatrics.* 2006;118(3):e859–e868. https://doi.org/10.1542/peds.2006-0239.
82. Coleman-Jensen A. Working for peanuts: nonstandard work and food insecurity across household structure. *J Fam Econ Issues.* 2011;32:84–97.
83. Montgomery BE, Rompalo A, Hughes J, et al. Violence against women in selected areas of the United States. *Am J Public Health.* 2015;(10):e1–e11.
84. Hernandez DC, Marshall A, Mineo C. Maternal depression mediates the association between intimate partner violence and food insecurity. *J Women's Health.* 2014;23(1):29–37. https://doi.org/10.1089/jwh.2012.4224.
85. Chilton MM, Rabinowich JR, Woolf NH. Very low food security in the USA is linked with exposure to violence. *Public Health Nutr.* 2014;17(1):73–82. https://doi.org/10.1017/S1368980013000281.
86. Sun J, Knowles M, Patel F, Frank DA, Heeren T, Chilton M. Childhood adversity and adult reports of food insecurity among households with children. *Am J Prev Med.* 2016;50(5):561–572. https://doi.org/10.1016/j.amepre.2015.09.024.
87. Davison KM, Marshall-Fabien GL, Tecson A. Association of moderate and severe food insecurity with suicidal ideation in adults: national survey data from three Canadian provinces. *Soc Psychiatry Psychiatr Epidemiol.* 2015;50(6):963–972. https://doi.org/10.1007/s00127-015-1018-1.
88. Kumanyika S. *Getting to Equity in Obesity Prevention: A New Framework.* Washington, DC: National Academy of Medicine; 2017.
89. Odoms-Young A, Bruce MA. Examining the impact of structural racism on food insecurity: implications for addressing racial/ethnic disparities. *Fam Community Health.* 2018;41(Suppl 2):S3–S6. https://doi.org/10.1097/FCH.0000000000000183.
90. Burke MP, Jones SJ, Frongillo EA, Fram MS, Blake CE, Freedman DA. Severity of household food insecurity and lifetime racial discrimination among African-American households in South Carolina. *Ethn Health.* 2018;23(3):276–292. https://doi.org/10.1080/13557858.2016.1263286.
91. Gallegos D, Chilton MM. Re-evaluating expertise: principles for food and nutrition security research, advocacy and solutions in high-income countries. *Int J Environ Res Public Health.* 2019;16(4). https://doi.org/10.3390/ijerph16040561.
92. Coleman-Jensen A, McFall W, Nord M. *Food Insecurity in Households With Children: Prevalence, Severity, and Household Characteristics, 2010-11.* USDA Economic Research Service. http://www.ers.usda.gov/publications/pub-details/?pubid=43765. Accessed 1 August 2019.
93. Huet C, Ford JD, Edge VL, et al. Food insecurity and food consumption by season in households with children in an Arctic city: a cross-sectional study. *BMC Public Health.* 2017;17(1):578. https://doi.org/10.1186/s12889-017-4393-6.

94. Drèze J, Sen A. *Hunger and Public Action*. Oxford: Clarendon Press Oxford; 1991. https://www.wider.unu.edu/publication/hunger-and-public-action. Accessed July 31, 2019.
95. Jones SJ, Draper CL, Bell BA, et al. Child hunger from a family resilience perspective. *J Hunger Environ Nutr*. 2018;13(3):340–361. https://doi.org/10.1080/19320248.2017.1364189.
96. Drucker ER, Liese AD, Sercy E, et al. Food insecurity, childhood hunger and caregiver life experiences among households with children in South Carolina, USA. *Public Health Nutr*. 2019:1–10. https://doi.org/10.1017/S1368980019000922.
97. Martin MS, Maddocks E, Chen Y, Gilman SE, Colman I. Food insecurity and mental illness: disproportionate impacts in the context of perceived stress and social isolation. *Public Health*. 2016;132:86–91. https://doi.org/10.1016/j.puhe.2015.11.014.
98. Temple JB. The association between stressful events and food insecurity: cross-sectional evidence from Australia. *Int J Environ Res Public Health*. 2018;15(11). https://doi.org/10.3390/ijerph15112333.
99. *In the Public Interest. How Privatization Increases Inequality. Section 3: Privatization of Critical Social Safety Net Services*; 2016. https://www.inthepublicinterest.org/wp-content/uploads/InthePublicInterest_Inequality_Sec3_Sept2016.pdf. Accessed July 31, 2019.
100. Eichner M. The privatized American family. *Notre Dame Law Rev*. 2017;93(1). https://www.ssrn.com/abstract=3060815.
101. Ziliak JP, Hardy B, Bollinger C. Earnings volatility in America: Evidence from matched CPS. *Labour Econ*. 2011;18(6):742–754. https://doi.org/10.1016/j.labeco.2011.06.015.
102. Hardy BL. Childhood income volatility and adult outcomes. *Demography*. 2014;51(5):1641–1665. https://doi.org/10.1007/s13524-014-0329-2.
103. Stuckler D, Reeves A, Loopstra R, Karanikolos M, McKee M. Austerity and health: the impact in the UK and Europe. *Eur J Public Health*. 2017;27(suppl_4):18–21. https://doi.org/10.1093/eurpub/ckx167.
104. Rodger III WM. *The Impact of a $15 Minimum Wage on Hunger in America*; 2016. https://tcf.org/content/report/the-impact-of-a-15-minimum-wage-on-hunger-in-america/. Accessed July 31, 2019.
105. Ingram J, Erickson P, Liverman D. *Food Security and Global Environmental Change*. 1st ed. London ; Washington, DC: Routledge; 2010.
106. Suweis S, Carr JA, Maritan A, Rinaldo A, D'Odorico P. Resilience and reactivity of global food security. *Proc Natl Acad Sci*. 2015;112(22):6902–6907. https://doi.org/10.1073/pnas.1507366112.
107. Paasch A. In: Garbers F, Hirsch T, eds. *Trade Policies and Hunger*. Geneva: Ecumenical Advocacy Alliance; 2007. https://www.etoconsortium.org/nc/en/main-navigation/library/documents/?tx_drblob_pi1%5BdownloadUid%5D=42. Accessed July 31, 2019.
108. Siegel A. NAFTA largely responsible for the obesity epidemic in Mexico. *Wash Univ J Law Policy*. 2016;50(1):195–226.
109. Svampa M. Resource extractivism and alternatives: Latin American perspectives on development. *J für Entwicklungspolitik*. 2012;28:117–143. https://doi.org/10.20446/JEP-2414-3197-28-3-43.
110. Bullock JM, Dhanjal-Adams KL, Milne A, et al. Resilience and food security: rethinking an ecological concept. *J Ecol*. 2017;105(4):880–884. https://doi.org/10.1111/1365-2745.12791.
111. Bindraban PS, van der Velde M, Ye L, et al. Assessing the impact of soil degradation on food production. *Curr Opin Environ Sustain*. 2012;4(5):478–488. https://doi.org/10.1016/j.cosust.2012.09.015.
112. Nagy GJ, Bidegain M, Caffera RM, Lagomarsino JJ, Ponce A, Sención G. *Adaptive Capacity for Responding to Climate Variability and Change in Estuarine Fisheries of the Rio de la Plata*: 16.
113. Bommarco R, Kleijn D, Potts SG. Ecological intensification: harnessing ecosystem services for food security. *Trends Ecol Evol*. 2013;28(4):230–238. https://doi.org/10.1016/j.tree.2012.10.012.
114. Sen A. Ingredients of famine analysis: availability and entitlements. *Q J Econ*. 1981;96(3):433–464.
115. National Commission on Hunger. *Freedom from Hunger: An Achievable Goal for the United States of America*. 2015.
116. *Rudd Links Food Bank Rise to Benefit Mess*; February 11, 2019. https://www.bbc.com/news/uk-politics-47203389. Accessed July 17, 2019.
117. *Austerity, Welfare Cuts, and the Right to Food in the UK | HRW*; 2017. https://www.hrw.org/report/2019/05/20/nothing-left-cupboards/austerity-welfare-cuts-and-right-food-uk.
118. Osborne H, Hopkins N. *Revealed: Ministers' Plan to Research Effect of Policies on Food Bank Use*. The Guardian; August 1, 2018. https://www.theguardian.com/society/2018/aug/01/revealed-ministers-plan-to-research-effect-of-policies-on-food-bank-use. Accessed July 17, 2019.
119. Riches G. Food banks and food security: welfare reform, human rights and social policy. Lessons from Canada? *Soc Policy Adm*. 2002;36(6):648–663. https://doi.org/10.1111/1467-9515.00309.
120. Chilton M, Rose D. A rights-based approach to food insecurity in the United States. *Am J Public Health*. 2009;99(7):1203–1211. https://www.ncbi.nlm.nih.gov/pmc/articles/PMC2696644/.
121. Salonen AS, Ohisalo M, Laihiala T. Undeserving, disadvantaged, disregarded: three viewpoints of charity food aid recipients in Finland. *Int J Environ Res Public Health*. 2018;15(12). https://doi.org/10.3390/ijerph15122896.
122. Poppendieck J. *Sweet Charity?* Penguin Random House; 1999. https://www.penguinrandomhouse.com/books/330861/sweet-charity-by-janet-poppendieck/9780140245561. Accessed July 17, 2019.
123. Synthesis Reportâ, Nyeleniâ, Via Campesinaâ, Newsletter, Bulletin, Boletin. https://nyeleni.org/spip.php?article334. Accessed 15 July 2019.
124. Nash R. *The Rights of Nature: A History of Environmental Ethics*. Vol. 11. Madison, WI: University of Wisconsin Press; 1989. https://doi.org/10.1177/027046769101100147. Accessed July 31, 2019.
125. Greene N. *The First Successful Case of the Rights of Nature implementation in Ecuadorâ, The Rights of Nature*; 2011. https://therightsofnature.org/first-ron-case-ecuador/. Accessed July 31, 2019.
126. Vidal J. *Bolivia Enshrines Natural World's Rights With Equal Status for Mother Earth*. The Guardian; April 10, 2011. https://www.theguardian.com/environment/2011/apr/10/bolivia-enshrines-natural-worlds-rights. Accessed July 17, 2019.
127. Barraclough T. *How Far Can the Te Awa Tupua (Whanganui River) Proposal e Said to Reflect the Rights of Nature in New Zealand?*. 2013.
128. Andrade PA. The government of nature: post-neoliberal environmental governance in Bolivia and Ecuador. In: de Castro F, Hogenboom B, Baud M, eds. *Environmental Governance in Latin America*. London: Palgrave Macmillan UK; 2016:113–136. https://doi.org/10.1007/978-1-137-50572-9_5.
129. The Emergence of Planetary Citizenship – Other News. http://www.other-news.info/2018/06/the-emergence-of-planetary-citizenship/. Accessed 17 July 2019.
130. Revkin AC. Ecuador constitution grants rights to nature. *New York Times, Dot Earth Blog*; September 29, 2008. https://dotearth.blogs.nytimes.com/2008/09/29/ecuador-constitution-grants-nature-rights/. Accessed July 17, 2019.
131. Eileen C. The affliction of human supremacy. *Ecol Citiz*. 2017;1(1):61–64. https://www.ecologicalcitizen.net/pdfs/v01n1-11.pdf.
132. Watts RJ, Diemer MA, Voight AM. Critical consciousness: current status and future directions. *New Dir Child Adolesc Dev*. 2011;2011(134):43–57. https://doi.org/10.1002/cd.310.
133. Baker P, Hawkes C, Wingrove K, et al. What drives political commitment for nutrition? A review and framework synthesis to inform the United Nations Decade of Action on Nutrition. *BMJ Glob Health*. 2018;3(1):e000485. https://doi.org/10.1136/bmjgh-2017-000485.

SECTION C

Clinical Nutrition

C H A P T E R

18

THE ROLE OF DIET IN CHRONIC DISEASE

Katherine L. Tucker, PhD

Department of Biomedical and Nutritional Sciences,
Zuckerberg College of Health Sciences, University of Massachusetts Lowell, Lowell, MA, United States

SUMMARY

Chronic disease incidence and prevalence has been growing rapidly throughout the globe over the past several decades. Many of these diseases, including obesity, diabetes, and cardiovascular diseases, are largely preventable with healthy lifestyle. Key lifestyle factors include physical activity, smoking, alcohol use, and dietary quality. This chapter provides a brief overview of the dietary factors known and hypothesized to relate to risk of these cardiometabolic diseases. Due to the complexity of nutrient effects on the body, interactions with other factors, and the long-term development of chronic disease, research to prove cause and effect for specific components of the diet is difficult. Numerous studies across differing populations are needed to obtain confidence in associations. There is a current debate regarding how to assess the evidence for creating dietary guidelines. Despite this, we do know a great deal about diet and health, and there is no doubt that overall quality of the dietary pattern, involving a variety of nutrients and foods in the right balance, has a major effort on chronic disease risk. There is general consensus that diets high in fruit, vegetables, whole grains, nuts and seeds, omega-3 fatty acids, and low-fat dairy and low in refined grains, sugary foods and beverages, salty snacks, and processed meats are protective against these conditions. Efforts to limit the rapidly increasing use of energy-dense, nutrient-poor foods at the expense of basic natural foods are critical to stem the tide of these chronic diseases.

Keywords: Cancer; Cardiovascular diseases; Chronic; Diabetes; Dietary intake; Dietary patterns; Obesity; Osteoporosis; Risk assessment.

I. INTRODUCTION

Over the past century, there has been a rapid shift in disease incidence, prevalence, and cause of death, from infectious disease to chronic conditions. This transition began in developed countries, particularly the United States, and has spread throughout the world with changes in technology, socioeconomic status, and particularly in the food supply. The Centers for Disease Control and Prevention (CDC) currently estimates that 60% of US adults have at least one chronic disease and that 40% have two or more.[1] Obesity has increased at an unprecedented rate over the past 40 years. Based on national survey data, the CDC estimates that fewer than 15% of US adults were obese between 1960 and 1980. Over successive National Health and Nutrition Examination Surveys (NHANESs) that prevalence jumped to 23% by 1994, 31% by 2000, 34% by 2008, and most recently was estimated at 40% in 2015–16.[2,3] This is of critical importance, as obesity is linked with subsequent cardiometabolic diseases, including type 2 diabetes, and cardiovascular diseases (CVDs). Not surprisingly, the prevalence of type 2 diabetes has increased rapidly in response to the increases in obesity. Based on data from the National Health Interview Survey, the CDC showed prevalence of diabetes as less than 2.5% of the US population prior to 1980, with increases to 3.0 by 1994, 4.4% by 2000, 6.3% by 2008, and 7.4% by 2015.[4]

While the United States has led the way, these trends are spreading globally. Changing dietary intake patterns are one, if not, major factor in these transitions. A 2010

Present Knowledge in Nutrition, Volume 2
https://doi.org/10.1016/B978-0-12-818460-8.00018-6

World Health Organization report notes that, in 2008, 63% of global deaths were due to noncommunicable diseases and that 80% of these were in low- and middle-income countries.[5] They emphasized that a large proportion of these deaths are preventable through four major behaviors: tobacco use, physical activity, excess alcohol, and unhealthy diet. A recent comprehensive look at the global health effects of poor diet across 195 countries, the Global Burden of Disease Study, concluded that dietary improvement could prevent one in every five deaths.[6] They estimated that, among diet-related outcomes, low intakes of whole grains, fruit, nuts and seeds, vegetables, and omega-3 fatty acids and high intakes of sodium accounted for most of the deaths and disability-adjusted life years, primarily due to CVD and type 2 diabetes.

II. THE NUTRITION TRANSITION

Diet has long been known to play a key role as a risk factor for chronic disease. During the post-World War II era in the United States, our food supply shifted rapidly from whole farm-based foods to highly processed foods (very refined foods with high energy density and relatively low nutrient density) that could reach the expanding urban population. Shortages during the war led the military to accelerate research into food processing, including canning, energy bars, restructured meat (e g., chicken nuggets, beef patties), shelf-stable bread, dehydrated cheese, TV dinners, and instant coffee.[7] Advances in food science fueled the food industry to expand choice with a rapidly increasing variety of shelf-stable foods, with high amounts of added sugars, fats, and refined grains. As more women entered the workforce, convenience became a priority and a proliferation of canned, dried, and instant products, such as frozen TV dinners, ensued. This focus on convenience and shelf life has continued. The Nielsen Homescan longitudinal study of foods purchased in the United States showed that more than 75% of dietary energy purchases were from moderately (16%) or highly processed (61%) foods and beverages in 2012, noting that these foods had higher saturated fat, sugar, and sodium than less processed foods.[8] This was confirmed with NHANES dietary intake data, where 60% of the reported US diet in 2011–12 came from high intake of highly processed foods, including breads, frozen or shelf-stable meals, confectionery, fruit drinks, milk drinks, cakes, cookies, pies, soft drinks, salty snacks, and breakfast cereals.[9] The proportion of the diet from these types of foods varied by sociodemographic variables, with inverse associations with age (highest in children, at 66%–67% of energy, and lowest in adults aged $\geq$60 y, at 53%), education, and family income.

While this movement began in the United States, it has continued to expand, first to other developed countries and now into less developed countries. In all of these cases, growth in chronic disease has followed this nutrition transition, where traditional, largely plant-based, diets have been replaced by high-fat, energy-dense diets with substantial inclusion of foods with added sugars and increasing use of animal-based foods.[10] A recent review[11] measured the increasing sales of ultraprocessed food and drink globally. They defined this category using the NOVA classification, which defines foods and drinks as "not modified foods but formulations made mostly or entirely from substances derived from foods and additives with little if any intact food."[12] Examples of such foods include sweet or salty packaged snacks and soft drinks. They estimated that between 2002 and 2016, sales in this category increased 67% for foods and 120% for drinks in South and Southeast Asia; 58% for foods in North Africa and the Middle East; and 71% for drinks in Africa. Lead contributors to these increases included baked goods and carbonated beverages. Importantly, they estimated that for each standard deviation (SD) increase in ultraprocessed drinks sold between 2002 and 2014, mean BMI increased by 0.20 kg/m^2 in men and 0.07 kg/m^2 in women, and for each SD increase in these ultraprocessed foods, BMI increased by 0.32 kg/m^2 in men, while the increase was not significant in women.[10]

Increases in risk of chronic diseases, particularly type 2 diabetes, have followed increases in obesity. Although decreases in physical activity also contribute to these risks, along with smoking, there is no doubt that dietary quality is of major importance. In addition to higher intakes of total energy, fat, and sugar associated with the nutrition transition, loss of specific nutrients associated with the replacement of basic foods with processed foods has differential effects on health. Here, we will briefly review the current knowledge on nutrients, foods, and dietary patterns in relation to obesity, type 2 diabetes, and CVD.

III. NUTRIENTS, FOODS, AND DIETARY PATTERNS IN RELATION TO OBESITY

As noted above, the prevalence of obesity in global populations has increased rapidly to a pandemic that has become the biggest health challenge of current times (Fig. 18.1). Although tremendous efforts have been put into research to better understand the etiology of obesity and its treatment, obesity has proven to be resistant to improvement, with continued increases in prevalence despite major public health efforts. From a simple perspective, weight gain is the balance of energy in

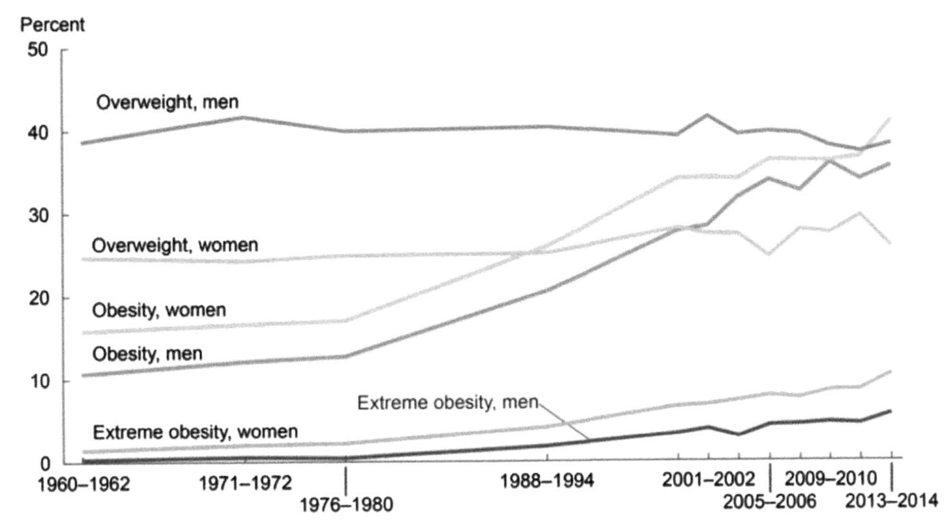

FIGURE 18.1 Trends in adult overweight, obesity, and extreme obesity among men and women aged 20–74: United States, 1960–62 through 2013–14. Notes: Age-adjusted by the direct method to the year 2000 US Census Bureau estimates using age groups 20–39, 40–59, and 60–74. Overweight is body mass index (BMI) of 25 kg/m^2 or greater but less than 30 kg/m^2; obesity is BMI greater than or equal to 30; and extreme obesity is BMI greater than or equal to 40. Pregnant females were excluded from the analysis. *Source: Fryar CD, Carroll MD, Ogden CL. Prevalence of Overweight, Obesity, and Extreme Obesity Among Adults Aged 20 and Over: United States, 1960–62 Through 2013–14. In: National Center for Health Statistics.*

versus energy out, and increases in energy intake, which have accompanied the adoption of more energy-dense foods, along with decreases in energy expenditure with changes in work and leisure activity toward more automation and computing, are the underlying reason for most population change in obesity. However, within these two major dynamics are complex details that need more research to fully understand. Given the sudden shift, many additional hypotheses emerged for the etiology of obesity, including sleep deprivation, decreased smoking, increased atmospheric carbon dioxide, control of ambient temperature, increased screen time, exposure to endocrine disruptors, pharmaceutical iatrogenesis, viral infection, dysbiosis of the gut microbiome, and sociopsychological factors.[13] New advances in genetics have provided some explanations for susceptibility to obesity and other chronic diseases in the face of dietary change. Specific polymorphisms that protected survival in a food-scarce environment may now promote weight retention in an environment of food excess.[14] Although few specific polymorphisms, on their own, have been proven to be major contributors to the rapid rise in obesity, they remain under investigation as likely contributors. After consideration of these diverse factors, the nutrition transition to refined energy-, fat- and sugar-dense, nutrient-poor foods and beverages, in interaction with other factors, remains the major likely cause of the obesity pandemic.

Importantly, the distribution of obesity is not equal across the population. NHANES data from 2015 to 2016 show that, although prevalence among all groups is high, it is greater among non-Hispanic black and Hispanic adults than non-Hispanic white or Asian adults, with more than 50% of black and Hispanic women in the obese category (Fig. 18.2). More research is needed to understand the possible interactions between genetic, cultural, and socioeconomic reasons for these disparities so that the gaps, currently increasing, may be closed.

A. Macronutrients

As the obesity problem escalated, there was consideration of individual nutrients as likely factors fueling weight gain. An early focus was dietary fat. Dietary guidelines, and the food guide pyramid, introduced in 1992, focused largely on reducing total and saturated fat intake, with grains as the base.[15] A proliferation of low-fat diets and low-fat consumer food products followed, both for weight loss and reduction of cardiovascular risk. However, despite the prevailing belief in these diets, weight gain continued to accelerate in the population.[16]

Eventually, the low-fat model was highly criticized, based on epidemiologic evidence that a focus on grains as the base of the pyramid, in their mostly highly refined form in US diets, and was not the best approach to controlling weight, and, when substituted for saturated fat, higher carbohydrates from grains and sugars were associated with higher triglycerides and lower HDL cholesterol.[17] In 2003, an analysis of the Nurses' Health Study (NHS) showed that weight gain over 12 y was inversely associated with intake of dietary fiber and

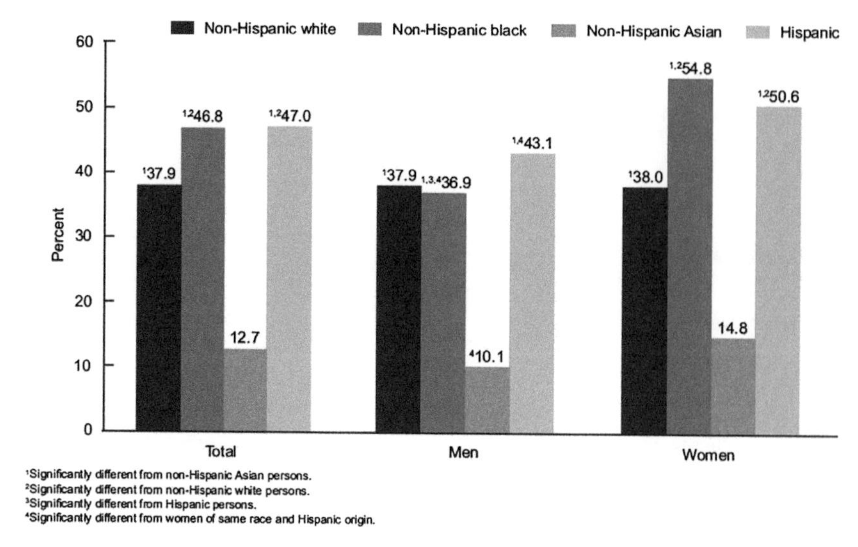

FIGURE 18.2 Age-adjusted prevalence of obesity among adults aged 20 and over, by sex and race and Hispanic origin: United States, 2015–16. Notes: All estimates are age-adjusted by the direct method to the 2000 US census population using the age groups 20–39, 40–59, and 60 and over. Access data table for Figure 2 at: **https://www.cdc.gov/nchs/data/databriefs/db288_table.pdf#2**. *Source: NCHS Data Brief No. 288 October 2017 Prevalence of Obesity Among Adults and Youth: United States, 2015–2016 US. Department of Health and Human Services Centers for Disease Control and Prevention National Center for Health Statistics Craig M. Hales, M.D., Margaret D. Carroll, M.S.P.H., Cheryl D. Fryar, M.S.P.H., and Cynthia L. Ogden, Ph.D.*

whole grain foods and positively associated with refined grain food products.[18] In addition, a clear correlation between the increase in sugar-sweetened beverages (SSB) and increases in obesity led many to shift the focus from fats to refined carbohydrates as the major factor in weight gain. A 2008 review showed that increases in soft drink consumption were coincident with the dramatic rise in obesity and noted that the evidence from observational studies and clinical trials suggested a link between the two.[19] A more recent review showed further support for the association between SSB and obesity.[20] Some scientists emphasized, in particular, the increased use of high-fructose corn syrup in the food supply as a major obesogenic driver, noting effects of fructose on leptin resistance and encouragement of increased food intake, as well as blocking of fatty acid oxidation and increased fat storage.[21]

Within the category of carbohydrates, there is considerable evidence that foods high in fiber, including whole grains, legumes, nuts, fruit, and vegetables, are protective against obesity. In a highly cited overview of this topic, Burton-Freeman explained how dietary fiber aids in energy intake regulation by providing early and prolonged satiety signals.[22] She notes that early signals are through physical bulking effects and later through viscosity-producing effects related to delays in fat absorption. More recently, emphasis has shifted to the important role of dietary fiber on maintaining a healthy gut microbiome. One recent study of longitudinal weight gain in women found significantly less gain among those with higher fiber intake and suggested that this was mediated by greater gut microbiota diversity.[23]

Given concerns about fat and refined carbohydrates in relation to obesity, some moved to recommending high-protein diets for weight control, noting that protein intake provides greater satiety than other macronutrients and preserves lean body mass during weight loss.[24] A recent review of dietary strategies for weight loss compared high-protein diets (12 studies), with other strategies, including diets focusing on low glycemic index or high fiber, and showed significant beneficial effect only of the high-protein diet in protecting against regain of weight after loss.[25]

B. Micronutrients

Others point to micronutrients and phytonutrients and the loss of exposure to these with processed foods as important. Antioxidants and other phytochemicals in plants may have antiobesogenic effects through pathways that affect appetite, lipid absorption and metabolism, insulin sensitivity, thermogenesis, and the gut microbiota.[26] A 2009 review of this topic pointed to antioxidants—including vitamins C and E and beta-carotene—vitamins A, B, and D, zinc, iron, and calcium as key micronutrients associated with obesity,[27] although they note that the direction of causality is unclear for most of these. They focus their causal argument primarily on leptin, suggesting that supplementation with vitamins A and D may reduce leptin expression and that the antioxidant nutrients are also associated with lower leptin concentration. An editorial[28] concurred that micronutrient deficiencies affect leptin and insulin metabolism, in turn, affecting appetite regulation and energy metabolism. They refer to a 26-week randomized trial in China with a multivitamin/mineral supplement versus placebo, where the supplement appeared to result in significant losses in body weight, fat mass, and waist circumference and increase resting energy expenditure.[29]

Most recently, a 2016 review points to dietary zinc and magnesium as important nutrients in preventing obesity, based on their roles in inflammation.[30] Regardless of the causal pathways, it is clear that obese individuals are more likely than the nonobese to have insufficient status for many micronutrients. The interrelationship is complex but may be due in large part to the fact that obesogenic foods tend to be high energy- and low nutrient-dense. Further concern is that the low nutrient status seen in obese individuals predisposes them to complications, including higher risk of type 2 diabetes.

C. Food Groups

Many argue that examination of individual micronutrients may be too reductionist and that whole foods delivering nutrients within the food matrix are more important. There have been investigations of numerous food groups and obesity. A recent comprehensive review, including 43 reports, showed inverse associations between obesity and whole grains, fruit, nuts, legumes, and fish and positive associations with refined grains, red meat, and SSB.[31] They noted that whole grains, fruit, and vegetables tend to be characterized by low glycemic load, while refined grains and sugar affect insulin resistance, which may contribute to weight gain.

In particular, SSB have received considerable attention. A 2008 review, including 14 prospective and 5 experimental studies, noted that the rise in obesity paralleled increases in soft drink consumption.[32] Three of the experimental studies found increases in body fat associated with SSB, while two did not. Most of the prospective studies found significant associations between SSB intake and obesity, even after adjusting for total energy intake. They conclude that SSB appear to contribute to obesity and that alternative biological associations, beyond higher energy intake, need to be studied.

Interestingly, nuts are high in fat and tend to be avoided by those trying to lose weight, but several studies, including both a prospective cohort with a median of 28 months and the NHS followed for 8 years, showed that frequent intake of nuts was associated with significantly less, not more, weight gain.[33]

D. Dietary Patterns

A tremendous amount of research has gone into understanding the obesity epidemic, and it is increasingly clear that its etiology is complex and that no single food or nutrient can be identified as responsible on its own. Therefore, thinking moved toward the entire dietary pattern. In response to concerns with the USDA diet pyramid and its associated Healthy Eating Index (HEI), which emphasized grains at the base, several groups began to examine the alternatives, with a focus on the Mediterranean diet. The Harvard School of Public Health, along with Oldways Preservation Trust, promoted a Mediterranean diet pyramid[34] and, later, an associated Alternative HEI, which included aspects of the Mediterranean diet, and was found to associate with health outcomes more strongly than the USDA HEI.[35] One systematic review[36] noted that the evidence pointed toward protection against obesity with a Mediterranean diet, although not all studies supported this conclusion. Mechanistic support for the Mediterranean diet includes more monounsaturated fatty acids (MUFAs), in the form of olive oil, which has many health benefits, including improved glucose metabolism increased postprandial fat oxidation, and overall energy expenditure, and encourages palatability of salads and vegetables. Further, there is increasing evidence for the beneficial effects of the Mediterranean diet through modulation of the gut microbiome and reducing systemic inflammation.[37]

Other dietary patterns have also been associated with obesity. Using data-driven dietary patterns, for example, one study showed that a diet high in meat and potatoes was associated with gains in BMI, while a pattern high in refined carbohydrates, mainly white bread, was associated with greater gains in central adiposity.[38] A recent review of dietary patterns[39] concluded that the evidence points to plant-based patterns rich in fruit, vegetables, and whole grains and limited in red and processed meat, refined grains, and added sugars as the most effective approach for prevention of obesity and other chronic conditions.

The USDA recently conducted a thorough systematic review of the evidence on dietary patterns and risk of obesity.[40] They concluded that there is moderate evidence that dietary patterns high in fruit, vegetables, whole grains, legumes, unsaturated oils, and fish; low in total meat, saturated fat, cholesterol, sugar-sweetened food and drinks, and sodium; and moderate in dairy and alcohol are associated with lower risk of obesity.

IV. NUTRIENTS, FOODS, AND DIETARY PATTERNS IN RELATION TO TYPE 2 DIABETES

A rapid sequela to the increase in obesity has been a parallel increase in prevalence of type 2 diabetes (Fig. 18.3). As noted above, the CDC showed that prevalence of diabetes increased from less than 2.5% of the US population prior to 1980 to 7.4% by 2015.[41] A more recent report estimates that prevalence further increased to 9.4% by 2017. Importantly, it is not distributed equally, being more common among American Indian/Alaskan Natives, non-Hispanic blacks, and Hispanics than among non-Hispanic whites or Asians.[41] Further, prevalence is associated with education and is highest among those with less than high school completion. It is also distributed unequally across states, with highest prevalence among adults, 18 y or older, in Mississippi (14%), West Virginia (13%), Alabama (12%), and Louisiana (12%). States with the lowest prevalence include Colorado (6%), Montana, New Hampshire, and Minnesota (each 7%).

Obesity, and more specifically central obesity, measured by waist circumference[42] is the strongest predictor of incident type 2 diabetes. Visceral obesity in the central abdomen is associated with metabolic abnormalities that increase risk beyond BMI, with higher insulinemic and glycemic responses with higher waist circumference. Clearly, the same foods and nutrients that contribute to obesity contribute through obesity to risk of type 2 diabetes.

Beyond obesity per se, one review article noted that dietary fat quality, carbohydrate quality, dietary fiber, and glycemic index, as well as with intakes of vitamin E, magnesium, chromium, and alcohol, affect glucose tolerance and insulin sensitivity, and therefore risk of type 2 diabetes.[43] Another review concurred that, beyond quantity of macronutrients, the quality of dietary fats and carbohydrates is of most importance.[44] In their summary of metaanalyses, they identified protective effects against type 2 diabetes with higher intakes of vitamin D, magnesium, and cereal fiber and risk with higher glycemic load and heme iron.

A. Macronutrients

Debate remains on the ideal macronutrient composition for diabetes prevention, with variation across global guidelines in the proportions from carbohydrate, protein, and fat. Carbohydrate intake has long been the focus of diabetes control and prevention. In 2004, the American Diabetes Association issued a statement that although diabetes has been seen as primarily a disorder of carbohydrate metabolism, a low carbohydrate diet is not recommended.[45] Rather, the focus should be on carbohydrate quality and glycemic load, as the glycemic

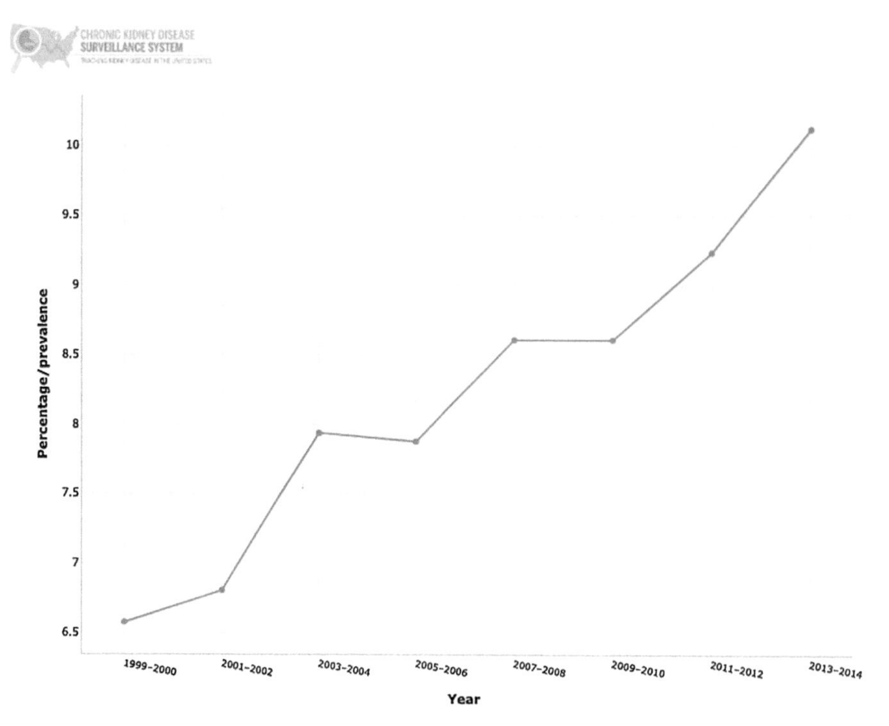

FIGURE 18.3 Percentage of US adults with diabetes by year. National Health and Nutrition Examination Survey. *Centers for Disease Control and Prevention. Chronic Kidney Disease Surveillance System—United States. Website: http://www.cdc.gov/ckd.*

index of the food is what determines the postprandial glucose response. Glycemic load is the sum of the carbohydrate in each food times their respective glycemic index. They noted that the use of glycemic load for blood glucose control has been supported by randomized controlled trials. Low glycemic index foods tend to be those high in fiber, while foods, with high sugar or refined grains, like white flour and white rice, contribute to higher glycemic load.

Although fat has received less focus than carbohydrates in diabetes prevention, one replacement analysis showed that high intake of saturated fat affects insulin sensitivity and risk of diabetes, while higher intake of polyunsaturated fatty acids reduces the risk.[46] A review of dietary fats and prevention of type 2 diabetes[47] concluded that replacing saturated and trans fats with polyunsaturated and/or monounsaturated fats is beneficial for insulin sensitivity and may reduce the risk of type 2 diabetes.

More recently, investigators have also examined the role of dietary protein in diabetes. A 2017 systematic review and metaanalysis of 11 cohort studies concluded that higher total protein was associated with higher risk, with a summary RR of 1.12(1.08−1.17), higher risks associated primarily with animal protein, and lower risk with plant protein.[48] A study from China concurred, noting that the association between protein and diabetes is not straightforward, and varies by dietary pattern, with plant protein inversely and animal protein positively associated.[49] As for obesity, it is increasingly clear that the absolute relative composition of fat, carbohydrate, and protein is less important than the quality of food choices within these categories.

As with many conditions, alcohol appears to be associated with risk of diabetes in a U-shaped curve, with a protective effect of moderate, but not high intake. A systematic review and metaanalysis concluded that risk for type 2 diabetes among men was lowest at 22 g/day of alcohol (RR = 0.87(0.76−1.0), but risk increased significantly at more than 60 g/day; while among women, risk was lowest at 24 g/day, RR = 0.60(0.62−0.69), and increased at more than 50 g/day.[50]

B. Micronutrients

Vitamin E is an important antioxidant that affects oxidative stress and insulin resistance. A study in New Zealand found that participants taking vitamin E, versus placebo, had lower plasma peroxides, blood glucose, and improved insulin sensitivity, suggesting that vitamin E could contribute to the delay in onset of diabetes.[51] A more recent review also concluded that vitamin E was related to significant reduction in plasma glucose and HbA1c, relative to placebo.[52] However, results from the Insulin Resistance Atherosclerosis Study (IRAS) showed that plasma alpha-tocopherol was protective against the development of type 2 diabetes among nonsupplement users, but not among supplement users, suggesting that the vitamin E from food sources may be most protective.[53]

Carotenoids also have important antioxidant activity and, similarly, may protect against diabetes by reducing oxidative stress. Examination of NHANES data showed inverse associations between serum beta-carotene ($P = .004$) and serum lycopene ($P = .044$) with newly diagnosed diabetes.[54] A more recent analysis from Australia showed that 2-hour postload plasma glucose and insulin concentrations were significantly lower with higher serum alpha- and beta-carotene, beta-cryptoxanthin, lutein/zeaxanthin, and lycopene.[55]

Vitamin D has also been linked with risk of diabetes and is involved with insulin secretion, resistance, and β-cell function, partially through increased parathyroid hormone with low vitamin D.[56] A review of this topic concluded that evidence suggests that although there are plausible mechanisms, and evidence of association between vitamin D deficiency and onset of diabetes, supplementation with vitamin D has not been shown to prevent incident diabetes or to improve glycemic control.[57] More work is needed in this area.

Magnesium is a nutrient that is lost during processing and, therefore, many people are at risk of inadequate intake with current dietary exposures. Magnesium serves as a cofactor for enzymes involved in glucose metabolism, and it is, therefore, of importance to prevention of type 2 diabetes.[58] Analysis of data with more than 85,000 women in the NHS and 42,800 men in the Health Professionals Follow-up Study (HPFS) showed significant association between magnesium intake and risk of diabetes.[59] A review of magnesium on health noted that trials with magnesium supplements have shown significant improvement in insulin sensitivity among individuals without diabetes, but with insulin resistance.[60] Food sources of magnesium include whole grains, dark green leafy vegetables, nuts, and legumes.

Chromium has been shown to be important in insulin signaling and sensitivity, and chromium tissue concentration has been associated with incident type 2 diabetes.[61] A review of the actions of chromium concluded that a large body of evidence, including both animal and human studies, shows that chromium is essential for insulin action but noted that the use of chromium supplementation for diabetes remains controversial.[62] Good sources of chromium include broccoli, green beans, apples, bananas, and whole grains.

C. Food Groups

Among food groups, Ley et al.[44] identified protection against diabetes with higher intakes of coffee, alcohol, dairy, and green leafy vegetables and risk with higher intakes of processed meat, red meat, white rice, and SSB. A recent systematic review and metaanalysis specifically examined relationships between 12 food groups with risk of type 2 diabetes.[63] They showed significant protective effects with greater intake of whole grains, vegetables, fruit, and dairy and significant negative effects with refined grains, eggs, red meat, processed meat, and SSB. They found no significant associations between risk of type 2 diabetes and intakes of nuts, legumes, or fish.

D. Dietary Patterns

With multiple nutrients and foods associated with diabetes, dietary patterns including these foods should be associated as well. Schulze et al. conducted a case–control study within the NHS comparing those with type 2 diabetes with those without this condition.[64] Using reduced rank regression, they identified a dietary pattern high in SSB, refined grains, diet soft drinks, and processed meat, while low in wine, coffee, cruciferous, and yellow vegetables with more than three times the likelihood of diabetes. They then examined incident cases and confirmed RR for extreme quintiles of 2.56(2.10–3.12) and 2.93(2.18–3.92) in the NHS and the NHSII, respectively. The identified pattern was strongly associated with inflammatory markers, suggesting that this mechanism may be responsible for the higher risk of diabetes.

A 2014 review[44] cited several studies showing lower risk of type 2 diabetes with the Mediterranean, Dietary Approaches to Stop Hypertension (DASH), and vegetarian diets. They further noted that higher scores on the alternative HEI and data-driven prudent dietary pattern (high in fruit, vegetables, whole grains, and vegetable oils and low in red meat, refined grains, and soft drinks) were associated with lower risk of type 2 diabetes. A more recent overview[65] concludes that there is general consensus that dietary patterns high in vegetables, fruit, whole grains, legumes, nuts, and dairy products including yogurt are useful in the prevention of type 2 diabetes, and that the Mediterranean diet is generally recommended.

Many agencies, including the CDC, have adopted a diabetes prevention plan for individuals with impaired glucose tolerance (prediabetes). This plan, which includes dietary and exercise lifestyle changes, was shown in a major trial[66] to be highly effective in a dose–response manner, reducing risk of incident diabetes by 58% overall, with greater results for compliant individuals. In addition to guidance on aerobic and resistance exercise, participants received tailored individual advice from a registered dietitian, with emphasis on reduction in total fat intake to <30% and saturated fat to <10% of energy and increases in dietary fiber to at least 15 g/1000 kcal. Whole grains, vegetables, fruit, low-fat milk and meat products, and monounsaturated-rich vegetable oils were encouraged.

The USDA conducted a systematic review on dietary patterns and risk of type 2 diabetes.[40] They concluded that there is evidence that a pattern high in fruit, vegetables, legumes, whole grains, nuts, fish, and unsaturated oils and low in meat and high-fat dairy is associated with lower risk of type 2 diabetes, based on dietary indices. They further note that dietary patterns identified by cluster or factor analysis also suggest that diets high in vegetables, fruit, and low-fat dairy were associated with lower risk, while those high in red meat, sugar-sweetened food and drinks, French fries, refined grains, and high-fat dairy were associated with higher risk. They reported, however, that there was insufficient evidence for Mediterranean or vegetarian dietary patterns in relation to incident type 2 diabetes, although the Mediterranean, DASH, and Nordic diets all have shown associations with better glucose tolerance and insulin resistance.

V. NUTRIENTS, FOODS, AND DIETARY PATTERNS IN RELATION TO TYPE CARDIOVASCULAR DISEASE

For the past 90 years, CVD has been the leading cause of death in the United States. Interestingly, despite the recent increases in obesity and diabetes described above, both of which are risk factors for CVD, mortality from CVD has declined in recent decades. However, the history of heart disease is also dramatic. Between the turn of the century in 1900 and the 1930s, heart disease went from an uncommon cause of death to the most common cause, due to increases in atherosclerosis.[67] It continued to rise, and reached 466 deaths/100,000 individuals at its peak in 1965, followed by a decline (Fig. 18.4). The magnitude of the problem led to considerable attention in the medical community and researchers, with efforts in identification of risk factors and development of new medical therapies. A major contributor to knowledge on this condition is the Framingham Heart Study, which began in 1948 in Massachusetts and has continued since that time.[68] Among their many findings, they confirmed that serum cholesterol predicted coronary heart disease (CHD). At the same time, they documented a 59% decrease in CHD mortality from 1950–69 to 1990–99, attributing this to improvements in both primary and secondary prevention, including reduction in smoking, increased use of aspirin, b-adrenergic receptor blockers, ACE

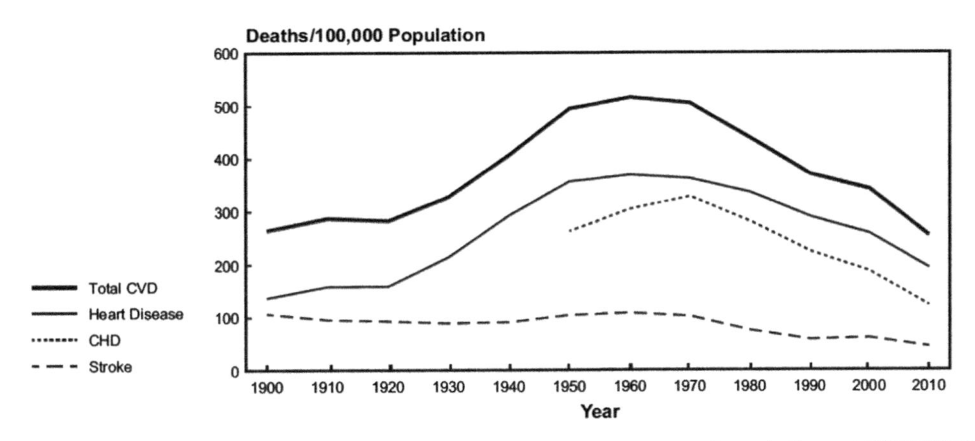

FIGURE 18.4 Death rates* for cardiovascular diseases: United States, 1900–2010. *Not age-adjusted. *Source: NHLBI FY 2012 Fact Book Chapter 4. Disease Statistics.*

inhibitors, lipid-lowering therapy, antiplatelet and thrombolytic treatment, and coronary surgery, as well as improvement in automated external defibrillators.[69] Importantly, CVD remains the number one cause of death in the United States. The lifetime risk of CHD after age 40 y has been estimated at 49% for men and 32% for women.[70] Globally, the risk of CHD continues to increase, therefore prevention is of critical importance and dietary intake is a major modifiable risk factor.

A. Macronutrients

As heart disease increased in the early part of the 20th century, little attention was initially paid to diet. However, the diet-heart health hypothesis became popular once serum cholesterol was clearly linked with atherosclerosis and incident CHD.[71] Famously, Ancel Keys presented ecological data from six countries, showing a correlation between total fat intake and death from heart disease.[72] Beginning in the late 1950s, researchers noted that serum cholesterol could be lowered by replacing saturated fat with vegetable oil.[73,74] In 1958, Dr. Keys launched the "Seven Countries Study," where they followed 12,500 middle aged men in Italy, Greece, Yugoslavia, Finland, Netherlands, Japan, and the United States and found strong associations between intake of saturated fat and heart disease.[75] Later, data from the seven countries study showed strong associations between 25-y CHD death rates and intake of the four major saturated fatty acids, lauric, myristic, palmitic, and stearic acid, of the trans fatty acid elaidic acid, and of dietary cholesterol.[76]

Along with limiting total and saturated fat to less than 30% and 10% of energy, and dietary cholesterol to less than 300 mg/day, the USDA food guide pyramid, designed in 1992, made grains the base, suggesting that people should eat the largest portion of the energy intake from the breads, cereals, rice, and pasta group.[77] This advice led to widespread messaging to lower fat in the diet, and food companies responded with a multitude of "low-fat" foods, mainly replacing the fat with carbohydrate which, in the US food supply, tended to be sugar and refined white flour. However, it was soon noted that replacing fat with refined carbohydrates led to increased triglyceride concentration and other health risks.[78] There has recently been considerable debate as to whether the early work on fat in the diet-heart hypothesis led to the focus on fat, in part, as a deflection away from sugar—as it appears that several important studies, including a highly influential 1967 review article in the New England Journal of Medicine by leading Harvard nutrition professors,[79] were funded by the sugar industry.[80] It has since been made clear that high intake of refined carbohydrates, including sugar, is also a major risk for heart disease. For example, the NHANES III–linked mortality cohort, with data from 1988 to 2006, showed that individuals consuming 10 – <25% or ≥25% of energy from sugar had hazard ratios (HR) (95% CI) for CVD mortality of 1.3(1.09–1.55) and 2.75(1.4–5.4), respectively, relative to those consuming <10% energy from sugar.[81]

In the meantime, along with lower fat food products, our food supply was increasingly replacing saturated fat with hydrogenated oils, in the misbelief that these were healthier alternatives. Margarines were recommended over butter, and processed baked goods with hydrogenated fats had the benefits of longer shelf life. It was not until the 1990s that trans fats were recognized as being worse for health than saturated fats. A New England Journal article in 1990[82] noted that trans fats not only raised LDL cholesterol, similarly to SFA, but also lowered HDL cholesterol, resulting in an overall more negative effect than the SFA. A subsequent NHS analysis showed a 50% greater relative risk for the highest versus lowest quartile of trans fat intake on incident CHD, 1.5(1.12–2.0).[83] Most recently, a systematic review showed significant associations between trans fat intake and all-cause mortality HR of 1.34(1.16–1.56) and CHD mortality of 1.28(1.09–1.5).

Although reducing saturated and trans fatty acids remains important for reducing heart disease, the actual effect depends on with what these fatty acids are replaced. MUFAs have recently emerged as heart healthy, primarily as part of the Mediterranean diet (see below), which has olive oil as the primary source of fat. It has been difficult to separate MUFAs from saturated fats in US and European studies, as MUFAs are commonly consumed along with SFA in meats. In a set of randomized crossover trials, where saturated fat was replaced with PUFA or MUFA, plasma LDL cholesterol was lowered by 22%, and HDL was lowered by 14% with PUFA, while LDL was lowered 15% and HDL by only 4% with MUFA.[84] They concluded that either replacement was equally effective. As recently as 2012, a review of the evidence concluded that results of MFA on CHD were inconsistent, but they noted protective effects on blood pressure and glycosylated hemoglobin.[85] Recent analyses of the NHS and HPFS found significant protective effects of MUFA from plant sources, in replacement of SFA and MUFA from animal sources, the HR(95%CI) for incident nonfatal myocardial infarction and fatal CHD, was 0.81(0.73–0.90).[86]

Although there is considerable evidence that replacing SFA with PUFA has benefit, there is also concern that due to greater unsaturation, there may be greater susceptibility to LDL oxidation with PUFA than MUFA.[87] Observation of lower heart disease risk among Greenland Eskimos,[88] who had high intakes of marine source long-chain omega-3 fatty acids, generated research to examine differences between omega-6 and omega-3 PUFA. Despite considerable attention and widespread belief of their protective effects, however, a recent Cochrane systematic review[89] concluded that moderate and high-quality evidence showed no protective effect of omega-3 fatty acids on CVD. However, this remains controversial, and most recently, the FDA has approved a new prescription drug, *icosapent ethyl*, an eicosapentaenoic acid ethyl ester, which contains 4 g/day of omega-3 fatty acids, after a major clinical trial, with 8000 patients showed significantly lower risk of ischemic events, including cardiovascular mortality RR = 0.80(0.66–0.98).[90]

Historical recommendations by the American Heart Association for the percent of energy from total fat evolved from 25%–30% in 1950, to <40% in 1968, and to <30% from 1982 to 2000. In 2006, this was changed to a range of 25%–35%,[91] with <7% as saturated and <1% as trans fat. Current AHA guidelines do not specify proportions of energy from fat, but simply state "Eat foods low in saturated and trans fat," encouraging intake of lean meats, tofu, fish, vegetables, beans, nuts, and low-fat dairy products and replacing saturated fats like butter with polyunsaturated or monounsaturated fats, like canola and olive oils.[92] They now also recommend limiting added sugars to no more than 100 kilocalories per day for women, and no more than 150 per day for men.[93] The 2015–2020 Dietary Guidelines for Americans also removed limitations on total fat and cholesterol intake, stating only to "consume an eating pattern low in added sugars, saturated fats and sodium."[94]

B. Micronutrients

Although the major focus on diet and heart disease has been on fats and sugars, many vitamins play important roles, including most of the B vitamins, vitamins C, D, and E, and previtamin A carotenoids. A major role of B vitamins is in the prevention of high homocysteine, a sulfur-containing intermediate metabolite that becomes elevated with insufficient intakes of folate, vitamin B12, and/or vitamin B6. Homocysteine has been associated with significantly higher risk of CHD. One review article estimated that every 5 umol/L of homocysteine was associated with 20% increase risk of CHD.[95] Numerous studies have also shown direct associations between B vitamin status and risk of heart disease. For example, in the Kuopio Heart Disease Risk Factor Study, the highest, versus lowest, quintile of plasma folate was associated with 65% lower risk of acute coronary events over 10 years, RR = 0.45(0.25–0.81).[96] In the Atherosclerosis Risk in Communities study, there was 72% lower risk HR = 0.28(0.10–0.70) of incident CHD in the highest, versus lowest, quintile of plasma pyridoxyl-5-phosphate (vitamin B6).[97] In the Netherlands, those in the lowest, versus highest, quartile of serum vitamin B12 were almost three times likely to develop coronary atherosclerosis, OR = 2.9(1.1–7.7).[98] Although numerous studies have shown associations of low B vitamin status with risk of CVD, a metaanalysis of B vitamin supplementation with CVD outcomes showed little or no protection against incidence of major cardiovascular events.[99] In contrast, another metaanalysis showed 10% lower risk of stroke and 4% lower risk of overall CVD with folic acid supplementation, but no effect on CHD.[100] It is likely that the effect of supplementation depends on baseline status.

Vitamin C is an effective antioxidant and free radical scavenger, which makes it a likely candidate for protection against CVD. Several, but not all, observational studies have shown protective effects. A 2016 review,[101] which considered both observational studies and randomized controlled trials, reported mixed results, with several cohort studies, including the European Prospective Investigation into Cancer and Nutrition, the Coronary Artery Development in Young Adults Study, and the Kuopio Ischemic Heart Disease Risk Factor Study showing protective effects, the NHS showing protective effects only with vitamin C supplements, no association in the HPFS, or IRAS, and increased risk with supplemental vitamin C in the Iowa Women's Health Study. Clinical trials generally showed no effect. They concluded that there is little support for the use of vitamin C supplements to reduce CVD risk, although evidence does exist for a protective effect of vitamin C intake on blood pressure and endothelial function. Consistently, a recent Cochrane review on vitamin C and primary prevention of CVD, including eight randomized clinical trials with 15,445 participants, concluded that there was no difference in major CVD events between vitamin C and placebo groups, although they noted that the quality of the evidence was low.[102] Further work is needed to separate effects of dietary vitamin C exposure from that of supplements.

Vitamin D has received considerable attention for multiple effects on health, including a potential role in CHD. Underlying mechanisms for this vitamin in CHD include inhibition of vascular smooth muscle proliferation, downregulation of pro- and upregulation of antiinflammatory cytokines, suppression of vascular calcification, and as a negative endocrine regulator of the renin-angiotensin system, the latter leading to insulin resistance and metabolic syndrome.[103] Several prospective cohort studies have shown protective effects in relation to CVD. For example, in the Framingham Offspring study,[104] participants with low 25(OH)D were 62% more likely to have an incident CVD event 1.62 (95% CI: 1.11–2.36, $P = .01$). In the HPFS, men with 25(OH)D ≤ 15 ng/mL had twice the risk of MI, relative to those with ≥ 30 ng/mL (RR = 2.09, 95% CI: 1.24–3.54, P-trend = 0.02).[105] Further, a recent review of several observational studies showed associations between low vitamin D status, hypertension, and higher CVD mortality.[106] However, several clinical trials have not supported vitamin D supplementation to prevent heart disease, including the recent large Vitamin D and Omega-3 Trial, with 2000 IU/day for more than 5 years, which showed no protection relative to placebo against CVD outcomes.[107] As with many nutrient health associations, results from observational studies, which suggest a long-term status based on food intake, and in this case sunlight exposure, show results that differ from interventions with supplements. More research is needed to clarify the meaning of these differences.

Vitamin E is a strong antioxidant that has been hypothesized to reduce risk of heart disease by protecting against the oxidation of LDL cholesterol, which contributes to heart disease through the release of inflammatory cytokines and enhanced adhesion to the endothelium, leading to atherosclerosis.[108] During the 1990s, considerable attention was given to the potential role of antioxidant intakes, including vitamin E, and CVD.

Several large cohort studies showed protective effects, including a large analysis involving 16 European populations, where plasma vitamin E showed a strong inverse correlation with mortality from ischemic heart disease ($r^2 = 0.63$, $P = 0.002$).[109] This was followed by evidence supportive of vitamin E intake and risk of CHD in the HPFS,[110] which showed a significant dose–response trend ($P = .01$) between total vitamin E intake and a 40% lower risk among those with the top quintile of vitamin E intake, versus the lowest, in fully adjusted models. Similarly, in the NHS,[111] higher vitamin E intake was associated with mortality from CHD over 8 years of follow-up, particularly among those not taking supplements (P trend = 0.004), and RR was 62% lower for women in the highest, versus lowest, quintile of intake. Several other cohort studies showed consistent results.[112–115] Together, these studies provided strong evidence for a protective effect of vitamin E, and many people began to take it.

In contrast to the promising results from observational studies, however, many subsequent clinical trials showed no effect of vitamin E supplementation on risk of heart disease,[116,117] Further, one metaanalysis of 19 trials showed increased risk with doses >150 IU/day.[118] There may be many reasons for this, but most importantly, there are important differences between long-term intake of a nutrient within the food matrix and dietary pattern and relatively short time intervention with supplementation with a single form. Most vitamin E supplements are provided as alpha-tocopherol, while vitamin E in foods presents with differing forms of the nutrient. There is evidence that gamma-tocopherol, the major form in the diet, may have important roles in health on its own, including in CVD.[119] Animal studies have shown greater effects on platelet aggregation, and inhibition of superoxide generation and LDL oxidation with gamma- than with alpha-tocopherol. This is consistent with results from the NHS, where dietary vitamin E, but not supplemental vitamin E, was protective against CVD mortality (Kushi 1996). Importantly, gamma-tocopherol concentration has been shown to be reduced among individuals taking alpha-tocopherol supplements, as in the Jackson Heart Study, where use of supplements was common.[120] High circulation of alpha-tocopherol from supplements may reduce gamma-tocopherol due to competition for hepatic transfer to protein carriers, leading to degradation of gamma-tocopherol.[121] This illustrates the complexity of differences between food sources of nutrients in observational studies and effects of supplements in clinical trials. Together, the evidence suggests that vitamin E from foods may be protective, but that supplements are not recommended. Good food sources of vitamin E include almonds and sunflower seeds.

Dietary carotenoids comprise numerous compounds in plants. In the human diet, the most common carotenoids are alpha-carotene, beta-carotene, and beta-cryptoxanthin, each precursers of vitamin A, and also lycopene, lutein, and zeaxanthin, found mainly in fruit and vegetables. In addition to their contribution to vitamin A, carotenoids act as important antioxidants. Among the major carotenoids, there is evidence for protective effects against heart disease for alpha- and beta-carotene. For example, in the NHS, after 12 years of follow-up, those in the highest, versus lowest, quintiles of intake for these two carotenoids had 20% and 25% lower risk of coronary artery disease, respectively.[122] Similarly, an Italian case–control study,[123] a Japanese study,[124] and the European Zutphen Elderly Study,[125] each showed protection against CVD, MI, or cardiovascular mortality with intake of carotenoids.

Other studies have shown greater protective associations against CVD with plasma lycopene.[126] For example, the Women's Health Study showed that those above, versus below, the median lycopene concentration had 34% lower risk. In the prospective Kuopio study in Finland, men in the lowest quartile, versus higher, of plasma lycopene had 3.3 times the risk of acute coronary events, and in a cross-sectional study, lycopene was significantly inversely associated with intima-media thickness of the carotid artery in men in fully adjusted models.[127,128] Similarly, in the Framingham Heart Study, lycopene intake was associated with lower incident CHD, HR = 0.74(0.58–0.94) for each 2.7 times difference in intake.[129] Most recently, a systematic review and metaanalysis concluded that high intake and serum status of lycopene were associated with 26% reduction in risk of stroke, 14% in CVD, and 37% in total mortality,[130] while another metaanalysis of 14 studies[131] also concluded that higher lycopene was associated with lower risk of CVD, CHD, and stroke. The major source of lycopene in the US diet is tomatoes, with cooked tomatoes having more bioavailable lycopene than raw. In addition to inverse associations with lycopene intake, Jacques et al.[129] found significant associations between tomato intake and heart disease in the Framingham Offspring Study; in fully adjusted models, the HR for intake of tomato products was 0.92(0.86–0.99). Mechanisms for lycopene against heart disease include protection of vascular function through prevention of atherosclerosis, antioxidant, antiinflammatory, antiplatelet, and antiapoptotic activities.[132] A recent review comparing lycopene versus tomato products in clinical trials showed that tomato provided better results against CVD risk factors than lycopene supplementation, with the exception of blood pressure, where lycopene appeared more effective.[133]

Lutein/zeaxanthin has also shown protective effects, based on an inhibitory effect of lutein on monocyte migration and on their inflammatory response to oxidized LDL in mice.[134,135] Although human studies have shown mixed results, a pooled analysis of nine cohorts showed a significant trend for lower risk of CHD events with higher lutein intake.[136] Lutein is found in yellow corn, egg yolk, oranges, and dark green leafy vegetables. It has been shown to inhibit lipid peroxidation[132] and therefore is likely to contribute to prevention of atherosclerosis. Zeaxanthin is an isomer of lutein, with similar food sources, which has been shown to protect against oxidative damage by regulating cellular antioxidant systems, and increasing glutathione concentrations in response to oxidative stress.[137]

As with vitamin E, despite evidence of protective effects in observational cohorts, RCT have not, for the most part, shown successful results with supplemental carotenoid intervention. The most common supplement has been in the form of beta-carotene. A metaanalysis of eight trials showed not only no benefit but also slight increase in risk of CVD and mortality. A systematic review of 12 trials subsequently confirmed significantly higher risk of mortality (7%) relative to placebo.[138,139] Together, this information again suggests caution in the use of a single nutrient supplements as an intervention, rather than a closer look at the complexity of food sources.

Among minerals, magnesium is a nutrient of importance for CVD. A recent overview[140] concluded that higher magnesium intake was associated with lower risk of metabolic syndrome, diabetes, hypertension, stroke, and CVD. They cite a pooled analysis of nine prospective cohorts showing inverse borderline associations of magnesium intake with CHD risk (RR = 0.90, 0.80–0.99) and a Japanese study showing protection against CHD in men in the fourth and fifth quintiles relative to the lowest (P-trend = 0.36). Further, several studies have shown associations between dietary magnesium intake and risk of CVD mortality, although not all are consistent. In one metaanalysis, protective effects were seen only in women.[141] However, a more recent metaanalysis[142] showed that those with higher, versus lowest, intakes of magnesium were 14% less likely to experience CVD mortality. Magnesium is important for numerous biological pathways that may affect CVD, including insulin resistance, dyslipidemia, oxidative stress, and inflammation.[140]

C. Food Groups

Despite questions regarding omega-3 fatty acids, there is considerable support for fish intake in prevention of heart disease. One metaanalysis of 11 studies over almost 12 y of follow-up showed that consumption of 2–4 fish meals/week was associated with 23% lower risk of CHD mortality.[143] A more recent review[144] confirms this finding and hypothesizes that the action is through antiinflammatory actions, inhibition of platelet aggregation, triglyceride lowering, enhancement of endothelial function, plaque stabilization, and antiarrhythmic effects. They note, however, that despite protective associations between fish intake and CVD in observational studies, trials of fish oil have been mixed, with some, but not all, showing protective effects, suggesting that fish, rather than supplements, is the preferred method of prevention.

There have been extensive reports of the benefits of fruit and vegetable intake for heart disease. A recent systematic review and metaanalysis[145] concluded that the RR/200 g/day of fruit and vegetable intake was 0.92(0.90–0.940) for CHD, 0.84(0.76–0.93) for stroke, and 0.92(0.90–0.95) for CVD. This, along with the results of numerous studies, leaves no doubt that increasing intake of fruit and vegetables is a priority to prevent heart disease.

D. Dietary Patterns

The evidence for the role of individual nutrients and foods in chronic disease prevention is important, but interpreting this evidence demands an understanding of how each nutrient or food interacts with the total diet. Therefore, the field has moved toward total dietary patterns as the important factor in health outcomes. Several approaches to dietary patterns have been used, including a priori scores, based on guidelines, and data-driven scores, based on population intake. These include the USDA HEI, the DASH diet, the Mediterranean diet, and data-driven Western versus Healthy diets.

Among these, the Mediterranean diet has risen to the top of protective patterns against heart disease. This dietary pattern emerged from the work of Ancel Keys and the Seven Countries study, where it was clear that populations living near the Mediterranean Sea had lower incidence of heart disease.[146] The main characteristics of the Mediterranean diet include consumption of olive oil as the primary source of fat, high intakes of unrefined cereals, vegetables and fruit, moderate intake of dairy products, wine, potatoes, fish, olives, legumes, and nuts, and lower intake of eggs, sweets, red meat, and meat products.[147] Since recognition of the Mediterranean diet, numerous studies have confirmed its utility. One metaanalysis of eight prospective studies showed that each 2-point increase in Mediterranean diet score was associated with 9% lower risk of CVD mortality.[148] Most recently, a careful review of the evidence concluded that there is "strong, plausible and consistent body of available prospective evidence to support the benefits of the Mediterranean diet on cardiovascular health."[149]

Another popular and evidence-based diet is the DASH diet. This diet focuses on maximizing intake of fruit, vegetables, and low-fat dairy, while limiting red meat, saturated fat, and sugars. The focus is on blood pressure, a major risk factor for CVD. In the initial RCT with 8 weeks of intervention, the DASH diet significantly reduced blood pressure.[150] Since then, multiple studies have shown protection from this dietary pattern against heart disease. A recent analysis of the Singapore Chinese Health Study[151] concluded that the DASH dietary pattern was associated with lower risk of coronary artery disease or stroke mortality. Similarly, analysis of data from the Million Veterans Program showed an inverse association between intake following the DASH score and incidence of coronary artery disease.[152] Similarly, in a British population, those with the highest DASH diets had 20% lower risk of incident CVD, and 28% lower risk of CVD related mortality, relative to those with the least DASH type diets.[153]

The USDA conducted a series of exhaustive evidence-based systematic reviews on dietary patterns and risk of CVD.[40] They concluded that there is strong or moderate evidence that dietary patterns high in fruit, vegetables, whole grains, nuts, legumes, unsaturated oils, low-fat diary, poultry, and fish and low in red and processed meat, high-fat dairy, and sugar-sweetened food and drinks, with moderate alcohol, are associated with lower risk of CVD including heart disease and stroke. They further concluded that there is strong evidence that the DASH diet results in lower blood pressure and limited evidence that vegetarian diets are associated with lower risk.

Together, evidence from dietary patterns supports the dietary recommendations to maximize intakes of fruit, vegetables, fish, whole grains, nuts, and seeds and to reduce intakes of meat, processed meat, and refined carbohydrates, including sugars and products from refined flour.

VI. CONCLUSION

Overall, the evidence is relatively consistent that the same healthful foods protect against obesity, type 2 diabetes, and CVDs. These include diets higher in fruit, vegetables, whole grains, nuts and seeds, and low-fat dairy products and lower in processed meat, SSB, refined baked products and other refined grains, and salty snacks. Dietary patterns, including the Mediterranean and DASH diets, appear to offer considerable evidence-based protection. Considerable efforts are needed not only in nutrition education to promote these diets but also with industry to reduce exposure to energy-rich, nutrient-poor foods that are attractive and affordable, but they contribute to the high burden of chronic disease in the United States and beyond.

RESEARCH GAPS

- Although much has been published on diet and chronic disease, it is becoming more apparent that these risks are dependent on interactions with other risks. More research is needed on these interactions, including other health behaviors and genetic variation to move toward personalized nutrition information.
- Current approaches to diet and health research are limited by existing statistical techniques. Innovation in complex data techniques, including machine learning, may lead to improved assessment of dietary risks in complex situations.
- While we have learned much about food groups and dietary patterns, dietary quality within food groups and patterns may be of even greater importance. Methods to examine this detail will require enhancements to current methods of dietary assessment.

VII. REFERENCES

1. Centers for Disease Control and Prevention. *About Chronic Diseases*. National Center for Chronic Disease Prevention and Health Promotion (NCCDPHP); 2019.
2. Hales CM, Fryar CD, Carroll MD, Freedman DS, Ogden CL. Trends in obesity and severe obesity prevalence in US Youth and adults by sex and age, 2007–2008 to 2015–2016. *J Am Med Assoc*. 2018;319(16):1723–1725.
3. Ogden CL, Carroll MD. *Prevalence of Overweight, Obesity, and Extreme Obesity Among Adults: United States, Trends 1960–1962 Through 2007–2008*. Centers for Disease Control and Prevention; 2010.
4. Centers for Disease Control and Prevention. *Long-term Trends in Diabetes Division of Diabetes Translation*. 2017.
5. WHO Library Cataloguing-in-Publication Data Global Status Report on Noncommunicable Diseases 2010 1.Chronic Disease – Prevention and Control. 2.Chronic Disease – Epidemiology. 3.Chronic Disease – Mortality. 4.Cost of Illness. 5.Delivery of Health Care. I.World Health Organization. ISBN 978 92 4 156422 9 (NLM classification: WT 500). ISBN 978 92 4 068645 8.
6. Afshin A, Sur PJ, Fay KA, et al. Health effects of dietary risks in 195 countries, 1990–2017: a systematic analysis for the Global Burden of Disease Study 2017. *Lancet*. 2019;393(10184):1958–1972.
7. Whelan L. 9 supermarket staples that were created by the military. In: *Mother Jones*. 2015. Food ed.
8. Poti JM, Mendez MA, Ng SW, Popkin BM. Is the degree of food processing and convenience linked with the nutritional quality of foods purchased by US households? *Am J Clin Nutr*. 2015; 101(6):1251–1262.
9. Baraldi LG, Martinez Steele E, Canella DS, Monteiro CA. Consumption of ultra-processed foods and associated sociodemographic factors in the USA between 2007 and 2012: evidence from a nationally representative cross-sectional study. *BMJ open*. 2018;8(3). e020574.
10. Popkin BM. The nutrition transition and obesity in the developing world. *J Nutr*. 2001;131(3):871S–873S.
11. Vandevijvere S, Jaacks LM, Monteiro CA, et al. Global trends in ultraprocessed food and drink product sales and their association with adult body mass index trajectories. *Obes Rev*. 2019;20.
12. Monteiro CA, Cannon G, Moubarac JC, Levy RB, Louzada MLC, Jaime PC. The UN decade of nutrition, the NOVA food classification and the trouble with ultra-processing. *Publ Health Nutr*. 2018; 21(1):5–17.
13. Davis RAH, Plaisance EP, Allison DB. Complementary hypotheses on contributors to the obesity epidemic. *Obesity*. 2018;26(1):17–21.
14. Franks PW, McCarthy MI. Exposing the exposures responsible for type 2 diabetes and obesity. *Science*. 2016;354(6308):69–73.
15. Welsh S, Davis C, Shaw A. Development of the food guide pyramid. *Nutr Today*. 1992;27(6):12–23.
16. La Berge AF. How the ideology of low fat conquered America. *J Hist Med Allied Sci*. 2008;63(2):139–177.
17. Willett WC, Leibel RL. Dietary fat is not a major determinant of body fat. *Am J Med*. 2002;113(9 Suppl 2):47–59.
18. Liu S, Willett WC, Manson JE, Hu FB, Rosner B, Colditz G. Relation between changes in intakes of dietary fiber and grain products and changes in weight and development of obesity among middle-aged women. *Am J Clin Nutr*. 2003;78(5):920–927.
19. Wolff E, Dansinger ML. Soft drinks and weight gain: how strong is the link? *Medscape J Med*. 2008;10(8):189.
20. Pereira MA. Sugar-sweetened and artificially-sweetened beverages in relation to obesity risk. *Adv Nutr*. 2014;5(6):797–808.
21. Johnson RJ, Sánchez-Lozada LG, Andrews P, Lanaspa MA. Perspective: a historical and scientific perspective of sugar and its relation with obesity and diabetes. *Adv Nutr*. 2017;8(3): 412–422.
22. Burton-Freeman B. Dietary fiber and energy regulation. *J Nutr*. 2000;130(2S Suppl):272s–275s.
23. Menni C, Jackson MA, Pallister T, Steves CJ, Spector TD, Valdes AM. Gut microbiome diversity and high-fibre intake are related to lower long-term weight gain. *Int J Obes*. 2017;41(7): 1099–1105.
24. Astrup A, Raben A, Geiker N. The role of higher protein diets in weight control and obesity-related comorbidities. *Int J Obes*. 2015; 39(5):721–726.
25. van Baak MA, Mariman ECM. Dietary strategies for weight loss maintenance. *Nutrients*. 2019;11(8):1916.
26. Martel J, Ojcius DM, Chang C-J, et al. Anti-obesogenic and antidiabetic effects of plants and mushrooms. *Nat Rev Endocrinol*. 2017; 13(3):149–160.
27. Garcia OP, Long KZ, Rosado JL. Impact of micronutrient deficiencies on obesity. *Nutr Rev*. 2009;67(10):559–572.
28. Astrup A, Bügel S. Micronutrient deficiency in the aetiology of obesity. *Int J Obes*. 2010;34(6):947–948.
29. Li Y, Wang C, Zhu K, Feng RN, Sun CH. Effects of multivitamin and mineral supplementation on adiposity, energy expenditure and lipid profiles in obese Chinese women. *Int J Obes*. 2010; 34(6):1070–1077.
30. Amp R. Role of micro-and macro-nutrients in obesity onset. *Global J Obes, Diabetes, Metab Syndrome*. 2016:011–014.
31. Schlesinger S, Neuenschwander M, Schwedhelm C, et al. Food groups and risk of overweight, obesity, and weight gain: a systematic review and dose-response meta-analysis of prospective studies. *Adv Nutr*. 2019;10(2):205–218.
32. Olsen NJ, Heitmann BL. Intake of calorically sweetened beverages and obesity. *Obes Rev*. 2009;10(1):68–75.
33. Bes-Rastrollo M, Wedick NM, Martinez-Gonzalez MA, Li TY, Sampson L, Hu FB. Prospective study of nut consumption, long-term weight change, and obesity risk in women. *Am J Clin Nutr*. 2009;89(6):1913–1919.

34. Willett WC, Sacks F, Trichopoulou A, et al. Mediterranean diet pyramid: a cultural model for healthy eating. *Am J Clin Nutr.* 1995;61(6):1402S–1406S.
35. McCullough ML, Feskanich D, Stampfer MJ, et al. Diet quality and major chronic disease risk in men and women: moving toward improved dietary guidance. *Am J Clin Nutr.* 2002;76(6): 1261–1271.
36. Buckland G, Bach A, Serra-Majem L. Obesity and the Mediterranean diet: a systematic review of observational and intervention studies. *Obes Rev.* 2008;9(6):582–593.
37. Bailey M, Holscher H. Microbiome-mediated effects of the Mediterranean diet on inflammation. *Adv Nutr.* 2018;9:193–206.
38. Newby P, Muller D, Hallfrisch J, Qiao N, Andres R, Tucker KL. Dietary patterns and changes in body mass index and waist circumference in adults. *Am J Clin Nutr.* 2003;77(6):1417–1425.
39. Medina-Remón A, Kirwan R, Lamuela-Raventós RM, Estruch R. Dietary patterns and the risk of obesity, type 2 diabetes mellitus, cardiovascular diseases, asthma, and neurodegenerative diseases. *Crit Rev Food Sci Nutr.* 2018;58(2):262–296.
40. United States Department of Agriculture. *A Series of Systematic Reviews on the Relationship Between Dietary Patterns and Health Outcomes.* 2014.
41. Centers for Disease Control and Prevention. *National Diabetes Statistics Report 2017.* Atlanta, GA: US Dept. of Health and Human Services; 2018.
42. Després J-P. Health consequences of visceral obesity. *Ann Med.* 2001;33(8):534–541.
43. Steyn NP, Mann J, Bennett PH, et al. Diet, nutrition and the prevention of type 2 diabetes. *Publ Health Nutr.* 2004;7(1A):147–165.
44. Ley SH, Hamdy O, Mohan V, Hu FB. Prevention and management of type 2 diabetes: dietary components and nutritional strategies. *Lancet.* 2014;383(9933):1999–2007.
45. Sheard NF, Clark NG, Brand-Miller JC, et al. Dietary carbohydrate (amount and type) in the prevention and management of diabetes: a statement by the american diabetes association. *Diabetes Care.* 2004;27(9):2266–2271.
46. Imamura F, Micha R, Wu JHY, et al. Effects of saturated fat, polyunsaturated fat, monounsaturated fat, and carbohydrate on glucose-insulin homeostasis: a systematic review and meta-analysis of randomised controlled feeding trials. *PLoS Med.* 2016;13(7). e1002087.
47. Riserus U, Willett WC, Hu FB. Dietary fats and prevention of type 2 diabetes. *Prog Lipid Res.* 2009;48(1):44–51.
48. Tian S, Xu Q, Jiang R, Han T, Sun C, Na L. Dietary protein consumption and the risk of type 2 diabetes: a systematic review and meta-analysis of cohort studies. *Nutrients.* 2017;9(9).
49. Ke Q, Chen C, He F, et al. Association between dietary protein intake and type 2 diabetes varies by dietary pattern. *Diabetol Metab Syndrome.* 2018;10:48.
50. Baliunas DO, Taylor BJ, Irving H, et al. Alcohol as a risk factor for type 2 diabetes: a systematic review and meta-analysis. *Diabetes Care.* 2009;32(11):2123–2132.
51. Manning PJ, Sutherland WHF, Walker RJ, et al. Effect of high-dose vitamin E on insulin resistance and associated parameters in overweight subjects. *Diabetes Care.* 2004;27(9):2166–2171.
52. Balbi ME, Tonin FS, Mendes AM, et al. Antioxidant effects of vitamins in type 2 diabetes: a meta-analysis of randomized controlled trials. *Diabetol Metab Syndrome.* 2018;10:18.
53. Mayer-Davis EJ, Costacou T, King I, Zaccaro DJ, Bell RA. Plasma and dietary vitamin E in relation to incidence of type 2 diabetes: the Insulin Resistance and Atherosclerosis Study (IRAS). *Diabetes Care.* 2002;25(12):2172–2177.
54. Ford ES, Will JC, Bowman BA, Narayan KM. Diabetes mellitus and serum carotenoids: findings from the Third National Health and Nutrition Examination Survey. *Am J Epidemiol.* 1999;149(2):168–176.
55. Coyne T, Ibiebele TI, Baade PD, et al. Diabetes mellitus and serum carotenoids: findings of a population-based study in Queensland, Australia. *Am J Clin Nutr.* 2005;82(3):685–693.
56. Chiu KC, Chu A, Go VLW, Saad MF. Hypovitaminosis D is associated with insulin resistance and β cell dysfunction. *Am J Clin Nutr.* 2004;79(5):820–825.
57. Nakashima A, Yokoyama K, Yokoo T, Urashima M. Role of vitamin D in diabetes mellitus and chronic kidney disease. *World J Diabetes.* 2016;7(5):89–100.
58. Paolisso G, Scheen A, D'Onofrio F, Lefebvre P. Magnesium and glucose homeostasis. *Diabetologia.* 1990;33(9):511–514.
59. Lopez-Ridaura R, Willett WC, Rimm EB, et al. Magnesium intake and risk of type 2 diabetes in men and women. *Diabetes Care.* 2004; 27(1):134–140.
60. Volpe SL. Magnesium in disease prevention and overall health. *Adv Nutr.* 2013;4(3):378S–383S.
61. Hummel M, Standl E, Schnell O. Chromium in metabolic and cardiovascular disease. *Horm Metab Res.* 2007;39(10):743–751.
62. Cefalu WT, Hu FB. Role of chromium in human health and in diabetes. *Diabetes Care.* 2004;27(11):2741–2751.
63. Schwingshackl L, Hoffmann G, Lampousi A-M, et al. Food groups and risk of type 2 diabetes mellitus: a systematic review and meta-analysis of prospective studies. *Eur J Epidemiol.* 2017;32(5): 363–375.
64. Schulze MB, Hoffmann K, Manson JE, et al. Dietary pattern, inflammation, and incidence of type 2 diabetes in women. *Am J Clin Nutr.* 2005;82(3):675–684. quiz 714-675.
65. Forouhi NG, Misra A, Mohan V, Taylor R, Yancy W. Dietary and nutritional approaches for prevention and management of type 2 diabetes. *BMJ.* 2018;361:k2234.
66. Tuomilehto J, Lindstrom J, Eriksson JG, et al. Prevention of type 2 diabetes mellitus by changes in lifestyle among subjects with impaired glucose tolerance. *N Engl J Med.* 2001;344(18): 1343–1350.
67. Dalen JE, Alpert JS, Goldberg RJ, Weinstein RS. The epidemic of the 20th century: coronary heart disease. *Am J Med.* 2014;127(9): 807–812.
68. Mahmood SS, Levy D, Vasan RS, Wang TJ. The Framingham Heart Study and the epidemiology of cardiovascular disease: a historical perspective. *Lancet.* 2014;383(9921):999–1008.
69. Fox CS, Evans JC, Larson MG, Kannel WB, Levy D. Temporal trends in coronary heart disease mortality and sudden cardiac death from 1950 to 1999: the Framingham Heart Study. *Circulation.* 2004;110(5):522–527.
70. Lloyd-Jones DM, Larson MG, Beiser A, Levy D. Lifetime risk of developing coronary heart disease. *Lancet.* 1999;353(9147): 89–92.
71. Kannel WB, Dawber TR, Kagan A, Revotskie N, Stokes III J. Factors of risk in the development of coronary heart disease—six-year follow-up experience: the Framingham study. *Ann Intern Med.* 1961;55(1):33–50.
72. Keys A. Atherosclerosis: a problem in newer public health. *J Mt Sinai Hosp N Y.* 1953;20(2):118–139.
73. Bronte-Stewart B, Antonis A, Eales L, Brock JF. Effects of feeding different fats on serum-cholesterol level. *Lancet.* 1956;270(6922): 521–526.
74. Keys A, Anderson JT, Grande F. Prediction of serum-cholesterol responses of man to changes in fats in the diet. *Lancet.* 1957; 273(7003):959–966.
75. Keys A. Coronary heart disease in seven countries. *Heart Assoc Monogr.* 1970;41(29):1–211.
76. Kromhout D, Menotti A, Bloemberg B, et al. Dietary saturated and transfatty acids and cholesterol and 25-year mortality from coronary heart disease: the seven countries study. *Prev Med.* 1995;24(3): 308–315.

77. Dixon LB, Cronin FJ, Krebs-Smith SM. Let the pyramid guide your food choices: capturing the total diet concept. *J Nutr.* 2001; 131(2):461S–472S.
78. Ma Y, Li Y, Chiriboga DE, et al. Association between carbohydrate intake and serum lipids. *J Am Coll Nutr.* 2006;25(2):155–163.
79. McGandy RB, Hegsted DM, Stare FJ. Dietary fats, carbohydrates and atherosclerotic vascular disease. *N Engl J Med.* 1967;277(5): 245–247.
80. Kearns CE, Schmidt LA, Glantz SA. Sugar industry and coronary heart disease research: a historical analysis of internal industry documents. *JAMA Intern Med.* 2016;176(11):1680–1685.
81. Yang Q, Zhang Z, Gregg EW, Flanders WD, Merritt R, Hu FB. Added sugar intake and cardiovascular diseases mortality among US adults. *JAMA Intern Med.* 2014;174(4):516–524.
82. Mensink RP, Katan MB. Effect of dietary trans fatty acids on high-density and low-density lipoprotein cholesterol levels in healthy subjects. *N Engl J Med.* 1990;323(7):439–445.
83. Willett WC, Stampfer MJ, Manson JE, et al. Intake of trans fatty acids and risk of coronary heart disease among women. *Lancet.* 1993;341(8845):581–585.
84. Hodson L, Skeaff CM, Chisholm WA. The effect of replacing dietary saturated fat with polyunsaturated or monounsaturated fat on plasma lipids in free-living young adults. *Eur J Clin Nutr.* 2001;55(10):908–915.
85. Schwingshackl L, Hoffmann G. Monounsaturated fatty acids and risk of cardiovascular disease: synopsis of the evidence available from systematic reviews and meta-analyses. *Nutrients.* 2012;4(12): 1989–2007.
86. Zong G, Li Y, Sampson L, et al. Monounsaturated fats from plant and animal sources in relation to risk of coronary heart disease among US men and women. *Am J Clin Nutr.* 2018;107(3): 445–453.
87. Schwab US, Sarkkinen ES, Lichtenstein AH, et al. The effect of quality and amount of dietary fat on the susceptibility of low density lipoprotein to oxidation in subjects with impaired glucose tolerance. *Eur J Clin Nutr.* 1998;52(6):452–458.
88. Bang HO, Dyerberg J, Hjøorne N. The composition of food consumed by Greenland Eskimos. *Acta Med Scand.* 1976;200: 69–73.
89. Abdelhamid AS, Brown TJ, Brainard JS, et al. Omega-3 fatty acids for the primary and secondary prevention of cardiovascular disease. *Cochrane Database Syst Rev.* 2018;7(7). CD003177.
90. Bhatt DL, Steg PG, Miller M, et al. Cardiovascular risk reduction with icosapent ethyl for hypertriglyceridemia. *N Engl J Med.* 2019; 380(1):11–22.
91. American Heart Association and American Stroke Association. *The Facts on Fats: 50 Years of American Heart Association Dietary Fats Recommendations.* June 2015.
92. Cigna. *American Heart Association Healthy Diet Guidelines;* 2017. Accessed November 18, 2019.
93. American Heart Association. *How much sugar is too much?.* https://www.heart.org/en/healthy-living/healthy-eating/eat-smart/sugar/how-much-sugar-is-too-much. Accessed 18 November 2019.
94. *Dietary Guidelines for Americans 2015–-2020.* 8th ed.; 2015. https://health.gov/dietaryguidelines/2015/guidelines/.
95. Humphrey LL, Fu R, Rogers K, Freeman M, Helfand M. Homocysteine level and coronary heart disease incidence: a systematic review and meta-analysis. *Mayo Clin Proc.* 2008;83(11): 1203–1212.
96. Voutilainen S, Virtanen JK, Rissanen TH, et al. Serum folate and homocysteine and the incidence of acute coronary events: the Kuopio Ischaemic Heart Disease Risk Factor Study. *Am J Clin Nutr.* 2004;80(2):317–323.
97. Folsom AR, Nieto FJ, McGovern PG, et al. Prospective study of coronary heart disease incidence in relation to fasting total homocysteine, related genetic polymorphisms, and B vitamins: the Atherosclerosis Risk in Communities (ARIC) Study. *Circulation.* 1998;98(3):204–210.
98. Siri PW, Verhoef P, Kok FJ. Vitamins B6, B12, and folate: association with plasma total homocysteine and risk of coronary atherosclerosis. *J Am Coll Nutr.* 1998;17(5):435–441.
99. Zhang C, Wang Z-Y, Qin Y-Y, Yu F-F, Zhou Y-H. Association between B vitamins supplementation and risk of cardiovascular outcomes: a cumulative meta-analysis of randomized controlled trials. *PLoS One.* 2014;9(9). e107060.
100. Li Y, Huang T, Zheng Y, Muka T, Troup J, Hu FB. Folic acid supplementation and the risk of cardiovascular diseases: a meta-analysis of randomized controlled trials. *J Am Heart Assoc.* 2016; 5(8):e003768.
101. Moser MA, Chun OK. Vitamin C and heart health: a review based on findings from epidemiologic studies. *Int J Mol Sci.* 2016;17(8).
102. Al-Khudairy L, Flowers N, Wheelhouse R, et al. Vitamin C supplementation for the primary prevention of cardiovascular disease. *Cochrane Database Syst Rev.* 2017;3:Cd011114.
103. Zittermann A, Schleithoff SS, Koerfer R. Putting cardiovascular disease and vitamin D insufficiency into perspective. *Br J Nutr.* 2005;94(4):483–492.
104. Judd SE, Tangpricha V. Vitamin D deficiency and risk for cardiovascular disease. *Am J Med Sci.* 2009;338(1):40–44.
105. Giovannucci E, Liu Y, Hollis BW, Rimm EB. 25-hydroxyvitamin D and risk of myocardial infarction in men: a prospective study. *Arch Intern Med.* 2008;168(11):1174–1180.
106. Kheiri B, Abdalla A, Osman M, Ahmed S, Hassan M, Bachuwa G. Vitamin D deficiency and risk of cardiovascular diseases: a narrative review. *Clin Hypertens.* 2018;24:9.
107. Lucas A, Wolf M. Vitamin D and health outcomes: then came the randomized clinical trials. *J Am Med Assoc.* 2019;322(19): 1866–1868.
108. Singh U, Devaraj S, Jialal I. Vitamin E, oxidative stress, and inflammation. *Annu Rev Nutr.* 2005;25:151–174.
109. Gey KF, Puska P, Jordan P, Moser UK. Inverse correlation between plasma vitamin E and mortality from ischemic heart disease in cross-cultural epidemiology. *Am J Clin Nutr.* 1991;53(1 Suppl): 326s–334s.
110. Rimm EB, Stampfer MJ, Ascherio A, Giovannucci E, Colditz GA, Willett WC. Vitamin E consumption and the risk of coronary heart disease in men. *N Engl J Med.* 1993;328(20):1450–1456.
111. Kushi LH, Folsom AR, Prineas RJ, Mink PJ, Wu Y, Bostick RM. Dietary antioxidant vitamins and death from coronary heart disease in postmenopausal women. *N Engl J Med.* 1996;334(18): 1156–1162.
112. Bolton-Smith C, Woodward M, Tunstall-Pedoe H. The Scottish Heart Health Study. Dietary intake by food frequency questionnaire and odds ratios for coronary heart disease risk. II. The antioxidant vitamins and fibre. *Eur J Clin Nutr.* 1992;46(2): 85–93.
113. Knekt P, Reunanen A, Jarvinen R, Seppanen R, Heliovaara M, Aromaa A. Antioxidant vitamin intake and coronary mortality in a longitudinal population study. *Am J Epidemiol.* 1994;139(12): 1180–1189.
114. Meyer F, Bairati I, Dagenais GR. Lower ischemic heart disease incidence and mortality among vitamin supplement users. *Can J Cardiol.* 1996;12(10):930–934.
115. Losonczy KG, Harris TB, Havlik RJ. Vitamin E and vitamin C supplement use and risk of all-cause and coronary heart disease mortality in older persons: the Established Populations for Epidemiologic Studies of the Elderly. *Am J Clin Nutr.* 1996;64(2): 190–196.
116. Eidelman RS, Hollar D, Hebert PR, Lamas GA, Hennekens CH. Randomized trials of vitamin E in the treatment and prevention

of cardiovascular disease. *Arch Intern Med.* 2004;164(14):1552–1556.
117. Shekelle PG, Morton SC, Jungvig LK, et al. Effect of supplemental vitamin E for the prevention and treatment of cardiovascular disease. *J Gen Intern Med.* 2004;19(4):380–389.
118. Miller 3rd ER, Pastor-Barriuso R, Dalal D, Riemersma RA, Appel LJ, Guallar E. Meta-analysis: high-dosage vitamin E supplementation may increase all-cause mortality. *Ann Intern Med.* 2005;142(1):37–46.
119. Jiang Q, Christen S, Shigenaga MK, Ames BN. γ-Tocopherol, the major form of vitamin E in the US diet, deserves more attention. *Am J Clin Nutr.* 2001;74(6):714–722.
120. Talegawkar SA, Johnson EJ, Carithers T, Taylor Jr HA, Bogle ML, Tucker KL. Total alpha-tocopherol intakes are associated with serum alpha-tocopherol concentrations in African American adults. *J Nutr.* 2007;137(10):2297–2303.
121. Huang HY, Appel LJ. Supplementation of diets with alpha-tocopherol reduces serum concentrations of gamma- and delta-tocopherol in humans. *J Nutr.* 2003;133(10):3137–3140.
122. Osganian SK, Stampfer MJ, Rimm E, Spiegelman D, Manson JE, Willett WC. Dietary carotenoids and risk of coronary artery disease in women. *Am J Clin Nutr.* 2003;77(6):1390–1399.
123. Tavani A, Gallus S, Negri E, Parpinel M, La Vecchia C. Dietary intake of carotenoids and retinol and the risk of acute myocardial infarction in Italy. *Free Radic Res.* 2006;40(6):659–664.
124. Ito Y, Kurata M, Suzuki K, Hamajima N, Hishida H, Aoki K. Cardiovascular disease mortality and serum carotenoid levels: a Japanese population-based follow-up study. *J Epidemiol.* 2006;16(4):154–160.
125. Buijsse B, Feskens EJ, Kwape L, Kok FJ, Kromhout D. Both alpha- and beta-carotene, but not tocopherols and vitamin C, are inversely related to 15-year cardiovascular mortality in Dutch elderly men. *J Nutr.* 2008;138(2):344–350.
126. Sesso HD, Buring JE, Norkus EP, Gaziano JM. Plasma lycopene, other carotenoids, and retinol and the risk of cardiovascular disease in women. *Am J Clin Nutr.* 2004;79(1):47–53.
127. Rissanen TH, Voutilainen S, Nyyssonen K, et al. Low serum lycopene concentration is associated with an excess incidence of acute coronary events and stroke: the Kuopio Ischaemic Heart Disease Risk Factor Study. *Br J Nutr.* 2001;85(6):749–754.
128. Rissanen TH, Voutilainen S, Nyyssonen K, Salonen R, Kaplan GA, Salonen JT. Serum lycopene concentrations and carotid atherosclerosis: the Kuopio Ischaemic Heart Disease Risk Factor Study. *Am J Clin Nutr.* 2003;77(1):133–138.
129. Jacques PF, Lyass A, Massaro JM, Vasan RS, D'Agostino Sr RB. Relationship of lycopene intake and consumption of tomato products to incident CVD. *Br J Nutr.* 2013;110(3):545–551.
130. Cheng HM, Koutsidis G, Lodge JK, Ashor AW, Siervo M, Lara J. Lycopene and tomato and risk of cardiovascular diseases: a systematic review and meta-analysis of epidemiological evidence. *Crit Rev Food Sci Nutr.* 2019;59(1):141–158.
131. Song B, Liu K, Gao Y, et al. Lycopene and risk of cardiovascular diseases: a meta-analysis of observational studies. *Mol Nutr Food Res.* 2017;61(9).
132. Mozos I, Stoian D, Caraba A, Malainer C, Horbańczuk JO, Atanasov AG. Lycopene and vascular health. *Front Pharmacol.* 2018;9:521.
133. Burton-Freeman B, Sesso HD. Whole food versus supplement: comparing the clinical evidence of tomato intake and lycopene supplementation on cardiovascular risk factors. *Adv Nutr.* 2014;5(5):457–485.
134. Dwyer JH, Paul-Labrador MJ, Fan J, Shircore AM, Merz CN, Dwyer KM. Progression of carotid intima-media thickness and plasma antioxidants: the Los Angeles Atherosclerosis Study. *Arterioscler Thromb Vasc Biol.* 2004;24(2):313–319.
135. Iribarren C, Folsom AR, Jacobs Jr DR, Gross MD, Belcher JD, Eckfeldt JH. Association of serum vitamin levels, LDL susceptibility to oxidation, and autoantibodies against MDA-LDL with carotid atherosclerosis. A case-control study. The ARIC Study Investigators. Atherosclerosis Risk in Communities. *Arterioscler Thromb Vasc Biol.* 1997;17(6):1171–1177.
136. Knekt P, Ritz J, Pereira MA, et al. Antioxidant vitamins and coronary heart disease risk: a pooled analysis of 9 cohorts. *Am J Clin Nutr.* 2004;80(6):1508–1520.
137. Gao S, Qin T, Liu Z, et al. Lutein and zeaxanthin supplementation reduces H_2O_2-induced oxidative damage in human lens epithelial cells. *Mol Vis.* 2011;17:3180–3190.
138. Vivekananthan DP, Penn MS, Sapp SK, Hsu A, Topol EJ. Use of antioxidant vitamins for the prevention of cardiovascular disease: meta-analysis of randomised trials. *Lancet.* 2003;361(9374):2017–2023.
139. Bjelakovic G, Nikolova D, Gluud LL, Simonetti RG, Gluud C. Mortality in randomized trials of antioxidant supplements for primary and secondary prevention: systematic review and meta-analysis. *J Am Med Assoc.* 2007;297(8):842–857.
140. Rosique-Esteban N, Guasch-Ferre M, Hernandez-Alonso P, Salas-Salvado J. Dietary magnesium and cardiovascular disease: a review with emphasis in epidemiological studies. *Nutrients.* 2018;10(2).
141. Xu T, Sun Y, Xu T, Zhang Y. Magnesium intake and cardiovascular disease mortality: a meta-analysis of prospective cohort studies. *Int J Cardiol.* 2013;167(6):3044–3047.
142. Fang X, Liang C, Li M, et al. Dose-response relationship between dietary magnesium intake and cardiovascular mortality: a systematic review and dose-based meta-regression analysis of prospective studies. *J Trace Elem Med Biol.* 2016;38:64–73.
143. He K, Song Y, Daviglus ML, et al. Accumulated evidence on fish consumption and coronary heart disease mortality: a meta-analysis of cohort studies. *Circulation.* 2004;109(22):2705–2711.
144. Kromhout D, Yasuda S, Geleijnse JM, Shimokawa H. Fish oil and omega-3 fatty acids in cardiovascular disease: do they really work? *Eur Heart J.* 2012;33(4):436–443.
145. Aune D, Giovannucci E, Boffetta P, et al. Fruit and vegetable intake and the risk of cardiovascular disease, total cancer and all-cause mortality-a systematic review and dose-response meta-analysis of prospective studies. *Int J Epidemiol.* 2017;46(3):1029–1056.
146. Feinleib M. Seven countries: a multivariate analysis of death and coronary heart disease. *J Am Med Assoc.* 1981;245(5):511–512.
147. Dontas AS, Zerefos NS, Panagiotakos DB, Vlachou C, Valis DA. Mediterranean diet and prevention of coronary heart disease in the elderly. *Clin Interv Aging.* 2007;2(1):109–115.
148. Sofi F, Cesari F, Abbate R, Gensini GF, Casini A. Adherence to Mediterranean diet and health status: meta-analysis. *BMJ.* 2008;337:a1344.
149. Martínez-González MA, Gea A, Ruiz-Canela M. The Mediterranean diet and cardiovascular health. *Circ Res.* 2019;124(5):779–798.
150. Conlin PR, Chow D, Miller 3rd ER, et al. The effect of dietary patterns on blood pressure control in hypertensive patients: results from the Dietary Approaches to Stop Hypertension (DASH) trial. *Am J Hypertens.* 2000;13(9):949–955.
151. Talaei M, Koh WP, Yuan JM, van Dam RM. DASH dietary pattern, mediation by mineral intakes, and the risk of coronary artery disease and stroke mortality. *J Am Heart Assoc.* 2019;8(5):e011054.
152. Djoussé L, Ho Y-L, Nguyen X-MT, et al. DASH score and subsequent risk of coronary artery disease: the findings from million Veteran Program. *J Am Heart Assoc.* 2018;7(9):e008089.
153. Jones NRV, Forouhi NG, Khaw KT, Wareham NJ, Monsivais P. Accordance to the Dietary Approaches to Stop Hypertension diet pattern and cardiovascular disease in a British, population-based cohort. *Eur J Epidemiol.* 2018;33(2):235–244.

CHAPTER

19

EATING DISORDERS

Renee D. Rienecke[1,2], *PhD, FAED*
Laura M. Nance[4], *MA, RDN*
Elizabeth M. Wallis[3], *MD, MS*

[1]Eating Recovery Center/Insight Behavioral Health Centers, Chicago, IL, United States
[2]Department of Psychiatry and Behavioral Sciences, Northwestern University, Chicago, IL, United States
[3]Department of Pediatrics, Medical University of South Carolina, Charleston, SC, United States
[4]MUSC Friedman Center for Eating Disorders, Charleston, SC, United States

SUMMARY

Eating disorders are associated with significant medical and psychiatric comorbidity and have among the highest mortality rates of any psychiatric disorder. In the case of anorexia nervosa (AN), the majority of medical complications are related to the direct effect of starvation and malnutrition on the body, whereas with bulimia nervosa (BN), complications are related primarily to purging or other compensatory behaviors. Treatment for eating disorders should involve a multidisciplinary team, with assessments addressing the medical, nutritional, and psychological components of the disorder. Family-based treatment (FBT) and cognitive behavioral therapy (CBT) are the leading evidence-based forms of treatment for eating disorders. Although the prognosis for those who receive treatment is promising, there is a need to improve access to evidence-based treatments and to remove barriers to care, as many individuals with eating disorders do not receive treatment.

Keywords: Anorexia nervosa; Assessment; Binge eating disorder; Bulimia nervosa; Nutritional assessment; Other specified feeing or eating disorder; Treatment.

I. INTRODUCTION

Eating disorders are serious mental illnesses associated with significant medical and psychiatric comorbidity.[1,2] Examples of eating disorders include AN, BN, and binge eating disorder (BED).

AN is characterized by significantly low body weight, fear of gaining weight or engaging in behavior that interferes with weight gain, and disturbance in the way one's body weight or shape is experienced, overvaluation of weight or shape, or lack of recognition of the serious nature of the low weight.[3] Two subtypes of AN are identified: restricting type and binge eating/purging type. Lifetime prevalence rates are estimated to be 0.9% for women and 0.3% for men.[4] Among adolescent girls, it has been identified as the third most common chronic condition after obesity and asthma.[5]

BN is characterized by binge eating, which involves eating a large amount of food in a discrete period of time and experiencing a loss of control over eating, and compensatory behaviors such as self-induced vomiting. These behaviors must occur at least weekly for 3 months and are accompanied by overvaluation of shape and weight.[3] Lifetime prevalence rates are estimated to be 1.5% for women and 0.5% for men.[4]

Individuals with BED engage in binge eating, at least weekly for 3 months, but do not engage in compensatory behaviors. The binge eating is associated with marked distress.[3] Lifetime prevalence rates for BED are 3.5% for women and 2.0% for men.[4] Those who

https://doi.org/10.1016/B978-0-12-818460-8.00019-8

experience clinically significant difficulties with eating or weight but do not meet full criteria for AN, BN, or BED may be given a diagnosis of other specified feeding or eating disorder (OSFED). The lifetime prevalence rate of OSFED has been found to be 7.64% among women.[6] Although not full threshold eating disorders, those with OSFED do not differ in terms of impairment[7] and several studies have found few differences between subthreshold and full threshold eating disorders in terms of symptomatology,[8] medical complications,[9] and response to treatment.[10]

Psychiatric comorbidities among eating disorders are common, with 56.2% of patients with AN, 94.5% of patients with BN, and 78.9% of patients with BED meeting criteria for at least one DSM-IV disorder,[4] most commonly mood and anxiety disorders. Eating disorders are associated with impaired quality of life[11] and elevated mortality rates.[12,13] AN in particular has mortality rates that are among the highest of any psychiatric disorder,[12] and individuals with AN are 31 times more likely to die by suicide than those in the general population.[14]

II. MEDICAL COMPLICATIONS OF EATING DISORDERS

AN and BN are associated with significant medical complications. In the case of AN, the majority of complications are related to the direct effects of starvation and malnutrition on the body, whereas with BN complications are related primarily to purging or other compensatory behaviors. Patients who do not meet full criteria for AN or BN or are diagnosed with OSFED often have the same severity of medical complications and need similarly detailed evaluation and management.[9] Fortunately, many of these complications are reversible with a return to a healthy weight and resumption of regular eating patterns and absence of purging behaviors. Although a comprehensive review of the medical complications associated with eating disorders is beyond the scope of this chapter, this section will provide an overview of some of the more common and most severe medical problems.

A. Anorexia Nervosa

Starvation impacts nearly every organ system in the body, and medical complications can occur within a relatively short time frame from onset of illness. Patients suffering from AN very often have bradycardia, hypotension, and dizziness, along with tachycardia associated with minor exertion.[15] A case series found that 69.6% of patients with AN presented with a heart rate under 50 beats per minute.[16] Vital signs typically normalize with refeeding once patients reach at least 85%–90% of their expected body weight (EBW)[17] and may occur more quickly with consistent early nutrition. One-third of deaths in AN are attributed to cardiac causes.[18] Longstanding AN can lead to thinning of the cardiac muscle[19] and myocardial fibrosis,[20] both of which can contribute to reduced cardiac function and arrhythmias. Although it is important to note that these changes are typically found in patients with longstanding AN, all patients with AN should be evaluated and monitored by a medical professional experienced in treating eating disorders.

Patients with AN almost universally report gastrointestinal (GI) symptoms during starvation and refeeding.[2] Gastroparesis, bloating, fullness, nausea, constipation, and abdominal pain are all common due to the altered motility that occurs with starvation.[21] Reassurance and supportive management, including small frequent meals, limiting fiber and legumes, and the use of liquid supplementation early in refeeding, are the mainstay of management. Medications targeted at symptom management may also be considered. These medications include promotility agents like erythromycin and metoclopramide, antispasmodic agents including hyoscyamine and dicyclomine, and medications for gastroesophageal reflux disease.

Hepatitis is another common finding in patients with AN during both starvation and refeeding. During starvation/malnutrition, elevations in liver transaminases (alanine aminotransferase and aspartate aminotransferase; AST and ALT) are common and relate to apoptosis (programmed cell death) of liver cells. During refeeding, this can also occur as nutrition is reintroduced and dextrose is converted to fat and deposited rapidly in the liver. Both these causes of transaminitis resolve with nutritional restoration, though patients with more severe AN are more likely to be affected.[22]

Endocrine abnormalities are also common with AN as starvation downregulates the hypothalamic–pituitary (HPA) axis. Amenorrhea occurs in 60%–85% of women with AN.[23] Additionally, low bone mineral density is common with AN and is a relatively early complication of starvation. Low bone mineral density is influenced by interruption of peak bone mass acquisition (usually between ages 17 and 22 years of age), as well as both increased bone resorption and decreased bone formation. Additionally, the downregulation of HPA axis leads to elevated hydrocortisone, low insulin-like growth factor-1, and low androgen levels (estrogen, progesterone, testosterone), all of which impact bone formation and resorption. Patients with AN who have longer durations of illness, later onset of menarche, and/or longer time frame of amenorrhea are at the highest risk of low bone mineral density.[24] Of note, hormonal therapy with estrogen (in the form of combined oral contraceptive pills) has not consistently demonstrated benefit in reversing bone mineral loss; rather nutritional restoration and adequate calcium and vitamin D are the mainstays of treatment.[25,26] Weight-bearing exercise is also not helpful in promoting skeletal development in patients who are not a healthy weight or are not menstruating and may increase risk of fracture.[27]

Finally, patients with AN may have a myriad of laboratory abnormalities including electrolyte disturbances, elevated transaminases, anemia, leukopenia, and in more severe cases, vitamin and micronutrient deficiencies. Anemia, including low ferritin and hemoglobin, and leukopenia from bone marrow suppression are a result of starvation and malnutrition. Patients with AN may have hypophosphatemia and hypoglycemia, but normal values of the other serum electrolytes are generally preserved even with severe malnutrition. Vitamin D deficiency is relatively common. Other deficiencies are sometimes seen in patients with particularly restrictive diets including very low-fat or vegan diets.

B. Bulimia Nervosa

Patients with BN have not only overlapping complications with AN including GI symptoms, abnormal vital signs, irregular menses, and others but also unique complications related to purging behaviors. Electrolyte abnormalities are common, and patients most typically have a metabolic alkalosis with hypokalemia, hypochloremia, and hyponatremia. Significant hypokalemia is associated with purging behavior but is not diagnostically sensitive, so it should not be used as a screening test for bulimia.[28] Patients are often asymptomatic or may present with weakness, fatigue, dizziness, and paresthesias. Severe hypokalemia ($K < 2.5$ mmol/L) can lead to muscle breakdown and cardiac arrhythmias that can be fatal. In severe cases, short-term electrolyte repletion may be warranted along with working toward cessation of purging behavior. Fluid resuscitation should be done judiciously, as rapid fluid rehydration can lead to edema, which can be painful and distressing to patients. It is also important to remember that many patients with purging behavior present with normal electrolytes, and this should not suggest that they are not engaging in serious eating disordered behavior. Additionally, in healthy patients presenting with isolated hypokalemia, covert purging behavior should be strongly considered in identifying the etiology.

GI symptoms are also very common in patients with BN. Patients engaging in self-induced vomiting often have significant reflux/heartburn, dysphagia, and chest pain. Reflux symptoms should be treated promptly as the acid over time damages the esophagus and can lead to chronic esophageal changes. BN patients often struggle with constipation, bloating, fullness, and delayed gastric motility. Patients who purge using laxatives may experience more significant symptoms, though there is little evidence to support gradual tapering off of laxatives.[19] Rather, use of nonstimulant laxatives, consistent fluid intake, and behavioral strategies are the main treatments for constipation. Patients also need reassurance that their symptoms will improve as bowel function returns to normal and their nutrition improves.

Patients with BN may have many other complications, including salivary gland swelling, sore throat, erosion of dental enamel, esophageal tears, and cardiac symptoms. Ongoing medical symptoms in patients with BN should be evaluated closely by a medical provider with expertise in eating disorders, even if symptoms seem fairly minor or not impairing.

C. Micronutrient Deficiencies

Vitamin and mineral deficiencies in patients with eating disorders are an area of ongoing study, and an individual's specific food and eating behaviors, as well as illness duration and severity, may help to identify individual risk. Patients may also be at risk for excessively high intake of certain micronutrients, depending on the type of restrictive diet the eating disorder prescribes. Generalized guidelines do not currently exist, but rather supplementation should focus on an individual's history and dietary intake.

Electrolyte abnormalities from purging behavior (vomiting and laxative abuse) are critical to identify and address. The most common electrolyte abnormality is elevated serum bicarbonate from chronic vomiting. This metabolic alkalosis can also result in low chloride (hypochloremia), low potassium (hypokalemia), and low sodium (hyponatremia). Hypokalemia, when severe (<2.5 mmol/L), can result in cardiac arrhythmias, muscle breakdown, and sudden death. Hypomagnesemia can also occur and contribute to cardiac abnormalities, particularly in the setting of hypokalemia.

Patients with chronic purging behavior (vomiting specifically) are persistently hypovolemic and often have upregulation of the renin–aldosterone–angiotensin axis. Increased aldosterone, in response to hypovolemia, acts to increase salt absorption and bicarbonate resorption, while wasting potassium and hydrogen. This phenomenon, known as *pseudo*-Bartter's syndrome from chronic vomiting or diuretic abuse, leads to the electrolyte disturbances described above.[29] Patients with laxative misuse can present with either a metabolic acidosis or alkalosis, depending on the type, chronicity, and stooling pattern, as well as any concurrent purging behaviors.

Common mineral deficiencies in patients with eating disorders include calcium, iron, and zinc. Serum calcium levels in patients with eating disorders are typically normal, as the body pulls calcium from bone to preserve serum calcium levels. Careful dietary history is important to identify whether patients are consuming adequate calcium. If possible, calcium should come from dietary sources, though supplementation is appropriate when needed. Patients with eating disorders may be at higher risk for iron deficiency, though data are mixed. In assessing patients with eating disorders, dietitians should identify iron sources in intake, consumption of beverages that inhibit iron absorption (coffee, tea, others), and whether amenorrhea is present. A plasma ferritin level can also help to identify early iron deficiency and whether supplementation is indicated.

Zinc deficiency in patients with eating disorders is an area of more robust study but no clear consensus. Patients may present with zinc deficiency due to low intake or impaired absorption. There is also some evidence that zinc deficiency may impair sense of taste, making increased nutrition and weight restoration more challenging for patients.[30] Empiric supplementation for all patients is likely not indicated, but all patients should be screened for zinc deficiency in dietary history and if indicated, serum testing, and supplemented if appropriate.

Vitamin deficiencies occur in patients with eating disorders and particularly in patients with comorbid alcohol use disorders. Thiamine (vitamin B1), pyridoxine (vitamin B6), and folic acid deficiencies are more common in patients with eating disorders and alcohol use disorders. Thiamine should also be supplemented empirically in patients with eating disorders who are hospitalized related to malnutrition, as deficiency can lead to irreversible Wernicke–Korsakoff syndrome.

Lastly, vitamin D deficiency is an area of intense study in many disease states, and no clear guidelines for supplementation exist. Patients with eating disorders should be screened for vitamin D deficiency (serum 25-hydroxy vitamin D <30 ng/mL) given its importance in bone health, and supplemented when deficient.

D. Refeeding Syndrome

Refeeding syndrome is a preventable but life-threatening complication of malnutrition among patients who are being refed and involves dangerous shifts in electrolytes and fluids,[31] which can lead to cardiovascular collapse and death.[15] In response to the initiation of nutrition, insulin is released leading to cellular shifts, primarily in potassium and phosphorus. The decrease in extracellular phosphorus leads to inadequate substrate for the production of adenosine triphosphate, which is necessary for muscle contraction. In severe cases, this can lead to respiratory and cardiac muscle weakness, heart failure, seizure, and death. Any patient at risk for refeeding syndrome should be hospitalized in an inpatient setting for initial medical and nutrition management. Patients most at risk are those who are below 70% of their EBW, have a body mass index (BMI) of <14, or have lost more than 5%–10% of their body weight within a short period of time.[32] The National Institute for Clinical Excellence guidelines for adult patients at risk of refeeding syndrome provide somewhat more comprehensive criteria (see Table 19.2).[33] Whether these same parameters should apply to younger patients, who generally have a lower risk of refeeding syndrome, is a topic of ongoing inquiry.

For patients at risk for refeeding syndrome, the longstanding approach of advancing nutrition *very* slowly for fear of refeeding complications (electrolyte disturbance, cardiovascular collapse) has been refuted, and several recent studies support more aggressive nutritional interventions and quicker calorie advancement.[34,35] Mehler and colleagues[32] provide an overview of methods for bringing about nutritional rehabilitation while avoiding medical complications. Prior to initiating nutritional rehabilitation, Mehler and colleagues recommend (1) identifying patients at risk and (2) measuring serum electrolytes and correcting any baseline abnormalities prior to nutrition. When initiating nutritional restoration, it is recommended to start at 30–45 kcal/kg/day and then advance by 300–400 kcal/day every other day as tolerated. Often patients without evidence of refeeding syndrome can then have a more aggressive calorie advance. Initially, practitioners should follow electrolytes closely (likely daily) for the first 5–7 days of nutritional restoration, specifically potassium, phosphorus, magnesium, and sodium. Correction of any abnormalities should be initiated early in deficiency, rather than waiting for a critically low value. Patients should be prescribed a low-fiber and low-lactose diet as needed, and protein generally should not exceed 2 g/kg/day. Additionally, attention to low-volume, high-density foods may help patients with feeling excessively full and distressed. At times, enteral nutrition via nasogastric tube may be required initially or as a supplement. There are isolated scenarios in which total parenteral nutrition may be indicated, but this is exceedingly rare and only in circumstances where enteral nutrition is not feasible.[36]

Calorie requirements for sustained weight gain vary among patients though are often higher than many providers expect, particularly in younger patients. Females may need 3500 kcal/day, and males may need in excess of 4000 kcal/day. Inpatients with AN may achieve weight gain of 3–4 pounds/week, while outpatients a more modest goal of 1–2 lb/week is appropriate. Patients not at risk for refeeding syndrome can have more liberal calorie escalation and can often be managed in an outpatient setting with a multidisciplinary team.

In summary, AN, BN, and OSFED have significant medical complications associated with illness, and patients should have close medical monitoring at onset of treatment and throughout their course. Fortunately, many of the medical complications will resolve with restored weight and nutrition, but the sooner nutrition is initiated, the less likely patients will have long-term sequelae of their illness.

III. ASSESSMENT

A. Medical Assessment

A thorough evaluation by a medical provider experienced in eating disorder care is an essential component of assessment and treatment planning. Patients with eating disorders often do not present with symptoms specifically attributable to the eating disorder or may attempt to mask their eating disorder behaviors. Commonly, patients present with nonspecific complaints like cold intolerance, fatigue, bloating or GI symptoms, numbness, and tingling or edema.

An initial assessment should include a thorough catalog of symptoms by organ system (see Table 19.1), specific questions to ascertain the type and frequency of eating disorder behaviors, physical exam, and laboratory evaluation. The physical exam should include careful measure of height, weight, and BMI. Resting pulse and blood pressure, temperature, and orthostatic vital signs should also be measured.[17] Patients with AN are often bradycardic, hypotensive, hypothermic, and may have orthostatic vital signs due to dehydration and altered autonomic tone. Physical exam findings in patients with AN may include changes in skin turgor, dry mucous membranes, dry skin, brittle hair and nails, fine lanugo on extremities and face, and hair loss on the scalp. Additionally, patients with AN may have cyanosis of their hands and feet, edema (generally nonpitting), cardiac murmurs, hypoactive bowel sounds, and generalized weakness.

In patients with BN, the physical exam findings are somewhat different. Patients may have a "normal" weight, pulse, and blood pressure but often have orthostatic vital signs from the chronic volume depletion associated with purging. Additionally, patients with BN may have dental erosions, enamel defects (particularly the lingual surface of upper teeth), angular cheilosis of the lips, periorbital petechiae, subconjunctival hemorrhage, and painless swelling of the parotid glands. Russell's sign, a well-known symptom of BN that describes callouses on the dorsum of the hand from repeated irritation from self-induced vomiting, is more commonly present early in the illness if at all.

TABLE 19.1 Medical signs and symptoms in patients with eating disorders.

Organ system	Anorexia nervosa	Bulimia nervosa
General	Weakness Dry skin	Swelling of feet/ankles Weakness/fatigue
Ear, nose, and throat		Swollen cheeks Nosebleed Sore throat Teeth sensitivity
Endocrine	Amenorrhea Cold intolerance Infertility	Irregular menses
Neurologic	Dizziness Headache	Numbness and tingling Dizziness Headache
Cardiovascular	Palpitations Chest Pain Syncope	Palpitations Chest Pain
Gastrointestinal	Nausea Heartburn Abdominal Pain Early satiety Constipation	Heartburn Difficulty swallowing Constipation/diarrhea Rectal bleeding Abdominal pain Abdominal bloating
Musculoskeletal	Low back pain	
Psychiatric	Irritability Poor sleep	Depression

TABLE 19.2 NICE guidelines for identification of adult patients at high risk for refeeding syndrome.[33]

Patient has one or more of the following:	OR Patient has two or more of the following:
• BMI < 16 kg/m^2 • Unintentional weight loss of $> 15\%$ in the previous 3-6 months • Little or no nutritional intake for > 10 days • Low levels of potassium, phosphorus, or magnesium before refeeding	• BMI < 18.5 kg/m^2 • Unintentional weight loss of $> 10\%$ in previous 3-6 months • Little or no nutritional intake for > 5 days • History of alcohol misuse or drugs, including insulin, chemotherapy, antacids or diuretics

As part of a comprehensive medical assessment, all patients should undergo laboratory testing. The following screening is recommended for all patients with eating disorders at initial assessment:

- complete blood count with differential,
- serum electrolytes including calcium, magnesium, and phosphorus, BUN, and creatinine,
- liver function tests,

- serum salivary amylase level,
- Vitamin D (25-hydroxy), and
- thyroid function.

Additionally, many patients also require electrocardiogram (EKG) and bone densitometry (DEXA).

B. Nutrition Assessment

The role of the dietitian as an essential component in the assessment and treatment of eating disorders is supported by the Academy of Nutrition and Dietetics (AND)[37] and the American Psychiatric Association.[38] The dietitian's role in eating disorder treatment begins with a thorough evaluation or assessment that adequately addresses the patient's nutritional status, knowledge base, motivation, and current eating and behavioral status.[39]

AND provides a framework for conducting nutrition assessments as part of the Nutrition Care Process Model.[40] This standardized practice of care has five domains for nutrition assessment, which includes anthropometric measurements, biochemical data and medical tests/procedures, food and nutrition-related history, client history, and nutrition-focused physical exam findings. While this model is intended to be used transdiagnostically, it can be tailored to eating disorders to help the team evaluate the physiologic effects of the disordered eating patterns and/or malnutrition and the severity of the eating disorder. The adapted nutrition assessment can also be instrumental in designing a nutrition plan.

Anthropometric measurements: These include current weight and height, BMI, growth chart percentiles, weight history (lowest and highest weights), and weight fluctuations (recent losses or gains). The dietitian can use this information to determine percent EBW and percent weight loss to help determine the presence and severity of malnutrition, especially in AN. Growth chart percentiles and historical growth patterns are of importance, particularly in the adolescent population, as they can be useful in helping the team determine a patient's restoration weight goal. This typically necessitates obtaining medical records from the patient's primary care practitioner.

Biochemical data and medical tests/procedures: Any relevant biochemical data or medical procedure results should be part of the nutrition assessment and interpreted along with other findings as part of the assessment. Commonly acquired laboratory markers of overall nutritional status (e.g., serum albumin, prealbumin, transferrin, and retinol-binding protein) may not be accurate in the eating disorder population. Several influencing factors common in patients with eating disorders, including under- or overhydration, may alter the results.[41] Although historically popular, studies are inconsistent in showing the validity of serum markers as determinants of patients' nutritional status.[42] Rock[41] recommends several biochemical measures of micronutrients that may be useful (and more reliable) as components of a nutrition assessment: vitamin E, vitamin D, folate, and ferritin. Laboratory measures of potassium and magnesium may reveal the presence of purging behaviors and/or laxative use.[43] Bhardwaj et al.[42] suggest that objective laboratory findings be used in conjunction with a nutrition-focused physical exam and other relevant clinical data to assess presence or level of malnutrition and guide intervention strategies. Newly diagnosed patients should have initial laboratory screening, but practitioners should be cautioned that normal results may not be unusual and should not rule out serious illness or medical instability from a diagnosis.[22,27] A dual-energy X-ray absorptiometry scan can be useful in assessing the bone mineral density of patients and can help determine the absence or presence of osteopenia. This type of procedure may be more appropriate for female patients with amenorrhea for more than 6–12 months[22] or male patients with AN who have had an abnormally low weight for >6 months.[27,44]

Food and nutrition-related history: The food and nutrition-related history portion of an assessment will likely be the most in-depth and time-consuming, yet most informative in terms of present and past disordered eating patterns and attitudes pertaining to weight, shape, and eating. Interviewing techniques that are nonjudgmental and nonleading are essential in this population and can lead to more truthful representation of intake. Because certain symptoms, such as binge eating, can be present across eating disorder diagnoses, the nutrition assessment is most useful in diagnosis and treatment if it is inclusive of all potential disordered eating behaviors. A thorough understanding of a patient's current food and nutrient intake patterns includes the frequency, volume, and physical environment of food (and beverage) consumption and the use of supplements (vitamins, minerals, herbals).

Clinically, knowing a patient's typical food intake may provide insight into potential micronutrient deficiencies that were not confirmed by laboratory measurement or provide support for the ordering of specific laboratory measurements. While there are several methods to establish intake, a 24-h food recall may be the most useful tool, and multiple 24-h food recalls may be better reflective of overall eating patterns.[41] Thirty-day food frequency questionnaires can be time-consuming and do not change the treatment model. To ensure accuracy of the 24-h food recall, it is important to either have parents complete it (for child and adolescent patients) or try to obtain collateral information from parents or other family members (for older patients).

Disordered eating patterns may vary from day to day, as in the case of BED (binge vs. nonbinge days) or BN (binge vs. restricting days). Questions about food rules and calorie and/or macronutrient restrictions are relevant in assessing the extent of disordered eating. Differentiating between a food restriction that is eating disorder-driven versus a religious, cultural, or personal preference (present prior to disordered eating behaviors) is important. In addition, known (or suspected) food allergies, sensitivities, and intolerances are relevant for creating a customized plan for treatment. Understanding a patient's daily activity patterns, including purposeful exercise, can help determine current energy expenditure. The presence and frequency of purging and other compensatory behaviors should be assessed, as should the use of laxatives, diuretics, weight loss aides, and coffee consumption.

Client history: Gaining perspective on a client's history related to disordered eating can help guide the development of a treatment plan. Reaching out to a past provider, with a release of information in place, may provide the current treating team with insight into what may or may not have been successful in the patient's past recovery process. A family history of eating disorders (treated or untreated) may be relevant, especially if the patient is currently residing with that person or the family member is a significant influence on the patient. Socioeconomic questions may help reveal the patient's financial security and access to food, knowledge of health, and level of support systems. Questions about oral health can rule out any barriers to food consumption and potentially prompt a referral to a dental health professional. Binge eating and purging behaviors, as well as nutritional deficiencies, may have detrimental effects on oral health, ranging from thermal sensitivity to periodontal disease.[45]

Nutrition-focused physical examination: Although a comprehensive eating disorder treatment team will have a medical practitioner to provide a thorough physical examination, the dietitian's exam remains helpful as a potential confirmation of the physician's findings. Additionally, the dietitian may be interacting with the patient more frequently than the medical provider and may have more opportunity to notice any physical changes that could be reflective of new disordered eating patterns or those not identified during initial diagnosis. Eating disorders of the restricting type (AN) may be quite visible during a nutrition-focused physical exam, as low body weight and muscle and fat wasting are often present. Observations of weakened nails and fragile, dry hair are not uncommon[43] and indicate a significant level of malnourishment. The dietitian should be familiar with the physical features commonly associated with BN as outlined in the Section IV.A of this chapter.

A comprehensive nutrition assessment, along with psychological and medical assessments, can help establish an eating disorder diagnosis and be instrumental in the development of a treatment plan for recovery. The process of assessment is an ongoing one, encompassing a need to reevaluate and reformulate treatment plans as more information comes to light, symptoms worsen or improve, and priorities shift.[46]

C. Psychological Assessment

The nature of the psychological portion of an assessment will vary depending on the treatment setting and the purpose of the assessment, e.g., screening, diagnosis, or treatment planning and outcome.[47] Although it is beyond the scope of this chapter to provide a comprehensive overview of the possible components of an assessment, this section will describe some important considerations when conducting a psychological assessment of an individual with an eating disorder.

Assessments should include a history of the current illness, including information on the onset and course of the disorder over time. Highest and lowest previous weights may provide helpful information on the degree of weight loss as well as a possible estimate of the target weight range for weight restoration. Current and past eating disordered behaviors should be assessed, including presence and frequency of binge eating, self-induced vomiting, laxative misuse, diuretic misuse, diet pill use, driven exercise, and fasting, as well as any other methods intended to result in weight loss (e.g., misuse of prescription medications, smoking). It may also be useful to inquire about other appearance-related activities such as body checking. A 24-h food recall will be useful in obtaining information on the degree of restriction and/or pattern of binge eating and purging. Information should also be obtained on current and past treatment received, including outpatient treatment, inpatient hospitalization, and other levels of care, such as partial hospitalization or intensive outpatient programs.

Although in certain settings it may not be possible to conduct a full structured diagnostic interview, it is important to inquire about mood and anxiety symptoms, as these are often comorbid with eating disorders.[4] Obtaining a timeline of symptoms is necessary to determine whether mood and anxiety symptoms are secondary to the eating disorder and may remit as the eating disorder improves or preceded the eating disorder and may require separate treatment. Information on self-harm and suicidality should also be gathered. A metaanalysis found that 27.3% of patients with eating disorders engage in nonsuicidal self-injury,[48] and one in five deaths in AN is due to suicide.[12] Substance use is important to assess, particularly as it may relate to disordered eating behavior and attempts at weight loss (e.g., misuse of stimulants). Asking patients about current work and/or educational status may provide a picture of their degree of functional impairment as a result of the eating disorder. Obtaining information about trauma history is also important, as patients with eating disorders, particularly those with binge/purge symptoms, often have a history of trauma.[49]

In addition to the content of the information gathered as part of the assessment, it is important to consider the ways in which this information is gathered. Those with eating disorders may minimize symptoms in a face-to-face interview, either because of shame or embarrassment, as is sometimes seen in BN,[50] or due to ambivalence about the prospect of recovery, as is often seen in AN.[51] Using both interviews and self-report measures may circumvent this challenge and provide more complete information. Interviews and self-report measures tend to provide similar information regarding unambiguous behaviors such as self-induced vomiting, but self-report measures result in higher scores on more complex concepts such as binge eating.[52] It is also important, particularly with children and adolescents, to gather collateral information from parents or other family members who are familiar with the patient's eating behaviors. In addition to being reluctant to share information, younger patients sometimes have difficulty articulating the reasons behind their engagement in certain eating disordered behaviors. For a more thorough overview of eating disorder assessment, as well as a description of commonly used interviews and self-report measures, see Mitchell and Peterson.[53]

A multidisciplinary assessment that addresses the medical, nutritional, and psychological components of eating disorders is critical for treatment planning.

IV. RISK FACTORS FOR EATING DISORDERS

Eating disorders are complex disorders with multiple factors contributing to their onset and development. Research has found a significant genetic component to AN and BN, with approximately 50%–80% of the variance in liability to the disorders, and disordered eating, being accounted for by genetic factors.[54,55] Risks of developing eating disorders are approximately 4–11 times higher among first-degree relatives of those with eating disorders than among controls.[56]

Perceived pressure to be thin and internalization of the Western "thinness ideal" can precede body dissatisfaction and weight and shape concerns,[57] which can lead to dieting, a significant risk factor for both AN and BN.[58–60] Additional risk factors for AN include female gender, childhood picky eating, adolescent age, early pubertal timing, obsessive-compulsive personality disorder, increased exposure to sexual abuse and other negative life events, and perfectionism. Additional risk factors for BN include female gender, higher BMI, higher levels of psychiatric morbidity or negative affect, adolescent age, early pubertal timing, and low self-esteem. Risk factors for BED include low self-esteem, high body concern, low perceived social support, and childhood experiences of sexual abuse and physical neglect. For a thorough review of risk factors for eating disorders, see Jacobi et al.[60] (Table 19.3).

While eating disorders are popularly viewed as a response to desire for control, there is little research to support this claim[61] and, in fact, those with eating disorders maintain very little control over their disordered eating behaviors without treatment. Another factor that has not consistently been found to put people at risk for eating disorders is poor family functioning. Although historically eating disorders have often been associated with dysfunctional families, research has not supported this and the idea that families cause eating disorders has largely fallen out of favor.[62] This is particularly relevant given the rise of family-based treatment (FBT) for adolescent eating disorders.

V. TREATMENT

A. Family-Based Treatment

FBT[63] has emerged as the first-line treatment for adolescents with AN,[33] and there is evidence to support its use for adolescents with BN,[64] as well as young adults with AN.[65] AN is an egosyntonic disorder—that is, those with AN often value their disorder and are ambivalent about recovery—so individuals with AN are often reluctant to engage in treatment. However, AN is a potentially fatal disorder and becomes more difficult to treat as time goes on, making early, effective intervention critical to recovery. FBT for AN avoids the difficulties associated with egosyntonicity and lack of motivation by putting parents in charge of the weight restoration process. This is done by temporarily asking parents to make all eating-related decisions for their child, much like a treatment team would do if the child

TABLE 19.3 Risk factors for eating disorders.

	Risk factor
Anorexia nervosa	Genetic factors
	Female gender
	Premature delivery Ethnicity
	Obstetric complications
	Picky eating
	Adolescent age
	Early pubertal timing
	Weight and shape concerns
	Dieting
Bulimia nervosa	Genetic factors
	Female gender
	Ethnicity
	Obstetric complications
	Early childhood health problems
	Higher BMI
	Childhood sexual abuse
	Negative affectivity
	Low interoceptive awareness
	Adolescent age
	Early pubertal timing
	Low self-esteem
	Weight and shape concerns
Binge eating disorder	Low self-esteem
	High body concern
	High use of escape-avoidance coping
	Low perceived social support
	Childhood sexual abuse

were on an inpatient unit. This is often met with considerable resistance, but the parents are empowered by the treatment team to manage this resistance and return their child to health. Once the patient has gained weight and his or her thinking is less clouded by the eating disorder, the patient is gradually given back more responsibility over his or her eating.

The rationale behind FBT's initial focus on weight restoration and a rapid return to physical health is based in part on the Minnesota Starvation Study, in which 36 healthy men who were conscientious objectors to World War II participated in an experiment in which they were put through a period of semistarvation and lost approximately 25% of their body weight.[66,67] In addition to profound physical changes, such as heart rate dropping from 55 to 35 beats per minute and a 40% decrease in basal metabolic rate, the men saw significant psychological changes. They became increasingly irritable and impatient, had difficulty concentrating, and became more socially withdrawn and apathetic. Some developed obsessive rituals around eating or started binge eating. These are all symptoms that are often present in patients with AN; part of the significance of the Minnesota Starvation Study was showing that the secondary symptoms often associated with AN are simply a result of malnutrition, and that with weight restoration, these symptoms can be reversed and the patient can recover.

The study also dispelled a popular myth about AN, that people suffering from it must "want to get better" before they can achieve recovery. In fact,

> The degree of apathy shown by the subjects, as well as their physical decline, led him to the conclusion that the mental attitude of starved persons cannot be changed for the better until they have been physically rehabilitated, [Keys] asserted.[68]

This is an important note to those treating AN: regaining weight generally precedes, rather than follows, a desire to recover.

The FBT treatment team consists primarily of a licensed mental health professional, a physician to manage medical complications, and a psychiatrist, if necessary, to manage medications. The team guides parents in accessing the knowledge that they have about nutrition and feeding their child to bring about rapid weight restoration, often with a guideline of 3000–5000 calories per day. This is also based in part on Keys et al.'s work,[67] who found that the study participants needed 4000 calories daily to achieve weight restoration. FBT does not use meal plans, and there is not a large focus on the exact nutritional breakdown of the calories provided; rather, parents are encouraged to find the solution that best fits their particular family. As Keys concluded

> The character of the rehabilitation diet is important also, but unless calories are abundant then extra proteins, vitamins and minerals are of little value.[68]

Treatment studies of FBT have not included registered dietitians (RDs) as part of the treatment team. However, RDs are an important part of many eating disorder teams and can support FBT tenets by meeting primarily with the parents, rather than the adolescent patient, and supporting parents to find their own solutions to the refeeding process rather than prescribing a specific approach.[69]

An important and useful part of FBT involves separating the disorder from the patient. Some families will name the eating disorder, often "Ed," to further emphasize the distinction between the illness and their healthy child and to highlight how it has taken over their healthy child when it comes to issues of food, eating, body shape, and weight. Parents are told that they must be firm with the disorder in setting expectations for eating, while remaining compassionate with their son or daughter and remembering the fear that he or she experiences when sitting down to a plate of food. It is helpful for all members of the treatment team to model this approach for parents and to remain patient with the sometimes difficult behavior associated with the eating disorder.

B. Cognitive Behavioral Therapy

Cognitive-behavioral therapy (CBT) is the first-line treatment for adults with BN and BED.[33,70] The CBT model of disordered eating states that cognitive and behavioral disturbances interact to maintain the disorder, and both need to be addressed in order for someone to fully recover.[71]

A common pattern of eating in BN is restricting one's diet due to overvaluation of the importance of body shape and weight. This dietary restriction leads to hunger, which can lead to binge eating and then purging. In the first of three phases of treatment, the focus is on helping patients establish a regular pattern of eating to reduce dietary restriction, thus reducing binge eating and breaking the binge/purge cycle. The second phase of treatment has a cognitive focus, in which patients' unhelpful and unrealistic thoughts about body shape and weight are challenged. The final phase focuses on maintaining treatment progress and addressing relapse prevention. An "enhanced" version of CBT (CBT-E) has been developed to improve treatment response by addressing four additional maintaining mechanisms: clinical perfectionism, mood intolerance, low self-esteem, and interpersonal difficulties.[72]

It is important to note that FBT and CBT, the two leading treatments for eating disorders, are quite behavioral in nature and focus on maintaining factors rather than on what may have caused the eating disorder in the first place. A common belief regarding eating disorders is that in order to recover from an eating disorder, the underlying "issues" that may have caused it need to be identified and worked through. However, research does not seem to support this belief, instead suggesting that a problem-focused approach, with an emphasis on the present rather than the past, is most effective.

FBT and CBT are the leading evidence-based forms of treatment for eating disorders.

C. Nutrition Therapy

The practice guideline for treatment of AN and BN recommends a normalization of nutrition and eating habits as a central goal in the treatment.[38] In BN specifically, establishing a regular eating pattern to break cycles of restriction and bingeing is key for treatment. The dietitian can play a significant role in this part of therapy as well as help patients expand their food choices, correct misguided notions about food, and dispel nutrition misinformation.[43]

In FBT and CBT, the primary therapist is responsible for working with the family to increase calories or with the individual patient to regulate eating patterns. Although RDs have not been included in many randomized controlled psychotherapy trials, many treatment teams have an RD to provide nutrition counseling as needed. This is determined on a case-by-case basis and may be sought when weight gain goals, especially in the case of AN, are not being met. In the case of FBT, it is important to avoid being too prescriptive, as meal plans are not used in this form of therapy. Rather, families are encouraged to decide for themselves what will work best for their child, with increasing guidance from the therapist and RD if parents seem to be struggling with what to feed their child or lack the expected basic knowledge about nutrition. Based on current intake, the RD provides suggestions for increasing caloric intake, being mindful of energy-dense choices to reduce volume. The treatment guideline of 3000–5000 calories per day in FBT to provide rapid weight restoration can be, at least initially, overwhelming for some families, so RDs may recommend that parents keep a daily food log to provide a more accurate reflection of actual caloric intake. This tool can be useful for the dietitian to assess and provide recommendations on the frequency of eating, portions, caloric density, and potential triggering foods for GI complications. Supplementing the diet with a liquid (oral) nutritional supplement in the early stages of refeeding to achieve the prescribed calorie goal is an effective strategy for weight gain, especially when a large calorie goal has been prescribed.[32] Caloric goals may need to be adjusted throughout treatment, and unusually high calorie diets may be necessary to provide continued weight gain, as many patients experience a plateau in the later stages of weight restoration.[32] It is suspected that an increase in Resting Energy Expenditure is responsible for this and is often clinically referred to as hypermetabolism. For this reason, the optimal treatment strategy should be based on regular monitoring of an individual's pattern of weight gain and adjusting the dietary plan.[32]

Similar to FBT models of treatment, weight restoration remains the first priority in most treatment modalities for AN. In non-FBT treatment, initial caloric needs can be determined individually by calculating Basal Energy Expenditure using the Harris–Benedict formula multiplied by a 1.5–2.0 activity factor. There may be a larger focus on macronutrient distribution, and oftentimes a structured meal plan is utilized to reach goals, using a food exchange list. This may be particularly important when treating adults with AN, for whom there is no first-line form of treatment. While caloric targets may vary among programs and treatment approaches, the need to monitor rate of weight gain and adjust the dietary plan as needed remains of vital importance. In any model of treatment, the dietitian has the expertise to assess and monitor caloric, macronutrient, and micronutrient intake for nutritional adequacy and provide evidence-based nutrition advice and strategies.

D. Pharmacotherapy

The use of medication or pharmacotherapy for patients with eating disorders is primarily reserved for refractory cases or in treating patients with comorbid psychiatric diagnoses. In patients with AN, small studies in adults have examined the use of second-generation (atypical) antipsychotics because of the potential benefit on anxiety and obsessive thinking with mixed results,[73–75] although a metaanalysis found that they were associated with an increase in anxiety.[76] Additionally, selective serotonin reuptake inhibitors (SSRIs) are of limited utility in malnourished patients at low weights,[77] as it is believed that the availability of serotonin is reduced and therefore there is limited substrate upon which the medication can act. In patients with AN who are weight restored or near weight restored, these and other psychiatric medications may be useful in treating comorbid conditions including major depressive disorder, anxiety, and obsessive–compulsive disorder. However, for patients without coexisting psychiatric illnesses, weight restoration and nutrition may improve their mood and anxiety significantly, leaving a limited role for medication.

In adult patients with BN, the use of SSRIs, particularly fluoxetine, has been shown to be useful in reducing the urge to binge and purge. Fluoxetine is the only FDA-approved drug for BN. Doses needed are typically at or above 60 mg and are higher than may be needed to treat depression or anxiety.[78] In adolescent patients, there are limited data, but the use of fluoxetine or another SSRI may have similar benefit[79] and is reasonable in patients who are not improving with traditional evidence-based therapies for BN.

E. Prognosis

A popular belief about eating disorders is that those who have them never fully recover; however, this is not supported by research. Those who receive effective, evidence-based interventions tend to do well. A study comparing systemic family therapy and FBT found that the percent of patients achieving remission (defined as >95% of EBW) for FBT at the end of treatment and 1-year follow-up was 33.1% and 40.7%, respectively.[80] A comparison of FBT and individual psychotherapy found that rates of remission (defined as >95% EBW, and scores on an eating disorder assessment measure that were within one standard deviation of community norms) were 42% at the end of treatment, 40% at 6-month follow-up, and 49% at 12-month follow-up.[81] Partial remission, defined as reaching >85% EBW, was reached by 89% of patients in FBT by the end of treatment. Thus, most patients receiving FBT improve with treatment, and some continue to improve even after treatment is over. Furthermore, gains made in FBT are maintained at 4- and 5-year follow-up.[82,83]

For CBT, remission rates (often defined as abstinence from binge eating and purging over the past 28 days) are generally 40%–50%.[84] One study defining remission as scores on an eating disorder assessment measure that were within one standard deviation of community norms found that 65.5% of patients receiving CBT-E had reached remission at the end of treatment.[85]

A long-term study of 228 patients with eating disorders found that after 22 years, 62.8% of patients with AN and 68.2% of patients with BN had recovered, with patients with BN recovering faster than patients with AN.[86] Although there is certainly room for improvement in the treatment of eating disorders, these findings suggest that there is hope for patients even after a protracted illness, and it is important for treatment providers to convey that hope to patients and their families.

However, many patients with eating disorders do not receive treatment. In a large nationally representative study of adults with eating disorders, 16% of patients with BN and 29% of patients with BED received treatment for emotional problems in the previous 12 months.[4] In a large study of adolescents, only

27.5%, 21.5%, and 11.4% had sought treatment for AN, BN, and BED, respectively.[87] Furthermore, when patients do receive treatment, they often do not receive evidence-based forms of treatment. Only 6%–36% of eating disorder clinicians report following a treatment manual,[88,89] despite evidence of the effectiveness and efficacy of evidence-based treatments.[90]

Although FBT and CBT have been shown to be effective, they do not work for all patients. There is a need for more effective forms of therapy for treatment nonresponders, as well as for adults with AN, for whom there is no first-line form of treatment. There is also a need to close the research-practice gap, so that those who receive treatment are receiving treatment that has been shown to work, and to close the treatment gap, removing barriers to receiving care.[91]

VI. CONCLUSION

Eating disorders are complicated, life-threatening illnesses that require prompt assessment, diagnosis, and treatment. Dietitians can play an important role in identifying and assisting in the treatment of eating disorders. Additionally, ensuring that patients receive comprehensive, multidisciplinary care is imperative in managing the medical and psychiatric facets of disease. Full recovery is achievable, and patients should be referred to evidence-based treatments whenever possible.

RESEARCH GAPS

- Identify effective forms of treatment for adults with AN
- Develop/enhance treatments for patients who are nonresponders to evidence-based forms of treatments
- Increase access to evidence-based treatments
- Reduce barriers to seeking treatment
- Optimize the role of caregivers/loved ones in the treatment of eating disorders

VII. REFERENCES

1. Halmi KA. Psychological comorbidities of eating disorders. In: Agras WS, Robinson A, eds. *The Oxford Handbook of Eating Disorders*. 2nd ed. New York, NY: Oxford University Press; 2018:229–243.
2. Westmoreland P, Krantz MJ, Mehler PS. Medical complications of anorexia nervosa and bulimia. *Am J Med*. 2016;129:30–37.
3. American Psychiatric Association. *Diagnostic and Statistical Manual of Mental Disorders*. 5th ed. Washington, DC: Author; 2013.
4. Hudson JI, Hiripi E, Pope Jr HG, Kessler RC. The prevalence and correlates of eating disorders in the National Comorbidity Survey Replication. *Biol Psychiatry*. 2007;61:348–358.
5. Lucas AR, Beard CM, O'Fallon WM, Kurland LT. 50-year trends in the incidence of anorexia nervosa in Rochester, Minn: a population-based study. *Am J Psychiatry*. 1991;148:917–922.
6. Micali N, Martini MG, Thomas JJ, et al. Lifetime and 12-month prevalence of eating disorders amongst women in mid-life: a population-based study of diagnoses and risk factors. *BMC Med*. 2017;15. https://doi.org/10.1186/s12916-016-0766-4.
7. Fairweather-Schmidt AK, Wade TD. DSM-5 eating disorders and other specified eating and feeding disorders: is there a meaningful differentiation? *Int J Eat Disord*. 2014;47:524–533.
8. Le Grange D, Crosby RD, Engel SG, et al. DSM-IV-defined anorexia nervosa versus subthreshold anorexia nervosa (EDNOS-AN). *Eur Eat Disord Rev*. 2013;21:1–7.
9. Peebles R, Hardy KK, Wilson JL, Lock JD. Are diagnostic criteria for eating disorders markers of medical severity? *Pediatrics*. 2010;125:e1193–e1201.
10. Lindstedt K, Kjellin L, Gustafsson SA. Adolescents with full or subthreshold anorexia nervosa in a naturalistic sample – characteristics and treatment outcome. *J Eat Disord*. 2017;5. https://doi.org/10.1186/s40337-017-0135-5.
11. Jenkins P, Hoste RR, Meyer C, Blissett J. Eating disorders and quality of life: a review of the literature. *Clin Psychol Rev*. 2011;31:113–121.
12. Arcelus J, Mitchell AJ, Wales J, Nielsen S. Mortality rates in patients with anorexia nervosa and other eating disorders: a meta-analysis of 36 studies. *Arch Gen Psychiatry*. 2011;68:724–731.
13. Chesney E, Goodwin GM, Fazel S. Risks of all-cause and suicide mortality in mental disorders: a meta-review. *World Psychiatry*. 2014;13:153–160.
14. Preti A, Rocchi MBL, Sisti D, Camboni MV, Miotto P. A comprehensive meta-analysis of the risk of suicide in eating disorders. *Acta Psychiatr Scand*. 2011;124:6–17.
15. Rome ES, Ammerman S. Medical complications of eating disorders: an update. *J Adolesc Health*. 2003;33:418–426.
16. Yahalom M, Spitz M, Sandler L, Heno N, Roguin N, Turgeman Y. The significance of bradycardia in anorexia nervosa. *Int J Angiol*. 2013;22:83–94.
17. Sachs KV, Harnke B, Mehler PS, Krantz MJ. Cardiovascular complication of anorexia nervosa: a systemic review. *Int J Eat Disord*. 2016;49:238–248.
18. Jáuregui-Garrido B, Jáuregui-Lobera I. Sudden death in eating disorders. *Vasc Health Risk Manag*. 2012;8:91–98.
19. Mehler PS. Medical complications of anorexia nervosa and bulimia nervosa. In: Agras WS, Robinson A, eds. *The Oxford Handbook of Eating Disorders*. 2nd ed. New York, NY: Oxford University Press; 2018:222–228.
20. Oflaz S, Yucel B, Oz F, et al. Assessment of myocardial damage by cardiac MRI in patients with anorexia nervosa. *Int J Eat Disord*. 2013;46:862–866.
21. Perez ME, Coley B, Crandall W, Di Lorenzo C, Bravender T. Effect of nutritional rehabilitation on gastric motility and somatization in adolescents with anorexia. *J Pediatr*. 2013;163:867–872.

22. Rosen D, The Committee on Adolescence. Clinical report - identification and management of eating disorders in children and adolescents. *Pediatrics*. 2010;126:1240–1253.
23. El Ghoch M, Bazzani P, Dalle Grave R. Management of ischiopubic stress fracture in patients with anorexia nervosa and excessive compulsive exercising. *BMJ Case Rep*. 2014. https://doi.org/10.1136/bcr-2014-206393.
24. Maimoun L, Guillaume S, Lefebvre P, et al. Role of sclerostin and dickkopf-1 in the dramatic alteration in bone mass acquisition in adolescents and young women with recent anorexia nervosa. *J Clin Edocr Metab*. 2014;99:E582–E590.
25. Gordon CM, Goodman E, Emans SJ, et al. Physiologic regulators of bone turnover in young women with anorexia nervosa. *J Pediatr*. 2002;141:64–70.
26. Sim LA, McGovern L, Elamin MB, Swiglo BA, Erwin PJ, Montori VM. Effect on bone health of estrogen preparations in premenopausal women with anorexia nervosa: a systematic review and meta-analyses. *Int J Eat Disord*. 2010;43:218–225.
27. Mehler PS, Anderson AE. *Eating Disorders: A Guide to Medical Care and Complications*. 3rd ed. Baltimore, MD: Johns Hopkins University Press; 2017.
28. Mehler PS, Walsh K. Electrolyte and acid-base abnormalities associated with purging behavior. *Int J Eat Disord*. 2016;49:311–318.
29. Bahia A, Mascolo M, Gaudiani JL, Mehler PS. PseudoBartter syndrome in eating disorders. *Int J Eat Disord*. 2012;45:150–153.
30. Setnick J. Micronutrient deficiencies and supplementation in anorexia and bulimia nervosa. *Nutr Clin Pract*. 2010;25:137–142.
31. Mehanna HM, Moledina J, Travis J. Refeeding syndrome: what it is, and how to prevent and treat it. *BMJ*. 2008;336:1495–1498.
32. Mehler PS, Winkelman AB, Andersen DM, Gaudiani JL. Nutritional rehabilitation: practical guidelines for refeeding the anorectic patient. *J Nutr Metab*. 2010. https://doi.org/10.1155/2010/625782.
33. National Institute for Health and Care Excellence. *Eating Disorders: Recognition and Treatment*. NICE guideline (NG69); 2017. https://www.nice.org.uk/guidance/ng69.
34. Golden NH, Keane-Miller C, Sainani KL, Kapphahn CJ. Higher calories in hospitalized adolescents with anorexia nervosa is associated with reduced length of stay and no increased rate of refeeding syndrome. *J Nutr Health*. 2013;53:573–575.
35. Redgrave GW, Coughlin JW, Schreyer CC, et al. Refeeding and weight restoration outcomes in anorexia nervosa: challenging current guidelines. *Int J Eat Disord*. 2015;48:866–873.
36. Mehler PS, Weiner KL. Use of total parenteral nutrition in the refeeding of selected patients with severe anorexia nervosa. *Int J Eat Disord*. 2007;40:285–287.
37. Ozier A, Henry B. Position of the American Dietetic Association: nutrition intervention in the treatment of eating disorders. *J Am Diet Assoc*. 2011;111:1236–1241.
38. Yager J, Devlin MJ, Halmi KA, et al. *Practice Guideline for the Treatment of Patients with Eating Disorders*. 3rd ed.; 2006. http://www.psychiatryonline.com/pracGuide/pracGuideTopic_12.aspx. Accessed March 17, 2019.
39. Henry B, Ozier A. Position of the American Dietetic Association: nutrition intervention in the treatment of anorexia nervosa, bulimia nervosa, and other eating disorders. *J Am Diet Assoc*. 2006;106:2073–2082.
40. Bueche J, Charney P, Pavlinac J, Skipper A, Thompson E, Myers E. Nutrition care process part II: using the international dietetics and nutrition terminology to document the nutrition care process. *J Am Diet Assoc*. 2008;108:1287–1293.
41. Rock CL. Nutritional assessment. In: Mitchell JE, Peterson CB, eds. *Assessment of Eating Disorders*. New York, NY: Guilford Press; 2005: 129–147.
42. Bharadwaj S, Ginoya S, Tandon P, et al. Malnutrition: laboratory markers vs. nutritional assessment. *Gastroenterol Rep*. 2016;4: 272–280.
43. Herrin M, Larkin M. *Nutrition Counseling in the Treatment of Eating Disorders*. 2nd ed. New York, NY: Routledge; 2013.
44. Drabkin A, Rothman MS, Wassenaar E, Mascolo M, Mehler PS. Assessment and clinical management of bone disease in adults with eating disorders: a review. *J Eat Disord*. 2017. https://doi.org/10.1186/s40337-017-0172-0.
45. Steinberg BJ. Medical and dental implications of eating disorders. *J Dent Hyg*. 2014;88:156–159.
46. Surgenor L, Maguire S. Assessment of anorexia nervosa: an overview of universal issues and contextual challenges. *J Eat Disord*. 2013;1:1–29.
47. Anderson DA, Donahue J, Ehrlich LE, Gorrell S. Psychological assessment of the eating disorders. In: Agras WS, Robinson A, eds. *The Oxford Handbook of Eating Disorders*. 2nd ed. New York, NY: Oxford University Press; 2018:211–221.
48. Cucchi A, Ryan D, Konstantakopoulos G, et al. Lifetime prevalence of non-suicidal self-injury in patients with eating disorders: a systematic review and meta-analysis. *Psychol Med*. 2016;46: 1345–1358.
49. Brewerton TD. Eating disorders, trauma, and comorbidity: focus on PTSD. *Eat Disord*. 2007;15:285–304.
50. Hayaki J, Friedman MA, Brownell KD. Shame and severity of bulimia symptoms. *Eat Behav*. 2002;3:73–83.
51. Couturier JL, Lock J. Denial and minimization in adolescents with anorexia nervosa. *Int J Eat Disord*. 2006;39:212–216.
52. Fairburn CB, Beglin SJ. Assessment of eating disorders: interview or self-report questionnaire? *Int J Eat Disord*. 1994;16:363–370.
53. Mitchell JE, Peterson CB, eds. *Assessment of Eating Disorders*. New York, NY: Guilford Press; 2005.
54. Berrettini W. The genetics of eating disorders. *Psychiatry*. 2004;1: 18–25.
55. Klump KL, Suisman JL, Burt SA, McGue M, Iacono WG. Genetic and environmental influences on disordered eating: an adoption study. *J Abnorm Psychol*. 2009;118:797–805.
56. Strober M, Freeman R, Lampert C, Diamond J, Kaye W. Controlled family study of anorexia nervosa and bulimia nervosa: evidence of shared liability and transmission of partial syndromes. *Am J Psychiatry*. 2000;157:393–401.
57. Stice E, Van Ryzin MJ. A prospective test of the temporal sequencing of risk factor emergence in the dual pathway model of eating disorders. *J Abnorm Psychol*. 2019;128:119–128.
58. Hilbert A, Pike K, Goldschmidt A. Risk factors across the eating disorders. *Psychiatry Res*. 2014;220:500–506.
59. Jacobi C, Hayward C, de Zwaan M, Kraemer HC, Agras WS. Coming to terms with risk factors for eating disorders: application of risk terminology and suggestions for a general taxonomy. *Psychol Bull*. 2004;130:19–65.
60. Jacobi C, Hütte K, Fittig E. Psychosocial risk factors for eating disorders. In: Agras WS, Robinson A, eds. *The Oxford Handbook of Eating Disorders*. 2nd ed. New York, NY: Oxford University Press; 2018:106–125.
61. Murray HB, Coniglio K, Hartmann AS, Becker AE, Eddy KT, Thomas JJ. Are eating disorders "all about control?" the elusive psychopathology of nonfat phobic presentations. *Int J Eat Disord*. 2017;50:1306–1312.
62. Le Grange D, Lock J, Loeb K, Nicholls D. Academy for eating disorders position paper: the role of the family in eating disorders. *Int J Eat Disord*. 2010;43:1–5.
63. Lock J, Le Grange D. *Treatment Manual for Anorexia Nervosa: A Family-Based Approach*. 2nd ed. New York: Guilford Press; 2013.
64. Le Grange D, Lock J, Agras WS, Bryson SW, Jo B. Randomized clinical trial of family-based treatment and cognitive-behavioral

therapy for adolescent bulimia nervosa. *J Am Acad Child Psychiatry.* 2015;54:886–894.
65. Chen EY, Weissman JA, Zeffiro TA, et al. Family-based therapy for young adults with anorexia nervosa restores weight. *Int J Eat Disord.* 2016;49:701–707.
66. Kalm LM, Semba RD. They starved so that others be better fed: remembering Ancel Keys and the Minnesota experiment. *J Nutr.* 2005;135:1347–1352.
67. Keys A, Brozek J, Henschel A, Mickelsen O, Taylor HL. *The Biology of Human Starvation I-II.* Minneapolis, MN: University of Minnesota Press; 1950.
68. Minnesota Star-Journal. *'U' Experiment Proves Starved People Can't Be Taught Democracy*; 1945. https://www.newspapers.com/clip/14823698/the_minneapolis_star/.
69. Lian B, Forsberg SE, Fitzpatrick KK. Adolescent anorexia: guiding principles and skills for the dietetic support of family-based treatment. *J Acad Nutr Diet.* 2019;119:17–25.
70. Linardon J, Wade TD, de la Piedad Garcia X, Brennan L. The efficacy of cognitive-behavioral therapy for eating disorders: a systematic review and meta-analysis. *J Consult Clin Psychol.* 2017;85:1080–1094.
71. Fairburn CG, Marcus MD, Wilson GT. Cognitive-behavioral therapy for binge eating and bulimia nervosa: a comprehensive treatment manual. In: Fairburn CG, Wilson GT, eds. *Binge Eating: Nature, Assessment, and Treatment.* New York, NY: Guilford Press; 1993:361–404.
72. Fairburn CG, Cooper Z, Shafran R, et al. Enhanced cognitive behavior therapy for eating disorders: the core protocol. In: Fairburn CG, ed. *Cognitive Behavior Therapy and Eating Disorders.* New York, NY: Guilford Press; 2008:45–193.
73. Bissada H, Tasca G, Barber A, Bradwejn J. Olanzapine in the treatment of low body weight and obsessive thinking in women with anorexia nervosa: a randomized, double-blind placebo controlled trial. *Am J Psychiatry.* 2008;165:1281–1288.
74. Mondraty N, Birmingham C, Touys W, Sundakov V, Chapman L, Beumont P. Randomized controlled trial of olanzapine in the treatment of cognitions in anorexia nervosa. *Australas Psychiatry.* 2005;13:72–75.
75. Hagman J, Gralla J, Sigel E, et al. A double-blind, placebo controlled study of risperidone for the treatment of adolescents and young adults with anorexia nervosa: a pilot study. *J Am Acad Child Psychiatry.* 2011;50:915–924.
76. Lebow J, Sim LA, Erwin PJ, Murad MH. The effect of atypical antipsychotic medications in individuals with anorexia nervosa : a systematic review and meta-analysis. *Int J Eat Disord.* 2013;46:332–339.
77. Marvanova M, Gramith K. Role of antidepressants in the treatment of adults with anorexia nervosa. *Ment Health Clin.* 2018;8:127–137.
78. Levine LR, Pope Jr HG, Enas GG, et al. Fluoxetine in the treatment of bulimia nervosa: a multicenter, placebo-controlled, double-blind trial. *Arch Gen Psychiatry.* 1992;49:139–147.
79. Couturier J, Lock J. A review of medication use for children and adolescents with eating disorders. *J Can Acad Child Adolesc Psychiatry.* 2007;16:173–176.
80. Agras WS, Lock J, Brandt H, et al. Comparison of 2 family therapies for adolescent anorexia nervosa: a randomized parallel trial. *JAMA Psychiatry.* 2014;71:1279–1286.
81. Lock J, Le Grange D, Agras WS, Moye A, Bryson SW, Jo B. Randomized clinical trial comparing family-based treatment with adolescent-focused individual therapy for adolescents with anorexia nervosa. *Arch Gen Psychiatry.* 2010;67:1025–1032.
82. Eisler I, Dare C, Russell GFM, et al. Family and individual therapy in anorexia nervosa: a 5-year follow-up. *Arch Gen Psychiatry.* 1997;54:1025–1030.
83. Lock J, Couturier J, Agras WS. Comparison of long-term outcomes in adolescents with anorexia nervosa treated with family therapy. *J Am Acad Child Psychiatry.* 2006;45:666–672.
84. Hay P. A systematic review of evidence for psychological treatments in eating disorders: 2005-2012. *Int J Eat Disord.* 2013;46:462–469.
85. Fairburn CG, Bailey-Straebler S, Basden S, et al. A transdiagnostic comparison of enhanced cognitive behaviour therapy (CBT-E) and interpersonal psychotherapy in the treatment of eating disorders. *Behav Res Ther.* 2015;70:64–71.
86. Eddy KT, Tabri N, Thomas JJ, et al. Recovery from anorexia nervosa and bulimia nervosa at 22-year follow-up. *J Clin Psychiatry.* 2017;78:184–189.
87. Swanson SA, Crow SJ, Le Grange D, Swendsen J, Merikangas KR. Prevalence and correlates of eating disorders in adolescents: results from the national comorbidity survey replication adolescent supplement. *Arch Gen Psychiatry.* 2011;68:714–723.
88. Tobin DL, Banker JD, Weisberg L, Bowers W. I know what you did last summer (and it was not CBT): a factor analytic model of international psychotherapeutic practice in the eating disorders. *Int J Eat Disord.* 2007;40:754–757.
89. Wallace LM, von Ranson KM. Treatment manuals: use in the treatment of bulimia nervosa. *Behav Res Ther.* 2011;49:815–820.
90. Waller G. Treatment protocols for eating disorders: clinicians' attitudes, concerns, adherence and difficulties delivering evidence-based psychological interventions. *Curr Psychiatry Rep.* 2016;18. https://doi.org/10.1007/s11920-016-0679-0.
91. Kazdin AE, Fitzsimmons-Craft EE, Wilfley DE. Addressing critical gaps in the treatment of eating disorders. *Int J Eat Disord.* 2017;50:170–189.

CHAPTER

20

DIABETES AND INSULIN RESISTANCE

Kirstine J. Bell, APD, CDE, PhD
Stephen Colagiuri, MBBS, FRACP
Jennie Brand-Miller, PhD, FAA, FAIFST, FNSA
University of Sydney, Sydney, NSW, Australia

SUMMARY

Diabetes can be classified into four categories, type 1 diabetes (T1D), type 2 diabetes (T2D), gestational diabetes (GDM), and diabetes due to other causes. Insulin resistance is a physiological phenomenon that raises insulin levels and is primarily associated with T2D and GDM. T1D results from severe insulin deficiency and requires exogenous insulin therapy to manage the condition. In contrast, T2D and GDM are metabolic disorders characterized by hyperglycemia resulting from a combination of insulin resistance and impaired insulin secretion. Prevention and management include lifestyle interventions with and without medications that achieve normal glucose levels and reduce the risk of complications. The molecular basis of insulin resistance, its role in health and disease, and the optimal diet composition for improving insulin sensitivity present continuing challenges to research scientists around the world.

Keywords: Diabetes; Diet; Insulin resistance; Obesity; Pregnancy.

I. BACKGROUND

Four classes of diabetes are currently recognized by the American Diabetes Association (ADA).[1] *Type 1 diabetes (T1D),* formerly known as insulin-dependent or juvenile diabetes, *type 2 diabetes (T2D),* formerly known as non–insulin-dependent or adult-onset diabetes, *gestational diabetes (GDM),* which is defined as hyperglycemia first identified during pregnancy, and diabetes resulting from genetic defects (monogenic diabetes), diabetes secondary to other diseases, or drug- or chemically induced diabetes (See Table 20.1).

Diabetes affects 1 in 11 adults (463 million people worldwide), with T2D accounting for 90% of all cases.[2] However, approximately 1 in 2 adults with diabetes are undiagnosed (~232 million people). With the current trends, it is estimated that by 2030, there will be 578 million people living with diabetes in the world.[2] The prevalence of insulin resistance, and associated health conditions, however, varies markedly around the world. It has strong lifestyle determinants, which are in turn influenced by socioeconomic status, culture, and education. It is increasingly common in younger age groups and in developing nations.

II. NORMAL FUNCTION AND PHYSIOLOGY

A. Glucose Utilization and Transport

Glucose oxidation is the primary mechanism used by cells to generate energy for metabolism. Many tissues also oxidize fatty acids, but the human brain, fetus, red cell, and the kidney medulla rely on glucose alone except in special circumstances, e.g., fasting for >24 h or a glucose-free diet. Glucose availability is driven primarily by carbohydrates in the diet, but gluconeogenesis is a secondary source, utilizing amino acids (derived from endogenous or exogenous protein), glycerol (derived from dietary fat), or lactic acid (derived from glycolysis)

Present Knowledge in Nutrition, Volume 2
https://doi.org/10.1016/B978-0-12-818460-8.00020-4

TABLE 20.1 Definitions of prediabetes and diabetes.[3]

Tests	Impaired glucose tolerance (IGT)[a]	Impaired fasting glucose (IFG)[a]	Prediabetes (intermediate hyperglycemia)[b]	Diabetes[b]
Fasting plasma glucose	<126 mg/dL (<7.0 mmol/L)	110–125 mg/dL (6.1 –6.9 mmol/L)	110–125 mg/dL[b] (6.1 –6.9 mmol/L)	≥126 mg/dL (≥7.0 mmol/L)
2-Hour plasma glucose following 75 g glucose load (oral glucose tolerance test; OGTT)	140–199 mg/dL (7.8 –11.0 mmol/L)	<140 mg/dL (<7.8 mmol/L)	140–199 mg/dL (7.8 –11.0 mmol/L)	≥200 mg/dL (≥11.1 mmol/L)
Random plasma glucose in symptomatic patient				≥200 mg/dL (≥11.1 mmol/L)
Hemoglobin A1c (HbA1c)				≥6.5% (≥48 mmol/ mol)

[a]*Diagnosis based on presence of* both *criteria listed.*
[b]*Diagnosis based on presence of* one *of the four. Note: The American Diabetes Association uses a different definition of prediabetes.*
Adapted from International Diabetes Federation.

as precursors. Depending on the type of tissue, glucose uptake into cells takes place via mass action, facilitated diffusion, or an active process involving specialized glucose transporters. In the context of diabetes and insulin resistance, GLUT4 transporters found on the surface of muscle and adipose tissue cells are the most sensitive to the concentration of blood insulin.[4] After a meal, circulating blood insulin levels rise and bind to insulin receptors on the cell surface, precipitating a series of reactions that result in glucose uptake into the cell and oxidation within mitochondria. If sufficient glucose is available, glucose is also converted into glycogen within muscle and liver cells. This limited storage form of glucose will be utilized when glucose availability falls, e.g., during prolonged strenuous exercise (muscle glycogen) or after 12 h of fasting (liver glycogen).

B. Actions of Insulin

Insulin is synthesized in the β-cells of the Islets of Langerhans inside the pancreas and stored until the cell is stimulated to release the insulin into circulation. Insulin, the most potent anabolic hormone in the body, exerts its main effects on carbohydrate, lipid, and protein metabolism and also contributes to the regulation of ion and amino acid transport, cell cycle and proliferation, cell differentiation, and nitric oxide (NO) synthesis.[5] Physiologically, insulin is released from the pancreatic β-cells after eating in order to reestablish euglycaemia and acts predominantly on the insulin-sensitive metabolic tissues, i.e., skeletal muscle, liver, and adipose tissue. Insulin promotes glucose uptake in skeletal muscle by stimulating translocation of glucose transporter 4 (GLUT4) from the cytosol to the plasma membrane where it facilitates glucose transport into the cell. Concomitantly, insulin stimulates intracellular utilization of glucose in other tissues. In the fed state, insulin stimulates liver glycogen synthesis and suppresses glycogenolysis and gluconeogenesis, reducing glucose production by the liver. In adipose tissue, insulin suppression of lipolysis can also reduce liver glucose output by limiting glycerol availability for gluconeogenesis—a novel example of an indirect mechanism of insulin contributing to coordination of whole-body metabolic flux.

The β-cell is exquisitely designed to detect and respond to the ingestion of carbohydrate predominantly and also protein, fat, gut hormones (glucagon-like peptide 1 and gastric inhibitory polypeptide), neural stimulation, and pharmacological agents to stimulate and/or amplify insulin secretion[6] (See Fig. 20.1).

C. Mechanisms of Insulin Action and Glucose Transport at the Cellular Level

In healthy individuals, blood glucose concentration is maintained within a narrow range. After an overnight fast or between meals, blood glucose normally falls within the range of 3.5–5.5 mM. Immediately after a meal containing carbohydrate, blood glucose concentration rises to a peak of 6–10 mM followed by a sharp decline back to baseline within 60 min. This fine control is achieved by the balance between glucose absorption from the gut, suppression of glucose production by the liver, and glucose extraction from the blood into the cells and tissues.[7] Insulin also regulates the final balance between the synthesis of glycogen, protein, and fat versus their catabolism and oxidation.

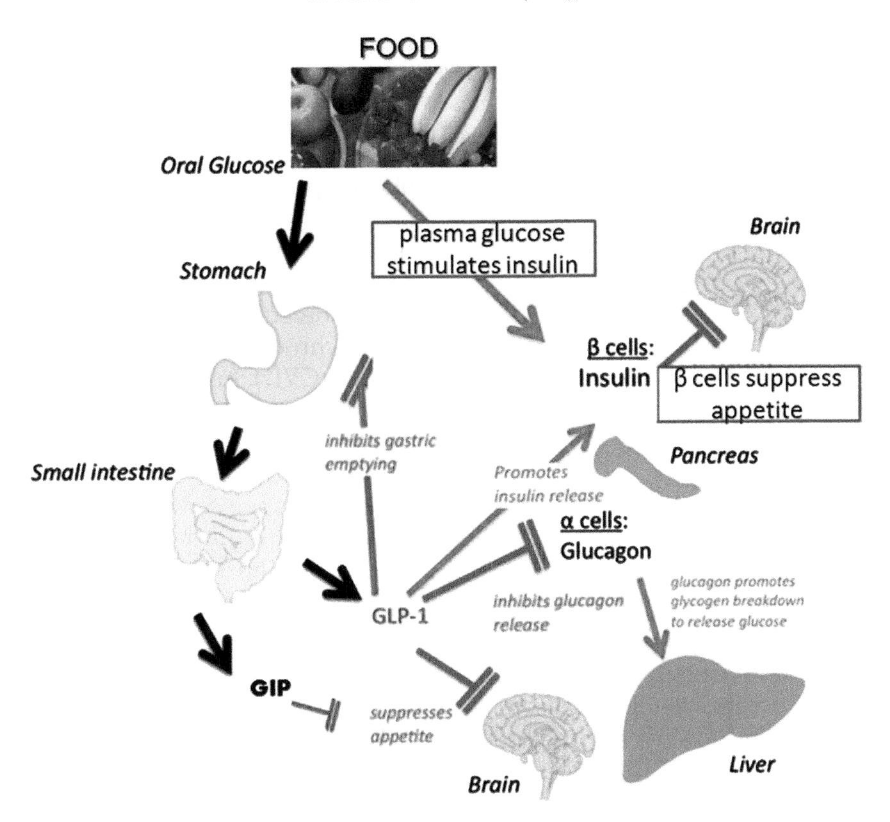

FIGURE 20.1 β-Cell and insulin function. In healthy subjects, food stimulates the release of gastrointestinal peptides, including GLP-1 (glucagon-like peptide 1) and GIP (gastric inhibitory peptide) in addition to the pancreatic β-cell hormone insulin. GLP-1 is released from L cells located in the small bowel and colon. Following the absorption of food, GLP-1 promotes insulin secretion. In diabetes, these steps are disrupted. GLP-1 acts to lower plasma glucose levels by several mechanisms, including inhibiting gastric emptying, and appetite. *Adapted from incretin.com.tw.*

Glucose uptake into the cell is the rate-limiting step in glucose utilization and/or storage, playing a key role in glucose homeostasis. In all tissues except the brain, glucose promotes its own utilization in a concentration-dependent manner (i.e., by mass action). However, in insulin-sensitive tissues, specific glucose transporters shuttle glucose from outside to the inner surface of the cell membrane. Glucose transporters vary in structure from tissue to tissue, with at least 14 different types.[8] GLUT4 is the insulin-dependent carrier that is specific to muscle and adipose tissue. Residing in an intracellular compartment in resting cells, it translocates to the cell surface when insulin receptors on the cell membrane detect a rise in insulin. This master hormone regulates energy metabolism by initiating signaling cascades that control cell growth and survival, as well as glucose, amino acid, and fat uptake. In muscle and adipose tissue, glucose transport is highly dependent on the phosphoinositide 3-kinase (PI3K) signaling cascade that initiates exocytosis of GLUT4 from intracellular storage sites.[9] Failure of GLUT4 to translocate to the plasma membrane in response to insulin is an early step in the development of insulin resistance and T2D.[10]

D. Insulin Sensitivity

Insulin resistance (poor insulin sensitivity) is defined as a condition in which cells fail to respond as expected to normal levels of insulin. It may be a normal physiological response to changes in metabolic circumstances such as in late pregnancy[10] or pathological in nature (e.g., obesity). Energy restriction or carbohydrate restriction causes a decline in insulin sensitivity. Indeed, insulin resistance in one set of tissues may facilitate the redirection of fuels around the body to the tissues in greatest need. During lactation, the mammary glands become extremely insulin sensitive, while muscles remain insulin resistant, thus driving uptake of glucose for the synthesis of lactose.[11] Insulin resistance also appears at birth in infants born small or large for gestational age.[12]

Insulin resistance is associated with excess visceral fat in the abdomen but not excess subcutaneous fat.[13] Surgical removal of visceral fat swiftly restores insulin sensitivity.[14] Because skeletal muscle is the largest insulin sensitive tissue, higher proportions of lean mass are associated with greater insulin sensitivity.

Within a normal healthy population, the amount of physical activity is the main determinant of variation in insulin sensitivity.[15] Both resistance exercise and aerobic exercise increase insulin sensitivity. Insulin sensitivity also varies from one ethnic group to another. Young European Caucasians are more insulin sensitive than those of Asian, South Asian, or SE Asian origins.[16] Pima Indians, distinguished by having the highest recorded rate of T2D in the world, are among the most insulin resistant.[17]

III. ABNORMAL PHYSIOLOGY AND FUNCTION

A. Characteristics of Diabetes

The most common form of diabetes, type 2, is characterized by an inadequate β-cell response to the progressive resistance to insulin that accompanies aging, inactivity, and weight gain. Genetic studies suggest that mutations in at least 40 genes related to β-cell physiology and function are the primary determinants.[18] Weight gain and severe insulin resistance are usually present, yet only a fraction of overweight and obese individuals go on to develop T2D.

Much less common is T1D, an autoimmune disorder in which the β-cells are essentially destroyed, leading to unrestrained lipolysis and free fatty acid oxidation, precipitating the life-threatening state of ketoacidosis. Like T2D, T1D also has a strong genetic component although an environmental trigger is also present.[19] Exogenous insulin therapy is required for life, although there is often a "honeymoon" period after diagnosis during which partial β-cell function is regained.[20] Insulin resistance does not play a role in the development of T1D but may develop slowly over time, resulting in the need for higher insulin doses.[21]

The third form of diabetes, GDM, occurs when the disease is diagnosed for the first time during pregnancy.[1] In developed nations, most pregnant women undergo a glucose tolerance test at the beginning of the third trimester (26–28 weeks gestation). Like T2D, prevalence is increasing, in some countries affecting 15%–25% of all pregnancies.[22]

Other forms of diabetes have also been described, including MODY—maturity onset diabetes of the young—but are relatively uncommon. MODY is a dominantly inherited condition similar to T2D but is typically diagnosed before 25 years of age.[18] Mutations in different genes are responsible, producing differences in clinical presentation. GCK, the gene encoding the pancreatic glucose sensor, glucokinase, is often responsible, but mutations in HNF1A are also recognized.[18]

B. Insulin Resistance

In 1936, Harold Himsworth introduced the concept of "insulin sensitivity," separating diabetes into two main types, an insulin-sensitive and an insulin-resistant phenotype.[23] He developed the first method for measuring insulin resistance and began studies to show that diet might influence glucose tolerance by altering insulin sensitivity. Today, being insulin sensitive is considered fundamental to good health and prevention of chronic diseases, such as T2D and cardiovascular disease (CVD). Insulin resistance, the opposite of insulin sensitivity, is a physiological phenomenon that describes impairments of insulin action, usually in respect to glucose metabolism rather than fatty acids or amino acids.[9] Compared with insulin sensitive individuals, those with insulin resistance require higher concentrations of insulin to facilitate the disposal of glucose in tissues. Insulin-resistant humans and animals therefore develop compensatory hyperinsulinemia in order to ensure normal utilization of glucose by the insulin target tissues. As a consequence, hyperinsulinaemia and insulin resistance go hand in hand.[7]

Insulin resistance can be a normal, physiological state or pathologically severe. Insulin resistance increases naturally at puberty[24] and during pregnancy,[25] but it is more extreme in people who are overweight or obese, have T2D and prediabetes, and often in those with CVD.[26] Recent research links insulin resistance to many conditions, including fatty liver disease, polycystic ovarian syndrome, sleep apnea, and cancer.[6]

Insulin resistance is the most accepted unifying theory explaining the origins of the "metabolic syndrome."[27] The metabolic syndrome is a widely recognized yet controversial concept that refers to a clustering of metabolic risk factors, such as high waist circumference, low HDL cholesterol, high serum triacylglycerol, hypertension, and impaired glucose tolerance (IGT) in the one individual.[28] There is lack of consensus on its practical utility, as either a diagnostic or management tool, and even its definition and diagnostic criteria vary around the world (Table 20.2).

While there is general agreement on four of the central components, there is disagreement on waist circumference and how this should be adjusted for use in different ethnic groups. A World Health Organization Expert Consultation concluded that it was a premorbid condition rather than a clinical diagnosis.[29]

Molecular mechanisms of insulin resistance

Although great strides are being made in understanding, the molecular mechanisms of insulin resistance still

TABLE 20.2 International Diabetes Federation criteria for diagnosis of the metabolic syndrome.

Measure	Categorical cut points[a]
Elevated waist circumference	Population and country-specific definitions (e.g., Europid ≥94 cm in males, and ≥80 cm in females; China ≥85 cm in males, ≥80 cm in females)
Elevated triacylglycerol	>150 mg/dL or 1.7 mmol/L
Reduced HDL cholesterol	<40 mg/dL or 1.0 mmol/L in males, <50 mg/dL or <1.3 mmol/L in females
Elevated blood pressure	Systolic ≥130 and/or diastolic ≥85 mm Hg
Elevated fasting glucose	≥100 mg/dL or 5.5 mmol/L

[a]*Drug treatment for any specific parameter is an alternative indicator.*
Data from Alberti et al.[28]

remain unclear. On a cellular level, insulin stimulates carbohydrate, protein, and lipid synthesis, cell growth, and differentiation, while also inhibiting lipolysis, protein degradation, and apoptosis. However, selective insulin resistance is possible and may explain why in the liver, insulin resistance to glucose metabolism coexists and is often seen alongside liver fat accumulation and development of nonalcoholic fatty liver disease.[30] Differential responses to insulin signaling from the insulin receptor downstream to the final substrates of insulin action involved in metabolic and mitogenic aspects of cellular function may contribute to tissue-specific situations of selective insulin resistance.

Initial attempts to unravel the molecular mechanisms of insulin resistance suggest that the defect in most people lies *downstream* of the insulin receptor. The number and function of insulin receptors are usually normal in patients with T2D, but magnetic resonance spectroscopy studies indicate that there is a defect in insulin-stimulated glucose transport into skeletal muscle.[31] Studies consistently show reduced signaling in the insulin receptor substrate 1 (IRS-1)/PI3K pathway, resulting in diminished glucose uptake and utilization in target tissues.[9] However, the nature of the culprit that initiates and sustains impaired insulin signaling along this pathway is still unclear.

Recent research in this field has produced candidate genes, proteins, and metabolites that have altered expression or activity in insulin-resistant states.[6] Beyond associations between these mediators and insulin action, the causal factors contributing to insulin resistance require demonstration that they are both necessary and sufficient to generate insulin resistance.

Inducing insulin resistance

Insulin resistance can be experimentally induced in several ways in animals and cells. Hyperinsulinemia per se is enough to downregulate expression of the insulin receptor at the cell surface. Models of overnutrition and lipotoxicity are often associated with blunted insulin action. Increased lipid accumulation in muscle and liver has long been associated with insulin resistance. Lipidomic studies are helping to identify individual intracellular lipid species that respond to diet and mediate insulin action. Increased diacylglycerol and ceramide lipid intermediates are associated with activation of protein kinase C (PKC) and antagonism of insulin signaling.[18]

Increased activity of serine kinases, such as PKC, could diminish insulin signal transduction by phosphorylating serine residues on IRS-1. Other triggering mechanisms such as mitochondrial dysfunction, hyperinsulinemia, or hyperglycemia have been proposed. Excessive serine phosphorylation of IRS proteins interferes with normal conductance of the insulin signal and may represent the negative feedback machinery regulating insulin signal transduction.[18] Insulin resistance is also induced by endoplasmic reticulum stress, mitochondrial defects, and oxidative stress, leading some to propose that insulin resistance of the cell is a protective mechanism to limit nutrient flux into the cell.[18] Activation of the transcription factor NF-κB in response to oxidative stress or proinflammatory molecules (including hyperglycemia within the normal range) also produces insulin resistance via a mechanism that involves impairments in the PI3K pathway.[32]

While a number of mechanisms at the molecular level have been proposed and tested in cell culture, interactions between tissues in the whole body in response to nutrient excess, hyperglycemia, hyperinsulinemia, body composition, body fat distribution, and inflammation must also be considered. Although adipose tissue is responsible for less than 10% of insulin-stimulated glucose disposal, adipokines, cytokines, and other molecules derived from adipocytes can also affect insulin sensitivity in peripheral tissues.[33]

The second molecular mechanism that could lead to insulin resistance is a disruption in the balance between the amounts of the two PI3K subunits.[9] The regulatory subunit, p85, is tightly associated with a catalytic subunit, p110. Insulin-resistant states could be associated with decreases in the expression of the p85 monomer, causing decreased PI3K activity. Pregnancy appears to be associated with increased expression of skeletal muscle p85 in response to increasing concentrations of human placental growth hormone.

Determining insulin resistance

Insulin plays a central role in the regulation of blood glucose concentration by suppressing glucose production and stimulating glucose uptake. Most methods used to measure any impairment in insulin action (i.e., insulin resistance) therefore assess the quantitative relationship between a given plasma insulin concentration and some measurable insulin-dependent process, usually at the whole-body level. A simple and common marker of insulin resistance is called HOMA-IR (homeostasis modeling assessment for insulin resistance) or HOMA-IS (HOMA insulin sensitivity), simply calculated as the product of the fasting glucose in mM and the fasting insulin in U/mL divided by 22.5.[34] In young, lean healthy individuals, this value approximates 1, but the range within the normal adult population is around 1–4 units. The top quartile is regarded as being relatively insulin resistant. Obese people and individuals with T2D show values in the range 4–8 units. However, HOMA reflects mostly hepatic insulin resistance and not the ability to deal with an oral carbohydrate challenge. Others have endeavored to improve on HOMA by using the quantitative insulin sensitivity check index (QUICKI) and the fasting glucose-to-insulin ratio. Techniques such as the frequently sampled intravenous glucose tolerance test or minimal modeling endeavor to measure how quickly blood glucose levels return to normal after injection of a given amount of insulin.[35] The "gold standard" method for measuring insulin resistance is the euglycemic-hyperinsulinemic clamp,[36] in which a constant intravenous infusion of insulin is balanced by a simultaneous infusion of glucose in a clinical research setting. Because of the invasive, time-consuming nature of the clamp procedure, it is difficult to use in routine clinical practice or in large epidemiological studies.

C. Type 1 Diabetes

T1D is characterized by severe insulin deficiency requiring exogenous insulin to prevent ketoacidosis, coma, and death. Although T1D may occur at any age, onset usually occurs during childhood, adolescence, or early adulthood, with peak age of diagnosis at age 10–14 years. The SEARCH for Diabetes in Youth Study is a population-based, multicenter observational study of youth with clinically diagnosed diabetes in the United States.[37] Based on data from 2002 to 2003, approximately 15,000 youth are newly diagnosed with T1D annually.[37] The incidence of T1D is higher in Caucasians than in other ethnic/racial groups, with the greatest discrepancy at younger ages.[37]

Prevention

Currently, there are no established approaches for primary prevention of T1D; studies are ongoing to better understand environmental triggers as well as the potential role of immunosuppressive therapy and various other approaches.

Etiology and diagnosis

T1D is characterized by T cell–mediated autoimmune destruction of the β-cells in the islets of Langerhans within the pancreas. Markers of this destruction include islet cell autoantibodies, autoantibodies to insulin, autoantibodies to GAD (GAD65, the enzyme that converts glutamate to gamma-aminobutyrate or GABA), and autoantibodies to the tyrosine phosphatases IA-2 and IA-2β.[38] Furthermore, T1D appears to be associated with particular histocompatibility leukocyte antigen alleles.[39] Often these antibodies can be found in the serum prior to the onset of clinical disease, and so it is important when considering the etiology of T1D to distinguish between the onset of autoimmunity, which can occur years before the onset of hyperglycemia, and the onset of the clinical disease.[39,40] Testing for the presence of these antibodies can be used in a clinical setting to confirm a T1D diagnosis.

D. Type 2 Diabetes

T2D is a metabolic disorder characterized by hyperglycemia resulting from insulin resistance and impaired insulin secretion from the pancreatic β-cells. Prediabetes (also known as "intermediate hyperglycemia") occurs when glucose levels become elevated but not to the diagnostic criteria for T2D—impaired fasting glucose (IFG), IGT, and/or elevated glycated hemoglobin A1c (HbA1c) (see Table 20.1). Individuals with prediabetes are at a higher risk of T2D. The prevention and management of T2D focuses on lifestyle modification (i.e., diet and physical activity) to reduce insulin resistance.

Cardiovascular disease and type 2 diabetes

Under normal circumstances, insulin exerts antiatherogenic and antiinflammatory actions in the endothelial cells and vascular smooth muscle cells lining the blood vessels.[41] Insulin inhibits the expression of adhesion molecules, monocyte chemoattractant protein 1, and the inflammatory transcription factor, NF-κB. However, in the presence of insulin resistance (i.e., with impaired PI3K signaling), hyperinsulinemia appears to exert adverse effects on the arterial wall.[40] Compensatory hyperinsulinemia becomes proatherogenic by stimulating both the MAP-kinase signaling pathway and excessive prenylation of Ras and Rho proteins (Fig. 20.2). Hence, management of insulin-resistant individuals must include effective measures to improve insulin sensitivity as well as decrease ambient insulinemia. The metabolic stages in the transition from normal glucose tolerance to β-cell failure and T2D are described in Box 20.1.

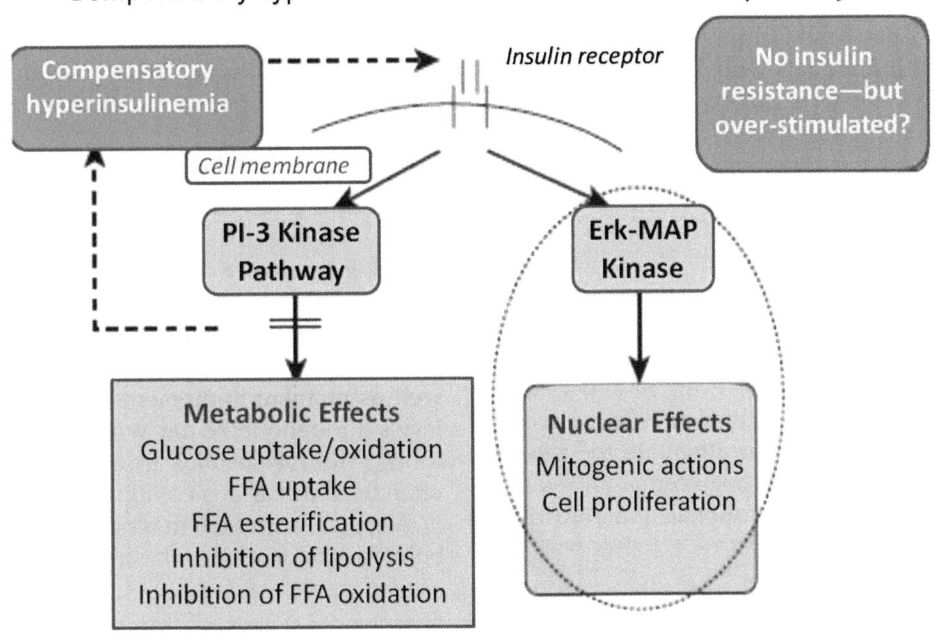

FIGURE 20.2 Two major pathways are stimulated when insulin binds to insulin receptors on cell membranes of insulin-sensitive tissues: phosphatidyl inositol-3 kinase and MAP-kinase. Insulin resistance appears to originate downstream of the insulin receptor in the PI3K pathway involved in the metabolism of carbohydrates, fats, and proteins but not in the MAP kinase pathway. Compensatory hyperinsulinemia resulting from insulin resistance in the PI3K pathway can mean overstimulation of the MAP kinase pathway, with implications for cell growth, multiplication, and differentiation. *Modified from Draznin.*[9]

BOX 20.1

How worsening insulin resistance contributes to the development of type 2 diabetes in individuals with insufficient β-cell reserve

Stage 1: Normal glucose tolerance, mild insulin resistance, compensatory hyperinsulinemia
Stage 2: Glucose tolerance begins to deteriorate; postprandial hyperglycemia becomes common
Stage 3: Impaired glucose tolerance (IGT) worsens, in fasting and postprandial hyperinsulinemia
Stage 4: β-Cells begin to fail, fasting and postprandial insulinemia declines, marked fasting and postprandial hyperglycemia
Stage 5: β-Cell mass declines, insulin replacement may be necessary

IV. PRIMARY TREATMENTS FOR DIABETES

A. Type 1 Diabetes

Dietary management

For individuals with T1D, intensive insulin therapy using multiple daily injections (MDI) or continuous subcutaneous infusion requires instruction on how to adjust insulin doses based on planned carbohydrate intake. Medical nutrition therapy is therefore focused on general healthy eating principles and individualized carbohydrate counting to improve glycemic control.[42] Adjustments to the dose may be needed to account for differences in glycemic index (GI), fat, and protein in the meal.[43,44] There is little high-quality evidence that a specific eating pattern (e.g., vegetarian, low-fat, low-carbohydrate, Mediterranean) is superior.[42]

Achieving glycemic control

Glycemic control and restoration of normal metabolism is the major treatment goal for all classes of diabetes. This task is accomplished using several modalities including a variety of pharmacological agents, close personal and laboratory monitoring (e.g., self-blood glucose testing, HbA1c, and renal function testing), and careful assessment by a variety of health professionals. All these elements, integrated and coordinated, are essential in the management of diabetes (Box 20.2).

The Diabetes Control and Complications Trial (DCCT) was conducted in individuals with T1D to compare the effects of intensive versus standard glycemic control.[45] Intensive treatment reduced the mean HbA1c from 9% to 7.2%, and greater attention to dietary strategies accounted for almost one-fourth of the glycemic improvement.[46] The risk of development and progression of retinopathy, albuminuria, and neuropathy was reduced by between 50% and 75% over 8 years. Reduction in the risk of complications was linearly related to the reduction in HbA1c, indicating that risk reduction can be achieved by improving glycemic control, even if a perfect or normal metabolic state is not achieved.[46] These accomplishments, as well as efforts to attenuate the two- to three fold increase in severe hypoglycemia and weight gain, were largely due to educational and nutritional strategies.[45,47]

Most recently, long-term follow-up of the DCCT cohort in the Epidemiology of Diabetes Interventions and Complications study has documented a continued differential in the risk of microvascular[48] and macrovascular[49] complications, even though HbA1c levels in the two groups have been similar for approximately 8 years.

Medical nutrition therapy

For all classes of diabetes, the first goal of medical nutrition therapy (MNT) is to assist in the achievement and maintenance of metabolic normality, including blood glucose, lipid, and lipoprotein levels (Box 20.3). For T1D, this means coordinating an individual's insulin regimen with his/her food choices and physical activity,[42] as well as moment-to-moment measures of blood glucose levels throughout the day with self–blood glucose monitoring. Multiple insulins are available (Table 20.3) and are often used in various combinations.

A typical approach in terms of insulin use is a "basal-bolus" regimen, either via subcutaneous insulin infusion

BOX 20.2

Summary of current American Diabetes Association (ADA) consensus nutrition recommendations regarding type 1 diabetes

- Macronutrient distribution should be based on individualized assessment of current eating patterns, preferences, and metabolic goals.
- Increasing fiber intake, preferably through food (vegetables, pulses [beans, peas, and lentils], fruits, and whole intact grains) or through dietary supplements, may help in modestly lowering HbA1c.
- Reducing overall carbohydrate intake for improving glycemia is recommended.
- People with diabetes and prediabetes should be screened and evaluated during DSMES and MNT encounters for disordered eating, and nutrition therapy should accommodate these disorders.
- Adults with diabetes or prediabetes who drink alcohol do so in moderation (one drink or less per day for adult women and two drinks or less per day for adult men) and be counseling about the signs, symptoms, and self-management of delayed hypoglycemia after drinking alcohol, especially when using insulin or insulin secretagogues.
- For individuals with type 1 diabetes, it is recommended to use carbohydrate counting approach in intensive insulin therapy to improve glycemia.
- For adults using fixed daily insulin doses, consistent carbohydrate intake with respect to time and amount, while considering the insulin action time, can result in improved glycemia and reduce the risk for hypoglycemia.
- When consuming a mixed meal that contains carbohydrate and is high in fat and/or protein, insulin dosing should not be based solely on carbohydrate counting. A cautious approach to increasing mealtime insulin doses is suggested; continuous glucose monitoring (CGM) or self-monitoring of blood glucose (SMBG) should guide decision-making for administration of additional insulin.
- Correcting hyperglycemia is one strategy for the management of gastroparesis, as acute hyperglycemia delays gastric emptying.
- Use of CGM and/or insulin pump therapy may aid the dosing and timing of insulin administration in people with type 1 or type 2 diabetes with gastroparesis.

Adapted from American Diabetes Association.[42]

BOX 20.3

Summary of medical nutrition therapy (MNT) implementation strategies for Type 1 Diabetes (T1D)

- When counseling people with diabetes, a key strategy to achieve glycemic targets should include an assessment of current dietary intake followed by individualized guidance to optimize meal timing and food choices and to guide medication and physical activity recommendations.
- All RDNs providing MNT in diabetes care should assess and monitor medication changes in relation to the nutrition care plan. Insulin therapy should be planned to match insulin action to lifestyle.
- Blood glucose levels should be monitored while keeping lifestyle consistent.
- Create algorithms for adjusting insulin for lifestyle flexibility and to correct blood glucose levels that are not in the target range.

Adapted from 2019 American Diabetes Association recommendations.[42]

TABLE 20.3 Insulin preparations: onset, peak, and duration of action.

Insulin	Brand name	Onset of action	Peak action	Duration of action
Rapid acting				
Insulin aspart analog	Fiasp	4 min	−1 h	3–5 h
Insulin aspart analog	NovoLog	10–20 min	0.5–2.5 h	3–5 h
Insulin lispro analog	Humalog			
Insulin glulisine	Apidra	20 min	1–2 h	3–6 h
Regular insulin	Humulin R	30–60 min	2–4 h	6–10 h
	Novolin R			
Intermediate acting				
NPH insulin	Humulin N	2–4 h	4–8 h	14–24 h
	Novolin N			
	ReliOn			
Lente insulin	Humulin L	2–4 h	4–15 h	16–24 h
Long acting				
Ultralente insulin	Humulin U	3–4 h	8–14 h	18–24 h
Insulin glargine	Lantus	1–2 h	No peak	Up to 24 h
	Basaglar	1–2 h	No peak	Up to 24 h
	Toujeo	6 h	No peak	24–36 h
Detemir	Levemir	1–2 h	Minimal	Up to 24 h
Degludec	Tresiba	1–4 h	No significant peak	Approx. 42 h

Data from Wylie-Rosett et al. (2006), Bennett JA; RPh, FACA, CDE.

(or pump therapy) or MDI in which insulin is delivered as a bolus before meals in amounts matched to total carbohydrate intake, with basal insulin on board consistently over time. There are other approaches to MDI, which utilize different types of insulin. Patients can either vary their insulin dose to match the amount of food consumed, with additional considerations for physical activity, or meals and physical activity can be held constant in order to match a constant dosing of insulin from day to day. Reduction of insulin dosage is the preferred method of preventing hypoglycemia during and/or after exercise, but this requires planning physical activity ahead of time. For unplanned exercise, increased carbohydrate intake may be needed.[42] Self–blood glucose monitoring, education, and experience allow the individual to learn how to keep all of this in balance.

B. Type 2 Diabetes

How to maximize insulin sensitivity to decrease risk of type 2 diabetes

The most important environmental and modifiable factors that worsen an individual's resistance to insulin are excessive body weight, physical inactivity, smoking, and poor sleep. Increased muscle mass and lower abdominal fat mass each markedly improve insulin sensitivity.[14,50] Hence, a combination of weight loss and physical activity, particularly resistance exercise, is the ideal lifestyle intervention to reduce the risk of T2D and CVD.

However, diet composition has been shown to have a separate additional effect. Observational studies and intervention trials have shown the macronutrient distribution (i.e., the ratio of fat, carbohydrate, protein energy) and the quality of individual macronutrients directly influence insulin sensitivity. In particular, the amount and quality of fat and carbohydrate are factors involved in the development of insulin resistance and T2D.

Diet composition and type 2 diabetes

Dietary fat and insulin sensitivity; The effects of dietary fat and carbohydrate on insulin sensitivity have been debated for decades. Some of the controversy stems from divergent findings in animals versus humans and in differing study designs. Insulin resistance can be induced in animal models by diets high in fat, sucrose, or fructose. However, a single bout of exercise or high starch meal can completely reverse the defect within 24 h. In humans, some studies suggest that a high intake of fat is associated with impaired insulin sensitivity but is modified by the type of fat and by the type of subject. Using clamp studies in humans, Vessby[36] was the first to show that insulin resistance was related to high proportions of saturated fatty acids and low proportions of unsaturated fatty acids in the serum cholesterol esters of healthy men who later developed T2D.

Later, fatty acid composition of the phospholipids in the skeletal muscle cell membrane was found to be directly related to insulin sensitivity in healthy males.[51] Specifically, the proportions of long-chain fatty acids with 20–22 carbon atoms correlated strongly with insulin sensitivity. However, the fatty acid pattern of skeletal muscle is influenced not just by diet but also by the amount of physical activity and by muscle fiber composition.[51]

The most convincing evidence of the effect of the role of fat type on insulin sensitivity comes from a metaanalysis of over 100 randomized controlled trials (totaling 4,220 adults) of isocaloric replacement of SFA, MUFA, and PUFA with carbohydrate, adjusted for protein, *trans* fat, and dietary fiber.[52] In the final analysis, replacing 5% energy from carbohydrate with SFA had no significant effect on fasting glucose but lowered fasting insulin by a trivial amount. Replacing carbohydrate with MUFA lowered HbA1c, 2 h postchallenge insulin, and HOMA-IR by a modest amount. However, replacing SFA with PUFA improved fasting glucose, HbA1c, C-peptide, and HOMA. Based on the gold standard method of acute insulin response, PUFA significantly improves insulin secretory capacity. Feeding studies showing that polyunsaturated fats produced the highest insulin sensitivity, followed by monounsaturated, and then saturated fat.[52]

Dietary carbohydrates and insulin sensitivity; Controversies surrounding the optimal intake of carbohydrate have increased in recent years. In healthy, young persons, isocaloric substitution of carbohydrates (to 57%E) in place of saturated fat improved insulin sensitivity within 4 weeks.[53] Similarly, well-designed studies have shown that optimal insulin sensitivity occurs at 41% carbohydrate energy (E%) in young men and 85%E in elderly men[54]

Like fat, the quality of carbohydrate, i.e., the content of whole grains, dietary fiber, proportion of simple sugars, and dietary GI of a high-carbohydrate diet, may be critical, each with independent effects on insulin sensitivity. Indeed, carbohydrates consumed without fiber may produce detrimental effects. In individuals with diabetes, higher carbohydrate intake has the potential to raise postprandial glucose and increase insulin demand, an effect that might worsen insulin resistance. Under metabolic ward conditions for 21 days, hepatic and peripheral insulin sensitivity as judged by the glucose clamp remained unchanged in 10 type 2 patients on either a high-carbohydrate (60%E) or low-carbohydrate (35%E) diet, matched for fiber.[55] However, the patients in this study were treated with insulin, a factor that may fundamentally affect the ability to metabolize a high carbohydrate meal.

In a cross-sectional analysis of ~3,000 individuals in the Framingham Offspring Study, whole grains, total fiber from all sources, and fiber from cereals and fruit were inversely related to HOMA-IR.[56] There was no relationship with total carbohydrate intake or intake of refined grains.

Higher whole-grain intake has also been directly correlated with insulin sensitivity in cross-sectional studies in which insulin sensitivity was assessed by FSIGTT (frequently sampled insulin-modified intravenous glucose tolerance test).[57] Findings from metaanalyses of prospective studies with high intakes of dietary fiber and whole grains were complementary, with striking dose–response evidence that suggests (but does not prove) causal relationships with T2D and total all-cause mortality.[58] The lowest risk was observed with fiber intakes of 25–29 g per day and whole grains of 40–50 g per day.

Unfortunately, these strong observational findings on carbohydrate quality are not well supported by randomized controlled trials (RCTs) with clinical outcomes.[59,60] A small but well-designed intervention study incorporated 6–10 servings of breakfast cereal, bread, rice, pasta, muffins, cookies, and snacks from either whole or refined grains (in both cases mostly ground into flour) in a diet containing 55%E from carbohydrate and 30%E from fat. Using the glucose clamp, insulin sensitivity was higher after 6 weeks on the whole grain diet compared with a similar period on the refined grain diet.[59] Unfortunately, this finding was not confirmed in the larger WHOLEheart Study in which 60–120 g/day whole-grain foods were ingested by 316 subjects for up to 16 weeks.[60]

Sucrose and fructose; The effects of fructose and sucrose (a disaccharide of glucose and fructose) on insulin sensitivity remains controversial. Studies in animals, often fed extremely high intakes (e.g., 70% of total calories) or in solution in place of water, have shown a detrimental effect of fructose and sucrose compared with starch or glucose.[61] When fructose and glucose were compared directly, fructose was found to be the culpable moiety.

The evidence in humans also suggests that fructose and sucrose in very high amounts produce an increase in insulin resistance.[62] However, the relevance of these findings to typical consumption has been questioned.[63] In more realistic amounts, fructose and sucrose may have beneficial effects on insulin sensitivity. In lean, young healthy males, a diet containing 25% sucrose produced higher insulin sensitivity as assessed in a two-step clamp procedure than a diet containing 1% sucrose.[64] Similarly, a study in patients with T2D showed that a diet with 10% of total energy as fructose produced a 34% improvement in insulin sensitivity measured by the euglycemic-hyperinsulinemic clamp.[65] In this study, patients lived in a hospital environment and all food was provided. Finally, using the glucokinase clamp, no effects on insulin sensitivity were noted after 3 months of a 13% fructose versus sucrose diet.[66] It is conceivable however that at very high intakes (>30%E), sucrose and fructose have adverse effects on insulin sensitivity.

Low-GI diets; Low-GI diets in which the carbohydrates are more slowly digested and absorbed, resulting in lower postprandial glycemia, have been associated with improved insulin sensitivity in some studies but not others. In the Framingham cohort, dietary GI and glycemic load (GL) were directly related to insulin resistance with approximately 10% more insulin resistance in the highest quintile of GI than in the lowest.[56] Glucose uptake from blood was 45% higher during the clamp procedure in T2D patients who ate a low-GI diet for 4 weeks compared with a macronutrient-matched high-GI diet.[67]

The alpha-glucosidase inhibitor, acarbose, which slows carbohydrate digestion but is not absorbed into the systemic circulation, also produces improvements in insulin sensitivity, thereby providing proof of principle.[68] Low-GI diets improved insulin sensitivity in women with polycystic ovarian syndrome as judged by the glucose tolerance test–based insulin sensitivity index,[69] but not in lean, active young males as judged by the glucose clamp.[64] In older, obese individuals, a 7 day low-GI diet combined with exercise training improved clamp-derived insulin sensitivity just as well as a high-GI diet + exercise, but there were greater benefits of the low-GI diet on systolic BP and VO_2 max.[70] In children and adolescents, low-GI diets resulted in more significant improvements in HOMA-IR compared with the respective high GI counterparts .[71] Finally, in a meta-analysis of RCTs comparing high versus low-GI diets in overweight and obese adults undergoing weight loss, fasting insulin was significantly lower on the low GI/GL arms.[72] In contrast, 3–5 weeks of a low-GI diet did not result in improvements in insulin sensitivity, lipid levels, or systolic blood pressure over a high-GI diet in 163 overweight adults (without diabetes).[73]

Micronutrients and insulin resistance; Insulin sensitivity has also been related to intake of specific micronutrients. Magnesium is an important cofactor for enzymes involved in carbohydrate metabolism and magnesium deficiency as judged by serum, and dietary magnesium concentration is associated with insulin resistance and increased risk of T2D.[74] Across 4 major cohorts, with over 240,000 participants and over 17,000 cases of T2D, higher magnesium intake was associated with a lower risk of T2D.[75] This association was stronger in those with lower carbohydrate quality (i.e., high GI or low cereal fiber) diets versus higher quality carbohydrate diets. Clinical evidence for magnesium supplementation in the treatment of T2D (through improved glucose tolerance) is limited and results vary, often due to underpowered studies. In RCTs, magnesium supplements given to deficient subjects with T2D have improved HOMA-IR.[76]

The ability of chromium to improve insulin sensitivity remains controversial. Chromium is clearly essential for carbohydrate metabolism, but it is widely available in the diet and deficiency states are rare. There is growing evidence that chromium supplementation, particularly at higher doses (1000 μg/day) in the form of chromium picolinate, is safe and may improve insulin sensitivity and glucose tolerance.[77] In a metaanalysis, chromium supplementation improved HOMA-IR in women with polycystic ovarian syndrome (a group with intrinsic insulin resistance) and patients with diabetes. However, the magnitude was small and the clinical relevance uncertain.[78]

Vitamin intake and status may also play a role in maintenance of insulin sensitivity. Lipid oxidation, for example, might be a mechanism contributing to impaired mitochondrial function. Variations in insulin-mediated glucose disposal were observed in healthy individuals relative to plasma concentrations of lipid-soluble antioxidant vitamins and compounds, including lutein, carotenoids, and tocopherols.[79] However, in other cross-sectional studies, antioxidant vitamins C and E showed no relationship to insulin sensitivity as judged by the FSIGTT.[80] The concentration of 25(OH) vitamin D correlated independently with clamp-derived insulin sensitivity in a study of 126 healthy, glucose-tolerant individuals in California.[81] Those with hypovitaminosis D were also three times more likely to have insulin resistance.

Blood pressure salt sensitivity, as judged by the difference in blood pressure after a high-versus low-sodium diet, was also strongly associated with insulin resistance in lean, essential-hypertensive patients.[82]

Diet and type 2 diabetes

There is no single diet that is ideal for all individuals with, or at risk of, T2D. Instead, metaanalysis suggests a range of evidence-based dietary approaches can be beneficial, including high-carbohydrate/low-fat, low-carbohydrate/high-fat low-glycemic index, Mediterranean, and high-protein diets.[83] For those at high risk of T2D, vegetarian and vegan diets,[84] the Dietary Approaches to Stop Hypertension diet,[85] and the Nordic diet[86] have also been associated with a reduced risk of T2D.

High- versus low-carbohydrate diets; The best evidence that dietary changes can improve insulin resistance and/or β-cell function comes from landmark studies in which intensive lifestyle interventions prevented or delayed progression from IGT to T2D mellitus.[87,88] Both studies employed low-fat, high-carbohydrate diets (30% of energy from fat, 10% from saturated fat) in combination with physical activity to achieve the goal of weight loss. These findings have since been perceived as a rational basis for recommending low-fat, high-carbohydrate diets. In all probability, weight loss per se likely played the most important role, and the superiority of low-fat diets for those with the metabolic syndrome is questionable.

Low-carbohydrate diets have also been shown to be effective for glycemic control in T2D in the short term. Three metaanalyses were published in 2017–18 and all showed greater reductions in HbA1c at 6 months with low-carbohydrate diets (<45% total energy) versus high-carbohydrate diets (>45% total energy), with greater improvements when carbohydrate was restricted to <26% total energy. However, the benefit of one diet over the other was no longer evident at 12 months. Similarly, reductions in body weight were greater at 6 months with low-carbohydrate diets, however, and only one of the three metaanalyses showed a continued benefit at 12 months compared with a traditional high-carbohydrate diet.

One concern about low-carbohydrate diets is the resulting increase in the proportion of dietary fat and thus the potential impact on CVD biomarkers. To address this, a hypocaloric very low-carbohydrate (14% total energy), high–unsaturated fat diet was compared to an energy-matched, low-fat, high-carbohydrate (53% total energy) diet in 115 overweight and obese adults with T2D. At 2 years, both diets induced statistically and clinically meaningful reductions in body weight and HbA1c, with no differences between the two diets.[89]

GI/GL; Metaanalyses have shown low-GI/GL diets can improve glycemic control (glycated hemoglobin), fasting glucose, BMI, total cholesterol, and LDL cholesterol in those with T1D or T2D or with IGT (prediabetes).[90,91]

In prospective observational studies, carbohydrate intake (whether high or low) is not usually an independent predictor of the development of T2D mellitus or CVD. In metaanalyses, however, the quality of carbohydrate intake (as assessed as the higher GI or GL) shows a consistent positive relationship to the risk of T2D mellitus[92,93] and CVD.[94] The highest relative risks (>2) were observed among those with both a higher dietary GI or GL and lower cereal fiber intake.[95] Some population studies have demonstrated that higher intake of high GI carbohydrates, but not low GI carbohydrates, is associated with greater risk of developing CVD.[96]

Mediterranean diet; The Mediterranean diet has grown in popularity over recent years as a dietary approach to assist with a range of health concerns, including obesity and the prevention and management of T2D. As its name suggests, the diet is based on traditional foods and eating patterns in the Mediterranean region, including vegetables, fruit, fish, legumes, nuts, olive, and wine. Metaanalysis has shown adoption of the Mediterranean diet decreases the risk of the metabolic syndrome[97,98] and T2D.[99,100] Metaanalysis of two long-term RCTs showed a 49% increased probability of remission from the metabolic syndrome during the 2–5 year follow-up.[101] For those already diagnosed with T2D, HbA1c was significantly reduced by an additional −0.31% points (−0.61 to −0.03) compared to usual care.[102]

Very-low-calorie diets (VLCD); Low-calorie diets (800–1200 kcal/day) and VLCD (500–800 kcal/day) are achieved using specially formulated, nutritionally complete, meal replacement products, along with medical supervision and dietetic support. They have been shown to induce weight loss of approximately 15% of initial body weight over 12 weeks and a significant reduction in blood glucose levels after 6 months in obese adults with prediabetes and T2D.[103] The PREVIEW study showed that 84% of overweight adults with prediabetes achieved the targeted ≥8% body weight loss within 8 weeks using VLCD meal replacements .[104] Of the study participants, 64% had IFG-only, 13% had IGT-only, and 23% had both IFG and IGT. The mean weight loss was 11 kg (11% total body weight) and was accompanied by significant improvements in risk factors for prediabetes, including fat mass, hip circumference, HOMA-IR, and metabolic syndrome z-score.

Similar findings have been found with T2D in the DiRECT trial.[105] The trial enrolled 149 participants to receive either a structured weight management program (including 12–20 weeks of total meal replacements) or standard care. At 1 year, 46% of intervention participants had remission of their T2D and 24% had maintained at least 15 kg weight loss. At 2 years, 36% of intervention participants had maintained remission of their T2D and 11% had maintained at least 15 kg weight loss.

Taken together, these studies imply that dietary approaches that reduce the risk of developing or improve management of T2D share a unifying mechanism of reducing postprandial glycemia and insulinemia despite variable macronutrient distribution. Thus, it is possible that any diet that facilitates reduced glycemia without increasing dyslipidemia is likely to improve insulin sensitivity and relieve the burden on the β-cell.

C. Gestational Diabetes

In late pregnancy, maternal insulin resistance develops and helps make more fuel, glucose and lipid, available to the growing fetus. Growth hormone secreted by the placenta has been shown to best relate to changes in insulin sensitivity in pregnancy.[106] In addition to directly reducing expression of the insulin receptor, growth hormone reduces insulin signaling and decreases GLUT4 translocation to the plasma membrane in muscle. It also stimulates the expression of IGF2 by the placenta which lowers the threshold for glucose-stimulated insulin production in β-cells and increases maternal circulating insulin.

D. Implications for Management

The triad of metabolic syndrome, insulin resistance, and overweight/obesity is strongly associated with each other.[10] Reducing weight in people who are overweight/obese compared with their population norm results in improvement in insulin resistance and the clinical manifestations of the metabolic syndrome. Therefore, the aim of management should be weight reduction and sustained weight-loss maintenance through increased physical activity and dietary modification. Reduction in total energy intake is usually required to achieve weight loss.

E. Resolving Unanswered Questions

Despite much new knowledge about the effects of diet on insulin resistance and prevention and management of diabetes, many questions remain unanswered.[63] Dietary guidelines are still based on data derived from observational studies, and therefore affected by confounding and other methodological problems. Most randomized controlled trials are short, rely on proxy measures, lack blinding, do not control for treatment intensity between dietary groups, and have limited compliance. Additional relevant considerations in effectiveness studies include the behavioral and environmental factors (e.g., food availability and affordability) affecting compliance. The resolution of these controversies will require mechanistically oriented feeding studies and long term clinical trials, prospective observational research, and examination of economic and environmental impacts.

While insulin resistance plays an important role in the development of T2D and GDM, the underlying mechanisms and molecular pathways remain obscure. Poor diets, including the quantity and quality of macronutrients, are considered a major risk factor for obesity and T2D. However, the optimal diet for treatment and prevention remains controversial. Past emphasis on the amount, type of fat, and proportion of fat has given way to questions about the amount and type of carbohydrate.

Carbohydrate quality, particularly in relation the type of fiber (soluble vs. insoluble), GI, sugars (added vs. free vs. naturally occurring in fruit and vegetables), and starch (rapidly digested, slowly digested, resistant starch), defies attempts to summarize in simple metrics.

The rate of carbohydrate digestion and postprandial effect on glycemia as reflected in the GI and GL of the diet requires further research. Current evidence indicates that GI and GL are substantial, causal food markers that predict the development of T2D in Europe, North America, and some Asian countries.[92,93] However, there is relatively little research from Africa, South America, India, and China.

With the increasing global burden of obesity and of GDM and T2D, there is a need to identify those aspects of the diet that can be manipulated by the food industry while still acceptable to consumers. Increasing intake of whole grain foods, fiber, and plant proteins has been documented in some countries but may not be acceptable to most consumers.

RESEARCH GAPS

- Would a reduction in total carbohydrate intake (currently typically 45%–65% of total energy) help control body weight in general population and susceptible subgroups?
- What is the role of a low-carbohydrate diet in treatment of metabolic syndrome and T2D and in management of T1D?
- In T1D, can we improve on "carbohydrate counting" and current insulin dosage adjustment algorithms to incorporate other nutrient information (e.g., fat and protein content of the meal)?
- Does ketosis induced by severe carbohydrate restriction provide any unique metabolic benefits and, if so, in what clinical settings would this diet be advisable?
- To what level should added (or free) sugars be restricted for optimum individual health and for the population as a whole?
- Would substitution of fructose in added sugars with glucose-based sweeteners provide metabolic benefit or harm?
- Would substitution of free sugars with poorly digestible sugars, sugar alcohols, or artificial sweeteners provide health benefits or harms (e.g., unexpected effects on the microbiome)?
- Is there benefit in replacing fructose containing sugars with other processed carbohydrates?
- Would increased intake of resistant starch provide health benefits?
- What are the health effects of substituting whole grains with other high-carbohydrate (fruits, legumes) or high-fat (nuts, seeds, avocado) whole plant foods?
- What are the long-term effects of different types of carbohydrates on population risk of cancer, neurodegenerative diseases, and cognitive function?
- Which carbohydrate-based foods will provide an optimal combination of health benefits, environmental sustainability, cost, and public acceptability?

**Modified from.*[63]

Acknowledgments

This chapter includes an update of the chapters titled Diabetes by Jacks LM, Wylie-Rosett J, and Mayer-Davis EJ and of Insulin Resistance and the Metabolic Syndrome by Brand-Miller J and Colaguiri S in *Present Knowledge in Nutrition*, 10th Edition, edited by Erdman JW, Macdonald IA, and Zeisel SH and published by Wiley-Blackwell. © 2012 International Life Sciences Institute. Portions of this update are from the previously published chapters, and the contributions of the previous authors are acknowledged.

V. REFERENCES

1. American Diabetes Association. Diagnosis and classification of diabetes mellitus. *Diabetes Care.* 2014;37(Suppl. 1):S81–S90.
2. International Diabetes Federation. *IDF Diabetes Atlas.* 9th edn. Brussels, Belgium: International Diabetes Federation; 2019.
3. International Diabetes Federation. 2019 (Atlas. to be published).
4. Shepherd PR, Kahn BB. Glucose transporters and insulin action — implications for insulin resistance and diabetes mellitus. *N Engl J Med.* 1999;341(4):248–257.
5. Wang CCL, Goalstone ML, Draznin B. Molecular mechanisms of insulin resistance that impact cardiovascular biology. *Diabetes.* 2004a;53:2735.
6. Petersen MC, Shulman GI. Mechanisms of insulin action and insulin resistance. *Physiol Rev.* 2018;98(4):2133–2223.
7. DeFronzo RA, Ferrannini E. Pathogenesis of NIDDM: a balanced overview. *Diabetes Care.* 1992;15:318–368.
8. Thorens B, Mueckler M. Glucose transporters in the 21st century. *Am J Physiol Endocrinol Metab.* 2009;298(2):E141–E145.
9. Draznin B. Molecular mechanisms of insulin resistance. In: Zeitler P, Nadeau K, eds. *Insulin Resistance. Childhood Precursors and Adult Disease.* Humana Press; 2008.
10. Defronzo RA. From the triumvirate to the ominous octet: a new paradigm for the treatment of type 2 diabetes mellitus. *Diabetes.* 2009;58:773–795.
11. Vernon R. Endocrine control of metabolic adaptation during lactation. *Proc Nutr Soc.* 1989;48:23–32.
12. McMillen I, Robinson JC. Developmental origins of the metabolic syndrome: prediction, plasticity, and programming. *Physiol Rev.* 2005;85:571–633.
13. Cnop M, Landchild MJ, Vidal J, et al. The concurrent accumulation of intra-abdominal and subcutaneous fat explains the association

between insulin resistance and plasma leptin concentrations: distinct metabolic effects of two fat compartments. *Diabetes*. 2002; 51:1005–1015.

14. Barzilai N, She L, Liu BQ, et al. Surgical removal of visceral fat reverses hepatic insulin resistance. *Diabetes*. 1999;48:94–98.
15. Helmerhorst HJF, Wijndaele K, Brage SR, et al. Objectively measured sedentary time may predict insulin resistance independent of moderate- and vigorous-intensity physical activity. *Diabetes*. 2009;58(8):1776–1779.
16. Dickinson S, Colagiuri S, Faramus E, et al. Postprandial hyperglycemia and insulin sensitivity differ among lean young adults of different ethnicities. *J Nutr*. 2002;132:2574–2579.
17. Bogardus C. Insulin resistance in the pathogenesis of NIDDM in Pima Indians. *Diabetes Care*. 1993;16:228–231.
18. McCarthy MI. Genomics, type 2 diabetes, and obesity. *N Engl J Med*. 2010;363(24):2339–2350.
19. Concannon P, Rich SS, Nepom GT. Genetics of type 1a diabetes. *N Engl J Med*. 2009;360:1646–1654.
20. Abdul-Rasoul M, Habib H, Al-Khouly M. The honeymoon phase' in children with type 1 diabetes mellitus: frequency, duration, and influential factors. *Pediatr Diabetes*. 2006;7:101–107.
21. Fourlanos S, Narendran P, Byrnes GB, et al. Insulin resistance is a risk factor for progression to Type 1 diabetes. *Diabetologia*. 2004; 47(10):1661–1667.
22. Ferrara A. Increasing prevalence of gestational diabetes mellitus. *Diabetes Care*. 2007;30:S141–S146.
23. Himsworth H. Diabetes mellitus: its differentiation into insulin-sensitive and insulin-insensitive sub-types. *Lancet*. 1936;227:127–130.
24. Goran M, Gower B. Longitudinal study on pubertal insulin resistance. *Diabetes*. 2001;50:2444–2450.
25. Butte N. Carbohydrate and lipid metabolism in pregnancy: normal compared with gestational diabetes mellitus. *Am J Clin Nutr*. 2000;71:1256S–1261S.
26. Facchini F, Hua N, Abbasi F, Reaven G. Insulin resistance as a predictor of age-related diseases. *J Clin Endocrinol Metab*. 2001;86(8): 3574–3578.
27. Mikhail N. The metabolic syndrome: insulin resistance. *Curr Hypertens Rep*. 2009;11:156–158.
28. Alberti KG, Eckel RH, Grundy SM, et al. Harmonizing the metabolic syndrome: a joint interim statement of the International Diabetes Federation Task Force on Epidemiology and Prevention; National Heart, Lung, and Blood Institute; American Heart Association; World Heart Federation; International Atherosclerosis Society; and International Association for the Study of Obesity. *Circulation*. 2009;120:1640–1645.
29. Simmons R, Alberti K, Gale E, et al. The metabolic syndrome: useful concept or clinical tool? Report of a WHO Expert Consultation. *Diabetologia*. 2010;53:600–605.
30. Dyson JK, Anstee QM, McPherson S. Republished: non-alcoholic fatty liver disease: a practical approach to treatment. *Postgrad Med J*. 2015;91:92–101.
31. Semenkovich CF. Insulin resistance and a long, strange trip. *N Engl J Med*. 2016;374(14):1378–1379.
32. Barnes PJ, Karin M. Nuclear factor-kappaB: a pivotal transcription factor in chronic inflammatory diseases. *N Engl J Med*. 1997;336: 1066–1071.
33. Rabe K, Lehrke M, Parhofer KG, et al. Adipokines and insulin resistance. *Mol Med*. 2008;14(11):741–751.
34. Matthews DR, Hosker J, Redenski A, et al. Homeostasis model assessment: insulin resistance and beta-cell function from fasting plasma glucose and insulin concentrations in man. *Diabetologia*. 1985;28:412–419.
35. Bergman RN, Zaccaro DJ, Watanabe RM, et al. Minimal model-based insulin sensitivity has greater heritability and a different genetic basis than homeostasis model assessment or fasting insulin. *Diabetes*. 2003;52:2168–2174.
36. Vessby B. Dietary fat and insulin action in humans. *Br J Nutr*. 2000; 83:S91–S96.
37. Hamman RF, Bell RA, Dabelea Jr D, et al. The SEARCH for diabetes in youth study: rationale, findings, and future directions. *Diabetes Care*. 2014;37:3336–3344.
38. American Diabetes Association. Position statement: diagnosis and classification of diabetes mellitus. *Diabetes Care*. 2010;33: S62–S69.
39. Atkinson MA. ADA Outstanding Scientific Achievement Lecture 2004: thirty years of investigating the autoimmune basis for type 1 diabetes: why can't we prevent or reverse this disease? *Diabetes*. 2005;54:1253–1263.
40. Muntoni S, Muntoni S. Epidemiological association between some dietary habits and the increasing incidence of type 1 diabetes worldwide. *Ann Nutr Metab*. 2006;50:11–19.
41. Wang CCL, Goalstone ML, Draznin B. Molecular mechanisms of insulin resistance that impact cardiovascular biology. *Diabetes*. 2004b;53:2735–2740.
42. Evert AB, Dennison M, Gardner CD, Garvey WT, Lau KH, MacLeod J, Mitri J, Pereira RF, Rawlings K, Robinson S, Saslow L, Uelmen S, Urbanski PB, Yancy WS. Nutrition therapy for adults with diabetes or prediabetes: a consensus report. *Diabetes Care*. 2019;42(5):731–754.
43. Bell KJ, Fio CZ, Twigg S, et al. Amount and type of dietary fat, postprandial glycemia, and insulin requirements in type 1 diabetes: a randomized within-subject trial. *Diabetes Care*. 2020;43: 59–66.
44. Bell KJ, Smart CE, Steil GM, et al. Impact of fat, protein, and glycemic index on postprandial glucose control in type 1 diabetes: implications for intensive diabetes management in the continuous glucose monitoring era. *Diabetes Care*. 2015;38:1008–1015.
45. Diabetes Control and Complications Trial Research Group. The effect of intensive treatment of diabetes on the development and progression of long-term complications in insulin-dependent diabetes mellitus. *N Engl J Med*. 1993;329:977–986.
46. Diabetes Control and Complications Trial Research Group. Weight gain associated with intensive therapy in the diabetes control and complications trial. *Diabetes Care*. 1988;1:567–573.
47. Delahanty LM, Nathan DM, Lachin JM, et al. *Am J Clin Nutr*. 2009; 89:518–524.
48. Genuth S, Sun W, Cleary P, et al. Glycation and carboxymethyllysine levels in skin collagen predict the risk of future 10-year progression of diabetic retinopathy and nephropathy in the diabetes control and complications trial and epidemiology of diabetes interventions and complications participants with type 1 diabetes. *Diabetes*. 2005;54:3103–3111.
49. Nathan DM, Cleary PA, Backlund JY, et al. Intensive diabetes treatment and cardiovascular disease in patients with type 1 diabetes. *N Engl J Med*. 2005;353:2643–2653.
50. Balkau B, Mhamdi L, Oppert JM, et al. Physical activity and insulin sensitivity: the RISC study. *Diabetes*. 2008;57:2613–2618.
51. Borkman M, Storlien L, Pan D, et al. The relationship between insulin sensitivity and the fatty acid composition of skeletal-muscle phospholipids. *N Engl J Med*. 1993;32:238–244.
52. Imamura F, Micha R, Wu JH, et al. Effects of saturated fat, polyunsaturated fat, monounsaturated fat, and carbohydrate on glucose-insulin homeostasis: a systematic review and meta-analysis of randomised controlled feeding trials. *PLoS Med*. 2016;13: E1002087.
53. Perez-Jimenez F, Lopez-Miranda J, Pinillos M, et al. A Mediterranean and a high carbohydrate diet improve glucose metabolism in healthy young persons. *Diabetologia*. 2002;44: 2038–2043.
54. Chen M, Bergman RN, Porte Jr D. Insulin resistance and beta-cell dysfunction in aging: the importance of dietary carbohydrate. *J Clin Endocrinol Metab*. 1988;67:951–957.

55. Garg A, Bonanome A, Grundy SM, et al. Comparison of a high-carbohydrate diet with a high-monounsaturated-fat diet in patients with non-insulin-dependent diabetes mellitus. *N Engl J Med*. 1988;319:829–834.
56. McKeown N, Meigs J, Liu S, et al. Carbohydrate nutrition, insulin resistance, and the prevalence of the metabolic syndrome in the Framingham offspring cohort. *Diabetes Care*. 2004;27:538–546.
57. Liese AD, Roach AK, Sparks KC, et al. Whole-grain intake and insulin sensitivity: the insulin resistance atherosclerosis study. *Am J Clin Nutr*. 2003;78(5):965–971.
58. Reynolds A, Mann J, Cummngs J, et al. Carbohydrate quality and human health: a series of systematic reviews and meta-analyses. *Lancet*. 2019;393:434–445.
59. Pereira M, Jacobs D, Pins J, et al. Effect of whole grains on insulin sensitivity in overweight hyperinsulinemic adults. *Am J Clin Nutr*. 2002;75:848–855.
60. Brownlee I, Moore C, Chatfield M, et al. Markers of cardiovascular risk are not changed by increased whole-grain intake: the WHOLEheart study, a randomised, controlled dietary intervention. *Br J Nutr*. 2010;104:125–134. https://doi.org/10.1017/S0007114510000644.
61. Daly ME, Vale C, Walker M. Dietary carbohydrates and insulin sensitivity. *Am J Clin Nutr*. 1997;66:1072–1085.
62. Tappy L. Fructose-containing caloric sweeteners as a cause of obesity and metabolic disorders. *J Exp Biol*. 2018;221(Pt suppl 1).
63. Ludwig DS, Hu FB, Tappy L, et al. Dietary carbohydrates: role of quality and quantity in chronic disease. *BMJ*. 2018;361:k2340.
64. Kiens B, Richter E. Types of carbohydrate in an ordinary diet affect insulin action and muscle substrates in humans. *Am J Clin Nutr*. 1996;63:47–53.
65. Koivisto VA, Yki-Harvinen H. Fructose and insulin sensitivity in patients with type 2 diabetes. *J Intern Med*. 1993;233:145–153.
66. Thorburn A, Crapo P, Griver K, Henry R. Insulin action and triglyceride turnover after long-term fructose feeding in subjects with non-insulin diabetes mellitus (NIDDM). *FASEB J*. 1988;2(5). A1201 (Abstract).
67. Rizkalla S, Taghrid L, Laromiguiere, et al. Improved plasma glucose control, whole-body glucose utilization, and lipid profile on a low-glycemic index diet in type 2 diabetic men: a randomized controlled trial. *Diabetes Care*. 2004;27:1866–1872.
68. Holman RR, Cull CA, Turner RC. A randomized double-blind trial of acarbose in type 2 diabetes shows improved glycemic control over 3 years (UKPDS 44). *Diabetes Care*. 1999;22(6): 960–964.
69. Marsh KA, Steinbeck KS, Atkinson FS, et al. Effect of a low glycemic index compared with a conventional healthy diet on polycystic ovary syndrome. *Am J Clin Nutr*. 2010;92(1):83–92.
70. Solomon TP, Haus JM, Kelly KR, et al. Randomized trial on the effects of a 7-d low-glycemic diet and exercise intervention on insulin resistance in older obese humans. *Am J Clin Nutr*. 2009;90(5): 1222–1229.
71. Schwingshackl L, Hobl LP, Hoffman G. Effects of low glycaemic index/low glycaemic load vs. high glycaemic index/ high glycaemic load diets on overweight/obesity and associated risk factors in children and adolescents: a systematic review and meta-analysis. *Nutrition Journal*. 2015;14:87.
72. Schwingshackl L, Hoffman G. Long-term effects of low glycemic index/load vs. high glycemic index/load diets on parameters of obesity and obesity-associated risks: a systematic review and meta-analysis. *Nutr Metab Cardiovasc Dis*. 2013;23(8):699–706.
73. Sacks FM, Carey VJ, Anderson CA, Miller 3rd ER, Copeland T, Charleston J, Harshfield BJ, Laranjo N, McCarron P, Swain J, White K, Yee K, Appel LJ. Effects of high vs low glycemic index of dietary carbohydrate on cardiovascular disease risk factors and insulin sensitivity: the OmniCarb randomized clinical trial. *JAMA*. 2014;312(23):2531–2541.
74. Huerta MG, Roemmich JN, Kington ML, et al. Magnesium deficiency is associated with insulin resistance in obese children. *Diabetes Care*. 2005;28(5):1175–1181.
75. Hruby A, Guasch-Ferre M, Bhupathiraju SN, Manson JE, Willett WC, McKeown NM, Hu FB. Magnesium intake, quality of carbohydrates, and risk of type 2 diabetes: results from three U.S. Cohorts. *Diabetes Care*. 2017;40(12):1695–1702.
76. Rodríguez-Morán M, Guerrero-Romero F. Oral magnesium supplementation improves insulin sensitivity and metabolic control in type 2 diabetic subjects: a randomized double-blind controlled trial. *Diabetes Care*. 2003;26(4):1147–1152.
77. Cefalu WT, Hu FB. Role of chromium in human health and in diabetes. *Diabetes Care*. 2004;27:2741–2751.
78. Heshmati J, Omani-Samani R, Vesali S, et al. The effects of supplementation with chromium on insulin resistance indices in women with polycystic ovarian syndrome: a systematic review and meta-analysis of randomized clinical trials. *Horm Metab Res*. 2018;50: 193–200.
79. Facchini FS, Humphreys MH, DoNascimento C, et al. Relation between insulin resistance and plasma concentrations of lipid hydroperoxides, carotenoids, and tocopherols. *Am J Clin Nutr*. 2000;72(3):776–779.
80. Sanchez-Lugo L, Mayer-Davis E, Howard G, et al. Insulin sensitivity and intake of vitamins E and C in african American, hispanic, and non-hispanic white men and women: the insulin resistance and atherosclerosis study (IRAS). *Am J Clin Nutr*. 1997;66(5): 1224–1231.
81. Chiu KC, Chu A, Go VLW, et al. Hypovitaminosis D is associated with insulin resistance and {beta} cell dysfunction. *Am J Clin Nutr*. 2004;79:820–825.
82. Yatabe MS, Yatabe J, Yoneda M, et al. Salt sensitivity is associated with insulin resistance, sympathetic overactivity, and decreased suppression of circulating renin activity in lean patients with essential hypertension. *Am J Clin Nutr*. 2010;92(1):77–82.
83. Ajala O, English P, Pinkney J. Systematic review and meta-analysis of different dietary approaches to the management of type 2 diabetes. *Am J Clin Nutr*. 2013;97:505–516.
84. Tonstad S, Stewart K, Oda K, et al. Vegetarian diets and incidence of diabetes in the adventist health study-2. *Nutr Metab Cardiovasc Dis*. 2013;23:292–299.
85. Liese AD, Nicols M, Sun XD, Agostino Jnr RB, Haffner SM. Adherence to the DASH Diet is inversely associated with incidence of type 2 diabetes: the insulin resistance atherosclerosis study. *Diabetes Care*. 2009;32(8):1434–1436.
86. Lacoppidan SA, Kyro C, Loft S, et al. Adherence to a healthy Nordic food index is associated with a lower risk of type-2 diabetes–The Danish Diet, Cancer and Health Cohort Study. *Nutrients*. 2015;7:8633–8644.
87. Diabetes Prevention Program Research Group. Reduction in the incidence of type 2 diabetes with lifestyle intervention or metformin. *N Engl J Med*. 2002;346:393–403.
88. Tuomilehto J, Lindstr√∂m J, Eriksson, et al. Prevention of type 2 diabetes mellitus by changes in lifestyle among subjects with impaired glucose tolerance. *N Engl J Med*. 2001;344(18):1343–1350.
89. Tay J, Thompson CH, Luscombe-Marsh ND, et al. Effects of an energy-restricted low-carbohydrate, high unsaturated fat/low saturated fat diet versus a high-carbohydrate, low-fat diet in type 2 diabetes: a 2-year randomized clinical trial. *Diabetes Obes Metab*. 2018;20:858–871.
90. Zafar MI, Mills KE, Zheng J, et al. Low-glycemic index diets as an intervention for diabetes: a systematic review and meta-analysis. *Am J Clin Nutr*. 2019;110(4):891–902.
91. Thomas D, Elliott EJ. Low glycaemic index, or low glycaemic load, diets for diabetes mellitus. *Cochrane Database Syst Rev*. 2009;1. CD006296.

92. Livesey G, Taylor R, Livesey FH, et al. Dietary glycemic index and load and the risk of type 2 diabetes: a systematic review and updated meta-analyses of prospective cohort studies. *Nutrients.* 2019a;11(6):e1280.
93. Livesey G, Taylor R, Livesey FH, et al. Dietary glycemic index and load and the risk of type 2 diabetes: assessment of causal relations. *Nutrients.* 2019b;11(6):1436.
94. Livesey G, Livesey H. Coronary heart disease and dietary carbohydrate, glycemic index, and glycemic load: dose-response meta-analyses of prospective cohort studies. *Mayo Clin Proc Inno Qual Outcomes.* 2019;3(1):52–69.
95. Ley SH, Hamdy O, Mohan V, Hu FB. Prevention and management of type 2 diabetes: dietary components and nutritional strategies. *Lancet.* 2014;383(9933):1999–2007.
96. Sieri S, Krogh V, Berrino F, et al. Dietary glycemic load and index and risk of coronary heart disease in a large Italian cohort: the EPICOR Study. *Arch Intern Med.* 2010;170(7):640–647.
97. Garcia M, Bihuniak JD, Shook J, et al. The effect of the traditional Mediterranean-style diet on metabolic risk factors: a meta-analysis. *Nutrients.* 2016;15:168.
98. Godos J, Zappala G, Bernardini S, et al. Adherence to the Mediterranean diet is inversely associated with metabolic syndrome occurrence: a meta-analysis of observational studies. *Int J Food Sci Nutr.* 2017;68:138–148.
99. Koloverou E, Esposito K, Giugliano D, et al. The effect of Mediterranean diet on the development of type 2 diabetes mellitus: a meta-analysis of 10 prospective studies and 136,846 participants. *Metabolism.* 2014;63:903–911.
100. Schwingshackl L, Missbach B, Dias S, et al. Impact of different training modalities on glycaemic control and blood lipids in patients with type 2 diabetes: a systematic review and network meta-analysis. *Diabetologia.* 2014;57(9):1789–1797.
101. Esposito K, Maiorino MI, Bellastella G, Chiodini P, Panagiotaskos D, Giugliano D. A journey into a Mediterranean diet and type 2 diabetes: a systematic review with meta-analyses. *BMJ Open.* 2015;5(8):e008222.
102. Carter P, Achana F, Troughton J, et al. A Mediterranean diet improves HbA1c but not fasting blood glucose compared to alternative dietary strategies: a network meta-analysis. *J Hum Nutr Diet.* 2014;27:280–297.
103. Li Z, Tseng CH, Li Q, et al. Clinical efficacy of a medically supervised outpatient high-protein, low-calorie diet program is equivalent in prediabetic, diabetic and normoglycemic obese patients. *Nutr Diabetes.* 2014;4:e105.
104. Christensen P, Meinert Larsen T, Westerterp-Plantenga M, et al. Men and women respond differently to rapid weight loss: metabolic outcomes of a multi-centre intervention study after a low-energy diet in 2500 overweight, individuals with pre-diabetes (PREVIEW). *Diabetes Obes Metab.* 2018;20:2840–2851.
105. Lean ME, Leslie W, Barnes AC, et al. Primary care-led weight management for remission of type 2 diabetes (Direct): an open-label, cluster-randomised trial. *Lancet.* 2018;391:541–551.
106. Napso T, Yong HE, Lopez-Tello J, et al. The role of placental hormones in mediating maternal adaptations to support pregnancy and lactation. *Front Physiol.* 2018:17–1091.

CHAPTER

21

HYPERTENSION

Thomas A.B. Sanders, PhD, DSc

King's College London, London, United Kingdom

SUMMARY

Hypertension is a major risk factor for cardiovascular disease (CVD) and if untreated can lead to renal failure. The cause of hypertension (raised blood pressure [BP]) is uncertain but is determined by diet and lifestyle and may have its origins in early development. Improvements in maternal pregnancy outcomes and improved infant nutrition may partially explain the secular decline in BP seen in many affluent communities. This chapter reviews the evidence for the relationship between specific dietary factors and hypertension. Decreasing the intake of salt, restricting alcohol intake to fewer units per day, losing excess weight, and increasing the intake of fruit, and vegetables in a combination diet can lower systolic/diastolic BP by up to 8/4 mmHg in those with hypertension and but about half as much in those with normal/high normal BP. However, it is difficult to restrict salt intake without the cooperation of the food industry. The strategy of encouraging the food industry to decrease the addition of salt to food and the use salt substitutes such as potassium chloride in processed food can make an important contribution to reducing salt intakes and lowering population BP. Even small changes in population BP are likely to substantially reduce the burden of CVD in the population.

Keywords: Alcohol; Birth weight; Blood pressure; Obesity; Potassium; Salt.

I. NORMAL FUNCTION AND PHYSIOLOGY

A. Measurement of Blood Pressure

Blood pressure (BP), which enables the perfusion of tissues with oxygenated blood, is determined by cardiac output and systemic vascular resistance. Arterial BP is normally estimated by measuring peripheral BP in the forearm using a sphygmomanometer, which is a device consisting of an inflatable cuff connected to a manometer. The cuff is placed around the upper and inflated and then gradually deflated while recording sounds from the brachial artery. The systolic blood pressure (SBP) marks the reappearance of pulse sounds following arterial occlusion, and the diastolic blood pressure (DBP) is recorded as either muffling or disappearance of the pulse sounds.

Normal SBP/DBP is typically 120/80 mm Hg or less. Low BP is typically below 90/60 mm Hg. Mean arterial pressure (MAP) is estimated by dividing the sum of SBP + (2 × DBP) by 3. MAP is preferred for monitoring BP in sepsis, where there is hypotension, and a MAP of less than 65 mm Hg is likely to result in hypoxia.

BP can be subject to substantial measurement error and bias. The use of automated sphygmomanometers reduces bias such as digit preference and cutoffs for DBP associated with the older mercury devices. Automated devices are very convenient and quick to provide results to detect low BP, for example, following a collapse, sepsis, or trauma or very high BP. However, in order to detect hypertension, most protocols[1] suggest three readings are taken with the patient seated following 15 min rest with intervals of 1–2 min between readings, the first reading is discarded and the mean of the second and third readings averaged (these are often lower than the first reading). However, elevated readings may be obtained when the subject is stressed ("white-coat hypertension"), and confirmation of the presence of hypertension is required with measurements on several different occasions. For this reason, ambulatory BP monitoring devices are preferred for confirming hypertension. The

Present Knowledge in Nutrition, Volume 2
https://doi.org/10.1016/B978-0-12-818460-8.00021-6

device is typically programmed to make measurements every 30 min in daytime (16 h) and every hour at night (8 h). The first three readings are usually ignored, and average taken of the remaining readings. The values obtained by this method typically are 5 mm Hg lower than clinic-seated BP, and nighttime BP is lower than daytime BP. The devices are relatively costly, and training is required to identify erroneous readings. Home measurement of BP, which is cheaper, can also be used with automated devices to confirm the presence of hypertension or to monitor treatment. The techniques used to measure BP and appropriate placebos are particularly relevant when evaluating the effects of changes in diet and lifestyle effects on BP.

B. Role of the Renin–Angiotensin–Aldosterone System

The renin–angiotensin system (RAS) plays a major role in the BP regulation and fluid balance. Renin is secreted by the kidneys when blood volume is low, the level of sodium in blood is low, or the level of potassium is high. Renin catalyzes the conversion of angiotensinogen produced in the liver into angiotensin I. Angiotensin I is subsequently converted into angiotensin II by the action of angiotensin-converting enzyme (ACE) that is expressed by endothelial cells, especially in the lung. Angiotensin II causes vasoconstriction of resistance arterioles and acutely elevates BP; it stimulates the secretion of aldosterone from the adrenal glands, which acts on the renal tubules to retain sodium and excrete potassium; it also has effects on the central nervous system to stimulate thirst and on the pituitary gland to secrete the antidiuretic hormone (ADH) (also known as vasopressin) to retain water. These actions are opposed by atrial natriuretic peptide, a hormone which is secreted by the heart in response to increased BP and volume and which promotes the excretion of sodium and water by the kidneys. Thus, the normal role of the RAS is to maintain BP and restore the balance of sodium, potassium, and fluids. However, if the RAS becomes overactive, it results in high BP. This can occur in response to decreased renal perfusion or excessive sympathetic nerve activation.

C. Normal Autonomic Nervous System Control

BP is regulated by autonomic nervous system based in the cardiovascular center of the medulla oblongata but is influenced by signaling between the hypothalamus and the pituitary gland, which responds by secreting hormones such ADH. The cardiovascular center comprises three components: the cardiovascular accelerator center, which increases heart rate and stroke volume via the cardiac accelerator nerve; the cardiac inhibitor center, which has the opposite effect mediated via parasympathetic stimulation of the vagus nerve; and the vasomotor center, which stimulates vasoconstriction of resistance arteries regulating blood flow. Baroreceptors in blood vessels detect change in BP and chemoreceptors that detect changes in pH (which falls when CO_2 accumulates) to allow for maintenance of normal BP via a feedback loop. Norepinephrine secreted by sympathetic nervous system neurons plays a central role in the neural regulation of BP.

D. Role of Nitric Oxide

Nitric oxide (NO) produced from arginine by the endothelium cells causes vasodilation and plays an important role in the regulation of vascular tone. NO production is stimulated by arterial shear stress. Impaired NO-dependent vasodilation is associated with the development of hypertension[2]; arginine supplements acutely lower BP,[3] and conversely, inhibitors of arginine metabolism such as N^G-monomethyl-L-arginine raise BP.

E. Age-Related Changes in BP

Younger women on average have lower BP than men, typically SBP/DBP is 10/5 mm Hg lower in women. However, around/following the menopause BP increases, indicating that ovarian hormones, especially estrogen, have a protective effect. SBP increases with age, whereas DBP tends to increase in line with SBP until the sixth decade and then tends to fall. It is thought that some of this age-related increase in SBP is in part due to decreased activity of the RAS as well as increased sympathetic nervous system activity.

II. PATHOPHYSIOLOGY

A. Abnormal Physiology or Function

Hypertension is classified as a systolic BP > 140 mm Hg and/or diastolic BP of >90 mm Hg[1] (Table 21.1). Hypertension usually results from increased resistance to blood flow by small arterioles (resistance vessels) rather than increased cardiac output. Hypertension is a self-amplifying process in which the arterioles develop thicker, more muscular walls in response to the increased pressure; these more muscular arterial walls when stimulated further increase peripheral vascular resistance.

TABLE 21.1 Classification of blood pressure (mm Hg) based on seated clinic blood pressure.

Condition	Systolic BP	Diastolic BP
Ideal	<120	<80
Normal	120–129	80–84
High normal (prehypertension)	130–139	85–89
Hypertension	140–159	90–99
Grade 1	140–159	90–99
Grade 2	160–179	100–109
Grade 3	>180	>110
Isolated systolic hypertension	>140	>90

Source: Williams et al.[1]

Impaired nitric oxide production

Impaired nitric oxide generation results in an impaired capacity of arteries to dilate (endothelial dysfunction), is associated with aging and type 2 diabetes, and blunts the normal attenuation of the increase in BP during physical exertion.[4] Conversely, increased NO generation lowers BP and excessive NO generation is why BP falls in sepsis. Impaired nitric oxide production is also associated with aging while stiffening of the large arteries also occurs with aging.[5]

Role of the central nervous system

The acute effects of stress on increasing BP are well known, such as increased heart rate and increased vascular resistance. However, the long-term effects of increased sympathetic nervous system activity on BP are now recognized as important in the genesis of hypertension. The term neurogenic hypertension is defined as high BP with sympathetic overdrive, loss of parasympathetically mediated cardiac variability, and excessive angiotensin II activity.[6,7] Increased sympathetic nervous system activity increases with age, obesity, salt intake, and excess alcohol intake. There is also more limited evidence that regular exercise reduces sympathetic nervous system activity.

Hypertensive effect of alcohol

Alcohol abuse is a known cause of hypertension. It acutely raises BP, and binge drinking can lead to large, more persistent increases.[1] Alcohol acutely suppresses vasopressin (ADH) secretion, thereby having a diuretic effect, but this is followed by a transient increase in renin secretion as a compensatory reaction to the vasodilatation and diuresis caused by alcohol. The BP-raising effect of alcohol is rapidly reversible and can be inhibited by alpha-adrenergic blockade.[8] However, one of the effects of chronic, high intakes of alcohol is to increase sympathetic nervous system activity.

Clinical consequences of raised blood pressure

Most hypertension usually develops over decades and is not easily reversed. By the age of 60 years, most adults are hypertensive.[1] Untreated hypertension results in end-organ damage, particularly to the microvasculature of the retina, brain, and kidney, and is an important cause of blindness, dementia, and chronic renal failure (Box 21.1).

Stroke; Severe hypertension as a major cause of stroke can be clearly seen from a large cohort study in China,[9] which shows the substantially increased risk with Grade 2 and Grade 3 hypertension (Figs. 21.1 and 21.2).

Impact on other risk factors; The hazards of cardiovascular disease (CVD) associated with BP extend well into the normal range of BP and are greater in the presence of other risk factors (increasing age, high blood cholesterol, smoking, diabetes mellitus, and target organ damage). Data from a metaanalysis of prospective cohort studies[10] show that all-cause mortality, stroke, and coronary heart disease (CHD) incidence increase on a doubling scale (log-linear) with increasing BP.

BOX 21.1

Major Hazards of Hypertension

- Cardiovascular disease
  - Stroke—increased risk of vascular hemorrhage, atherosclerotic plaque rupture
  - Coronary heart disease—increased risk of atherosclerotic plaque rupture
  - Peripheral vascular disease—increased risk of atherosclerotic plaque rupture
- Renal failure—microvascular damage
- Retinal damage—microvascular damage
- Eclampsia of pregnancy—impaired placental function resulting in impaired fetal growth and severe hypertension

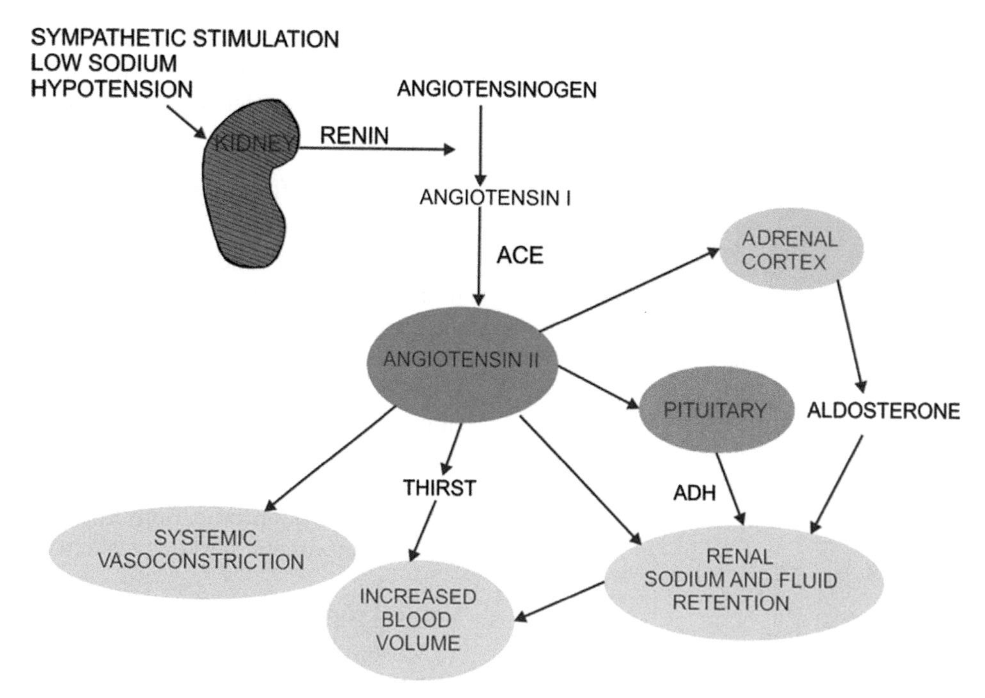

FIGURE 21.1 The renin–angiotensin system (RAS) and its effects on systemic vasoconstriction, sodium, and fluid balance. *ACE*, angiotensin-converting enzyme; *ADH*, antidiuretic hormone (vasopressin). *Taken from Sanders and Emery.*[11]

Regression dilution in measurement; Furthermore, the association of BP with risk of CVD tends to be underestimated because of regression dilution bias. It is well known that BP falls in response to repeat measurement, regressing toward the mean. Adjusting for regression dilution bias by using multiple measures of BP on different days or by using ambulatory BP monitoring gives a better estimate of true BP and strengthens the relationship with risk.[12]

Effect of lowering BP on risk; Treating hypertension with drugs reduces mortality, especially from stroke but also from CHD.[13] The clearest benefit is seen in those with the highest initial BP. It has been difficult to demonstrate benefit from lowering BP below 120/80 mm Hg in high-risk groups, such as people with type 2 diabetes.[14] Consequently, ideal BP is below 120/80 mm Hg.

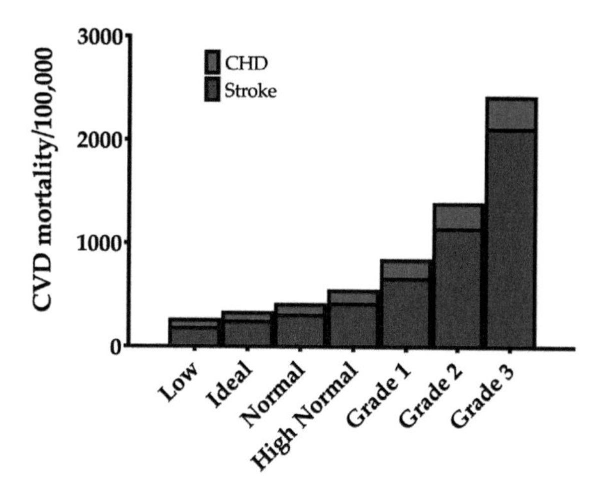

FIGURE 21.2 Effect of stage of hypertension on risk of stroke and cardiovascular disease in a large Chinese population.[9]

Hypertension in pregnancy; Hypertension can develop during pregnancy which can, if untreated, result in eclampsia, but BP usually returns to normal postpartum. Such elevations in BP are thought to be due to increased inflammation and other substances produced by the placenta. It is estimated that 3%–10% of all pregnancies worldwide are affected.[15] Moderate increases in BP can be managed by diet and lifestyle changes, but more severe elevations of BP may require pharmacological intervention.

B. Role of Diet and Lifestyle in the Onset Hypertension

Prevalence of hypertension internationally

Fig. 21.3 shows the worldwide prevalence of hypertension in 2015 according to the World Health Organization.[16] The prevalence of hypertension is high in most communities, with a few exceptions such as the Tsimané, a Bolivian population living a subsistence lifestyle of hunting, gardening, and fishing.[17] Hypertension is more prevalent in sub-Saharan Africa and rates are higher in urban than in rural areas. For example, migrants from rural areas of Kenya were found to show large increases in BP when they moved into cities.[18]

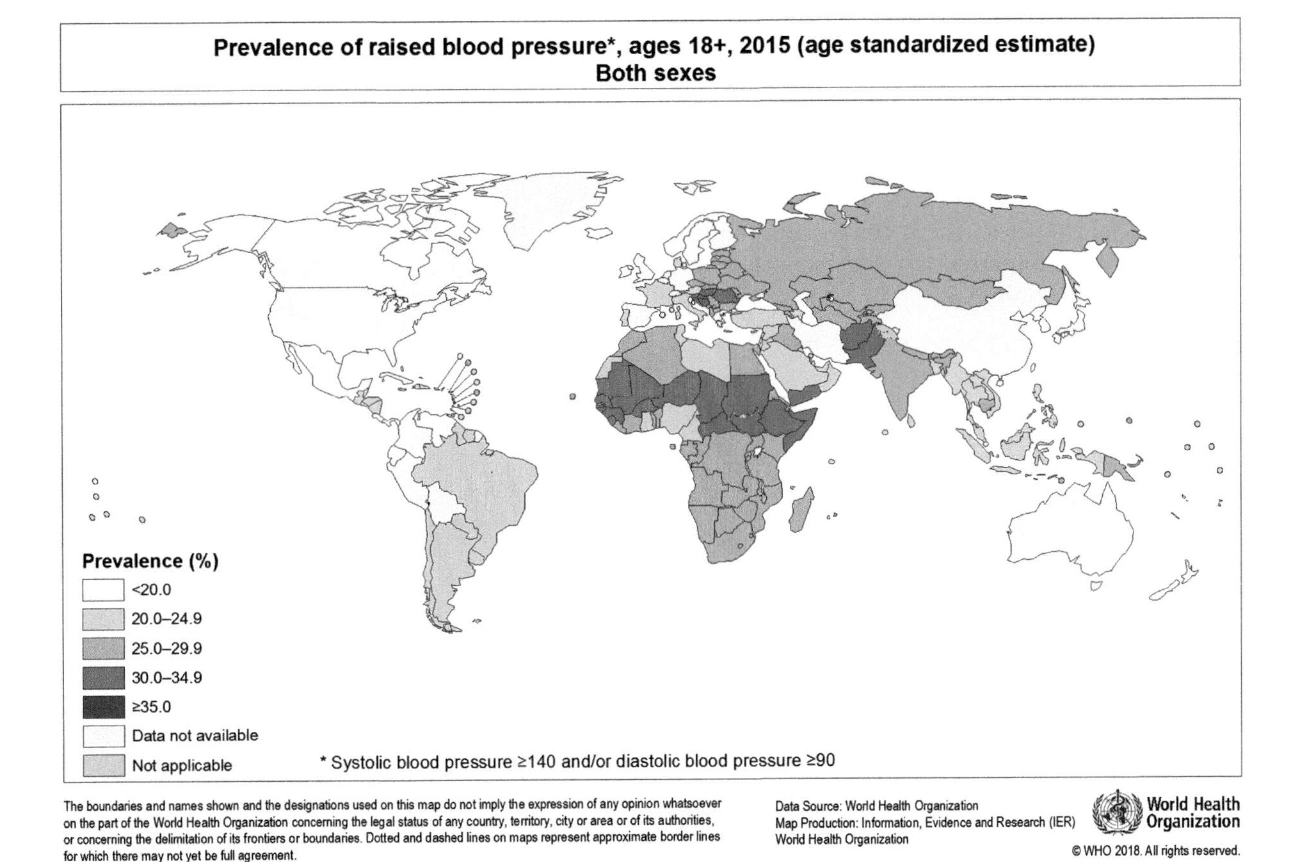

FIGURE 21.3 Global prevalence of hypertension (World Health Organization).

The burden of hypertension in emerging economies is likely to grow as populations become urbanized and live longer. In contrast, BP and the prevalence of hypertension is falling in many richer countries (e.g., North America, Western Europe, Japan, Australasia) for reasons that are uncertain, while the opposite is occurring in middle-income (e.g., Russia and former Eastern Bloc countries).[19]

The population approach to controlling BP focuses on lowering the average population BP, not just in those with hypertension. It aims to decrease exposure to factors that increase risk and to empower individuals to make healthier lifestyle choices. Frost et al.[20] argue that lowering the BP of the whole population is likely to have a greater impact on cardiovascular mortality than just focusing on individuals with high BP because larger numbers are exposed to risk.

Contributing risk factors

Cross-sectional studies find a high salt intake, obesity, excess alcohol, and a low fruit and vegetable intake (associated with low potassium intake) are all linked to raised BP. The INTERSALT investigators[21] showed that the age-related increase in BP across a large number of different communities was independently related to body mass index, alcohol intake, and the urinary ratio of sodium/potassium. An increase in sodium intake of 100 mmol/day (about 6 g salt/d) was associated with an increase in SBP/DBP of 3–6/0–3 mm Hg. This relationship was found to be true for both men and women, young and old people, and hypertensive and normotensive subjects.[21] There have been substantial changes in salt intake in some countries, notably in Japan,[22] as the consumption of salted and pickled foods declined while the consumption of fresh, chilled, and frozen food has increased.

Fatty acid intake; The INTERMAP study[23,24] has provided some evidence for a weak negative relationship between polyunsaturated fatty acid intake and BP by using four 24 hour dietary recalls to assess dietary intake and eight clinic BP measurements over 3 weeks in 17 populations in Japan, China, the United Kingdom, and the United States ($n = 4680$). This study concluded that dietary linoleic acid intake may contribute to prevention and control of adverse BP levels in the general population. It was estimated that the SBP/DBP differences with 2 SD higher linoleic acid intake (3.77% kcal) were −1.42/−0.91 mm Hg ($P < .05$ for both) for participants not being treated for hypertension. Similar findings were made for total polyunsaturated fatty acids intake. The same study reported small effects <1 mm Hg for SBP for n-3 PUFA, especially those derived from oily fish.

Body mass index; More robust evidence is provided by prospective cohort studies. These consistently show a relationship between hypertension and increased body mass index[25] and alcohol intake.[26]

Sodium intake; On the other hand, studies have revealed mixed conclusions regarding salt per se.[27] However, estimates of salt intake from dietary records are generally unreliable compared with measures of intake based on the collection of 24 hour urine samples. The PURE study[28] measured BP and the sodium content of a morning sample of urine following an overnight fast in over 95,000 individuals in 369 communities defined as middle-income and emerging economies internationally. Overall, mean systolic BP increased by 2.86 mm Hg per 1 g increase in mean sodium intake. Communities in China had the highest sodium intakes (5.58 g/d), and there were strong associations with BP and stroke in that country. However, the association of sodium intake with CVD was less clear in other countries.

Potassium intake; Prospective epidemiological studies consistently show a relationship between low potassium intake from foods and raised BP as well as increased risk of stroke.[29] Potassium in the diet is mainly provided by fruits and vegetables but also by potatoes, which are not classified as fruit and vegetables in some dietary guidelines. About 80% of dietary potassium is excreted in urine, the remainder being in feces. Recommended intakes for potassium are typically 90 mmol/d, which corresponds to a urine excretion of about 72 mmol/d. Diets high in refined cereals such as white rice are particularly low in potassium. The PURE study[28] found urinary potassium excretion to be consistently associated with a lower BP and a lower risk of CVD in all countries.

Origins in early development; The evolution of raised BP may have its origins in early development. It is well established that hypertension is more likely to develop in the offspring of mothers who develop preeclampsia or gestational diabetes. Low birth weight and rapid weight gain in early life are also associated with higher adult BP. The US. Collaborative Perinatal Project (1959–74) studied 55,908 pregnancies and found that for each 1 kg increase in birth weight, the odds increased by 2.19 for raised SBP at 7 years of age and confirmed the finding that those who crossed growth centiles over the intervening 7 years were most at risk.[30] Animal studies suggest that diet in early life may program the hypothalamic–pituitary axis in a way that modifies stress responses that impact on BP in adult life.[31] Improvements in pregnancy outcomes and infant nutrition may in part explain the secular decline in BP seen in many affluent countries.

III. PRIMARY TREATMENT MODALITIES

A. Surgical Treatment

Stenosis of one of the renal arteries, which can be diagnosed by ultrasound, can result in hypertension and can be treated by angioplasty/stenting of the affected artery.[32] Catheter-based renal denervation for uncontrolled hypertension using the radiofrequency ablation of the main renal arteries was claimed to be effective in lowering BP. Further larger randomized controlled trials using sham-controlled patients have produced mixed results.[33] Bariatric surgery for the management of obesity lowers BP, which is related to the amount of weight lost (see section on obesity).

B. Pharmacological Treatment

Hypertension is more usually managed with medication often used in combination. As the health risk of hypertension increases markedly with age, it is the older age groups that are most like to see benefit from treatment.[10] This in part explains why BP-lowering medication (e.g., ACE inhibitors, diuretics, beta-blockers, calcium channel antagonists) are mainly prescribed for groups over the age of 45 years where the absolute risk of a CVD event increases. ACE inhibitors and sartans inhibit the vasoconstriction caused by angiotensin, beta-blockers slow heart rate, diuretics increase sodium excretion, and calcium channel blockers and alpha-blockers have direct effects on vascular musculature causing vasodilation. While the prevalence of severe hypertension (Grade 3) and the population BP has been falling in most affluent countries,[19] untreated severe hypertension remains common in many emerging economies.[16]

Until recently, BP-lowering medication was not widely available in emerging economies, but the advent inexpensive reliable automated sphygmomanometers and generic drugs have allowed for better management of hypertension. The management of hypertension preeclampsia in economically developed countries has had a substantial impact on reducing maternal mortality. However, drug treatment is not recommended for women with SBP less than 160 mm Hg in pregnancy based on a risk/benefit analysis due to hypothetical/potential adverse effects of the medication on the fetus.

Drug treatment of hypertension is usually recommended for patients with BP greater than 160/

100 mm Hg, as well as for patients with lower BP but with preexisting conditions, e.g., type 2 diabetes or previous CVD events. For individuals without preexisting conditions with moderately elevated BP (Grade 1), risk stratification is used to determine a patient's absolute risk of suffering a cardiovascular event over the next 10 years. This approach is used in the European[1] and US guidelines.[34] In Europe, medication is considered when the risk is greater than 20% in patients without preexisting CVD or diabetes. In contrast, the United States has adopted a 10% absolute risk over 10 years.[34] ACE inhibitors or sartans are first line therapies, especially for younger patients. In elderly patients, diuretics or calcium channel blockers are more usually recommended, but the latter can have the side effect of pedal edema. With increasing BP, a combination of medications is often needed to meet the treatment target. It usually takes several years for the full effects of BP medication to have their maximal effects, as was demonstrated in the ALLHAT study.[35]

A low-cost "polypill" has been developed for treatment of hypertension in low-income countries using a combination of half the standard dose of generic BP-lowering drugs because the different drugs have synergistic effects and can lower SBP/DBP 9.8/5 mm Hg in patients with predominantly Grade 1 hypertension.[36]

C. Lifestyle and Dietary Management

A high proportion of the population has "prehypertension" or "mild hypertension" where the risk profile does not favor drug treatment. Diet and lifestyle are considered to have their most important influence on the prevention of high BP rather than on the management of established hypertension, and early intervention in the hypertensive process almost certainly helps prevent BP becoming severely elevated. The guidelines of the joint committee of the European Society of-ardiology and the European Society of Hypertension include regular physical exercise to maintain normal BP, smoking cessation, advice regarding controlling body weight, salt reduction, moderation of alcohol intake, and an increased intake of fruit and vegetables.[1]

Obesity

Obesity is strongly related to increases in BP and the effects are reversible; in the United States, it may account for 60%–70% of hypertension in adults.[37] However, obesity accounts for a much lower proportion of hypertension in China and Japan. For each kilogram of weight lost, BP falls by about 1 mm Hg over a range of weight loss of 1–5 kg.[38] There is no clear evidence to indicate the superiority of low-calorie diets that contain a higher proportion of fat than carbohydrate in reducing elevated BP. It would appear that the accumulation of abdominal visceral fat rather than subcutaneous adipose tissue is related to augmented sympathetic activity. Chronically high levels of insulin due to insulin resistance and high levels of leptin and/or obstructive sleep apnea may be responsible for sympathetic overactivity in obesity-related hypertension.[37] Part of this effect appears to be mediated via the melanocortin-4 receptor independent of insulin.[39]

Dietary lipids

In contrast to the effects of body fatness, it appears that dietary fat composition has minimal effects on population BP within the normal ranges of dietary intake. The OMNIHEART study[40] provided some evidence to suggest that replacement of carbohydrate with unsaturated fatty acids or protein lowers SBP by 1.3 and 1.4 mm Hg, respectively, compared with carbohydrate, without any change in body weight. However, a metaanalysis comparing diets high in monounsaturated fatty acids versus ones high in carbohydrates was unable to demonstrate superiority of monounsaturated fatty acids.[41] A later large randomized multicenter controlled trial was unable to show any effect of replacing saturated fatty acids with MUFA or carbohydrate (either of high or low glycemic index) on clinic BP.[42] Pharmacological intake of long-chain n-3 polyunsaturated fatty acids lowered BP with intakes above 3 g/d,[43] but lower intakes had no effect.[44]

Salt (sodium chloride)

As previously discussed, there is consistent evidence both between populations and within populations that dietary salt (sodium chloride) intake is associated with the age-related increase in BP. Many trials have also show that restricting salt intake lowers BP, particularly in those with hypertension. A Cochrane review of these trials by He and MacGregor[45] concluded that a 4.4 g reduction in salt intake (equivalent to 75 mmol [1725 mg] sodium excretion/24 h) resulted in falls in SBP/DBP of 4.18/2.06 mm Hg. The reductions in SBP/DBP in mm Hg were 5.39/2.82 in hypertensive and 2.42/1.0 in normotensive individuals, respectively.

There are large cultural differences with regard to the use of salt in domestic food preparation and the addition of salt at table. A metaanalysis[46] reported that advice to reduce salt intake was limited in efficacy in lowering BP; the average reduction in 24 hour urinary sodium excretion of 35.5 mmol/day (equivalent to about 2 g of salt/day) resulted in the fall in SBP and DBP of mm Hg of 1/0.6.

When most of the salt is supplied by commercially processed foods (e.g., bread and sauces), it is likely to be more effective to engage with the food industry to reduce the amount of salt in food.[47] The UK Food Standards Agency persuaded food manufacturers to reduce the salt content of processed foods, particularly bread and ready prepared meals, and launched a media campaign to make consumers aware of the salt in processed food in 2004.[48] This initial success of this policy is corroborated by evidence showing 24 h urine sodium excretion fell in the United Kingdom and has remained lower (Public Health England). In contrast, a review of measures of salt intake by 24 h urinary excretion in the United States showed little change in salt intake over the past 50 years.[49]

Current dietary guidelines for adults in Europe advocate that salt intakes should not exceed 6 g/day (100 mmol), levels that are readily achievable. WHO guidelines suggest an intake of no more than 5 g/d. However, in the United States, there is a more stringent target of less than 4 g/day (65 mmol/day) in adults over 51 years of age and those with hypertension.[34]

Sucrose

A metaanalysis conducted for the WHO[50] suggested that high intakes of sucrose increase SBP by 6.9 and DBP by 5.6 mm Hg, but this included many poorly controlled studies with unreliable methods of BP measurement. A later metaanalysis comparing the effects of substituting free sugars for complex carbohydrate found no effect.[51]

Alcohol

Alcohol consumption increases BP acutely, and binge drinking can lead to large, more persistent increases. As mentioned previously, alcohol acutely suppresses vasopressin (ADH) secretion, thereby having a diuretic effect, but this is followed by a transient increase in renin secretion. It is believed that plasma renin activity increases as a compensatory reaction to the vasodilatation and diuresis caused by alcohol. The BP-raising effect of alcohol is rapidly reversible and can be inhibited by alpha-adrenergic blockade. One of the effects of chronic, high intakes of alcohol is to increase sympathetic nervous system activity.

The BP-raising effects of alcohol may decrease with increasing age, at least at low/moderate intakes. However, excess intake remains an important cause of hypertension in the elderly.

A metaanalysis of 15 randomized controlled clinical trials of hypertensive and normotensive heavy drinkers (>3 drinks daily) found that alcohol reduction was associated with a significant reduction in mean systolic BP of 3.3 mm Hg and diastolic BP of 2.0 mm Hg.[52] A more recent analysis[53] showed that the reductions in BP are proportional to initial intake with the greatest falls occurring with the highest intakes, and with no effect on BP with a reduction from low to moderate intakes up to 2 drinks per day. SBP/DBP falls of 5.5/3.97 mm Hg were observed among heavy drinkers (>6 drinks daily) who halve their alcohol intake (Fig. 21.4).

Fruit and vegetables

It had been argued that the beneficial effects of increased fruit and vegetable intake may be a consequence of an increased potassium intake. Researchers in the United Kingdom conducted a cross-over study to address this issue.[54] Free-living subjects with prehypertension or grade 1 hypertension were followed for four 6 week periods on four dietary protocols with their usual diets: control (a placebo capsules), +20 mmol (0.8 g) potassium from additional fruits and vegetables, +40 mmol (1.6 g) potassium from fruits and vegetables, and +40 mmol (1.6 g) potassium as potassium chloride. Using ambulatory BP monitoring, they were unable to show that intakes of additional potassium-rich fruit and vegetables from either fruits and vegetables or the equivalent as potassium chloride lowered BP.

A subsequent literature search of available studies on the effectiveness of advice to increase fruit and vegetable consumption (four studies) or provision of fruits and vegetables (six studies) to participants showed that such advice lowered SBP by 3 mm Hg, but provision of fruits and vegetables had little effect.[55]

Dairy products

A metaanalysis of prospective cohort studies supports the inverse association between low-fat dairy foods and fluid dairy foods and the risk of elevated BP while no relationship was found with cheese.[56] As milk products are a major source of dietary calcium, it is not surprising that a similar relationship has been found with calcium intake and BP. It has also been proposed that vitamin D status may influence BP, but the

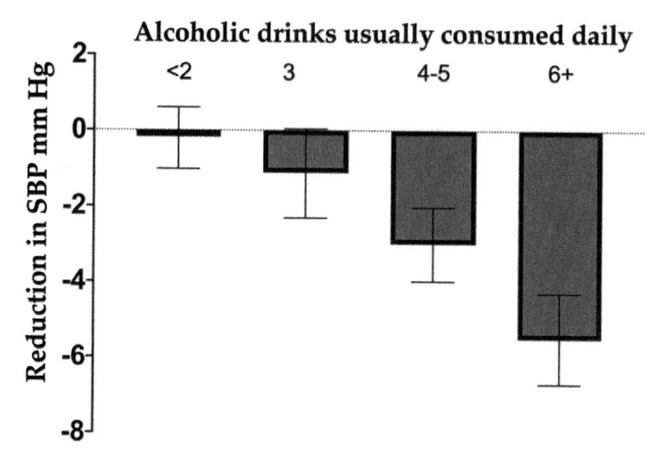

FIGURE 21.4 Effect of advice to decrease alcohol consumption on subsequent blood pressure reduction grouped by baseline alcohol intake.[53]

few randomized controlled trials to date provide no clear evidence.[57] However, a systematic review of combined vitamin D and calcium supplementation[58] concluded that supplementation lowered SBP but not DBP by 2–4 mm Hg. Furthermore, a metaanalysis also concluded that calcium supplementation had a beneficial effect in pregnancy on preventing hypertensive disorders.[59]

Peptides produced through the fermentation of dairy products with *Lactobacillus helveticus* have BP-lowering properties.[60] These peptides appear to partially inhibit ACE and thereby reduce BP. Foods containing these peptides were first marketed in Japan, then Finland, and some other European countries. However, using ambulatory BP monitoring as the outcome, two large multicenter studies were unable to confirm the BP-lowering effects of dairy peptides.[61] At present, the evidence from cohort studies suggests a possible beneficial effect of liquid milk products in protecting against hypertension, but there is a lack of data supporting this effect from randomized controlled trials.

Potassium intake

A metaanalysis of 33 randomized controlled trials of oral potassium supplements[62] revealed significant heterogeneity between studies, and *post hoc* analyses indicate a reduction in BP that was only apparent when salt intakes were high (>165 mmol [3800 mg] sodium/d). Potassium supplementation in China, an area where salt intakes are high and potassium intakes (primarily from fruits and vegetables) are low, lowered SBP by about 5 mm Hg.[63]

In a 12 week cross-over trial, 42 individuals with hypertension, some with Class 1 and 2, were fed a placebo diet and two potassium supplements (64 mmol or 2.5 g potassium/d) of either potassium chloride or potassium bicarbonate each for 4 weeks. Using ambulatory BP monitoring, there were no significant differences in BP between the supplements and the placebo, although other measures of endothelial function were improved on the potassium supplements, with no difference in the form of supplement.[64]

As mentioned earlier, a second randomized controlled trial using ambulatory BP monitoring[58] also failed to show any BP-lowering effect of an additional 40 mmol potassium (1.6 g) provided as a potassium citrate supplement to UK subjects with early hypertension. These findings are in agreement with a Cochrane review[65] that found no benefit of potassium supplementation for the treatment of hypertension. However, another review found benefit, particularly where potassium intake at baseline was less than 90 mmol (3.6g)/d and sodium intake was greater than 4 g (175 mmol)/d.[66]

Salt substitutes

It seems likely there is a threshold effect of supplementary potassium intake above which potassium has no effect on BP; this may be as high as 90 mmol (3.6 g)/d in Southern Europe[66] or as low as 40 mmol (1.6 g)/d especially when salt intakes are high as observed in China. However, several trials[67] have demonstrated that the partial replacement of salt with potassium chloride is effective in lowering BP. The UK Scientific Advisory Committee on Nutrition and Committee on Toxicity[68] conducted a risk–benefit analysis. Based on the recommendations of the European Union BRAFO project, it estimated that the use of salt substitutes containing potassium as potassium chloride, potassium bicarbonate, or potassium citrate replacing 15%–25% of dietary sodium would contribute to reducing sodium intake while not exceeding the dietary recommendation for potassium.

Plant bioactive materials

Caffeine; Caffeine has a short-term, BP-raising effect, which is mainly a consequence of its effect on heart rate. A metaanalysis of chronic caffeine/coffee intake in randomized controlled trials[69] found that caffeine intake increased SBP by 2.04 mm Hg and DBP by 0.73 mm Hg without affecting heart rate. However, a metaanalysis of the effects of coffee intake, which is the major dietary source of caffeine, found no effect on BP.[70]

Flavonoids; A recent metaanalysis[71] of the effect of cocoa flavonoids suggests a reduction of SBP/DBP by 1.76/1.76 mm Hg, but a later analysis found no effect.[72] The soy isoflavone genistein, when infused into the forearm has a similar effect to estradiol on forearm blood flow, which could be attributed to differences in nitric oxide bioavailability.[73] A metaanalysis of soy isoflavones and BP reported a 1.92 mm lower SBP with intakes ranging between 25 and 375 mg soy isoflavones.[74] However, this level of isoflavone intake is well above the typical exposure of people consuming Western diets. There is a lack of reliable data to support claims for a BP-lowering effect of other flavonoids and anthocyanins.

Arginine and nitrate; A systematic review[75] of the effect of protein intake on BP in observational prospective cohort studies and randomized intervention trials indicated a small BP-lowering effect, especially in the case of plant protein. Plant foods have a higher nonprotein nitrogen content than foods of animal origin, mainly due to the presence of nitrate, which is well known to lower BP in animals. The BP-lowering effects of organic nitrates are well established, but evidence has emerged to show that dietary inorganic nitrate can acutely lower BP by generating NO.[76] This effect is apparently a consequence of some bacterial conversion of nitrate to nitrite in the mouth that subsequently results in increased NO.[77,78] A metaanalysis of short-term randomized controlled trials[79] of beetroot juice, high in nitrate, reported mean reduction in SBP/DBP of 4.4/1.1 mm Hg. Currently, there is a lack of high quality randomized controlled trials of more widely consumed vegetables with high nitrate content on BP in humans. The potential benefits from increased nitrate consumption from vegetables on lowering BP needs to be weighed against the potential harm, including nitrosamine formation resulting from conversion to nitrite.

D. An Integrated Dietary Approach to Prevent Hypertension

From the above, it can be seen that several dietary factors can influence BP, and in most cases, the effects on SBP are in the range of 2–4 mm Hg (Table 21.2). However, these small differences have additive/synergistic effects when dietary advice is combined. The Dietary Approaches to Stop Hypertension (DASH) study[80] compared three diets in 459 subjects (of whom 133 had grade 1 hypertension) each for a period of 3 weeks: a control diet that was low in fruit, vegetables, and dairy products with a fat content typical of the American diet; a diet rich in fruit and vegetables; and a "combination diet" rich in fruits and vegetables and low in saturated fats and added sugars (the diet comprised whole grains, low-fat dairy products, fish, and poultry, with restrictions on the consumption of red meat, sugary drinks, cakes, and biscuits). BP was measured using ambulatory monitoring on multiple occasions, and the study was statistically well-powered. SBP was 3–4 mm Hg lower for the high fruit and vegetable group compared with the control group and a much greater reduction in SBP of 5.5 mm Hg overall with the combination diet. The average decrease in SBP in the hypertensive subgroup was 11.4 mm Hg.

Since the initial DASH study, several further studies have examined the effects of a DASH-style eating plan in combination with other lifestyle interventions. The DASH-2 study[81] examined the effects of different levels of dietary salt reduction in conjunction with the DASH diet. The benefits of the DASH diet for BP reduction were enhanced with a reduction in salt intake. Combined effects on BP of a low salt intake and the DASH diet were greater than the effects of either intervention alone. The combined effect of the DASH diet with a low salt intake resulted in a reduction in SBP of 7.1 mm Hg in normotensive subjects and 11.5 mm Hg in the hypertensive subjects. The effect of full-fat dairy products in the DASH eating plan, shown to be as effective in lowering BP as with low fat items, had the adverse effect of an increase in low-density lipoprotein cholesterol concentrations.[82]

TABLE 21.2 Summary of the size effects of the reductions in blood pressure (mm Hg) by diet based on metaanalysis of randomized controlled trials.

Dietary factor	Systolic BP	Diastolic BP
5 kg weight loss	−4.4	−3.3
1.7 g less sodium/d	−4.2	−2.0
<2 alcohol units/d	−3.3	−2.0
Combination diet	−8.0	−4.3

The DASH studies, however, were tightly controlled dietary interventions as opposed to tests of the effectiveness of dietary advice. The PREMIER study[83] was designed for this purpose and compared the effect of lifestyle advice with and without behavioral therapy on BP in free-living subjects after 6 months of intervention. Participants were given the lifestyle advice with the DASH diet alone or with behavioral therapy, and a third group received standard dietary advice (reduce salt intake, lose weight, and cut back on alcohol intake) and behavioral therapy. Dietary advice alone resulted in a reduction in SBP/DBP of 3.7/1.7 mm Hg. However, if advice was accompanied by behavioral therapy, reductions in SBP/DBP of 8.0/4.3 mm Hg were observed in patients with hypertension.

In this study, similar reductions in BP were obtained with standard advice (reduce salt intake, lose weight, and cut back on alcohol intake) compared with the DASH diet. Most of the changes in BP in the groups that received behavioral intervention could be attributed to changes in weight (4–5 kg weight loss difference compared with advice alone which would be predicted to lower SBP by 4–5 mm Hg) as intakes of alcohol were low at baseline and sodium intake as estimated from urinary excretion of sodium was only 10 mmol/day lower.

The approach adopted by the DASH investigators has been replicated in other countries and currently appears to be the most effective dietary intervention. For example, a dietary intervention trial in older men and women with normal/high normal/stage 1 hypertension, who were of average body weight and not receiving hypertensive medication,[84] compared a diet complying with UK dietary guidelines versus a traditional UK diet and reported reductions of 4.2/2.5 mm and 2.9/1.9 mm Hg in daytime and nighttime ambulatory BPs, respectively, compared with the intervention. Causal-mediated effects analysis based on urinary sodium excretion indicated that sodium reduction explained 2.4 mm Hg of the fall in daytime BP, which is close to the reduction predicted from metaanalysis of salt reduction trials.[45]

The genesis of hypertension still remains poorly understood with a number of key issues that need to be addressed in future research.

RESEARCH GAPS

- What are the mechanisms causing arterial stiffening and can such stiffening be modified by diet?
- How is adult BP programmed in early life?
- Why does weight gain cause increased BP?
- Does sugar/fructose affect BP?
- What are the central nervous mechanisms for regulating BP?
- What are the mechanisms causing arterial stiffening and can it be modulated by diet?

IV. REFERENCES

1. Williams B, Mancia G, Spiering W, , et alfor the ESC Scientific Document Group. 2018 ESC/ESH guidelines for the management of arterial hypertension. *Eur Heart J*. 2018;39:3021–3104.
2. Weil BR, Stauffer BL, Greiner JJ, et al. Prehypertension is associated with impaired nitric oxide-mediated endothelium-dependent vasodilation in sedentary adults. *Am J Hypertens*. 2011;24:976–981.
3. Vasdev S, Gill V. The antihypertensive effect of arginine. *Int J Angiol*. 2008;17:7–22.
4. Brett SE, Ritter JM, Chowienczyk PJ. Diastolic blood pressure changes during exercise positively correlate with serum cholesterol and insulin resistance. *Circulation*. 2000;101:611–615.
5. Safar ME, Asmar R, Benetos A, et al. French study group on arterial stiffness. Interaction between hypertension and arterial stiffness. *Hypertension*. 2018;72:796–805.
6. Joyner MJ, Charkoudian N, Wallin BG. Sympathetic nervous system and blood pressure in humans: individualized patterns of regulation and their implications. *Hypertension*. 2010;56:10–16.
7. Fisher JP, Paton JF. The sympathetic nervous system and blood pressure in humans: implications for hypertension. *J Hum Hypertens*. 2012;26:63–75.
8. Randin D, Vollenweider P, Tappy L, et al. Suppression of alcohol-induced hypertension by dexamethasone. *N Engl J Med*. 1995;332: 1733–1737.
9. Gu D, Kelly TN, Wu X, et al. Blood pressure and risk of cardiovascular disease in Chinese men and women. *Am J Hypertens*. 2008;21: 265–272.
10. Lewington S, Clarke R, Qizilbash N, et al. Age-specific relevance of usual blood pressure to vascular mortality: a meta-analysis of individual data for one million adults in 61 prospective studies. *Lancet*. 2002;360:1903–1913.
11. Sanders T, Emery P. *The Molecular Basis of Human Nutrition*. London: Taylor Frances; 2003.
12. Lewington S, Lacey B, Clarke R, , et alFor the China Kadoorie Biobank Consortium. The burden of hypertension and associated risk for cardiovascular mortality in China. *JAMA Intern Med*. 2016;176: 524–532.
13. Czernichow S, Zanchetti A, Turnbull F, et al. The effects of blood pressure reduction and of different blood pressure-lowering regimens on major cardiovascular events according to baseline blood pressure: meta-analysis of randomized trials. *J Hypertens*. 2011;29: 4–16.
14. Cushman WC, Evans GW, Byington RP, et al. Effects of intensive blood-pressure control in type 2 diabetes mellitus. *N Engl J Med*. 2010;362:1575–1585.
15. Jeyabalan A. Epidemiology of preeclampsia: impact of obesity. *Nutr Rev*. 2013;71(Suppl 1):S18–S25.
16. World Health Organization. *World: Prevalence of Raised Blood Pressure, Ages 18+, Age Standardized: Both Sexes, 2015*; 2018. Available from: http://gamapserver.who.int/mapLibrary/Files/Maps/Global_BloodPressurePrevalence_2015_BothSexes.png. Accessed August 14, 2019.
17. Kaplan H, Thompson RC, Trumble BC, et al. Coronary atherosclerosis in indigenous South American Tsimane: a cross-sectional cohort study. *Lancet*. 2017;389:1730–1739.
18. Poulter NR, Khaw KT, Hopwood BE, et al. The Kenyan Luo migration study: observations on the initiation of a rise in blood pressure. *BMJ*. 1990;300:967–972.
19. NCD Risk Factor Collaboration (NCD-RisC). Worldwide trends in blood pressure from 1975 to 2015: a pooled analysis of 1479 population-based measurement studies with 19·1 million participants. *Lancet*. 2017;389:37–55.
20. Frost CD, Law MR, Wald NJ. By how much does dietary salt reduction lower blood pressure? II – analysis of observational data within populations. *BMJ*. 1991;302:815–818.
21. Elliott P, Stamler J, Nichols R, , et alfor the Intersalt Cooperative Research Group. Intersalt revisited: further analyses of 24 hour sodium excretion and blood pressure within and across populations. *BMJ*. 1996;312:1249–1253.
22. Ueda K, HasuoY, Kiyohara Y, et al. Intracerebral hemorrhage in a Japanese community, Hisayama: incidence, changing pattern during long-term follow-up, and related factors. *Stroke*. 1988;19:48–52.
23. Ueshima H, Stamler J, Elliott P, et al. Food omega-3 fatty acid intake of individuals (total, linolenic acid, long-chain) and their blood pressure: INTERMAP study. *Hypertension*. 2007;50:313–319.
24. Miura K, Stamler J, Nakagawa H, et al. Relationship of dietary linoleic acid to blood pressure. The international study of macro-micronutrients and blood pressure study. *Hypertension*. 2008;52: 408–414.
25. Whitlock G, Lewington S, Sherliker P, et al. Body-mass index and cause-specific mortality in 900,000 adults: collaborative analyses of 57 prospective studies. *Lancet*. 2009;373:1083–1096.
26. Millwood IY, Walters RG, Mei XW, , et alFor the China Kadoorie Biobank Collaborative Group. Conventional and genetic evidence on alcohol and vascular disease aetiology: a prospective study of 500 000 men and women in China. *Lancet*. 2019;393:1831–1842.
27. Strazzullo P, D'Elia L, Kandala NB, et al. Salt intake, stroke, and cardiovascular disease: meta-analysis of prospective studies. *BMJ*. 2009;339. b4567.
28. Mente A, O'Donnell M, Rangarajan S, et al. Urinary sodium excretion, blood pressure, cardiovascular disease, and mortality: a community-level prospective epidemiological cohort study. *Lancet*. 2018;392:496–506.
29. Vinceti M, Filippini T, Crippa A, de Sesmaisons A, Wise LA, Orsini N. Meta-analysis of potassium intake and the risk of stroke. *J Am Heart Assoc*. 2016;5. pii:e004210.

30. Hemachandra AH, Howards PP, Furth SL, et al. Birth weight, postnatal growth, and risk for high blood pressure at 7 years of age: results from the Collaborative Perinatal Project. *Pediatrics*. 2007;119: e1264–e1270.
31. *British Nutrition Foundation Task Force on Nutrition and Development —Short- and Long-Term Consequences for Health*. Chichester: Wiley-Blackwell; 2013.
32. Jaff MR, Bates M, Sullivan T, et al. Significant reduction in systolic blood pressure following renal artery stenting in patients with uncontrolled hypertension: results from the HERCULES trial. *Cathet Cardiovasc Interv*. 2012;80:343–350.
33. Weber MA, Mahfoud F, Schmieder RE, et al. Renal denervation for treating hypertension: current scientific and clinical evidence. *JACC Cardiovasc Interv*. 2019;24:1095–1105.
34. Whelton PK, Carey RM, Aronow WS, et al. ACC/AHA/AAPA/ABC/ACPM/AGS/APhA/ASH/ASPC/NMA/PCNA guideline for the prevention, detection, evaluation, and management of high blood pressure in adults: a report of the American College of Cardiology/American Heart Association Task Force on clinical practice guidelines. *J Am Coll Cardiol*. 2018;71:e127–e248.
35. ALLHAT Investigators. Major outcomes in high-risk hypertensive patients randomized to angiotensin-converting enzyme inhibitor or calcium channel blocker vs diuretic: the Antihypertensive and Lipid-Lowering Treatment to Prevent Heart Attack Trial (ALLHAT). *J Am Med Assoc*. 2002;288:2981–2997.
36. Webster R, Salam A, de Silva HA, et al. Fixed low-dose triple combination antihypertensive medication vs usual care for blood pressure control in patients with mild to moderate hypertension in Sri Lanka: a randomized clinical trial. *J Am Med Assoc*. 2018;320:566–579.
37. Fu Q. Sex differences in sympathetic activity in obesity and its related hypertension. *Ann N Y Acad Sci*. 2019;1454:31–41. https://doi.org/10.1111/nyas.14095.
38. Neter JE, Stam BE, Kok FJ, et al. Influence of weight reduction on blood pressure: a meta-analysis of randomized controlled trials. *Hypertension*. 2003;42:878–884.
39. Greenfield JR. Melanocortin signalling and the regulation of blood pressure in human obesity. *J Neuroendocrinol*. 2011;23:186–193.
40. Appel LJ, Sacks FM, Carey VJ, et al. Effects of protein, monounsaturated fat, and carbohydrate intake on blood pressure and serum lipids: results of the Omni Heart randomized trial. *J Am Med Assoc*. 2005;294:2455–2464.
41. Shah M, dams-Huet B, Garg A. Effect of high-carbohydrate or high-cis-monounsaturated fat diets on blood pressure: a meta-analysis of intervention trials. *Am J Clin Nutr*. 2007;85:1251–1256.
42. Jebb SA, Lovegrove JA, Griffin BA, et al. Effect of changing the amount and type of fat and carbohydrate on insulin sensitivity and cardiovascular risk: the RISCK (Reading, Imperial, Surrey, Cambridge, and Kings) trial. *Am J Clin Nutr*. 2010;92:748–758.
43. Geleijnse JM, Giltay EJ, Grobbee DE, et al. Blood pressure response to fish oil supplementation: metaregression analysis of randomized trials. *J Hypertens*. 2002;20:1493–1499.
44. Sanders TAB, Hall WL, Maniou Z, et al. Effect of low doses of long chain n-3 polyunsaturated fatty acids on endothelial function and arterial stiffness: a randomized, controlled trial. *Am J Clin Nutr*. 2011;94:973–980.
45. He FJ, Li J, MacGregor GA. Effect of longer term modest salt reduction on blood pressure: Cochrane systematic review and meta-analysis of randomized trials. *BMJ*. 2013;346. f1325.
46. Hooper L, Bartlett C, Davey SG, et al. Advice to reduce dietary salt for prevention of cardiovascular disease. *Cochrane Database Syst Rev*. 2004. CD003656.
47. Anderson CA, Appel LJ, Okuda N, et al. Dietary sources of sodium in China, Japan, the United Kingdom, and the United States, women and men aged 40 to 59 years: the INTERMAP study. *J Am Diet Assoc*. 2010;110:736–745.
48. Shankar B, Brambila-Macias J, Traill B, et al. An evaluation of the UK Food Standards Agency's salt campaign. *Health Econ*. 2013; 22:243–250.
49. Bernstein AM, Willett WC. Trends in 24-h urinary sodium excretion in the United States, 1957–2003: a systematic review. *Am J Clin Nutr*. 2010;92:1172–1180.
50. Te Morenga LA, Howatson AJ, Jones RM, Mann J. Dietary sugars and cardiometabolic risk: systematic review and meta-analyses of randomized controlled trials of the effects on blood pressure and lipids. *Am J Clin Nutr*. 2014;100:65–79.
51. Fattore E, Botta F, Agostoni C, Bosetti C. Effects of free sugars on blood pressure and lipids: a systematic review and meta-analysis of nutritional isoenergetic intervention trials. *Am J Clin Nutr*. 2017;105:42–56.
52. Xin X, He J, Frontini MG, et al. Effects of alcohol reduction on blood pressure: a meta-analysis of randomized controlled trials. *Hypertension*. 2001;38:1112–1117.
53. Roerecke M, Kaczorowski J, Tobe SW, et al. The effect of a reduction in alcohol consumption on blood pressure: a systematic review and meta-analysis. *Lancet Public Health*. 2017;2:e108–e120.
54. Berry SE, Mulla UZ, Chowienczyk PJ, et al. Increased potassium intake from fruit and vegetables or supplements does not lower blood pressure or improve vascular function in UK men and women with early hypertension: a randomised controlled trial. *Br J Nutr*. 2010;104:1839–1847.
55. Hartley L, Igbinedion E, Holmes J, et al. Increased consumption of fruit and vegetables for the primary prevention of cardiovascular diseases. *Cochrane Database Syst Rev*. 2013;6. https://doi.org/10.1002/14651858.CD009874.pub2. CD009874.
56. Ralston RA, Lee JH, Truby H, Palermo CE, Walker KZ. A systematic review and meta-analysis of elevated blood pressure and consumption of dairy foods. *J Hum Hypertens*. 2012;26: 3–13.
57. Geleijnse JM. Vitamin D and the prevention of hypertension and cardiovascular diseases: a review of the current evidence. *Am J Hypertens*. 2011;24:253–262.
58. Chung M, Balk EM, Brendel M, et al. Vitamin D and calcium: a systematic review of health outcomes. *Evid Rep Technol Assess (Full Rep)*. 2009;183:1–420.
59. Hofmeyr GJ, Lawrie TA, Atallah AN, et al. Calcium supplementation during pregnancy for preventing hypertensive disorders and related problems. *Cochrane Database Syst Rev*. 2010. CD001059.
60. Seppo L, Jauhiainen T, Poussa T, et al. A fermented milk high in bioactive peptides has a blood pressure-lowering effect in hypertensive subjects. *Am J Clin Nutr*. 2003;77:326–330.
61. van Mierlo LA, Koning MM, van der Zander K, et al. Lactotripeptides do not lower ambulatory blood pressure in untreated whites: results from 2 controlled multicenter crossover studies. *Am J Clin Nutr*. 2009;89:617–623.
62. Whelton PK, He J, Cutler JA, et al. Effects of oral potassium on blood pressure. Meta-analysis of randomized controlled clinical trials. *J Am Med Assoc*. 1997;277:1624–1632.
63. Gu D, He J, Wu X, et al. Effect of potassium supplementation on blood pressure in Chinese: a randomized, placebo-controlled trial. *J Hypertens*. 2001;19:1325–1331.
64. He FJ, Marciniak M, Carney C, et al. Effects of potassium chloride and potassium bicarbonate on endothelial function, cardiovascular risk factors, and bone turnover in mild hypertensives. *Hypertension*. 2010;55:681–688.
65. Dickinson HO, Nicolson DJ, Campbell F, et al. Potassium supplementation for the management of primary hypertension in adults. *Cochrane Database Syst Rev*. 2006. CD004641.
66. Filippini T, Violi F, D'Amico R, et al. The effect of potassium supplementation on blood pressure in hypertensive subjects: a systematic review and meta-analysis. *Int J Cardiol*. 2017;230:127–135.

67. Peng YG, Li W, Wen XX, et al. Effects of salt substitutes on blood pressure: a meta-analysis of randomized controlled trials. *Am J Clin Nutr*. 2014;100:1448–1454.
68. SACN/COT. *Potassium-based Sodium Replacers: Assessment of the Health Benefits and Risks of Using Potassium-Based Sodium Replacers in Foods in the UK*; 2017. A Joint Statement by the Scientific Advisory Committee on Nutrition and the Committee on Toxicity in Food, Consumer Products and the Environment. Available from: https://assets.publishing.service.gov.uk/government/uploads/system/uploads/attachment_data/file/660526/SACN_COT_-_Potassium-based_sodium_replacers.pdf. Accessed August 14, 2019.
69. Noordzij M, Uiterwaal CS, Arends LR, et al. Blood pressure response to chronic intake of coffee and caffeine: a meta-analysis of randomized controlled trials. *J Hypertens*. 2005;23:921–928.
70. Poole R, Kennedy OJ, Roderick P, Fallowfield JA, Hayes PC, Parkes J. Coffee consumption and health: umbrella review of meta-analyses of multiple health outcomes. *BMJ*. 2017;359. j5024. BMJ. 2018 Jan 12;360:k194.
71. Ried K, Fakler P, Stocks NP. Effect of cocoa on blood pressure. *Cochrane Database Syst Rev*. 2017;4. https://doi.org/10.1002/14651858.CD008893.pub3. CD008893.
72. Godos J, Vitale M, Micek A, et al. Dietary polyphenol intake, blood pressure, and hypertension: a systematic review and meta-analysis of observational studies. *Antioxidants (Basel)*. 2019;8(6):152. https://doi.org/10.3390/antiox8060152. Published 2019 May 31.
73. Walker HA, Dean TS, Sanders TA, et al. The phytoestrogen genistein produces acute nitric oxide-dependent dilation of human forearm vasculature with similar potency to 17beta-estradiol. *Circulation*. 2001;103:258–262.
74. Taku K, Lin N, Cai D, et al. Effects of soy isoflavone extract supplements on blood pressure in adult humans: systematic review and meta-analysis of randomized placebo-controlled trials. *J Hypertens*. 2010;28:1971–1982.
75. Altorf-van der Kuil W, Engberink MF, Brink EJ, et al. Dietary protein and blood pressure: a systematic review. *PLoS One*. 2010;5. e12102.
76. Webb AJ, Patel N, Loukogeorgakis S, et al. Acute blood pressure lowering, vasoprotective, and antiplatelet properties of dietary nitrate via bioconversion to nitrite. *Hypertension*. 2008;51:784–790.
77. Lundberg JO, Gladwin MT, Ahluwalia A, et al. Nitrate and nitrite in biology, nutrition and therapeutics. *Nat Chem Biol*. 2009;5: 865–869.
78. Kapil V, Milsom AB, Okorie M, et al. Inorganic nitrate supplementation lowers blood pressure in humans: role for nitrite-derived NO. *Hypertension*. 2010;56:274–281.
79. Siervo M, Lara J, Ogbonmwan I, Mathers JC. Inorganic nitrate and beetroot juice supplementation reduces blood pressure in adults: a systematic review and meta-analysis. *J Nutr*. 2013;143:818–826.
80. Appel LJ, Moore TJ, Obarzanek E, , et alfor the DASH Collaborative Research Group. A clinical trial of the effects of dietary patterns on blood pressure. *N Engl J Med*. 1997;336:1117–1124.
81. Sacks FM, Svetkey LP, Vollmer WM, , et alfor the DASH-Sodium Collaborative Research Group. Effects on blood pressure of reduced dietary sodium and the Dietary Approaches to Stop Hypertension (DASH) diet. *N Engl J Med*. 2001;344:3–10.
82. Chiu S, Bergeron N, Williams PT, et al. Comparison of the DASH (Dietary Approaches to Stop Hypertension) diet and a higher-fat DASH diet on blood pressure and lipids and lipoproteins: a randomized controlled trial. *Am J Clin Nutr*. 2016;103:341–347.
83. Appel LJ, Champagne CM, Harsha DW, et al. Effects of comprehensive lifestyle modification on blood pressure control: main results of the PREMIER clinical trial. *J Am Med Assoc*. 2003;289:2083–2093.
84. Reidlinger DP, Darzi J, Hall WL, et al. How effective are current dietary guidelines for cardiovascular disease prevention in healthy middle-aged and older men and women? A randomized controlled trial. *Am J Clin Nutr*. 2015;10:922–930.

CHAPTER

22

NUTRITION AND ATHEROSCLEROTIC CARDIOVASCULAR DISEASE

Philip A. Sapp, MS
Terrence M. Riley, BSc
Alyssa M. Tindall, PhD, RDN
Valerie K. Sullivan, RDN
Emily A. Johnston, MPH, RDN, CDE
Kristina S. Petersen, PhD, BNutDiet(Hons)
Penny M. Kris-Etherton, PhD, RDN
The Pennsylvania State University, University Park, PA, United States

SUMMARY

Key functions of the heart and circulatory system are to supply oxygen and nutrients to all organs and tissues and remove carbon dioxide and waste products from peripheral tissues and organs. A healthy blood flow promotes the normal functions of all cells, tissues, and organs. Atherosclerosis impedes blood flow thereby initiating the onset and accelerating the progression of many cardiovascular diseases (CVDs). Atherosclerotic CVD (ASCVD) is initiated by a nonresolving inflammatory response and later develops into a chronic disease in which genetic predisposition, diet, and lifestyle promote onset and progression. Interventions targeting diet and lifestyle are the primary means of prevention and reduce the risk of ASCVD. Modifiable ASCVD risk factors are many and include overweight/obesity, elevated total cholesterol, low-density lipoprotein cholesterol, elevated triglycerides, high non–high-density lipoprotein cholesterol, low high-density lipoprotein cholesterol, elevated blood pressure, hyperglycemia, physical inactivity, cigarette smoking, stress, and an unhealthy dietary pattern. There is a strong evidence base for the current food-based dietary recommendations and specific nutrient targets (e.g., lower saturated fat, sodium, added sugars) that collectively contribute to a healthy vasculature and reduced CVD risk.

Keywords: Atherosclerotic cardiovascular disease; Diet; Dyslipidemia; Hypertension; Lifestyle; Nutrition; Risk factors.

I. NORMAL VASCULAR FUNCTION AND PHYSIOLOGY

The structural composition of blood vessels plays an active role in normal vascular function and contributes to overall cardiovascular homeostasis.[1] Arteries have a trilaminar structure situated in three layers as concentric circles. The tunica intima is the interface between the vasculature and the blood; the tunica media is the middle layer comprising smooth muscle to regulate vessel tone; the outermost layer, the tunica adventitia, acts as a mechanical support consisting of fibroblasts and connective tissue. The layers of blood vessels are subject to changing environmental conditions, which, in large part, influence homeostatic signaling through the endothelial cells of the intima.[2]

https://doi.org/10.1016/B978-0-12-818460-8.00022-8

The endothelium acts as a mediator for normal vascular function by establishing a semipermeable barrier between the lumen and smooth muscle. At the luminal surface, a meshlike extracellular network of proteoglycans, glycosaminoglycans, and glycoproteins collectively called the glycocalyx exists.[3] This glycocalyx helps maintain homeostasis by mediating coagulation, cell adhesion, and shear stress from blood flow. In addition, the glycocalyx functions as an anionic "charge barrier" assisting in the regulation of endothelial permeability alongside other structural barriers such as interendothelial junctions, fenestrae, and transcellular receptor mediators.[4] A variety of molecular signals can propagate through these extracellular structures. For example, prevention of oxidative damage occurs through endothelial expression of superoxide dismutase (SOD), which acts to protect cells from damage by reactive oxygen species.[5] Expression of SOD increases in the presence of excess physiologic levels of reactive oxygen species. Extracellular SOD bound to proteoglycans of the extracellular matrix and glycocalyx establish a structural complex to reduce the presence of reactive oxygen species in the basement membrane or luminal environment, respectively.[6] Oxidative products circulating in the blood or internalized into the basement membrane of vessels contribute to important steps in the progression of atherosclerotic cardiovascular disease (ASCVD); the expression of SOD alongside a variety of other chemical signals is important in preventing disease development.

Mechanical stimuli also help regulate inflammation, tone, and homeostasis. Shear stress, the frictional force from pulsatile blood flow, induces a signal cascade that promotes cellular differentiation and maintenance of the glycocalyx.[5] Increased expression of endothelial transcription factors, such as Krüppel-like factors (KLFs), in response to shear stress is a form of mechanotransduction that helps maintain normal vascular function. KLFs upregulate homeostatic mechanisms including the activation of endothelial nitric oxide synthase resulting in reduced local vascular pressure through nitric oxide (NO) synthesis.[5,7]

The importance of circulating serum lipids in normal vascular function also contributes to vascular homeostasis since many of the associated risk factors for ASCVD are present in the blood. Traditional measurements of ASCVD risk target low-density lipoprotein cholesterol (LDL-C) due to the causal relationship between elevated LDL-C and CVD events.[8] However, in vitro studies suggest there is limited atherogenicity of unmodified (native) LDL-C.[5] Modifications to native LDL-C are implicated in ASCVD risk; this includes changes to the lipoprotein composition of specific membrane-bound apolipoproteins (Apo-B, Apo-E, and Apo-C) and cholesterol particle number (LDL-P). Lipids and lipoproteins of native LDL-C can also be directly modified by lipid oxidation, desialylation, and particle charge acquisition resulting in the accumulation of modified LDL-C in the subendothelial space and initiation of an atherosclerotic lesion.[9] Elevated circulating LDL-C concentration is a major risk factor for ASCVD, and LDL-C lowering by pharmacologic therapy or lifestyle modification reduces rates of coronary events.[8] The National Lipid Association and 2018 Guideline on the Management of Blood Cholesterol recommend keeping LDL-C below 100 mg/dL (see guidelines for more information).[10,11]

II. PATHOPHYSIOLOGY OF ATHEROSCLEROTIC CARDIOVASCULAR DISEASE

ASCVD initiation and progression is a multifactorial process in which chronic inflammation is mediated by endothelial dysfunction, cellular damage, and circulating cardiometabolic risk factors (e.g., LDL-C, LDL-P, oxidized LDL-C [oxLDL-C]). The clinical manifestations of ASCVD, therefore, present in a variety of forms listed and described in detail in the following section.

A. Coronary Heart Disease, Stroke, and Peripheral Vascular Disease

Cardiovascular disease (CVD) is defined as any disease of the heart and its associated blood vessels, most commonly coronary heart disease (CHD), stroke, and peripheral vascular disease.

CHD, also known as coronary artery disease, is a disease of the coronary arteries, which provide the heart's oxygen and nutrient requirements.[12] These arteries are at high risk for narrowing when cholesterol deposits (i.e., plaques) build up inside the artery. With significant narrowing of the coronary arteries, blood supply to the heart is significantly decreased, resulting in pain or angina. If the plaque ruptures, a thrombus (blood clot) forms and may obstruct the artery, thereby decreasing blood flow and frequently causing a myocardial infarction or stroke. The stoppage of blood flow to the heart also causes necrosis of the affected muscle, resulting in diminished function of the heart. CHD accounts for 43.2% of CVD deaths and is the leading cause of CVD-related deaths in the United States.[13]

Stroke, also known as a cerebrovascular accident (CVA), is another form of CVD that exists in two forms. Ischemic stroke results when the formation of a plaque blocks the blood flow within the artery leading to the brain, while hemorrhagic stroke results after the rupture of a blood vessel and is characterized by uncontrolled bleeding into the surrounding brain tissue. In 2016, deaths attributable to CVAs totaled 5.5 million worldwide with 2.7 million and 2.8 million deaths linked to ischemic and hemorrhagic stroke, respectively.[13] Stoppage of blood flow for more than a few seconds leads to the loss of oxygen to cells within the brain, causing cell death and permanent brain damage.

Peripheral vascular disease is disease of the blood vessels outside of the brain and heart.[14] Inflammation, tissue damage, and plaque accumulation cause narrowing of the blood vessels leading to the periphery—the arms, legs, stomach, and kidneys—and result in damage to these organs and tissues.

B. Endothelial Injury

Initiation of endothelial injury can occur through a variety of conditions including physical and mechanical factors, oxidation, and LDL modification. These pathophysiological states result in endothelial dysfunction and are the initial conditions in fatty streak formation. Chronic inflammation and dysregulation of macromolecular permeability, vascular remodeling, or oxidation promote plaque formation and progression, which can be attenuated through diet and lifestyle changes described in subsequent sections.

Physical/mechanical factors

Endothelial dysfunction provides a generalized characterization of ASCVD initiation; however, fatty lesion formation and atherogenesis are generally focal in nature. Specific regions of the cardiovascular system are considered thrombogenic, partly due to the physical and mechanical forces of blood flow on the endothelium.[5] Shear stress at arterial bifurcations and curvatures creates a unique hemodynamic state at the blood–endothelial interface.[6] Flow-related irregularities develop at these locations and include disturbed blood flow and oscillatory or low shear stress that promotes atherogenesis.[15] Counterintuitively, areas of increased laminar flow that also provide regular, high shear stress are resistant to fatty streak formation, whereas disturbed blood flow regions create atherogenic pathologies.[6] Such is the case at the sinus bifurcation of the carotid artery (Fig. 22.1), which is a common atherogenic locus.[5] One explanation for the protective effect of high shear stress is related to increased glycocalyx maintenance and cell signaling as a result of mechanotransduction.[1] Investigation of atherogenic susceptible regions shows alterations to cellular morphology and irregular expression of glycocalyx proteoglycans.[17] Lipoprotein particles (e.g., LDL-C) and other plasma molecules can then traverse the damaged endothelium into the intima or subendothelial space.[1] Within the intima, the lipoproteins are sequestered and modified, thereby contributing to their chemotaxic, proinflammatory, cytotoxic, and proatherogenic properties.[1,5]

Oxidative stress

The role of oxidation in fatty streak formation occurs in tandem with endothelial dysfunction.[18] Passage of LDL-Ps into the subendothelial space can occur in areas of disturbed laminar flow or abnormal glycocalyx formation.[1] Internalization and retention of LDL-C increases the oxidative potential of the fatty acids that exist in the lipoprotein particles. While in vitro studies suggest

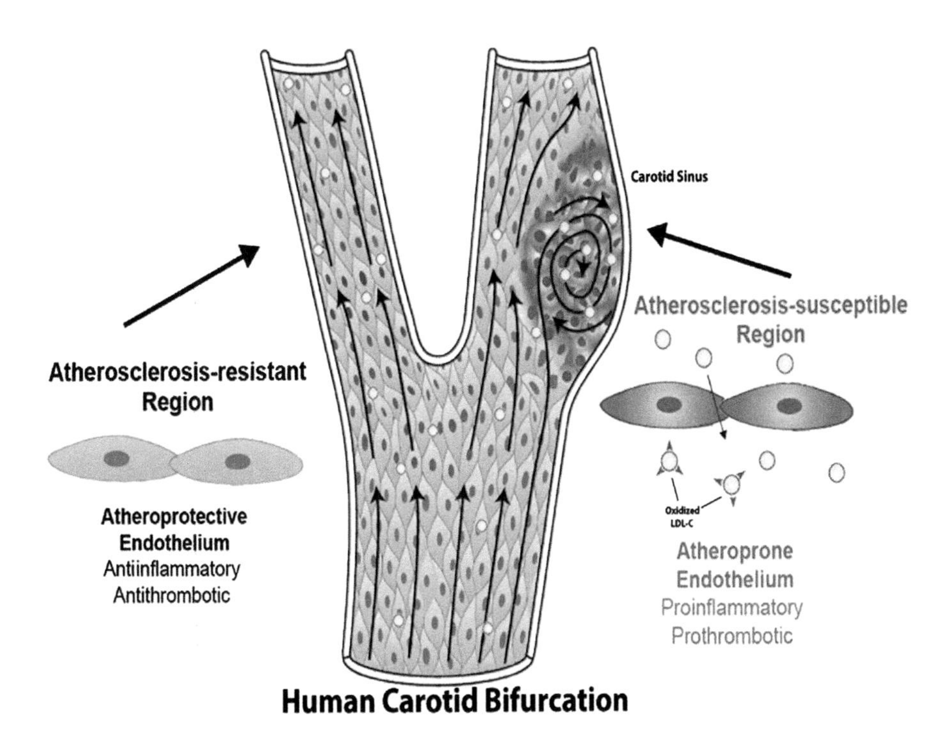

FIGURE 22.1 Focal nature of atherosclerosis at the human carotid bifurcation. Atherosclerosis-resistant regions are mediated by high shear stress and maintenance of luminal structures. Mechanotransduction increases homeostatic mechanisms such as antiinflammatory and antithrombotic signals (KLFs, glycocalyx maintenance) preventing conditions of atherogenesis. Hemodynamic factors including disturbed flow at the carotid sinus contribute to an atheroprone endothelium. Impaired endothelial barrier function increases LDL-C extravasation resulting in subendothelial retention and modification in the tunica intima. *Adapted from: Tabas et al.*[16]

native LDL-C is insufficient to elicit an inflammatory response, a retention hypothesis has been proposed as a mechanism for lipid oxidation in the vessels.[5] Positively charged sites along an Apo-B100–containing LDL-C originating from the liver have an ionic interaction with the negatively charged proteoglycans of the subendothelial space.[19] Binding induces a conformational shift to the Apo-B100 and the lipoprotein particle creating the potential for oxidation and retention within the subendothelial space. The peripheral layer of phospholipids surrounding LDL-C contains varying degrees of polyunsaturated fatty acids (PUFAs) that are vulnerable targets for peroxidation by free radicals.[5] Reactive by-products of oxidation initiate the inflammatory response by activating endothelial cells to recruit leukocytes from the lumen into the subendothelial space. An unresolved inflammatory response promotes foam cell and plaque formation described in detail in the next section and depicted in Figs. 22.2 and 22.3 below.

Elevated cholesterol and lipoprotein modification

Elevated serum concentrations of cholesterol and its lipoprotein carriers are associated with ASCVD. In particular, cholesterol carried by apoB-containing lipoproteins, collectively referred to as non–high-density lipoproteins (non-HDL-C), are considered atherogenic.[20] These include low-density (LDL-C), intermediate-density (IDL-C), very–low-density lipoproteins (VLDL-C), and lipoprotein(a), plus chylomicrons and their remnants in the postprandial state. Elevation of apoB-containing lipoproteins is directly associated with atherosclerosis and contributes to cardiovascular events. Infiltration of the arterial intima by these lipoprotein particles (especially from small, dense LDL-P) causes intimal thickening—a marker of subclinical atherosclerosis—and low-grade inflammation.[21]

LDL-C modification, particularly by oxidation, contributes importantly to atherogenesis. Intrinsic factors such as antioxidant content (e.g., vitamin C and vitamin E), fatty acid composition, particle size (small and dense subfractions of LDL-C are more susceptible to oxidation), and extrinsic factors, including the surrounding pH, local antioxidant concentrations, and transition metal availability, increase the susceptibility of LDL-C to oxidation.[22]

Native LDL-C does not substantially contribute to lipid accumulation in the arterial wall, but modifications of LDL-C in the bloodstream may increase its atherogenicity. Specifically, desialylation (removal of sialyic acid groups) appears to be one of the first modifications, followed by physical and chemical modifications that change the lipid composition, decrease size, increase density, increase electrical charge, and oxidize LDL-C (oxLDL) particles.[9,23,24] Such modified LDL-C precipitates an immune response within the arterial wall,[25] leading to foam cell development and plaque progression (Fig. 22.2).[26]

C. Inflammatory Response

The endothelium is activated by several atherogenic and proinflammatory particles found in the circulation.

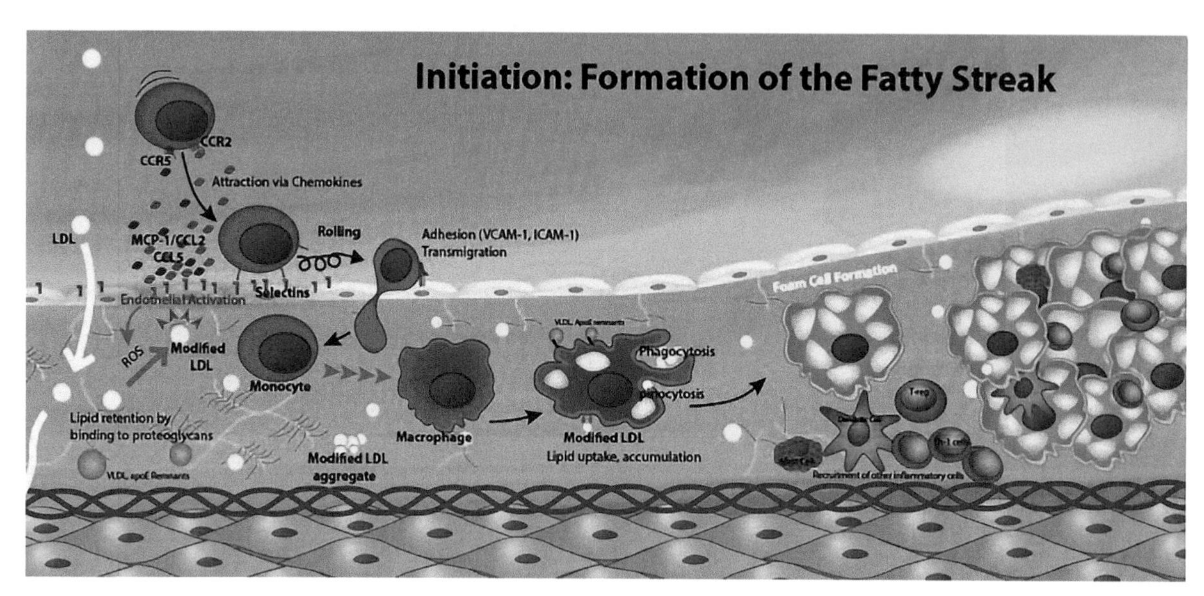

FIGURE 22.2 Initiation of the atherosclerotic lesion. The fatty streak phase of atherosclerosis begins with dysfunctional endothelial cells and the retention of apoB-containing lipoproteins (LDL-C, VLDL-C, and apoE remnants) in the subendothelial space. Retained lipoproteins are modified (oxidation, glycation, enzymatic), which, along with other atherogenic factors, promotes activation of endothelial cells. Activated endothelial cells have increased expression of monocyte interaction/adhesion molecules (selectins, VCAM-1) and chemoattractants (MCP-1, CCR2, CCR5, CCL2, CCL5) leading to attachment and transmigration of monocytes into the intimal space. The monocytes differentiate into macrophages and express receptors that mediate the internalization of VLDL-C, apoE remnants, and modified LDL to become foam cells. Macrophage chemokine release signals additional inflammatory leukocytes including T-helper 1, T-regulatory, mast, and dendritic cells. *Courtesy of Linton et al.*[5]

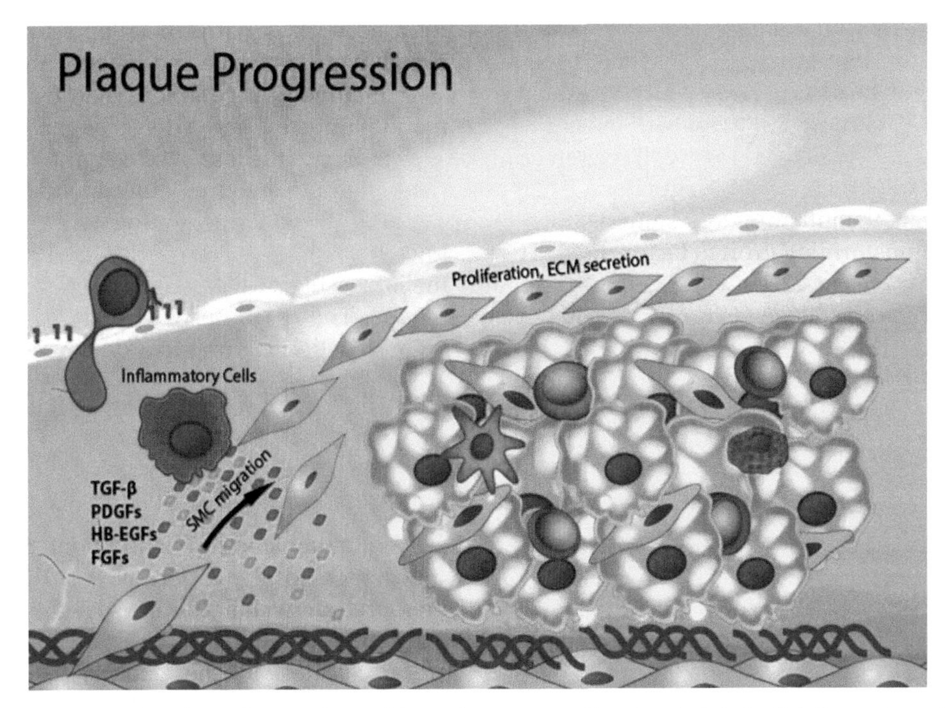

FIGURE 22.3 Progression of the atherosclerotic plaque. Macrophage foam cell and endothelial cell inflammatory signaling continues to promote the recruitment of more monocytes and immune cells into the subendothelial space. Transition from a fatty streak to a fibrous fatty lesion occurs with the infiltration and proliferation of tunica media smooth muscle cells. Macrophage foam cells and other inflammatory cells produce a number of chemoattractant and proliferation factors, including transforming growth factor beta (TGF-β), platelet-derived growth factor (PDGF) isoforms, matrix metalloproteinases, fibroblast growth factors (FGF), and heparin-binding epidermal growth factor (HB-EGF). Smooth muscle cells are recruited to the luminal side of the lesion to proliferate and generate an extracellular matrix network to form a barrier between lesional prothrombotic factors and blood platelets and procoagulant factors. A subset of smooth muscle cells express macrophage receptors and internalize lipoproteins to become foam cells. *Courtesy of Linton et al.*[5]

LDL-C modification allows for its cellular uptake via the scavenger receptor and consequent promotion of atherogenesis. Lipid peroxidation is mediated in part by 15-lipoxygenase, myeloperoxidase, or nitric oxide synthase.[5] OxLDL-C is atherogenic and is a direct and indirect chemoattractant for circulating monocytes,[27] with the latter occurring via the release of monocyte chemoattractant protein 1 (MCP-1) from the endothelium.[5] OxLDL-C polarizes macrophage phenotype toward M1- or M2-like macrophage cells that increase inflammatory cytokine signaling.[5] The endothelium in turn has increased expression of various cell adhesion molecules, such as the vascular cell adhesion molecule 1, which results in the recruitment and migration of monocytes and T-lymphocytes from the blood.[5] Other molecules also participate in the recruitment of blood-borne cells to the atherosclerotic lesion, including intercellular adhesion molecule 1 (ICAM-1), E selectin, and P selectin.[28,29]

Adhesion to the endothelium is followed by transendothelial migration mediated via one or more chemotactic cytokines.[5] In the intima, the attracted monocytes differentiate into macrophages and undergo receptor-mediated phagocytosis of VLDL-C, ApoE remnants, and modified LDL-C. Phagocytosis continues in an abundance of lipoproteins until the activated macrophages undergo apoptosis or necrosis.[5] Death of the foam cells leads to the formation of a soft and unstable lipid-rich core within the atherosclerotic plaque.[30]

In conditions of low LDL-C and high HDL-C plasma levels, the foam cells may shrink through the efflux of cellular cholesterol to extracellular HDL-C mediated by membrane transporters,[31,32] creating the initial step in reverse cholesterol transport (RCT). Moderate to high levels of HDL-C have been found to be cardioprotective since the risk of atherosclerosis is inversely related to HDL-C levels[33] with the protective effect due to the mediation of RCT by HDL-C.[34] In this process, HDL-C particles remove free cholesterol from the macrophages and transport it to the liver for excretion in the bile.[34] The presence of HDL-C also inhibits smooth muscle chemokine expression and proliferation.[5] Since HDL-mediated RCT contributes to a decrease in tissue cholesterol levels, increased RCT stimulates atheroregression and decreases the risk of atherosclerotic plaque development.

D. Plaque Progression and Stabilization

The fibroproliferative response mediated by vascular smooth muscle cells produces a collagen-rich matrix that stabilizes atherosclerotic plaques. In addition, foam cell clearance of accumulating cholesteryl esters is diminished due to compromised lysosomal function further contributing to plaque formation.[5] Breakdown of the foam cell elicits migration of smooth muscle cells to aggregate around the damaged foam cell core creating a fragile, fibrous cap (see Fig. 22.3).[5] Regulatory T-helper cells (T-reg) mediate the inflammatory status of the plaque by releasing transforming growth factors beta (TGF-β) and interleukins (see Fig. 22.4[5]). T-Reg cells also signal cell death and increased collagen expression to help stabilize the plaque.[5]

Continuation of foam cell breakdown is detrimental in that several matrix-degrading (proteolytic) enzymes are released, such as matrix metalloproteinases, which further destabilize the plaque and induce thrombogenesis.[5]

A relatively large atherosclerotic plaque is prone to plaque rupture where a defect or gap occurs in the fibrous cap leading to the loss of the separation between its lipid-rich core and the circulating blood.[35] This results in a cascade of events beginning with plaque rupture followed by platelet aggregation to the exposed subendothelial tissue and fibrin formation over the ruptured plaque. The rapid onset of platelet aggregation creates an obstruction leading to a decrease in blood flow.[30]

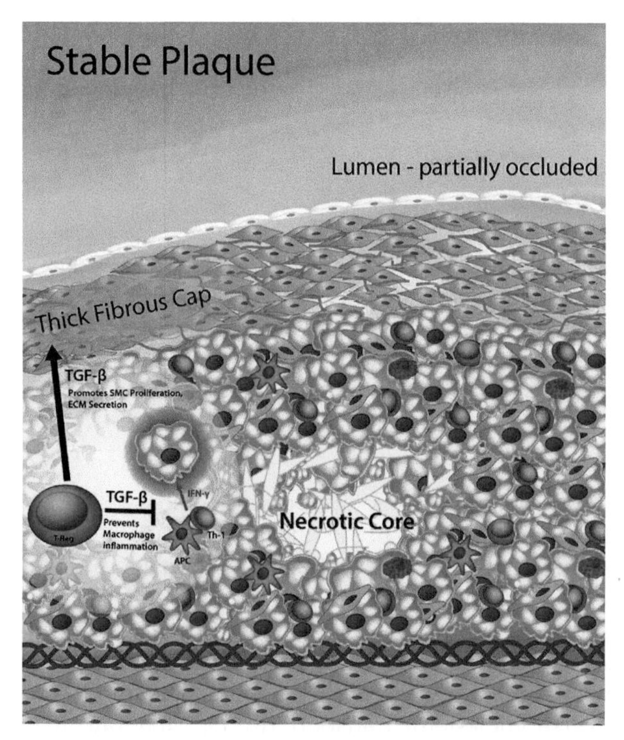

FIGURE 22.4 Features of the stable fibrous plaque. As the cell volume of the intima increases, there is vascular remodeling so that the lumen is only partially occluded, substantially lessening clinical events resulting from occlusion. The stable plaque contains a generous thick fibrous cap composed of layers of smooth muscle cells ensconced in a substantial extracellular matrix network of collagen, proteoglycans, and elastin. The thick fibrous cap of the stable plaque provides an effective barrier preventing plaque rupture and exposure of lesion prothrombotic factors to blood, thereby limiting thrombus formation and clinical events. Maintenance of a thick fibrous cap is enabled by regulation of the inflammatory status of the foam cell core of the lesion. Regulatory T (T-reg) cells produce transforming growth factor beta (TGF-β). In addition, T-reg cells inhibit antigen-specific activation of T helper 1 (Th-1) cells to produce interferon gamma (IFNg). Increased TGF-β reduces the proinflammatory macrophage phenotype leading to reduced cell death, effective efferocytosis (phagocytosis of dead cells), and anti-inflammatory cytokine production (i.e., TGF-β). Thus, stable plaques have small necrotic cores containing macrophage debris and extracellular lipid resulting from secondary necrosis of noninternalized apoptotic macrophage foam cells. The production of TGF-β by T-reg cells and macrophages maintains fibrous cap quality by being a potent stimulator of collagen production in smooth muscle cells. *Courtesy of Linton et al.*[5]

III. RISK FACTORS FOR ATHEROSCLEROSIS

Abnormal blood lipid and lipoprotein levels are major contributors to atherosclerosis. In addition, elevated blood pressure, overweight/obesity, dysglycemia, physical inactivity, smoking, stress, and an unhealthy dietary pattern are implicated in the etiology of atherosclerosis.[13,36] Approximately 20%–25% of initial vascular events occur in patients with one major CVD risk factor, with about one-half of those having elevated LDL-C.[37] Moreover, overweight and obesity, physical inactivity, and an unhealthy diet are associated with elevated LDL-C, blood pressure, and glucose. Recommended nutrition and medical interventions target modifiable risk factors and can significantly reduce the progression of atherosclerosis and CVD. These modifiable and nonmodifiable risk factors are presented in Table 22.1.[11,36,38]

A. Smoking

Cigarette smoking is a major risk factor for the development of atherosclerosis through the inhalation of many toxic chemicals (e.g., nicotine, carbon monoxide, polycyclic aromatic hydrocarbons).[39] The main mechanisms involve endothelial dysfunction, inflammation, and an unfavorable lipid profile.[39] Smoking is associated with increased triglyceride (TG) and decreased HDL-C concentrations.[39] Similarly, electronic cigarette (e-cigarette or vaping) usage is associated with increased odds of myocardial infarction and stroke.[40] Although the mechanisms are not fully understood, the aerosolized vapor may contain toxic materials (e.g., nicotine, heavy metals, ultrafine particles) that promote atherosclerosis.[41,42]

Another major risk factor for atherosclerosis, high blood pressure, causes endothelial injury through shear stress and microtears in the artery wall.[43] Other risk factors, such as overweight and obesity, elevated blood glucose, physical inactivity, and an unhealthy dietary pattern, play a major role in the progression of atherosclerosis. A chronic state of inflammation, induced by excess adiposity, dysglycemia, and/or poor diet, presented as

TABLE 22.1 Modifiable and nonmodifiable risk factors for primary prevention of atherosclerosis.

Nonmodifiable	Modifiable	Goals for modifiable risk factors
Age	Weight[b]	Weight loss is recommended if BMI is $\geq$25 kg/m^2
Sex	Lipid profile[a]	Total cholesterol: <150 mg/dL (3.8 mmol/L)
Family history/ genetics		LDL-C: <100 mg/dL (2.6 mmol/L)
Race and ethnicity		Triglycerides: <150 mg/dL (3.8 mmol/L)
		HDL-C: Men: $\geq$40 mg/dL (1.0 mmol/L) Women: $\geq$50 mg/dL (1.3 mmol/L)
	Blood pressure[c]	Systolic: <120 mmHg Diastolic: <80 mmHg
	Glycemic control[a]	Fasting blood glucose: <100 mg/dL (5.6 mmol/L)
	Physical activity[b]	150 min of moderate-intensity activity or 75 min of vigorous-intensity activity per week (or an equivalent combination of both)
	Tobacco use[b]	Cessation of all types of tobacco use
	Diet[a,b]	Follow a heart-healthy diet

Please see 2018 Guideline on the Management of Blood Cholesterol for clinical management in high-risk and secondary prevention.[11]
[a]*2018 AHA/ACC/AACVPR/AAPA/ABC/ACPM/ADA/AGS/APhA/ASPC/NLA/PCNA Guideline on the Management of Blood Cholesterol: Executive Summary.*[11]
[b]*2019 ACC/AHA Guideline on the Primary Prevention of Cardiovascular Disease.*[36]
[c]*2017 ACC/AHA/AAPA/ABC/ACPM/AGS/APhA/ASH/ASPC/NMA/PCNA Guideline for the Prevention, Detection, Evaluation, and Management of High Blood Pressure in Adults: A Report of the American College of Cardiology/American Heart Association Task Force on Clinical Practice Guidelines.*[38]

elevated levels of C-reactive protein and other proinflammatory cytokines, along with decreased levels of antiinflammatory cytokines, has also been found to promote atherosclerotic plaque development.[44] Targeting these risk factors is central to reducing ASCVD.

B. Blood Pressure

Elevated blood pressure is a major risk factor for atherosclerosis. Thus, it is a clinical target for lifestyle and pharmacological therapies to reduce ASCVD risk. The current definition of hypertension in the United States is blood pressure $\geq$130/80 mmHg.[38] Individuals with elevated blood pressure (120–129/<80 mmHg) and individuals with hypertension who are not at high ASCVD risk are prescribed nonpharmacological interventions, including dietary modification. Pharmacological treatment is recommended for individuals with hypertension and high ASCVD risk.

Hypertension can both cause and perpetuate atherosclerosis. Hypertension is implicated in the development of endothelial dysfunction, oxidative stress, vascular remodeling, and fibrosis, contributing to atherosclerosis.[45] The narrowing of arteries due to atherosclerotic plaque formation can also increase blood pressure. The complex interrelations between atherosclerosis and blood pressure are important in preventing and treating CVD (See Chapter 21, Hypertension).

Elevated blood pressure is also both a cause and consequence of arterial stiffening, a degenerative process in which elastic arteries undergo structural changes that affect extracellular matrix proteins in the vessel wall.[46,47] Arterial stiffening is caused by changes in the media (the middle layer of the arteries) and is characterized by reductions in elastin and increases in collagen deposition. The greater pressure needed to eject blood during systole can also cause a reduction in aortic diastolic blood pressure (DBP). Stiffening of the arteries increases the likelihood of atherosclerosis, although the atherosclerotic process occurs in the arterial intima as a result of lipid accumulation, oxidation, and inflammation.[46]

Vascular stiffening and atherosclerosis often co-occur and share some risk factors, such as elevated blood pressure and chronic inflammation.[48–50] Arterial stiffness is an independent predictor of CVD events, as well as an additional risk factor that improves risk prediction information when coupled with the traditional risk predictor models such as Framingham Risk Score.[51]

C. Blood Glucose

Impaired glycemic regulation results from insufficient or absent insulin production and/or resistance to insulin signaling. The former is a classic feature of type 1 diabetes, whereas type 2 diabetes is characterized by insulin resistance with or without insufficient compensatory insulin production. Dysglycemia resulting from insulin resistance is also a common feature of metabolic syndrome, defined as having at least three out of the five criteria (elevated fasting glucose [$\geq$100 mg/dL], TGs [$\geq$150 mg/dL], waist circumference [men: $\geq$102 cm or $\geq$40 in and women: $\geq$88 cm or $\geq$35 in], blood pressure [$\geq$130 mmHg SBP or $\geq$85 mmHg DBP), and low HDL-C (men:<40 mg/dL and women:<50 mg/dL).[52] Regardless of etiology, hyperglycemia increases atherosclerotic risk.[53] Additionally, elevated fasting glucose, in the absence of diabetes mellitus, may increase CVD risk.[54]

Hyperglycemia damages the vasculature through several mechanisms. Acute hyperglycemia increases expression of vascular adhesion molecules and proinflammatory markers (e.g., ICAM, VCAM, IL-6, E-selectin) and promotes accumulation of reactive oxygen species, resulting in vascular inflammation and endothelial dysfunction.[55,56] Glycation of LDL-C is also increased by hyperglycemia, thereby increasing its atherogenicity.[57] People with metabolic syndrome and/or diabetes are more likely to have atherosclerosis and are at higher risk for CVD events than individuals free of these conditions.[58–60] Lifestyle factors that promote blood glucose control and insulin sensitivity, and reduce glycemic excursions, can slow the development and progression of ASCVD.[61]

The foundation for reducing CVD risk is a healthy lifestyle, including a high-quality diet. A suboptimal diet leads to metabolic and physiological aberrations involved in the pathogenesis of CVD. This section discusses the role of diet in the onset of CVD.

D. Role of Diet in Onset of CVD

Poor-quality diet

Globally, approximately 53% of CVD deaths and 58% of CVD-related disability are because of poor diet quality, making it the leading risk factor for CVD-related morbidity and mortality.[62] Poor diet quality is defined as suboptimal intake of fruits, vegetables, whole grains, seafood, nuts and seeds, fiber, legumes, polyunsaturated fatty acids, and milk coupled with the overconsumption of sodium, *trans* fats, sugar-sweetened beverages, and processed meats.[62] Recent research has reported that high consumption of sodium and low intake of whole grains and fruits account for more than half of all diet-related deaths and 66% of diet-related disability worldwide (predominantly from CVD).[62] These findings are representative of diet-related death and disability in the United States, Canada, and many other high- and middle-income countries.

The diets of fewer than 0.5% of adults in the United States met the criteria for an ideal Healthy Diet Score, while ~82% of adults aged 20–49 years and ~73% of individuals aged 50+ had a poor score.[13] The Healthy Diet Score, as defined by the AHA, is calculated based on intake of fruits and vegetables; fish and shellfish; sodium; sugar-sweetened beverages; whole grains; nuts, legumes, and seeds; processed meats; and saturated fat (Table 22.2).[63] Since 2003, there has been little improvement in the percentage of US adults with an ideal Healthy Diet Score.[13]

TABLE 22.2 The definition of ideal, intermediate, and poor levels of AHA's Healthy Diet Score.

Component	
Primary*	
Fruits and vegetables	≥4.5 cups/day
Fish 3.5 oz servings (preferably oily fish)	≥2 servings/week
Sodium	1500 mg/day
Sweets/sugar-sweetened beverages	≤450 kcal (36 oz.)/week
Whole grains	≥3 1-oz equivalent servings/day
Secondary	
Nuts, legumes, seeds	≥4 servings/wk
Processed meats	≤2 servings/wk
Saturated fat	≤7% of kcal

Healthy Diet Score: Ideal = 4–5 components, intermediate = 2–3 components, and poor = 0–1 component. *Scaled for 2000 kcal/day.
Adapted from Lloyd–Jones et al.[63]

Observational studies consistently show a dose–response relationship between better diet quality (indices based on adherence to dietary recommendations) and lower CVD morbidity and mortality in diverse populations studied.[64–69] An analysis from the Nurses' Health Study and the Health Professionals Follow-up Study showed per 20 percentile increase in diet quality, total mortality was reduced by 8%–17% (depending on the diet quality index used), and risk of cardiovascular mortality was reduced by 7%–15% during the follow-up period.[69] However, declining diet quality over the 16 years of follow-up was associated with a 22%–24% increase in total mortality and a 24%–33% increase in cardiovascular mortality (depending on the diet quality index used). This is consistent with evidence showing that poor-quality diets, often referred to as "Western-style diets," are associated with metabolic dysfunction and increased risk of CVD.[70–72] Western-style diets are typically characterized by higher intakes of red meats, processed meats, refined grains, sweets and desserts, French fries, and high-fat dairy products.[70]

Findings from clinical trials are supportive of the poor diet–disease relationships identified in epidemiologic research. The PREDIMED trial showed that Mediterranean diets (high in either extra virgin olive oil or mixed nuts) reduced CVD events by approximately 30% compared to a control diet lower in fat in participants (55–80 years of age) at high risk of CVD.[73] Notably, in PREDIMED, the Mediterranean diet score difference between the Mediterranean diet groups and the control group ranged from 1.4 to 1.8 points (out of 14) over the approximate 5 years of follow-up, demonstrating that small improvements in diet quality conferred clinically significant cardiovascular benefit.[73]

The cardiovascular risk reduction observed with improved diet quality is mediated by improvements in cardiovascular risk factors. Meta-analyses of randomized controlled trials have shown that healthy dietary patterns lower blood pressure[74] and LDL-C[75] and reduce systemic inflammation.[76] The Mediterranean diet lowers blood pressure and modestly reduces LDL-C and TG,[77] reduces fasting plasma glucose,[78] and improves arterial stiffness and endothelial function.[79,80] Similarly, the Dietary Approaches to Stop Hypertension (DASH) diet, defined below (see Table 22.3), improves a number of risk factors for CVD such as blood pressure, total cholesterol, and LDL-C.[75,84]

TABLE 22.3 Healthy dietary patterns for atherosclerotic cardiovascular disease (ASCVD) prevention and management, amounts to include based on 2000 kcal/day.

Food group	Healthy US-style eating pattern[81]	Healthy Mediterranean-style eating pattern[81]	Healthy vegetarian eating pattern[81]	DASH diet[81]
Vegetables	2½ c-eq/day	2½ c-eq/day	2½ c-eq/day	2–5 c/day
Dark green	1½ c-eq/wk	1½ c-eq/wk	1½ c-eq/wk	–
Red and orange	5½ c-eq/wk	5½ c-eq/wk	5½ c-eq/wk	–
Legumes (beans and peas)	1½ c-eq/wk	1½ c-eq/wk	3 c-eq/wk	2–2½ c/wk
Starchy	5 c-eq/wk	5 c-eq/wk	5 c-eq/wk	–
Other	4 c-eq/wk	4 c-eq/wk	4 c-eq/wk	–
Fruits	2 c-eq/day	2½ c-eq/day	2 c-eq/day	2–2½ c/day
Grains	6 oz-eq/day	6 oz-eq/day	6½ oz-eq/day	6–8 oz/day
Whole grains	≥3 oz-eq/day	≥3 oz-eq/day	≥3½ oz-eq/day	–
Refined grains	≤3 oz-eq/day	≤3 oz-eq/day	≤3 oz-eq/day	–
Dairy	3 c-eq/day	2 c-eq/day	3 c-eq/day	2–3 c/day
Protein foods	5½ oz-eq/day	6½ oz-eq/day	3½ oz-eq/day	≤6 oz/day
Seafood	8 oz-eq/wk	15 oz-eq/wk	Not applicable	–
Meat, poultry, eggs	26 oz-eq/wk	26 oz-eq/wk	3 oz-eq/wk (eggs)	–
Nuts, seeds, soy	5 oz-eq/wk	5 oz-eq/wk	15 oz-eq/wk (7 oz nuts/seeds, 8 oz soy)	6–7½ oz/wk
Oils	27 g/day	27 g/day	27 g/day	8–12 g/day
Limit calories from other sources (% of calories)	270 kcal/day (14%)	260 kcal/day (13%)	290 kcal/day (15%)	–
Saturated fat	<8% or 18 g/day[a]	<8% or 18 g/day[a]	<8% or 18 g/day[a]	<7%[b]
Added sugars	<30 g/day (6%)	<30 g/day (6%)	<30 g/day (6%)	~35 g/day
Sodium	≤2300 mg/day	≤2300 mg/day	≤2300 mg/day	≤2300 mg/day

[a]*SFA estimates derived from ACC/AHA recommendations.*[82]
[b]*SFA estimates derived from DASH trial.*[83]

While overall poor diet quality is the leading contributor to CVD development, specific dietary components make a significant contribution to the CVD burden. In the subsequent sections, the contributions of sodium, macronutrients, and omega-3 (n-3) fatty acids will be discussed.

Role of sodium in the onset of CVD

High sodium intake causes a greater proportion of CVD-related deaths and disability than any other dietary factor. Recent global estimates show high sodium intake accounts for 28% of diet-related CVD deaths.[62] Concordant and high-level evidence shows a positive linear relationship between sodium intake and blood pressure.[85] On the basis of a comprehensive literature review, the 2019 review of Dietary Reference Intakes for sodium[85] reported that systolic and DBPs are lowered by 2.4–2.7 mmHg and 1.2–1.7 mmHg per 1000 mg/day reduction in sodium intake (where baseline sodium intake is in the range of 1000–5000 mg), respectively. Furthermore, reducing sodium by 1000 mg/day is associated with a 27% reduction in CVD risk and a 20% reduction in hypertension risk.

In addition to inducing dose–response increases in blood pressure, sodium also acts on the vasculature, causing micro- and macrovascular impairment.[86–88] In a 7-day randomized crossover-controlled feeding study, a high sodium intake (5313 mg/day) reduced endothelium-dependent dilation by 32%, compared with a low-sodium diet (667 mg/day), in healthy normotensive subjects; this endothelial impairment occurred independently of changes in blood pressure.[87] In a similar experiment, high sodium consumption (5359 mg/day) for 7 days impaired cutaneous microvascular function independently of blood pressure, compared to a low-sodium diet (741 mg/day). Finally, a meta-analysis of 11 randomized controlled trials showed that sodium reduction of ~2000 mg/day lowered carotid-femoral pulse wave velocity (PWV), the gold standard for noninvasive assessment of arterial stiffness, by 2.8%.[88] This improvement in PWV appeared to be independent of changes in blood pressure. The mechanism(s) responsible for the endothelial dysfunction, microvascular impairment, and arterial stiffening induced by high sodium intake is still incompletely understood. However, it has been established that sodium promotes oxidative stress by increasing the generation of reactive oxygen species, which reduces nitric oxide bioavailability, a potent vasodilator[89] and antiatherogenic agent.

Role of macronutrients in the onset of CVD

Dietary macronutrient composition affects CVD risk, and because intake of single macronutrients cannot be changed in isolation, current research focuses on how macronutrient substitutions affect CVD risk.[10,36,82] This is principally because examinations of the relationships between single macronutrients (fats, carbohydrate [CHO], and protein) and CVD risk have yielded inconsistent results since the associations observed are dependent on what is used as the replacement macronutrient.[90]

Replacement analyses consistently show that isocaloric replacement of 5% of calories from saturated fatty acids (SFAs) with PUFAs, monounsaturated fatty acids (MUFAs), or whole grains reduces CVD risk by 25%, 15%, and 9%, respectively.[90,91] In contrast, replacement of SFAs with *trans* fat and refined grains/added sugars does not change CVD risk. Isocaloric substitution of 5% of calories from refined grains/added sugars with PUFAs, MUFAs, or whole grains lowers CVD risk by 22%, 5%, and 11%, respectively, with no risk reduction observed for *trans* fat or SFA replacement.[91] Thus, replacement of SFAs with PUFAs appears to confer the greatest CVD risk reduction.

Heterogeneity exists in the CVD risk conferred by SFAs from particular food sources, which may be because of the types of SFAs in the food sources or effects of the food matrix.[92] Dairy is a rich source of SFA; however, data from prospective cohort studies show dairy has a favorable or neutral association with CVD risk.[93] Importantly, though, isocaloric replacement of 5% of calories from dairy fat with vegetable fat, PUFAs, or whole grains lowers CVD risk by 10%, 24%, and 28%, respectively.[94] Replacement of 5% of calories from dairy fat with other animal fat is associated with a 6% increase in CVD risk. Thus, replacement of dairy fat with sources of unsaturated fats or whole grains is preferable to lower CVD risk, although consumption of dairy fat confers less risk than other animal fats.

Intake of macronutrients principally affects CVD risk by modulation of lipids and lipoproteins. Lowering intake of SFAs is the primary target for CVD risk reduction because increased intake increases atherogenic cholesterol levels, particularly LDL-C. Strong and consistent evidence shows that replacing SFAs with PUFAs confers the greatest LDL-C and TG lowering and minimizes HDL-C reductions. Replacement of 5% of calories from SFAs with PUFAs lowers LDL-C and TGs by approximately 9 and 2 mg/dL, respectively.[10] In comparison, replacement of 5% of calories from SFAs with MUFAs or CHO lowers LDL-C by 6.5 and 6 mg/dL, respectively, and increases TGs by 1 and 9.5 mg/dL, respectively. If SFAs are replaced with CHO, whole grain sources should be chosen, since whole grains confer greater LDL-C reductions (3.5 mg/dL) compared with refined grains.[95] Replacement of 5% of calories from SFAs with PUFA, MUFA, or CHO lowers HDL-C by 1, 6, and 2 mg/dL, respectively. To lower TG levels, replacement of CHO with MUFA or PUFA is recommended; replacement of 5% of calories from CHO with MUFA or PUFA will lower TGs by 6.7 and 9.3 mg/dL, respectively.[96]

With regard to individual SFAs, replacement of 1% of calories from CHO with lauric acid (C12:0), myristic acid (C14:0), or palmitic acid (C16:0) increases LDL-C by 0.7, 1.7, and 1.4 mg/dL, respectively.[96] In contrast, stearic acid (C18:0) has a relatively neutral effect on LDL-C and no change occurs when it replaces CHO. Tropical oils, including coconut oil and palm oil, are sources of the medium chain SFA (C12:0), and while they increase LDL-C less than longer chain SFAs found in animal products, the increases observed are greater than with MUFA- or PUFA-rich food sources.[97,98] Therefore, to lower CVD risk, sources of SFAs should be replaced with unsaturated fats including nontropical oils such as those found in nuts and seeds.

Role of n-3 fatty acids (also known as omega-3 fatty acids) in the onset of CVD

Plant-based n-3 fatty acids: α-linolenic acid; Evidence suggests that higher intakes of the n-3 fatty acid, α-linolenic acid (ALA), measured by self-reported dietary intake methods and plasma/serum/whole blood biomarkers, are associated with a modestly lower risk of CVD.[99–101] Consistently, higher ALA intake is associated with lower risk of fatal CHD.[99,100] In a meta-analysis of five prospective cohort studies, the relative risk of CHD death was lowered by 10% per 1 g/day increase in ALA.[100] In addition, a Cochrane Collaboration systematic review of randomized controlled trials reported that higher ALA intake was associated with a nonsignificant 5%–10% reduction in CVD.[102] The mechanism(s) by which ALA may lower CVD risk is incompletely understood; however, evidence shows ALA does not directly affect lipids/lipoproteins but has antiarrhythmic properties.[90]

Marine-derived n-3 fatty acids; Strong and consistent evidence suggests that consumption of 1–2 servings/week (3.5 oz./serving) of nonfried fish (especially types that are high in long-chain n-3 fatty acids, such as eicosapentaenoic acid [EPA] and docosahexaenoic acid [DHA]) lowers the risk of CVD.[103] There is mixed evidence about whether n-3 supplements containing EPA and/or DHA are beneficial for primary and secondary prevention of CVD.[104] Recently, three large randomized controlled trials were completed, and an updated meta-analysis that included these trials and previously conducted studies (13 trials and

127,477 participants) showed marine-derived n-3 supplementation was associated with significantly lower risk of myocardial infarction, CHD death, total CHD, CVD death, and total CVD.[105] However, there are currently no recommendations for use of supplemental n-3 fatty acids for primary and secondary prevention of CVD.

N-3 fatty acids have demonstrated efficacy for lowering TGs. In patients with high (200–499 mg/dL) or very high TG levels (>500 mg/dL), 4 g/day of prescription n-3 fatty acids lowered TGs by 20%–30% and ≥30%, respectively.[106] In REDUCE-IT, a multicenter, randomized, double-blinded, placebo-controlled trial in patients with CVD or at high risk of CVD with statin-controlled LDL-C but elevated TGs, 4 g/day of icosapent ethyl (EPA in ethyl ester form) lowered TGs by ~14%. Furthermore, the risk of cardiovascular events (CVD death, myocardial infarction, stroke, revascularization, or unstable angina) was reduced by 25%.[107] This risk reduction is larger than would be expected on the basis of TG lowering alone, suggesting other mechanisms of action.

In addition to TG lowering, n-3 fatty acids (marine-derived) have been shown to affect a number of factors implicated in the etiology of CVD, including inflammation, thrombosis, arrhythmia, endothelial and autonomic function, blood pressure, myocardial efficiency, and plaque stability suggestive of cardiovascular benefit.[103,108]

Summary: role of diet in onset of CVD

Poor diet quality is responsible for a substantial proportion of CVD worldwide. While traditionally diet and CVD risk has been viewed through an individual nutrient lens, contemporary efforts are focused on dietary patterns. The focus on dietary patterns reflects the totality of the diet—specifically the combinations and quantities of foods and nutrients consumed.[109] Importantly, dietary patterns account for the cumulative, interactive, and synergistic effects of the many nutrients and other dietary factors that contribute to human health and disease risk.[110] The greatest contributors to poor diet quality related CVD are suboptimal intake of fruits, vegetables, whole grains, seafood, nuts and seeds, fiber, legumes, and PUFAs, with concurrent overconsumption of sodium, added sugars, and SFAs.[62]

IV. PRIMARY NUTRITIONAL TREATMENT MODALITIES

A. Dietary Patterns for Prevention of Atherosclerotic Cardiovascular Disease

A healthy lifestyle is the foundation of ASCVD prevention.[36] A cornerstone of a healthy lifestyle is a healthy dietary pattern. While there are many healthy dietary patterns, they all have commonalities and shared principles. In general, healthy dietary patterns are abundant in fruits, vegetables, legumes, whole grains, nuts and seeds, plant or lean animal protein, and fish. In addition, *trans* fats, sodium, processed meats, added sugars, and sugar-sweetened beverages are limited. Research has demonstrated that a healthy dietary pattern followed throughout the life course will lower ASCVD risk to a clinically significant extent. This is true for both individuals with high genetic risk and those who do not have a genetic predisposition. In an analysis of three large prospective cohorts and one cross-sectional study, following a healthy lifestyle (meeting at least three of the four criteria [no smoking, not obese, regular physical activity, and a healthy diet]) compared to an unhealthy lifestyle (≤1 of the four criteria) lowered risk of CAD by 46% in individuals with high genetic predisposition; this is comparable to the risk reduction observed in individuals at low genetic risk following a healthy lifestyle compared to an unhealthy lifestyle (45%).[111,112]

Three eating patterns for general health and reducing chronic disease risk were recommended in the 2015–2020 Dietary Guidelines for Americans: the healthy US-style eating pattern, the healthy Mediterranean-style eating pattern, and the healthy vegetarian eating pattern (Table 22.3).[81] These eating patterns were derived using food pattern modeling and each meet the 2015–2020 US Dietary Guidelines food-based and nutrient recommendations.

DASH diet

The DASH dietary pattern is rich in fruits, vegetables, and low-fat dairy, is low in saturated fat, and is high in calcium, potassium, and magnesium (Table 22.3). A recent umbrella review of systematic reviews and meta-analyses, including 15 prospective cohorts and 31 controlled trials, found decreased incidence of CVD (RR 0.80, 95% CI:0.76–0.85), CHD (0.79, 95% CI: 0.71–0.88), and significant reductions in both systolic blood pressure (SBP) (mean difference = −5.2 mmHg, 95% CI: −7.0 to −3.4) and DBP (−2.60 mmHg, 95% CI: −3.50 to −1.70) with consumption of the DASH dietary pattern (both with and without reductions in sodium).[75]

In the original clinical trial, the DASH diet (~3000 mg/day sodium) lowered SBP −5.5 mmHg and DBP −3.0 mmHg in all populations compared to the typical American diet (also held to ~3000 mg/day sodium) with greater reduction in minority groups but no differences between sexes.[83] Individuals with stage 1 hypertension (SBP: 130–139 or DBP: 80–89 mmHg) had the greatest blood pressure reductions (SBP: −11.4 mm Hg and DBP: −5.5 mmHg) compared to normotensive individuals (SBP: −3.5 mm Hg and DBP: −2.1 mm Hg) when consuming the DASH diet.[83] Furthermore, there were significant reductions in total cholesterol (−13.5 mg/dL) and LDL-C (−10.8 mg/dL) in the DASH diet group with no significant differences by race or baseline lipid levels.[113]

In the DASH Sodium Trial, compared with a typical American diet the DASH diet significantly lowered blood pressure at three sodium levels (1150, 2300, and 3450 mg/day), with more significant reductions in the lowest sodium group.[114] A recent systematic review and meta-analysis of randomized controlled trials including 20 articles (and 1917 participants) estimated that the DASH diet reduced CVD risk by 13%, based on the blood pressure and lipid/lipoprotein improvements observed with the DASH diet, which were independent of differences in dietary sodium intake.[115]

Mediterranean diet

The Mediterranean diet refers to the traditional dietary patterns of the countries that border the Mediterranean Sea. While there are some differences by country or region, these diets are rich in olive oil, vegetables, fruits, nuts, legumes, seafood, and whole grains with lower intakes of processed meats, red meats, dairy, and added sugar (Table 22.3). This dietary pattern generally has a higher monounsaturated fatty acids/polyunsaturated fatty acids to saturated fatty acids ratio (MUFA/PUFA: SFA) because it is low in saturated fat and higher in unsaturated fats.

Observational cohort studies such as the Nurses Health Study[116] showed a 22% lower CVD risk (CHD and stroke) and ~40% reduced risk of a fatal CVD event in women with higher adherence to a Mediterranean dietary pattern compared to women with the lowest adherence.[116–118] A recent systematic review and meta-analysis of 29 observational studies showed reduced risk of CVD in those following a Mediterranean diet: the pooled RR for those with the highest compared to lowest Mediterranean diet score for CHD/acute myocardial infarction based on 11 studies was 0.70 (95% CI: 0.62 to 0.80), for unspecified stroke based on six studies 0.73 (95% CI: 0.59 to 0.91), and ischemic stroke based on five studies 0.82 (95% CI: 0.73 to 0.92).[119]

PREDIMED (discussed previously), a large clinical trial conducted in Spain, assessed the effects of the Mediterranean diet supplemented with extra virgin olive oil (≥50 g/day) or with mixed nuts (30 g/day [15 g walnuts, 7.5 g hazelnuts, and 7.5 g almonds]) compared to a control lower fat (<30% of calories) diet on CVD events in high-risk individuals >55 years at onset of the study. The primary endpoint of total cardiovascular events (a composite of MI, stroke, and death from CVD causes) was lower in the intervention groups after approximately 5 years of follow-up. The hazard ratio for the olive oil group compared to the lower fat group was 0.69 (95% CI: 0.53 to 0.91) and for the nut group compared to the lower fat diet 0.72 (95% CI: 0.54 to 0.95), demonstrating that a Mediterranean-style eating pattern, supplemented with extra virgin olive oil or mixed nuts, compared to the control diet, reduced CVD risk.[73] Significant reductions were observed in fasting glucose, blood pressure, and total cholesterol in both intervention groups compared to the lower fat group. Overall, there was an approximate 30% reduction in risk of major cardiovascular events for individuals following the Mediterranean diet.[73] Furthermore, a meta-analysis of 27 prospective cohort studies and clinical trials showed an 11% relative risk reduction in CVD outcomes for each two-point increase in adherence to a Mediterranean diet (on a nine-point scale).[117] The results of these studies show consistent benefits of a Mediterranean dietary pattern on CVD risk reduction.

Vegetarian diet (includes vegan)

Vegetarian diets are characterized by fruits, vegetables, whole grains, nuts, legumes, and seeds. A vegan diet excludes all animal products, notably meat, eggs, dairy, and fish, but for some, also animal-derived ingredients (e.g., honey, gelatin, whey, etc.), while the pesco-vegetarian diet includes fish, but not meat.[81] A lactoovo vegetarian diet includes eggs and dairy, but no meat or fish,[81] with other variations depending on beliefs and preferences, such as a flexitarian diet or semivegetarian—mainly a vegetarian diet with occasional incorporation of meat and fish. Individuals following a healthy vegetarian diet will also likely have higher intakes of fiber and unsaturated fat, both MUFA and PUFA, with decreased SFA, cholesterol, and sodium, compared to a typical American diet.[120] However, care must be taken to ensure vegetarian/vegan diets are appropriately planned and nutritionally adequate.[121]

Epidemiologic evidence shows decreased risk of CVD with consumption of healthy vegetarian eating patterns compared to a typical American diet. A North American cohort of Seventh-day Adventists consuming a vegetarian diet had a standard mortality ratio of 0.74 (95% CI: 0.63 to 0.88) for ischemic heart disease (IHD) when compared to nonvegetarians and overall lower all-cause mortality (HR: 0.88 [95% CI: 0.80 to 0.97]).[122] While questions about the impact that other lifestyle factors related to Seventh-day Adventist philosophy may have on such metrics, a systematic review and meta-analysis of prospective cohort studies comparing vegetarians to nonvegetarians estimated a 29% reduction in mortality from IHD.[123] Furthermore, vegetarian diets are associated with more desirable lipid and lipoprotein levels when compared to a poor-quality American diet. A recent systematic review and metaanalysis of 30 observational and 19 intervention trials compared vegetarian-style diets with omnivorous diets; vegetarian-style diets were associated with lower total cholesterol (−29.2 and −12.5 mg/dL) and LDL-C (−22.9 and −12.2 mg/dL) in the observational studies and in the clinical trials, respectively.[124]

The 2015–2020 Dietary Guidelines for Americans include a healthy vegetarian-style eating pattern (see Table 22.2). The importance of following a healthy plant-based diet (rich in fruits/vegetables, whole grains, nuts/legumes) compared to an unhealthy plant-based diet (high in sugar-sweetened beverages, refined grains, and sweets) is highlighted in recent analyses from large prospective cohorts in the United States.[125] Using an assessment instrument and assigning diet scores for degree of dietary alignment with different plant-based diets, greater adherence to a healthy plant-based diet was inversely associated with CHD (HR: 0.75, 95% CI: 0.68–0.83); however, an unhealthy plant-based diet was associated with greater risk of CHD (HR: 1.32, 95% CI: 1.20–1.46). Thus, these findings indicate that following a healthy vegetarian diet, such as the USDA's healthy vegetarian diet[81] that includes recommended intakes of macro- and micronutrients (which can be inadequate or in excess if following a low-quality vegetarian diet), decreases risk of CHD.

B. Dietary Guidance in the Management of ASCVD

A healthy dietary pattern is essential in the management of ASCVD risk, regardless of pharmacotherapy.[10] The healthy dietary patterns discussed in the previous section are appropriate for management of ASCVD[10,36,38,82]; however, additional specific recommendations are important for the management of dyslipidemias and hypertension. These recommendations focus on weight management and the addition of specific nutrient targets for those with dyslipidemia or hypertension. Additionally, referral to a Registered Dietitian Nutritionist (RDN) is recommended to increase adherence to a healthy dietary pattern.

To lower elevated LDL-C (and non-HDL-C)

- Adopt saturated fat (SFA) intake goal of <7% of total energy (<15 g or 140 kcal based on a 2000 kcal/day diet).[10] A greater reduction of SFA intake to 5%–6% of total energy results in further LDL-C lowering.[82] Currently, the average intake of SFA in the United States is ~11%[126] and reducing intake to <7% is expected to lower LDL-C by up to 10%.[127] To achieve the SFA goal, recommendations are to replace dietary SFA with MUFA/PUFA and/or whole grains.[10] To reduce intake of SFA, choose lean cuts of meat and low- or no-fat dairy, avoid processed meats, and choose nontropical vegetable oils.
- Consume 5–10 g of viscous, or soluble, fiber daily reduces LDL-C by 3%–5%.[10] To achieve LDL-C lowering, individuals following a 2000 kcal/day Healthy US-Style eating pattern should consume 31 g of fiber/day[128] with 5–10 g being viscous fiber. Good sources of viscous fiber include legumes, oats, fruits (e.g., oranges and apples), and vegetables (e.g., broccoli and Brussels sprouts).
- Achieve a clinically meaningful weight loss of ≥5% of initial body weight.[36] A systematic review of 13 studies demonstrated that weight loss of 10 kg was associated with ~9 mg/dL reduction in total cholesterol and ~8 mg/dL reduction in LDL-C.[129]

To manage hypertriglyceridemia

- Intensive lifestyle change can lower TG levels by as much as 50% in individuals with hypertriglyceridemia.[130] Interventions vary based on severity of hypertriglyceridemia (moderate hypertriglyceridemia: 150–499 mg/dL (fasting or nonfasting); severe hypertriglyceridemia: > 500 mg/dL (fasting); suspected cause such as uncontrolled diabetes mellitus, enzyme deficiency, or medications; and risk of pancreatitis.[10]
- Intake of added sugars should be limited to <10% if TG <500 mg/dL or <5% if TG >500 mg/dL of total energy and would be expected to lower TG by 10%–25%.[10,131–133] The primary sources of added sugars in the American diet are sugar-sweetened beverages, baked goods, and desserts including candy.[134]
- Major sources of refined grains are white bread, pasta, processed breakfast cereals, snack/meal bars, and white rice; they should be replaced with fiber-rich whole grains.
- Consumption of alcohol should be reduced when TGs are 150–500 mg/dL or eliminated if TGs are >500 mg/dL,[135] especially in obese individuals to reduce the risk of pancreatitis.[10,82] Consuming 30 g of ethanol, or ~2 standard drinks[105] per day, is expected to increase TG by 6 mg/dL.[136]
- Intake of 1–4 g/day n-3 fatty acids from EPA and DHA has been shown to lower TG 3%–45% depending upon baseline TG levels and the quantity of n-3 fatty acids consumed.[10] The recommended intake for individuals with high TG (200–499 mg/dL) and very high TG (≥500 mg/dL) is 4 g/day of prescription EPA or EPA + DHA.[106] This dose may confer ~20%–30% reduction in patients with high TG and ≥30% reductions in patients with very high TG.[106] The available evidence indicates that just 10% of Americans consume 0.5 g of EPA + DHA per day from diet,[137] which is the population-based dietary recommendation issued by the Academy of Nutrition and Dietetics.[138] Over-the-counter fish oil supplements are available; however, prescription capsules contain higher amounts of EPA and DHA and are necessary to obtain these higher therapeutic doses recommended for the treatment of hypertriglyceridemia.[81]
- Weight loss of 5%–10% is recommended for individuals who are overweight or obese to reduce TG.[10] Reductions of 5%–15% of body weight are associated with 20%–30% reductions in TG.

To decrease hypertension

- Lower body weight; a meta-analysis of 25 intervention trials reported a −4.44 mmHg reduction in SBP and −3.57 mmHg reduction in DBP with a mean weight loss of 5.1 kg, but greater weight loss was associated with greater BP improvements.[139] For individuals with a BMI >25 kg/m^2 and elevated BP or hypertension, weight loss is recommended.

- Consume a DASH diet which has been shown to lower SBP ~11 mmHg and DBP ~5 mmHg in individuals with hypertension.[83]
- Sodium should be reduced if daily consumption exceeds 2300 mg/day.[85] Reducing sodium by 1000 mg/day with an optimal goal of ~1500 mg/day may lower SBP 5–6 mmHg.[38] To achieve this goal, a low sodium DASH dietary pattern is recommended. Approximately 70% of sodium consumed is added outside the home[140]; therefore, care should be taken to select lower sodium foods based on the Nutrition Facts Panel, and lower sodium options should be selected when eating out.
- Dietary sources of potassium should be increased with a goal of >2600 mg.[85] Intake of 3500–5000 mg may lower SBP by 4–5 mmHg.[38] Consuming a diet abundant in fruits and vegetables such as the DASH diet will aid in achieving increased potassium intake with reductions in dietary sodium intake.

Overweight and obesity

- In patients who are overweight or obese, weight loss is recommended to reduce ASCVD risk.[11,36,38] To achieve weight loss, negative energy balance is required; an approximate calorie deficit of 500 kcal/day is expected to result in weight loss of one pound per week. Weight loss of as little as 3%–5% of body weight can result in clinically meaningful improvements in ASCVD risk factors.[141]
- Current evidence does not define one diet or a "best diet" that patients should be counseled on to decrease energy intake.[141] Therefore, for a prescribed daily calorie deficit, a number of dietary approaches can be implemented to achieve weight loss, including the dietary patterns outlined in the previous section or diets with specific targets for macronutrients (carbohydrate, fat, protein) (see Chapter 9, Eating Behavior and Strategies to Promote Weight Loss and Maintenance).

Role of the Registered Dietitian Nutritionist

Adherence to a healthy dietary pattern is critical for the management of ASCVD. The current guidelines for prevention of CVD, management of dyslipidemia, and management of hypertension recommend a team-based health care approach, and central is the involvement of a RDN.[10,36,38] Patients may see improvements in total cholesterol, LDL-C, and TG with only two to four medical nutrition therapy sessions with a RDN.[142] Additionally, such therapy sessions are associated with reduced need for pharmacotherapy interventions for dyslipidemia and better LDL-C lowering outcomes.[142,143] Overall, working closely with an RDN may increase adherence to a heart-healthy diet, improve CVD risk factors, and help maintain weight loss.

RESEARCH GAPS

- The crucial role of diet in the prevention of CVD is established beyond doubt. Despite the strong evidence of the benefits of healthy dietary patterns, the diet quality gap for all population groups has not tangibly closed (i.e., what people are eating vs. what they should be eating). The daunting challenge that lies ahead is to identify population-based strategies that elicit measurable improvements in diet quality.
- As recently recommended by Anderson et al.[144] to enable healthier food choices consistent with ideal cardiovascular health, the following are critically needed:
  - healthy and innovative system-level approaches that improve food consumption behaviors on an individual and on a population basis,
  - stronger industry and community efforts, and
  - policies aligned with evidence-based recommendations.
- There is a pressing need for research to identify effective system-level approaches that markedly improve diet quality.
- There is a need to improve the understanding of how to more precisely characterize dietary patterns by their food constituents and the implications of the food constituents on nutrient adequacy through the use of Food Pattern Modeling; more precise characterization, particularly of protein foods, is needed.[81]
- Effective strategies that individualize and align one of the recommended healthy dietary patterns to an individual's culture and food preferences are needed to increase the probability of long-term adoption of a healthy dietary pattern that improves CVD health.

Acknowledgments

This chapter is an update of the chapter titled "Atherosclerotic Cardiovascular Disease" by Simone D. Holligan, Claire E. Berryman, Li Wang, Michael R. Flock, Kristina A. Harris, and Penny M. Kris-Etherton, in Present Knowledge in Nutrition, 10th Edition, edited by Erdman JW, Macdonald IA, and Zeisel SH and published by Wiley-Blackwell. © 2012 International Life Sciences Institute. Portions of this update are from the previously published chapter and the contributions of previous authors are acknowledged.

V. REFERENCES

1. Cahill PA, Redmond EM. Vascular endothelium – Gatekeeper of vessel health. *Atherosclerosis*. 2016;248:97–109. https://doi.org/10.1016/j.atherosclerosis.2016.03.007.
2. Murakami M. Signaling required for blood vessel maintenance: molecular basis and pathological manifestations. *Int J Vasc Med*. 2012;2012. https://doi.org/10.1155/2012/293641.
3. Abdel-Sater K. Pathophysiology of the endothelium. *EC Cardiol*. 2015;1:17–26.
4. Ono S, Egawa G, Kabashima K. Regulation of blood vascular permeability in the skin. *Inflamm Regen*. 2017;37(1):11. https://doi.org/10.1186/s41232-017-0042-9.
5. Linton MF, Yancey PG, Davies SS, et al. The role of lipids and lipoproteins in atherosclerosis. *Endotext [Internet]*. 2019. MDText.com, Inc.
6. Gouverneur M, Van Den Berg B, Nieuwdorp M, Stroes E, Vink H. Vasculoprotective properties of the endothelial glycocalyx: effects of fluid shear stress. *J Intern Med*. 2006;259(4):393–400. https://doi.org/10.1111/j.1365-2796.2006.01625.x.
7. Chang E, Nayak L, Jain MK. Kruppel-like factors in endothelial cell biology. *Curr Opin Hematol*. 2017;24(3):224–229. https://doi.org/10.1097/MOH.0000000000000337.
8. Silverman MG, Ference BA, Im K, et al. Association between lowering LDL-C and cardiovascular risk reduction among different therapeutic interventions. *J Am Med Assoc*. 2016;316(12):1289. https://doi.org/10.1001/jama.2016.13985.
9. Zakiev ER, Sukhorukov VN, Melnichenko AA, Sobenin IA, Ivanova EA, Orekhov AN. Lipid composition of circulating multiple-modified low density lipoprotein. *Lipids Health Dis*. 2016;15(1):134. https://doi.org/10.1186/s12944-016-0308-2.
10. Jacobson TA, Maki KC, Orringer CE, et al. National lipid association recommendations for patient-centered management of dyslipidemia: Part 2. *J Clin Lipidol*. 2015;9(6). https://doi.org/10.1016/J.JACL.2015.09.002. S1-S122.e1.
11. Grundy SM, Stone NJ, Bailey AL, et al. 2018 AHA/ACC/AACVPR/AAPA/ABC/ACPM/ADA/AGS/APhA/ASPC/NLA/PCNA guideline on the management of blood cholesterol: a report of the American College of Cardiology/American Heart Association Task Force on Clinical Practice Guidelines. *J Am Coll Cardiol*. 2019;73(24):e285–e350.
12. Morrow DA, Gersh BJ. Chronic coronary artery disease. In: *Braunwald's Heart Disease: A Textbook of Cardiovascular Medicine*. 8th ed. Philadelphia: Elsevier; 2007.
13. Benjamin EJ, Muntner P, Alonso A, et al. Heart disease and stroke statistics—2019 update: a report from the American Heart Association. *Circulation*. 2019;139(10):e56–e528. https://doi.org/10.1161/CIR.0000000000000659.
14. Nguyen M, Cohen J. Peripheral vascular disease. In: *Pain Medicine*. Springer; 2017:495–496.
15. Chiu J-J, Chien S. Effects of disturbed flow on vascular endothelium: pathophysiological basis and clinical perspectives. *Physiol Rev*. 2011;91(1):327–387. https://doi.org/10.1152/physrev.00047.2009.
16. Tabas I, Garcia-Cardena G, Owens GK. Recent insights into the cellular biology of atherosclerosis. *J Cell Biol*. 2015;209(1):13–22. https://doi.org/10.1083/jcb.201412052.
17. van den Berg BM, Spaan JAE, Rolf TM, Vink H. Atherogenic region and diet diminish glycocalyx dimension and increase intima-to-media ratios at murine carotid artery bifurcation. *Am J Physiol Heart Circ Physiol*. 2006;290(2):H915–H920. https://doi.org/10.1152/ajpheart.00051.2005.
18. Victor VM, Rocha M, Sola E, Banuls C, Garcia-Malpartida K, Hernandez-Mijares A. Oxidative stress, endothelial dysfunction and atherosclerosis. *Curr Pharmaceut Des*. 2009;15(26):2988–3002.
19. Borén J, Olin K, Lee I, Chait A, Wight TN, Innerarity TL. Identification of the principal proteoglycan-binding site in LDL. A single-point mutation in apo-B100 severely affects proteoglycan interaction without affecting LDL receptor binding. *J Clin Invest*. 1998;101(12):2658–2664.
20. Abdullah SM, Defina LF, Leonard D, et al. Long-Term association of low-density lipoprotein cholesterol with cardiovascular mortality in individuals at low 10-year risk of atherosclerotic cardiovascular disease: results from the Cooper Center Longitudinal Study. *Circulation*. 2018;138(21):2315–2325.
21. Ivanova EA, Myasoedova VA, Melnichenko AA, Grechko AV, Orekhov AN. Small dense low-density lipoprotein as biomarker for atherosclerotic diseases. *Oxid Med Cell Longev*. 2017;2017.
22. Young IS, McEneny J. Lipoprotein oxidation and atherosclerosis. *Biochem Soc Trans*. 2001;29:358–362.
23. Tertov VV, Kaplun VV, Sobenin IA, Orekhov AN. Low-density lipoprotein modification occurring in human plasma possible mechanism of in vivo lipoprotein desialylation as a primary step of atherogenic modification. *Atherosclerosis*. 1998;138(1):183–195.
24. Nikifirov NG, Zakiev ER, Elizova N, Sukhorukov VN, Orekhov AN. Multiple-modified low-density lipoprotein as atherogenic factor of patients'; blood: development of therapeutic approaches to reduce blood atherogenicity. *Curr Pharmaceut Des*. 2017;23(6):932–936. https://doi.org/10.2174/1381612823666170124112918.
25. Orekhov AN, Oishi Y, Nikiforov NG, et al. Modified LDL particles activate inflammatory pathways in monocyte-derived macrophages: transcriptome analysis. *Curr Pharmaceut Des*. 2018;24(26):3143–3151. https://doi.org/10.2174/1381612824666180911120039.
26. Orekhov AN, Ivanova EA, Melnichenko AA, Sobenin IA. Circulating desialylated low density lipoprotein. *Cor Vasa*. 2017;59(2):e149–e156.
27. Gimbrone Jr MA, García-Cardeña G. Endothelial cell dysfunction and the pathobiology of atherosclerosis. *Circ Res*. 2016;118(4):620–636.
28. Libby P. Inflammation in atherosclerosis. *Nature*. 2002;420(6917):868–874. https://doi.org/10.1038/nature01323.
29. Hansson GK. Inflammation, atherosclerosis, and coronary artery disease. *N Engl J Med*. 2005;352(16):1685–1695.
30. Falk E. Pathogenesis of atherosclerosis. *J Am Coll Cardiol*. 2006;47(suppl 8):C7–C12.
31. Glass CK, Witztum JL. Atherosclerosis: the road ahead. *Cell*. 2001;104(4):503–516.

32. Lewis GF, Rader DJ. New insights into the regulation of HDL metabolism and reverse cholesterol transport. *Circ Res*. 2005; 96(12):1221–1232.
33. Tall AR, Jiang X, Luo Y, Silver D. 1999 George Lyman Duff memorial lecture: lipid transfer proteins, HDL metabolism, and atherogenesis. *Arterioscler Thromb Vasc Biol*. 2000;20(5):1185–1188.
34. Burgess JW, Sinclair PA, Chretien CM, Boucher J, Sparks DL. Reverse cholesterol transport. In: *Biochemistry of Atherosclerosis*. Springer; 2006:3–22.
35. Schaar JA, Muller JE, Falk E, et al. Terminology for high-risk and vulnerable coronary artery plaques. *Eur Heart J*. 2004;25(12): 1077–1082.
36. Arnett DK, Blumenthal RS, Albert MA, et al. 2019 ACC/AHA guideline on the primary prevention of cardiovascular disease: executive summary: a report of the American College of Cardiology/American Heart Association Task Force on Clinical Practice Guidelines. *J Am Coll Cardiol*. 2019;74(10):1376–1414. https://doi.org/10.1161/CIR.0000000000000678.
37. Ridker PM, Brown NJ, Vaughan DE, Harrison DG, Mehta JL. Established and emerging plasma biomarkers in the prediction of first atherothrombotic events. *Circulation*. 2004;109(25_suppl_1). IV-6.
38. Whelton PK, Carey RM, Aronow WS, et al. 2017 ACC/AHA/AAPA/ABC/ACPM/AGS/APhA/ASH/ASPC/NMA/PCNA guideline for the prevention, detection, evaluation, and management of high blood pressure in adults: a report of the American College of Cardiology/American Heart Association Task Force on Clinical Pr. *J Am Coll Cardiol*. 2018;71(19):e127–e248. https://doi.org/10.1016/J.JACC.2017.11.006.
39. Roy A, Rawal I, Jabbour S, Prabhakaran D. Tobacco and cardiovascular disease: a summary of evidence. In: *Cardiovascular, Respiratory, and Related Disorders*. 3rd ed. The International Bank for Reconstruction and Development/The World Bank; 2017.
40. Vindhyal MR, Ndunda P, Munguti C, Vindhyal S, Okut H. Impact on cardiovascular outcomes among e-cigarette users: a review from national health interview surveys. *J Am Coll Cardiol*. 2019;73(9 Suppl 2):11. https://doi.org/10.1016/S0735-1097(19)33773-8.
41. Darville A, Hahn EJ. E-cigarettes and atherosclerotic cardiovascular disease: what clinicians and researchers need to know. *Curr Atherosclerosis Rep*. 2019;21(5):15.
42. Centers for Disease Control and Prevention. *About Electronic Cigarettes (E-Cigarettes)*; 2019. https://www.cdc.gov/tobacco/basic_information/e-cigarettes/about-e-cigarettes.html.
43. American Heart Association. My Life Check-Life's Simple 7. http://mylifecheck.heart.org/Multitab.aspx?NavID=3.
44. Rafieian-Kopaei M, Setorki M, Doudi M, Baradaran A, Nasri H. Atherosclerosis: process, indicators, risk factors and new hopes. *Int J Prev Med*. 2014;5(8):927.
45. Ambale Venkatesh B, Volpe GJ, Donekal S, et al. Association of longitudinal changes in left ventricular structure and function with myocardial fibrosis: the Multi-Ethnic Study of Atherosclerosis study. *Hypertension (Dallas)*. 2014;64(3):508–515. https://doi.org/10.1161/HYPERTENSIONAHA.114.03697.
46. Palombo C, Kozakova M. Arterial stiffness, atherosclerosis and cardiovascular risk: pathophysiologic mechanisms and emerging clinical indications. *Vasc Pharmacol*. 2016;77:1–7. https://doi.org/10.1016/J.VPH.2015.11.083.
47. Lacolley P, Regnault V, Segers P, Laurent S. Vascular smooth muscle cells and arterial stiffening: relevance in development, aging, and disease. *Physiol Rev*. 2017;97(4):1555–1617. https://doi.org/10.1152/physrev.00003.2017.
48. Torzewski M, Rist C, Mortensen RF, et al. C-reactive protein in the arterial intima: role of C-reactive protein receptor-dependent monocyte recruitment in atherogenesis. *Arterioscler Thromb Vasc Biol*. 2000;20(9):2094–2099.
49. Kozakova M, Morizzo C, Guarino D, et al. The impact of age and risk factors on carotid and carotid-femoral pulse wave velocity. *J Hypertens*. 2015;33(7):1446–1451. https://doi.org/10.1097/HJH.0000000000000582.
50. AlGhatrif M, Strait JB, Morrell CH, et al. Longitudinal trajectories of arterial stiffness and the role of blood pressure: the Baltimore Longitudinal Study of Aging. *Hypertension (Dallas)*. 2013;62(5):934–941. https://doi.org/10.1161/HYPERTENSIONAHA.113.01445.
51. Ben-Shlomo Y, Spears M, Boustred C, et al. Aortic pulse wave velocity improves cardiovascular event prediction: an individual participant meta-analysis of prospective observational data from 17,635 subjects. *J Am Coll Cardiol*. 2014;63(7):636–646. https://doi.org/10.1016/j.jacc.2013.09.063.
52. Grundy SM, Cleeman JI, Daniels SR, et al. Diagnosis and management of the metabolic syndrome: an American heart association/national heart, lung, and blood institute scientific statement. *Circulation*. 2005;112(17):2735–2752.
53. The Emerging Risk Factors Collaboration. Diabetes mellitus, fasting blood glucose concentration, and risk of vascular disease: a collaborative meta-analysis of 102 prospective studies. *Lancet*. 2010;375(9733):2215–2222. https://doi.org/10.1016/S0140-6736(10)60484-9.
54. Jin C, Chen S, Vaidya A, et al. Longitudinal change in fasting blood glucose and myocardial infarction risk in a population without diabetes. *Diabetes Care*. 2017;40(11). https://doi.org/10.2337/dc17-0610, 1565 LP - 1572.
55. Madonna R, De Caterina R. Cellular and molecular mechanisms of vascular injury in diabetes — Part I: pathways of vascular disease in diabetes. *Vasc Pharmacol*. 2011;54(3–6):68–74. https://doi.org/10.1016/j.vph.2011.03.005.
56. Perkins JM, Joy NG, Tate DB, Davis SN. Acute effects of hyperinsulinemia and hyperglycemia on vascular inflammatory biomarkers and endothelial function in overweight and obese humans. *Am J Physiol Endocrinol Metab*. 2015;309(2):E168–E176. https://doi.org/10.1152/ajpendo.00064.2015.
57. Younis N, Charlton-Menys V, Sharma R, Soran H, Durrington PN. Glycation of LDL in non-diabetic people: small dense LDL is preferentially glycated both in vivo and in vitro. *Atherosclerosis*. 2009; 202:162–168. https://doi.org/10.1016/j.atherosclerosis.2008.04.036.
58. Malik S, Budoff MJ, Katz R, et al. Impact of subclinical atherosclerosis on cardiovascular disease events in individuals with metabolic syndrome and diabetes: the multi-ethnic study of atherosclerosis. *Diabetes Care*. 2011;34(10):2285–2290. https://doi.org/10.2337/dc11-0816.
59. Bertoni AG, Kramer H, Watson K, Post WS. Diabetes and clinical and subclinical CVD. 2016;11(3):337–342. https://doi.org/10.1016/j.gheart.2016.07.005.
60. Liu L, Simon B, Shi J, Mallhi AK, Eisen HJ. Impact of diabetes mellitus on risk of cardiovascular disease and all-cause mortality: evidence on health outcomes and antidiabetic treatment in United States adults. *World J Diabetes*. 2016;7(18):449. https://doi.org/10.4239/wjd.v7.i18.449.
61. Glechner A, Keuchel L, Affengruber L, et al. Effects of lifestyle changes on adults with prediabetes: a systematic review and meta-analysis. *Prim Care Diabetes*. 2018;12(5):393–408. https://doi.org/10.1016/j.pcd.2018.07.003.
62. Afshin A, Sur PJ, Fay KA, et al. Health effects of dietary risks in 195 countries, 1990–2017: a systematic analysis for the Global Burden of Disease Study 2017. *Lancet*. 2019;393(10184): 1958–1972. https://doi.org/10.1016/S0140-6736(19)30041-8.
63. Lloyd-Jones DM, Hong Y, Labarthe D, et al. Defining and setting national goals for cardiovascular health promotion and disease reduction. *Circulation*. 2010;121(4):586–613. https://doi.org/10.1161/CIRCULATIONAHA.109.192703.

64. George SM, Ballard-Barbash R, Manson JE, et al. Comparing indices of diet quality with chronic disease mortality risk in postmenopausal women in the women's health initiative observational study: evidence to inform national dietary guidance. *Am J Epidemiol*. 2014; 180(6):616–625. https://doi.org/10.1093/aje/kwu173.
65. Harmon BE, Boushey CJ, Shvetsov YB, et al. Associations of key diet-quality indexes with mortality in the multiethnic cohort: the dietary patterns methods project. *Am J Clin Nutr*. 2015; 101(3):587–597. https://doi.org/10.3945/ajcn.114.090688.
66. Reedy J, Krebs-Smith SM, Miller PE, et al. Higher diet quality is associated with decreased risk of all-cause, cardiovascular disease, and cancer mortality among older adults. *J Nutr*. 2014; 144(6):881–889. https://doi.org/10.3945/jn.113.189407.
67. Yu D, Sonderman J, Buchowski MS, et al. Healthy eating and risks of total and cause-specific death among low-income populations of African-Americans and other adults in the Southeastern United States: a prospective cohort study. *PLoS Med*. 2015;12(5):e1001830. https://doi.org/10.1371/journal.pmed.1001830.
68. Schwingshackl L, Hoffmann G. Diet quality as assessed by the healthy eating index, the alternate healthy eating index, the dietary approaches to stop hypertension score, and health outcomes: a systematic review and meta-analysis of cohort studies. *J Acad Nutr Diet*. 2015;115(5):780–800. https://doi.org/10.1016/j.jand.2014.12.009.
69. Sotos-Prieto M, Bhupathiraju SN, Mattei J, et al. Association of changes in diet quality with total and cause-specific mortality. *N Engl J Med*. 2017;377(2):143–153. https://doi.org/10.1056/NEJMoa1613502.
70. Hu FB, Rimm EB, Stampfer MJ, Ascherio A, Spiegelman D, Willett WC. Prospective study of major dietary patterns and risk of coronary heart disease in men. *Am J Clin Nutr*. 2000;72(4): 912–921. https://doi.org/10.1093/ajcn/72.4.912.
71. Fung TT, Willett WC, Stampfer MJ, Manson JE, Hu FB. Dietary patterns and the risk of coronary heart disease in women. *Arch Intern Med*. 2001;161(15):1857–1862. http://www.ncbi.nlm.nih.gov/pubmed/11493127.
72. Drake I, Sonestedt E, Ericson U, Wallström P, Orho-Melander M. A Western dietary pattern is prospectively associated with cardio-metabolic traits and incidence of the metabolic syndrome. *Br J Nutr*. 2018;119(10):1168–1176. https://doi.org/10.1017/S000711451800079X.
73. Estruch R, Ros E, Salas-Salvadó J, et al. Primary prevention of cardiovascular disease with a Mediterranean diet supplemented with extra-virgin olive oil or nuts. *N Engl J Med*. June 2018. https://doi.org/10.1056/NEJMoa1800389. Epub ahead of print.
74. Ndanuko RN, Tapsell LC, Charlton KE, Neale EP, Batterham MJ. Dietary patterns and blood pressure in adults: a systematic review and meta-analysis of randomized controlled trials. *Adv Nutr*. 2016; 7(1):76–89. https://doi.org/10.3945/an.115.009753.
75. Chiavaroli L, Viguiliouk E, Nishi SK, et al. DASH dietary pattern and cardiometabolic outcomes: an umbrella review of systematic reviews and meta-analyses. *Nutrients*. 2019;11(2):338. https://doi.org/10.3390/nu11020338.
76. Neale EP, Batterham MJ, Tapsell LC. Consumption of a healthy dietary pattern results in significant reductions in C-reactive protein levels in adults: a meta-analysis. *Nutr Res*. 2016;36(5):391–401. https://doi.org/10.1016/j.nutres.2016.02.009.
77. Rees K, Takeda A, Martin N, et al. Mediterranean-style diet for the primary and secondary prevention of cardiovascular disease. *Cochrane Database Syst Rev*. 2019;3:CD009825. https://doi.org/10.1002/14651858.CD009825.pub3.
78. Nordmann AJ, Suter-Zimmermann K, Bucher HC, et al. Meta-analysis comparing mediterranean to low-fat diets for modification of cardiovascular risk factors. *Am J Med*. 2011;124(9). https://doi.org/10.1016/j.amjmed.2011.04.024, 841-851.e2.
79. Jennings A, Berendsen AM, de Groot LCPGM, et al. Mediterranean-style diet improves systolic blood pressure and arterial stiffness in older adults. *Hypertension*. 2019;73(3): 578–586. https://doi.org/10.1161/HYPERTENSIONAHA.118.12259.
80. Davis CR, Hodgson JM, Woodman R, Bryan J, Wilson C, Murphy KJ. A Mediterranean diet lowers blood pressure and improves endothelial function: results from the MedLey randomized intervention trial. *Am J Clin Nutr*. 2017;105(6). https://doi.org/10.3945/ajcn.116.146803. ajcn146803.
81. Dietary Guidelines Advisory Committee. *Scientific Report of the 2015 Dietary Guidelines Advisory Committee: Advisory Report to the Secretary of Health and Human Services and the Secretary of Agriculture. Washington (DC)*. 2015.
82. Eckel RH, Jakicic JM, Ard JD, et al. 2013 AHA/ACC guideline on lifestyle management to reduce cardiovascular risk: a report of the American College of Cardiology/American Heart Association Task Force on Practice Guidelines. *J Am Coll Cardiol*. 2014;63(25 Pt B):2960–2984. https://doi.org/10.1016/j.jacc.2013.11.003.
83. Appel LJ, Moore TJ, Obarzanek E, et al. A clinical trial of the effects of dietary patterns on blood pressure. *N Engl J Med*. 1997; 336(16):1117–1124. https://doi.org/10.1056/NEJM199704173361601.
84. Soltani S, Chitsazi MJ, Salehi-Abargouei A. The effect of dietary approaches to stop hypertension (DASH) on serum inflammatory markers: a systematic review and meta-analysis of randomized trials. *Clin Nutr*. 2018;37(2):542–550. https://doi.org/10.1016/j.clnu.2017.02.018.
85. National Academies of Science Engineering and Medicine. *Dietary Reference Intakes for Sodium and Potassium*. Washington, DC: National Academies Press; 2019.
86. Greaney JL, DuPont JJ, Lennon-Edwards SL, Sanders PW, Edwards DG, Farquhar WB. Dietary sodium loading impairs microvascular function independent of blood pressure in humans: role of oxidative stress. *J Physiol*. 2012;590(21):5519–5528.
87. DuPont JJ, Greaney JL, Wenner MM, et al. High dietary sodium intake impairs endothelium-dependent dilation in healthy salt-resistant humans. *J Hypertens*. 2013;31(3):530.
88. D'Elia L, Galletti F, La Fata E, Sabino P, Strazzullo P. Effect of dietary sodium restriction on arterial stiffness: systematic review and meta-analysis of the randomized controlled trials. *J Hypertens*. 2018;36(4):734–743.
89. Edwards DG, Farquhar WB. Vascular effects of dietary salt. *Curr Opin Nephrol Hypertens*. 2015;24(1):8.
90. Sacks FM, Lichtenstein AH, Wu JHY, et al. Dietary fats and cardiovascular disease: a presidential advisory from the American Heart Association. *Circulation*. 2017;136(3):e1–e23.
91. Li Y, Hruby A, Bernstein AM, et al. Saturated fats compared with unsaturated fats and sources of carbohydrates in relation to risk of coronary heart disease: a prospective cohort study. *J Am Coll Cardiol*. 2015;66(14):1538–1548. https://doi.org/10.1016/j.jacc.2015.07.055.
92. Mozaffarian D. Dairy foods, obesity, and metabolic health: the role of the food matrix compared with single nutrients. *Adv Nutr*. 2019; 10(5):917S–923S.
93. Drouin-Chartier J-P, Brassard D, Tessier-Grenier M, et al. Systematic review of the association between dairy product consumption and risk of cardiovascular-related clinical outcomes. *Adv Nutr*. 2016;7(6):1026–1040.
94. Chen M, Li Y, Sun Q, et al. Dairy fat and risk of cardiovascular disease in 3 cohorts of US adults. *Am J Clin Nutr*. 2016;104(5): 1209–1217.
95. Hollænder PLB, Ross AB, Kristensen M. Whole-grain and blood lipid changes in apparently healthy adults: a systematic review and meta-analysis of randomized controlled studies1-3. *Am J Clin Nutr*. 2015. https://doi.org/10.3945/ajcn.115.109165.

96. Mensink RP. *Effects of Saturated Fatty Acids on Serum Lipids and Lipoproteins: A Systematic Review and Regression Analysis.* World Heal Organ; 2016.
97. Eyres L, Eyres MF, Chisholm A, Brown RC. Coconut oil consumption and cardiovascular risk factors in humans. *Nutr Rev.* 2016; 74(4):267–280.
98. Sun Y, Neelakantan N, Wu Y, Lote-Oke R, Pan A, van Dam RM. Palm oil consumption increases LDL cholesterol compared with vegetable oils low in saturated fat in a meta-analysis of clinical trials. *J Nutr.* 2015;145(7):1549–1558.
99. Del Gobbo LC, Imamura F, Aslibekyan S, et al. ω-3 polyunsaturated fatty acid biomarkers and coronary heart disease: pooling project of 19 cohort studies. *J Am Med Assoc Intern Med.* 2016; 176(8):1155–1166.
100. Pan A, Chen M, Chowdhury R, et al. α-Linolenic acid and risk of cardiovascular disease: a systematic review and meta-analysis. *Am J Clin Nutr.* 2012;96(6):1262–1273.
101. Chowdhury R, Warnakula S, Kunutsor S, et al. Association of dietary, circulating, and supplement fatty acids with coronary risk: a systematic review and meta-analysis. *Ann Intern Med.* 2014; 160(6):398–406.
102. Abdelhamid AS, Brown TJ, Brainard JS, et al. Omega-3 fatty acids for the primary and secondary prevention of cardiovascular disease. *Cochrane Database Syst Rev.* 2018;11.
103. Rimm EB, Appel LJ, Chiuve SE, et al. Seafood long-chain n-3 polyunsaturated fatty acids and cardiovascular disease: a science advisory from the American Heart Association. *Circulation.* 2018;138(1):e35–e47.
104. Siscovick DS, Barringer TA, Fretts AM, et al. Omega-3 polyunsaturated fatty acid (fish oil) supplementation and the prevention of clinical cardiovascular disease: a science advisory from the American Heart Association. *Circulation.* 2017;135(15):e867–e884.
105. Hu Y, Hu FB, Manson JE. Marine omega-3 supplementation and cardiovascular disease: an updated meta-analysis of 13 randomized controlled trials involving 127 477 participants. *J Am Heart Assoc.* 2019;8(19):e013543. https://doi.org/10.1161/JAHA.119.013543.
106. Skulas-Ray AC, Wilson PWF, Harris WS, et al. Omega-3 fatty acids for the management of hypertriglyceridemia: a science advisory from the American Heart Association. *Circulation.* 2019; 140(12):e673–e691.
107. Bhatt DL, Steg PG, Miller M, et al. Cardiovascular risk reduction with icosapent ethyl for hypertriglyceridemia. *N Engl J Med.* 2019; 380(1):11–22.
108. Mozaffarian D, Wu JH. Omega-3 fatty acids and cardiovascular disease: effects on risk factors, molecular pathways, and clinical events. *J Am Coll Cardiol.* 2011;58(20):2047–2067. https://doi.org/10.1016/j.jacc.2011.06.063.
109. Tapsell LC, Neale EP, Satija A, Hu FB. Foods, nutrients, and dietary patterns: interconnections and implications for dietary guidelines. *Adv Nutr.* 2016;7(3):445–454.
110. Cespedes EM, Hu FB. Dietary patterns: from nutritional epidemiologic analysis to national guidelines. *Am J Clin Nutr.* 2015;101(5): 899–900.
111. Khera AV, Emdin CA, Drake I, et al. Genetic risk, adherence to a healthy lifestyle, and coronary disease. *N Engl J Med.* 2016; 375(24):2349–2358. https://doi.org/10.1056/NEJMoa1605086.
112. Li Y, Pan A, Wang DD, et al. Impact of healthy lifestyle factors on life expectancies in the US population. *Circulation.* 2018;138(4): 345–355. https://doi.org/10.1161/CIRCULATIONAHA.117.032047.
113. Obarzanek E, Sacks FM, Vollmer WM, et al. Effects on blood lipids of a blood pressure-lowering diet: the dietary approaches to stop hypertension (DASH) trial. *Am J Clin Nutr.* 2001;74(1): 80–89.
114. Sacks FM, Svetkey LP, Vollmer WM, et al. Effects on blood pressure of reduced dietary sodium and the dietary approaches to stop hypertension (DASH) diet. *N Engl J Med.* 2001;344(1):3–10. https://doi.org/10.1056/NEJM200101043440101.
115. Siervo M, Lara J, Chowdhury S, Ashor A, Oggioni C, Mathers JC. Effects of the Dietary Approach to Stop Hypertension (DASH) diet on cardiovascular risk factors: a systematic review and meta-analysis. *Br J Nutr.* 2015;113(1):1–15. https://doi.org/10.1017/S0007114514003341.
116. Fung TT, Rexrode KM, Mantzoros CS, Manson JE, Willett WC, Hu FB. Mediterranean diet and incidence of and mortality from coronary heart disease and stroke in women. *Circulation.* 2009; 119(8):1093–1100. https://doi.org/10.1161/CIRCULATIONAHA.108.816736.
117. Martínez-González M, Hershey M, Zazpe I, Trichopoulou A. Transferability of the Mediterranean diet to non-Mediterranean countries. What is and what is not the Mediterranean diet. *Nutrients.* 2017;9(11):1226. https://doi.org/10.3390/nu9111226.
118. Sofi F, Cesari F, Abbate R, Gensini GF, Casini A. Adherence to Mediterranean diet and health status: meta-analysis. *BMJ.* 2008; 337:a1344. https://doi.org/10.1136/BMJ.A1344.
119. Rosato V, Temple NJ, La Vecchia C, Castellan G, Tavani A, Guercio V. Mediterranean diet and cardiovascular disease: a systematic review and meta-analysis of observational studies. *Eur J Nutr.* 2019;58(1):173–191. https://doi.org/10.1007/s00394-017-1582-0.
120. Clarys P, Deliens T, Huybrechts I, et al. Comparison of nutritional quality of the vegan, vegetarian, semi-vegetarian, pesco-vegetarian and omnivorous diet. *Nutrients.* 2014;6(3):1318–1332. https://doi.org/10.3390/nu6031318.
121. Melina V, Craig W, Levin S. Position of the Academy of nutrition and Dietetics: vegetarian diets. *J Acad Nutr Diet.* 2016;116(12): 1970–1980. https://doi.org/10.1016/j.jand.2016.09.025.
122. Le LT, Sabaté J. Beyond meatless, the health effects of vegan diets: findings from the Adventist cohorts. *Nutrients.* 2014;6(6): 2131–2147. https://doi.org/10.3390/nu6062131.
123. Huang T, Yang B, Zheng J, Li G, Wahlqvist ML, Li D. Cardiovascular disease mortality and cancer incidence in vegetarians: a meta-analysis and systematic review. *Ann Nutr Metab.* 2012; 60(4):233–240. https://doi.org/10.1159/000337301.
124. Yokoyama Y, Levin SM, Barnard ND. Association between plant-based diets and plasma lipids: a systematic review and meta-analysis. *Nutr Rev.* 2017;75(9):683–698. https://doi.org/10.1093/nutrit/nux030.
125. Satija A, Bhupathiraju SN, Spiegelman D, et al. Healthful and unhealthful plant-based diets and the risk of coronary heart disease in U.S. Adults. *J Am Coll Cardiol.* 2017;70(4):411–422. https://doi.org/10.1016/j.jacc.2017.05.047.
126. USDA Agricultural Research Service. *Usual Nutrient Intake from Food and Beverges, by Gender and Age, what We Eat in America.* 2019. NHANES 2013-2016.
127. Appel LJ, Sacks FM, Carey VJ, et al. Effects of protein, monounsaturated fat, and carbohydrate intake on blood pressure and serum lipids. *J Am Med Assoc.* 2005;294(19):2455. https://doi.org/10.1001/jama.294.19.2455.
128. Van Horn L, Carson JAS, Appel LJ, et al. Recommended dietary pattern to achieve adherence to the American Heart Association/American College of Cardiology (AHA/ACC) guidelines: a scientific statement from the American Heart Association. *Circulation.* 2016;134(22):e505–529. https://doi.org/10.1161/CIR.0000000000000462.
129. Poobalan A, Aucott L, Smith WCS, et al. Effects of weight loss in overweight/obese individuals and long-term lipid outcomes – a systematic review. *Obes Rev.* 2004;5(1):43–50. https://doi.org/10.1111/j.1467-789X.2004.00127.x.

130. Miller M, Stone NJ, Ballantyne C, et al. Triglycerides and cardiovascular disease. *Circulation*. 2011;123(20):2292–2333. https://doi.org/10.1161/CIR.0b013e3182160726.
131. Sacks FM, Carey VJ, Anderson CAM, et al. Effects of high vs low glycemic index of dietary carbohydrate on cardiovascular disease risk factors and insulin sensitivity: the OmniCarb randomized clinical trial glycemic index, cardiovascular disease, and insulin sensitivity glycemic index, cardiovascul. *J Am Med Assoc*. 2014; 312(23):2531–2541. https://doi.org/10.1001/jama.2014.16658.
132. Maki KC, Palacios OM, Lindner E, Nieman KM, Bell M, Sorce J. Replacement of refined starches and added sugars with egg protein and unsaturated fats increases insulin sensitivity and lowers triglycerides in overweight or obese adults with elevated triglycerides. *J Nutr*. 2017;147(7):1267–1274. https://doi.org/10.3945/jn.117.248641.
133. Te Morenga LA, Howatson AJ, Jones RM, Mann J. Dietary sugars and cardiometabolic risk: systematic review and meta-analyses of randomized controlled trials of the effects on blood pressure and lipids. *Am J Clin Nutr*. 2014;100(1):65–79. https://doi.org/10.3945/ajcn.113.081521.
134. Steele EM, Baraldi LG, Da Costa Louzada ML, Moubarac JC, Mozaffarian D, Monteiro CA. Ultra-processed foods and added sugars in the US diet: evidence from a nationally representative cross-sectional study. *BMJ Open*. 2016;6(3):e009892. https://doi.org/10.1136/bmjopen-2015-009892.
135. Klop B, do Rego AT, Cabezas MC. Alcohol and plasma triglycerides. *Curr Opin Lipidol*. 2013;24(4):321–326. https://doi.org/10.1097/MOL.0b013e3283606845.
136. Rimm EB, Williams P, Fosher K, Criqui M, Stampfer MJ. Moderate alcohol intake and lower risk of coronary heart disease: meta-analysis of effects on lipids and haemostatic factors. *BMJ*. 1999;319(7224):1523–1528. https://doi.org/10.1136/bmj.319.7224.1523.
137. Richter CK, Bowen KJ, Mozaffarian D, Kris-Etherton PM, Skulas-Ray AC. Total long-chain n-3 fatty acid intake and food sources in the United States compared to recommended intakes: NHANES 2003–2008. *Lipids*. 2017;52(11):917–927. https://doi.org/10.1007/s11745-017-4297-3.
138. Vannice G, Rasmussen H. Position of the Academy of nutrition and dietetics: dietary fatty acids for healthy adults. *J Acad Nutr Diet*. 2014;114(1):136–153. https://doi.org/10.1016/j.jand.2013.11.001.
139. Neter JE, Stam BE, Kok FJ, Grobbee DE, Geleijnse JM. Influence of weight reduction on blood pressure: a meta-analysis of randomized controlled trials. *Hypertension*. 2003;42(5):878–884. https://doi.org/10.1161/01.HYP.0000094221.86888.AE.
140. Harnack LJ, Cogswell ME, Shikany JM, et al. Sources of sodium in US adults from 3 geographic regions. *Circulation*. 2017;135(19): 1775–1783. https://doi.org/10.1161/CIRCULATIONAHA.116.024446.
141. Jensen MD, Ryan DH, Apovian CM, et al. 2013 AHA/ACC/TOS guideline for the management of overweight and obesity in adults: a report of the American College of Cardiology/American Heart Association Task Force on Practice Guidelines and the Obesity Society. *J Am Coll Cardiol*. 2014;63(25 Pt B):2985–3023. https://doi.org/10.1016/j.jacc.2013.11.004.
142. Academy of Nutrition and Dietetics. Academy of Nutrition and Dietetics Evidence Analysis library. "Medical Nutrition Therapy and disorders of Lipid Metabolism" https://www.andeal.org/topic.cfm?menu=5300&cat=4402. Accessed 13 January 2019.
143. Sikand G, Cole RE, Handu D, et al. Clinical and cost benefits of medical nutrition therapy by registered dietitian nutritionists for management of dyslipidemia: a systematic review and meta-analysis. *J Clin Lipidol*. 2018;12(5):1113–1122. https://doi.org/10.1016/j.jacl.2018.06.016.
144. Anderson CAM, Thorndike AN, Lichtenstein AH, et al. Innovation to create a healthy and sustainable food system: a science advisory from the American Heart Association. *Circulation*. 2019. CIR-0000000000000686.

C H A P T E R

23

NUTRITION AND GASTROINTESTINAL DISORDERS

Carolyn Newberry[1,2], MD
Elizabeth Prout Parks[3,4], MD, MSCE
Asim Maqbool[3,4], MD

[1]Gastroenterology and Hepatology, New York-Presbyterian Hospital
[2]Medicine, Weill Cornell Medical College, Cornell University
[3]Gastroenterology, Hepatology and Nutrition, The Children's Hospital of Philadelphia, Philadelphia, PA, United States
[4]Pediatrics, University of Pennsylvania Perelman School of Medicine, Philadelphia, PA, United States

SUMMARY

In this chapter, we discuss disorders of the gastrointestinal track from 2 aspects, firstly from the perspective of the impact diseases and disorders on digestion and absorption, and secondly from the influence of diet and nutrition on diseases and disorders themselves. Nutritional considerations and risks for specific deficiencies are discussed in detail in the setting of bariatric surgery, exocrine pancreatic insufficiency and for functional gastrointestinal disorders. This effects of the diet and nutrition on disease processes as well as from therapeutic aspects for conditions including gastroesophageal reflux, eosinophilic esophagitis, celiac disease, inflammatory bowel disease and for functional gastrointestinal disorders are also discussed.

Keywords: Celiac Disease; Eosinophilic esophagitis; Exocrine pancreatic insufficiency; Functional Gastrointestinal Disorders; Gastroesophageal reflux; Inflammatory Bowel Disease.

I. INTRODUCTION

In this chapter, we review disorders involving the alimentary tract. We will specifically focus on the nutritional aspects of etiology as well as management of these disorders. Selected examples are used to highlight the roles of each part of the alimentary tract in the digestion and absorption of nutrients. Comprehensive discussion of disorders is beyond the scope of this chapter.

Disorders of the alimentary tract pertinent to digestion and absorption can be organized by anatomical aspects as well as from a functional perspective (Fig. 23.1). The entire gastrointestinal tract acts in concert in the digestion and absorption of nutrients, as exemplified by vitamin B_{12} (Fig. 23.2). Specific diseases also encompass the entirety of the GI tract from a digestive, absorptive, and nutritional perspective, with cystic fibrosis (CF) being the example. Overall, nutrition plays a key role in pathogenesis and management of gastrointestinal disease and will be discussed accordingly. It additionally may help define the relationship between metabolomics, the gut microbiome, and health.

II. ESOPHAGEAL DISORDERS

Although the esophagus plays a minor role in the digestion and absorption of nutrients, esophageal disorders can be managed with nutritional therapy. Prime examples are gastroesophageal reflux disease (GERD) and eosinophilic esophagitis (EoE).

Present Knowledge in Nutrition, Volume 2
https://doi.org/10.1016/B978-0-12-818460-8.00023-X

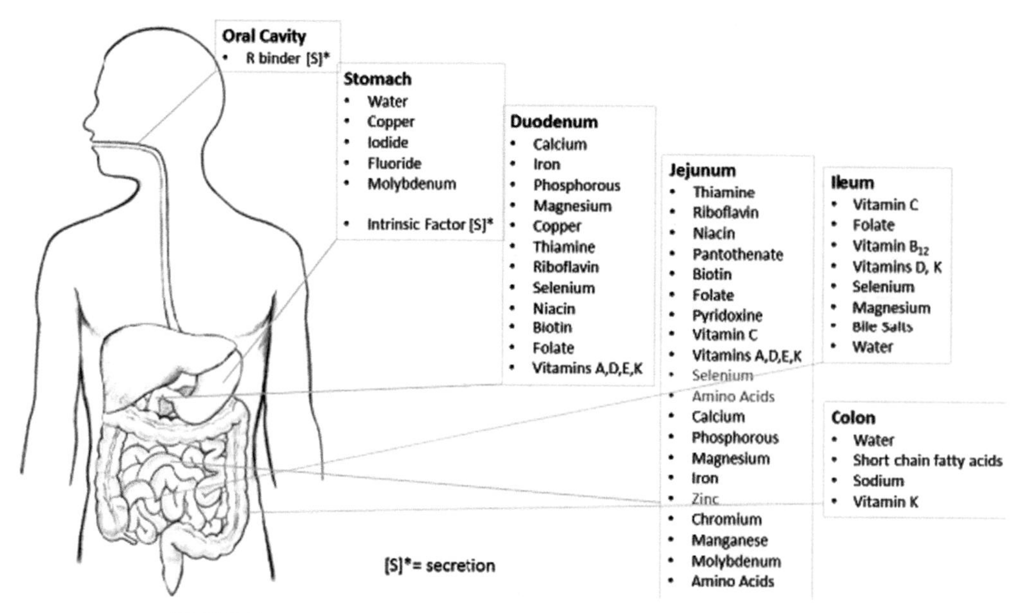

FIGURE 23.1 The alimentary tract: organs, secretion, and absorption.

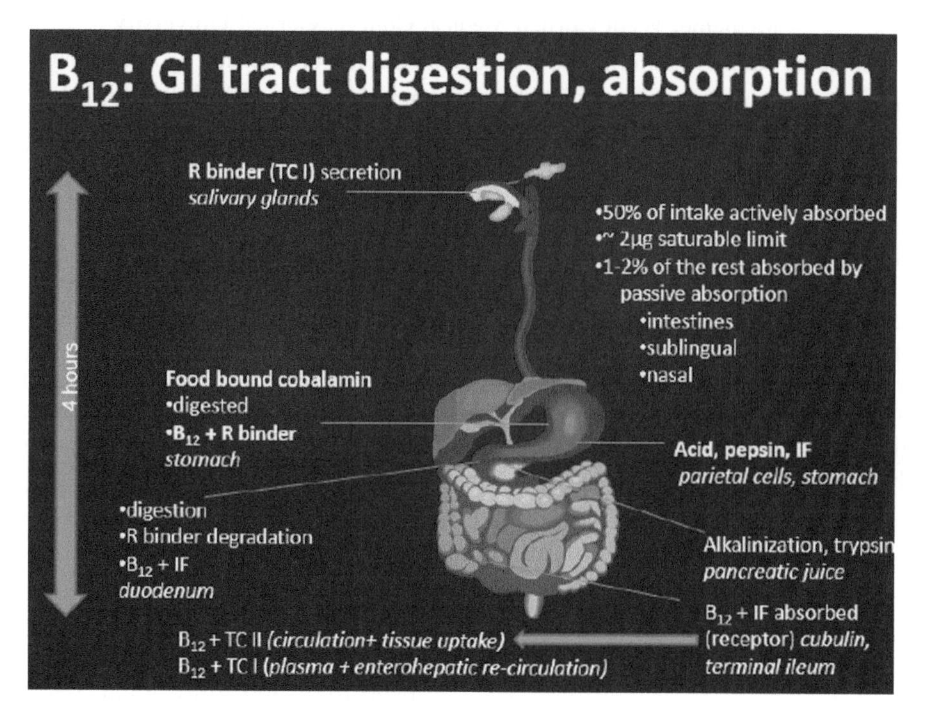

FIGURE 23.2 Vitamin B_{12}: digestion and absorption.

A. Gastroesophageal Reflux Disease

GERD is a common gastrointestinal disorder defined by troublesome symptoms secondary to increased esophageal acid exposure.[1] The disease occurs in the setting of an incompetent gastroesophageal barrier, which is composed of the lower esophageal sphincter (LES), angle of His, and crural diaphragm.[2] Risk factors include smoking, central adiposity, and medical conditions that slow gastrointestinal motility.[3] GERD can lead to esophageal and extraesophageal symptoms, mucosal disease, and esophageal dysmotility.[4] Lifestyle factors are implicated and are considered first line therapy in addition to acid suppression medications such as hydrogen receptor antagonists and proton pump inhibitors (PPIs). Considering adverse effects associated with PPIs including increased risk of infections, kidney dysfunction, and changes in micronutrient absorption (i.e., B_{12}, iron, and calcium), nonpharmacological therapies are often preferred by patients and providers.[5] Although cessation of smoking and weight loss are primary intervention targets, the role of dietary therapy continues to be explored. Late night eating patterns and increased size and/or caloric density of meals have been linked to worsening GERD symptoms.[6–8] Specific foods may also be related, although evidence remains sparse to make definitive recommendations. For example, patients are often instructed to avoid acidic or carbonated beverages, spicy foods, caffeine, chocolate, mint, and alcohol to control symptoms. Proposed mechanisms of disease include direct esophageal mucosal irritation (acid, spice), increased gastric distention (carbonation), and reduction in LES tone (caffeine, chocolate, mint, alcohol).[4] More recently, macronutrient manipulation has been studied, with some research supporting reduction in overall fat and simple sugar intake in favor of fiber and protein.[9]

B. Eosinophilic Esophagitis

EoE is an increasingly common allergic disease defined by characteristic inflammatory changes in the esophagus, which may lead to fibrosis and swallowing dysfunction.[10] Pathogenesis includes environmental stimuli like food allergens and antibiotics as well as genetic predisposition. The condition occurs most commonly in young males with history of atopic diseases, though it can develop in any age group or sex.[11] Cornerstones of therapy include acid blockers (specifically PPI), oral glucocorticoids, endoscopic dilations for strictures, and dietary manipulation. Depending on approach, dietary therapy can be as equally efficacious as steroids and has fewer adverse effects. The three most common dietary interventions are the use of commercial elemental diets (ELED), six food elimination diets (SFED), and allergen-directed diets.[12] ELED is the most effective option, resolving eosinophilic-predominant inflammation in 90% of patients; however, this approach is rarely used in adult patients secondary to poor tolerability associated with tube feed use.[13,14] SFED is also effective, boosting histological remission rates in 68% –76% of patients, and is easier to implement. This diet requires complete elimination of the six most common food allergens (wheat, soy, dairy, eggs, nuts/tree nuts, and fish/shellfish) with sequential reintroduction to identify triggers.[14,15] Newer research shows up to half of patients may respond to elimination of only four food groups (wheat, soy, dairy, and eggs), indicating optimal treatment approaches are still unknown.[16] The least effective dietary approach is allergen-directed therapy, which relies on skin prick and allergy patch testing to identify culprit foods. Although initially promising and less restrictive than other options, allergen-directed therapy has lower reported rates of histological remission ranging from 13% to 77%.[17–20] Additionally, long-term restrictive diets are challenging for patients to follow.

III. GASTRIC DISORDERS

The stomach plays an important role in the mechanical and enzymatic digestion of food. It also contributes intrinsic factor to aid vitamin B_{12} absorption. Therefore, gastric disorders may affect digestion and absorption of nutrients in a variety of ways. For example, inflammation of the proximal gastrointestinal tract (including the stomach) can present with protein-losing enteropathy (PLE) as seen in Ménétrier disease and Crohn's disease.[21] The etiology of PLE can include primary GI diseases including erosive gastrointestinal disorders, nonerosive gastrointestinal disorders, and disorders involving increased central venous pressure or mesenteric lymphatic obstruction.[21,22]

Bariatric surgery presents a good model to understand and appreciate the impact of surgical modifications in nutrition and calls attention to management of disease.

A. Bariatric Surgery

Bariatric surgery presents a good model to understand and appreciate the impact of surgical modifications in nutrition and calls attention to management of disease.

<u>Nutritional considerations in bariatric surgery</u>

Weight loss surgeries (WLS) modify the gastrointestinal tract by restricting caloric intake, reducing absorption of nutrients, and altering hormonal secretion of anorexic and orexigenic hormones.[23] These same mechanisms leading to successful weight loss can also result in nutritional derangements. There are four major surgical procedures that are currently utilized in adults: the Roux-en-Y gastric bypass (RYGB), the laparoscopic adjustable gastric band (LAGB), the vertical sleeve gastrectomy (VSG), and least commonly the biliopancreatic diversion with duodenal switch (BPD/DS). Only RYGB and VSG are FDA approved for use in adolescents.[24] Patients with obesity or a body mass index (BMI ≥ 30) often have micronutrient deficiencies prior to surgery, and the current recommendation is to screen and supplement when indicated.[25,26] The most common preoperative micronutrient deficiencies include vitamin D (25OH < 75 nmol/L) 92%, folate (<5.3 mg/mL) 63%, iron (ferritin <15 μg/L) 10%, vitamin A (<1.05 μmol/L) 6.2%, and vitamin B_{12} (<188 pg/mL) 5.1%.[25,27] Understanding surgical alterations to the gastrointestinal tract and their effects on the absorption of macronutrients and micronutrients is important to predict and avoid deficiencies (Table 23.3).

Roux-en-Y gastric bypass (Fig. 23.3); Until 2011, the laparoscopic RYGB was the most commonly performed surgery in the United States in adults and adolescents.[28] The RYGB involves the creation of a small gastric pouch (20–30 mL) with a small outlet that results in early

Procedures	Description	Figures
Malabsorptive		
Roux-en-Y gastric bypass (RYGB)	15–30-mL gastric pouch with gastro-jejunal anastomosis	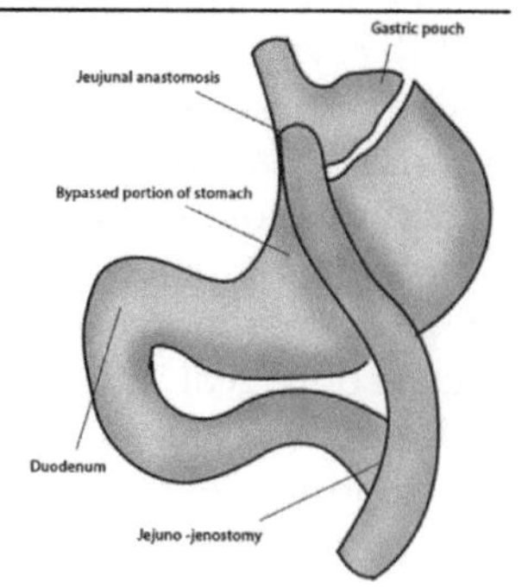
Biliopancreatic diversion with duodenal switch (BPD/DS)	Distal gastrectomy with anastomoses to distal ileum; proximal ileum is anastomosed to terminal ileum	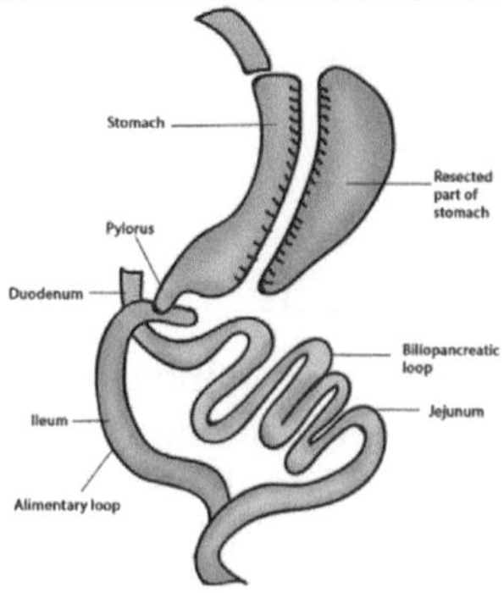
Restrictive		
Laparoscopic adjustable gastric banding (LAGB)	Adjustable silicone band is positioned around the stomach to create a 15-mL pouch	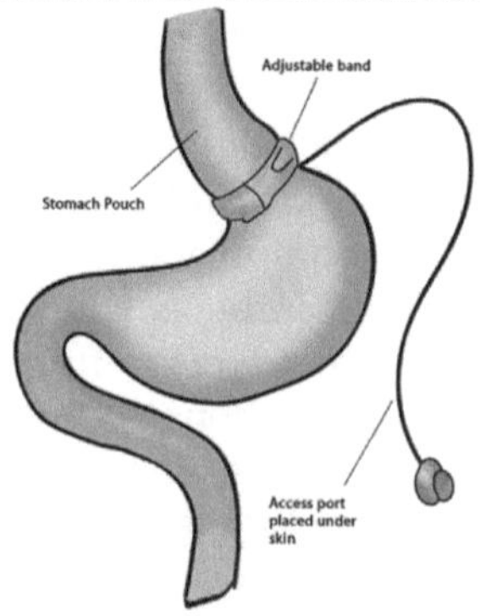
Sleeve gastrostomy (SG)	Removal of greater curvature to create a tubular stomach	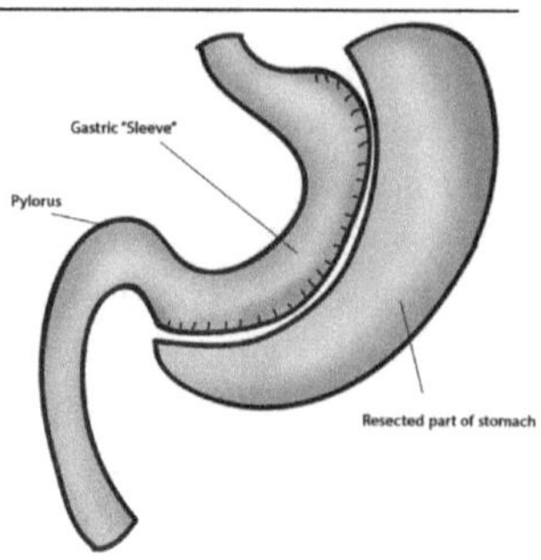

FIGURE 23.3 **Restrictive and mixed restrictive-malabsorptive bariatric procedures.** (A) Laparoscopic band (restrictive). (B) Sleeve gastrectomy (restrictive). (C) Roux-en-Y gastric bypass (mixed restrictive and malabsorptive). (D) Biliopancreatic diversion with duodenal switch (mixed restrictive and malabsorptive).

satiety. This pouch is anastomosed with a roux limb of distal jejunum. The fundus of the stomach, the entire duodenum, and about 40 cm of proximal jejunum is bypassed. The standard Roux limb is 100 cm. The surgery on average achieves 20%–30% total body weight loss or 65%–70% of excess weight loss. Excess weight is defined as weight that exceeds the ideal body weight (BMI 25 kg/m^2).[23]

TABLE 23.1 Common sources of gluten: dietary and nondietary.

Gluten-Containing grains	Rye, wheat (Bulgur, Durum, Einkorn, Emmer, Farro, Farina, Kamut, Semolina, Spelt, Kamut, Khorasan), barley
Hidden food gluten sources	Beer, food coloring, malt, soy sauce, dressings, starch, processed meats, soups
Nonfood gluten sources	Cosmetics, toothpaste, medications, sunscreens

The RYGB anatomy increases the risk for micronutrient deficiencies including vitamins B_{12}, A, D, E, K, and B6, thiamine, zinc, folate, and copper. The creation of a gastric pouch also results in parietal cell dysfunction leading to reduced secretion of intrinsic factor, and subsequent vitamin B_{12} deficiency. Bypass of the duodenum results in fat-soluble vitamins (A, D, E, K), malabsorption, and most commonly vitamins D and A. Blood thiamine, iron, calcium, and folate levels may also be affected due to reduced duodenal absorption. Reduction in jejunal length affects blood zinc and vitamin B6. The American Society for Metabolic and Bariatric Surgery recommends screening and correcting micronutrient deficiencies prior to RYGB and VSG.[26] Presurgery screening includes thiamine, complete blood count, vitamin B_{12}, (B_{12} levels and methyl malonic acid), folate, iron (ferritin, iron, total iron-binding capacity [TIBC]), calcium, fat-soluble vitamins (A, D, E, K), zinc, and copper (copper and ceruloplasmin).[23,29]

Laparoscopic adjustable gastric band; The LAGB is the least invasive of the bariatric surgical procedures and was historically the most common procedure performed in. More recently, adverse outcomes have limited its use, and as of 2016, this procedure accounted for <3.5% of WLS performed.[30] This procedure was designed to recreate the restrictive element of the RYGB surgery. A silicone inflatable band is placed around the uppermost stomach to create a small pouch (20–30 mL) with a narrow outlet. Gastric restriction can be adjusted via saline injections into a subcutaneous reservoir. The stomach is

TABLE 23.2 Nutrient absorption and affected bariatric surgeries.

Stomach	**Duodenum**	**Jejunum**	**Ileum**
• VSG[a], RYGB[b], BP/DS[c]	• RYGB, BP/DS	• RYGB • BP/DS	
Water	*Calcium	*Calcium	Vitamin C
Ethyl alcohol	*Iron	*Iron	Folate
		*Zinc	
Copper	Phosphorus	Phosphorus	Vitamin B_{12}[d]
Iodide	Magnesium	Magnesium	Vitamin D
Fluoride	Copper	Copper	Vitamin K
Molybdenum	Selenium		Magnesium
	Thiamin	Thiamin	Bile salts/acids
Intrinsic factor	Riboflavin	Riboflavin	
HCL[e]	Niacin		
	Biotin	Biotin	
	Folate	Folate	
	Vitamins A, D, E, K	Vitamins A, D, E, K	
		Vitamin B_6	
		Manganese	
		Molybdenum	
		Amino acids	

[a]*vertical sleeve gastrectomy*
[b]*Roux-en-Y gastric bypass*
[c]*biliopancreatic biliodiversion*
[d]*SG, RYGB, BP/DS affected secondary to decreased intrinsic factor production*
** Requires HCL for absorption.*
Adapted from Shikora S. 2007.[23]

TABLE 23.3 Supporting evidence for proposed IBD structured diets.

Diet	Description	Supporting evidence
Exclusive enteral nutrition (EEN)[184–186,189–192]	Polymeric, semielemental, or elemental formula taken as the sole source of nutrition.	Multiple prospective studies support the use of EEN for • induction of remission • mucosal healing • growth impairment in pediatric Crohn's. Effective for maintenance of remission in adult Crohn's.
Partial enteral nutrition (PEN)[194]	Same as EEN, except that formula is not the exclusive source for nutrition.	Retrospective and prospective studies support the use of PEN for induction of remission and maintenance therapy in pediatric CD. Amount of nonformula varies across studies for induction and maintenance of remission.
Specific carbohydrate diet (SCD)[217]	Allows for consumption of monosaccharides but not di-, oligo-, and polysaccharides	Limited evidence. Small retrospective study demonstrated improved clinical disease activity scores. Small prospective study showed improvement in mucosal healing.
IBD antiinflammatory diet[218]	Multiple-phase diet derived from the SCD. Certain carbohydrates and fats are restricted, and intake of pre- and probiotics is encouraged.	Limited evidence; small retrospective case series of adult subjects with IBD demonstrated improvement in disease activity scores.
Crohn's Disease exclusion diet[219,220]	Structured diet that reduces or eliminates exposure to animal fats, dairy products, gluten, and processed foods.	Limited evidence; retrospective study demonstrated improvement in disease activity and mucosal healing in adult and pediatric Crohn's. Has been used in conjunction with PEN.
Semivegetarian diet[221]	Diet containing fruits, vegetables, dairy, and eggs with limited fish and meat.	Limited evidence. Prospective study showed improvement in symptom-based remission compared to free diet.

Modified from[198].

not cut or stapled, and no anastomoses are made.[23] It is important to note that there are no hormonal alterations with this procedure. Thus although there is restriction, there is no subsequent changes in the counter effects of hunger and satiety that are seen with other procedures. Reasons for decreased use include inadequate weight loss or weight regain and complications like dysphagia, chronic emesis, band slippage, and gastric and esophageal tissue erosion leading to high rates of surgical revisions (33%–65%).[31,32]

Nutritional deficiencies do not occur as commonly with the LAGB as with other bariatric procedures as there is no change in nutrient absorption. However, some patients may develop deficiencies from decreased consumption and complications like prolonged vomiting. Reported deficiencies with vomiting include thiamine, vitamin B_{12}, and iron.[23]

Vertical sleeve gastrectomy; The VSG is the most commonly performed surgery in adults and adolescents and involves a 60%–75% irreversible gastrectomy.[28,30] Weight loss effects are from restriction of gastric content, decrease in production of the appetite stimulating hormone ghrelin, and decreased production of the appetite suppressing hormone GLP-1 and peptide YY. VSG was originally conceived in 2002 as the first stage of a two-stage operative approach for high-risk patients undergoing BPD/DS or RYGB. It was thought a two-stage approach would confer the advantages of technical facility, shorter operative times, and interval weight loss between stages, which in turn would result in decreased morbidity in this high-risk group. The VSG gained popularity as a stand-alone procedure secondary to improved tolerance and reduced complications in comparison to RYGB and LABG.[26] Nutrition deficiencies can be seen as early as 4 months (protein, vitamin D), with greatest decreases seen 12 months postoperatively (vitamin B_{12}, folate, calcium, vitamin D).[27]

Bileopancreatic diversion with duodenal switch; BPD/DS involves (1) the removal of 80% of the stomach leaving a tubular pouch (a sleeve gastrectomy), (2) transection of the small intestine halfway between the ligament of Treitz and the ileocecal valve, (3) a RYGB from the stomach pouch to the distal bowel loop creating an alimentary limb, and (4) a biliopancreatic limb anastomosed with the alimentary limb 50 cm before the ileocecal valve.[33] The BPD/DS results in weight loss through the restriction of food consumption, malabsorption of fat, carbohydrates, and protein, and alterations in hormonal regulation. The creation of a gastric sleeve results in the restrictive effects. The bypass of the duodenum and jejunum and disconnect with pancreatic juices results in malabsorption of carbohydrate, fat, and protein.[23] The BPD/DS is the most extensive bariatric procedure, with the most postoperative complications and nutrition deficiencies that have led to infrequent use.

Nutritional deficiencies

Macronutrients; Macronutrient alterations are most prevalent in RYGB and BPD/DS. Malabsorption of carbohydrate and fat occurs as a result of bypass of the duodenum. Protein malabsorption occurs mainly in BPD/DS (21%), but it can be seen in RYGB (13%) and less commonly in VSG and LABG secondary to reduced dietary intake.[34] Patients with decreased dietary consumption of protein or who have prolonged vomiting have increased risk of protein malnutrition. Prevention requires a protein intake of at least 1.1 g/kg of ideal body weight or 60–120 g/day.[34] Dietary protein is important for satiety, energy expenditure, and wound healing, and an intake of greater than 60 g/day has been associated with a preservation of lean body mass after WLS.[35] For this reason, it is important to monitor protein intake through dietary tracking and protein stores (albumin and prealbumin) after any WLS.

Micronutrients

Fat-soluble vitamins: Fat-soluble vitamin deficiencies are most prevalent in RYGB and BPD/DS secondary to delayed mixing of dietary fat with pancreatic enzymes and bile salts leading to fat malabsorption and maldigestion.[36] Vitamin A deficiency is seen after RYGB in 10% of patients within 4 years of surgery. Vitamin E deficiency is rarely encountered with screening and usually presents without clinical manifestations. Vitamin K deficiency is mainly seen after BPD/DS, occurring in 50%–70% of patients within 2–4 years of surgery.[36] Vitamin D deficiency is seen within the first 4 months after all WLS with the lowest levels in those who were deficient prior to their procedure. Decreased sun exposure leading to decreased intrahepatic circulation of vitamin D can occur. Low serum vitamin D levels may contribute to calcium malabsorption and deficiency resulting in a secondary hyperparathyroidism. This causes release of calcium from bone and increases risk for bone loss.[36] Therefore, a bone density scan is recommended at 2 years postsurgery.[37]

Water-soluble vitamins Thiamine (vitamin B1) deficiency can be seen after all WLS types. Thiamine deficiency occurs in the setting of decreased wholegrain consumption (AGB, VSG, RYGB, BPD/DS) and/or decreased absorption in the duodenum and jejunum (RYGB, BPD/DS).[36] This deficiency presents in the first 1–3 months after surgery, usually with prolonged nausea and vomiting. It can also present with peripheral neuropathy (dry beriberi), neuropsychiatric symptoms (encephalopathy), unstable gait (ataxia), eye changes (opthalmoplegia), confusion, and rarely high-output heart failure (wet beriberi).[36]

Folate is absorbed throughout the gastrointestinal tract, but decreased intake of green leafy vegetables increases the risk of this deficiency in all WLS.[27,36] Vitamin B_{12} is absorbed in the terminal ileum (TI), but this requires gastric acid, intrinsic factor, and pancreatic proteases to be effectively absorbed. Meat intolerance, aversion, and prolonged vomiting can increase the risk of deficiency. Vitamin B_{12} deficiency is seen in 18%–22% of patients after SG and BPD/DS and 60% after RYGB.[36] Screening with serum methyl malonic acid is the most sensitive means of detection with concentrations >500 nmol indicative of vitamin B_{12} deficiency. Vitamin B_6 is absorbed in the jejunum and requires riboflavin, niacin, and zinc for its metabolism. Folate and carnitine require vitamin B_6 as a cofactor for their metabolism.[38]

Trace minerals Iron is the most common micronutrient deficiency after bariatric surgery. Iron is generally well-absorbed in the duodenum and jejunum, but only in the presence of sufficient gastric acid. Iron deficiency is seen in 30% of RYGB and VSG patients within 5 years after surgery using serum ferritin as the biomarker.[34]

Zinc is absorbed in the jejunum in the presence of sufficient gastric acid; therefore, deficiency is mainly seen after BPD/DS and RYGB. Deficiency also occurs with postoperative diets limited in protein and whole grains. Zinc absorption is regulated by metallothionein. Metallothionein binds to zinc and other divalent cations such as copper, therefore zinc supplementation may worsen copper deficiency.[36]Copper is absorbed throughout the gastrointestinal tract, so deficiencies are rarely seen.[39]

In a prospective study of micronutrient deficiencies were detected the time of surgery: vitamin D (63%), iron (29%), folate (24%), calcium (18%), vitamin B_{12} (32%), and increased PTH concentration (12%).[27] Vitamin D, iron, and folate deficiencies were seen by 4 months, but calcium and vitamin B_{12} deficiency and elevated PTH concentrations were not detected until 12 months postoperatively.[27]

IV. DUODENAL AND PROXIMAL SMALL BOWEL DISORDERS

A. Celiac Disease

Celiac disease is an autoimmune disorder that develops in response to gluten exposure and is characterized by small intestinal inflammation. It is common, affecting about 1% of the general population,[40] but may be underdiagnosed.[41] Gluten is a polymeric protein found in wheat, barley, and rye. Its unique chemical composition renders it resistant to enzyme degradation and enhances immunogenicity.[42] Gluten induces an innate immune response in genetically susceptible patients, which leads to changes in small intestinal permeability and inflammatory mediators. Continued exposure furthers inflammatory cascade pathways and results in altered immunity and development of chronic inflammation.[40] Proximal small bowel mucosa is disproportionately affected by ingested gluten, although the entire intestinal tract can be implicated. Inflammation leads to reduction in nutrient absorption with subsequent development of micronutrient deficiencies, weight loss, and gastrointestinal symptoms (bloating, abdominal pain, and diarrhea).[43,44] There is a wide range of disease presentations, from subtle laboratory findings like mild iron deficiency anemia to severe diarrhea, symptomatic vitamin deficiencies, and loss of bone and muscle mass.[40,45] The disease may have extraintestinal manifestations including infertility, neurological symptoms, and skin findings of dermatitis herpetiformis.[43,46,47] Patients with celiac disease are also at increased risk for autoimmune disorders when compared with the general population.

Celiac disease is diagnosed by a combination of blood tests and enteric biopsies. Options for blood tests include antitissue transglutaminase IgA antibodies (most sensitive and specific), antiendomysial IgA antibodies, and antigliadin IgG and IgA antibodies.[48] The latter are useful in the setting of IgA deficiency but otherwise have lower specificity and are not used as first-line diagnostic tests.[49] Enteric biopsies are necessary to confirm diagnosis in adults, though endoscopy may be avoided in high-risk children who present with characteristic symptoms, positive genetic testing, and high antibody titers. Distinctive pathology defines the disease and is classified based on Marsh criteria, which grades villous architectural distortion, crypt hyperplasia, and intraepithelial lymphocyte density.[48] After confirmation of diagnosis, a dietician consultation is required, as the only approved therapy is strict gluten avoidance. Nearly all patients who avoid gluten will have resolution of both symptoms and intestinal mucosal abnormalities. The small percentage (1% −2%) who are nonresponsive to a gluten-free diet are termed "refractory" and have higher risks of disease complications like ulcerative jejunitis and enteropathy-associated T-cell lymphoma.[40] Refractory patients may respond to high-dose oral steroids after a detailed history confirms dietary compliance. Many refractory patients are later found to have inadvertent gluten exposures through cross-contamination with other closely related grains (i.e., oats) or nonfood sources. Removal of gluten and other inciting agents restores normal villous architecture and eliminates associated symptoms.[50]

Complications of celiac disease are avoided with a gluten-free diet; however, this dietary restriction can lead other complications, which need to be addressed. The gluten-free diet is inherently restrictive and challenging to follow. Close monitoring by a physician and dietician is encouraged to assess understanding of the food and beverage composition and discuss barriers to diet adherence including food choice and availability. Patients require education on reading food labels and determining safety of food when eating outside the home. The highest risk food items (i.e., those with unrecognized gluten) includes sauces, seasoned foods, and complex dishes.[51] Nonfood sources of gluten include toothpaste, mouthwash, and medication capsules, and these are common sources of inadvertent exposures.[43]

The nutritional quality of the gluten-free diet varies by patient, but on average, it is found to be lower in fiber and B vitamins such as niacin, thiamine, and folate, as well as calcium and iron.[52] It additionally may be higher in total fat and added sugar content.[53] Some of the adverse nutritional effects can be reduced with promotion of naturally gluten-free foods such as fruits, vegetables, and proteins and incorporation of alternative gluten-free grains such as millet, buckwheat, and amaranth.[54]

There is a small subset of patients who have clinical manifestations of celiac disease when ingesting gluten but have negative blood tests and small bowel mucosal biopsies. These patients are thought to have "nonceliac gluten sensitivity," which may have some overlap with irritable bowel syndrome (IBS).[55,56] Currently, no diagnostic testing exists to identify this condition. Patients may benefit from gluten restriction after celiac disease rules out, with similar therapeutic approaches to avoid nutritional deficits and dietary limitations.[40]

V. LIVER, GALLBLADDER AND PANCREAS

The digestive functional units of the pancreas are the ducts, which primarily secrete bicarbonate, and the acini, which primarily secrete digestive enzymes, including proteases, amylase, and lipase in an inactive or proenzyme form (Fig. 23.4A). Chyme (the semidigested pulpy and acid food mass) exiting the stomach and entering the duodenum stimulates the pancreas and gallbladder via endocrine and neurocrine pathways. Pancreatic ducts are stimulated by secretion, whereas the acini are stimulated by secretin and cholecystokinin (CCK; Fig. 23.4B). CCK is stimulated by intraluminal fat and certain amino acids in chyme. CCK in turn stimulates not only pancreatic secretions but also gallbladder contraction and secretion of bile acids (which are secreted by the liver and stored in the gallbladder) into the duodenum. Duodenal luminal brush border enzymes cleave proenzymes into active forms optimally at a pH of 5–6 afforded by pancreatic bicarbonate secretion (Fig. 23.4B). It is in this milieu that digestion occurs. Pancreatic enzymes are also subsequently degraded in this environment after facilitating digestion. Bile acids are required to further solubilize enzymatically hydrolyzed fats for absorption at the level of the TI. Bile acids further undergo enterohepatic circulation (reabsorption at the TI), with ~5% losses in the stool. People with normally functioning digestive tracts absorb about 93% of dietary fat.

A. Pancreas

Exocrine pancreatic insufficiency

While pancreatic lipase constitutes only ~2% of pancreatic enzyme output, the consequences of lipase deficiency clinically results in GI signs and symptoms including gas, abdominal distention, steatorrhea, weight loss, and/or lack of weight gain (particularly in children). CF and Shwachman–Diamond syndrome (both hereditary in etiology) are leading causes of EPI in children, while chronic pancreatitis secondary to alcohol or biliary disease causes EPI in adults.

CF is one of the most common heritable diseases in Caucasians and occurs secondary to impairments in the CF transmembrane regulator (CFTR). The initial CF gene mutation described was a frameshift error on chromosome 7 (delta F508); subsequently, there have been about 2000 additional mutations associated with CF symptoms.[57] Mutations are categorized by functional or phenotypic class (five classes) with variable degrees of function. CFTR functions as both a chloride and bicarbonate transporter; impairments in function result in inspissated secretions, which result in impaired fluid transport, obstructions in susceptible organs, inflammation, damage, and destruction of these tissues to various degrees. Whilee CF is often considered to be primarily a sinopulmonary disease, the pancreas, hepatobiliary system, and GI tract are also intimately involved, to variable degrees.

CFTR is expressed in both ductal and acinar pancreatic tissue. The more severe class mutations result in early pancreatitis and loss of acinar tissue, rendering >80% of patients with exocrine pancreatic insufficiency (EPI) in utero, the neonatal period, or early in life. Conversely, patients with CF who have milder class mutations may have residual CFTR function and are at risk for acute, recurrent, or chronic pancreatitis. Patients with CF are therefore classified as having either pancreatic insufficiency or pancreatic sufficiency (PS). PS is a relative term, as patients with PS do not have normal exocrine pancreatic function as compared to healthy people.[58] CF is the pancreatic disease model that has advanced the understanding of EPI.

The consequences of EPI include chronic dietary fat malabsorption (lost calories), fat-soluble vitamin, and essential fatty acid deficiencies. Recall that both the ducts and acini are affected by pancreatitis, and the ducts primarily secrete bicarbonate, which helps to neutralize gastric acid at the level of the duodenum. This acid–base balance is important for the optimal functioning of brush border and pancreatic enzymes and allows for the digestion and absorption of multiple micronutrients, including vitamin B_{12} (Fig. 23.4B). Pancreatic secretions, luminal pH, and bile acids all work in concert to digest and solubilize fats for downstream absorption. A TI is required to actively absorb B_{12}, and patients without a TI, including

(A)

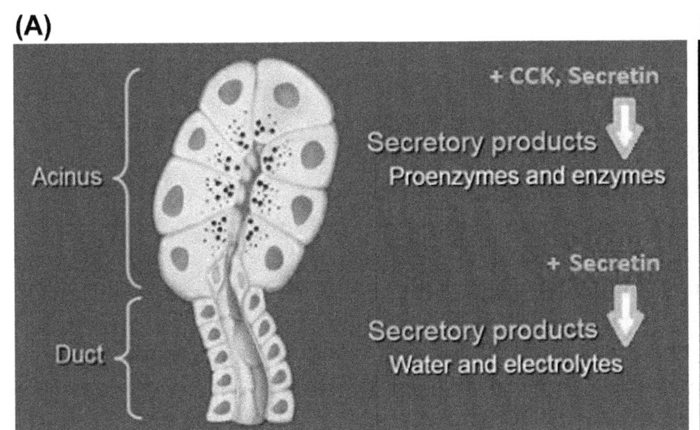

(B)

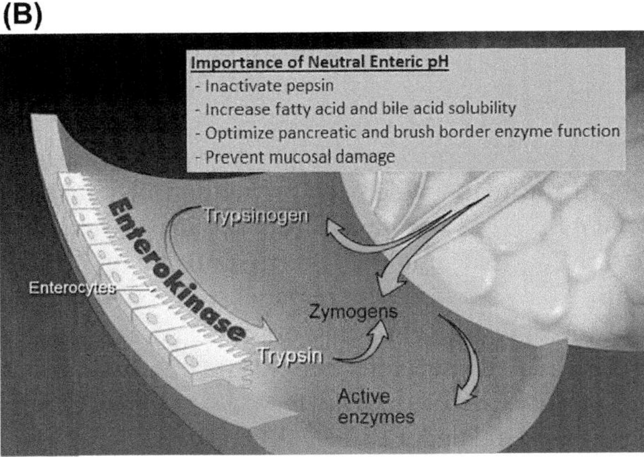

FIGURE 23.4 (A) Major functional units and endocrine regulation of the exocrine pancreas. (B) Site of zymogen activation: duodenum.

those with Crohn's disease, short bowel syndrome, and CF following ileal resection, are at risk for B_{12} deficiency.

Less common causes of EPI include history of pancreatic resections such as for pancreatic tumors or congenital hyperinsulinism. Pancreatitis may also result in EPI. The etiology of pancreatitis varies somewhat by whether or not it is acute, acute recurrent, or chronic. Nutritionally relevant risk factors for acute pancreatitis include hypertriglyceridemia and hypercalcemia. Alcohol exposure is the best known environmental/dietary trigger for the development of pancreatitis, particularly in adults, followed by tobacco use. Gallstone is a common risk factor for pancreatitis adults and children; the etiology of gallstones is reviewed elsewhere.[59] CF is the most common cause of recurrent hereditary pancreatitis and may occur without the classical presentation, affecting both children and adults.[60–63]

Regardless of the etiology of pancreatitis, nutritional management has moved away from the historical "resting the pancreas" to more evidence-based "recovering the pancreas" approach. Early and aggressive hydration (1.5–2x maintenance fluid needs) is recommended to reduce risk for pancreatic necrosis, which carries significantly higher risk for morbidity and mortality for adults. Lactated Ringer's (LR) intravenous solution currently is recommended over normal saline solution. LR hastens recovery and may reduce risk for complications from pancreatitis. Early enteral nutrition [EN] feeding resumption (oral, nasogastric, or nasojejunal) is also recommended to reduce risk for gut bacterial translocation and for sepsis.[64–69] It is not unusual to have an adynamic ileus with pancreatitis, which can confound abdominal pain and delay recovery. Narcotics therefore should be used sparingly as they reduce GI motility and can make EN challenging.[66–72] EN is preferable over parenteral nutrition (PN) due to decrease in infectious complications and enhanced recovery. PN has a limited role in acute pancreatitis and is reserved for patients for whom EN is not feasible.[73,74] In appropriate patients (i.e., who do not tolerate EN or are not candidates for EN), PN should be initiated 4–5 days after admission. After the first week of hospitalization, tolerance issues that result in hypocaloric enteral feeding for energy requirements may necessitate the addition of supplemental PN.

There is insufficient evidence to recommend low-fat diets in the management or prevention of pancreatitis. Dietary fat does not have a known adverse effect and does not confer any benefit to patients in terms of inflammation.[75,76] The use of pancreatic enzyme replacement therapy (PERT) is only appropriate in limited settings. PERT is not effective in preventing recurrent pancreatitis. PERT is useful in management of chronic pancreatitis–related EPI.[77–79] PERT is not effective for managing pancreatitis-related pain independent of its effect on managing EPI. Pancreatitis severity and chronicity dictates degree and duration of EPI from progressive destruction leading to loss of ductal and acinar tissue.

The management of EPI includes the use of PERT (mostly porcine derived), the dosing of which varies by degree of EPI, dietary fat intake, and by underlying etiology of EPI. PERT is dosed by lipase units, either as a function of patient weight (500–2000 lipase units/kg/meal, up to 10,000 lipase units/kg/day) or by grams of fat per meal (practical for children with more predictable dietary intake). Dose ranges vary by underlying disorder, with patients with CF usually receiving higher range doses than for patients with EPI from other causes. It is critical to note that there is an upper limit to PERT dosing. PERT, pH, and bile as well as other factors act in concert to facilitate fat absorption, and there is a ceiling to fat absorption. High-dose PERT use exceeding this ceiling dose has historically been associated with risk for fibrosing colonopathy in patients with CF, a serious adverse effect.[80–82] If PERT is at maximal safe dosing, additional measures can be considered to further enhance fat digestion and absorption. Increasing duodenal pH may be helpful to increase efficacy of PERT for fat maldigestion.[83] In patients with CF and mild CF–related liver disease, addition of ursodeoxycholic acid may enhance dietary fat digestion and absorption.[84] Newer developments to improve fat absorption include a bacteriophage-derived lipase component of an in line feeding cartridge for tube feeding and an organized lipid matrix that bypasses chylomicron formation and enhances fat absorption with our without the need for PERT.[85–87]

EPI may be transient and of varying severity in patients with acute, recurrent, and chronic pancreatitis. EPI status should therefore be followed over time in these patients.[88] Given risks of high-dose PERT and the burden of using PERT (cost, adherence, and compliance considerations), recommendations advise against open-ended use of PERT in patients with pancreatitis and EPI unless permanent EPI.[65] Clinical guidelines for the evaluation and management of EPI, including use of PERT, have been published elsewhere and are available online.[89]

B. Liver and Gallbladder

As reviewed prior, bile acids aid in digestion of fats in the duodenum at an optimal pH between 5 and 6, providing a detergent-like effect to solubilize digested fats. They are critical components of micelle formation and facilitate absorption of fats at the TI. Approximately 95% of luminal bile acids are reabsorbed at the level of the TI and return to the liver (enterohepatic circulation).[90] Bile acids are synthesized from cholesterol, with some entering circulation, the others stored in the gallbladder, and a small fraction not reabsorbed are excreted in the stool.

A number of different conditions present with alterations—reductions—in bile flow, including biliary atresia, TPN cholestasis, and obstruction (i.e., malignancies, primary biliary cirrhosis, primary sclerosing cholangitis). Alagille syndrome is a hereditary vasculopathy associated with the Jagged 1 mutation affecting the Notch2 signaling pathway.[91] The hepatic manifestation is a paucity of intrahepatic bile ducts starting in utero, at/after birth. Patients with Alagille syndrome are at risk for fat-soluble vitamin deficiencies and may be at risk for essential fatty acid deficiencies.[92–100] Patients with Alagille's syndrome do not have EPI; impaired bile flow and associated cholestasis result in pruritus and xanthoma formation.[101]

Other causes of cholestatic liver disease include CF and TI diseases or resections (such as in patients with CF with ileal perforation, Crohn's disease of the TI, and short bowel syndrome). The etiology of disease is impaired enterohepatic bile acid excretion and increased fecal fat, fat-soluble vitamin, bile acid, and vitamin B_{12} losses. In patients with CF, altered duodenal pH related to EPI alters bile acid solubility in the duodenum and affects function.

VI. DISORDERS OF THE COLON

A. Inflammatory Bowel Disease

Inflammatory bowel disease [IBD] is a form of chronic inflammation of the GI tract that broadly follows three patterns:

- Ulcerative colitis (UC), with mucosal inflammation limited to the colon.
- Crohn's disease, which can be present in a continuous or discontinuous fashion from mouth to anus and has the potential to have transmural inflammation. Crohn's disease can present with structuring or fistulizing disease and can have different disease phenotypes/clinical course based on what parts of the GI tract are involved.
- Indeterminate colitis, which is defined as chronic inflammation that cannot be classified as UC or Crohn's.

Classification and GI tract distribution of IBD impacts both clinical course and management decisions. In addition to chronic inflammation and blood loss, sites of disease involvement can result in specific nutritional risks and deficiencies. IBD can occur in all ages, and in children, it can present with malnutrition and failure to thrive. Nutritional compromise and stunting is more common in pediatric Crohn's disease compared to UC.[102]

Diet as a risk factor for IBD

The etiology of IBD is likely multifactorial and involves interactions between intestinal mucosal barrier function, immune function, and the environment (including the diet and microbiota) in genetically susceptible individuals.[103]

There is genetic predisposition for IBD such as in Ashkenazi Jews and people with Northern European ancestry.[104,105] The NOD 2 gene defect was the first of nearly 200 genes that have now been identified in association with IBD.[106] While our genes have not changed significantly over the past 10,000 years, the global incidence and prevalence of IBD has been increasing, expanding beyond previously established high-risk populations, which suggests additional risk factors are at play.[105,107–111] Globally, trends in developing countries undergoing the nutrition transition have been linked to increased incidence of first UC and then Crohn's disease (Fig. 23.5).[105,110–112] Several environmental risk factors have been identified and include tobacco exposure,[113,114] changes diet, lifestyle, and the gastrointestinal microbiome.[115–120]

The dietary risk factors for developing chronic, noncommunicable diseases including IBD relate to the nutrition transition, which marks a departure from traditional diets to the modern Westernized diet. Alterations in dietary fat intake, specifically increases in saturated fats (from animal proteins and dairy products) and omega 6 polyunsaturated fatty acids (red meat, poultry, eggs, vegetable oils) and decreases in omega 3 polyunsaturated fatty acids (fish), have been identified as risk factors.[121] A change in carbohydrate intake, with decreases in complex carbohydrates and fiber and increases in added simple sugars, has also been identified as risk factors. Iron intake in heme form (from animal protein) has also thought to increase oxidative damage in IBD.[122–124] Additives in food such as maltodextrin, emulsifiers (carboxymethylcellulose and polysorbate-80 in particular), and the emulsifier and dairy-thickening agent carrageenan (derived from red and purple seaweed) are thought to contribute to inflammation.[125–133] Gluten intake (wheat, barley, rye) has been implicated as a risk factor for IBD presumably by impairing mucosal barriers and enhancing permeability, as is the case for celiac disease.[134,135]

The contributions of the diet to the pathogenesis of diet and IBD occurs by different mechanisms, including alterations to the microbiota, immune functioning (both to innate immunity and the adaptive immune systems), and host luminal/mucosal barrier function at the intestinal epithelial interface.[103] There are differential effects of these dietary changes and microbiota profiles in terms of the risk for developing UC versus Crohn's.[136]

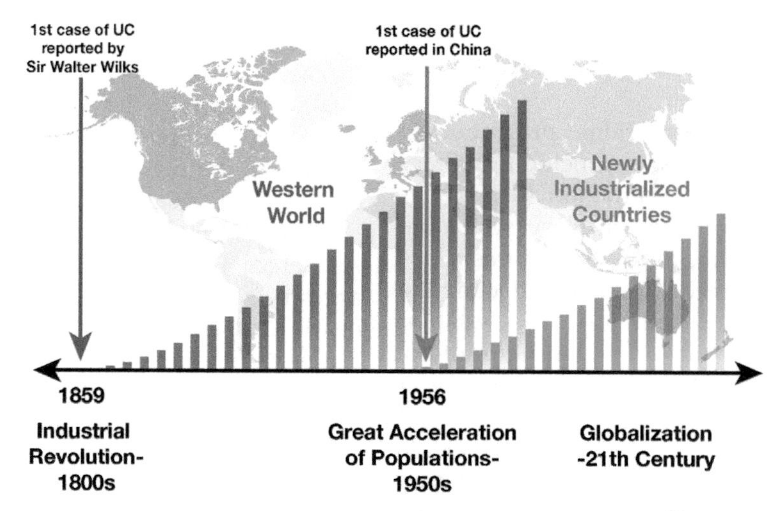

FIGURE 23.5 **Understanding and preventing the global increase of inflammatory bowel disease.**[112] Increasing trend of IBD in industrialized countries since the 19th century and in industrializing countries since the 20th century.

The term "microbiome" refers to organisms and their genomes/functions, whereas "microbiota" refers to the organisms themselves. The difference is very subtle, and sometimes they are used interchangeably. The metabolome specifically refers to the collection of metabolites that organisms produce.

In patients with IBD, the composition of the gut microbiome is altered. There is decreased species diversity and richness in the IBD microbiota. There is a decrease in Firmicutes (including clostridia), *Faecalibacterium prausnitzii, Bilophila wadsworthia,* and *Bifidobacterium adolescentis* and an increase in Actinobacteria and enterobacteriae proteobacteria, including adherent invasive *Escherichia coli.* These microbiota profiles are different than unaffected individuals within the same geographic populations.[137–141] Furthermore, there are some differences in the microbiota in patients with UC versus Crohn's.[136] It remains unclear if these changes to the microbiota are causative or correlated with having IBD.[142] Research tools such as heat maps are used to describe microbiome differences in subjects with Crohn's and how they compare to nonaffected controls (Fig. 23.6).[143]

Dietary intake influences the intestinal luminal environment, and there is dynamic interplay between this intestinal substrate and the microbiota. These differences occur in the neonatal period, with differences in the metabolome developing between breastfed and formula-fed infants.[144] Breastfed infants support a microbiome rich in *Bifidobacterium,* which has antiinflammatory properties thought to against Crohn's disease in particular.[139,145,146] Diets high in animal fat and low in fiber have increased concentrations of *Bacteroides* species, whereas those diets rich in carbohydrates and low in fat have predominance of *Prevotella* species. This is suggestive of a bidirectional relationship between the microbiota and nutrition, further influenced by host genetic susceptibility from an immune regulation and/or intestinal barrier function perspective.[140,147,148]

Short-chain fatty acids, including butyric acid, are the preferred energy source for colonocytes and are produced by the bacteria clostridia, which ferments dietary fiber. This is the preferred substrate for Firmicutes. A lack of dietary fiber results in less fermentation of this substrate by gut bacteria to short-chain fatty acids. Furthermore, lack of fiber ingestion results in intestinal bacteria targeting an alternative substrate in the absence of fiber, namely the unstirred mucus layer. The unstirred mucus layer serves a barrier between the lumen and enterocytes. When the unstirred mucus layer is targeted and permeated, this contributes to inflammation of the mucosa that is exposed underneath. Studies suggest that dietary fiber may have more benefit in patients with Crohn's disease than UC.[149,150] Emulsifiers also found in the diet also impact the intestinal unstirred mucus layer and permeability to *E. coli*, which may drive inflammation.[125]

General nutritional considerations with IBD

Generalized protein-calorie malnutrition with weight loss is common in patients with Crohn's disease and may affect those with UC. In general, patients with Crohn's disease, in the absence of an intestinal obstruction, should consume a diet sufficient in protein and calories to gain back lost weight and maintain a normal weight status. There is no benefit to a low-carbohydrate or low-residual diet except in the presence of an intestinal obstruction. There is also no proven benefit from an increased unrefined carbohydrate.[151] Potentially, higher complex carbohydrates and soluble fiber diets may be beneficial to patients with colitis because of the effects on colonic mucosa of short-chain fatty acids derived from fermentation. Enteral nutritional support studies have suggested diets or formulas high in long-chain triglycerides may be associated with an increased relapse risk of Crohn's disease.[152] Fiber supplementation may be of benefit in Crohn's disease, but not in UC.[153,154]

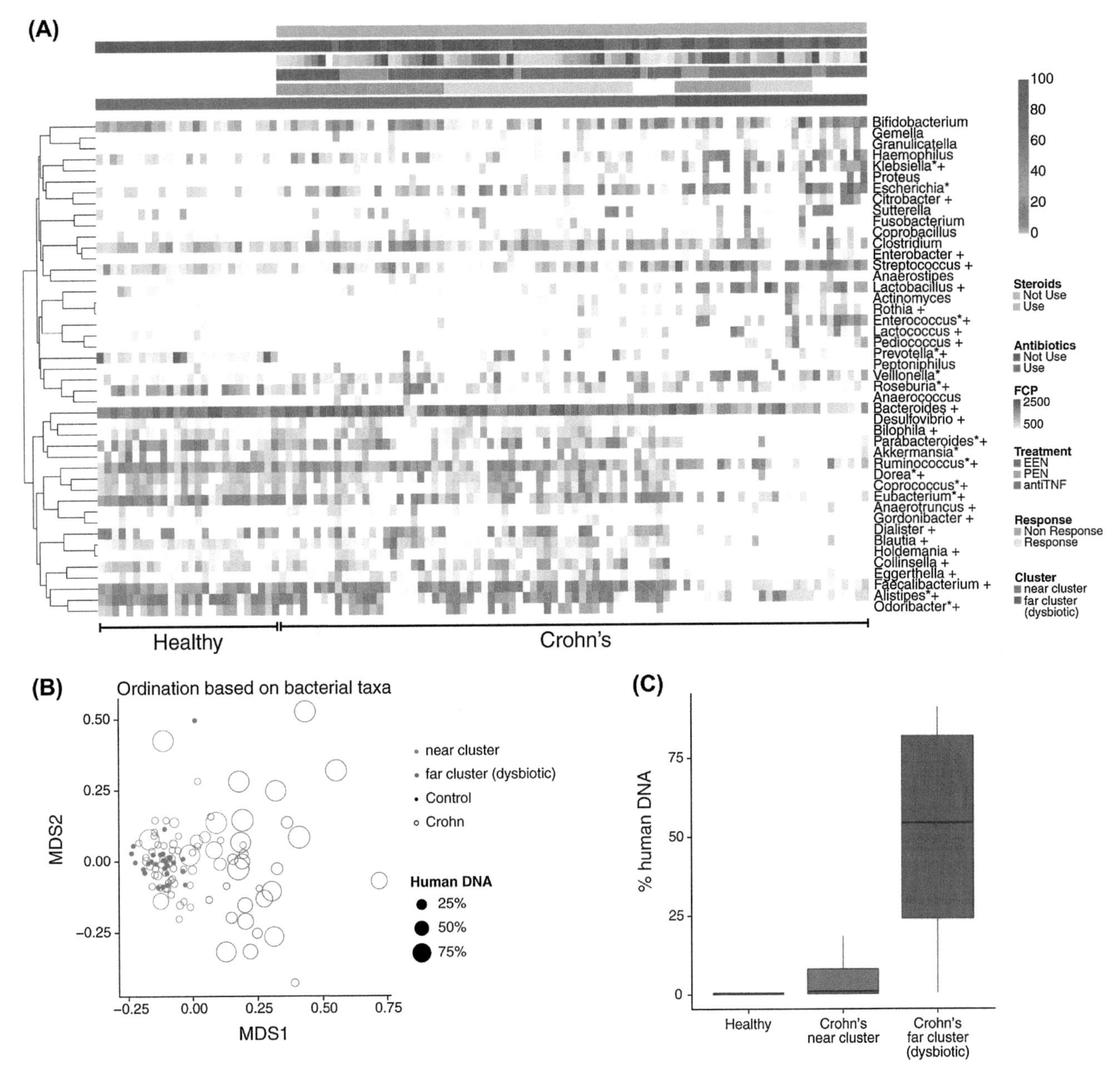

FIGURE 23.6 **Heat map depicting differences in the microbiota in subjects with Crohn's disease as compared to healthy controls.** Bacterial composition in samples from children with Crohn's disease and healthy controls. (A) A heat map demonstrating relative abundance of bacterial taxa prior to therapy according to presence or absence of Crohn's disease, cluster assignment, use of corticosteroids and antibiotics, FCP concentration, and response to therapy. Metadata is indicated by the color code at the top of the figure. White cells indicate missing data. Taxa that were statistically different in abundance between Crohn's disease and healthy controls are identified by *; taxa that were statistically different in abundance between the two Crohn's disease clusters are identified by † ($q < 0.05$). FCP in this and subsequent figures indicates fecal calprotectin. Samples were ordered by the metadata (healthy vs. Crohn's samples, and cluster 1 vs. cluster 2, then other forms of metadata). (B) Multidimensional scaling (MDS) analysis of samples from children with Crohn's disease and healthy controls. Bacterial taxa present were quantified by MetaPhlAn, distances were calculated using binary Jaccard index, and samples were plotted based on MDS. Samples from healthy controls are shown by the filled circles and Crohn's disease as open circles. Clusters were defined by partitioning around medoids with estimation of number of clusters (PAMK) and are colored blue (healthy associated) and red (dysbiotic). The size of the dot is scaled by the proportion of human DNA in the sample. (C) Percentage of human DNA reads in each metagenomic sequence sample. Near cluster (blue, associated with healthy controls) and far cluster (red, dysbiotic) refer to the groups shown in 1B. *Lewis JD, et al.* Cell Host Microbe. *October 14, 2015; 18(4):489–500.*[143]

Specific nutrient concerns in IBD

Vitamin B_{12} deficiency may develop in those patients with chronically active terminal ileal disease or in those with terminal and distal ileal resections totaling >60 cm.[155]

The reduced bile salt pool that occurs with terminal ileal disease or resection leads to fat maldigestion and can result in deficiency of fat-soluble vitamins (A, D, E).[156–158] Vitamin D deficiency has implications regarding

IBD disease activity, and correction of vitamin D deficiency is advised, although the optimal way to achieve this has not been clearly established.[109,159,160] Essential fatty acid deficiency has been described in IBD, and this may relate to terminal ileal disease/resection, increased fatty acid derived eicosanoid utilization in inflammatory cascades, or associated with zinc deficiency, as zinc is an essential nutrient in these specific metabolic pathways.[161,162] Zinc deficiency may be observed in upwards of 40% of patients with Crohn's disease secondary to luminal and malabsorptive losses.[163] Deficiency is difficult to determine on the basis of serum zinc concentration because zinc is bound to serum albumin, other proteins, and amino acids, and these may be depressed in active Crohn's disease and including protein-losing enteropathy. Similarly, conventional measures of iron deficiency may not be optimal in patients with active Crohn's disease or UC because ferritin, as an acute phase reactant, is often elevated, and TIBC may be decreased. Newer approaches to assessment and management of anemia in IBD are reviewed elsewhere.[164,165]

Bacterial overgrowth may occur proximal to intestinal strictures, and these compete with the enterocytes for nutrient absorption. Folate deficiency has been described in upwards of a third of patients with Crohn's disease[166] and in those patients taking folic acid antagonists such as methotrexate or medications that decrease folic acid uptake (i.e., sulfasalazine).

Dietary oxalate should be restricted in patients with steatorrhea from chronically active disease or resection involving the TI. Normally, dietary oxalate is bound to calcium. However, in the setting of steatorrhea, calcium binds preferentially to free fatty acids. Dietary oxalate then passes into the colon where it is absorbed; this may be related to enhanced colonic permeability caused by the presence of bile salts, which normally would have been reabsorbed in the TI. The oxalate is then filtered in the kidneys where it binds to calcium and may lead to calcium oxalate nephrolithiasis as a complication of IBD.[167–169]

Specific nutrient supplementation in IBD

Iron supplementation to prevent or treat anemia secondary to iron deficiency is recommended, with the oral route preferred over intravenous in states of active inflammation.[170] However, given concerns for enteral iron as increasing oxidative stress, and that parenteral iron is not known to promote intestinal luminal inflammation, there is disagreement about the optimal manner in which to provide iron.[122,164,165,170–173]

Specific nutritional supplements have also been studied in patients with IBD. Omega 3 rich fish oils have been studied in patients with IBD, and despite early encouraging earlier studies, larger and controlled studies are equivocal.[174–176] Curcumin derived from spice turmeric is known to have both antiinflammatory and antioxidant properties. There have been improvements in both patient reported disease activity scores and inflammatory markers in a small study in five subjects with Crohn's disease supplemented with curcumin.[177] A double-blinded placebo-controlled trial in 82 subjects with UC demonstrated curcumin to be superior to placebo for maintenance of remission.[178] Furthermore, in combination with mesalamine (a 5-aminosalicylate used to treat IBD), curcumin was shown to be superior to mesalamine + placebo for both clinical and endoscopic improvements/remission.[179] The doses of curcumin used in these studies exceeds that of typical dietary intake. Several small studies of glutamine as therapy for Crohn's disease did not support its use as a therapeutic agent; one rodent study suggested inflammation was worsened with glutamine supplementation.[180,181]

Probiotic therapy, specifically using *E. coli* Nissle 1917 or VSL#3 (specific *Vibrio*, *Saccharomyces*, and *Lactobacillus reuteri* species)—but not necessarily other probiotics—has been used in patients with mild to moderate UC for the induction of remission. The studies using *Lactobacillus* were used for mild distal colitis and were provided in enema form.[182] Probiotics have not been shown to be for the induction or maintenance of remission in Crohn's disease,[183] and their use is not recommended.[170]

Diet therapy for IBD: structured diets

Dietary approaches to establish and maintain clinical remission in patients with IBD have been conducted. Of these, exclusive enteral nutrition (EEN) has been the most studied and effective modality. EEN has been shown in metaanalyses to achieve clinical remission in 60%–86% of pediatric subjects with Crohn's and has also been shown to be superior to corticosteroids in achieving mucosal healing.[184–189] EEN has no known side effects. EEN has also been demonstrated to improve growth in pediatric patients with IBD. European Pediatric Gastroenterology, Hepatology, and Nutrition Guidelines endorse use of EEN as a first-line therapy for Crohn's disease.[170] Time to remission with EEN varies between 3 and 12 weeks across these studies.

Recent advances in our understanding of EEN include that the type of formula seems less relevant than previously thought (polymeric, elemental, etc.). EEN can be administered orally or by tube feeds, or by some combination of approaches. While EEN was thought to be have the strongest response for Crohn's disease predominantly affecting the small bowel, more recent studies have not demonstrated differences based on disease location.[190]

One of the issues with EEN relates to tolerance of enteral feeding and adherence with both tube feeding and a restrictive, monotonous diet. The use of partial enteral nutrition (PEN) is defined by providing >50% of calories from EN with formula. More recent studies suggest >65% to 80%–90% of calories from EN are required to induce remission.[191] PEN has also been demonstrated as an effective treatment to maintain remission in Crohn's in both pediatric and adult patients, with as little as 50% of calories from formula.[192] In adult Crohn's patients, PEN is as effective as 6-mercaptopurine in maintaining remission.[193]

Comparing EEN and PEN, the former is more effective in pediatric Crohn's, even when used in combination with biologics like infliximab.[185,194]

For both EEN and PEN, the precise mechanism of action is unclear and may have to do with carbohydrate monotony and downregulation of the gastrointestinal immune response to feeds, among other potential mechanisms.[195,196] There are several limitations to EEN and PEN, which include difficulty with enteral tolerance to tube feeds (volume, symptoms such as bloating, nausea, etc.), palatability, adherence, and taste fatigue.[196] Other investigators have studied food based-approaches that attempt to mimic or replicate EEN and have promising results.[197]

Current recommendations support the use of EEN or PEN even in the setting of a history of intestinal strictures or stenosis, provided that there are no active obstructive symptoms, and if feeds can be administered beyond the level of the stricture/stenosis.[170] There are appropriate indications for PN in IBD including intestinal obstruction, bowel perforation, prolonged postoperative ileus, short bowel syndrome, anastomotic leak, or high-output fistula.[170]

There are other diets that have been studied in patients with IBD. Gluten increases intestinal permeability in patients both with and without celiac disease.[135] There is currently insufficient evidence to restrict gluten as part of care for IBD. Other diets that are less well studied in IBD include the specific carbohydrate diet, the IBD antiinflammatory diet, the Crohn's disease exclusion diet, the semivegetarian diet, and the Paleolithic diet. A gluten-free diet may improve symptoms in subjects with IBD and possibly active disease activity in Crohn's. These diets are reviewed in detail elsewhere and are summarized in Table 23.3.[198]

In summary, the diet has significant implications for the etiology and management of IBD. IBD is associated with specific nutrient deficiencies that may impact nutritional and growth status particularly in children with Crohn's disease. There are nutritional approaches for both inducing and maintaining clinical remission for IBD, some of which are well established. These are as effective as immunosuppressants, without many side effects and with subsequent improvement of growth for specific patterns of IBD, especially Crohn's disease affecting the small bowel.

VII. FUNCTIONAL GASTROINTESTINAL DISORDERS

Functional gastrointestinal disorders (FGID) comprise a group of conditions that relate to the gastrointestinal tract that cannot be completely explained by anatomical or biochemical abnormalities (infectious, inflammatory). FGID afflict both children and adults and are defined on the basis of symptoms. These symptom-based criteria have been developed by expert consensus and opinion under the auspices of the Rome Foundation and are referred to Rome Criteria. Definitions were updated most recently in 2016, known as the Rome IV criteria.[199–201] FGID pose diagnostic challenges as there is no anatomical or laboratory-based diagnosis. These disorders can coexist across the spectrum of GI disorders, such as with IBD or celiac disease and IBS. Many FGID occur concomitantly with psychosocial, emotional, and behavior stressors. The brain–gut axis plays a role in the pathophysiology of many FGID. Some FGID manifestations may relate to dysbiosis and the intestinal microbiota. FGID may have genetic basis. Early life stressors may manifest later as FGID. Maladaptive responses and lack of adequate coping skills in patients may complicate the management of FGID and often require comanagement with behavioral health providers.

IBS is an FGID. Pediatric and adult IBS is similarly classified by symptoms: IBS with predominant constipation, IBS with predominant diarrhea, and IBS with constipation and diarrhea. IBS includes findings of abdominal pain four or more days per month associated with defecation and/or a change in frequency of stool from baseline and/or a change in form/appearance of stool. Pain may or may not resolve following resolution of constipation; if it does, it is then reclassified as functional constipation. As with other FGIDs, IBS cannot be explained by another underlying medical condition. The pathophysiology of IBS is thought to involve the brain–gut axis and includes a psychosocial stressor component. Visceral hypersensitivity may be attenuated or amplified by psychosocial stressors. Abdominal or rectal pain may occur. A postinfectious (such as with viral infections) IBS phenomenon is known to occur in children, adolescents, and adults and may be driven by inflammatory cytokines. Perturbations in the intestinal microbiota may be coincident, with causality or consequence not clearly established. The GI differential diagnosis includes anatomical, infectious, inflammatory, and motility disorders as well as conditions associated with malabsorption. Differentiation between those GI disorders and IBS is guided by the history and physical, and markers of inflammation—and particularly in the stool—such as fecal calprotectin, are becoming more clinically useful.[199–201]

Aerophagia is more common in patients with impairments in neurocognition. Air swallowing is described as excessive, occurring throughout the day with progressive abdominal distention and with associated passage of gas via belching and/or flatus. Symptoms may be more severe in those children who cannot pass gas once it is swallowed (such as those following gastric fundoplication as a reflux control measure). Chewing gum and gulping down liquids may be risk factors. Symptoms are not attributable to other causes such as partial obstructions, small bowel bacterial overgrowth, gastrointestinal dysmotility (pseudoobstruction), or malabsorptive disorders. Abdominal pain, nausea, and early satiety are reportedly associated GI symptoms, with sleeping issues, headaches, and dizziness also of concern. Anxiety is a frequent comorbidity and may contribute to the behavior. Treatment is mostly supportive and multidisciplinary, including with clinical nutrition, gastroenterology, and behavior psychology.[199]

Beyond addressing aerophagia, gas is a common GI complaint for patients with FGID, including IBS. Dietary approaches are important in management of gas, including reduction or restriction of foods that may provoke symptoms. Some carbohydrates are poorly digested in the small intestine and promote the gas, distention, bloating, and loose stools observed in patients with IBS. These gas forming carbohydrates go by the acronym FODMAPS (fermentable oligo-, di-, monosaccharides, and polyols). High-FODMAP foods cause symptoms, and management strategies include shifting the diet to low-FODMAP foods. Examples of high-FOMAP fruits may include apples and cherries, whereas grapes and strawberries are low-FODMAP foods.[202] Limiting other symptom-provoking foods may also be helpful, either empirically or preferably following specific evaluations, such as for lactose or dietary fructose intolerance. Use of supplemental enzymes such as lactase for lactose intolerance or alpha galactosidase for some plant-based food intake may help symptoms. Switching from fiber with high-FODMAP to low-FODMAP profiles may be helpful in managing symptoms. Confounding variables may include altered GI motility and constipation, which can promote small bowel bacterial overgrowth or dysbiosis.[203–206] Altering gut microbiota by use of probiotics in children and antibiotics in adults has been studies, though with inconclusive results.[207] Behavioral psychology is important to identify possible psychosocial stressors in patients with FGID and to help identify coping mechanisms as part of clinical care.

IBS can coexist with IBD and celiac disease. Low-FODMAP diets may help patients with IBD and celiac disease (gluten-free); while adherence to these specific dietary approaches has been linked to reduction in functional pain symptoms, there is no effect on underlying inflammatory processes in patients.[208–216]

VIII. SUMMARY

The conditions and diseases highlighted in this chapter provide examples of digestive tract physiology and pathophysiology pertinent to nutritionally related pathology and clinical care. Digestion and absorption requires not only an intact and functional gastrointestinal tract but also a dynamic interplay with the metabolome, which is shaped by nutrient intake and external environment and can promote health and disease states.

RESEARCH GAPS

The role of food and pH for gastroesophageal reflux requires further investigation. Alterations and perturbations in pH may have significant impact on gastroesophageal reflux, digestion, and absorption of nutrients, on the microbiome, and possibly also for risk for chronic noncommunicable diseases, including some cancers, and warrant further investigation. There are inadequate data regarding types of fiber intake and clinical outcomes across various GI disease states, including IBD. The role of antiinflammatory diets and antioxidants in pancreatitis and IBD is understudied. The microbiota and metabolome constitute an important bidirectional interface in both health and disease states and need to be further explored and understood, for the prevention and management of disease.

Acknowledgments

This chapter is an update of the chapter titled "52. Nutrition and Gastrointestinal Illness" by Alan L. Buchman and Stephen A. McClave, in *Present Knowledge in Nutrition, 10th Edition*, edited by Erdman JW, Macdonald IA, and Zeisel SH and published by Wiley-Blackwell. © 2012 International Life Sciences Institute. Portions of this update are from the previously published chapter, and the contributions of previous authors are acknowledged.

IX. REFERENCES

1. Vakil N, van Zanten SV, Kahrilas P, Dent J, Jones R. The montreal definition and classification of gastroesophageal reflux disease: a global evidence-based consensus. *Am J Gastroenterol*. 2006;101: 1900–1920. quiz 43.
2. Spechler SJ. Clinical manifestations and esophageal complications of GERD. *Am J Med Sci*. 2003;326:279–284.
3. Argyrou A, Legaki E, Koutserimpas C, et al. Risk factors for gastroesophageal reflux disease and analysis of genetic contributors. *World J Clin Cases*. 2018;6:176–182.
4. *Practical Manual of Gastroesophageal Reflux Disease*. Portland: John Wiley & Sons, Ltd.; 2013.
5. Ness-Jensen E, Hveem K, El-Serag H, Lagergren J. Lifestyle intervention in gastroesophageal reflux disease. *Clin Gastroenterol Hepatol*. 2016;14:175–182.e1–3.
6. Kaltenbach T, Crockett S, Gerson LB. Arel lifestyle measures effective in patients with gastroesophageal reflux disease? An evidence-based approach. *Arch Intern Med*. 2006;166:965–971.
7. Piesman M, Hwang I, Maydonovitch C, Wong RK. Nocturnal reflux episodes following the administration of a standardized meal. Does timing matter? *Am J Gastroenterol*. 2007;102: 2128–2134.
8. Colombo P, Mangano M, Bianchi PA, Penagini R. Effect of calories and fat on postprandial gastro-oesophageal reflux. *Scand J Gastroenterol*. 2002;37:3–5.
9. Newberry C, Lynch K. Can we use diet to effectively treat esophageal disease? A review of the current literature. *Curr Gastroenterol Rep*. 2017;19:38.
10. Furuta GT, Liacouras CA, Collins MH, et al. Eosinophilic esophagitis in children and adults: a systematic review and consensus recommendations for diagnosis and treatment. *Gastroenterology*. 2007;133:1342–1363.
11. Furuta GT, Katzka DA. Eosinophilic esophagitis. *N Engl J Med*. 2015;373:1640–1648.
12. Gonsalves N, Kagalwalla AF. Dietary treatment of eosinophilic esophagitis. *Gastroenterol Clin N Am*. 2014;43:375–383.
13. Peterson KA, Byrne KR, Vinson LA, et al. Elemental diet induces histologic response in adult eosinophilic esophagitis. *Am J Gastroenterol*. 2013;108:759–766.
14. Arias A, Gonzalez-Cervera J, Tenias JM, Lucendo AJ. Efficacy of dietary interventions for inducing histologic remission in patients with eosinophilic esophagitis: a systematic review and meta-analysis. *Gastroenterology*. 2014;146:1639–1648.
15. Kagalwalla AF, Sentongo TA, Ritz S, et al. Effect of six-food elimination diet on clinical and histologic outcomes in eosinophilic esophagitis. *Clin Gastroenterol Hepatol*. 2006;4:1097–1102.
16. Molina-Infante J, Arias A, Barrio J, Rodriguez-Sanchez J, Sanchez-Cazalilla M, Lucendo AJ. Four-food group elimination diet for adult eosinophilic esophagitis: a prospective multicenter study. *J Allergy Clin Immunol*. 2014;134, 1093-9 e1.
17. Spergel JM, Andrews T, Brown-Whitehorn TF, Beausoleil JL, Liacouras CA. Treatment of eosinophilic esophagitis with specific food elimination diet directed by a combination of skin prick and patch tests. *Ann Allergy Asthma Immunol*. 2005;95:336–343.
18. Paquet B, Begin P, Paradis L, Drouin E, Des Roches A. Variable yield of allergy patch testing in children with eosinophilic esophagitis. *J Allergy Clin Immunol*. 2013;131:613.
19. Al-Hussaini A, Al-Idressi E, Al-Zahrani M. The role of allergy evaluation in children with eosinophilic esophagitis. *J Gastroenterol*. 2013;48:1205–1212.
20. Molina-Infante J, Martin-Noguerol E, Alvarado-Arenas M, Porcel-Carreno SL, Jimenez-Timon S, Hernandez-Arbeiza FJ. Selective elimination diet based on skin testing has suboptimal efficacy for adult eosinophilic esophagitis. *J Allergy Clin Immunol*. 2012;130:1200–1202.
21. Braamskamp MJ, Dolman KM, Tabbers MM. Clinical practice. Protein-losing enteropathy in children. *Eur J Pediatr*. 2010;169: 1179–1185.
22. Umar SB, DiBaise JK. Protein-losing enteropathy: case illustrations and clinical review. *Am J Gastroenterol*. 2010;105:43–49. quiz 50.
23. Shikora SA, Kim JJ, Tarnoff ME. Nutrition and gastrointestinal complications of bariatric surgery. *Nutr Clin Pract*. 2007;22:29–40.
24. Pratt JSA, Browne A, Browne NT, et al. ASMBS pediatric metabolic and bariatric surgery guidelines, 2018. *Surg Obes Relat Dis*. 2018;14:882–901.
25. Krzizek EC, Brix JM, Herz CT, et al. Prevalence of micronutrient deficiency in patients with morbid obesity before bariatric surgery. *Obes Surg*. 2018;28:643–648.
26. Parrott J, Frank L, Rabena R, Craggs-Dino L, Isom KA, Greiman L. American society for metabolic and bariatric surgery integrated health nutritional guidelines for the surgical weight loss patient 2016 update: micronutrients. *Surg Obes Relat Dis*. 2017;13:727–741.
27. Al-Mulhim AS. Laparoscopic sleeve gastrectomy and nutrient deficiencies: a prospective study. *Surg Laparosc Endosc Percutaneous Tech*. 2016;26:208–211.
28. Abraham A, Ikramuddin S, Jahansouz C, Arafat F, Hevelone N, Leslie D. Trends in bariatric surgery: procedure selection, revisional surgeries, and readmissions. *Obes Surg*. 2016;26:1371–1377.
29. Stroh C, Manger T, Benedix F. Metabolic surgery and nutritional deficiencies. *Minerva Chir*. 2017;72:432–441.
30. Griggs CL, Perez Jr NP, Goldstone RN, et al. National trends in the use of metabolic and bariatric surgery among pediatric patients with severe obesity. *JAMA Pediatr*. 2018;172:1191–1192.
31. Jaber J, Glenn J, Podkameni D, Soto F. A 5-year history of laparoscopic gastric band removals: an analysis of complications and associated comorbidities. *Obes Surg*. 2019;29:1202–1206.
32. Tammaro P, Hansel B, Police A, et al. Laparoscopic adjustable gastric banding: predictive factors for weight loss and band removal after more than 10 years' follow-up in a single university unit. *World J Surg*. 2017;41:2078–2086.
33. Anderson B, Gill RS, de Gara CJ, Karmali S, Gagner M. Biliopancreatic diversion: the effectiveness of duodenal switch and its limitations. *Gastroenterol Res Pract*. 2013;2013:974762.
34. Lupoli R, Lembo E, Saldalamacchia G, Avola CK, Angrisani L, Capaldo B. Bariatric surgery and long-term nutritional issues. *World J Diabetes*. 2017;8:464–474.
35. Ito MK, Goncalves VSS, Faria S, et al. Effect of protein intake on the protein status and lean mass of post-bariatric surgery patients: a systematic review. *Obes Surg*. 2017;27:502–512.
36. Patel JJ, Mundi MS, Hurt RT, Wolfe B, Martindale RG. Micronutrient deficiencies after bariatric surgery: an emphasis on vitamins and trace minerals [formula: see text]. *Nutr Clin Pract*. 2017;32:471–480.
37. Mechanick JI, Youdim A, Jones DB, et al. Clinical practice guidelines for the perioperative nutritional, metabolic, and nonsurgical

support of the bariatric surgery patient–2013 update: cosponsored by American Association of Clinical Endocrinologists, the Obesity Society, and American Society for Metabolic & Bariatric Surgery. *Obesity.* 2013;21(Suppl 1):S1–S27.

38. *Nutrition and Bariatric Surgery.* Boca Raton, FL: CRC PRess; 2015.
39. Pellitero S, Martinez E, Puig R, et al. Evaluation of vitamin and trace element requirements after sleeve gastrectomy at long term. *Obes Surg.* 2017;27:1674–1682.
40. Leonard MM, Sapone A, Catassi C, Fasano A. Celiac disease and nonceliac gluten sensitivity: a review. *JAMA.* 2017;318:647–656.
41. Fasano A, Berti I, Gerarduzzi T, et al. Prevalence of celiac disease in at-risk and not-at-risk groups in the United States: a large multicenter study. *Arch Intern Med.* 2003;163:286–292.
42. Guandalini S, Gokhale R. Update on immunologic basis of celiac disease. *Curr Opin Gastroenterol.* 2002;18:95–100.
43. See J, Murray JA. Gluten-free diet: the medical and nutrition management of celiac disease. *Nutr Clin Pract.* 2006;21:1–15.
44. Bardella MT, Fredella C, Prampolini L, Molteni N, Giunta AM, Bianchi PA. Body composition and dietary intakes in adult celiac disease patients consuming a strict gluten-free diet. *Am J Clin Nutr.* 2000;72:937–939.
45. Mora S, Barera G, Beccio S, et al. A prospective, longitudinal study of the long-term effect of treatment on bone density in children with celiac disease. *J Pediatr.* 2001;139:516–521.
46. Bolotin D, Petronic-Rosic V. Dermatitis herpetiformis. Part II. Diagnosis, management, and prognosis. *J Am Acad Dermatol.* 2011;64:1027–1033. quiz 33-4.
47. Bolotin D, Petronic-Rosic V. Dermatitis herpetiformis. Part I. Epidemiology, pathogenesis, and clinical presentation. *J Am Acad Dermatol.* 2011;64:1017–1024. quiz 25-6.
48. Rubio-Tapia A, Hill ID, Kelly CP, Calderwood AH, Murray JA. ACG clinical guidelines: diagnosis and management of celiac disease. *Am J Gastroenterol.* 2013;108:656–676. quiz 77.
49. Lebwohl B, Rubio-Tapia A, Assiri A, Newland C, Guandalini S. Diagnosis of celiac disease. *Gastrointest Endosc Clin N Am.* 2012; 22:661–677.
50. Malamut G, Murray JA, Cellier C. Refractory celiac disease. *Gastrointest Endosc Clin N Am.* 2012;22:759–772.
51. Fine KD, Meyer RL, Lee EL. The prevalence and causes of chronic diarrhea in patients with celiac sprue treated with a gluten-free diet. *Gastroenterology.* 1997;112:1830–1838.
52. Shepherd SJ, Gibson PR. Nutritional inadequacies of the gluten-free diet in both recently-diagnosed and long-term patients with coeliac disease. *J Hum Nutr Diet.* 2013;26:349–358.
53. Babio N, Alcazar M, Castillejo G, et al. Patients with celiac disease reported higher consumption of added sugar and total fat than healthy individuals. *J Pediatr Gastroenterol Nutr.* 2017;64:63–69.
54. Lee AR, Ng DL, Dave E, Ciaccio EJ, Green PH. The effect of substituting alternative grains in the diet on the nutritional profile of the gluten-free diet. *J Hum Nutr Diet.* 2009;22:359–363.
55. Matuchansky C. Gluten-free diet and irritable bowel syndrome-diarrhea. *Gastroenterology.* 2013;145:692–693.
56. Sapone A, Bai JC, Ciacci C, et al. Spectrum of gluten-related disorders: consensus on new nomenclature and classification. *BMC Med.* 2012;10:13.
57. Sosnay PR, Raraigh KS, Gibson RL. Molecular genetics of cystic fibrosis transmembrane conductance regulator: genotype and phenotype. *Pediatr Clin N Am.* 2016;63:585–598.
58. Ahmed N, Corey M, Forstner G, et al. Molecular consequences of cystic fibrosis transmembrane regulator (CFTR) gene mutations in the exocrine pancreas. *Gut.* 2003;52:1159–1164.
59. Lammert F, Gurusamy K, Ko CW, et al. Gallstones. *Nat Rev Dis Primers.* 2016;2:16024.
60. Gelrud A, Sheth S, Banerjee S, et al. Analysis of cystic fibrosis gener product (CFTR) function in patients with pancreas divisum and recurrent acute pancreatitis. *Am J Gastroenterol.* 2004;99: 1557–1562.
61. Schneider A, Larusch J, Sun X, et al. Combined bicarbonate conductance-impairing variants in CFTR and SPINK1 variants are associated with chronic pancreatitis in patients without cystic fibrosis. *Gastroenterology.* 2011;140:162–171.
62. Ravnik-Glavac M, Glavac D, di Sant' Agnese P, Chernick M, Dean M. Cystic fibrosis gene mutations detected in hereditary pancreatitis. *Pflüg Arch.* 1996;431:R191–R192.
63. Bishop MD, Freedman SD, Zielenski J, et al. The cystic fibrosis transmembrane conductance regulator gene and ion channel function in patients with idiopathic pancreatitis. *Hum Genet.* 2005;118:372–381.
64. Theodoridis X, Grammatikopoulou MG, Petalidou A, et al. Nutrition interventions in pediatric pancreatitis: in guidelines we can trust. *J Pediatr Gastroenterol Nutr.* 2019;69(1):120–125.
65. Abu-El-Haija M, Uc A, Werlin SL, et al. Nutritional considerations in pediatric pancreatitis: a position paper from the NASPHAN pancreas committee and ESPHAN cystic fibrosis/pancreas working group. *J Pediatr Gastroenterol Nutr.* 2018;67:131–143.
66. Janisch NH, Gardner TB. Advances in management of acute pancreatitis. *Gastroenterol Clin N Am.* 2016;45:1–8.
67. Conwell DL, Lee LS, Yadav D, et al. American pancreatic association practice guidelines in chronic pancreatitis: evidence-based report on diagnostic guidelines. *Pancreas.* 2014;43:1143–1162.
68. IAP/APA evidence-based guidelines for the management of acute pancreatitis. *Pancreatology.* 2013;13:e1–15.
69. Mirtallo JM, Forbes A, McClave SA, Jensen GL, Waitzberg DL, Davies AR. International consensus guidelines for nutrition therapy in pancreatitis. *JPEN J Parenter Enteral Nutr.* 2012;36:284–291.
70. AGA Institute medical position statement on acute pancreatitis. *Gastroenterology.* 2007;132:2019–2021.
71. Goldenberg DE, Gordon SR, Gardner TB. Management of acute pancreatitis. *Expert Rev Gastroenterol Hepatol.* 2014;8:687–694.
72. Giger U, Stanga Z, DeLegge MH. Management of chronic pancreatitis. *Nutr Clin Pract.* 2004;19:37–49.
73. Sax HC, Warner BW, Talamini MA, et al. Early total parenteral nutrition in acute pancreatitis: lack of beneficial effects. *Am J Surg.* 1987;153:117–124.
74. Al-Omran M, Albalawi ZH, Tashkandi MF, Al-Ansary LA. Enteral versus parenteral nutrition for acute pancreatitis. *Cochrane Database Syst Rev.* 2010:CD002837.
75. Larino-Noia J, Lindkvist B, Iglesias-Garcia J, Seijo-Rios S, Iglesias-Canle J, Dominguez-Munoz JE. Early and/or immediately full caloric diet versus standard refeeding in mild acute pancreatitis: a randomized open-label trial. *Pancreatology.* 2014;14:167–173.
76. Jacobson BC, Vander Vliet MB, Hughes MD, Maurer R, McManus K, Banks PA. A prospective, randomized trial of clear liquids versus low-fat solid diet as the initial meal in mild acute pancreatitis. *Clin Gastroenterol Hepatol.* 2007;5:946–951. quiz 886.
77. D'Haese JG, Ceyhan GO, Demir IE, et al. Pancreatic enzyme replacement therapy in patients with exocrine pancreatic insufficiency due to chronic pancreatitis: a 1-year disease management study on symptom control and quality of life. *Pancreas.* 2014;43: 834–841.
78. Walkowiak J, Sands D, Nowakowska A, et al. Early decline of pancreatic function in cystic fibrosis patients with class 1 or 2 CFTR mutations. *J Pediatr Gastroenterol Nutr.* 2005;40:199–201.
79. Czako L, Takacs T, Hegyi P, et al. Quality of life assessment after pancreatic enzyme replacement therapy in chronic pancreatitis. *Can J Gastroenterol.* 2003;17:597–603.
80. Schwarzenberg SJ, Wielinski CL, Shamieh I, et al. Cystic fibrosis-associated colitis and fibrosing colonopathy. *J Pediatr.* 1995;127: 565–570.

81. FitzSimmons SC, Burkhart GA, Borowitz D, et al. High-dose pancreatic-enzyme supplements and fibrosing colonopathy in children with cystic fibrosis. *N Engl J Med*. 1997;336:1283–1289.
82. Borowitz DS, Grand RJ, Durie PR. Use of pancreatic enzyme supplements for patients with cystic fibrosis in the context of fibrosing colonopathy. Consensus Committee. *J Pediatr*. 1995;127:681–684.
83. Ng SM, Moore HS. Drug therapies for reducing gastric acidity in people with cystic fibrosis. *Cochrane Database Syst Rev*. 2016: CD003424.
84. Drzymala-Czyz S, Jonczyk-Potoczna K, Lisowska A, Stajgis M, Walkowiak J. Supplementation of ursodeoxycholic acid improves fat digestion and absorption in cystic fibrosis patients with mild liver involvement. *Eur J Gastroenterol Hepatol*. 2016;28:645–649.
85. Stevens J, Wyatt C, Brown P, Patel D, Grujic D, Freedman SD. Absorption and safety with sustained use of RELiZORB evaluation (ASSURE) study in patients with cystic fibrosis receiving enteral feeding. *J Pediatr Gastroenterol Nutr*. 2018;67:527–532.
86. Lepage G, Yesair DW, Ronco N, et al. Effect of an organized lipid matrix on lipid absorption and clinical outcomes in patients with cystic fibrosis. *J Pediatr*. 2002;141:178–185.
87. Stallings VA, Schall JI, Maqbool A, et al. Effect of oral lipid matrix supplement on fat absorption in cystic fibrosis: a randomized placebo-controlled trial. *J Pediatr Gastroenterol Nutr*. 2016;63: 676–680.
88. Huang W, de la Iglesia-Garcia D, Baston-Rey I, et al. Exocrine pancreatic insufficiency following acute pancreatitis: systematic review and meta-analysis. *Dig Dis Sci*. 2019;64(7):1985–2005.
89. *Inititating Pancreatic Enzyme Replacement Therapy [PERT] Clinical Pathway*. 2019.
90. Monte MJ, Marin JJ, Antelo A, Vazquez-Tato J. Bile acids: chemistry, physiology, and pathophysiology. *World J Gastroenterol*. 2009; 15:804–816.
91. Krantz ID, Piccoli DA, Spinner NB. Alagille syndrome. *J Med Genet*. 1997;34:152–157.
92. Babin F, Lemonnier F, Goguelin A, Alagille D, Lemonnier A. Plasma fatty acid composition and lipid peroxide levels in children with paucity of interlobular bile ducts. *Ann Nutr Metab*. 1988;32:220–230.
93. Rovner AJ, Schall JI, Jawad AF, et al. Rethinking growth failure in Alagille syndrome: the role of dietary intake and steatorrhea. *J Pediatr Gastroenterol Nutr*. 2002;35:495–502.
94. Moisseiev E, Cohen S, Dotan G. Alagille syndrome associated with xerophthalmia. *Case Rep Ophthalmol*. 2013;4:311–315.
95. Amedee-Manesme O, Furr HC, Alvarez F, Hadchouel M, Alagille D, Olson JA. Biochemical indicators of vitamin A depletion in children with cholestasis. *Hepatology*. 1985;5:1143–1148.
96. Alvarez F, Cresteil D, Lemonnier F, Lemonnier A, Alagille D. Plasma vitamin E levels in children with cholestasis. *J Pediatr Gastroenterol Nutr*. 1984;3:390–393.
97. Davit-Spraul A, Cosson C, Couturier M, et al. Standard treatment of alpha-tocopherol in Alagille patients with severe cholestasis is insufficient. *Pediatr Res*. 2001;49:232–236.
98. Alagille D, Estrada A, Hadchouel M, Gautier M, Odievre M, Dommergues JP. Syndromic paucity of interlobular bile ducts (Alagille syndrome or arteriohepatic dysplasia): review of 80 cases. *J Pediatr*. 1987;110:195–200.
99. Venkat VL, Shneider BL, Magee JC, et al. Total serum bilirubin predicts fat-soluble vitamin deficiency better than serum bile acids in infants with biliary atresia. *J Pediatr Gastroenterol Nutr*. 2014;59:702–707.
100. Alvarez F, Landrieu P, Feo C, Lemmonier F, Bernard O, Alagille D. Vitamin E deficiency is responsible for neurologic abnormalities in cholestatic children. *J Pediatr*. 1985;107:422–425.
101. Kamath BM, Piccoli DA, Magee JC, Sokol RJ. Pancreatic insufficiency is not a prevalent problem in Alagille syndrome. *J Pediatr Gastroenterol Nutr*. 2012;55:612–614.
102. Shamir R. Nutritional aspects in inflammatory bowel disease. *J Pediatr Gastroenterol Nutr*. 2009;48(suppl 2):S86–S88.
103. Levine A, Sigall Boneh R, Wine E. Evolving role of diet in the pathogenesis and treatment of inflammatory bowel diseases. *Gut*. 2018;67:1726–1738.
104. Loftus Jr EV, Sandborn WJ. Epidemiology of inflammatory bowel disease. *Gastroenterol Clin N Am*. 2002;31:1–20.
105. Molodecky NA, Soon IS, Rabi DM, et al. Increasing incidence and prevalence of the inflammatory bowel diseases with time, based on systematic review. *Gastroenterology*. 2012;142:46–54. e42; quiz e30.
106. Ogura Y, Bonen DK, Inohara N, et al. A frameshift mutation in NOD2 associated with susceptibility to Crohn's disease. *Nature*. 2001;411:603–606.
107. Ng SC, Bernstein CN, Vatn MH, et al. Geographical variability and environmental risk factors in inflammatory bowel disease. *Gut*. 2013;62:630–649.
108. M'Koma AE. Inflammatory bowel disease: an expanding global health problem. *Clin Med Insights Gastroenterol*. 2013;6:33–47.
109. Schultz M, Butt AG. Is the north to south gradient in inflammatory bowel disease a global phenomenon? *Expert Rev Gastroenterol Hepatol*. 2012;6:445–447.
110. Ng SC, Shi HY, Hamidi N, et al. Worldwide incidence and prevalence of inflammatory bowel disease in the 21st century: a systematic review of population-based studies. *Lancet*. 2018;390: 2769–2778.
111. Kaplan GG. The global burden of IBD: from 2015 to 2025. *Nat Rev Gastroenterol Hepatol*. 2015;12:720–727.
112. Kaplan GG, Ng SC. Understanding and preventing the global increase of inflammatory bowel disease. *Gastroenterology*. 2017;152: 313–321 e2.
113. Yadav P, Ellinghaus D, Remy G, et al. Genetic factors interact with tobacco smoke to modify risk for inflammatory bowel disease in humans and mice. *Gastroenterology*. 2017;153:550–565.
114. Salih A, Widbom L, Hultdin J, Karling P. Smoking is associated with risk for developing inflammatory bowel disease including late onset ulcerative colitis: a prospective study. *Scand J Gastroenterol*. 2018;53:173–178.
115. Dolan KT, Chang EB. Diet, gut microbes, and the pathogenesis of inflammatory bowel diseases. *Mol Nutr Food Res*. 2017;61.
116. Lakatos PL. Environmental factors affecting inflammatory bowel disease: have we made progress? *Dig Dis*. 2009;27: 215–225.
117. Niewiadomski O, Studd C, Wilson J, et al. Influence of food and lifestyle on the risk of developing inflammatory bowel disease. *Intern Med J*. 2016;46:669–676.
118. Harper JW, Zisman TL. Interaction of obesity and inflammatory bowel disease. *World J Gastroenterol*. 2016;22:7868–7881.
119. Cosnes J. Smoking, physical activity, nutrition and lifestyle: environmental factors and their impact on IBD. *Dig Dis*. 2010;28: 411–417.
120. Shouval DS, Rufo PA. The role of environmental factors in the pathogenesis of inflammatory bowel diseases: a review. *JAMA Pediatr*. 2017;171:999–1005.
121. Shoda R, Matsueda K, Yamato S, Umeda N. Epidemiologic analysis of Crohn disease in Japan: increased dietary intake of n-6 polyunsaturated fatty acids and animal protein relates to the increased incidence of Crohn disease in Japan. *Am J Clin Nutr*. 1996;63:741–745.
122. Constante M, Fragoso G, Calve A, Samba-Mondonga M, Santos MM. Dietary heme induces gut dysbiosis, aggravates colitis, and potentiates the development of adenomas in mice. *Front Microbiol*. 2017;8:1809.
123. Khalili H, de Silva PS, Ananthakrishnan AN, et al. Dietary iron and heme iron consumption, genetic susceptibility, and risk of Crohn's disease and ulcerative colitis. *Inflamm Bowel Dis*. 2017; 23:1088–1095.

124. Reifen R, Matas Z, Zeidel L, Berkovitch Z, Bujanover Y. Iron supplementation may aggravate inflammatory status of colitis in a rat model. *Dig Dis Sci*. 2000;45:394–397.
125. Lock JY, Carlson TL, Wang CM, Chen A, Carrier RL. Acute exposure to commonly ingested emulsifiers alters intestinal mucus structure and transport properties. *Sci Rep*. 2018;8:10008.
126. Nickerson KP, McDonald C. Crohn's disease-associated adherent-invasive *Escherichia coli* adhesion is enhanced by exposure to the ubiquitous dietary polysaccharide maltodextrin. *PLoS One*. 2012; 7:e52132.
127. Lewis JD, Abreu MT. Diet as a trigger or therapy for inflammatory bowel diseases. *Gastroenterology*. 2017;152:398–414 e6.
128. Pfeffer-Gik T, Levine A. Dietary clues to the pathogenesis of Crohn's disease. *Dig Dis*. 2014;32:389–394.
129. Viennois E, Chassaing B. First victim, later aggressor: how the intestinal microbiota drives the pro-inflammatory effects of dietary emulsifiers? *Gut Microb*. 2018:1–4.
130. Roberts CL, Rushworth SL, Richman E, Rhodes JM. Hypothesis: increased consumption of emulsifiers as an explanation for the rising incidence of Crohn's disease. *J Crohns Colitis*. 2013;7:338–341.
131. Marion-Letellier R, Amamou A, Savoye G, Ghosh S. Inflammatory bowel diseases and food additives: to add fuel on the flames!. *Nutrients*. 2019;11.
132. Munyaka PM, Sepehri S, Ghia JE, Khafipour E. Carrageenan gum and adherent invasive *Escherichia coli* in a piglet model of inflammatory bowel disease: impact on intestinal mucosa-associated microbiota. *Front Microbiol*. 2016;7:462.
133. Martino JV, Van Limbergen J, Cahill LE. The role of carrageenan and carboxymethylcellulose in the development of intestinal inflammation. *Front Pediatr*. 2017;5:96.
134. Aziz I, Branchi F, Pearson K, Priest J, Sanders DS. A study evaluating the bidirectional relationship between inflammatory bowel disease and self-reported non-celiac gluten sensitivity. *Inflamm Bowel Dis*. 2015;21:847–853.
135. Hollon J, Puppa EL, Greenwald B, Goldberg E, Guerrerio A, Fasano A. Effect of gliadin on permeability of intestinal biopsy explants from celiac disease patients and patients with non-celiac gluten sensitivity. *Nutrients*. 2015;7:1565–1576.
136. Schaffler H, Kaschitzki A, Alberts C, et al. Alterations in the mucosa-associated bacterial composition in Crohn's disease: a pilot study. *Int J Colorectal Dis*. 2016;31:961–971.
137. Fujimoto T, Imaeda H, Takahashi K, et al. Decreased abundance of Faecalibacterium prausnitzii in the gut microbiota of Crohn's disease. *J Gastroenterol Hepatol*. 2013;28:613–619.
138. Machiels K, Joossens M, Sabino J, et al. A decrease of the butyrate-producing species Roseburia hominis and Faecalibacterium prausnitzii defines dysbiosis in patients with ulcerative colitis. *Gut*. 2014;63:1275–1283.
139. Joossens M, Huys G, Cnockaert M, et al. Dysbiosis of the faecal microbiota in patients with Crohn's disease and their unaffected relatives. *Gut*. 2011;60:631–637.
140. Sartor RB. Gut microbiota: diet promotes dysbiosis and colitis in susceptible hosts. *Nat Rev Gastroenterol Hepatol*. 2012;9:561–562.
141. Tawfik A, Flanagan PK, Campbell BJ. Escherichia coli-host macrophage interactions in the pathogenesis of inflammatory bowel disease. *World J Gastroenterol*. 2014;20:8751–8763.
142. Ni J, Wu GD, Albenberg L, Tomov VT. Gut microbiota and IBD: causation or correlation? *Nat Rev Gastroenterol Hepatol*. 2017;14: 573–584.
143. Lewis JD, Chen EZ, Baldassano RN, et al. Inflammation, antibiotics, and diet as environmental stressors of the gut microbiome in pediatric Crohn's disease. *Cell Host Microbe*. 2015;18: 489–500.
144. Saavedra JM, Dattilo AM. Early development of intestinal microbiota: implications for future health. *Gastroenterol Clin N Am*. 2012; 41:717–731.
145. Imaoka A, Shima T, Kato K, et al. Anti-inflammatory activity of probiotic Bifidobacterium: enhancement of IL-10 production in peripheral blood mononuclear cells from ulcerative colitis patients and inhibition of IL-8 secretion in HT-29 cells. *World J Gastroenterol*. 2008;14:2511–2516.
146. LoCascio RG, Desai P, Sela DA, Weimer B, Mills DA. Broad conservation of milk utilization genes in *Bifidobacterium longum* subsp. infantis as revealed by comparative genomic hybridization. *Appl Environ Microbiol*. 2010;76:7373–7381.
147. Goldsmith JR, Sartor RB. The role of diet on intestinal microbiota metabolism: downstream impacts on host immune function and health, and therapeutic implications. *J Gastroenterol*. 2014;49: 785–798.
148. Ray A, Dittel BN. Interrelatedness between dysbiosis in the gut microbiota due to immunodeficiency and disease penetrance of colitis. *Immunology*. 2015;146:359–368.
149. Amre DK, D'Souza S, Morgan K, et al. Imbalances in dietary consumption of fatty acids, vegetables, and fruits are associated with risk for Crohn's disease in children. *Am J Gastroenterol*. 2007;102: 2016–2025.
150. Ananthakrishnan AN, Khalili H, Konijeti GG, et al. A prospective study of long-term intake of dietary fiber and risk of Crohn's disease and ulcerative colitis. *Gastroenterology*. 2013;145:970–977.
151. Ritchie JK, Wadsworth J, Lennard-Jones JE, Rogers E. Controlled multicentre therapeutic trial of an unrefined carbohydrate, fibre rich diet in Crohn's disease. *Br Med J*. 1987;295:517–520.
152. Middleton SJ, Rucker JT, Kirby GA, Riordan AM, Hunter JO. Long-chain triglycerides reduce the efficacy of enteral feeds in patients with active Crohn's disease. *Clin Nutr*. 1995;14: 229–236.
153. Burisch J, Pedersen N, Cukovic-Cavka S, et al. Environmental factors in a population-based inception cohort of inflammatory bowel disease patients in Europe–an ECCO-EpiCom study. *J Crohns Colitis*. 2014;8:607–616.
154. Andersen V, Chan S, Luben R, et al. Fibre intake and the development of inflammatory bowel disease: a European prospective multi-centre cohort study (EPIC-IBD). *J Crohns Colitis*. 2018;12: 129–136.
155. Behrend C, Jeppesen PB, Mortensen PB. Vitamin B_{12} absorption after ileorectal anastomosis for Crohn's disease: effect of ileal resection and time span after surgery. *Eur J Gastroenterol Hepatol*. 1995;7:397–400.
156. Bousvaros A, Zurakowski D, Duggan C, et al. Vitamins A and E serum levels in children and young adults with inflammatory bowel disease: effect of disease activity. *J Pediatr Gastroenterol Nutr*. 1998;26:129–135.
157. Schaffler H, Schmidt M, Huth A, Reiner J, Glass A, Lamprecht G. Clinical factors are associated with vitamin D levels in IBD patients: a retrospective analysis. *J Dig Dis*. 2018;19:24–32.
158. Frigstad SO, Hoivik M, Jahnsen J, et al. Vitamin D deficiency in inflammatory bowel disease: prevalence and predictors in a Norwegian outpatient population. *Scand J Gastroenterol*. 2017;52: 100–106.
159. Del Pinto R, Pietropaoli D, Chandar AK, Ferri C, Cominelli F. Association between inflammatory bowel disease and vitamin D deficiency: a systematic review and meta-analysis. *Inflamm Bowel Dis*. 2015;21:2708–2717.
160. Richman E, Rhodes JM. Review article: evidence-based dietary advice for patients with inflammatory bowel disease. *Aliment Pharmacol Ther*. 2013;38:1156–1171.
161. Socha P, Ryzko J, Koletzko B, et al. Essential fatty acid depletion in children with inflammatory bowel disease. *Scand J Gastroenterol*. 2005;40:573–577.
162. Solomons NW, Rosenberg IH. Zinc and inflammatory bowel disease. *Am J Clin Nutr*. 1981;34:1447–1448.

163. Valberg LS, Flanagan PR, Kertesz A, Bondy DC. Zinc absorption in inflammatory bowel disease. *Dig Dis Sci*. 1986;31:724–731.
164. Murawska N, Fabisiak A, Fichna J. Anemia of chronic disease and iron deficiency anemia in inflammatory bowel diseases: pathophysiology, diagnosis, and treatment. *Inflamm Bowel Dis*. 2016; 22:1198–1208.
165. Martin J, Radeke HH, Dignass A, Stein J. Current evaluation and management of anemia in patients with inflammatory bowel disease. *Expert Rev Gastroenterol Hepatol*. 2017;11:19–32.
166. Elsborg L, Larsen L. Folate deficiency in chronic inflammatory bowel diseases. *Scand J Gastroenterol*. 1979;14:1019–1024.
167. Dobbins JW, Binder HJ. Importance of the colon in enteric hyperoxaluria. *N Engl J Med*. 1977;296:298–301.
168. Dharmsathaphorn K, Freeman DH, Binder HJ, Dobbins JW. Increased risk of nephrolithiasis in patients with steatorrhea. *Dig Dis Sci*. 1982;27:401–405.
169. Sangaletti O, Petrillo M, Bianchi Porro G. Urinary oxalate recovery after oral oxalic load: an alternative method to the quantitative determination of stool fat for the diagnosis of lipid malabsorption. *J Int Med Res*. 1989;17:526–531.
170. Forbes A, Escher J, Hebuterne X, et al. ESPEN guideline: clinical nutrition in inflammatory bowel disease. *Clin Nutr*. 2017;36: 321–347.
171. Nielsen OH, Ainsworth M, Coskun M, Weiss G. Management of iron-deficiency anemia in inflammatory bowel disease: a systematic review. *Medicine (Baltim)*. 2015;94:e963.
172. Massironi S, Rossi RE, Cavalcoli FA, Della Valle S, Fraquelli M, Conte D. Nutritional deficiencies in inflammatory bowel disease: therapeutic approaches. *Clin Nutr*. 2013;32:904–910.
173. Dignass AU, Gasche C, Bettenworth D, et al. European consensus on the diagnosis and management of iron deficiency and anaemia in inflammatory bowel diseases. *J Crohns Colitis*. 2015;9:211–222.
174. Belluzzi A, Brignola C, Campieri M, Pera A, Boschi S, Miglioli M. Effect of an enteric-coated fish-oil preparation on relapses in Crohn's disease. *N Engl J Med*. 1996;334:1557–1560.
175. Hawthorne AB, Daneshmend TK, Hawkey CJ, et al. Treatment of ulcerative colitis with fish oil supplementation: a prospective 12 month randomised controlled trial. *Gut*. 1992;33:922–928.
176. Feagan BG, Sandborn WJ, Mittmann U, et al. Omega-3 free fatty acids for the maintenance of remission in Crohn disease: the EPIC Randomized Controlled Trials. *JAMA*. 2008;299: 1690–1697.
177. Holt PR, Katz S, Kirshoff R. Curcumin therapy in inflammatory bowel disease: a pilot study. *Dig Dis Sci*. 2005;50:2191–2193.
178. Hanai H, Iida T, Takeuchi K, et al. Curcumin maintenance therapy for ulcerative colitis: randomized, multicenter, double-blind, placebo-controlled trial. *Clin Gastroenterol Hepatol*. 2006;4: 1502–1506.
179. Lang A, Salomon N, Wu JC, et al. Curcumin in combination with mesalamine induces remission in patients with mild-to-moderate ulcerative colitis in a randomized controlled trial. *Clin Gastroenterol Hepatol*. 2015;13:1444–1449.e1.
180. Akobeng AK, Miller V, Stanton J, Elbadri AM, Thomas AG. Double-blind randomized controlled trial of glutamine-enriched polymeric diet in the treatment of active Crohn's disease. *J Pediatr Gastroenterol Nutr*. 2000;30:78–84.
181. Shinozaki M, Saito H, Muto T. Excess glutamine exacerbates trinitrobenzenesulfonic acid-induced colitis in rats. *Dis Colon Rectum*. 1997;40:S59–S63.
182. Oliva S, Di Nardo G, Ferrari F, et al. Randomised clinical trial: the effectiveness of Lactobacillus reuteri ATCC 55730 rectal enema in children with active distal ulcerative colitis. *Aliment Pharmacol Ther*. 2012;35:327–334.
183. Bousvaros A, Guandalini S, Baldassano RN, et al. A randomized, double-blind trial of Lactobacillus GG versus placebo in addition to standard maintenance therapy for children with Crohn's disease. *Inflamm Bowel Dis*. 2005;11:833–839.
184. Dziechciarz P, Horvath A, Shamir R, Szajewska H. Meta-analysis: enteral nutrition in active Crohn's disease in children. *Aliment Pharmacol Ther*. 2007;26:795–806.
185. Lee D, Baldassano RN, Otley AR, et al. Comparative effectiveness of nutritional and biological therapy in north American children with active Crohn's disease. *Inflamm Bowel Dis*. 2015;21: 1786–1793.
186. Levine A, Turner D, Pfeffer Gik T, et al. Comparison of outcomes parameters for induction of remission in new onset pediatric Crohn's disease: evaluation of the porto IBD group "growth relapse and outcomes with therapy" (GROWTH CD) study. *Inflamm Bowel Dis*. 2014;20:278–285.
187. Cohen-Dolev N, Sladek M, Hussey S, et al. Differences in outcomes over time with exclusive enteral nutrition compared with steroids in children with mild to moderate Crohn's disease: results from the GROWTH CD study. *J Crohns Colitis*. 2018;12: 306–312.
188. Connors J, Basseri S, Grant A, et al. Exclusive enteral nutrition therapy in paediatric Crohn's disease results in long-term avoidance of corticosteroids: results of a propensity-score matched cohort analysis. *J Crohns Colitis*. 2017;11:1063–1070.
189. Grover Z, Burgess C, Muir R, Reilly C, Lewindon PJ. Early mucosal healing with exclusive enteral nutrition is associated with improved outcomes in newly diagnosed children with luminal Crohn's disease. *J Crohns Colitis*. 2016;10:1159–1164.
190. Buchanan E, Gaunt WW, Cardigan T, Garrick V, McGrogan P, Russell RK. The use of exclusive enteral nutrition for induction of remission in children with Crohn's disease demonstrates that disease phenotype does not influence clinical remission. *Aliment Pharmacol Ther*. 2009;30:501–507.
191. Gupta K, Noble A, Kachelries KE, et al. A novel enteral nutrition protocol for the treatment of pediatric Crohn's disease. *Inflamm Bowel Dis*. 2013;19:1374–1378.
192. Wilschanski M, Sherman P, Pencharz P, Davis L, Corey M, Griffiths A. Supplementary enteral nutrition maintains remission in paediatric Crohn's disease. *Gut*. 1996;38:543–548.
193. Hanai H, Iida T, Takeuchi K, et al. Nutritional therapy versus 6-mercaptopurine as maintenance therapy in patients with Crohn's disease. *Dig Liver Dis*. 2012;44:649–654.
194. Johnson T, Macdonald S, Hill SM, Thomas A, Murphy MS. Treatment of active Crohn's disease in children using partial enteral nutrition with liquid formula: a randomised controlled trial. *Gut*. 2006;55:356–361.
195. Britto S, Kellermayer R. Carbohydrate monotony as protection and treatment for inflammatory bowel disease. *J Crohns Colitis*. 2019;13(7):942–948.
196. Ashton JJ, Gavin J, Beattie RM. Exclusive enteral nutrition in Crohn's disease: evidence and practicalities. *Clin Nutr*. 2019;38: 80–89.
197. Svolos V, Hansen R, Nichols B, et al. Treatment of active Crohn's disease with an ordinary food-based diet that replicates exclusive enteral nutrition. *Gastroenterology*. 2019;156:1354–13567 e6.
198. Stein R, Baldassano RN. Dietary therapies for inflammatory bowel disease. In: Mamula P, Grossman AB, Baldassano RN, Kelsen JR, Markowitz JE, eds. *Pediatric Inflammatory Bowel Disease*. 3rd ed. Cham, Switzerland: Springer International Publishing AG; 2017:473–483.
199. Hyams JS, Di Lorenzo C, Saps M, Shulman RJ, Staiano A, van Tilburg M. *Functional Disorders: Children and Adolescents*. Gastroenterology; 2016.
200. Koppen IJ, Nurko S, Saps M, Di Lorenzo C, Benninga MA. The pediatric Rome IV criteria: what's new? *Expert Rev Gastroenterol Hepatol*. 2017;11:193–201.

201. Benninga MA, Faure C, Hyman PE, St James Roberts I, Schechter NL, Nurko S. Childhood functional gastrointestinal disorders: Neonate/Toddler. *Gastroenterology.* 2016;130(5):1519–1526.
202. *FODMAP Food List.* Monash University; 2019.
203. Craig RM. Low FODMAP diet for IBS. *Gastroenterology.* 2018;154:1547.
204. Staudacher HM, Ralph FSE, Irving PM, Whelan K, Lomer MCE. Nutrient intake, diet quality, and diet diversity in irritable bowel syndrome and the impact of the low FODMAP diet. *J Acad Nutr Diet.* 2019. https://doi.org/10.1016/j.jand.2019.01.017.
205. Eswaran S, Farida JP, Green J, Miller JD, Chey WD. Nutrition in the management of gastrointestinal diseases and disorders: the evidence for the low FODMAP diet. *Curr Opin Pharmacol.* 2017;37:151–157.
206. Chumpitazi BP. Update on dietary management of childhood functional abdominal pain disorders. *Gastroenterol Clin N Am.* 2018;47:715–726.
207. Horvath A, Dziechciarz P, Szajewska H. Meta-analysis: lactobacillus rhamnosus GG for abdominal pain-related functional gastrointestinal disorders in childhood. *Aliment Pharmacol Ther.* 2011;33:1302–1310.
208. Testa A, Imperatore N, Rispo A, et al. Beyond irritable bowel syndrome: the efficacy of the low fodmap diet for improving symptoms in inflammatory bowel diseases and celiac disease. *Dig Dis.* 2018;36:271–280.
209. Roncoroni L, Bascunan KA, Doneda L, et al. Correction: Roncoroni, L. et al. A Low FODMAP Gluten-Free Diet Improves Functional Gastrointestinal Disorders and Overall Mental Health of Celiac Disease Patients: a Randomized Controlled Trial. Nutrients 2018, 10, 1023. *Nutrients.* 2019;11.
210. Roncoroni L, Bascunan KA, Doneda L, et al. A low FODMAP gluten-free diet improves functional gastrointestinal disorders and overall mental health of celiac disease patients: a randomized controlled trial. *Nutrients.* 2018;10.
211. Roncoroni L, Elli L, Doneda L, et al. A retrospective study on dietary FODMAP intake in celiac patients following a gluten-free diet. *Nutrients.* 2018;10.
212. Barbalho SM, Goulart RA, Aranao ALC, de Oliveira PGC. Inflammatory bowel diseases and fermentable oligosaccharides, disaccharides, monosaccharides, and polyols: an overview. *J Med Food.* 2018;21:633–640.
213. Colombel JF, Shin A, Gibson PR. AGA clinical practice update on functional gastrointestinal symptoms in patients with inflammatory bowel disease: expert review. *Clin Gastroenterol Hepatol.* 2019;17:380–390 e1.
214. Damas OM, Garces L, Abreu MT. Diet as adjunctive treatment for inflammatory bowel disease: review and update of the latest literature. *Curr Treat Options Gastroenterol.* 2019;17:313–325.
215. Duff W, Haskey N, Potter G, Alcorn J, Hunter P, Fowler S. Non-pharmacological therapies for inflammatory bowel disease: recommendations for self-care and physician guidance. *World J Gastroenterol.* 2018;24:3055–3070.
216. Hou JK, Lee D, Lewis J. Diet and inflammatory bowel disease: review of patient-targeted recommendations. *Clin Gastroenterol Hepatol.* 2014;12:1592–1600.
217. Obih C, Wahbeh G, Lee D, et al. Specific carbohydrate diet for pediatric inflammatory bowel disease in clinical practice within an academic IBD center. *Nutrition.* 2016;32:418–425.
218. Olendzki BC, Silverstein TD, Persuitte GM, Ma Y, Baldwin KR, Cave D. An anti-inflammatory diet as treatment for inflammatory bowel disease: a case series report. *Nutr J.* 2014;13:5.
219. Levine A, Wine E, Assa A, et al. Crohn's disease exclusion diet plus partial enteral nutrition induces sustained remission in a randomized controlled trial. *Gastroenterology.* 2019;157(2):440–450.e8.
220. Sigall Boneh R, Sarbagili Shabat C, Yanai H, et al. Dietary therapy with the Crohn's disease exclusion diet is a successful strategy for induction of remission in children and adults failing biological therapy. *J Crohns Colitis.* 2017;11:1205–1212.
221. Chiba M, Abe T, Tsuda H, et al. Lifestyle-related disease in Crohn's disease: relapse prevention by a semi-vegetarian diet. *World J Gastroenterol.* 2010;16:2484–2495.

CHAPTER

24

KIDNEY DISEASE AND NUTRITION IN ADULTS AND CHILDREN

Namrata G. Jain[1], MD
Hilda E. Fernandez[2], MD, MS
Thomas L. Nickolas[2], MD, MS

[1]Columbia University Irving Medical Center, Department of Pediatrics, Pediatric Nephrology, New York, NY, United States

[2]Columbia University Irving Medical Center, Department of Medicine, Nephrology, New York, NY, United States

SUMMARY

Chronic kidney disease (CKD) affects over 20 million individuals in the United States and 752 million individuals worldwide.[1] Progressive kidney disease that leads to the need for dialysis (end-stage renal disease or ESRD) or transplantation affects over 700,000 individuals in the United States. CKD is defined as abnormalities of kidney structure or function present for >3 months, with stratification based on estimated glomerular filtration rate category and the magnitude of albuminuria.[2] The Kidney Disease: Improving Global Outcomes group has updated the classification of CKD and changed the term "stage" to "grade," as not all kidney disease is progressive, and noted that the presence or absence of albuminuria can greatly influence prognosis.[3] In this chapter, we describe in brief the primary nutritional and metabolic derangement in children and adults with CKD.

Keywords: Growth hormone; Mineral and bone disease; Nutritional supplementation; Pediatric and adult chronic kidney disease; Protein energy wasting; Renal transplant.

I. INTRODUCTION

In both children and adults, the kidneys are critical for the maintenance of fluid and electrolyte homeostasis, excretion of metabolic waste products, and the regulation of various hormonal and metabolic pathways. Even a slight reduction in kidney function may have metabolic and nutritional consequences. Patients with chronic kidney disease (CKD) consequently display a variety of metabolic and nutritional abnormalities (Fig. 24.1, Table 24.1). Metabolic and nutritional abnormalities arise in CKD from both pathophysiological (e.g., uremic toxicity, altered metabolism) and iatrogenic (e.g., polypharmacy and the prescription of a low-protein diet to slow disease progression) causes. In the late stage of CKD, defined by the need to start renal replacement therapy (RRT) (dialysis or kidney transplantation), some of these abnormalities are attenuated, while novel ones may occur.

In children with CKD, nutritional derangements are common and are associated with significant morbidity and mortality. Prenatal factors play a role in the development of future CKD, especially in preterm infants and those with congenital anomalies of the kidney and urinary tract. Studies have reported a prevalence of 20%–45% of malnutrition in children with CKD.[4] Malnutrition in CKD is not entirely explained by reduced nutritional intake. A complex combination of different factors, including hormonal imbalances, decreased appetite, inflammation, increased catabolism, and metabolic derangements, all predispose these patients to malnutrition.[5–8] The exact mechanisms leading to malnutrition, including the timing and trajectory

https://doi.org/10.1016/B978-0-12-818460-8.00024-1

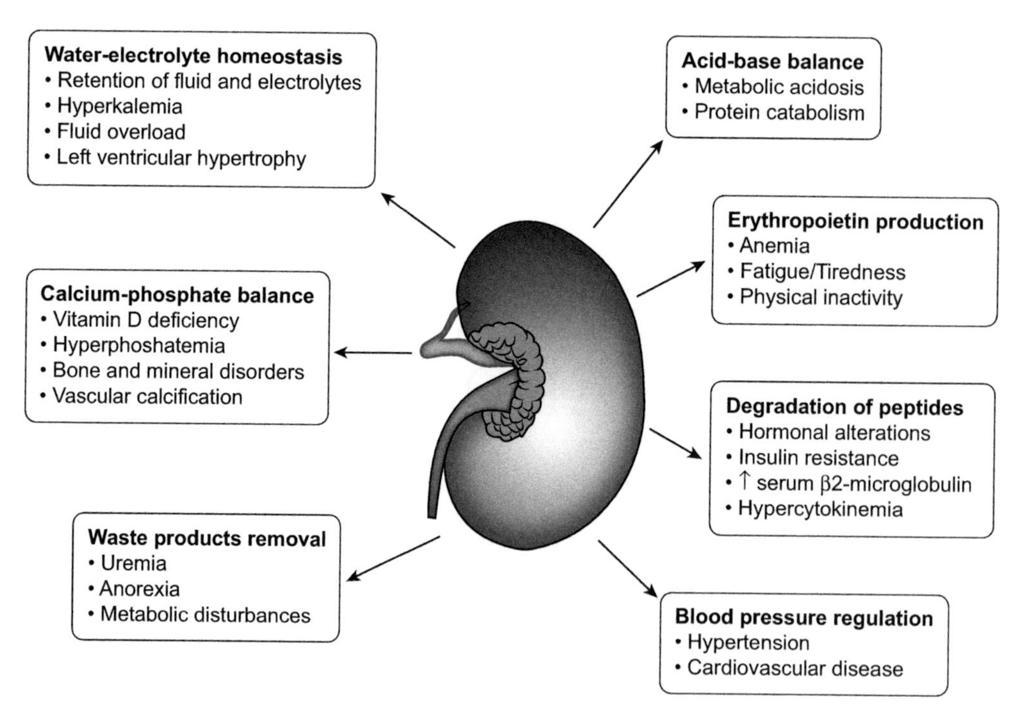

FIGURE 24.1 Major roles of the kidney in metabolic regulation. *Reproduced with permission from Axelsson, T.G., Chmielewski, M. and Lindholm, B. (2012). Kidney Disease. In Present Knowledge in Nutrition (eds J.W. Erdman, I.A. Macdonald and S.H. Zeisel). doi: https://doi.org/10.1002/9781119946045.ch53*

TABLE 24.1 Stages of chronic kidney disease[a].

Stage 1: >90	Mild CKD
Stage 2: 60–90	
Stage 3: 30–60	Moderate CKD
Stage 4: 15–30	Advanced CKD
Stage 5: <15	

[a]*By estimated glomerular filtration rate (eGFR) mL/min/1.73 m².*

TABLE 24.2 Nutritional aberrations that are associated with CKD.

Growth impairment (pediatrics)
Metabolic acidosis
Anemia from ineffective erythropoiesis
CKD—mineral bone disease Decreased formation of 1,25-OH_2 vitamin D Secondary hyperparathyroidism Hyperphosphatemia
Electrolyte derangements
Hyperuricemia leading to increase cardiovascular risks
Protein-energy wasting

of weight loss, slow weight gain, and poor linear growth in children with CKD with suboptimal nutritional status, are not well understood.

II. PROTEIN-ENERGY WASTING: PREVALENCE, MECHANISMS, AND SIGNIFICANCE

Among the complications of CKD, progressive loss of body protein mass and energy reserves is one of the most typical and detrimental. This loss has been termed protein-energy wasting (PEW).[9] It is most prevalent in patients with advanced stages of CKD and may affect up to 75% of subjects with end-stage renal disease. The term PEW was proposed by the International Society of Renal Nutrition and Metabolism to describe a state of decreased body stores of protein and fat. Criteria for PEW are listed in Table 24.2.[10]

Unlike protein-energy malnutrition, which describes deficient protein energy explained purely by inadequate dietary protein intake, PEW describes deficient protein energy that cannot be corrected by increasing energy and protein intake alone. The pathogenesis of PEW is not well understood and is shown to be related to many complex factors, including hypermetabolism, hypercatabolism, retention of uremic toxins, acidosis, insulin resistance, elevated circulating proinflammatory cytokines, depression, and imbalance in hormonal regulatory pathways for hunger and satiety (Table 24.3).[4,11,12]

PEW is to a large extent caused by undernutrition. Impaired food intake is a consequence of several overlapping processes. A low-protein diet is advocated in CKD subjects as it has been shown to reduce uremic symptoms

TABLE 24.3 Clinical criteria of PEW in CKD.

- ≥ Three out of the four listed categories along with at least one test in each of the selected category must be satisfied for the diagnosis of kidney disease–related PEW.
- Each criterion should be documented on at least three occasions, preferably 2–4 weeks apart.

Serum chemistry
• Serum albumin <3.8 g/dL • Serum prealbumin <30 mg/dL (for maintenance dialysis patients only) • Serum cholesterol < 100 mg/dL
Body mass
• Body mass index (edema free) < 23 • Unintentional weight loss over time: 5% over 3 months or 10% over 6 months • Total body fat percentage < 10%
Muscle mass
• Reduced muscle mass 5% over 3 months or 10% over 6 months • Reduced midarm muscle circumference area (reduction >10% in relation to 50th percentile of reference population)[a] • Creatinine appearance[b]
Dietary mass
• Unintentional low DPI <0.80 g/kg/day for at least 2 months for dialysis patients or < 0.6 g/kg/day for patients with CKD stages 2–5 • Unintentional low DEI <25 kcal/kg/day for at least 2 months

CKD, chronic kidney disease; *DEI*, Dietary energy intake; *DPI*, Dietary protein intake; *GFR*, glomerular filtration rate; PEW, protein-energy wasting.
[a]*Measured by a trained anthropometrist*
[b]*Estimated by measurement of creatinine in 24 h urine collection and in collected spent dialysate.*
Adapted from Obi et al.[10]

and retard the progression of the disease.[13] However, it may result in negative protein balance, especially in subjects not receiving amino acid and/or ketoacid supplementation. As CKD progresses, anorexia develops.[14] This is due to uremic intoxication and hormonal derangements, including an increase in circulating levels of multiple anorexigens such as leptin. Finally, as patients progress toward end-stage renal disease, dialysis is introduced, which is associated with significant losses of nutrients into the dialysate in both types of dialysis treatment. Decreased food intake is not the only culprit for PEW occurrence. Chronic low-grade inflammation seems to be of equal importance.[9,15] This prevalent complication of CKD has been shown in several studies to decrease protein generation and to increase protein breakdown, resulting in a highly negative protein balance. Other disturbances predispose CKD patients to deteriorations of nutritional status. These include, for example, oxidative stress, acidosis, nutrient losses, social factors such as loneliness and poverty, and comorbid conditions such as diabetes mellitus, cardiovascular disease, and infections, which are all highly prevalent in CKD patients.[9]

PEW is associated with impaired growth and development in children with CKD, as well as increased risk of hospitalizations and death.[16] PEW has been well studied in adults with CKD and shown to be a risk factor for cardiovascular complications and death, but it is not well characterized in children.[17] Of the diagnostic PEW biochemical marker adult criteria, such as albumin, prealbumin, transferrin, cholesterol, triglyceride, retinol-binding protein, hemoglobin, and total lymphocyte count, none have reliably demonstrated utility in assessing PEW in children.

In general, none of the currently favored biomarkers for malnutrition (i.e., albumin, prealbumin, and transferrin) have been demonstrated to accurately reflect nutritional status in CKD[18–20] Instead, strong associations between biomarkers and mortality seem to derive, at least in part, from their close association with inflammation and from the important role of the kidney in metabolizing circulating inflammatory peptides.[18,21] The serum *albumin* concentration is determined by its synthesis, breakdown, and volume of distribution.[22,23] In CKD patients, factors such as overhydration, proteinuria, and protein losses into the dialysate and urine may cause a decrease in serum protein concentration—thus albumin is not an ideal biomarker in this population. Hypoalbuminemia in CKD patients is more associated with chronic inflammatory state than with insufficient food intake.[24]

Like serum albumin, *prealbumin* is mainly synthesized in the liver, and a reduced dietary protein intake is associated with a decline in serum concentrations that are more quickly restored by nutritional therapy, due to its lower concentration and shorter half-life (2–3 days).[25–27] However, serum prealbumin concentrations are also greatly affected by inflammation.[28] In CKD, reduced renal catabolism of prealbumin also contributes to altered serum prealbumin concentrations.[29] Lastly, serum *transferrin* is a visceral protein that transports iron in the circulation. Its concentration is affected by iron metabolism, much altered in CKD, and inflammation.[30] Thus, serum transferrin is not a reliable marker of nutritional status in CKD. Despite the prevailing use of these biomarkers in CKD, circulating concentrations of albumin, prealbumin, and transferrin are in fact *not* appropriate indicators of the nutritional status in patients with CKD.

Studies identifying novel biochemical markers of PEW, such as unacylated ghrelin, obestatin, and leptin, are in progress.[12,31] Abraham et al. adapted the PEW definition from adult populations to pediatric populations.[16] It includes biochemical markers used in the adult criterion of PEW, as well as the pediatric-focused criterion (e.g., poor growth defined as short stature or poor linear growth velocity). By including pediatric-focused criterion, the modified PEW definition was better able to predict rates of hospitalization in children with CKD. Most recently, metabolomics has been usedto identify biomarkers of dietary acid load (i.e., balance of acid and base–producing foods) in CKD. The Modification of Diet in Renal Disease (MDRD) and the African American Study of Kidney Disease and Hypertension metabolomic profiling demonstrated 13 common metabolites associated with dietary acid load.[32]

Cross-sectional studies in adults suggest that weight loss begins around an estimated glomerular filtration rate (eGFR) of 40 mL/min/1.73 m^2.[33] A pediatric study in CKD suggests that weight loss accelerated when eGFR decreases to <35 mL/min/1.73 m^2. The rate of weight loss was also associated with higher risk for ESRD.[5] However, weight and body mass index (BMI) do not accurately reflect nutritional status in CKD. Fluid overload in CKD leads to inaccurate estimation of lean body mass. Children with CKD also tend to have a stunted growth velocity and short stature, which leads to a falsely reassuring BMI status. Also, body weight does not accurately reflect changes in body composition caused by PEW, which is characterized by decreasing protein and fat mass status. Therefore, Kidney Disease Outcomes Quality Initiative (KDOQI) recommends including several additional anthropometric measurements in evaluation of PEW in children, including height-for-age-percentile or standard deviation scores (SDS), height velocity-for-age or SDS, and estimated dry weight-for-age or SDS.[4]

Obesity is a frequent finding in CKD, reflecting the growing prevalence of overweight and obesity in the general population. In fact, obesity is one of the most frequent risk factors for CKD progression.[34] However, PEW is equally frequent and equally detrimental in obese as it is in lean patients with CKD.[35] PEW is a strong and independent predictor of cardiovascular and noncardiovascular mortality in CKD patients. Decreased indices of nutritional status, as serum albumin, prealbumin, or cholesterol, have been associated with increased risk of death.[36] Similarly, decrease in muscle mass and dietary protein and energy intake have been linked to worse outcomes.

III. INSULIN RESISTANCE AND DYSLIPIDEMIA

Diabetes mellitus is the leading cause of CKD all over the world, accounting for up to 40% of cases of ESRD in some countries. Insulin resistance is a typical finding in moderate-to-severe CKD.[37] Insulin resistance has been associated with progression of renal disease by worsening renal hemodynamics by various mechanisms, including activation of the sympathetic nervous system, sodium retention, and downregulation of the natriuretic peptide system.[38]

Hypertriglyceridemia appears in early stages of CKD with the highest concentrations in patients on dialysis and in those with nephrotic syndrome. The ratio of triglycerides to cholesterol in LDL and HDL particles is increased in patients with CKD, with hypertriglyceridemia resulting from delayed catabolism of triglyceride-rich lipoproteins.[39] Mechanistically, an accumulation of triglyceride-rich lipoproteins in CKD appears mainly to be a result of a decreased catabolism of lipids.[40] As decreased insulin sensitivity occurs (commonly in patients with GFR < 30 mL/min/1.73 m^2), an overproduction of insulin-sensitive very–low-density lipoproteins is likely to contribute to hypertriglyceridemia in CKD patients. Patients with moderate CKD have a highly prevalent dyslipidemic phenotype consisting of increased triglyceride-rich lipoproteins, which is strongly associated with a high burden of subclinical atherosclerosis and has also been shown to be associated with increased risk of coronary heart disease.[41–43]

IV. CKD—MINERAL AND BONE DISEASE

Parathyroid hormone (PTH), fibroblast growth factor 23 (FGF23), 1,25-dihydroxyvitamin D (1,25(OH)2D), and α-klotho regulate serum calcium and phosphorus concentrations via feedback loops. In addition to the maintenance of normal extracellular and intracellular levels of calcium and phosphorus, the long-term goal is to ensure adequate availability of these ions for bone that is growing (modeling) or remodeling and to minimize extraskeletal calcification in soft tissues and vasculature. The kidney is involved in all of these homeostatic loops, and thus, it is not surprising that mineral homeostasis is disrupted in patients with CKD. Abnormalities begin early in the course of CKD (Fig. 24.2). At eGFR near 60 mL/min/1.73 m^2, levels of 1,25(OH)2D are decreased and PTH and FGF23 increased (Fig. 24.2). It is believed that with progression of CKD, the body attempts to maintain normal serum concentrations of calcium and phosphorus via increased PTH and FGF23. The elevated FGF23 also leads to increased catabolism of both 25(OH)D and 1,25(OH)2D. Thus, as early as eGFR <60 mL/min/m^2, there is evidence of the biochemical abnormalities of CKD-MBD. In contrast to the early rise in FGF23 and PTH and decrease in 1,25(OH)2D, serum levels of calcium and phosphorus are abnormal only when the eGFR is < 30 mL/min/m^2. There is decreased calcium absorption in the intestine that can be corrected with the administration of 1,25(OH)2D. However, in CKD stages 3 and 4, there is also a marked reduction in urine calcium excretion. The mechanism by which this occurs is not well understood. It is possible that increased PTH leads to reabsorption; however, the urine calcium does not change in response to treatments with 1,25(OH)2D or its analogs, while the concentration of PTH is lowered

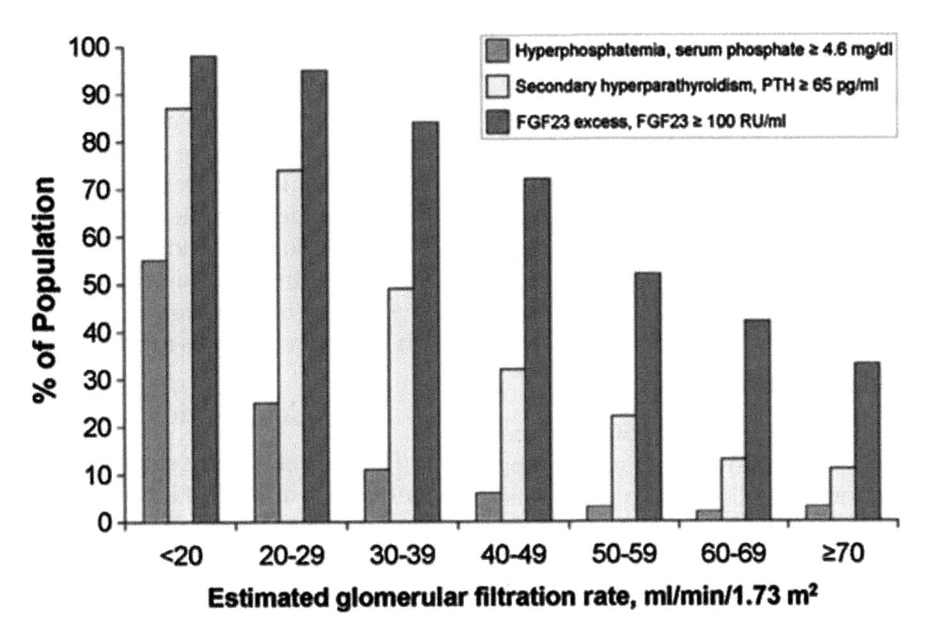

FIGURE 24.2 Prevalence of hyperphosphatemia, secondary hyperparathyroidism, and elevated FGF23 in relation to eGFR. Hyperphosphatemia was defined as serum phosphate >4.6 mg/dL, secondary hyperparathyroidism as parathyroid hormone (PTH) > 65 pg/mL, and fibroblast growth hormone-23 (FGF23) excess as FGF23 > 100 RU/mL. *eGFR*, estimated glomerular filtration rate.[54]

by 30%.[44] These decreases in calcium intestinal absorption and kidney excretion with CKD put patients at risk of positive calcium balance. Two recent calcium balance studies have demonstrated positive calcium with oral intake from diet and supplements/binders of 800–1000 mg/day.[45,46] The potential adverse consequences of positive calcium balance or excess calcium intake include suppression of bone remodeling rates and extraskeletal calcium deposition, at least in patients with ESRD.[47] Thus, indiscriminate use of calcium supplements in patients with CKD should be avoided. Epidemiologic data suggest that serum phosphate concentrations above the normal range are associated with increases in morbidity and all-cause and cardiovascular mortality in patients with CKD. Furthermore, several studies have demonstrated that treatment of patients undergoing dialysis with phosphate binder therapy is associated with a 20%–40% lower risk of death.[48–52] Vitamin D deficiency (<20 ng/mL) and insufficiency (<30 ng/mL) are common in patients with CKD, only 29% and 17% of those with stage 3 and 4 disease, respectively, have sufficient vitamin D, and the prevalence of frank deficiency (<10 mg/mL) was 14% and 26% in patients with stage 3 and 4 CKD, respectively.[53]

In pediatrics, there are age-specific goals for serum calcium, phosphorous, and PTH from the 2008 KDOQI Guidelines (see Table 24.4).[55] It is important to note what may be considered "hyperphosphatemia" for an adult patient may be within the serum phosphorous ranges for infants who need more phosphorous for bone growth in this particular time period.[55]

V. NUTRITIONAL ASSESSMENT IN CKD PATIENTS

Many methods have been created to identify malnourished and wasted CKD patients and to grade different degrees of PEW. Unfortunately, there is no single method that can be used for this purpose; with so

TABLE 24.4 Age-specific normal ranges of blood ionized calcium, total calcium, and phosphorus.

Age	Ionized calcium (mmol/L)	Calcium (mg/dL)	Phosphorus (mg/dL)
0–5 months	1.22–1.40	8.7–11.3	5.2–8.4
6–12 months	1.20–1.40	8.7–11.0	5.0–7.8
1–5 years	1.22–1.32	9.4–10.8	4.5–6.5
6–12 years	1.15–1.32	9.4–10.3	3.6–5.8
13–20 years	1.12–1.30	8.8–10.2	2.3–4.5

Conversion factor for calcium and ionized calcium: mg/dL × 0.25 = mmol/L.
Conversion factor for phosphorus: mg/dL × 0.323 = mmol/L.
Adapted with permission Ref. 55; Specker.[55]

many concurrent metabolic and nutritional abnormalities, such an effective clinical tool has remained elusive. The National Kidney Foundation Clinical Practice Guidelines for Nutrition in Chronic Renal Failure thus recommends that nutritional status should be evaluated using a combination of valid, complementary measures.[29] These measures may include biological assessment of protein-energy status, subjective global assessment (SGA), dietary intake assessment, and anthropometry measurements.[29]

A. Subjective Global Assessment

With limited usefulness of biomarkers, SGA has been proposed as a simple, inexpensive, and easy-to-apply method of assessing nutritional status in this patient group. SGA is a reliable indicator of PEW in uremic patients.[29,56,57] Furthermore, SGA uses scoring of the patient's medical history and physical examination to differentiate nutritional status categories: well-nourished slightly malnourished, and severely malnourished patients. The attributes scored in the SGA include the following: gastrointestinal symptoms, dietary intake, body weight, disease state, and functional capacity. Owing to its strong correlations between PEW and important clinical outcomes, SGA is recommended as a component of longitudinal monitoring of chronic dialysis patients by the National Kidney Foundation Kidney Disease/Dialysis Outcomes and Quality Initiative.[29,58,59] Although SGA is a useful tool in CKD, it should be kept in mind that SGA is a subjective score that may be biased by inter- and intrapersonal differences.[60,61] As such, it is perhaps best employed in a longitudinal manner by the same trained clinician to follow patients over time.

B. Dietary Intake Records

The estimation of dietary intake is of central importance in CKD patients. The most commonly used to quantify individual intake of nutrients are the dietary interview, the 24-h dietary recall, and the prospective dietary record. These tools are useful for the estimation of macronutrient intake in the clinical setting. While under- or overestimation of dietary intake is common. These methods have been successfully used in the CKD patient population. In hemodialysis patients, dietary protein intake assessed by prospectively collected 7 -day food records correlated with intake estimated by normalized protein catabolic rate, and there were significant differences in diets between dialysis and nondialysis days.[62] In a study investigating the accuracy of food records with regard to energy consumption, energy intake was evaluated using 4-day food record and resting energy expenditure (REE) was measured by indirect calorimetry; energy intake based on 4-day food diaries was underestimated.[63]

C. Hand Grip

Handgrip strength testing is a validated noninvasive modality to evaluate nutrition status in CKD with an advantage of not being affected by hydration status.[64–66] In adults, handgrip strength has been demonstrated to be an independent predictor of mortality in hemodialysis patients.[67] Further study in children demonstrated that hand grip strength was below the 10% for age and sex in ~70% of the children with CKD, thus exhibiting that this may have utility as a tool for nutritional assessment.[68]

D. Body Composition

Theoretically, body composition and the whole body content of muscle, fat, protein, mineral, and water should reflect long-term dietary intake and nutritional status. While several methods have been employed to assess body composition in CKD patients, they each suffer from the impact of variation of body water seen commonly in this patient group.

E. Bioelectrical Impedance Analysis

Bioelectrical impedance analysis (BIA) and bioelectrical impedance spectrometry (BIS) have been proposed as noninvasive, simple, and quick techniques for measuring body composition. BIA and BIS use measured variations in electrical currents of one or more frequencies passed through the body to estimate body water, fat, and fat-free mass. However, the difficulty of determining the amount and distribution of intra- and extracellular water in CKD patients limits the usefulness of this method for nutritional assessment. A recent pediatric study on hemodialysis patients demonstrated that BIA overestimated fat mass in malnourished children and underestimated fat mass in obese children.[69]

F. Dual-Energy X-ray Absorptiometry

A more reliable tool to estimate body composition is dual-energy X-ray absorptiometry (DXA). DXA passes low-energy X-rays through the body to measure fat mass, fat-free mass, and bone mineral mass.[70] While DXA is good at measuring fat mass, it is not used routinely in the CKD clinical setting because of its high cost and inaccuracy in severely overhydrated patients.[63,71]

G. Anthropometric Measurement

Midarm muscle circumference area is used to determine muscle mass reduction in diagnostic criteria of PEW. Skinfold thickness is an anthropometric measurement widely used in clinical practice because of its low cost, simplicity, and noninvasive nature. It is used to estimate both fat mass and fat-free mass.[72] However, skinfold thickness measurements require skilled anthropometrists or the measurement may suffer from a large intra- and interobserver variability and are modestly reliable.[63] Another marker used to determine body fat mass is waist circumference. It is a simple and easy method and suggested to predict survival in CKD patients.[73]

VI. PEDIATRIC NUTRITION AND MALNUTRITION STATUS IN CKD

The second trimester and third trimester of pregnancy see a significant increase in the number of fetal nephrons, the functional working units of the kidney, completion of human renal development is by 36 weeks.[74] For full-term infants, on average, each kidney has an average of 1 million nephrons.[75] By 20 weeks of gestational age, 90% of amniotic fluid volume comes from the fetal kidneys[76] In some children with congenital anomalies of the kidney urinary tract, oligohydramnios may be present in utero and also affecting lung size and maturity (i.e., Potter sequence). Children who survive may have different electrolyte needs when the obstruction is corrected surgically and the postobstructive diuresis occurs.

Wong et al. demonstrated that for every one standard deviation score decline height in children with CKD compared to healthy children, there was a 14% increased risk in mortality.[77] Using participant data from the Chronic Kidney Disease in Children study, Ayesteran et al. determined that worsening renal function (CKD stages 4–5) was associated with significant worse appetite and quality of life and increased emergency room visits and hospitalization.[78] Additional studies show that children with lower BMI prior to kidney transplant and those who require clean intermittent catheterization of urine posttransplant remain at highest risk of posttransplant failure to thrive.[79]

Malnutrition is associated not only with increased hospitalizations and mortality in children but also with increase arterial stiffness via pulse wave velocity (PWV measurements) with potential for cardiovascular risks and decreased 25-OH Vitamin D concentrations.[80,81]

VII. TREATING NUTRITIONAL DEFICIENCIES IN PEDIATRIC AND ADULT CKD PATIENTS

During stages of childhood, growth is influenced by different parameters: in infancy, growth is primary driven by nutrition, whereas growth hormone (GH) and sex hormones play important roles in growth during childhood and adolescence.[82] Poor growth may affect the youngest children with CKD the hardest, when they should be growing rapidly. The primary nutrition for these infants remains breast milk or formula.[83] In some cases, tubular renal dysfunction leading to salt wasting may predominate leading to growth abnormalities.[84] Thus, special renal formulas are available with low potassium and phosphorous compositions for children with CKD in infants without access to breast milk.

To treat failure to thrive, one can increase calories but simply adding extra scoops of formula may not be ideal—since this can increase protein and solute load. Thus, we also recommend use of modular nutrient components including fats, carbohydrates, etc. Modular additives with only calories and no protein are also utilized to supplement calories without significant potassium and sodium affecting renal solute load. Microlipids are used as calorie additives to enhance nutrition without adding protein.[85] Please refer to Table 24.4 regarding recommended protein intake per KDOQI.[55]

In clinical practice, kayexalate, an oral medication, is utilized to further help lower potassium content in formulas via a method of decanting: liquid or powder kayexalate is utilized in a titrated ratio (grams of kayexalate per milliequivalents of potassium to be removed) and this is refrigerated for 30 min. The precipitate contains the bound potassium and some calcium and is discarded. Monitoring for hypokalemia, hypernatremia, and hypocalcemia is recommended.[86]

Some formula supplements can be used in children >1 year of age in the United States, but may be used earlier in other countries, but it is not intended to be the sole source of nutrition (Tables 24.5 and 24.6). For children with motility issues, more elemental formulas (decanted with kayexyalate it needed) can also be considered. For older children and adults, there are some renal formulas that provide primary source nutrition; Coleman et al. demonstrated that gastrostomy tubes (G-tubes) were integral for infants and children with CKD to achieve catch-up growth. In this study, children received 61% of their feeds via G-tube and able to achieve 116% caloric needs and support enabling catch-up growth for weight and height.[87] Children ages <2 years have been noted to have the best response to nutrition interventions while on a dialysis modality.[87] In 2019, the Pediatric Renal Nutrition Rask Force published guidelines regarding energy and protein requirements for infants, children and adolescents with CKD stages 2–5 (Table 24.7).[88]

Megestrol acetate has been shown to improve weight gain in pediatric patients with CKD as well as adult hemodialysis patients with few side effects reported.[89,90]

TABLE 24.5 Recommended dietary protein intake in children with CKD stages 3–5 and 5D.

	DRI				
Age	DRI (g/kg/day)	Recommended for CKD stage 3 (g/kg/day) (100%–140% DRI)	Recommended for CKD stages 4–5 (g/kg/day) (100%–120% DRI)	Recommended for HD (g/kg/day)[a]	Recommended for PD (g/kg/day)[b]
0–6 months	1.5	1.5–2.1	1.5–1.8	1.6	1.8
7–12 months	1.2	1.2–1.7	1.2–1.5	1.3	1.5
1–3 years	1.05	1.05–1.5	1.05–1.25	1.15	1.3
4–13 years	0.95	0.95–1.35	0.95–1.15	1.05	1.1
14–18 years	0.85	0.85–1.2	0.85–1.05	0.95	1.0

[a]*DRI + 0.1 g/kg/day to compensate for dialytic losses.*
[b]*DRI + 0.15–0.3 g/kg/day depending on patient age to compensate for peritoneal losses.*

TABLE 24.6 Renal formulas and supplementation to optimize nutrition for patients with CKD.

Supplements	
Modular: Duocal[B] (Nutricia North America)	492 kcal/100 g
Modular: Solcarb[B] (Medica Nutrition)	376 kcal/100 g
Modular: Renastart[B] (Nestle)	477 kcal/100 g
Not a sole source of nutrition:	
Microlipid[B] (Nestle)	67.5kcal/15 mL
Specialized renal formulas	
Infant: Similac[B] PM 60/40 (Abbott Nutrition)	0.68 cal/1 mL
Children/adult: Suplena[B] (Abbott Nutrition)	1.8 cal/1 mL
Children/adult: Nepro[B] (Abbott Nutrition)	1.8 cal/1 mL

VIII. GROWTH HORMONE IN PEDIATRIC CKD PATIENTS

At least one-third of children with pediatric onset of CKD have demonstrated impairment in linear growth despite advances in care over the years.[91] Growth insufficiency has been associated with an increase in mortality when height is less than one standard deviation with significant increase in death when height for age is persistently <first percentile on the growth curve.[92] Studies have demonstrated a partial resistance to GH in CKD due to alternations in phosphorylation of the JACK2/STAT pathway.[93,94] This GH insensitivity can be treated with more than physiological doses of recombinant human GH to stimulate functional insulin-like growth factor 1.[95]

The 2008 KDOQI guidelines recommend initiation of GH therapy if linear catch-up growth has not been achieved within 3 months of optimized nutrition management.[55] A Consensus Statement from the European Society of Pediatric Nephrology defined persistent growth failure as length/height below the 3rd percentile or height velocity less than the 25th percentile for a period of 3 months for infants and more than 6 months in children. Children with CKD stages 3–5 who are greater than 6 months of age should be prescribed GH after optimization of nutrition, electrolytes, thyroid status, dialysis, anemia, and bone disease.96 GH is typically prescribed at starting doses of 0.05 mg/kg/day as nightly subcutaneous infusions and continued until renal transplant. For some children with persistent growth failure postrenal transplant in steroid-free regimens, children should be considered for GH therapy for 1 year posttransplant.[96]

IX. CONTRAINDICATIONS FOR GROWTH HORMONE THERAPY

GH should not be used in patients with diabetic retinopathy, recent trauma or heart/abdominal surgeries, and active malignancy.[96] In particular, GH should be avoided in severe secondary hyperparathyroidism with PTH levels >500 pg/mL due to increases risk of slipped capital femoral epiphysis in children.[97]

TABLE 24.7 Energy and protein requirements for infants, children and adolescents with CKD2-5D aged 0-18 years.

SDI for energy and protein: birth[a] to 18 years				
Month	SDI[b] energy (kcal/kg/day)	SDI protein (g/kg/day)	SDI protein (g/day)	
0	93-107	1.52-2.5	8-12	
1	93-120	1.52-1.8	8-12	
2	93-120	1.4-1.52	8-12	
3	82-98	1.4-1.52	8-12	
4	82-98	1.3-1.52	9-13	
5	72-82	1.3-1.52	9-13	
6-9	72-82	1.1-1.3	9-14	
10-11	72-82	1.1-1.3	9-15	
12	72-120	0.9-1.14	11-14	
Year	SDI energy (kcal/kg/day)		SDI protein (g/kg/day)	SDI protein (g/day)
	Male	Female		
2	81-95[c]	79-92[c]	0.9-1.05	11-15
3	80-82	76-77	0.9-1.05	13-15
4-6	67-93	64-90	0.85-0.95	16-22
7-8	60-77	56-75	0.9-0.95	19-28
9-10	55-69	49-63	0.9-0.95	26-40
11-12	48-63	43-57	0.9-0.95	34-42
13-14	44 63	39-50	0.8-0.9	34-50
15-17	40-55	36-46	0.8-0.9	Male: 52-65 Female: 45-49

For children with poor growth, reference to the SDI for height age may be appropriate. Height age is the age that corresponds to an individual's height when plotted on the 50th centile on a growth chart

[a]*Thirty-seven/40 weeks gestation. Premature infants have higher energy and protein requirements. The increased need for these and other particular nutrients (sodium, potassium, calcium, and phosphorus) must be balanced against the nutritional interventions to control the effects of CKD. This is outside the scope of this CPR*

[b]*Suggested Dietary Intake (SDI) is based on the Physical Activity Level (PAL) used by the international bodies: 1-3 year PAL 1.4; 4-9 year PAL 1.6; and 10-17 year PAL 1.8. Where guidelines have given a range of energy requirements for different levels of PAL, the lowest PAL has been taken for SDI energy in consideration that children with CKD are likely to have low activity levels*

[c]*Scientific Advisory Committee on Nutrition (9) reports energy requirements as kcal/day: male 1040 kcal/day; female 932 kcal/day*

X. RENAL REPLACEMENT THERAPY

When patients reach ESRD, RRT is introduced to improve uremia to a different degree, depending on the RRT. While renal transplantation is by far the best RRT, dialysis has its drawbacks and limitations. Both the dialyzer membrane in hemodialysis and the peritoneal membrane in peritoneal membrane patients are far less selective than the kidney's glomerular barrier. Therefore, many essential nutrients are lost into the dialysate, and the dialysis procedure itself may cause a transitory inflammatory response stimulating protein catabolism. Nevertheless, dialysis can improve nutritional status, and that adequate dialysis supports PEW prevention. It has been demonstrated that adequate dialysis is a prerequisite for PEW prevention.[98] In patients in whom the dialysis dose does not meet their requirements, uremic intoxication and volume overload evolve. These factors play an important role in PEW development. In patients undergoing kidney transplantation, the immunosuppressive therapy, in particular corticosteroids, may lead to metabolic and nutritional alterations including metabolic syndrome and PEW.[99]

XI. DIETARY COMPOSITION IN CKD

A. Protein

The European Society of Parenteral and Enteral Nutrition (ESPEN) and the National Kidney Foundation (NKF) guidelines recommend that CKD patients stages 4–5 (GFR < 30 mL/min) consume a moderately reduced protein intake of 0.55–0.60 g/kg/day.[100] A very–low-protein diet with protein intake of 0.3–0.4 g/kg/day is used in several countries, and patients receiving such a diet must be monitored and supported by essential amino acids or keto acids supplements to avoid a negative nitrogen balance.[100] The progression of CKD may slow significantly when following introduction of a low-protein diet.[101–104] Low-protein diets may have additional benefits in CKD patients and lead to a decrease risk in hyperkalemia, hyperphosphatemia, metabolic acidosis, and other electrolyte disorders.[105] Furthermore, many of the clinical and metabolic disturbances characteristic of uremia may be delayed or prevented by the reduction of nitrogenous wastes and inorganic ions from a diet rich in protein. There is more variation in protein requirements in CKD patients than in healthy patients, as a result of additional sources of variability such as endocrine and biochemical abnormalities, anemia, medications, physical inactivity, and comorbid conditions. In addition, some nonessential amino acids become conditionally essential in CKD because of the loss of amino acid conversion in the kidney and specific effects of the dialytic process.[106] Owing to these factors, it is recommended that CKD patients starting dialysis discontinue a low-protein diet and have a protein intake of 1.2–1.3 g/kg/day, of which a large part should be protein of high biological value.[29] It is, however, interesting to note that recent findings suggest that a protein intake of 0.6–0.8 g of protein/kg/day may lead to improved preservation of residual renal function without adverse consequences in dialysis patients.[106,107] Thus, whereas many patients may require less than 1.2 g/kg/day to maintain nitrogen equilibrium, some patients, e.g., those who develop PEW, may require higher amounts of protein and energy.[106,108] Indeed, studies have suggested that some patients may benefit from eating as much as 1.4–2.1 g protein/kg/day, especially during the initial months of dialysis treatment.[106]

B. Fat

Fat is the most energy-dense macronutrient and possibly beneficial to malnourished CKD patients, especially those on a low-protein diet. However, there are no studies to indicate optimal amount of fat in the CKD diet. The ESPEN and NKF KDOQI Guidelines, respectively, for CKD patients recommend a total energy intake for adults, which is similar to that of the general population, i.e., 35 kcal/kg/day, and for older adults (>60 years) 30–35 kcal/kg/day.[100,109] For patients at CKD stages 1–3, the energy requirement is based on energy expenditure and depends on the underlying nutritional status of the patient. Thus, those who are underweight need a high-calorie intake for weight gain than patients who are of healthy weight or overweight.[109] Not only the quantity but also the type of the dietary fat is important. In one study, unsaturated fat supplementation in hemodialysis patients was associated with improved blood lipids, reduced systemic inflammation, and improved nutritional status.[110]

C. Carbohydrates

There is no evidence that energy requirements of CKD patients are systematically different from those of normal subjects. While most studies have shown normal REE in both early and late CKD, one study reported decreased REE in nondialyzed CKD patients.[63,111] Thus, an energy intake of at least 35 kcal/kg body weight is currently recommended in CKD patients.[29] Importantly, studies show that most CKD patients have a lower energy intake, and this may contribute to PEW.[63] In dialysis patients, HD is mostly energy neutral, while PD patients may absorb about 60% of the dialysate glucose load (100–200 g glucose/24 h), and this contributes to energy intake.[29,112]

D. Vitamins

CKD patients commonly suffer from micronutrient deficiencies.[8] Of the water-soluble vitamins that have been studied, serum ascorbic acid, thiamine (B1), pyridoxine (B6), and folic acid have all been reported to be low in dialysis patients.[113] Thiamin deficiency with associated encephalopathy has been described in dialysis patients and may be confounded by other neurologic diseases. A typical thiamine intake of 0.5–1.5 mg/day may be supplemented with 1–5 mg/day of thiamin hydrochloride. Vitamin B6 coenzymes play a vital role in several aspects of amino acid utilization, and the need for vitamin B6 is particularly critical if protein and amino acid intake is limited.[114] Indeed, changes in fasting plasma amino acid and serum HDL concentration after correction of the vitamin B6 deficiency in dialysis patients indicate its role in the pathogenesis of the abnormal amino acid and lipid metabolism of CKD.[115] The daily requirement of pyridoxine may be higher in dialysis patients than in normal subjects, and dialysis patients should be supplemented with a minimum of 10 mg of vitamin B6 per day.[116] As a water-soluble vitamin, folate is lost in dialysate. Because serum folate levels have been reported to be reduced in CKD, 1 mg folic acid daily supplement is recommended. High doses of folic acid (5–10 mg/day) have been shown to reduce elevated plasma homocysteine in dialysis patients by about two-thirds, and the value was still above the normal range.[117] The question whether high dose folate should be prescribed in order to lower plasma homocysteine to reduce cardiovascular morbidity and mortality in CKD is still open, and prospective studies are needed. Furthermore, while supplementation with vitamin C has also been recommended in CKD, a high intake of vitamin C may aggravate hyperoxalemia in dialysis patients, and controlled trials are also lacking to support this recommendation. Unlike water-soluble vitamins, supplementation of the fat-soluble vitamins A, D, E, and K is not recommended on a routine basis to CKD patients.[113,118,119] Vitamin A tends to accumulate in CKD patients and can potentially have harmful effects. Vitamin D is converted in the kidney from 25-hydroxyvitamin D to its active form, 1,25-dihydroxyvitamin D. Most patients with advanced CKD, especially stages 4 and 5, are deficient in 1,25-dihydroxyvitamin D and 25-hydroxyvitamin D, and supplementation of active 1-25 vitamin D is often given based on bone metabolic status and taking the risks of hyperphosphatemia and hypercalcemia into consideration.[120] In most studies of uremic patients, blood vitamin E concentrations have been found to be normal and stable.[121] As vitamin K deficiency may play a role in the development of vascular calcification in CKD patients, supplementation of vitamin K might be beneficial, but there are no data to support this. Vitamin E is an antioxidant compound, and it may reduce cardiovascular disease. This was tested in a randomized controlled trial with a high dose of vitamin E supplementation in CKD patients with high cardiovascular risk. This study found a significant 50% decrease in cardiovascular incidents as compared with placebo.[122]

E. Trace Elements

Dietary requirements for trace elements are not well defined in CKD patients.[123] Trace element metabolism is frequently altered in CKD, and high blood concentrations have been attributed to impaired renal elimination or mineral contamination of dialysis fluids. Low concentrations of trace elements may occur as a result of inadequate dietary intake or loss of protein-bound trace elements into the dialysate.[113] Zinc deficiency has been reported to be common in CKD, and it may be effectively treated by zinc administration in one study.[124] These results have not been confirmed and the prevalence of zinc deficiency and requirements for extra zinc in CKD patients remain controversial.[113]

F. Nutrition Counseling

The goal of nutritional management of CKD patients is to delay the need for dialysis by using low-protein diets while maintaining good nutrient intake and nutritional status.[125] Thus, the specialized renal dietitian has a fundamental role in the assessment and treatment of CKD patients, and counseling is a part of a multidisciplinary care team approach.[50] In CKD, both regular dietary counseling and protein-energy status assessment are needed. In order to avoid a decline in nutritional status during CKD progression, a regular schedule with follow-up evaluations by dietitians and nephrologists is recommended.[126] According to the KDOQI K/DOQI Recommendations for Nutritional Management guidelines, dietary interviews and counseling in adults should be provided performed every 3–4 months.[127] Multidisciplinary care and counseling should be conducted monthly.[54] In addition, serum albumin (although value as a CKD nutritional biomarker is questionable), together with body weight and SGA, should be monitored every 1–3 months in adults and monitored monthly in children with advanced CKD. A key reason for monitoring protein-energy status is to adjust nutritional intakes to the patient's nutritional needs, including optimizing growth in children, to detect signs of PEW and to identify patients requiring nutritional support.

G. Intradialytic Nutritional Support

In order to compensate for nutrient losses related to dialysis treatment and to further improve nutritional status of dialysis patients, intradialytic nutritional support in the form of intravenous (in HD) and intraperitoneal (in PD) infusions can be part of the nutritional care plan. Intradialytic parenteral nutrition (IDPN) is an objective method of protein and energy supplementation in HD patients. Typically composed of a mixture of amino acids, dextrose, and lipids, IDPN has been shown to increase protein synthesis and decrease protein degradation, resulting in a highly positive protein balance.[128] However, studies have demonstrated no clear benefit of effective IDPN over effective oral nutritional support.[129] Guidelines recommend the use of IDPN for wasted subjects in whom oral nutritional support is ineffective in improving nutritional status.[125] Protein losses into the dialysate in PD patients are greater than those occurring in HD. Protein intake ought therefore to be increased in these PD patients. Moreover, amino acid based peritoneal dialysis fluids have been developed. In this case, amino acids serve also as an osmotic factor, instead of the common osmotic agent, glucose, and can improve protein balance. One PD exchange with amino acid–based dialysate in malnourished subjects treated with PD is usually enough to replace 24 h of losses of protein and amino acids in PD patients.

H. Preparation for Kidney Transplantation in Children With CKD/ESRD

Transplantation remains the goal for pediatric CKD patients; transplantation is associated with increased survival as well as improvement in neurocognitive development and growth.[130–132] Prior to renal transplant, many renal transplant centers aim to increase linear growth velocity as well as reach a weight goal of ~15 kg.[133–135] Ku et al. demonstrated that poor height states and obesity were associated with reduced chances of receiving kidney transplants.[136] In our particular center, we aim for a 10 kg weight goal and 65 cm height goal, which typically can occur between 1 and 2 years for these children. Feltran et al. recently found no significant difference in time to preparation for renal transplant for children 7–15 kg versus this children >15 kg (except in those children who required procedures for urinary tract malformations).[137] Thus, in the future, there may be a shift toward transplantation at lower weight thresholds.

XII. FUTURE DIRECTIONS

PEW has demonstrated to be important in determining clinical outcomes in patients with CKD, and clinical research could focus on effective PEW prevention and treatment in children and adults. It is essential that nutritional requirements be met, but this may not be sufficient for prevention and treatment of PEW. As malnutrition is not the main determinant of PEW in CKD patients who suffer from so many other catabolic conditions, e.g., chronic systemic inflammation and comorbidities, contributing to PEW and—by other mechanisms—to poor clinical outcomes. The number of adequately powered RCTs in this field is very limited. New trials could verify the usefulness of nutritional initiatives in CKD patients. Such trials should aim at evaluating the impact of particular nutritional interventions, not only on nutrition indices but also on mortality of CKD patients. PEW is a multifactorial process, and interventions targeted against several factors responsible for PEW could have a significant impact on patient outcomes. Improvement in nutritional assessments and ideal nutritional support in patients with kidney diseases will lead to improvements in clinical outcomes.

Acknowledgments

This chapter is an update of the chapter titled "53. Kidney Disease" by Thiane G. Axelsson, Michal Chmielewski and Bengt Lindholm, in *Present Knowledge in Nutrition, 10th Edition*, edited by Erdman JW, Macdonald IA, and Zeisel SH and published by Wiley-Blackwell. © 2012 International Life Sciences Institute. Portions of this update are from the previously published chapter, and the contributions of previous authors are acknowledged.

XIII. REFERENCES

1. Bikbov B, Perico N, Remuzzi G, on behalf of the, G.B.D Genitourinary Diseases Expert Group. Disparities in chronic kidney disease prevalence among males and females in 195 countries: analysis of the global burden of disease 2016 study. *Nephron*. 2018:1–6.
2. Group, K.D.I.G.O.K.C.W. KDIGO 2012 clinical practice guideline for the evaluation and management of chronic kidney disease. *Kidney Int Suppl*. 2013;3:1–150.
3. Levin A, Stevens PE. Summary of KDIGO 2012 CKD Guideline: behind the scenes, need for guidance, and a framework for moving forward. *Kidney Int*. 2014;85:49–61.
4. Iorember FM. Malnutrition in chronic kidney disease. *Front Pediatr*. 2018;6:161.
5. Ku E, Kopple JD, McCulloch CE, et al. Associations between weight loss, kidney function decline, and risk of ESRD in the chronic kidney disease in children (CKiD) cohort study. *Am J Kidney Dis*. 2018;71:648–656.
6. Patel HP, Saland JM, Ng DK, et al. Waist circumference and body mass index in children with chronic kidney disease and metabolic, cardiovascular, and renal outcomes. *J Pediatr*. 2017;191:133–139.
7. Oliveira EA, Cheung WW, Toma KG, Mak RH. Muscle wasting in chronic kidney disease. *Pediatr Nephrol*. 2018;33:789–798.
8. Kalantar-Zadeh K, Ikizler TA, Block G, Avram MM, Kopple JD. Malnutrition-inflammation complex syndrome in dialysis patients: causes and consequences. *Am J Kidney Dis*. 2003;42:864–881.
9. Fouque D, Kalantar-Zadeh K, Kopple J, et al. A proposed nomenclature and diagnostic criteria for protein-energy wasting in acute and chronic kidney disease. *Kidney Int*. 2008;73:391–398.
10. Obi Y, Qader H, Kovesdy CP, Kalantar-Zadeh K. Latest consensus and update on protein-energy wasting in chronic kidney disease. *Curr Opin Clin Nutr Metab Care*. 2015;18:254–262.
11. Nourbakhsh N, Rhee CM, Kalantar-Zadeh K. Protein-energy wasting and uremic failure to thrive in children with chronic kidney disease: they are not small adults. *Pediatr Nephrol*. 2014;29: 2249–2252.
12. Monzani A, Perrone M, Prodam F, et al. Unacylated ghrelin and obestatin: promising biomarkers of protein energy wasting in children with chronic kidney disease. *Pediatr Nephrol*. 2018;33: 661–672.
13. Fouque D, Laville M. Low protein diets for chronic kidney disease in non diabetic adults. *Cochrane Database Syst Rev*. 2009;(3). CD001892.
14. Carrero JJ, Yilmaz MI, Lindholm B, Stenvinkel P. Cytokine dysregulation in chronic kidney disease: how can we treat it? *Blood Purif*. 2008;26:291–299.
15. Stenvinkel P, Heimburger O, Lindholm B, Kaysen GA, Bergstrom J. Are there two types of malnutrition in chronic renal failure? Evidence for relationships between malnutrition, inflammation and atherosclerosis (MIA syndrome). *Nephrol Dial Transplant*. 2000;15:953–960.
16. Abraham AG, Mak RH, Mitsnefes M, et al. Protein energy wasting in children with chronic kidney disease. *Pediatr Nephrol*. 2014;29: 1231–1238.
17. Carrero JJ, Stenvinkel P, Cuppari L, et al. Etiology of the protein-energy wasting syndrome in chronic kidney disease: a consensus statement from the International Society of Renal Nutrition and Metabolism (ISRNM). *J Ren Nutr*. 2013;23:77–90.
18. de Mutsert R, Grootendorst DC, Indemans F, et al. Association between serum albumin and mortality in dialysis patients is partly explained by inflammation, and not by malnutrition. *J Ren Nutr*. 2009;19:127–135.
19. Ikizler TA, Wingard RL, Harvell J, Shyr Y, Hakim RM. Association of morbidity with markers of nutrition and inflammation in chronic hemodialysis patients: a prospective study. *Kidney Int*. 1999;55:1945–1951.
20. Stenvinkel P, Barany P, Chung SH, Lindholm B, Heimburger O. A comparative analysis of nutritional parameters as predictors of outcome in male and female ESRD patients. *Nephrol Dial Transplant*. 2002;17:1266–1274.
21. Naseeb U, Shafqat J, Jagerbrink T, et al. Proteome patterns in uremic plasma. *Blood Purif*. 2008;26:561–568.
22. Jeejeebhoy KN. Nutritional assessment. *Nutrition*. 2000;16: 585–590.
23. Klein S. The myth of serum albumin as a measure of nutritional status. *Gastroenterology*. 1990;99:1845–1846.
24. Mak RH, Cheung W. Energy homeostasis and cachexia in chronic kidney disease. *Pediatr Nephrol*. 2006;21:1807–1814.

25. Measurement of visceral protein status in assessing protein and energy malnutrition: standard of care. Prealbumin in Nutritional Care Consensus Group. *Nutrition*. 1995;11:169–171.
26. Chertow GM, Ackert K, Lew NL, Lazarus JM, Lowrie EG. Prealbumin is as important as albumin in the nutritional assessment of hemodialysis patients. *Kidney Int*. 2000;58:2512–2517.
27. Neyra NR, Hakim RM, Shyr Y, Ikizler TA. Serum transferrin and serum prealbumin are early predictors of serum albumin in chronic hemodialysis patients. *J Ren Nutr*. 2000;10:184–190.
28. Ingenbleek Y, De Visscher M, De Nayer P. Measurement of prealbumin as index of protein-calorie malnutrition. *Lancet*. 1972;2: 106–109.
29. Kopple JD, National Kidney Foundation, K.D.W.G. The National Kidney Foundation K/DOQI clinical practice guidelines for dietary protein intake for chronic dialysis patients. *Am J Kidney Dis*. 2001;38:S68–S73.
30. Ferrari P, Kulkarni H, Dheda S, et al. Serum iron markers are inadequate for guiding iron repletion in chronic kidney disease. *Clin J Am Soc Nephrol*. 2011;6:77–83.
31. Canpolat N, Sever L, Agbas A, et al. Leptin and ghrelin in chronic kidney disease: their associations with protein-energy wasting. *Pediatr Nephrol*. 2018;33:2113–2122.
32. Rebholz CM, Surapaneni A, Levey AS, et al. The serum metabolome identifies biomarkers of dietary acid load in 2 studies of adults with chronic kidney disease. *J Nutr*. 2019;149:578–585.
33. Kopple JD, Greene T, Chumlea WC, et al. Relationship between nutritional status and the glomerular filtration rate: results from the MDRD study. *Kidney Int*. 2000;57:1688–1703.
34. Zoccali C. The obesity epidemics in ESRD: from wasting to waist? *Nephrol Dial Transplant*. 2009;24:376–380.
35. Honda H, Qureshi AR, Axelsson J, et al. Obese sarcopenia in patients with end-stage renal disease is associated with inflammation and increased mortality. *Am J Clin Nutr*. 2007;86:633–638.
36. Kovesdy CP, Kalantar-Zadeh K. Why is protein-energy wasting associated with mortality in chronic kidney disease? *Semin Nephrol*. 2009;29:3–14.
37. de Boer IH, Zelnick L, Afkarian M, et al. Impaired glucose and insulin homeostasis in moderate-severe CKD. *J Am Soc Nephrol*. 2016;27:2861–2871.
38. Spoto B, Pisano A, Zoccali C. Insulin resistance in chronic kidney disease: a systematic review. *Am J Physiol Renal Physiol*. 2016;311: F1087–F1108.
39. Ferro CJ, Mark PB, Kanbay M, et al. Lipid management in patients with chronic kidney disease. *Nat Rev Nephrol*. 2018;14: 727–749.
40. Prinsen BH, de Sain-van der Velden MG, de Koning EJ, Koomans HA, Berger R, Rabelink TJ. Hypertriglyceridemia in patients with chronic renal failure: possible mechanisms. *Kidney Int Suppl*. 2003;84. S121-124.
41. Lamprea-Montealegre JA, McClelland RL, Astor BC, et al. Chronic kidney disease, plasma lipoproteins, and coronary artery calcium incidence: the Multi-Ethnic Study of Atherosclerosis. *Arterioscler Thromb Vasc Biol*. 2013;33:652–658.
42. Lamprea-Montealegre JA, Astor BC, McClelland RL, et al. CKD, plasma lipids, and common carotid intima-media thickness: results from the multi-ethnic study of atherosclerosis. *Clin J Am Soc Nephrol*. 2012;7:1777–1785.
43. Lamprea-Montealegre JA, McClelland RL, Grams M, Ouyang P, Szklo M, de Boer IH. Coronary heart disease risk associated with the dyslipidaemia of chronic kidney disease. *Heart*. 2018; 104:1455–1460.
44. Coyne D, Acharya M, Qiu P, et al. Paricalcitol capsule for the treatment of secondary hyperparathyroidism in stages 3 and 4 CKD. *Am J Kidney Dis*. 2006;47:263–276.
45. Spiegel DM, Brady K. Calcium balance in normal individuals and in patients with chronic kidney disease on low- and high-calcium diets. *Kidney Int*. 2012;81(11):1116–1122.
46. Hill KM, Martin BR, Wastney ME, et al. Oral calcium carbonate affects calcium but not phosphorus balance in stage 3-4 chronic kidney disease. *Kidney Int*. 2012;83(5):959–966.
47. Barreto DV, Barreto FC, Carvalho AB, Cuppari L, Draibe SA, Dalboni MA. Association of changes in bone remodeling and coronary calcification in hemodialysis patients: a prospective study. *Am J Kidney Dis*. 2008;52.
48. Komaba H, Wang M, Taniguchi M, et al. Initiation of sevelamer and mortality among hemodialysis patients treated with calcium-based phosphate binders. *Clin J Am Soc Nephrol*. 2017;12:1489–1497.
49. Isakova T, Gutierrez OM, Chang Y, et al. Phosphorus binders and survival on hemodialysis. *J Am Soc Nephrol*. 2009;20:388–396.
50. Locatelli F, Fouque D, Heimburger O, et al. Nutritional status in dialysis patients: a European consensus. *Nephrol Dial Transplant*. 2002;17:563–572.
51. Cannata-Andia JB, Fernandez-Martin JL, Locatelli F, et al. Use of phosphate-binding agents is associated with a lower risk of mortality. *Kidney Int*. 2013;84:998–1008.
52. Lopes AA, Tong L, Thumma J, et al. Phosphate binder use and mortality among hemodialysis patients in the Dialysis Outcomes and Practice Patterns Study (DOPPS): evaluation of possible confounding by nutritional status. *Am J Kidney Dis*. 2012;60:90–101.
53. LaClair RE, Hellman RN, Karp SL, et al. Prevalence of calcidiol deficiency in CKD: a cross-sectional study across latitudes in the United States. *Am J Kidney Dis*. 2005;45:1026–1033.
54. Isakova T, et al. Fibroblast growth factor 23 is elevated before parathyroid hormone and phosphate in chronic kidney disease. *Kidney Int*. 2011;79:1370–1378.
55. Group KW. KDOQI clinical practice guideline for nutrition in children with CKD: 2008 update. Executive summary. *Am J Kidney Dis*. 2009;53. S11-104.
56. Detsky AS, McLaughlin JR, Baker JP, et al. What is subjective global assessment of nutritional status? *J Parenter Enter Nutr*. 1987;11:8–13.
57. Toigo G, Aparicio M, Attman PO, et al. Expert Working Group report on nutrition in adult patients with renal insufficiency (part 1 of 2). *Clin Nutr*. 2000;19:197–207.
58. Cooper BA, Bartlett LH, Aslani A, Allen BJ, Ibels LS, Pollock CA. Validity of subjective global assessment as a nutritional marker in end-stage renal disease. *Am J Kidney Dis*. 2002;40:126–132.
59. Yang FL, Lee RP, Wang CH, Fang TC, Hsu BG. A cohort study of subjective global assessment and mortality in Taiwanese hemodialysis patients. *Ren Fail*. 2007;29:997–1001.
60. Campbell KL, Ash S, Bauer JD, Davies PS. Evaluation of nutrition assessment tools compared with body cell mass for the assessment of malnutrition in chronic kidney disease. *J Ren Nutr*. 2007; 17:189–195.
61. Steiber A, Leon JB, Secker D, et al. Multicenter study of the validity and reliability of subjective global assessment in the hemodialysis population. *J Ren Nutr*. 2007;17:336–342.
62. Chauveau P, Grigaut E, Kolko A, Wolff P, Combe C, Aparicio M. Evaluation of nutritional status in patients with kidney disease: usefulness of dietary recall. *J Ren Nutr*. 2007;17:88–92.
63. Avesani CM, Draibe SA, Kamimura MA, Colugnati FA, Cuppari L. Resting energy expenditure of chronic kidney disease patients: influence of renal function and subclinical inflammation. *Am J Kidney Dis*. 2004;44:1008–1016.
64. Leal VO, Stockler-Pinto MB, Farage NE, et al. Handgrip strength and its dialysis determinants in hemodialysis patients. *Nutrition*. 2011;27:1125–1129.

65. Wang AY, Sea MM, Ho ZS, Lui SF, Li PK, Woo J. Evaluation of handgrip strength as a nutritional marker and prognostic indicator in peritoneal dialysis patients. *Am J Clin Nutr.* 2005;81:79–86.
66. Amparo FC, Cordeiro AC, Carrero JJ, et al. Malnutrition-inflammation score is associated with handgrip strength in nondialysis-dependent chronic kidney disease patients. *J Ren Nutr.* 2013;23:283–287.
67. Vogt BP, Borges MCC, Goes CR, Caramori JCT. Handgrip strength is an independent predictor of all-cause mortality in maintenance dialysis patients. *Clin Nutr.* 2016;35:1429–1433.
68. Abd El Basset Bakr AM, Hasaneen BM, AbdelRasoul Helal Bassiouni D. Assessment of nutritional status in children with chronic kidney disease using hand grip strength tool. *J Ren Nutr.* 2018;28:265–269.
69. Wong Vega M, Srivaths PR. Air displacement plethysmography versus bioelectrical impedance to determine body composition in pediatric hemodialysis patients. *J Ren Nutr.* 2017;27:439–444.
70. Gotfredsen A, Jensen J, Borg J, Christiansen C. Measurement of lean body mass and total body fat using dual photon absorptiometry. *Metabolism.* 1986;35:88–93.
71. Bhatla B, Moore H, Emerson P, et al. Lean body mass estimation by creatinine kinetics, bioimpedance, and dual energy x-ray absorptiometry in patients on continuous ambulatory peritoneal dialysis. *Am Soc Artif Intern Organs J.* 1995;41:M442–M446.
72. Durnin JV, Womersley J. Body fat assessed from total body density and its estimation from skinfold thickness: measurements on 481 men and women aged from 16 to 72 years. *Br J Nutr.* 1974;32:77–97.
73. Postorino M, Marino C, Tripepi G, Zoccali C, Group CW. Abdominal obesity and all-cause and cardiovascular mortality in end-stage renal disease. *J Am Coll Cardiol.* 2009;53:1265–1272.
74. Osathanondh V, Potter EL. Development of human kidney as shown by microdissection. Iii. Formation and interrelationship of collecting tubules and nephrons. *Arch Pathol.* 1963;76:290–302.
75. Hoy WE, Douglas-Denton RN, Hughson MD, Cass A, Johnson K, Bertram JF. A stereological study of glomerular number and volume: preliminary findings in a multiracial study of kidneys at autopsy. *Kidney Int Suppl.* 2003:S31–S37.
76. Vanderheyden T, Kumar S, Fisk NM. Fetal renal impairment. *Semin Neonatol.* 2003;8:279–289.
77. Wong CS, Gipson DS, Gillen DL, et al. Anthropometric measures and risk of death in children with end-stage renal disease. *Am J Kidney Dis.* 2000;36:811–819.
78. Ayestaran FW, Schneider MF, Kaskel FJ, et al. Perceived appetite and clinical outcomes in children with chronic kidney disease. *Pediatr Nephrol.* 2016;31:1121–1127.
79. Sgambat K, Cheng YI, Charnaya O, Moudgil A. The prevalence and outcome of children with failure to thrive after pediatric kidney transplantation. *Pediatr Transplant.* 2019;23:e13321.
80. Karava V, Printza N, Dotis J, et al. Body composition and arterial stiffness in pediatric patients with chronic kidney disease. *Pediatr Nephrol.* 2019;34:1253–1260.
81. Kumar J, McDermott K, Abraham AG, et al. Prevalence and correlates of 25-hydroxyvitamin D deficiency in the chronic kidney disease in children (CKiD) cohort. *Pediatr Nephrol.* 2016;31:121–129.
82. Karlberg J. On the construction of the infancy-childhood-puberty growth standard. *Acta Paediatr Scand Suppl.* 1989;356:26–37.
83. Nelms CL. Optimizing enteral nutrition for growth in pediatric chronic kidney disease (CKD). *Front Pediatr.* 2018;6:214.
84. Akchurin OM. Chronic kidney disease and dietary measures to improve outcomes. *Pediatr Clin N Am.* 2019;66:247–267.
85. Amissah EA, Brown J, Harding JE. Fat supplementation of human milk for promoting growth in preterm infants. *Cochrane Database Syst Rev.* 2018;6. CD000341.
86. Le Palma K, Pavlick ER, Copelovitch L. Pretreatment of enteral nutrition with sodium polystyrene sulfonate: effective, but beware the high prevalence of electrolyte derangements in clinical practice. *Clin Kidney J.* 2018;11:166–171.
87. Coleman JE, Watson AR, Rance CH, Moore E. Gastrostomy buttons for nutritional support on chronic dialysis. *Nephrol Dial Transplant.* 1998;13:2041–2046.
88. Weaver Jr DJ, Somers MJG, Martz K, Mitsnefes MM. Clinical outcomes and survival in pediatric patients initiating chronic dialysis: a report of the NAPRTCS registry. *Pediatr Nephrol.* 2017;32:2319–2330.
89. Hobbs DJ, Bunchman TE, Weismantel DP, et al. Megestrol acetate improves weight gain in pediatric patients with chronic kidney disease. *J Ren Nutr.* 2010;20:408–413.
90. Zheng Z, Chen J, He D, Xu Y, Chen L, Zhang T. The effects of megestrol acetate on nutrition, inflammation and quality of life in elderly haemodialysis patients. *Int Urol Nephrol.* 2019;51:1631–1638.
91. Franke D, Winkel S, Gellermann J, et al. Growth and maturation improvement in children on renal replacement therapy over the past 20 years. *Pediatr Nephrol.* 2013;28:2043–2051.
92. Furth SL, Stablein D, Fine RN, Powe NR, Fivush BA. Adverse clinical outcomes associated with short stature at dialysis initiation: a report of the North American Pediatric Renal Transplant Cooperative Study. *Pediatrics.* 2002;109:909–913.
93. Fernandez-Iglesias A, Lopez JM, Santos F. Growth plate alterations in chronic kidney disease. *Pediatr Nephrol.* 2020;35(3):367–374.
94. Schaefer F, Chen Y, Tsao T, Nouri P, Rabkin R. Impaired JAK-STAT signal transduction contributes to growth hormone resistance in chronic uremia. *J Clin Investig.* 2001;108:467–475.
95. Rees L. Growth hormone therapy in children with CKD after more than two decades of practice. *Pediatr Nephrol.* 2016;31:1421–1435.
96. Drube J, Wan M, Bonthuis M, et al. Clinical practice recommendations for growth hormone treatment in children with chronic kidney disease. *Nat Rev Nephrol.* 2019;15:577–589.
97. Watkins SL. Does renal osteodystrophy develop and/or progress during the course of rhGH treatment? *Br J Clin Pract Suppl.* 1996;85:59–60.
98. Azar AT, Wahba K, Mohamed AS, Massoud WA. Association between dialysis dose improvement and nutritional status among hemodialysis patients. *Am J Nephrol.* 2007;27:113–119.
99. Ward HJ. Nutritional and metabolic issues in solid organ transplantation: targets for future research. *J Ren Nutr.* 2009;19:111–122.
100. Cano N, Fiaccadori E, Tesinsky P, et al. ESPEN guidelines on enteral nutrition: adult renal failure. *Clin Nutr.* 2006;25:295–310.
101. Fouque D, Laville M, Boissel JP, Chifflet R, Labeeuw M, Zech PY. Controlled low protein diets in chronic renal insufficiency: meta-analysis. *BMJ.* 1992;304:216–220.
102. Klahr S, Levey AS, Beck GJ, et al. The effects of dietary protein restriction and blood-pressure control on the progression of chronic renal disease. Modification of Diet in Renal Disease Study Group. *N Engl J Med.* 1994;330:877–884.
103. Levey AS, Adler S, Caggiula AW, et al. Effects of dietary protein restriction on the progression of advanced renal disease in the Modification of Diet in Renal Disease Study. *Am J Kidney Dis.* 1996;27:652–663.
104. Pedrini MT, Levey AS, Lau J, Chalmers TC, Wang PH. The effect of dietary protein restriction on the progression of diabetic and nondiabetic renal diseases: a meta-analysis. *Ann Intern Med.* 1996;124:627–632.
105. Mitch WE, Remuzzi G. Diets for patients with chronic kidney disease, still worth prescribing. *J Am Soc Nephrol.* 2004;15:234–237.
106. Bergstrom J, Lindholm B. Nutrition and adequacy of dialysis. How do hemodialysis and CAPD compare? *Kidney Int Suppl.* 1993;40:S39–S50.

107. Jiang N, Qian J, Sun W, et al. Better preservation of residual renal function in peritoneal dialysis patients treated with a low-protein diet supplemented with keto acids: a prospective, randomized trial. *Nephrol Dial Transplant*. 2009;24:2551–2558.
108. Kopple JD, Bernard D, Messana J, et al. Treatment of malnourished CAPD patients with an amino acid based dialysate. *Kidney Int*. 1995;47:1148–1157.
109. Kent PS. Integrating clinical nutrition practice guidelines in chronic kidney disease. *Nutr Clin Pract*. 2005;20:213–217.
110. Ewers B, Riserus U, Marckmann P. Effects of unsaturated fat dietary supplements on blood lipids, and on markers of malnutrition and inflammation in hemodialysis patients. *J Ren Nutr*. 2009;19:401–411.
111. Monteon FJ, Laidlaw SA, Shaib JK, Kopple JD. Energy expenditure in patients with chronic renal failure. *Kidney Int*. 1986;30:741–747.
112. Heimburger O, Waniewski J, Werynski A, Lindholm B. A quantitative description of solute and fluid transport during peritoneal dialysis. *Kidney Int*. 1992;41:1320–1332.
113. Gilmour ER, Hartley GH, Goodship THJ. Trace elements and vitamins in renal disease. In: Mitch WE, Klahr S, eds. *Nutrition and the Kidney*. Vol. 468. Boston, Little, Brown; 1993:114–127. pp xiii.
114. Kopple JD. Nutritional therapy in kidney failure. *Nutr Rev*. 1981;39:193–206.
115. Frohling PT, Schmicker R, Vetter K, et al. Conservative treatment with ketoacid and amino acid supplemented low-protein diets in chronic renal failure. *Am J Clin Nutr*. 1980;33:1667–1672.
116. Kopple JD. Role of diet in the progression of chronic renal failure: experience with human studies and proposed mechanisms by which nutrients may retard progression. *J Nutr*. 1991;121:S124.
117. Arnadottir M, Brattstrom L, Simonsen O, et al. The effect of high-dose pyridoxine and folic acid supplementation on serum lipid and plasma homocysteine concentrations in dialysis patients. *Clin Nephrol*. 1993;40:236–240.
118. Booth ML. Introducing fluidics. *Eng Med*. 1976;5:3–5.
119. Canavese C, Petrarulo M, Massarenti P, et al. Long-term, low-dose, intravenous vitamin C leads to plasma calcium oxalate supersaturation in hemodialysis patients. *Am J Kidney Dis*. 2005;45:540–549.
120. Jean G, Terrat JC, Vanel T, et al. Daily oral 25-hydroxycholecalciferol supplementation for vitamin D deficiency in haemodialysis patients: effects on mineral metabolism and bone markers. *Nephrol Dial Transplant*. 2008;23:3670–3676.
121. Clermont G, Lecour S, Lahet J, et al. Alteration in plasma antioxidant capacities in chronic renal failure and hemodialysis patients: a possible explanation for the increased cardiovascular risk in these patients. *Cardiovasc Res*. 2000;47:618–623.
122. Boaz M, Smetana S, Weinstein T, et al. Secondary prevention with antioxidants of cardiovascular disease in endstage renal disease (SPACE): randomised placebo-controlled trial. *Lancet*. 2000;356:1213–1218.
123. Kalantar-Zadeh K, Kopple JD. Trace elements and vitamins in maintenance dialysis patients. *Adv Ren Replace Ther*. 2003;10:170–182.
124. Rashidi AA, Salehi M, Piroozmand A, Sagheb MM. Effects of zinc supplementation on serum zinc and C-reactive protein concentrations in hemodialysis patients. *J Ren Nutr*. 2009;19:475–478.
125. Fouque D, Aparicio M. Eleven reasons to control the protein intake of patients with chronic kidney disease. *Nat Clin Pract Nephrol*. 2007;3:383–392.
126. Aparicio M, Chauveau P, Combe C. Low protein diets and outcome of renal patients. *J Nephrol*. 2001;14:433–439.
127. National Kidney Foundation K/DOQI clinical practice guidelines for nutrition in chronic renal failure. *Am J Kidney Dis*. 2000;35. S1-140.
128. Pupim LB, Flakoll PJ, Brouillette JR, Levenhagen DK, Hakim RM, Ikizler TA. Intradialytic parenteral nutrition improves protein and energy homeostasis in chronic hemodialysis patients. *J Clin Investig*. 2002;110:483–492.
129. Cano NJ, Fouque D, Roth H, et al. Intradialytic parenteral nutrition does not improve survival in malnourished hemodialysis patients: a 2-year multicenter, prospective, randomized study. *J Am Soc Nephrol*. 2007;18:2583–2591.
130. Rana A, Gruessner A, Agopian VG, et al. Survival benefit of solid-organ transplant in the United States. *J Am Med Assoc Surg*. 2015;150:252–259.
131. Chen K, Didsbury M, van Zwieten A, et al. Neurocognitive and educational outcomes in children and adolescents with CKD: a systematic review and meta-analysis. *Clin J Am Soc Nephrol*. 2018;13:387–397.
132. Icard P, Hooper SR, Gipson DS, Ferris ME. Cognitive improvement in children with CKD after transplant. *Pediatr Transplant*. 2010;14:887–890.
133. Neipp M, Offner G, Luck R, et al. Kidney transplant in children weighing less than 15 kg: donor selection and technical considerations. *Transplantation*. 2002;73:409–416.
134. Mickelson JJ, MacNeily AE, Leblanc J, White C, Gourlay WA. Renal transplantation in children 15 Kg or less: the British Columbia Children's Hospital experience. *J Urol*. 2006;176:1797–1800.
135. Vitola SP, Gnatta D, Garcia VD, et al. Kidney transplantation in children weighing less than 15 kg: extraperitoneal surgical access-experience with 62 cases. *Pediatr Transplant*. 2013;17:445–453.
136. Ku E, Glidden DV, Hsu CY, Portale AA, Grimes B, Johansen KL. Association of body mass index with patient-centered outcomes in children with ESRD. *J Am Soc Nephrol*. 2016;27:551–558.
137. Feltran LS, Cunha MF, Perentel SM, et al. Is preoperative preparation time a barrier to small children being ready for kidney transplantation? *Transplantation*. 2020;104(3):591–596.

CHAPTER

25

ALCOHOL: THE ROLE IN NUTRITION AND HEALTH

Paolo M. Suter, MD, MS

Clinic and Policlinic of Internal Medicine, University Hospital, Zurich, Switzerland

SUMMARY

Alcohol is globally a major component of daily life and nutrition. Presently, about 61% of US adults are current drinkers. Due to its metabolic characteristics, alcohol as a function of the absolute amount consumed, consumption frequency, genetic factors etc., has a high potential to affect most metabolic pathways and cell and organ function including the metabolism and nutriture of all macro- and micronutrients. In this chapter, the present knowledge of the effects of alcohol on selected nutrients as well as health and disease burden will be summarized.

Keywords: Alcohol; Cardiovascular disease risk; Disease risk; Ethanol; Metabolism; Nutrition; Safe intake level; Vitamins.

I. INTRODUCTION

Alcohol[a] is globally a major component of daily life, contributing with it's Janus-faced characteristics a perceived pleasure and at the same time contributing to 5% of the Global Burden of Disease (GBD).[1] Presently, about 61% of US adults (67% of men and 55% of women) are current drinkers, about 14% were former drinkers, 24% of the adults were lifetime abstainers, and approximately 5% of the adults were classified as heavier drinkers.[2,3] According to a modeling study, global per capita alcohol consumption (pure alcohol per adult ≥15 years) increased between 1990 and 2017 from 5.9 L (95% CI 5·8–6·1) to 6·5 L (6·0–6·9), further increasing till 2030 to 7·6 L (6·5–10·2).[4] Similarly, several representative US surveys reported an increased consumption during the last decades.[5] In the United States, the prevalence of 12 month DSM-IV alcohol use disorders (AUD) among alcohol users increased between 2001–02 and 2012–13 from 12.9% to 17.5%; the increase was mainly seen in women, older adults, and socioeconomically disadvantaged individuals.[6] Currently, alcohol-related health inequalities increase and the gender gap in AUD closes and alcohol-related emergency department consultations increase.[7] Despite the wide acceptance of alcohol, it remains an important cause and modulator of disease risk and modulator of life expectancy[8]: the harmful use of alcohol is a causal factor in more than 200 disease states leading worldwide to about 3 million (5.3% of total) deaths[1] and 132.6 million (5.2% of total) of disability-adjusted life years.[1] The alcohol consumption patterns vary greatly from one country or geographic areas to the other. For instance, in China, heavy alcohol consumption showed in <20 years a 70-fold increase creating a new health challenges, due to Asian unique characteristics in alcohol metabolism, lifestyle and behavior, consumption patterns, and last but not least nutrition.[9] Among adults younger than 69 years, alcohol was responsible for 7.2% of premature mortality, affecting disproportionally more often individuals at younger age.[1] With approximately 88,000 deaths per year attributable to excessive drinking,

[a] The terms "alcohol" and "ethanol" are used interchangeably denoting ethyl alcohol (C_2H_5-OH).

Present Knowledge in Nutrition, Volume 2
https://doi.org/10.1016/B978-0-12-818460-8.00025-3

alcohol consumption represents the third leading cause of death after tobacco and poor diet and physical inactivity.[10] In view of the aging population, alcohol as a risk factor for dementia should not be underestimated. 57% of individuals with the diagnosis of early onset dementia had also an AUD.[11]

Compared with other food items, alcohol has three characteristic features: depending on the absolute amount and frequency of consumption, it can be regarded as a nutrient, a toxin, or a psychoactive drug. Alcohol consumption is a very complex behavior, and each society (including the political decision makers) and each consumer determines which aspect of alcohol will prevail.

For the purposes of this discussion, one "standard" drink (or one alcohol drink equivalent) corresponds to approximately 14 g (range 12–15g) of pure alcohol, which is contained in approximately 12 fl did (fl) ounces (350 mL) of beer (5% alcohol by volume), 8–9 fl ounces (235–260 mL) of malt liquor (7%), 5 fl ounces of wine (150 mL) of table wine (12%–13%), or 1.5 fl ounces (45–50 mL) of distilled spirits (40%)[12,13] (Fig. 25.1). The definition of a standard drink is getting increasingly complicated, since newly designed beverages contain varying amounts of alcohol, and many product names and designations are (often intentionally) misleading for most consumers.[14] Presently, moderate drinking is defined as up to one drink per day for women and two drinks per day for men. A review of alcohol's effects on selected nutrients and on health and disease risk follows.

II. ALCOHOL METABOLISM

Alcohol is rapidly absorbed from the stomach and the jejunum and is distributed in the total water compartment of the body. Alcohol can be metabolized via three different enzyme systems (depending on the dose and frequency of consumption) (Fig. 25.2). In light-moderate consumers, alcohol is metabolized in the liver catalyzed by the cytosolic alcohol dehydrogenase (ADH); however, a small amount may be metabolized in the stomach mucosa (i.e., during the first-pass metabolism)[15] or by a nonoxidative pathway leading to fatty acid ethyl esters (FAEEs), ethyl glucuronide (EtG), and phosphatidylethanol,[16] which might be useful as biomarkers for alcohol intake.[17] Alcohol metabolism by peroxisomal catalase is only of minor importance. The first-pass metabolism in the stomach is higher in men than in women, declines with age, and is reduced by bariatric surgery[18] and certain drugs, e.g., aspirin. For higher levels of intake, alcohol is predominantly metabolized in the inducible microsomal ethanol oxidizing system (MEOS),[19] which depends on different cytochrome P450 isoenzymes[20] (Fig. 25.2). The oxidation of alcohol in both the ADH and the MEOS pathway leads to the production of acetaldehyde, which is further metabolized to acetate by acetaldehyde dehydrogenase (ALDH). Acetate is shuttled to the peripheral tissues and used as a source of energy.

Because of its potential toxicity and the inability of the body to store alcohol, it has to be eliminated as quickly as

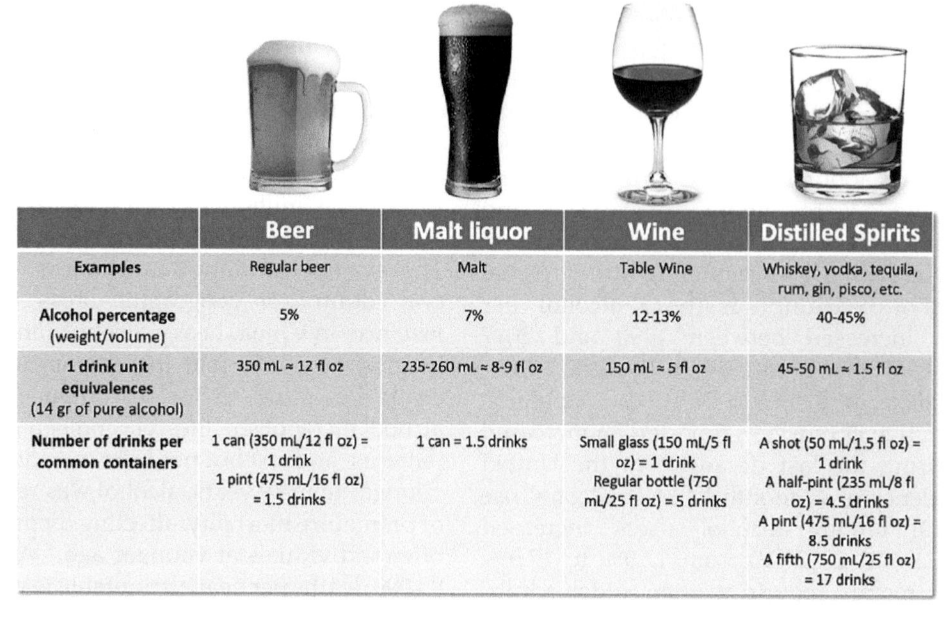

	Beer	Malt liquor	Wine	Distilled Spirits
Examples	Regular beer	Malt	Table Wine	Whiskey, vodka, tequila, rum, gin, pisco, etc.
Alcohol percentage (weight/volume)	5%	7%	12-13%	40-45%
1 drink unit equivalences (14 gr of pure alcohol)	350 mL ≈ 12 fl oz	235-260 mL ≈ 8-9 fl oz	150 mL ≈ 5 fl oz	45-50 mL ≈ 1.5 fl oz
Number of drinks per common containers	1 can (350 mL/12 fl oz) = 1 drink 1 pint (475 mL/16 fl oz) = 1.5 drinks	1 can = 1.5 drinks	Small glass (150 mL/5 fl oz) = 1 drink Regular bottle (750 mL/25 fl oz) = 5 drinks	A shot (50 mL/1.5 fl oz) = 1 drink A half-pint (235 mL/8 fl oz) = 4.5 drinks A pint (475 mL/16 fl oz) = 8.5 drinks A fifth (750 mL/25 fl oz) = 17 drinks

FIGURE 25.1 Equivalences between different alcoholic beverages, amount of alcohol, and number of drinks per common containers. *From Arab et al.*[38]

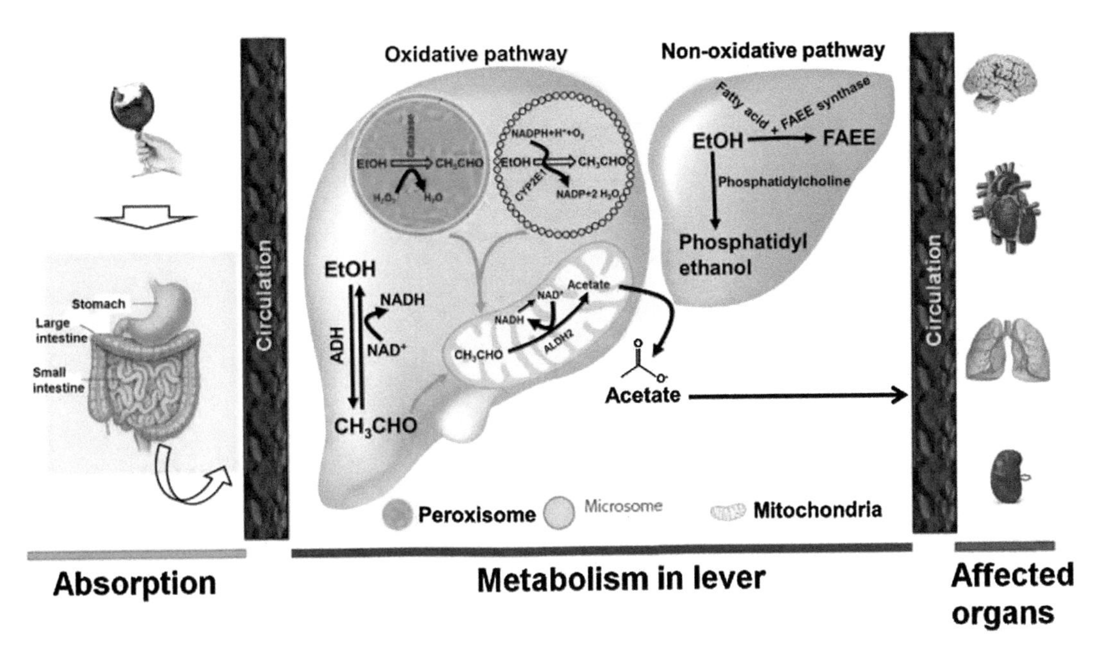

FIGURE 25.2 Alcohol metabolism. *From Mandal et al.*[493]

possible from the body. This absolute priority in metabolism is a major cause of the metabolic effects of alcohol on nearly all nutrients, metabolic pathways, on all organ systems, and, finally, on disease risks. Many societal, individual, and genetic factors determine the health and nutritional effects of alcohol[21–24] (Figs. 25.3 and 25.4). The metabolism of alcohol induces a change in the redox potential in the liver, reactive oxygen and nitrogen species, cofactor depletion (e.g., NAD+), an impaired cellular energy homeostasis, alterations in membrane fluidity, and acetaldehyde toxicity (Figs. 25.2 and 25.4).[24] These changes contribute to different metabolic and clinical consequences and to functional abnormalities such as suppression of the Krebs cycle, with an increased transformation of pyruvate to lactate, impaired gluconeogenesis and hypoglycemia, greater fatty acid (FA) synthesis, reduced urate excretion, and hyperuricemia[25]. Acetaldehyde leads to many different effects, such as increased free radical production and lipid peroxidation, inhibition of protein synthesis, and impaired vitamin metabolism.[26,27] Indirect mechanisms include pathologies due to extracellular vesicles such as exosomes or microvesicles,[28] altered methylation,[29] or mitochondrial dysfunction to mention just a few.[30]

Alcohol metabolism shows a wide interindividual variability (Fig. 25.3) that is modulated by different genotypes of the alcohol-metabolizing enzymes ADH and ALDH.[22,31] Depending on the ADH genotype, higher maximal alcohol and acetaldehyde concentrations and a slower alcohol elimination are found, a situation that may lead to increased direct and indirect alcohol toxicity and thus a different alcohol-related disease pattern. In many people of Asian origin, the activity of ALDH may be low and thus cause a typical facial flushing reaction and headaches after ingestion of even small amounts of alcohol.

Although the capacity to metabolize alcohol varies widely, a healthy person metabolizes 5–7 g/h alcohol on average. There is no useful and safe strategy (except a high fructose intake leading to a reduced nicotinamide adenine dinucleotide reoxidation) known to increase the rate of alcohol degradation.

III. THE NUTRITIONAL ASSESSMENT OF THE ALCOHOLIC PATIENT

Nutritional assessment of the alcoholic patient is a challenging task with risk of over- and underreporting of alcohol intake.[32] In (heavy) alcohol consumers, a nutritional evaluation is a mandatory complementary procedure to the usual medical care[33–35]; however, the ideal screening tool is controversial[36] and depends on the clinical setting and different guidelines for patients with alcoholic liver disease (ALD) are available.[35,37–39] The clinical signs of alcohol-related malnutrition depend on the stage of alcoholism, the level of socioeconomic integration, social and familial networks, associated alcohol- and non–alcohol-related diseases (especially liver disease), and concomitant medication intake[40] (Figs. 25.3 and 25.4). Socioeconomically integrated heavy drinkers without clinically visible somatic diseases rarely show signs of malnutrition,[41] although the dietary pattern may be already affected.[42] With the

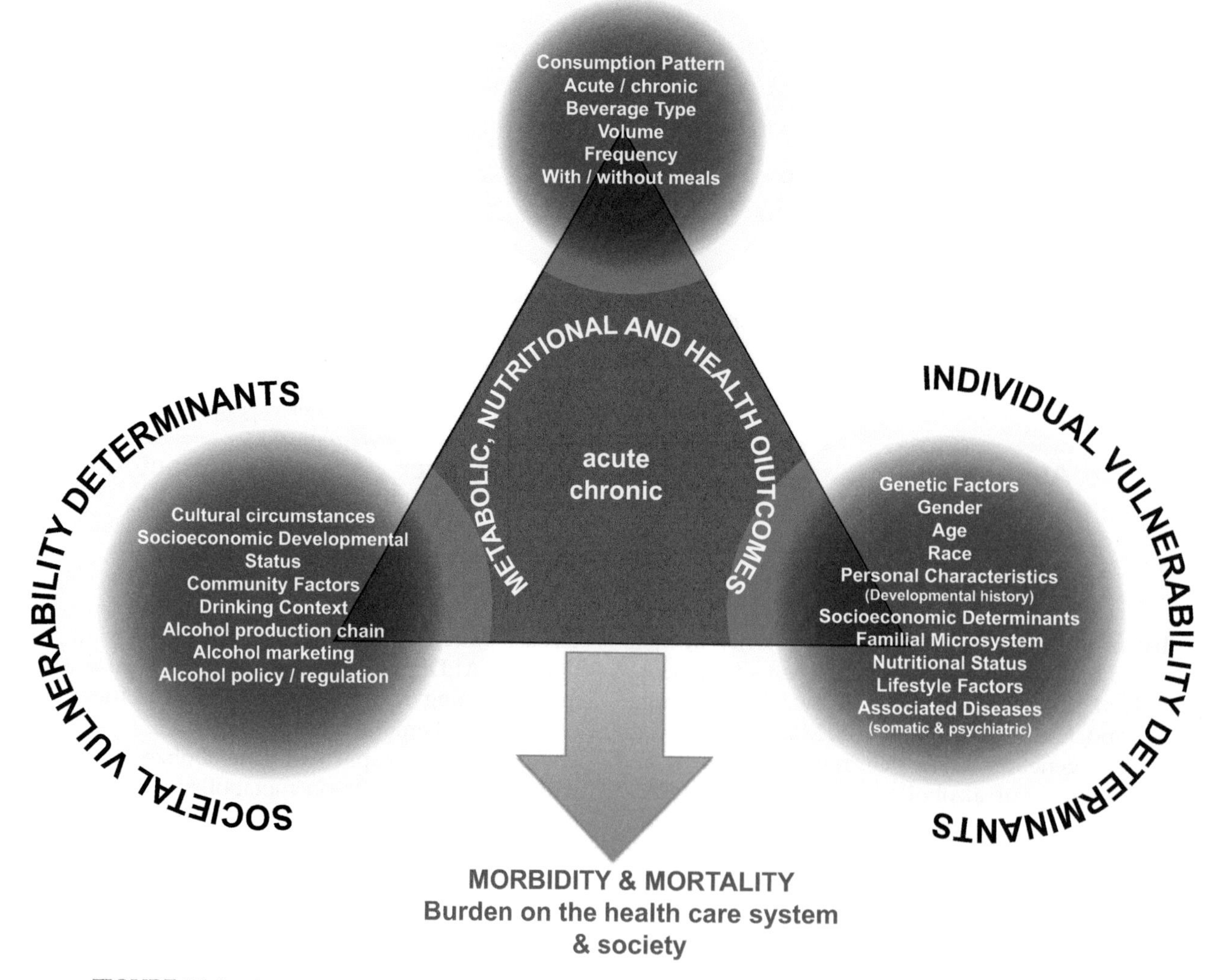

FIGURE 25.3 Conceptual causal model of alcohol consumption and health outcomes. *Adapted from Gilmore et al.*[494]

progression of alcoholism, different clinical signs of malnutrition may be found; for example, thin arms and legs due to muscle wasting[43] and myopathy,[44–47] edema (protein deficiency), glossitis (vitamin B deficiency), and scaly, dry skin (zinc and essential FA deficiency). Spider naevi and multiple hematomas due to easy bruising (vitamin C and K deficiency) may occur.[48,49] The parotid glands are often enlarged due to chronic parotitis. The patients may present with new bone fractures and several old costal fractures, and advanced osteoporosis (especially in men).[50] Alcohol-associated endocrine pathologies may lead to gynecomastia, testicular atrophy, and loss of body hair. Neurological signs may be limited to peripheral neuropathy (vitamin B deficiency), different central nervous system impairments (see Section IX.A), or the full clinical picture of stroke or dementia. An impaired dark adaptation due to zinc deficiency is fairly common and should not be misinterpreted as vitamin A deficiency. In general, the nutritional assessment of the alcoholic patient is not different from the assessment of other patients. The biochemical assessment includes measurement of the conventional alcohol markers (i.e., liver transaminase levels and red blood cell mean cell volume) in combination with biochemical markers of nutritional status.[34] Other biochemical markers for alcohol consumption (such as carbohydrate-deficient transferrin [CDT] or FAEEs or EtG), ethyl sulfate in blood/urine, may be helpful.[51–55] The measurement of FAEE or EtG in hair allows the assessment of alcohol intake over a period of up to 6 months.[55] A chronic alcohol consumption (>7 days) in the range of 50–70 g/d induces the hepatocyte to produce a transferrin molecule that is deficient in carbohydrates. The CDT is a marker for sustained and harmful alcohol consumption and normalizes slowly upon cessation of alcohol intake. Elevated

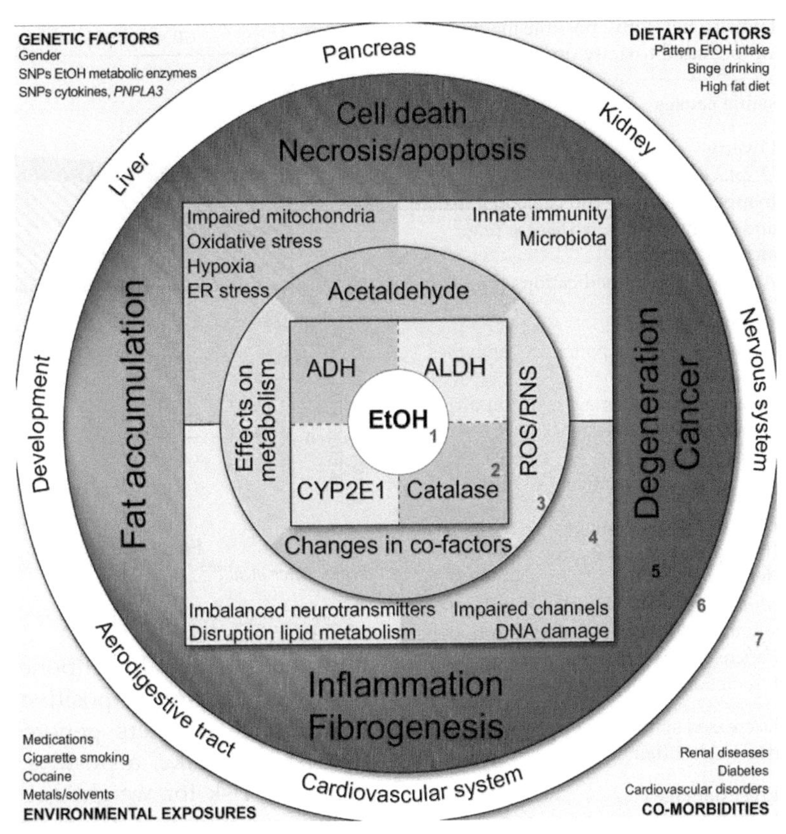

FIGURE 25.4 Determinants, modulators, and mechanisms of the metabolic and toxic effects of alcohol. *From Rusyn et al.*[24]

levels of high-density lipoprotein (HDL) cholesterol, uric acid, and fasting triacylglycerol levels without other explanation may be signs of excessive alcohol intake.

The assessment of alcohol intake at either the population or individual level is still very difficult. Although heavy alcohol intake is detected sooner or later by typical clinical signs or laboratory test results, there is no reliable clinical sign of biochemical marker for the assessment of light-to-moderate alcohol intake. Intentional or unintentional underreporting and overreporting occurs frequently. The difficulty in assessing low-to-moderate levels of alcohol consumption represents probably one of the most important causes for inconsistent research findings. New technologies such as wearable electrochemical biosensors[56,57] might be a promising and reliable approach in the not-too-distant future.

IV. ALCOHOL AND NUTRITION

As a function of the amount of alcohol consumed, the duration of intake, and any associated diseases and medication intake, drinking can impair the nutritional status of all nutrients (Figs. 25.3 and 25.4). Alcohol-associated malnutrition includes both primary and secondary malnutrition.[58] At low levels of alcohol intake, appetite and food intake is enhanced ("apéritif effect").[59,60] At higher consumption levels, due to many direct and indirect effects on food intake regulation, alcohol displaces other energy sources and thus many essential nutrients in the diet, thereby lowering the intake of most nutrients (primary malnutrition). Gastrointestinal and metabolic complications of heavy alcohol intake (especially liver dysfunction) lead to so-called secondary malnutrition. Anorexia and vomiting from alcoholic gastritis further promote inadequate intakes of food. Malabsorption of nearly all nutrients can develop as a result of mucosal dysfunction, liver insufficiency, and pancreatic insufficiency.[61] Alcoholic liver dysfunction causes a reduced capacity to transport nutrients in the blood, a reduced storage capacity, and an insufficient activation of nutrients such as vitamins. In addition, alcohol increases the excretion of nutrients in the urine and bile. In alcoholic patients, several mechanisms for the development of malnutrition usually occur simultaneously (Table 25.1).[61]

TABLE 25.1 Alcohol and nutritional status: possible mechanisms of the alcohol-mediated toxicity on nutrition.

Mechanisms	Possible causes
Reduced dietary intake	• Poverty • Displacement of normal food • Inappetence due to direct alcohol toxicity and secondary due to disease (e.g., alcoholic gastritis) • Anorexia due to medications
Impaired digestion	• Alcoholic gastritis • Impaired bile and pancreatic enzymes secretion • Direct mucosal damage and impairment of mucosal enzymes (e.g., folyl conjugase) • Altered gastrointestinal mobility
Malabsorption	• Direct mucosal damage • Indirect damage (e.g., due to folate deficiency) • Motility changes including accelerated small intestinal transit time and diarrhea • Pancreatic insufficiency • Interactions with medications
Impaired transport in the circulation	• Decreased synthesis of transport proteins due to liver damage
Impaired activation	• Liver damage • Inadequate supply of cofactors • Cellular dysfunction
Decreased storage	• Liver pathology • Alcoholic myopathy/sarcopenia/ cachexia
Increased losses	• Increased excretion in urine and bile • Increased urinary losses due to medications • Increased fecal losses
Increased requirements	• Due to the above factors • Increased metabolic rate

V. ALCOHOL AND ENERGY METABOLISM

The energy content of alcohol, compared with other energy sources, is rather high (1 g alcohol = 7.1 kcal = 29.7 kJ), thus representing an important source of energy contributing to about 4.3% of the total energy intake at the whole population level depending on age, sex, and socioeconomic status and contributing 17.2% of the energy intake in alcohol consumers.[62] In heavy drinkers, alcohol may contribute up to 50% of the daily energy intake, thus having a high potential to displace other food (Fig. 25.5). Alcohol's calories are unregulated, empty calories.[63,64] For weight maintenance, the energy balance has to be equilibrated, and alcohol has been reported to affect all components of the energy balance negatively, favoring a positive energy balance.[65]

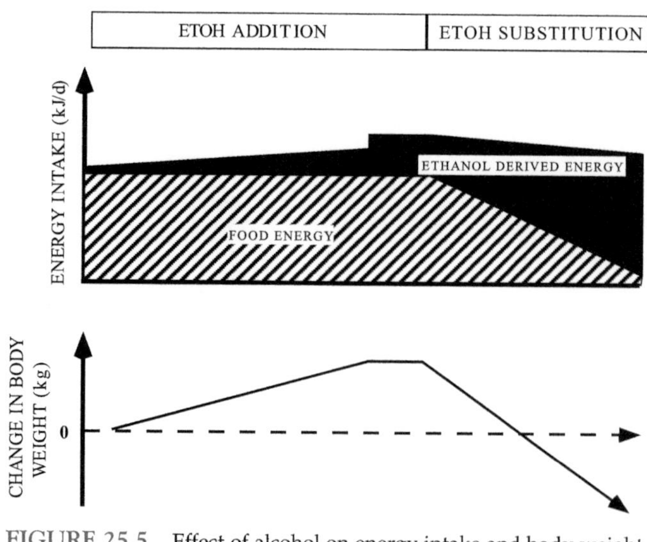

FIGURE 25.5 Effect of alcohol on energy intake and body weight. *From Suter et al.*[495]

Moderate drinkers generally add alcohol to their usual food intake, a positive energy balance with an increased risk for weight gain, and obesity will result unless compensated for by other means. This risk is increased by the combination of a high-fat diet and even in the moderate intake range due to the hyperphagic effect of alcohol.[66] Alcohol substitution (i.e., the usual food energy sources are substituted by alcohol) is the typical feature of the heavy drinker and will result in malnutrition and weight loss.

Alcohol leads to an increase of energy expenditure. In an indirect calorimetry study in young, moderate drinkers, the addition and the substitution of 25% of their energy requirements (corresponding to 96 ± 4 g alcohol) by alcohol leads to increasing energy expenditures of 7% ± 1% and 4% ± 1%, respectively.[67] The increase of energy expenditure corresponds to a thermic effect of 20%–25% of the energy content of the ingested alcohol. Other studies[65,68] reported a similar thermic effect of alcohol in healthy, moderate consumers in the range of 15%–25%, which is rather high compared with other energy sources (e.g., the thermic effect of a mixed meal is approximately 12%).

Presently, it is not completely clear what fraction of the alcohol energy could be used for adenosine triphosphate (ATP) production. In their classical studies nearly 120 years ago, Atwater and Benedict[69] suggested that alcohol energy seems to be equivalent to the energy of carbohydrates or fat. However, subsequent studies revealed that as a function of the pathway of the metabolic degradation of alcohol (i.e., ADH vs. MEOS), lower amounts of ATP are produced than theoretical calculations would suggest.[70] Despite some energy wastage, alcohol calories are largely a useable energy source in the moderate consumer.

Alcohol also affects the energy balance equation by its effects on substrate balance. Independently, whether alcohol is added to or substituted for usual food, lipid oxidation is suppressed approximately by a third,[67] producing a positive fat balance. The positive fat balance is not caused by a de novo lipogenesis from alcohol, but due to acetate being used in the peripheral organs as a source of energy at the expense of a lower fat oxidation. Use of stable isotope mass spectrometry techniques has shown that most (98%) of the carbons of a moderate alcohol load (25 g) are transported as acetate to the peripheral tissues, and only a negligible amount of the ingested dose (<1%) is used for de novo lipogenesis.[71]

Despite these effects of alcohol on energy balance, some epidemiological and experimental studies were unable to identify moderate alcohol consumption as a risk factor for obesity.[72–76] Cross-sectional studies described positive or null associations between alcohol intake and body weight in men and inverse or null in women. There are only a few prospective studies about this association, and they are equally controversial. Data from a 13 year follow-up in the Women's Health Study[74] found that initially normal weight light-to-moderate alcohol consuming women gained less weight and had a lower risk of becoming overweight and/or obese as compared with nondrinking women. These controversial findings are not surprising in view of the difficulty in assessing alcohol intake and other lifestyle parameters that may compensate for some of the effects of alcohol. Further on, socioeconomic factors determine alcohol consumption pattern and health behaviors[2] including coping with factors affecting body weight changes that explain the controversial outcomes in most if not all studies.[77] Because of the suppression of lipid oxidation and the resulting positive energy balance, even moderate amounts of alcohol have to be regarded as a risk factor for weight gain and obesity when not counterbalanced by other means (i.e., reduced energy intake and/or increased energy expenditure by physical activity). To counteract the effects of alcohol on fat oxidation, fat intake should be kept as low as possible, and whenever alcohol is consumed, fat intake has to be reduced ideally in proportion to the amount of alcohol ingested to remain in substrate balance. In agreement with data from well-controlled metabolic studies, different intervention studies (including the Look AHEAD trial) showed that alcohol consumption was related to a worse long-term weight loss outcome.[78] Regular heavy alcohol intake in young adults leads to a higher risk for weight gain and higher chances of transitioning to overweight/obesity.[79]

Alcohol enhances the abdominal deposition of fat,[80,81] representing a typical feature of the metabolic syndrome, which is associated with several adverse health outcomes such as hypertension or dyslipi demia.[82,83] Again, the later relationship is complicated by epidemiologic findings reporting a lower prevalence of the typical features of the metabolic syndrome in mild-to-moderate alcohol consumers.[84,85] Based on the present evidence, it seems to be warranted to conclude that alcohol consumption is a risk factor for obesity in many individuals.[86]

VI. EFFECTS OF ALCOHOL ON LIPID METABOLISM

As a function of the amount consumed, the frequency of drinking, presence of concomitant diseases (especially liver disease, overweight, and obesity, diabetes mellitus type 2), and other characteristics of the consumer (such as gender, age, polypmorphisms of alcohol-metabolizing enzymes, beverage choice, or overall lifestyle),[87,88] alcohol affects all lipoprotein fractions in the blood.[89–91] The development of alcohol-related fatty liver (hepatic steatosis) disease, a common characteristic early sign of ALD, is caused by many mechanisms affecting nearly all pathways and aspects of hepatic lipid metabolism[92] such as increased expression of hepatic FA transporters, the alcohol-induced suppression of lipid oxidation in the liver, by an increased influx of fat from the peripheral tissues,[93] alcohol-induced alterations of transcriptional controls of lipid metabolism,[93] endoplasmatic reticulum stress, direct effects on lipogenic enzymes,[92] disturbances in hepatic circadian clock,[94,95] or alterations of the gut microbiome.[96] Alcohol affects the hepatic FA pool so that hepatic lipidomic studies might assist to elucidate the pathway to understand the alcohol-associated pathway to liver disease.[97] Already early changes in liver function are associated with the typical constellations of alcoholic hyperlipidemia, which include elevated serum triacylglycerol levels caused by an increased hepatic secretion of very low-density lipoproteins (VLDL) mediated by an upregulation of apolipoprotein B synthesis[98] and alcohol-induced injury to peripheral removal of the VLDLs resulting from an impaired lipoprotein lipase activity[99] and suppression of lipid oxidation.

The alcohol-induced rise in triacylglycerol levels is potentiated by a high-fat diet. The effects of alcohol on triacylgylcerol levels are also seen during the postprandial phase; however, they can be partially counteracted by a concomitant reduction in fat intake and/or higher physical activity before or after the meal.[100] Obviously, the response to alcohol might vary in certain subgroups of the population as a function of genetic and/or environmental factors, and a even a J-shaped relation between alcohol intake and plasma triacylglycerol levels has been reported,[101,102] which cannot be readily explained and which might be due to other lifestyle factors. Most of the evidence shows that the triglyceride-rising effect is beverage-type independent.

Except in the setting of severe liver disease, the chronic *moderate* ingestion of alcohol leads to a dose–response-dependent increase in HDL cholesterol[103,104] and is associated with a smaller longitudinal decline in HDL cholesterol concentration.[103] Alcohol could accelerate cholesterol clearance by PPARγ and SR-B1–mediated increased reverse cholesterol transport.[105] However, heavier alcohol consumption is associated with lower HDL cholesterol due to an impaired liver function.[106] The HDL cholesterol–increasing effects are regarded as a potential mechanism for the cardioprotective effects of alcohol,[107,108] although HDL function might be more important than the absolute HDL concentration.[109] The alcohol-associated increase in HDL cholesterol may have multiple causes, including an increased hepatic production and secretion of apoproteins AI and AII,[110] an increased peripheral production due to lipid exchange within the different lipoprotein fractions, and a decreased catabolism of the HDL particle caused by alcohol's effects on specific enzymes involved in lipid transfer or effects on postprandial lipemia.[93,111] The HDL-raising effects of alcohol are nonlinear, showing a threshold effect on HDL cholesterol,[112] and depend on different factors such as gender, body mass index (BMI), smoking habits, and genotype (e.g., ADH or apolipoprotein E genotype)[113] and also affect all HDL subfractions. One study[113] reported that only in women with the apolipoprotein E genotype ε4/3 does alcohol consumption intensify the increase in low-density lipoprotein (LDL) cholesterol and the decrease in HDL cholesterol associated with increasing BMI. In this context, it should be recalled that obesity (besides physical inactivity and smoking and genetics) represents one of the major causes of low HDL cholesterol.

The effects of alcohol on LDL cholesterol are only minor and less consistent[110] than the effects on the other lipoprotein fractions. In animal studies, alcohol led to a decrease in LDL clearance due to a decreased hepatic LDL receptor expression and specific effects on signaling pathways in lipid metabolism.[93] Alcohol may unfavorably affect the size of the lipoprotein particles, especially also increase the proatherogenic small dense LDL particles.[110,114] The role of certain polyphenolic compounds of wine as modulators of LDL oxidation rates in vivo is uncertain,[115] especially given the strong prooxidative effects of alcohol and the extremely variable bioavailability and bioefficacy of these compounds.[116,117] The effect of alcohol on the atherogenic lipoprotein (a) is controversial[118]: moderate consumption led to a lowering, heavy consumption had no effect; the effect according to the beverage type is also not clear. A minor fraction of ethanol is metabolized by the formation of FAEEs,[119] and they may be of pathophysiologic relevance in the development of alcohol-related pathologies.[120] Synthetically produced omega-3-fatty acid ethyl esters might be therapeutically useful for triglyceride lowering and control of cardiovascular risk.[121,122]

VII. ALCOHOL AND CARBOHYDRATE METABOLISM

The effects of alcohol on glucose handling are multiple and a function of the dosage, duration of alcohol intake, and overall nutritional status.[123,124] In healthy, moderate drinkers with normal food intake, alcohol's effects on carbohydrate metabolism are hardly of any clinical relevance. By contrast, excessive alcohol consumption may be associated with the typical clinical entity of alcoholic pancreatitis,[125] which results in exocrine pancreatic insufficiency with maldigestion and malabsorption. The reduced forms of nicotinamide adenine dinucleotide (NADH) and acetate produced during alcohol metabolism represent major modulators of glucose metabolism.

The increased production of reducing equivalents caused by the oxidation of alcohol leads to a decrease in gluconeogenesis.[126] This decrease may bring about clinically dangerous and life-threatening hypoglycemia, especially in the heavy drinker with an overall inadequate diet and poor intake of carbohydrates (and thus low glycogen stores).[127] This effect is being reinforced in people with diabetes by the ingestion of oral hypoglycaemic agents, insulin, or both[128] and after longer fasting periods. The alcohol-induced reduction in gluconeogenesis also occurs in the fed state but is usually compensated for by the glucose in the ingested food. The clinical features of hypoglycemia may share some of the signs of alcohol intoxication and could thus be misdiagnosed as simple alcohol intoxication with deleterious health consequences. In addition, alcohol produces changes in the secretory response of different counterregulatory hormones (such as epinephrine or growth hormone), thus resulting in an absence of the potential clinical warning signs of hypoglycemia.[128] Alcohol also inhibits the storage of glycogen, further increasing the predisposition to hypoglycemia when carbohydrate intake is insufficient. Light-to-moderate amounts of alcohol are inversely related to fasting and postload insulin levels.[129]

VIII. EFFECT OF ALCOHOL ON FAT-SOLUBLE VITAMINS

A. Vitamin A

Alcohol may interfere with the metabolism of all fat-soluble vitamins. Retinol (vitamin A), also an alcohol, shares some metabolic pathways with ethanol and thus leading to a high potential of interaction.[130] In light to moderate drinkers, vitamin A metabolism is not altered. Despite low intakes, frank vitamin A deficiency is rarely seen in alcoholics, probably because of the rather large hepatic stores of this vitamin. However, chronic alcohol consumption may lead to low levels of vitamin A in plasma, and when ALD is present, decreased hepatic vitamin A levels are found. These lower liver levels are a result of an initial rapid mobilization of the hepatic stores (leading to increased levels in extrahepatic tissues), followed by an increased degradation of the vitamin as a consequence of the induction of microsomal enzymes[131,132] and the alcohol-induced decreased synthesis of retinol-binding protein.[133] This condition may lead to the prescription of vitamin A supplements; however, higher levels of vitamin A intake (independent of alcohol intake) are associated with considerable hepatotoxicity,[131] and alcohol represents one of the most important modulators of vitamin A toxicity, especially in the presence of liver disease. In the setting of chronic alcohol consumption, an increased production of polar retinol metabolites seems to be a central mechanism of hepatocellular damage.[134] A tissue-specific increase in endogenous all-trans retinoic acid may contribute to chronic ethanol toxicity.[135,136] Further, alcohol affects the expression and activation of retinoic acid receptors, thus impairing different signaling pathways.[137] Alcohol stimulates retinyl ester hydrolysis associated with an initial increased retinyl ester synthesis, but with an altered composition of the hepatic retinyl esters.[138]

Although the vitamin A precursor beta-carotene is thought to bear no toxicity in humans, one epidemiological study reported an increased lung cancer rate in beta-carotene–supplemented smokers, especially in those who were also drinking alcohol, an increase most likely due to alcohol-induced alterations in the beta-carotene metabolism.[139] The negative effects of alcohol observed in this study were seen at rather low consumption levels, starting at $\geq$12.9 g/d. Although heavy drinkers ($\geq$200 g/d) show lower beta-carotene plasma concentrations than do control subjects, they show higher beta-carotene serum levels than those drinking less.[140] These higher levels may be caused by an impaired utilization or excretion of beta-carotene due to liver damage or a partial shift in the degradation of beta-carotene from central cleavage to eccentric cleavage.[131,141] Chronic alcohol intake upregulates the hepatic expression of the carotenoid cleavage enzymes (15,15′-monooxygenase 1 (CMO1)) and to a lesser extend also CMO2.[141] Despite some contradictory results,[142] it is not advisable to routinely prescribe either high-dose beta-carotene, other carotenoids (e.g., lycopene),[143,144] or vitamin A supplements to (heavy) alcohol consumers. Retinoic acid, a metabolite of dietary vitamin A, functions as a ligand for different nuclear receptor transcription factors. Alcohol might interfere with these signaling pathways, and it was suggested that acetaldehyde-induced altered retinoic acid signaling pathways may be involved in the fetal alcohol syndrome disorders[145] and other pathologies.

B. Vitamin E

Vitamin E intake and plasma and hepatic levels of vitamin E are reduced in chronic alcohol consumers independent of cirrhosis as a result of reduced intake and higher requirements.[146,147] The effects of alcohol on lowering antioxidant status are already seen at moderate consumption levels.[148,149] Vitamin E supplementation may reduce alcohol-induced lipid peroxidation; however, it is not clear how vitamin E supplementation will affect laboratory or clinical outcomes,[150–152] and presently, vitamin E therapy has not yet found its way into the guidelines for ALD[35,153] (contrary to NASH).[37] Recently, RRR-alpha-tocopherol[154] was reported to decrease hepatic de novo lipogenesis. Tocotrienol,[155] an isoform of vitamin E, has been reported to have protective effects in a rat model on the development of alcoholic neuropathy,[156] neuroinflammation,[157] or also alcohol-induced small intestinal damage.

C. Vitamin K

Data about the effect of alcohol on vitamin K nutriture is scarce. Acute and chronic alcohol consumption has been reported to lead to alterations in gamma-carboxylated molecules such as osteocalcin[158] or prothrombin.[159] In the setting of ALD, vitamin K might have favorable effects on bone health.[160] Alcohol consumption is a risk factor for bleeding in patients under treatment with vitamin K antagonists.[161]

D. Vitamin D

Heavier drinkers have a lower vitamin D intake, malabsorption, lower rate of sun exposure, lower hepatic and renal activation of vitamin D,[162] and an increased degradation leading to lower serum/plasma vitamin D (metabolites) levels.[163,164] Moderate alcohol intake does most likely not affect vitamin D nutriture.[165] Heavier alcohol consumption (with and without liver disease) may be associated with an increased fracture risk due to indirect and direct alcohol effects on bone metabolism and on vitamin D metabolism.[166–168] In addition, because of alcohol's effects on the target organs, tissue-specific vitamin D effects may be impaired. An inverse association between vitamin D status and alcoholic steatohepatitis[169] or vascular calcifications[170] has been reported. There may be a relationship between vitamin D deficiency and alcoholic myopathy.[170–172].

IX. EFFECTS OF ALCOHOL ON WATER-SOLUBLE VITAMINS

All water-soluble vitamins may be affected by the ingestion of alcohol, and the effects on water-soluble vitamin metabolism are dose dependent. In the range of light-to-moderate alcohol intake in healthy subjects eating a balanced diet, no adverse effects are expected. In heavy drinkers, a deficiency of several vitamins is usually present,[173] so the typical clinical signs of vitamin deficiency are not necessarily seen.

A. Thiamin

Heavy alcohol intake represents a major cause and predictor of thiamin deficiency in the US population.[174] Up to 80% of heavy drinkers have impaired thiamin nutriture independent of the presence of liver disease. Insufficient dietary intake, malabsorption,[175] increased metabolic demands, insufficient activation, reduced hepatic stores, and an increased urinary excretion are the major causes of thiamin deficiency in alcoholics.[176] Low doses of thiamin are absorbed by a carrier-mediated active process or at high concentrations by passive diffusion.[177,178] Among chronic alcohol consumers, vitamin B_1 intake is generally low so that the vitamin is principally absorbed by the active rate-limited, carrier-mediated process. The cellular transport (e.g., uptake into the brain or any other organ)[179] of thiamin is mediated by two specific thiamin transporters (THTR1 and THTR2), which are also negatively affected by chronic alcohol consumption.[180,181] Even in nonalcoholic subjects, active thiamin absorption is inhibited by an acute single dose of alcohol and abstinence leads to improved absorption.[182] Alcohol also induces a reduction in the activation of thiamin by phosphorylation and an increase in the dephosphorylation of phosphorylated thiamin; these effects are potentiated in the presence of liver disease. Thiamin losses in urine may increase by alcohol intake due to a decreased and impaired transport across the renal epithelia.[180] The thiamin storage capacity is reduced due to liver abnormalities and decreased muscle mass.[183] Alcohol induces specific alterations of thiamin metabolism in the central nervous system,[184,185] thereby producing the typical clinical symptoms of Wernicke-Korsakoff syndrome. Wernicke-Korsakoff syndrome is probably the only medical emergency situation involving vitamin deficiencies: the neurological condition has to be treated immediately with parenteral thiamin.[186] The syndrome shows typical clinical features including encephalopathy (altered consciousness, psychosis), oculomotor dysfunction (eye muscle paralysis), and gait ataxia.[186–189] The combination of pregnancy and thiamin deficiency potentiates synergistically the negative effects of alcohol on the fetal brain development.[190] Bariatric patients drinking alcohol are at increased risk for thiamin deficiency.[191–193] Other at-risk population is psychiatric patients[194] or patients with a (septic) shock.[195]

Although no prospective evidence supports the routine preventive administration of several vitamins to alcoholic patients, there is enough rationale for a benefit of vitamin B supplementation in these patients.[196] Research has shown that the neurotoxic effects of alcohol may be potentiated even in subclinical thiamin deficiency,[197] and a strong synergism[198,199] for the negative effects on the brain is known. Accordingly, if alcohol abuse cannot be controlled, the preventive supplementation of thiamin and other B vitamins is indicated.[11,196] An adequate supply of magnesium is crucial[200–203] to assure optimal utilization of thiamin. In the alcoholic patient (even when alcohol intake is reduced), thiamin deficiency may represent an important cause for heart failure, especially in combination with diuretics with increased urinary thiamin losses.[204,205]

B. Riboflavin

Riboflavin deficiency is found in up to 50% of chronic alcohol consumers and is due to low intakes, decreased absorption resulting from an alcohol-induced impairment of intraluminal hydrolysis of flavin adenine dinucleotide (FAD) in food sources,[206] inhibition of the specific carrier-mediated riboflavin absorption,[207] and a hyperriboflavinuria. In addition, alcohol inhibits the transformation of the vitamin into its coenzyme forms; impaired activation; and uptake of the vitamin in the intestine and also in peripheral tissues (e.g., renal tissue).[207,208] Riboflavin is an essential cofactor in the conversion of vitamin B6 and folate, and thus it represents an important modulator of the overall nutritional status of the B vitamins. Usually, riboflavin deficiency does not occur in isolation but in combination with a deficiency of other B-complex vitamins resulting in an atypical clinical entity.

C. Niacin

Light-to-moderate alcohol consumption hardly interferes with niacin nutriture. A deficiency in niacin (vitamin B_3) is mainly found in the setting of chronic excessive alcohol consumption and AUD,[209] usually together with deficiencies of other B-complex vitamins[210,211] and other nutrients such as zinc. Niacin deficiency might be encountered in AUD in combination with poverty, however often remaining undiagnosed due to the atypical clinical presentation.[209] The prevalence of low plasma niacin levels in chronic alcohol consumers varies widely, probably due to fact that niacin can be obtained preformed from food and from synthesis in the liver from tryptophan. In chronic liver disease as well as in the presence of specific nutrient deficiencies (e.g., vitamin B1, B2, B6 or protein malnutrition), the synthetic pathway is impaired.[212] In excessive alcohol consumers, a low intake, decreased synthesis from tryptophan, lack of essential cofactors, an increased urinary excretion, and an increased requirement might be of pathophysiological importance for the development of deficiency. The coenzyme forms of this vitamin (NAD and NADH) play an important role in alcohol metabolism,[213] and the increased production of NADH changes the NAD/NADH+ ratio in the liver, which might be a key factor in the pathogenesis of fatty liver disease.[214] In clinical practice, niacin deficiency symptoms (diarrhea, dermatitis, and dementia) might be confused with the Wernicke-Korsakoff syndrome[215] and eventually other severe neuropsychiatric conditions[216,217] alone or in combination with thiamin deficiency. Niacin supplementation might lead to an increase in liver transaminase levels, which could be misinterpreted as an alcohol-induced increase. Further pharmacological doses of niacin in the form of a supplement may exacerbate gastric ulcer disease and gout, both conditions that are often found in chronic alcohol consumers.

D. Vitamin B6

Low-to-moderate alcohol intake has been associated with an improved vitamin B6 status, especially in beer consumers,[218] due to the vitamin B6 content in beer. In chronic high(er) alcohol consumption and depending on liver function, between 50% and 90% of alcoholics show low pyridoxal-5′-phosphate (PLP) serum levels as well as a reduced ratio of serum alpha-aminobutyrate:cystathionine.[219] The PLP content in liver tissue is reduced in heavy alcohol consumers independent of the presence of liver disease. As for most nutrients, the pathogenesis of the impaired vitamin B6 nutriture is multifactorial. The formation of the active vitamin (PLP) in the liver is reduced or even completely blocked by the ingestion of alcohol.[220,221] Acetaldehyde increases the degradation of the vitamin by displacing the vitamin from binding sites and this, in turn, leads to an increased catabolism of the free vitamin and consecutively an increased urinary loss.[206] Since the vitamin has to be activated in the liver, supplementation of this vitamin does not necessarily lead to an improved vitamin B6 nutriture in alcoholics if they continue alcohol consumption. Vitamin B6 might play a role in alcohol-related peripheral neuropathy.[222]

E. Folic Acid

Folate deficiency is one of the most prevalent deficiencies in alcohol consumers. Before the grain fortification period, up to 80% of heavy alcohol consumers showed low concentrations of serum folate and/or low red blood cell folate.[223] The prevalence declined after introduction of folate food fortification strategies to 10%–25%.[224] Beer consumers may show higher plasma folate levels than other beverage consumers because of the folic acid content of this beverage. Alcohol-induced folate deficiency is caused by low folate intakes, malabsorption, altered hepatobiliary metabolism (including abnormal enterohepatic circulation), decreased liver uptake and storage, increased degradation, and an increased urinary excretion[223,225,226] and increased requirements. The clinical hallmark of folate deficiency is a megaloblastic anemia caused by damaged cell replication. It is found in all tissues, but especially in those with a high turnover rate, including the gastrointestinal mucosa[227] resulting in functional abnormalities and clinical symptoms such as diarrhea and due to an interference with the folate transporters malabsorption of folate itself as well as of other nutrients (e.g., water-soluble vitamins). Further the hepatic metabolic transformation to different active folate metabolites is impaired as a consequence of altered liver function and toxic alcohol and acetaldehyde effects on different enzymes.

The inhibition of the specific carrier-mediated folate uptake in different tissues (e.g., intestinal absorption, kidney, brain) or organelles[228,229] is in part due to effects at the transcriptional level.[229] Folate is absolutely essential for a normal brain and spinal cord development, and the folate metabolic pool of the fetus of alcohol consuming mothers is reduced in part also due am impaired folate transport across the placenta; the combination of pregnancy and alcohol intake should be completely avoided.[230] Because of an alcohol-induced rise in free radical production, the degradation of the vitamin is increased and may cause a tissue-specific deficiency. Alcohol consumption is an established risk factor for colorectal cancer (CRC), and the effects are due to direct alcohol effects and also folate metabolism related pathways leading to DNA hypomethylation and aberrant DNA synthesis.[231,232] The alcohol-associated risk of colorectal carcinogenesis (as well as other cancer sites) varies as a function of folate site-specific effects and in part according to the genetic polymorphisms of the 5,10-methylenetetrahydrofolate reductase (MTHFR) related to DNA methylation.[233] Due to multiple dose-dependent effects of alcohol on different vitamins involved in the homocysteine metabolism, elevated homocysteine levels are found in chronic alcohol consumers.[234,235]

X. EFFECTS OF ALCOHOL ON MINERAL AND TRACE ELEMENT METABOLISM

A. Magnesium

Low serum and tissue levels of magnesium are a typical feature in heavy drinkers, and these alterations are more prevalent in the presence of liver disease.[236] Magnesium deficiency in chronic alcoholism is due to reduced intake, malabsorption, decreased exchangeable magnesium (decreased magnesium content in the muscle), increased urinary losses, secondary hyperaldosteronism, hypocalcemia and increased fecal losses due to diarrhea.[237,238] Chronic alcohol consumption is associated with other electrolyte and mineral disturbances further aggravating magnesium deficiency.[239] A reduction of alcohol intake is associated with an improvement of magnesium nutriture. The decreased magnesium content of tissues may play a role in the development and progression of alcohol-associated pathologies[240,241] including liver damage.[242,243] Magnesium content is especially decreased in heart tissue predisposing to cardiac arrhythmias (prolongation of the QT interval). Because of magnesium's effects in the maintenance of membranes, a deficiency may exacerbate the development of organ damage, including liver damage. Magnesium plays a central role in over 300 biochemical reactions, one of them being thiamin phosphorlylation. Although magnesium can function as an inhibitor or neurotransmitter release, it is unclear whether magnesium is useful in the treatment of an alcohol withdrawal syndrome[244] but may result in a lower 1 year mortality in alcohol withdrawal.[245]

B. Zinc

Heavy alcohol consumption is associated with deceased serum zinc and lower hepatic zinc concentrations.[246] The deficient zinc status results from low intakes, a reduced absorption, an increased urinary excretion, altered hepatic zinc metabolism, and an alteration of zinc distribution. The zinc malabsorption is caused by direct and indirect alcohol effects, such as mucosal damage[247] and altered synthesis of zinc ligands (such as metallothionein), owing to alcohol-induced impaired protein synthesis. The presence and the degree of exocrine pancreatic insufficiency is an additional modulator of zinc status. The lower zinc levels are correlated with the degree of alcoholic liver damage, but low zinc levels in serum are also found in less-advanced liver disease, such as fatty liver disease.[246,248] In ALD, hepatic zinc levels are up to 50% lower,[249] and liver disease represents one of the major predictors for metabolic perturbations in zinc nutriture.[248] Chronic alcohol consumption alters the expression of hepatic zinc transporters most likely due to oxidative stress.[250] The increased urinary excretion of zinc correlates with the degree of liver damage[251] and is caused by decreased peripheral tissue zinc uptake and decreased serum levels of albumin. Further, low plasma zinc levels were a prognostic marker for liver transplantation free survival[252]; however, such associations should be not overestimated. Upon abstention, the increased urinary zinc excretion returned to normal.[253] However, in patients with liver cirrhosis, the increased urinary zinc excretion persists even after cessation of alcohol intake. In chronic alcoholism also the handling of zinc at the level of the endoplasmatic reticulum and mitochondria is disturbed.[254] The acute ingestion of alcohol among moderate drinkers causes increased urinary zinc excretion, a consequence that suggests direct effects of alcohol on zinc homeostasis at the level of the kidney.[251] A disruption of the epithelial barrier in the distal small intestine plays an important role in alcohol-induced gut leakiness and consecutively also alcoholic endotoxemia and hepatitis. Zinc deficiency may interfere with the intestinal barrier function by a direct action on tight junction proteins or by sensitizing to the effects of alcohol[247,255] and alcoholic steatosis.[256] In the experimental setting, zinc supplementation reduced the gut leakiness and endotoxinemia.[257,258] Zinc deficiency has further been implicated in the alcohol-induced alveolar epithelial and macrophage dysfunction,[259,260] and zinc supplementation might correct the dysfunction.[261]

Malnutrition (for instance, due to exocrine pancreatic insufficiency) in combination with alcohol leads to a higher degree of zinc depletion. It has been suggested that alcohol-induced alterations in zinc metabolism may increase alcohol-associated carcinogenesis.[262,263] In view of the multiple effects of zinc, clinical signs of zinc deficiency abnormalities of taste and smell, hypogonadism, infertility, and an impaired dark adaptation - are often seen in alcoholics. An impaired dark adaptation is a characteristic symptom in alcohol consumers, which is generally not caused by vitamin A deficiency but by zinc deficiency.[264,265] Defective zinc nutriture may increase alcohol toxicity given that the rate-limiting enzyme ADH is a zinc metalloenzyme.

XI. ALCOHOL, MORTALITY, AND CARDIOVASCULAR DISEASE

During the last few years, the knowledge around the alcohol-related morbidity and mortality pattern increased further; however, one has to be aware that there will never be an ideal study, which is accepted by all players in this field.[266,267] A protective effect of alcohol on coronary disease risk has been reported in earlier studies in men and women.[268–277] In these studies, the effect of alcohol on morbidity and mortality was biphasic, showing a J-shaped relationship: moderate consumption was found to be associated with a protection, but abstinence and higher consumption levels with an increased risk of cardiovascular and noncardiovascular mortality due to different cancers, ALD, and cardiovascular diseases such as arrhythmias, alcoholic cardiomyopathy, hypertension, and stroke.[268,270,272,274,276,278–281] The intake levels related to the nadir of risk vary widely in different studies[282] and are debated, but might be lower than presently recommended.[283–285] It is important to recognize that several studies found the protective effects mainly in older people and/or those who do have one or more of the classical cardiovascular risk factors,[269,271,273,286,287] suggesting that alcohol might modulate those risks. The reduced mortality risk at lower intakes has been explained by a reduced risk of coronary artery disease[268–270,278,279,288] and reduced a reduced risk of ischemic stroke.[289] However, several[283–285] recent studies cast some doubt on these potential protective health effects of moderate amounts of alcohol on mortality risk and cardiovascular health. In the China Kadoorie Biobank study[283] (a prospective observational study over 10 years, n = 512,715), using *conventional epidemiology* self-reported alcohol intake (mainly in form of spirits) showed a J-shaped association between the incidence of ischemic stroke, intracerebral hemorrhage, and myocardial infarction: men with an intake of around 100 g/week showed a protection for all three conditions as compared to nondrinkers or heavier drinkers. However, using the same data set but applying *genetic epidemiology*, no significant association was found regarding myocardial infarction,[283] and the protective association with stroke disappeared. In the Global Burden of Disease Study (GBD study),[290] alcohol-associated health outcomes were assessed in 195 countries. In this study, all-cause mortality (especially also cancer mortality) was higher than in earlier studies and rises with increasing alcohol consumption, and the study was not able to identify a safe consumption level.[290] The minimal health risk was at zero intake. The study found a minor protective effect for ischemic heart disease and diabetes, an association that disappeared by considering overall risk. For all other diseases, the risk increased in a nearly linear manner with increasing alcohol intake even in the low consumption range.[290] It is difficult to interpret the GBD study regarding any vascular benefit, since the study was based on data from developed and developing nations (with quite different lifestyles, nutritional habits, environmental factors, socioeconomic factors, and morbidity and mortality patterns, which all are modulated by alcohol intake). This constellation makes the interpretation and generalization of the data regarding vascular protection challenging. In another study[285] pooling UK data including 599, g/week of pure alcohol. This curvilinear relationship was due to different effects of alcohol on cardiovascular disease entities: for cardiovascular diseases other than myocardial infarction, no clear lower threshold was identified and the risk for coronary artery disease excluding myocardial infarction, heart failure, fatal hypertensive disease, and fatal aortic aneurysm increased more or less linearly; however, alcohol consumption was log-linearly associated with a lower risk of myocardial infarction (HR 0·94, 0·91–0·97).[285] The potential protective amounts for myocardial infarction were found to be lower than in earlier studies and currently recommended. These data suggest that some consumers might eventually get a protection regarding the risk of myocardial infarction as long as they are able to consume only small amounts (0–>100 g/week). The low or lower level of consumption might also be favorable regarding the risk of atrial fibrillation (AF)[291] and other conditions. Different mechanisms[77,275,279,288,292–301] for the potential cardioprotective effects of alcohol have been suggested (Table 25.2). Based on these new data, those who want to drink alcohol should not target at moderate, but only at "low" consumption levels, which might be associated with "coronary vascular protection." This is in agreement with the older data that occasional and low-volume "drinkers" might have a chance for a reduced CV risk. The problem with any recommendation around alcohol is that many consumers cannot balance their consumption behavior between risk and benefit due to environmental, societal, many personal factors, and also their genotype.[283] Form the public health and societal view, the burden of disease by alcohol outweighs any potential health benefit. The hallmark of excessive alcohol intake are metabolic and structural alterations at the level of the liver, and liver cirrhosis is the leading cause of death in heavy drinkers, and in the United States, mortality due to liver cirrhosis and cancer is increasing since 1999,[290,302] especially in younger adults. In addition, approximately one-third of all traffic crash fatalities in the United States are alcohol related.[10]

Whether alcohol and exercise result in a higher protection on CV morality is controversial, and it was reported that the daily deviation from the usual physical

TABLE 25.2 Summary (order of factors is not related to any theoretical relevance) and classification of possible cardioprotective mechanisms of alcohol.

Category	Potential mechanisms
Lipid effects	• HDL cholesterol ↑ • LDL particle number ↓; LDL particle size ↑, concentration of LDL cholesterol ↓ • LDL oxidation ↓ • Lipoprotein (a) ↓ • LDL receptor effects • Modified fatty acids
Blood coagulation	• Hypercoagulability ↓ • Platelet reactivity ↓ • Fibrinolysis ↑
Endocrine effects	• Improved insulin sensitivity (insulin mediated glucose uptake ↑) • Estrogen metabolism • Steroid metabolism • Adiponectin ↓
Nonnutritive compounds	• Bioactive components in, e.g., wine (flavonoids, nonflavonoids; phytoalexins [e.g., resveratrol])
Miscellaneous effects	• Endothelial function andvasoreactivity (NO release ↑, coronary flow ↑) • Ischemic preconditioning • Membrane fluidity • Liver structure (liver sieve) • Paraoxonase↑ • Associated health-promoting behaviors • Antiinflammatory effects (CRP ↓, leukocyte adhesion ↓) • Antioxidation
Psychological effects	• Control of type A behavior • Antianxiety effects • Stress control • Personality type

HDL, High-density lipoprotein; *LDL*, Low-density lipoprotein.

activity pattern was associated with daily total alcohol use.[88,303,304] In the Cooper Center Longitudinal Study (observation period of 17 years), alcohol did not modify the association between fitness and all-cause mortality and cardiovascular mortality,[305] suggesting that if heart protection is wished, the priority should be put in exercise and not on alcohol,[286] contradicting some older data.[304,306]

Despite the potentially favorable effects of alcohol on coronary artery disease risk, alcohol represents an important cause of hypertension,[307,308] hemorrhagic stroke,[309,310] alcoholic cardiomyopathy, heart insufficiency, and arrhythmias.[280,311]

In view of the present research evidence, alcohol has to be regarded as a risk factor to overall and also cardiovascular health,[277] but for *certain* consumers, a light intake might elicit a cardiovascular protection. However, there is presently no mean to identify those who might benefit without risk. Accordingly, a nondrinker should not be encouraged to consume alcohol for any health reason. There is no doubt that high-dose consumption is deleterious for cardiovascular and overall heart health. The theoretically protective dose is most likely lower than presently recommended.

A. Alcohol and Type II Diabetes Mellitus

Most, but not all,[312,313] observational studies[129,314–323] reported a lower risk for type 2 diabetes mellitus (T2DM) in light-to-moderate alcohol consumers. This protection was apparent till an intake level of approximately 60 g/d[324] might depend on gender,[312,325] ethnicity,[323] the beverage type,[318] and body weight status (BMI). [321,323–325] The gender differences might be due to sex-specific drinking patterns or could also be confounded by different reporting characteristics. The lowest risk was seen in light-to-moderate consumers, whereas heavier alcohol consumption and binge drinking led to a higher risk for type II diabetes.[129,314–316] Data using 18 year alcohol consumption trajectories from the China Health and Nutrition Survey were not able to find a risk reduction for T2DM,[312] but they showed that heavy alcohol consumption in early adulthood was significantly associated with an increased risk of T2DM, which remained high even with a reduction of alcohol consumption later in life. The latter constellation was also found in US studies[326] and deserves special attention in view of the increasing alcohol consumption among young adults. Assessing the causality between alcohol intake and diabetes risk using a Mendelian randomization approach, a higher and even moderate consumption level was causally related to diabetes risk and worsened traits.[313] In the contrary, a 2 year randomized trial[319] (control with water) suggests that initiating moderate wine intake in well-controlled diabetic patients might have favorable effects on different components of the metabolic syndrome. However, only in patients with the ADH allele ADH1B*1 (slow alcohol metabolizers), wine elicits a beneficial effect on glycemic control (although not affecting the number of antidiabetic medications, which rises questions regarding a true benefit).[319] Moderate alcohol intake may lead to a decrease in fasting insulin and HbA1c concentrations among nondiabetic individuals.[327] Further, insulin sensitivity might improve inconsistently among women. It is conceivable that the alcohol-induced higher estradiol levels might modulate the diabetes risk in women[328] and explain in part the gender differences. In patients with sulfonylurea or insulin treatment, alcohol might increase the risk for hypoglycemia.[329] In a recent study from Finland, treated diabetic patients (especially those on insulin) had an increased risk for alcohol-related deaths,[330] and there is always a risk for an alcohol-induced exacerbation of diabetic complications.[331] Alcohol and components of the metabolic syndrome exert synergistic effects in the pathogenesis and promotion of liver injury and cirrhosis.[332]

B. Alcohol and Hypertension

The first description of a nearly linear relationship between alcohol and blood pressure in heavy alcohol consumers was published by Lian in 1915. Cross-sectional, prospective, and interventional studies have reported an increase in systolic and diastolic blood pressure with increasing alcohol intake[333–337]; however, some studies reported no effect or even a protective blood pressure–lowering effect in low-level consumers (defined as <20 g/d)[338]; however, this potentially protective effect might be limited to women only.[337] Cessation of alcohol intake in heavy consumers led to a reduction in blood pressure,[339] and there seems to be a dose-dependent association between the baseline alcohol consumption and consecutive blood pressure reduction upon a reduced consumption.[336] The decline in blood pressure upon cessation of heavier alcohol consumption[340] shows a wide variability due to many individual endogenous and exogenous factors,[341] consumption patterns,[342] and gender. A 10 year follow-up study with several time points of alcohol intake assessments showed a linear association between baseline and long-term alcohol consumption and incident hypertension as related to baseline intake.[343] Further, a Mendelian randomization study from Southeast China showed a causal effect of alcohol on blood pressure in current and previous consumers as compared to never drinkers[75]; similar results were reported in another Chinese Mendelian randomization study[283] showing a strong positive association over the whole consumption spectrum. Blood pressure effects are more pronounced in daily alcohol consumers and binge drinkers. A concomitant blood pressures lowering pharmacological therapy might modulate the pressure effects of alcohol.[344] The effect of the timing of blood pressure measurements after alcohol intake on the magnitude and direction of the blood pressure change[345] could affect study outcomes, and this may also be an additional reason for inconsistent effects of alcohol on blood pressure in epidemiological and some experimental studies. Further on, polymorphisms in the alcohol-metabolizing enzymes modify the pressor effects of alcohol and also the effects of an unhealthy dietary pattern.[346,347] The pathophysiologic mechanisms for the pressor effects of alcohol are not exactly known, and multiple mechanisms involving direct and indirect effects of alcohol on autonomic regulation, neurohumoral effects, altered baroreceptor function, endothelial dysfunction, nitric oxide availability, effects on peripheral resistance, calcium handling in the vascular smooth muscle cells, oxidative stress, and altered stress perception have been suggested. Alterations in liver function may affect the metabolism of antihypertensive drugs. Heavier alcohol consumption is one of the most important reasons for resistant and difficult to treat hypertension.

C. Alcohol and Stroke

Alcohol has been identified as an independent risk factor for hemorrhagic stroke.[283,310,339,348] The increased stroke risk is partly caused by the pressure effects of alcohol as well as effects on cerebrovascular vasculature.[283,309,310,339] Several older and newer studies reported that alcohol had a protective effects on ischemic stroke[283,349,350] due to shared pathophysiological features and 1–2 drinks/d could have a protective effect as compared to nondrinkers or heavy drinkers.[283] When analyzing the same data[283] using genetic epidemiology for two ADH variants, a continuous log-linear association was found between genotype-predicted mean alcohol intake and stroke risk, which was stronger for hemorrhagic stroke (relative risk [RR] per 280 g/week 1.58, CI 1.36–1.84, $P < .0001$) than for ischemic stroke (RR 1.27, CI 1.13–1.43, $P = .0001$).[283] This *genetic epidemiology* study shows that the apparent stroke protection by moderate amounts of alcohol is most likely noncausal[283] and that the usual blood pressure is linearly related to both entities of stroke.[351] According to this study, even small amounts of alcohol increase the stroke risk and there is no safe consumption threshold. Similarly, a Mendelian randomization analysis in 261,991 individuals with European descent concluded that a reduction of alcohol intake might be favorable regarding the cardiovascular risk profile, including hypertension, even in moderate or light consumers,[352] suggesting that the data from the large Chinese studies are most likely generalizable to all ethnicities. The cumulative alcohol consumption has been identified as an independent risk factor for total and also ischemic stroke.[353] Further, the risk of ischemic stroke onset is transiently elevated in the hour immediately after alcohol ingestion.[354] The role of alcohol as a poststroke functional prognostic modifier is unclear.[355] The role of alcohol in the promotion of AF, an important risk factor for ischemic stroke, is controversial[356,357]; however, based on epidemiologic data and also potential mechanisms, a lower intake might be advantageous.[291] It is important to remember that moderate alcohol consumption (especially wine consumption) is associated with a healthier lifestyle such as increased fruit and vegetable consumption,[358–360] and an increased fruit and vegetable intake is associated with a reduced risk of stroke,[361–364] besides others also due to a lower blood pressure.

Several studies reported that moderate alcohol consumption is associated with better cognitive functioning and a reduced risk of a cognitive decline with aging.[365–368] The data are controversial and vary besides others according to the time point where alcohol consumption was initiated and the baseline cognitive function.[366,369,370] Once again, it is not completely clear whether light alcohol drinking or the behavior of the drinker is the protective principle. Nevertheless, heavier alcohol intake is a risk factor for (premature) dementia.[11,371]

XII. ALCOHOL AND LIVER DISEASE

ALD includes a wide spectrum of injury, ranging from steatosis, alcoholic hepatitis, and cirrhosis till liver cancer. Worldwide each year about 2 millions individuals die due to ALD and 50% of the cirrhosis mortality is caused by alcohol,[372,373] further accounting for 30% of hepatocellular carcinoma (HCC) cases and HCC-specific mortality.[374] Alcohol is the major cause of liver disease, and liver cirrhosis death rate shows a direct relationship with the per capita alcohol consumption (independent of the beverage type and already at moderate intake levels [especially in women]).[375,376] Besides a genetic and epigenetic predisposition, different modifiable individual factors might modulate the alcohol-related risk of liver disease (e.g., an elevated BMI,[372] consuming alcohol without meals,[375] or also circadian misalignment[377]). For instance, women who drank alcohol with meals experienced a risk reduction by half.[375] Irrespective of the absolute amount of alcohol intake, consumption frequency is another risk determinant: in the UK Million Women Study,[375] daily drinkers had a considerably increased risk (1.61, 95% CI 1.40–1.85) as compared to nondaily drinkers.[375] There is an additive and/or even synergistic interaction between nonalcoholic fatty liver disease and alcohol-related liver disease.[378–380] The mechanisms of alcohol-induced liver injury are complex, multiple and incompletely understood, and include factors such as altered hepatic lipid metabolism and hepatic steatosis,[381] acetaldehyde-mediated toxicity, oxidative stress, altered redox potential (NADH/NAD+), alcohol-induced leaky gut and microbiome dysbiosis-related factors (gut-liver-adipose tissue axis), cross talk between adipose tissue and the liver, cytokine- and chemokine-induced hepatic inflammation and immune cell mediated mechanisms (e.g., mast cells), extracellular vesicle-related mechanisms, endocrine- and cytokine-related mechanisms, associated infections (e.g., hepatitis C), and last but not least an impaired liver regeneration capacity[382–385] to mention just a few pathogenetic factors, which are usually more pronounced in women (Fig. 25.6). One key mechanism (even in non-ALD) is the induction of Cyp2E1, which leads to the generation of reactive oxygen species[386,387] and thus enhanced biotransformation[372] and increased production of toxic metabolites.[388] Further, alcohol enhances the generation of inflammatory cytokines (e.g., TNF-α, IL-1 or IL-6) with local as well as systemic effects.[388,389]

As with other alcohol-related pathologies, susceptibility to developing alcoholic cirrhosis varies from one individual to another as a function of the amount and duration of alcohol intake, drinking pattern and the beverage type, gender, genetic predisposition, age, race/ethnicity, characteristics of alcohol metabolism, previous hepatitis B or C,[390] obesity, smoking, drug intake, and potential nutritional factors.[372,375,391,392] The quantity of alcohol consumed and consumption frequency are the most important risk factors for ALD.[375,393] Heavy episodic drinking (binge drinking) is an often forgotten risk factor for ALD. In view of the many factors modulating the risk, it is difficult to define a no-risk consumption level regarding the ALD risk.[394,395] Despite all the limitations of ecological studies,[396] it seems that populations with a daily consumption of >21 g/d of pure alcohol (1.5 standard drinks) showed a significantly higher cirrhosis morality rate as compared to countries with a lower consumption level.[397] For women, the threshold dose of alcohol is about half the threshold dosage of men, i.e., they are twice as sensitive to alcohol-induced hepatotoxicity.[375] Further, women develop more severe ALD and within a shorter duration of alcohol exposure. The nutritional deficiencies (ranging from protein energy malnutrition and multiple micronutrient deficiencies) described in this chapter are commonly found in alcoholic patients and should be corrected by a combination of normal food, evidence-based nutrient supplementation, and alcohol abstinence.[35] Mortality in ALD increases directly proportional to the degree of malnutrition.[398] It is possible that dietary strategies (e.g., pre- or probiotics) targeted at the microbiome might be of therapeutic relevance in ALD.[96] The maintenance of muscle mass is an important determinant of the disease course in liver disease.[399] The role of alcohol in non-ALD is still unclear, some studies found a decreased NASH disease severity in low and moderate consumers.[400] A recent Mendelian randomization study[401] suggests that the association

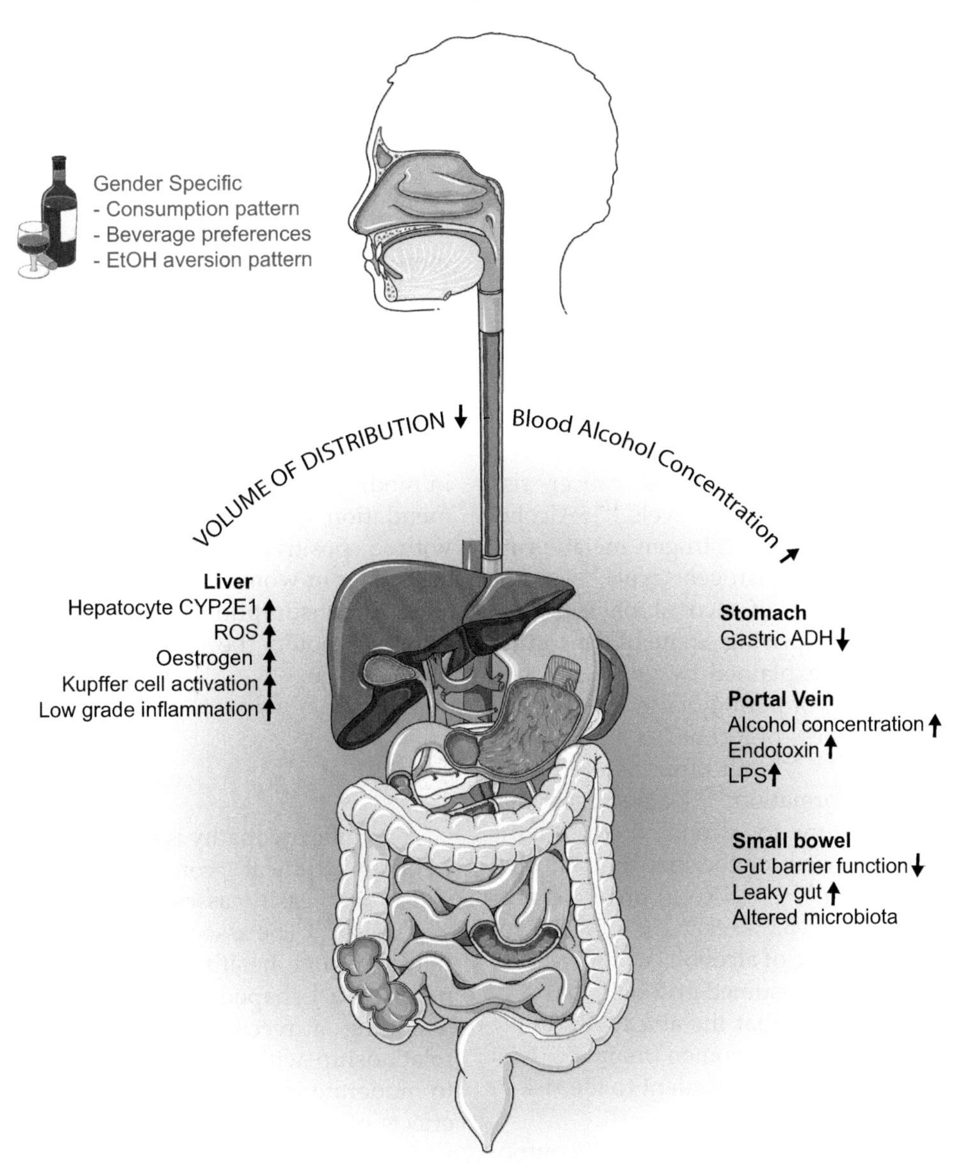

FIGURE 25.6 Mechanisms of the increased vulnerability of women for alcoholic liver disease. *Adapted from Szabo et al.*[403]

between a high BMI and alcohol intake with liver injury and with the risk of liver disease warrants a concomitant control of the BMI and of alcohol intake.

XIII. ALCOHOL AND CANCER

Alcohol consumption[402] is related to an increased prevalence of head and neck cancer (oropharyngeal[403,404]), esophageal, liver,[374] CRCs,[405] and female breast (pre- and postmenopausal).[406,407] The evidence for the latter carcinomas is convincingly strong. Less-consistent evidence suggests a role of alcohol in the pathogenesis of stomach[408,409] and pancreatic cancers.[410] Alcohol and it's first metabolite acetaldehyde are classified as carcinogens,[411,412] although some authors claim that pure alcohol per se is not a carcinogen.[413] Often, a dose–response relationship between alcohol intake and cancer risk can be found[414]; however, for some cancers (such as CRC), also a J-shaped relationship has been described.[405] The risk of kidney cancer[415] and non-Hodgkin lymphoma[416] might be reduced by alcohol. These potentially protective effects cannot be explained at present and other alcohol-related risks outweight most likely an observed protection. The pathophysiologic bases of the alcohol-induced cancers are multiple, might vary according to the location, are potentiated by smoking, and include effects of acetaldehyde (e.g., DNA damage)[413,417] and/or effects of alcohol on methyl group metabolism,[418] retinoic acid metabolism,[406] inflammatory phenomena, oxidative damage, hormone (e.g., estrogen)-related mechanisms, effects on gene expression, enhanced/increased activation of procarcinogens, membrane effects, interference in signaling pathways, and others. The increased alcohol intake, in combination with a low/deficient micronutrient nutriture increases cancer risk.

Alcohol consumption is associated with an increased risk of breast cancer (especially hormone-sensitive cancer types) and varies in a complex manner according to the estrogen and progesterone receptor status as well as breast cancer subtypes[419–422] and breast cancer recurrence particularly among postmenopausal and overweight/obese women.[423] Most studies showed a dose–response relationship with breast cancer risk already within light consumption levels.[424] Alcohol has a high potential to modulate estrogen metabolism, leading to higher circulating estrogen levels,[425] so the potential detrimental effects of alcohol on estrogen-sensitive cancers are not surprising. Some of the controversy of the data can be explained by genetic factors and/or menopausal status or period of life with alcohol consumption. The awareness of alcohol as a risk factor for breast cancer is low[426–428] and often ignored even due to intentional misinformation.[429] Data suggest that already early life exposure to alcohol increases the risk, a worrying fact in view of the increased alcohol intake of young women.[430,431] RR of breast cancer increased by 7.1% (95% CI 5.5%–8.7%; $P < .00001$) for each additional 10 g/d intake of alcohol, i.e., for each extra unit or drink of alcohol consumed on a daily basis.[432] A modeling study suggested that the absolute lifetime risk of alcohol-related cancers in women (mainly driven by breast cancer risk) would be equivalent to the risk of 10 cigarettes per week.[433]

Alcoholic beverages represent complex multicomponent mixtures containing potentially different chemicals with carcinogenic properties (e.g., acetaldehyde, aflatoxins, arsenic, cadmium, benzene, and others).[434] Based on the present evidence, it is the alcohol and its metabolite that causes the carcinogenicity and not these carcinogens. Accordingly, one cannot classify an alcoholic beverage as more/less carcinogenic than another.[434] However, globally about 25% of the consumed pure alcohol is unrecorded alcohol, which might bear a health threat due to these contaminants.[435]

The relation between alcohol and cancer is very complex, and many aspects are still a black box. The complexity is last but not least also caused by gene variants in the alcohol-metabolizing enzymes, which vary also by ethnicity modulating the risk by complex gene–environment interaction(s).[436,437] Thus, it is most likely impossible to make one consumption recommendation for all consumers. Individuals carrying the inactive aldehyde dehydrogenase 2*2 (ALDH 2*2) allele have an increased risk for alcohol-related esophageal cancer.[438] Carriers of other genetic variants (e.g., alcohol dehydrogenase 1C*1 [ADH1C*1] homozygotes or MTHFR 677CT variants) have also a higher risk for alcohol-related cancers.[22,418,439] Maybe, the further elucidation of these associations may result in more targeted and more successful preventive strategies. Further lifestyle factors (e.g., smoking, poor oral hygiene, physical activity pattern, certain dietary deficiencies [e.g., folate, vitamin B6, methyl donors]) or an excess of certain micronutrients (vitamin A/β-carotene) may potentiate the risk for alcohol-associated tumors.[406]

From the public health and clinical view "moderation in moderation" is at present most likely the best recommendation for all consumer (especially also for those with a positive personal history or family history, especially in women regarding breast cancer)[402,440] and a daily consumption, a binge drinking consumption pattern should be discouraged especially also at younger age.

XIV. ALCOHOL, BONE, AND MUSCLE

Alcoholic myopathy is one of the most prominent and frequent clinical comorbidity in heavy alcohol consumers easily assessable as muscle atrophy and weakness.[441] The association between alcohol consumption and bone health is inconsistent and some studies reported a J-shaped[442,443] relationship, whereas others including a recent metaanalysis showed a positive relationship with the risk of osteoporosis even at low to moderate intake.[444] The different direct and indirect effects of alcohol on bone and muscle metabolism are very complex[445] and multiple and depend on the amount, the duration of alcohol intake, the presence of liver disease,[50] gender, age, genetic factors and concomitant factors (such as smoking, dietary factors including protein intake or exercise pattern/resistance training), and many other factors. Light-to-moderate consumption may have favorable effects on bone health[445–449] in adults resulting in higher bone mineral density and reduced age-associated bone loss. Heavier alcohol intake has the opposite effects including an increased risk for fractures. It is crucial to be aware that the bone effects of alcohol in younger individuals might be different. Heavy episodic drinking (binge drinking) is associated with a poorer overall bone health in adolescent and young women,[450] an effect persisting for the whole life. Moderate wine intake has been reported to elicit a higher protection, although the data are gender specific and controversial[443,449,451] and might be caused by other behavioral factors.[452]

Acute and chronic effects of alcohol on bone have to be distinguished. Chronic alcohol intake affects all aspects of bone metabolism from bone growth, bone turnover, and remodeling till repair after fractures.[453,454] In heavy drinkers, the calcium balance is negatively affected by low intakes and malabsorption of calcium due to direct mucosal damage, an impaired vitamin D nutriture, increased urinary calcium losses,[455] and liver disease.[50] In heavy drinkers, different structural and functional changes occur in bone tissues. Low to moderate amounts of alcohol have no adverse effects[448] or even a protective effect[449,456] on bone mass in postmenopausal women, maybe because of alcohol's effects on endogenous (and exogenous) estrogens (see above) as well as the presence of other bone protective factors (e.g., silicon in beer). Different studies reported that light-to-moderate alcohol consumption was associated with a lower rate of (injurious) falls in older adults[457] and lower risk for hip fractures,[443] which might just be a reflection of a better overall health and also socioeconomic status in these consumers or also lower medication intakes.[458] In the clinical setting, any unexplained fracture, fall, or osteoporosis (especially in men) may point to alcohol-related problems.

Alcohol consumption leads to a dose-dependent negative effect on skeletal muscle, leading to progressive functional and structural alterations of skeletal muscle cells with a concomitant decline in lean body mass.[45,459,460] Alcohol reduces muscle protein mass by different mechanisms (e.g., decreasing protein synthesis due to oxidative stress and increased anabolic signaling, an increased protein breakdown (catabolism) due to oxidative stress and inflammation, reduced amino acid intake and other cosubstrates; reduced stretch stimulus of the protein synthesis).[441,461–463] The alcoholic myopathy is a typical clinical feature of the heavy alcohol consumer,[460] both fast and slow muscle fibers are affected, and seems to occur in female chronic alcohol abusers earlier than in men.[47] The pathogenesis involves alterations in different molecular signaling pathways (e.g., IGF-1).[47] Importantly, these effects are also seen at the level of the heart muscle in form of alcoholic cardiomyopathy.[464–466]

XV. FETAL ALCOHOL SPECTRUM DISORDER

Alcohol consumption during pregnancy increases the risk for impaired growth, stillbirth, and fetal alcohol spectrum disorder (FASD).[467,468] More than five decades ago, it was first reported that heavy alcohol intake during pregnancy may be associated with fetal alcohol syndrome, which is now summarized with the term FASD, which includes different clinical symptoms/entities characterized by growth deficiency, facial dysmorphology, central nervous system dysfunctions, and neurobehavioral features[3,468–470] alone or in combination. The consequences of alcohol exposure during pregnancy are the most important nonheritable cause of intellectually disability and are accordingly basically completely preventable.[471] The recent trends[472,473] of alcohol consumption during pregnancy are worrisome: in the United States, 11.5% of pregnant women reported current drinking and 3.9% reported binge drinking during the past 30 days,[474] representing an increase as compared to earlier surveys, although others reported a decline of alcohol use at least in certain age groups of pregnant women.[475] Certain subpopulation of women (e.g., unmarried women) might be at higher risk.[476,477] Alcohol is a teratogen, and the effects may occur well before a woman knows about her pregnancy with varying phenotypic expression of the FASD.[3,478] Children with FASD show a pre- and postnatal growth retardation, facial dysmorphy, and central nervous system dysfunctions that cause permanent cognitive impairment and learning disabilities.[476,479] FASD represents the severe end points of a vast spectrum of structural, behavioral, and neurodevelopmental abnormalities caused by exposure to alcohol in utero. Different pathogenetic models for the FASD have been suggested, and it seems that alcohol metabolism–induced altered retinoid signaling may represent a key mechanism.[480,481] Alcohol intake during pregnancy, and also preconceptionally increases the risk of early pregnancy loss and FASD.[482] In view of the irreversible lifelong effects of alcohol drinking during pregnancy on the unborn child, pregnancy (ideally also the preconception period) has to be a period of life during which alcohol intake should be completely avoided. There is no safe amount of alcohol during pregnancy[467] and preconception (most likely this applies even to men[483,484]).

XVI. ALCOHOL AND BARIATRIC PATIENTS

After a sleeve gastrectomy or Roux-en-Y gastric bypass, there is an increased risk for alcohol-related nutritional problems[485,486] as well as AUD. Many post-bariatric patients resume their usual (prebariatric) alcohol intake. However, long-term studies (13–15 years of follow-up) reported an increased risk for a higher consumption postoperatively and also a significantly higher risk for AUD.[193,487–489] The risk increases with time and with a greater weight loss. The metabolism of alcohol is altered postoperatively as a function of the surgical procedures (no changes after gastric banding) so that "one drink becomes two": there is a reduced first-pass metabolism in the stomach, a faster absorption rate, a higher peak blood alcohol concentration, and a slower elimination rate[490] leading to an aumentation of the alcohol effects. The risk of alcohol-related injuries, car accidents, and toxicity increases accordingly. Craving and alcohol reward signaling might also be changed after bariatric surgery. Despite the many benefits of bariatric surgery, different emerging risks, including AUD, call for a lifelong strict monitoring not only of nutritional disorders but also the risk of AUD. The CAGE test and AUDIT questionnaire (and other tools such as the Patient Health Questionnaire [491]) should be included in any pre- and postoperative assessment/monitoring.[492] The best strategy to avoid these difficult-to-control effects is complete abstinence from alcohol in bariatric patients, especially in the presence of other of risk factors for risky drinking and alcoholism.

XVII. CONCLUSION

The relationship between health, nutrition, and alcohol is very complex. As a function of the drinking pattern (amount/frequency of consumption) and many individual determinants (genetic factors, behavioral determinants, endogenous and environmental factors, including lifestyle and nutritional factors), the overall health and nutritional effects of alcohol may be in some consumers positive or negative (Fig. 25.3). Recent evidence shows that any potentially protective health effect is most likely outweighed by negative effects. In today's world, the art of any patient counseling and public health counseling about alcohol consumption is not to forbid alcohol consumption but to try to formulate strategies and recommendations to assure a lifelong safe consumption levels for those wishing to drink - probably at light consumption levels only. In any case, alcohol should not be recommended for health reasons or for health maintenance, especially as long as there are no specific and sensitive predictors for harmful alcohol use and abuse.

Evidence suggests that the safe amount may vary considerably from one individual to another, even for those whose alcohol intake is in the light-to-moderate range and the safe consumption level might be lower than the present recommendations, thus moderation in "moderate consumption" is most likely the best strategy to pursue.

RESEARCH GAPS

- Develop new tools to measure/assess alcohol intake reliably in epidemiological and clinical settings (e.g., alcohol skin biosensors).
- Settle the controversy around the alcohol-related burden of disease by using state-of-the-art genetic and molecular epidemiology and laboratory research.
- Study the neurophysiological basis of alcohol craving/dependence and develop behavioral and/or pharmacological means to avoid dependence and to reduce risk of AUD.
- Develop easy tools and strategies for evidence-based public health education around the role of alcohol in health and disease, which are comprehensible and implementable for all strata of the population.
- Fill research gaps about the role of alcohol in relation to specific conditions (e.g., specific metabolic pathways including nutrient metabolism, signaling effects, alcohol and dementia, metabolism in (young) women, specific ethnicities and/or specific genotypes, specific life circumstances (e.g., shift work), interactions with common medications including supplements, role of circadian desynchronization and sleep disturbances, and BMI and body weight status).
- Clarify interactions between environmental factors (e.g., pollutants, pesticides, nanoplastic, etc.) and alcohol in relation to health and disease risk. What is the role of the nutritional pattern and/or specific nutrients?
- Identify drivers of alcohol consumption in the modern world to create a society and lifestyle for everybody without the risk for increased alcohol craving and high disease burden due to alcohol. Develop burden of disease guided taxations and fees along the whole alcohol supply chain.

XVIII. REFERENCES

1. WHO (World-Health-Organization). *Global Status Report on Alcohol and Health 2018*. 2018.
2. Schoenborn CA, Adams PE. Health behaviors of adults: United States, 2005–2007. *Vital Health Stat*. 2010;245:1–132.
3. National Institute on Alcohol Abuse and Alcoholism (NIAAA). *Alcohol Across the Lifespan. Five Year Strategic Plan FY09-14*; 2009. http://pubsniaaanihgov/publications/strategicplan/niaaastrategicplanhtm (downloaded June 20th,2010).
4. Manthey J, Shield KD, Rylett M, Hasan OSM, Probst C, Rehm J. Global alcohol exposure between 1990 and 2017 and

forecasts until 2030: a modelling study. *Lancet*. 2019;393(10190): 2493–2502.
5. Dawson DA, Goldstein RB, Saha TD, Grant BF. Changes in alcohol consumption: United States, 2001–2002 to 2012–2013. *Drug Alcohol Depend*. 2015;148:56–61.
6. Grant BF, Chou SP, Saha TD, et al. Prevalence of 12-month alcohol use, high-risk drinking, and DSM-IV alcohol use disorder in the United States, 2001–2002 to 2012–2013: results from the national epidemiologic survey on alcohol and related conditions prevalence of alcohol use, high-risk drinking, and DSM-IV alcohol use disorder prevalence of alcohol use, high-risk drinking, and DSM-IV alcohol use disorder. *JAMA Psychiatry*. 2017;74:911–923.
7. Myran DT, Hsu AT, Smith G, Tanuseputro P. Rates of emergency department visits attributable to alcohol use in Ontario from 2003 to 2016: a retrospective population-level study. *Can Med Assoc J*. 2019;191:E804.
8. Trias-Llimós S, Kunst AE, Jasilionis D, Janssen F. The contribution of alcohol to the East-West life expectancy gap in Europe from 1990 onward. *Int J Epidemiol*. 2017;47:731–739.
9. Wang W-J, Xiao P, Xu H-Q, Niu J-Q, Gao Y-H. Growing burden of alcoholic liver disease in China: a review. *World J Gastroenterol*. 2019;25:1445–1456.
10. *Alcohol Facts and Statistics*. National Institute on Alcohol Abuse and Alcoholism (NIH); 2019. https://www.niaaa.nih.gov/alcohol-health/overview-alcohol-consumption/alcohol-facts-and-statistics.
11. Schwarzinger M, Pollock BG, Hasan OSM, et al. Contribution of alcohol use disorders to the burden of dementia in France 2008–13: a nationwide retrospective cohort study. *Lancet Public Health*. 2018;3:e124–e132.
12. *What is a Standard Drink?*; 2019. https://www.niaaa.nih.gov/alcohol-health/overview-alcohol-consumption/what-standard-drink.
13. Drinking patterns and their definitions. *Alcohol Res*. 2018;39: 17–18.
14. Creating Alcohol Labelling Chaos. at https://www.eurocare.org/cares.php?sp=labeling&ssp=creating-alcohol-labelling-chaos.).
15. Paton A. Alcohol in the body. *Br Med J*. 2005;330:85–87.
16. Sonderberg BL, Sicinska ET, Blodget E, et al. Preanalytical variables affecting the quantification of fatty acid ethyl esters in plasma and serum samples. *Clin Chem*. 1999;45:2183–2190.
17. De Vos A, De Troyer R, Stove C. Chapter 57 – Biomarkers of alcohol misuse. In: Preedy VR, ed. *Neuroscience of Alcohol*. Academic Press; 2019:557–565.
18. Acevedo MB, Eagon JC, Bartholow BD, Klein S, Bucholz KK, Pepino MY. Sleeve gastrectomy surgery: when 2 alcoholic drinks are converted to 4. *Surg Obes Relat Dis*. 2018;14:277–283.
19. Lieber CS, DeCarli LM. Hepatic microsomal ethanol-oxidizing system: in vitro characteristics and adaptive properties in vivo. *J Biol Chem*. 1970;245:2505–2512.
20. Teschke R. Microsomal ethanol-oxidizing system: success over 50 years and an encouraging future. *Alcohol Clin Exp Res*. 2019;43: 386–400.
21. Higuchi S, Matsushita S, Masaki T, et al. Influence of genetic variations of ethanol-metabolizing enzymes on phenotypes of alcohol-related disorders. *Ann N Y Acad Sci*. 2004;1025: 472–480.
22. Druesne-Pecollo N, Tehard B, Mallet Y, et al. Alcohol and genetic polymorphisms: effect on risk of alcohol-related cancer. *Lancet Oncol*. 2009;10:173–180.
23. Wall TL, Luczak SE, Hiller-Sturmhöfel S. Biology, genetics, and environment: underlying factors influencing alcohol metabolism. *Alcohol Res*. 2016;38:59–68.
24. Rusyn I, Bataller R. Alcohol and toxicity. *J Hepatol*. 2013;59: 387–388.
25. Watson RR, Preedy VR. *Nutrition and Alcohol: Linking Nutrient Interactions and Dietary Intake*. Boca Raton, FL: CRC Press; 2003.
26. Guo R, Ren J. Alcohol and acetaldehyde in public health: from marvel to menace. *Int J Environ Res Public Health*. 2010;7: 1285–1301.
27. Niemelä O. Acetaldehyde adducts in circulation. *Novartis Found Symp*. 2007;285:183–192.
28. Rahman MA, Patters BJ, Kodidela S, Kumar S. Extracellular vesicles: intercellular mediators in alcohol-induced pathologies. *J Neuroimmune Pharmacol*. 2019. https://doi.org/10.1007/s11481-019-09848-z.
29. Kruman II, Fowler AK. Impaired one carbon metabolism and DNA methylation in alcohol toxicity. *J Neurochem*. 2014;129:770–780.
30. Ratna A, Mandrekar P. Alcohol and cancer: mechanisms and therapies. *Biomolecules*. 2017;7:61. https://doi.org/10.3390/biom7030061.
31. Li TK. Pharmacogenetics of responses to alcohol and genes that influence alcohol drinking. *J Stud Alcohol*. 2000;61:5–12.
32. Ratteree K, Yang S, Courville AB, et al. Adults with alcohol use disorder may overreport dietary intake using the 1-year Diet History Questionnaire II. *Nutr Res*. 2019;67:53–59.
33. Teixeira J, Mota T, Fernandes JC. Nutritional evaluation of alcoholic inpatients admitted for alcohol detoxification. *Alcohol Alcohol*. 2011;46:558–560.
34. Chao A, Waitzberg D, de Jesus RP, et al. Malnutrition and nutritional support in alcoholic liver disease: a review. *Curr Gastroenterol Rep*. 2016;18:65.
35. European-Association for the Study of the Liver. EASL Clinical Practice Guidelines on nutrition in chronic liver disease. *J Hepatol*. 2019;70:172–193.
36. McFarlane M, Hammond C, Roper T, et al. Comparing assessment tools for detecting undernutrition in patients with liver cirrhosis. *Clin Nutr ESPEN*. 2018;23:156–161.
37. Plauth M, Bernal W, Dasarathy S, et al. ESPEN guideline on clinical nutrition in liver disease. *Clin Nutr*. 2019;38:485–521.
38. Arab JP, Roblero JP, Altamirano J, et al. Alcohol-related liver disease: clinical practice guidelines by the Latin American Association for the Study of the Liver (ALEH). *Ann Hepatol*. 2019;18:518–535.
39. Singal AK, Bataller R, Ahn J, Kamath PS, Shah VH. ACG clinical guideline: alcoholic liver disease. *Am J Gastroenterol*. 2018;113: 175–194.
40. Santolaria-Fernandez FJ, Gomez-Sirvent JL, Gonzalez-Reimers CE, et al. Nutritional assessment of drug addicts. *Drug Alcohol Depend*. 1995;38:11–18.
41. Salaspuro M. Nutrient intake and nutritional status in alcoholics. *Alcohol Alcohol*. 1993;28:85–88.
42. Fawehinmi TO, Ilomäki J, Voutilainen S, Kauhanen J. Alcohol consumption and dietary patterns: the FinDrink study. *PLoS One*. 2012;7:e38607.
43. Dasarathy J, McCullough AJ, Dasarathy S. Sarcopenia in alcoholic liver disease: clinical and molecular advances. *Alcohol Clin Exp Res*. 2017;41:1419–1431.
44. Urbano-Marquez A, Fernandez-Sola J. Effects of alcohol on skeletal and cardiac muscle. *Muscle Nerve*. 2004;30:689–707.
45. Fernandez-Solà J, Preedy VR, Lang CH, et al. Molecular and cellular events in alcohol-induced muscle disease. *Alcohol Clin Exp Res*. 2007;31:1953–1962.
46. González-Reimers E, Quintero-Platt G, González-Arnay E, Martín-González C, Romero-Acevedo L, Santolaria-Fernández F. Chapter 31 – Alcoholic myopathy. In: Walrand S, ed. *Nutrition and Skeletal Muscle*. Academic Press; 2019:529–547.
47. Shenkman BS, Zinovyeva OE, Belova SP, et al. Cellular and molecular signatures of alcohol-induced myopathy in women. *Am J Physiol Endocrinol Metab*. 2019;316:E967–E976.
48. Smith KE, Fenske NA. Cutaneous manifestations of alcohol abuse. *J Am Acad Dermatol*. 2000;43:1–18.

49. Dogra S, Jindal R. Cutaneous manifestations of common liver diseases. *J Clin Exp Hepatol*. 2011;1:177–184.
50. González-Reimers E, Quintero-Platt G, Rodríguez-Rodríguez E, Martínez-Riera A, Alvisa-Negrín J, Santolaria-Fernández F. Bone changes in alcoholic liver disease. *World J Hepatol*. 2015;7: 1258–1264.
51. Mancinelli R, Ceccanti M. Biomarkers in alcohol misuse: their role in the prevention and detection of thiamine deficiency. *Alcohol Alcohol*. 2009;44:177–182.
52. Delanghe JR, De Buyzere ML. Carbohydrate deficient transferrin and forensic medicine. *Clin Chim Acta*. 2009;406:1–7.
53. Das SK, Dhanya L, Vasudevan DM. Biomarkers of alcoholism: an updated review. *Scand J Clin Lab Investig*. 2008;68:81–92.
54. Borucki K, Schreiner R, Dierkes J, et al. Detection of recent ethanol intake with new markers: comparison of fatty acid ethyl esters in serum and of ethyl glucuronide and the ratio of 5-hydroxytryptophol to 5-hydroxyindole acetic acid in urine. *Alcohol Clin Exp Res*. 2005;29:781–787.
55. Staufer K, Yegles M. Biomarkers for detection of alcohol consumption in liver transplantation. *World J Gastroenterol*. 2016;22: 3725–3734.
56. Wang Y, Fridberg DJ, Leeman RF, Cook RL, Porges EC. Wrist-worn alcohol biosensors: strengths, limitations, and future directions. *Alcohol*. 2020;81:83–92.
57. Campbell AS, Kim J, Wang J. Wearable electrochemical alcohol biosensors. *Current Opin Electrochemistry*. 2018;10:126–135.
58. Vizzini A, Aranda-Michel J. Malnutrition in patients with cirrhosis. In: Keaveny AP, Cárdenas A, eds. *Complications of Cirrhosis: Evaluation and Management*. Cham: Springer International Publishing; 2015:289–294.
59. Poppitt SD, Eckhardt JW, McGonagle J, Murgatroyd PR, Prentice AM. Short-term effects of alcohol consumption on appetite and energy intake. *Physiol Behav*. 1996;60:1063–1070.
60. Caton SJ, Ball M, Ahern A, Hetherington MM. Dose-dependent effects of alcohol on appetite and food intake. *Physiol Behav*. 2004;81: 51–58.
61. Seitz HK, Suter PM. Ethanol toxicity and the nutritional status. In: Kotsonis FN, Mackey M, Hjelle J, eds. *Nutritional Toxicology*. New York, N.Y.: Raven Press; 1994:95–116.
62. Butler L, Poti JM, Popkin BM. Trends in energy intake from alcoholic beverages among US adults by sociodemographic characteristics, 1989–2012. *J Acad Nutr Diet*. 2016;116, 1087-100.e6.
63. Westerterp-Plantenga MS, Verwegen CRT. The appetizing effect of an apéritif in overweight and normal-weight humans. *Am J Clin Nutr*. 1999;69:205–212.
64. Caton SJ, Bate L, Hetherington MM. Acute effects of an alcoholic drink on food intake: aperitif versus co-ingestion. *Physiol Behav*. 2007;90:368–375.
65. Suter PM. Is alcohol consumption a risk factor for weight gain and obesity? *Crit Rev Clin Lab Sci*. 2005;42:1–31.
66. Yeomans MR, Hails NJ, Nesic JS. Alcohol and the appetizer effect. *Behav Pharmacol*. 1999;10:151–161.
67. Suter PM, Schutz Y, Jéquier E. The effect of ethanol on fat storage in healthy subjects. *N Engl J Med*. 1992;326:983–987.
68. Suter PM, Jéquier E, Schutz Y. The effect of ethanol on energy expenditure. *Am J Physiol*. 1994;266:R1204–R1212.
69. Atwater WD, Benedict FG. An experimental inquiry regarding the nutritive value of alcohol. *Mem Natl Acad Sci*. 1902;8: 235–272.
70. Lieber C. Perspectives: do alcohol calories count ? *Am J Clin Nutr*. 1991;54:976–982.
71. Siler SQ, Neese RA, Hellerstein MK. De novo lipogenesis, lipid kinetics, and whole-body lipid balances in humans after acute alcohol consumption. *Am J Clin Nutr*. 1999;70:928–936.
72. Liu S, Serdula MK, Williamson DF, Mokad AH, Byers T. A prospective study of alcohol intake and change in body weight among US adults. *Am J Epidemiol*. 1994;140:912–920.
73. Rohrer JE, Rohland BM, Denison A, Way A. Frequency of alcohol use and obesity in community medicine patients. *BMC Fam Pract*. 2005;6:17.
74. Wang L, Lee I-M, Manson JE, Buring JE, Sesso HD. Alcohol consumption, weight gain, and risk of becoming overweight in middle-aged and older women. *Arch Intern Med*. 2010;170:453–461.
75. Zhao P-P, Xu L-W, Sun T, et al. Relationship between alcohol use, blood pressure and hypertension: an association study and a Mendelian randomisation study. *J Epidemiol Community Health*. 2019;73(9):796–801. jech-2018-211185.
76. O'Donovan G, Stamatakis E, Hamer M. Associations between alcohol and obesity in more than 100 000 adults in England and Scotland. *Br J Nutr*. 2018;119:222–227.
77. Britton A, Marmot MG, Shipley M. Who benefits most from the cardioprotective properties of alcohol consumption–health freaks or couch potatoes? *J Epidemiol Community Health*. 2008;62:905–908.
78. Chao AM, Wadden TA, Tronieri JS, Berkowitz RI. Alcohol intake and weight loss during intensive lifestyle intervention for adults with overweight or obesity and diabetes. *Obesity*. 2019; 27:30–40.
79. Fazzino TL, Fleming K, Sher KJ, Sullivan DK, Befort C. Heavy drinking in young adulthood increases risk of transitioning to obesity. *Am J Prev Med*. 2017;53:169–175.
80. Dallongeville J, Marécaux N, Ducimetière P, et al. Influence of alcohol consumption and various beverages on waist girth and waist-to-hip ratio in a sample of French men and women. *Int J Obes Relat Metab Disord*. 1998;22:1778–1783.
81. Bendsen NT, Christensen R, Bartels EM, et al. Is beer consumption related to measures of abdominal and general obesity? a systematic review and meta-analysis. *Nutr Rev*. 2013;71:67–87.
82. Sakurai Y, Umeda T, Shinchi K, et al. Relation of total and beverage-specific alcohol intake to body mass index and waist-to-hip ratio: a study of self-defense officials in Japan. *Eur J Epidemiol*. 1997;13:893–898.
83. Suter PM, Maire R, Vetter W. Is an increased waist:hip ratio the cause of alcohol-induced hypertension. The AIR94 study. *J Hypertens*. 1995;13:1857–1862.
84. Alkerwi A, Boutsen M, Vaillant M, et al. Alcohol consumption and the prevalence of metabolic syndrome: a meta-analysis of observational studies. *Atherosclerosis*. 2009;204:624–635.
85. Freiberg MS, Cabral HJ, Heeren TC, Vasan RS, Curtis Ellison R. Alcohol consumption and the prevalence of the metabolic syndrome in the U.S.: a cross-sectional analysis of data from the third national health and nutrition examination. *Survey Diabetes Care*. 2004;27:2954–2959.
86. Traversy G, Chaput J-P. Alcohol consumption and obesity: an update. *Curr Obes Rep*. 2015;4:122–130.
87. Sasakabe T, Wakai K, Kawai S, et al. Modification of the associations of alcohol intake with serum low-density lipoprotein cholesterol and triglycerides by ALDH2 and ADH1B polymorphisms in Japanese men. *J Epidemiol*. 2018;28:185–193.
88. Soedamah-Muthu SS, De Neve M, Shelton NJ, Tielemans SM, Stamatakis E. Joint associations of alcohol consumption and physical activity with all-cause and cardiovascular mortality. *Am J Cardiol*. 2013;112:380–386.
89. Vu KN, Ballantyne CM, Hoogeveen RC, et al. Causal role of alcohol consumption in an improved lipid profile: the atherosclerosis risk in communities (ARIC) study. *PLoS One*. 2016;11:e0148765.
90. Barona E, Lieber CS. Alcohol and lipids. In: Galanter M, ed. *Recent Developments in Alcoholism*. New York (N.Y.): Plenum Press; 1998: 97–134. Consequences of Alcoholism; vol. 14.

91. Brinton EA. Effects of ethanol intake on lipoproteins and atherosclerosis. *Curr Opin Lipidol*. 2010;21:346–351. https://doi.org/10.1097/MOL.0b013e32833c1f41.
92. You M, Arteel GE. Effect of ethanol on lipid metabolism. *J Hepatol*. 2019;70:237–248.
93. Sozio M, Crabb DW. Alcohol and lipid metabolism. *Am J Physiol Endocrinol Metab*. 2008;295:E10–E16.
94. Zhou P, Ross RA, Pywell CM, Liangpunsakul S, Duffield GE. Disturbances in the murine hepatic circadian clock in alcohol-induced hepatic steatosis. *Sci Rep*. 2014;4:3725.
95. Udoh SU, Valcin AJ, Gamble LK, Bailey MS. The molecular circadian clock and alcohol-induced liver injury. *Biomolecules*. 2015;5.
96. Sarin SK, Pande A, Schnabl B. Microbiome as a therapeutic target in alcohol-related liver disease. *J Hepatol*. 2019;70:260–272.
97. Clugston RD, Gao MA, Blaner WS. The hepatic lipidome: a gateway to understanding the pathogenes is of alcohol-induced fatty liver. *Curr Mol Pharmacol*. 2017;10:195–206.
98. Kaibori M, Kwon AH, Oda M, Kamiyama Y, Kitamura N, Okumura T. Hepatocyte growth factor stimulates synthesis of lipids and secretion of lipoproteins in rat hepatocytes. *Hepatology*. 1998;27:1354–1361.
99. Zemánková K, Makoveichuk E, Vlasáková Z, Olivecrona G, Kovář J. Acute alcohol consumption downregulates lipoprotein lipase activity in vivo. *Metabolism*. 2015;64:1592–1596.
100. Suter PM, Gerritsen-Zehnder M, Häsler E, et al. Effect of alcohol on postprandial lipemia with and without preprandial exercise. *J Am Coll Nutr*. 2001;20:58–64.
101. Tolstrup J, Grønbaek M, Nordestgaard BG. Alcohol intake, myocardial infarction, biochemical risk factors, and alcohol dehydrogenase genotypes. *Circ Cardiovasc Genet*. 2009;2009:507–514.
102. Klop B, Rego ATd, Cabezas MC. Alcohol and plasma triglycerides. *Curr Opin Lipidol*. 2013;24:321–326.
103. Huang S, Li J, Shearer GC, et al. Longitudinal study of alcohol consumption and HDL concentrations: a community-based study. *Am J Clin Nutr*. 2017;105:905–912.
104. Wakabayashi I. Relationships between alcohol intake and cardiovascular risk factors in middle-aged men with hypo-HDL cholesterolemia. *Clin Chim Acta*. 2019;495:94–99.
105. Li M, Diao Y, Liu Y, et al. Chronic moderate alcohol intakes accelerate SR-B1 mediated reverse cholesterol transport. *Sci Rep*. 2016; 6:33032.
106. Devenyi P, Robinson GM, Kapur BM, Roncari DAK. High-density lipoprotein cholesterol in male alcoholics with and without severe liver disease. *Am J Med*. 1981;71:589–594.
107. Manttari M, Tenkanen L, Alikoski T, Manninen V. Alcohol and coronary heart disease: the roles of HDL-cholesterol and smoking. *J Intern Med*. 1997;214:157–163.
108. Muth ND, Laughlin GA, von Mühlen D, Smith SC, Barrett-Connor E. High-density lipoprotein subclasses are a potential intermediary between alcohol intake and reduced risk of cardiovascular disease: The Rancho Bernardo Study. *Br J Nutr*. 2010; 104:1034–1042.
109. Chiesa ST, Charakida M. High-density lipoprotein function and dysfunction in health and disease. *Cardiovasc Drugs Ther*. 2019; 33:207–219.
110. Tabara Y, Arai H, Hirao Y, et al. The causal effects of alcohol on lipoprotein subfraction and triglyceride levels using a Mendelian randomization analysis: the Nagahama study. *Atherosclerosis*. 2017;257:22–28.
111. Rye K-A, Barter PJ. Regulation of high-density lipoprotein metabolism. *Circ Res*. 2014;114:143–156.
112. Johansen D, Andersen PK, Jensen MK, Schnohr P, Gronbaek M. Nonlinear relation between alcohol intake and high-density lipoprotein cholesterol level: results from the Copenhagen city heart study. *Alcohol Clin Exp Res*. 2003;27:1305–1309.
113. Lussier-Cacan S, Bolduc A, Xhignesse M, Niyonsenga T, Sing CF. Impact of alcohol intake on measures of lipid metabolism depends on context defined by gender, body mass index, cigarette smoking, and apolipoprotein E genotype. *Arterioscler Thromb Vasc Biol*. 2002;22:824–831.
114. Ayaori M, Ishikawa T, Yoshida H, et al. Beneficial effects of alcohol withdrawal on LDL particle size distribution and oxidative susceptibility in subjects with alcohol induced hypertriglyceridemia. *Arterioscler Thromb Vasc Biol*. 1997;17:2540–2547.
115. Fuhrman B, Lavy A, Aviram M. Consumption of red wine with meals reduces the susceptibility of human plasma and low-density-lipoprotein to lipid peroxidation. *Am J Clin Nutr*. 1995; 61:549–554.
116. Ajmo JM, Liang X, Rogers CQ, Pennock B, You M. Resveratrol alleviates alcoholic fatty liver in mice. *Am J Physiol Gastrointest Liver Physiol*. 2008;295:G833–G842.
117. Manach C, Williamson G, Morand C, Scalbert A, Remesy C. Bioavailability and bioefficacy of polyphenols in humans. I. Review of 97 bioavailability studies. *Am J Clin Nutr*. 2005;81, 230S-42.
118. Enkhmaa B, Anuurad E, Berglund L. Lipoprotein (a): impact by ethnicity and environmental and medical conditions. *J Lipid Res*. 2016;57:1111–1125.
119. Lange LG. Nonoxidative ethanol metabolism: formation of fatty acid ethyl esters by cholesterol esterase. *Proc Natl Acad Sci USA*. 1982;79:3954–3957.
120. Petersen OH, Tepikin AV, Gerasimenko JV, Gerasimenko OV, Sutton R, Criddle DN. Fatty acids, alcohol and fatty acid ethyl esters: toxic Ca^{2+} signal generation and pancreatitis. *Cell Calcium*. 2009;45:634–642.
121. Bhatt DL, Steg PG, Miller M, et al. Cardiovascular risk reduction with icosapent ethyl for hypertriglyceridemia. *N Engl J Med*. 2018; 380:11–22.
122. Jia X, Koh S, Al Rifai M, Blumenthal RS, Virani SS. Spotlight on Icosapent Ethyl for cardiovascular risk reduction: evidence to date. *Vasc Health Risk Manag*. 2020;16:1–10.
123. Steiner LJ, Crowell TK, Lang HC. Impact of alcohol on glycemic control and insulin action. *Biomolecules*. 2015;5.
124. Rachdaoui N, Sarkar DK. Effects of alcohol on the endocrine system. *Endocrinol Metabol Clin*. 2013;42:593–615.
125. Apte M, Pirola R, Wilson J. New insights into alcoholic pancreatitis and pancreatic cancer. *J Gastroenterol Hepatol*. 2009;24:S51–S56.
126. Siler SQ, Neese RA, Chrstiansen MP, Hellerstein MK. The inhibition of gluconeogenesis following alcohol in humans. *Am J Physiol*. 1998;275:E897–E907.
127. Flanagan D, Wood P, Sherwin R, Debrah K, Kerr D. Gin and tonic and reactive hypoglycemia: what is important – the gin, the tonic, or both? *J Clin Endocrinol Metab*. 1998;83(3):796–800.
128. Pedersen-Bjergaard U, Reubsaet JL, Nielsen SL, et al. Psychoactive drugs, alcohol, and severe hypoglycemia in insulin-treated diabetes: analysis of 141 cases. *Am J Med Sci*. 2005; 118:307–310.
129. Crandall JP, Polsky S, Howard AA, et al. Alcohol consumption and diabetes risk in the diabetes prevention program. *Am J Clin Nutr*. 2009;90:595–601.
130. Blomhoff R, Blomhoff HK. Overview of retinoid metabolism and function. *J Neurobiol*. 2006;66:606–630.
131. Leo MA, Lieber CS. Alcohol, vitamin A, and beta-carotene: adverse interactions, including hepatotoxicity and carcinogenicity. *Am J Clin Nutr*. 1999;69:1071–1085.
132. Clugston RD, Huang L-S, Blaner WS. Chronic alcohol consumption has a biphasic effect on hepatic retinoid loss. *FASEB J*. 2015; 29:3654–3667.
133. Haaker MW, Vaandrager AB, Helms JB. Retinoids in health and disease: a role for hepatic stellate cells in affecting retinoid level. *BBA - Mol Cell Biol L*. 2020;1865:158674.

134. Dan Z, Popov Y, Patsenker E, et al. Hepatotoxicity of alcohol-induced polar retinol metabolites involves apoptosis via loss of mitochondrial membrane potential. *FASEB J.* 2005;19(7): 845–847.
135. Kane MA, Folias AE, Wang C, Napoli JL. Ethanol elevates physiological all-trans-retinoic acid levels in select loci through altering retinoid metabolism in multiple loci: a potential mechanism of ethanol toxicity. *FASEB J.* 2010;24:823–832.
136. Wolf G. Tissue-specific increases in endogenous all-trans retinoic acid: possible contributing factor in ethanol toxicity. *Nutr Rev.* 2010;68:689–692.
137. Kumar A, Singh CK, DiPette DD, Singh US. Ethanol impairs activation of retinoic acid receptors in cerebellar granule cells in a rodent model of fetal alcohol spectrum disorders. *Alcohol Clin Exp Res.* 2010;34:928–937.
138. Clugston RD, Jiang H, Lee MX, et al. Altered hepatic retinyl ester concentration and acyl composition in response to alcohol consumption. *Biochim Biophys Acta Mol Cell Biol Lipids.* 2013; 1831:1276–1286.
139. Albanes D, Heinonen OP, Taylor PR, et al. α-tocopherol and b-carotene supplements and lung cancer incidence in the alpha-tocopherol, beta-carotene cancer prevention study: effects of base-line characteristics and study compliance. *J Natl Cancer Inst.* 1996;88:1560–1570.
140. Ahmed S, Leo MA, Lieber CS. Interactions between alcohol and b-carotene in patients with alcoholic liver disease. *Am J Clin Nutr.* 1994;60:430–436.
141. Luvizotto RAM, Nascimento AF, Veeramachaneni S, Liu C, Wang X-D. Chronic alcohol intake upregulates hepatic expression of carotenoid cleavage enzymes and PPAR in rats. *J Nutr.* 2010; 140:1808–1814.
142. Stice CP, Wang X-D. Carotenoids and alcoholic liver disease. *Hepatobiliary Surg Nutr.* 2013;2:244–247.
143. Veeramachaneni S, Ausman LM, Choi SW, Russell RM, Wang X-D. High dose lycopene supplementation increases hepatic cytochrome P4502E1 protein and inflammation in alcohol-fed rats. *J Nutr.* 2008;138:1329–1335.
144. Stice CP, Xia H, Wang X-D. Tomato lycopene prevention of alcoholic fatty liver disease and hepatocellular carcinoma development. *Chronic Dis Transl Med.* 2018;4:211–224.
145. Shabtai Y, Fainsod A. Competition between ethanol clearance and retinoic acid biosynthesis in the induction of fetal alcohol syndrome. *Biochem Cell Biol.* 2017;96:148–160.
146. Bell H, Bjorneboe A, Eidsvoll B, et al. Reduced concentration of hepatic α-tocopherol in patients with alcoholic liver cirrhosis. *Alcohol Alcohol.* 1992;27:39–46.
147. Tanner AR, Bantock I, Hinks L, Lloyd B, Turner NR, Wright R. Depressed selenium and vitamin E levels in an alcoholic population. *Dig Dis Sci.* 1986;31:1307–1312.
148. Hartman TJ, Baer DJ, Graham LB, et al. Moderate alcohol consumption and levels of antioxidant vitamins and isoprostanes in postmenopausal women. *Eur J Clin Nutr.* 2005;59:161–168.
149. González-Reimers E, Fernández-Rodríguez CM, Candelaria Martín-González M, et al. Antioxidant vitamins and brain dysfunction in alcoholics. *Alcohol Alcohol.* 2013;49:45–50.
150. de-la-Maza MP, Petermann M, Bunout D, Hirsch S. Effects of long-term vitamin E supplementation in alcoholic cirrhotics. *J Am Coll Nutr.* 1995;14:192–196.
151. Sario AD, Candelaresi C, Omenetti A, Benedetti A. Vitamin E in chronic liver diseases and liver fibrosis. In: Gerald L, ed. *Vitamins & Hormones.* Academic Press; 2007:551–573.
152. Kolasani B, Sasidharan P, Kumar A. Efficacy of vitamin E supplementation in patients with alcoholic liver disease: an open-label, prospective, randomized comparative study. *Int J Nutr, Pharmacol, Neurol Dis.* 2016;6:101–110.
153. Perumpail JB, Li AA, John N, et al. The role of vitamin E in the treatment of NAFLD. *Diseases.* 2018;6.
154. Podszun MC, Rolt A, Garaffo M, et al. 22 – Vitamin E (RRR-α-tocopherol) decreases hepatic de novo lipogenesis. *Free Radic Biol Med.* 2017;112:30–31.
155. Shirpoor A, Barmaki H, Khadem Ansari M, lkhanizadeh B, Barmaki H. Protective effect of vitamin E against ethanol-induced small intestine damage in rats. *Biomed Pharmacother.* 2016;78:150–155.
156. Tiwari V, Kuhad A, Chopra K. Tocotrienol ameliorates behavioral and biochemical alterations in the rat model of alcoholic neuropathy. *Pain.* 2009;145:129–135.
157. Tiwari V, Kuhad A, Chopra K. Suppression of neuro-inflammatory signaling cascade by tocotrienol can prevent chronic alcohol-induced cognitive dysfunction in rats. *Behav Brain Res.* 2009;203:296–303.
158. Nyquist F, Ljunghall S, Berglund M, Oberant K. Biochemical markers of bone metabolism after short and long time ethanol withdrawal in alcoholics. *Bone.* 1996;19:51–54.
159. Iber FL, Shamszad M, Miller PA, Jacob R. Vitamin K deficiency in chronic alcoholic males. *Alcohol Clin Exp Res.* 1986;10: 679–681.
160. Shiomi S, Nishiguchi S, Kubo S, et al. Vitamin K2 (menatetrenone) for bone loss in patients with cirrhosis of the liver. *Am J Gastroenterol.* 2002;97:978–981.
161. Liabeuf S, Scaltieux L-M, Masmoudi K, et al. Risk factors for bleeding in hospitalized at risk patients with an INR of 5 or more treated with vitamin K antagonists. *Medicine.* 2015;94:e2366.
162. Laitinen K, Valimaki M, Lamberg-Allardt C, et al. Deranged vitamin D metabolism but normal bone mineral density in Finnish noncirrhotic male alcoholics. *Alcohol Clin Exp Res.* 1990; 14:551–556.
163. Ogunsakin O, Hottor T, Mehta A, Lichtveld M, McCaskill M. Chronic ethanol exposure effects on vitamin D levels among subjects with alcohol use disorder. *Environ Health Insights.* 2016;10: 191–199.
164. Tardelli VS, Lago MPPD, Silveira DXD, Fidalgo TM. Vitamin D and alcohol: a review of the current literature. *Psychiatry Res.* 2017;248:83–86.
165. Touvier M, Deschasaux M, Montourcy M, et al. Determinants of vitamin D status in Caucasian adults: influence of sun exposure, dietary intake, sociodemographic, lifestyle, anthropometric, and genetic factors. *J Investig Dermatol.* 2015;135:378–388.
166. Alvisa-Negrín J, González-Reimer sE, Santolaria-Fernández F, et al. Osteopenia in alcoholics: effect of alcohol abstinence. *Alcohol Alcohol.* 2009;44(5):468–475.
167. Nyquist F, Karlsson MK, Obrant KJ, Nilsson JA. Osteopenia in alcoholics after tibia shaft fractures. *Alcohol Alcohol.* 1997;32: 599–604.
168. Guañabens N, Parés A. Liver and bone. *Arch Biochem Biophys.* 2010;503:84–94.
169. Anty R, Canivet CM, Patouraux S, et al. Severe vitamin D deficiency may be an additional cofactor for the occurrence of alcoholic steatohepatitis. *Alcohol Clin Exp Res.* 2015;39: 1027–1033.
170. Quintero-Platt G, González-Reimers E, Martín-González MC, et al. Vitamin D, vascular calcification and mortality among alcoholics. *Alcohol Alcohol.* 2014;50:18–23.
171. González-Reimers E, Durán-Castellón MC, López-Lirola A, et al. Alcoholic myopathy: vitamin D deficiency is related to muscle fibre atrophy in a murine model. *Alcohol Alcohol.* 2010;45: 223–230.
172. Wijnia JW, Wielders JP, Lips P, van de Wiel A, Mulder CL, Nieuwenhuis KG. Is vitamin D deficiency a confounder in alcoholic skeletal muscle myopathy? *Alcohol Clin Exp Res.* 2013;37: E209–E215.
173. Jamieson CP, Obeid OA, Powell-Tuck J. The thiamin, riboflavin and pyridoxine status of patients on emergency admission to hospital. *Clin Nutr.* 1999;18:87–91.

174. Whitfield KC, Bourassa MW, Adamolekun B, et al. Thiamine deficiency disorders: diagnosis, prevalence, and a roadmap for global control programs. *Ann N Y Acad Sci.* 2018;1430:3–43.
175. Tomasulo PA, Kater RM, Iber FL. Impairment of thiamine absorption in alcoholism. *Am J Clin Nutr.* 1968;21:1341–1344.
176. Hoyumpa Jr AM. Mechanisms of thiamin deficiency in chronic alcoholism. *Am J Clin Nutr.* 1980;33:2750–2761.
177. Said HM, Nexo E. Gastrointestinal handling of water-soluble vitamins. *Comp Physiol.* 2018;8:1291–1311. https://doiorg/101002/cphyc1700542018.
178. Said Hamid M. Intestinal absorption of water-soluble vitamins in health and disease. *Biochem J.* 2011;437:357.
179. Srinivasan P, Subramanian VS, Said HM. Mechanisms involved in the inhibitory effect of chronic alcohol exposure on pancreatic acinar thiamin uptake. *Am J Physiol Gastrointest Liver Physiol.* 2014;306:G631–G639.
180. Subramanian VS, Subramanya SB, Tsukamoto H, Said HM. Effect of chronic alcohol feeding on physiological and molecular parameters of renal thiamin transport. *Am J Physiol Renal Physiol.* 2010; 299:F28–F34.
181. Subramanya SB, Subramanian VS, Said HM. Chronic alcohol consumption and intestinal thiamin absorption: effects on physiological and molecular parameters of the uptake process. *Am J Physiol Gastrointest Liver Physiol.* 2010;299:G23–G31.
182. Holzbach E. Thiamin absorption in alcoholic delirium patients. *J Stud Alcohol.* 1996;57:581–584.
183. Preedy V, Reilly ME, Patel VB, Richardson PJ, Peters TJ. Protein metabolism in alcoholism: effects on specific tissues and the whole body. *Nutrition.* 1999;15:604–608.
184. Ke ZJ, Wang X, Fan Z, Luo J. Ethanol promotes thiamine deficiency-induced neuronal death: involvement of double-stranded RNA-activated protein kinase. *Alcohol Clin Exp Res.* 2009;33:1097–1103.
185. Hazell AS. Astrocytes are a major target in thiamine deficiency and Wernicke's encephalopathy. *Neurochem Int.* 2009;55: 129–135.
186. Sinha S, Kataria A, Kolla BP, Thusius N, Loukianova LL. Wernicke encephalopathy—clinical pearls. *Mayo Clin Proc.* 2019;94: 1065–1072.
187. Martin PR, Singleton CK, Hiller-Sturmhofel S. The role of thiamine deficiency in alcoholic brain disease. *Alcohol Res Health.* 2003;27:134–142.
188. Harper C. The neuropathology of alcohol-related brain damage. *Alcohol Alcohol.* 2009;44:136–140.
189. Polegato BF, Pereira AG, Azevedo PS, et al. Role of thiamin in health and disease. *Nutr Clin Pract.* 2019;0.
190. Kloss O, Eskin NAM, Suh M. Thiamin deficiency on fetal brain development with and without prenatal alcohol exposure. *Biochem Cell Biol.* 2017;96:169–177.
191. Tang L, Alsulaim HA, Canner JK, Prokopowicz GP, Steele KE. Prevalence and predictors of postoperative thiamine deficiency after vertical sleeve gastrectomy. *Surg Obes Relat Dis.* 2018;14: 943–950.
192. Oudman E, Wijnia JW, van Dam M, Biter LU, Postma A. Preventing Wernicke encephalopathy after bariatric surgery. *Obes Surg.* 2018;28:2060–2068.
193. King WC, Chen J-Y, Courcoulas AP, et al. Alcohol and other substance use after bariatric surgery: prospective evidence from a U.S. multicenter cohort study. *Surg Obes Relat Dis.* 2017;13: 1392–1402.
194. Linder LM, Robert S, Mullinax K, Hayes G. Thiamine prescribing and Wernicke's encephalopathy risk factors in patients with alcohol use disorders at a psychiatric hospital. *J Psychiatr Pract.* 2018;24:317–322.
195. Holmberg MJ, Moskowitz A, Patel PV, et al. Thiamine in septic shock patients with alcohol use disorders: an observational pilot study. *J Crit Care.* 2018;43:61–64.
196. Chou W-P, Chang Y-H, Lin H-C, Chang Y-H, Chen Y-Y, Ko C-H. Thiamine for preventing dementia development among patients with alcohol use disorder: a nationwide population-based cohort study. *Clin Nutr.* 2019;38:1269–1273.
197. Crowe SF, Kempton S. Both ethanol toxicity and thiamine deficiency are necessary to produce long-term memory deficits in the young chick. *Pharmacol Biochem Behav.* 1997;58:461–470.
198. Gong Y-S, Hu K, Yang L-Q, et al. Comparative effects of EtOH consumption and thiamine deficiency on cognitive impairment, oxidative damage, and β-amyloid peptide overproduction in the brain. *Free Radic Biol Med.* 2017;108:163–173.
199. Toledo Nunes P, Vedder LC, Deak T, Savage LM. A pivotal role for thiamine deficiency in the expression of neuroinflammation markers in models of alcohol-related brain damage. *Alcohol Clin Exp Res.* 2019;43:425–438.
200. McLean J, Manchip S. Wernicke's encephalopathy induced by magnesium depletion. *Lancet.* 1999;353:1768.
201. Sharain K, May AM, Gersh BJ. Chronic alcoholism and the danger of profound hypomagnesemia. *Am J Med.* 2015;128:e17–e18.
202. Baroncini D, Annovazzi P, Minonzio G, Franzetti I, Zaffaroni M. Hypomagnesaemia as a trigger of relapsing non-alcoholic Wernicke encephalopathy: a case report. *Neurol Sci.* 2017;38:2069–2071.
203. Dingwall KM, Delima JF, Gent D, Batey RG. Hypomagnesaemia and its potential impact on thiamine utilisation in patients with alcohol misuse at the Alice Springs Hospital. *Drug Alcohol Rev.* 2015;34:323–328.
204. Suter PM, Vetter W. Diuretics and vitamin B1: are diuretics a risk factor for thiamin malnutrition? *Nutr Rev.* 2000;58:319–323.
205. Keith ME, Walsh NA, Darling PB, et al. B-vitamin deficiency in hospitalized patients with heart failure. *J Am Diet Assoc.* 2009; 109:1406–1410.
206. Pinto J, Huang YP, Rivlin RS. Mechanisms underlying the differential effects of ethanol on the bioavailability of riboflavin and flavin adenine dinucleotide. *J Clin Investig.* 1987;79: 1343–1348.
207. Subramanian VS, Subramanya SB, Ghosal A, Said HM. Chronic alcohol feeding inhibits physiological and molecular parameters of intestinal and renal riboflavin transport. *Am J Physiol Cell Physiol.* 2013;305:C539–C546.
208. Ono S, Takahashi H, Hirano H. Ethanol enhances the esterification of riboflavin in rat organ tissue. *Int J Vitam Nutr Res.* 1987;57:335.
209. Narasimha VL, Ganesh S, Reddy S, et al. Pellagra and alcohol dependence syndrome: findings from a tertiary care addiction treatment centre in India. *Alcohol Alcohol.* 2019;54:148–151.
210. Dastur DK, Santhadevi Q, Quadros EV. The B-vitamins in malnutrition with alcoholism. *Br J Nutr.* 1976;36:143–159.
211. Terada N, Kinoshita K, Taguchi S, Tokuda Y. Wernicke encephalopathy and pellagra in an alcoholic and malnourished patient. *BMJ Case Rep.* 2015;2015. bcr2015209412.
212. Badawy AA. Pellagra and alcoholism: a biochemical perspective. *Alcohol Alcohol.* 2014;49:238–250.
213. Hardman MJ, Page RA, Wiseman MS, Crow KE. Regulation of rates of ethanol metabolism and liver [NAD^+]/[NADH] ratio. In: Palmer NT, ed. *Alcoholism a Molecular Perspective.* New York, N.Y.: Plenum Press; 1991:27–33.
214. Masia R, McCarty WJ, Lahmann C, et al. Live cell imaging of cytosolic NADH/NAD^+ratio in hepatocytes and liver slices. *Am J Physiol Gastrointest Liver Physiol.* 2018;314:G97–G108.
215. Cook CCH, Hallwood PM, Thomson AD. B-Vitamin deficiency and neuropsychiatric syndromes in alcohol misuse. *Alcohol Alcohol.* 1998;33:317–336.

216. López M, Olivares JM, Berrios GE. Pellagra encephalopathy in the context of alcoholism: review and case report. *Alcohol Alcohol.* 2013;49:38–41.
217. Luthe SK, Sato R. Alcoholic pellagra as a cause of altered mental status in the emergency department. *J Emerg Med.* 2017;53: 554–557.
218. Ueland PM, Ulvik A, Rios-Avila L, Midttun Ø, Gregory JF. Direct and functional biomarkers of vitamin B6 status. *Annu Rev Nutr.* 2015;35:33–70.
219. Medici V, Peerson JM, Stabler SP, et al. Impaired homocysteine transsulfuration is an indicator of alcoholic liver disease. *J Hepatol.* 2010;53:551–557.
220. Walsh MP, Howorth PJN, Marks V. Pyridoxine deficiency and tryptophan metabolism in chronic alcoholics. *Am J Clin Nutr.* 1966;19:379–383.
221. Mitchell D, Wagner C, Stone WJ, Wilkinson GR, Schenker S. Abnormal regulation of plasma pyridoxal-5′-phosphate in patients with liver disease. *Gastroenterology.* 1976;71:1043–1049.
222. Julian T, Glascow N, Syeed R, Zis P. Alcohol-related peripheral neuropathy: a systematic review and meta-analysis. *J Neurol.* 2018;266: 2907–2919.
223. Medici V, Halsted CH. Folate, alcohol, and liver disease. *Mol Nutr Food Res.* 2013;57:596–606.
224. Sanvisens A, Zuluaga P, Pineda M, et al. Folate deficiency in patients seeking treatment of alcohol use disorder. *Drug Alcohol Depend.* 2017;180:417–422.
225. Hamid A, Wani NA, Kaur J. New perspectives on folate transport in relation to alcoholism-induced folate malabsorption – association with epigenome stability and cancer development. *FEBS J.* 2009;276:2175–2191.
226. Wani NA, Hamid A, Khanduja KL, Kaur J. Folate malabsorption is associated with down-regulation of folate transporter expression and function at colon basolateral membrane in rats. *Br J Nutr.* 2012;107:800–808.
227. Halsted CH. Alcohol and folate interactions: clinical implications. In: Bailey LB, ed. *Folate in Health and Disease.* New York (N.Y): Marcel Dekker Inc.; 1995:313–327.
228. Ross DM, McMartin KE. Effect of ethanol on folate binding by isolated rat renal brush border membranes. *Alcohol.* 1996;13:449–454.
229. Biswas A, Senthilkumar SR, Said HM. Effect of chronic alcohol exposure on folate uptake by liver mitochondria. *Am J Physiol Cell Physiol.* 2011;302:C203–C209.
230. Kapur BM, Baber M. FASD: folic acid and formic acid — an unholy alliance in the alcohol abusing mother. *Biochem Cell Biol.* 2017;96:189–197.
231. Svensson T, Yamaji T, Budhathoki S, et al. Alcohol consumption, genetic variants in the alcohol- and folate metabolic pathways and colorectal cancer risk: the JPHC Study. *Sci Rep.* 2016;6:36607.
232. Dumitrescu RG. Alcohol-induced epigenetic changes in cancer. In: Dumitrescu RG, Verma M, eds. *Cancer Epigenetics for Precision Medicine: Methods and Protocols.* New York, NY: Springer New York; 2018:157–172.
233. Mason JB, Tang SY. Folate status and colorectal cancer risk: a 2016 update. *Mol Asp Med.* 2017;53:73–79.
234. Chien Y-W, Chen Y-L, Peng H-C, Hu J-T, Yang S-S, Yang S-C. Impaired homocysteine metabolism in patients with alcoholic liver disease in Taiwan. *Alcohol.* 2016;54:33–37.
235. van der Gaag MS, Ubbink JB, Sillanaukee P, Nikkari S, Hendriks HF. Effect of consumption of red wine, spirits, and beer on serum homocysteine. *Lancet.* 2000;355:1522.
236. Kisters K, Schodjaian K, Nguyen SQ, et al. Effect of alcohol on plasma and intracellular magnesium status in patients with steatosis or cirrhosis of the liver. *Med Sci Res.* 1997;25:805–806.
237. Romani AM. Magnesium homeostasis and alcohol consumption. *Magnes Res.* 2008;21:197–204.
238. Rink EB. Magnesium deficiency in alcoholism. *Alcohol Clin Exp Res.* 1986;10:590–594.
239. de Baaij JH, Hoenderop JG, Bindels RJ. Magnesium in man: implications for health and disease. *Physiol Rev.* 2015;95:1–46.
240. Cheungpasitporn W, Thongprayoon C, Qian Q. Dysmagnesemia in hospitalized patients: prevalence and prognostic importance. *Mayo Clin Proc.* 2015;90:1001–1010.
241. Workinger LJ, Doyle PR, Bortz J. Challenges in the diagnosis of magnesium status. *Nutrients.* 2018;10.
242. Wu L, Zhu X, Fan L, et al. Magnesium intake and mortality due to liver diseases: results from the third national health and nutrition examination survey cohort. *Sci Rep.* 2017;7:17913.
243. Poikolainen K, Alho H. Magnesium treatment in alcoholics: a randomized clinical trial. *Subst Abus Treat Prev Policy.* 2008;3:1.
244. Sarai M, Tejani AM, Chan AHW, Kuo IF, Li J. Magnesium for alcohol withdrawal. *Cochrane Database Syst Rev.* 2013;(Issue 6), CD008358. https://doi.org/10.1002/14651858.CD008358.pub2.
245. Maguire D, Ross DP, Talwar D, et al. Low serum magnesium and 1-year mortality in alcohol withdrawal syndrome. *Eur J Clin Investig.* 2019;0:e13152.
246. Bode JC, Hanisch P, Henning H, Koenig W, Richter FW, Bode C. Hepatic zinc content in patients with various stages of alcoholic liver disease and in patients with chronic active and chronic persistent hepatitis. *Hepatology.* 1988;8:1605–1609.
247. Zhong W, McClain CJ, Cave M, Kang YJ, Zhou Z. The role of zinc deficiency in alcohol-induced intestinal barrier dysfunction. *Am J Physiol Gastrointest Liver Physiol.* 2010;298:G625–G633.
248. Stamoulis I, Kouraklis G, Theocharis S. Zinc and the liver: an active interaction. *Dig Dis Sci.* 2007;52:1595–1612.
249. Skalny AV, Skalnaya MG, Grabeklis AR, Skalnaya AA, Tinkov AA. Zinc deficiency as a mediator of toxic effects of alcohol abuse. *Eur J Nutr.* 2018;57:2313–2322.
250. Sun Q, Li Q, Zhong W, et al. Dysregulation of hepatic zinc transporters in a mouse model of alcoholic liver disease. *Am J Physiol Gastrointest Liver Physiol.* 2014;307:G313–G322.
251. Rodriguez MF, Gonzalez RE, Santolaria FF, et al. Zinc, copper, manganese, and iron in chronic alcoholic liver disease. *Alcohol.* 1997;14:39–44.
252. Sengupta S, Wroblewski K, Aronsohn A, et al. Screening for zinc deficiency in patients with cirrhosis: when should we start? *Dig Dis Sci.* 2015;60:3130–3135.
253. Sullivan JF, Lankford HG. Zinc metabolism and chronic alcoholism. *Am J Clin Nutr.* 1965;17:57–63.
254. Sun Q, Zhong W, Zhang W, et al. Zinc deficiency mediates alcohol-induced apoptotic cell death in the liver of rats through activating ER and mitochondrial cell death pathways. *Am J Physiol Gastrointest Liver Physiol.* 2015;308:G757–G766.
255. Zhong W, Zhao Y, McClain CJ, Kang YJ, Zhou Z. Inactivation of hepatocyte nuclear factor-4{alpha} mediates alcohol-induced downregulation of intestinal tight junction proteins. *Am J Physiol Gastrointest Liver Physiol.* 2010;299:G643–G651.
256. Kang X, Zhong W, Liu J, et al. Zinc supplementation reverses alcohol-induced steatosis in mice through reactivating hepatocyte nuclear factor-4α and peroxisome proliferator-activated receptor-α. *Hepatology.* 2009;50:1241–1250.
257. McClain C, Vatsalya V, Cave M. Role of zinc in the development/progression of alcoholic liver disease. *Curr Treat Options Gastroenterol.* 2017;15:285–295.
258. Zhong W, Zhou Z. Chapter 8 – Sealing the leaky gut represents a beneficial mechanism of zinc intervention for alcoholic liver disease. In: Watson RR, Preedy VR, eds. *Dietary Interventions in Gastrointestinal Diseases.* Academic Press; 2019:91–106.
259. Joshi PC, Guidot DM. The alcoholic lung: epidemiology, pathophysiology, and potential therapies. *Am J Physiol Lung Cell Mol Physiol.* 2007;292:L813–L823.

260. Mehta AJ, Yeligar SM, Elon L, Brown LA, Guidot DM. Alcoholism causes alveolar macrophage zinc deficiency and immune dysfunction. *Am J Respir Crit Care Med*. 2013;188:716–723.
261. Joshi PC, Mehta A, Jabber WS, Fan X, Guidot DM. Zinc deficiency mediates alcohol-induced alveolar epithelial and macrophage dysfunction in rats. *Am J Respir Cell Mol Biol*. 2009;41: 207–216.
262. Prasad AS, Beck FW, Snell DC, Kucuk O. Zinc in cancer prevention. *Nutr Cancer*. 2009;61:879–887.
263. Seitz HK, Pöschl G, Simanowski UA. Alcohol and cancer. In: Galanter M, ed. *Recent Advances in Alcoholism*. New York (NY): Plenum Press; 1998:67–134.
264. McClain CJ, van Thiel DH, Parker S, Badzin LK, Gilbert H. Alterations in zinc, vitamin A, and retinol-binding protein in chronic alcoholics: a possible mechanism for night blindness and hypogonadism. *Alcohol Clin Exp Res*. 1979;3:135–141.
265. Morrison SA, Russell RM, Carney EA, Oaks EV. Zinc deficiency: a cause of abnormal dark adaptation in cirrhotics. *Am J Clin Nutr*. 1978;31:276–281.
266. Stockwell T, Zhao J, Panwar S, Roemer A, Naimi T, Chikritzhs T. Do "moderate" drinkers have reduced mortality risk? A systematic review and meta-analysis of alcohol consumption and all-cause mortality. *J Stud Alcohol Drugs*. 2016;77:185–198.
267. Zeisser C, Stockwell TR, Chikritzhs T. Methodological biases in estimating the relationship between alcohol consumption and breast cancer: the role of drinker misclassification errors in meta-analytic results. *Alcohol Clin Exp Res*. 2014;38:2297–2306.
268. Hill JA. In vino veritas: alcohol and heart disease. *Am J Med Sci*. 2005;329:124–135.
269. Thun MJ, Peto R, Lopez AD, et al. Alcohol consumption and mortality among middle aged and elderly U.S. adults. *N Engl J Med*. 1997;337:1705–1714.
270. Mukamal KJ, Chen CM, Rao SR, Breslow RA. Alcohol consumption and cardiovascular mortality among U.S. Adults, 1987 to 2002. *J Am Coll Cardiol*. 2010;55:1328–1335.
271. Hvidtfeldt UA, Tolstrup JS, Jakobsen MU, et al. Alcohol intake and risk of coronary heart disease in younger, middle-aged, and older adults. *Circulation*. 2010;121:1589–1597.
272. Costanzo S, Di Castelnuovo A, Donati MB, Iacoviello L, de Gaetano G. Alcohol consumption and mortality in patients with cardiovascular disease: a meta-analysis. *J Am Coll Cardiol*. 2010; 55:1339–1347.
273. Sun W, Schooling CM, Chan WM, Ho KS, Lam TH, Leung GM. Moderate alcohol use, health status, and mortality in a prospective Chinese elderly cohort. *Ann Epidemiol*. 2009;19:396–403.
274. Sadakane A, Gotoh T, Ishikawa S, Nakamura Y, Kayaba K. Amount and frequency of alcohol consumption and all-cause mortality in a Japanese population: the JMS cohort study. *J Epidemiol Community Health*. 2009;19:107–115.
275. Rimm EB, Williams P, Fosher K, Criqui M, Stampfer MJ. Moderate alcohol intake and lower risk of coronary artery disease: meta-analysis of effects on lipids and haemostatic factors. *Br Med J*. 1999;319:1523–1528.
276. Kloner RA, Rezkalla SH. To drink or not to drink? That is the question. *Circulation*. 2007;116:1306–1317.
277. Fernández-Solà J. Cardiovascular risks and benefits of moderate and heavy alcohol consumption. *Nat Rev Cardiol*. 2015;12: 576.
278. Gaziano JM, Gaziano TA, Glynn RJ, et al. Light-to-moderate alcohol consumption and mortality in the physicians' health study enrollment cohort. *J Am Coll Cardiol*. 2000;35:96–105.
279. Djousse L, Lee I-M, Buring JE, Gaziano JM. Alcohol consumption and risk of cardiovascular disease and death in women: potential mediating mechanisms. *Circulation*. 2009;120:237–244.
280. Klatsky AL. Alcohol and cardiovascular health. *Physiol Behav*. 2010;100:76–81.
281. Kunzmann AT, Coleman HG, Huang W-Y, Berndt SI. The association of lifetime alcohol use with mortality and cancer risk in older adults: a cohort study. *PLoS Med*. 2018;15:e1002585.
282. White IR. The level of alcohol consumption at which all-cause mortality is least. *J Clin Epidemiol*. 1999;52:967–975.
283. Millwood IY, Walters RG, Mei XW, et al. Conventional and genetic evidence on alcohol and vascular disease aetiology: a prospective study of 500 000 men and women in China. *Lancet*. 2019;393: 1831–1842.
284. Janis IL. *Air War and Emotional Stress*. Westport (CT, USA): Greenwood Press Publishers; 1951.
285. Wood AM, Kaptoge S, Butterworth AS, et al. Risk thresholds for alcohol consumption: combined analysis of individual-participant data for 599912 current drinkers in 83 prospective studies. *Lancet*. 2018;391:1513–1523.
286. Martin J, Barry J, Goggin D, Morgan K, Ward M, O'Suilleabhain T. Alcohol-attributable mortality in Ireland. *Alcohol Alcohol*. 2010;45: 379–386.
287. Snow WM, Murray R, Ekuma O, Tyas SL, Barnes GE. Alcohol use and cardiovascular health outcomes: a comparison across age and gender in the Winnipeg Health and Drinking Survey Cohort. *Age Ageing*. 2009;38:206–212.
288. Rimm EB, Klatsky A, Grobbee D, Stampfer MJ. Review of moderate alcohol consumption and reduced risk of coronary heart disease: is the effect due to beer, wine, or spirits? *Br Med J*. 1996; 312:731–736.
289. Reynolds K, Lewis LB, Nolen JDL, Kinney GL, Sathya B, He J. Alcohol consumption and risk of stroke: a meta-analysis. *J Am Med Assoc*. 2003;289:579–588.
290. Griswold MG, Fullman N, Hawley C, et al. Alcohol use and burden for 195 countries and territories, 1990–2016: a systematic analysis for the Global Burden of Disease Study 2016. *Lancet*. 2018; 392:1015–1035.
291. Voskoboinik A, Wong G, Lee G, et al. Moderate alcohol consumption is associated with atrial electrical and structural changes: insights from high-density left atrial electroanatomic mapping. *Heart Rhythm*. 2019;16:251–259.
292. Pagel PS, Kersten JR, Warltier DC. Mechanisms of myocardial protection produced by chronic ethanol consumption. *Pathophysiology*. 2004;10:121–129.
293. Collins MA, Neafsey EJ, Mukamal KJ, et al. Alcohol in moderation, cardioprotection, and neuroprotection: epidemiological considerations and mechanistic studies. *Alcohol Clin Exp Res*. 2009;33: 206–219.
294. Zheng J-P, Ju D, Jiang H, Shen J, Yang M, Li L. Resveratrol induces p53 and suppresses myocardin-mediated vascular smooth muscle cell differentiation. *Toxicol Lett*. 2010;199:115–122.
295. Bertelli AA, Das DK. Grapes, wines, resveratrol, and heart health. *J Cardiovasc Pharmacol*. 2009;54:468–476.
296. Brown L, Kroon PA, Das DK, et al. The biological responses to resveratrol and other polyphenols from alcoholic beverages. *Alcohol Clin Exp Res*. 2009;33:1513–1523.
297. Spaak J, Merlocco AC, Soleas GJ, et al. Dose-related effects of red wine and alcohol on hemodynamics, sympathetic nerve activity, and arterial diameter. *Am J Physiol Heart Circ Physiol*. 2008;294: H605–H612.
298. Spaak J, Tomlinson G, McGowan CL, et al. Dose-related effects of red wine and alcohol on heart rate variability. *Am J Physiol Heart Circ Physiol*. 2010;298:H2226–H2231.
299. Hansel B, Thomas F, Pannier B, et al. Relationship between alcohol intake, health and social status and cardiovascular risk factors in the urban Paris-Ile-De-France Cohort: is the cardioprotective action of alcohol a myth[quest]. *Eur J Clin Nutr*. 2010;64: 561–568.
300. Mortensen EL, Jensen HH, Sanders SA, Reinisch JM. Better psychological functioning and higher social status may largely

explain the apparent health benefits of wine: a study of wine and beer drinking in young Danish adults. *Arch Intern Med*. 2001;161: 1844–1848.
301. Trevisan M, Krogh V, Farinaro E. Alcohol consumption, drinking pattern and blood pressure: analysis of data from the Italian National Research Council Study. *Int J Epidemiol*. 1987;16: 520–527.
302. Tapper EB, Parikh ND. Mortality due to cirrhosis and liver cancer in the United States, 1999–2016: observational study. *Br Med J*. 2018;362:k2817.
303. Conroy DE, Ram N, Pincus AL, et al. Daily physical activity and alcohol use across the adult lifespan. *Health Psychol*. 2015;34: 653–660.
304. Kopp M, Burtscher M, Kopp-Wilfling P, et al. Is there a link between physical activity and alcohol use? *Subst Use Misuse*. 2015; 50:546–551.
305. Shuval K, Barlow CE, Chartier KG, Gabriel KP. Cardiorespiratory fitness, alcohol, and mortality in men: the Cooper Center longitudinal study. *Am J Prev Med*. 2012;42:460–467.
306. Leasure JL, Neighbors C, Henderson CE, Young CM. Exercise and alcohol consumption: what we know, what we need to know, and why it is important. *Front Psychiatry*. 2015;6:156.
307. Taylor B, Irving HM, Baliunas D, et al. Alcohol and hypertension: gender differences in dose–response relationships determined through systematic review and meta-analysis. *Addiction*. 2009; 104:1981–1990.
308. Suter PM, Vetter W. The effect of alcohol on blood pressure. *Nutr Clin Care*. 2000;3:24–34.
309. Hillbom M, Numminen H. Alcohol and stroke: pathophysiologic mechanisms. *Neuroepidemiology*. 1998;17:281–287.
310. Patra J, Taylor B, Irving H, et al. Alcohol consumption and the risk of morbidity and mortality for different stroke types – a systematic review and meta-analysis. *BMC Public Health*. 2010;10:258.
311. Fogle RL, Lynch CJ, Palopoli M, Deiter G, Stanley BA, Vary TC. Impact of chronic alcohol ingestion on cardiac muscle protein expression. *Alcohol Clin Exp Res*. 2010;34:1226–1234.
312. Han T, Zhang S, Duan W, et al. Eighteen-year alcohol consumption trajectories and their association with risk of type 2 diabetes and its related factors: the China Health and Nutrition Survey. *Diabetologia*. 2019;62:970–980.
313. Peng M, Zhang J, Zeng T, et al. Alcohol consumption and diabetes risk in a Chinese population: a Mendelian randomization analysis. *Addiction*. 2019;114:436–449.
314. Joosten MM, Chiuve SE, Mukamal K, Hu FB, Hendriks HF, Rimm EB. Changes in alcohol consumption and subsequent risk of type 2 diabetes in men. *Diabetes*. 2011;60:74–79.
315. Bantle AE, Thomas W, Bantle JP. Metabolic effects of alcohol in the form of wine in persons with type 2 diabetes mellitus. *Metabolism*. 2008;57:241–245.
316. Pietraszek A, Gregersen S, Hermansen K. Alcohol and type 2 diabetes. a review. *Nutr, Metab Cardiovas Dis*. 2010;20:366–375.
317. Li X-H, Yu F-f, Zhou Y-H, He J. Association between alcohol consumption and the risk of incident type 2 diabetes: a systematic review and dose-response meta-analysis. *Am J Clin Nutr*. 2016;103: 818–829.
318. Koloverou E, Panagiotakos DB, Pitsavos C, et al. Effects of alcohol consumption and the metabolic syndrome on 10-year incidence of diabetes: the ATTICA study. *Diabetes Metab*. 2015; 41:152–159.
319. Gepner Y, Golan R, Harman-Boehm I, et al. Effects of initiating moderate alcohol intake on cardiometabolic risk in adults with type 2 diabetes: a 2-year randomized, controlled trial two-year moderate alcohol intervention in adults with type 2 diabetes. *Ann Intern Med*. 2015;163:569–579.
320. Lai Y-J, Hu H-Y, Lee Y-L, et al. Frequency of alcohol consumption and risk of type 2 diabetes mellitus: a nationwide cohort study. *Clin Nutr*. 2019;38:1368–1372.
321. Kerr WC, Ye Y, Williams E, Lui CK, Greenfield TK, Lown EA. Lifetime alcohol use patterns and risk of diabetes onset in the national alcohol survey. *Alcohol Clin Exp Res*. 2019;43:262–269.
322. Holst C, Becker U, Jørgensen ME, Grønbæk M, Tolstrup JS. Alcohol drinking patterns and risk of diabetes: a cohort study of 70,551 men and women from the general Danish population. *Diabetologia*. 2017;60:1941–1950.
323. Kerr WC, Williams E, Li L, et al. Alcohol use patterns and risk of diabetes onset in the 1979 national longitudinal survey of youth cohort. *Prev Med*. 2018;109:22–27.
324. Knott C, Bell S, Britton A. Alcohol consumption and the risk of type 2 diabetes: a systematic review and dose-response meta-analysis of more than 1.9 million individuals from 38 observational studies. *Diabetes Care*. 2015;38:1804.
325. He X, Rebholz CM, Daya N, Lazo M, Selvin E. Alcohol consumption and incident diabetes: The Atherosclerosis Risk in Communities (ARIC) study. *Diabetologia*. 2019;62:770–778.
326. Liang W, Chikritzhs T. Alcohol consumption during adolescence and risk of diabetes in young adulthood. *BioMed Res Int*. 2014;2014:6.
327. Schrieks IC, Heil AL, Hendriks HF, Mukamal KJ, Beulens JW. The effect of alcohol consumption on insulin sensitivity and glycemic status: a systematic review and meta-analysis of intervention studies. *Diabetes Care*. 2015;38:723–732.
328. Rohwer RD, Liu S, You N-C, Buring JE, Manson JE, Song Y. Interrelationship between alcohol intake and endogenous sex-steroid hormones on diabetes risk in postmenopausal women. *J Am Coll Nutr*. 2015;34:273–280.
329. Srinivasan MP, Shawky NM, Kaphalia BS, Thangaraju M, Segar L. Alcohol-induced ketonemia is associated with lowering of blood glucose, downregulation of gluconeogenic genes, and depletion of hepatic glycogen in type 2 diabetic db/db mice. *Biochem Pharmacol*. 2019;160:46–61.
330. Niskanen L, Partonen T, Auvinen A, Haukka J. Excess mortality in Finnish diabetic subjects due to alcohol, accidents and suicide: a nationwide study. *Eur J Endocrinol*. 2018;179:299.
331. Munukutla S, Pan G, Deshpande M, Thandavarayan RA, Krishnamurthy P, Palaniyandi SS. Alcohol toxicity in diabetes and its complications: a double trouble? *Alcohol Clin Exp Res*. 2016;40:686–697.
332. Boyle M, Masson S, Anstee QM. The bidirectional impacts of alcohol consumption and the metabolic syndrome: cofactors for progressive fatty liver disease. *J Hepatol*. 2018;68:251–267.
333. Sesso HD, Cook NR, Buring JE, Manson JE, Gaziano JM. Alcohol consumption and the risk of hypertension in women and men. *Hypertension*. 2008;51:1080–1087.
334. Klatsky AL, Friedman GD, Siegelaub AB, Gérard MJ. Alcohol consumption and blood pressure: Kaiser-Permanente multiphasic health examination data. *N Engl J Med*. 1977;296:1194–1200.
335. Huntgeburth M, Ten-Freyhaus H, Rosenkranz S. Alcohol consumption and hypertension. *Curr Hypertens Rep*. 2005;7:180–185.
336. Roerecke M, Kaczorowski J, Tobe SW, Gmel G, Hasan OSM, Rehm J. The effect of a reduction in alcohol consumption on blood pressure: a systematic review and meta-analysis. *Lancet Public Health*. 2017;2:e108–e120.
337. Roerecke M, Tobe Sheldon W, Kaczorowski J, et al. Sex-specific associations between alcohol consumption and incidence of hypertension: a systematic review and meta-analysis of cohort studies. *J Am Heart Assoc*. 2018;7:e008202.
338. Briasoulis A, Agarwal V, Messerli FH. Alcohol consumption and the risk of hypertension in men and women: a systematic review and meta-analysis. *J Clin Hypertens*. 2012;14:792–798.

339. Grobbee DE, Rimm EB, Keil U, Renauld S. Alcohol and the cardiovascular system. In: Macdonald I, ed. *Health Issues Related to Alcohol Consumption*. Washington D.C: ILSI; 1999.
340. Xin X, He J, Frontini MG, Ogden LG, Motsamai OI, Whelton PK. Effects of alcohol reduction on blood pressure. *Hypertension*. 2001; 38:1112–1117.
341. Bell S, Daskalopoulou M, Rapsomaniki E, et al. Association between clinically recorded alcohol consumption and initial presentation of 12 cardiovascular diseases: population based cohort study using linked health records. *Br Med J*. 2017;356:j909.
342. Piano Mariann R, Burke L, Kang M, Phillips Shane A. Effects of repeated binge drinking on blood pressure levels and other cardiovascular health metrics in young adults: national health and nutrition examination survey, 2011–2014. *J Am Heart Assoc*. 2018;7:e008733.
343. Yoo M-G, Park KJ, Kim H-J, Jang HB, Lee H-J, Park SI. Association between alcohol intake and incident hypertension in the Korean population. *Alcohol*. 2019;77:19–25.
344. Wakabayashi I. History of antihypertensive therapy influences the relationships of alcohol with blood pressure and pulse pressure in older men. *Am J Hypertens*. 2010;23:633–638.
345. McFadden CB, Brensinger CM, Berlin JA, Townsend RR. Systematic review of the effect of daily alcohol intake on blood pressure. *Am J Hypertens*. 2005;18:276–286.
346. Ma C, Yu B, Zhang W, Wang W, Zhang L, Zeng Q. Associations between aldehyde dehydrogenase 2 (ALDH2) rs671 genetic polymorphisms, lifestyles and hypertension risk in Chinese Han people. *Sci Rep*. 2017;7:11136.
347. Ota M, Hisada A, Lu X, Nakashita C, Masuda S, Katoh T. Associations between aldehyde dehydrogenase 2 (ALDH2) genetic polymorphisms, drinking status, and hypertension risk in Japanese adult male workers: a case-control study. *Environ Health Prev Med*. 2016;21:1–8.
348. Singer J, Gustafson D, Cummings C, et al. Independent ischemic stroke risk factors in older Americans: a systematic review. *Aging*. 2019;11:3392–3407.
349. Sacco RL, Elkind M, Boden-Albala B, et al. The protective effect of moderate alcohol consumption on ischemic stroke. *J Am Med Assoc*. 1999;281:53–60.
350. Larsson SC, Wallin A, Wolk A, Markus HS. Differing association of alcohol consumption with different stroke types: a systematic review and meta-analysis. *BMC Med*. 2016;14:178.
351. Lacey B, Lewington S, Clarke R, et al. Age-specific association between blood pressure and vascular and non-vascular chronic diseases in 0·5 million adults in China: a prospective cohort study. *Lancet Global Health*. 2018;6:e641–e649.
352. Holmes MV, Dale CE, Zuccolo L, et al. Association between alcohol and cardiovascular disease: Mendelian randomisation analysis based on individual participant data. *Br Med J*. 2014; 349:g4164.
353. Duan Y, Wang A, Wang Y, et al. Cumulative alcohol consumption and stroke risk in men. *J Neurol*. 2019;266(9):2112–2119.
354. Mostofsky E, Burger MR, Schlaug G, Mukamal KJ, Rosamond WD, Mittleman MA. Alcohol and acute ischemic stroke onset: the stroke onset study. *Stroke*. 2010;41: 1845–1849.
355. Shiotsuki H, Saijo Y, Ogushi Y, Kobayashi S. Relationships between alcohol intake and ischemic stroke severity in sex stratified analysis for Japanese acute stroke patients. *J Stroke Cerebrovasc Dis*. 2019;28:1604–1617.
356. Bazal P, Gea A, Martínez-González MA, et al. Mediterranean alcohol-drinking pattern, low to moderate alcohol intake and risk of atrial fibrillation in the PREDIMED study. *Nutr Metab Cardiovasc Dis*. 2019;29:676–683.
357. Conen D, Tedrow UB, Cook NR, Moorthy MV, Buring JE, Albert CM. Alcohol consumption and risk of incident atrial fibrillation in women. *J Am Med Assoc*. 2008;300:2489–2496.
358. Klatsky AL, Armstrong MA, Kipp H. Correlates of alcoholic beverage preference: traits of persons who choose wine, liquor or beer. *Br J Addict*. 1990;85:1279–1289.
359. Tjonneland A, Gronbæk M, Stripp C, Overvad K. Wine intake and diet in a random sample of 48763 Danish men and women. *Am J Clin Nutr*. 1999;69:49–54.
360. Rouillier P, Boutron-Ruault MC, Bertrais S, et al. Drinking patterns in French adult men—a cluster analysis of alcoholic beverages and relationship with lifestyle. *Eur J Nutr*. 2004;43: 69–76.
361. Mizrahi A, Knekt P, Montonen J, Laaksonen MA, Heliövaara M, Järvine R. Plant foods and the risk of cerebrovascular diseases: a potential protection of fruit consumption. *Br J Nutr*. 2009;102: 1075–1083.
362. Lock K, Pomerleau J, Causer L, Altmann DR, McKee M. The global burden of disease attributable to low consumption of fruit and vegetables: implications for the global strategy on diet. *Bull World Health Organ*. 2005;83:100–108.
363. Du H, Li L, Bennett D, et al. Fresh fruit consumption and major cardiovascular disease in China. *N Engl J Med*. 2016;374: 1332–1343.
364. Aune D, Giovannucci E, Boffetta P, et al. Fruit and vegetable intake and the risk of cardiovascular disease, total cancer and all-cause mortality-a systematic review and dose-response meta-analysis of prospective studies. *Int J Epidemiol*. 2017;46:1029–1056.
365. Stampfer MJ, Kang JH, Chen J, Cherry R, Grodstein F. Effects of moderate alcohol consumption on cognitive function in women. *N Engl J Med*. 2005;352:245–253.
366. Brust JCM. Ethanol and cognition: indirect effects, neurotoxicity and neuroprotection: a review. *Int J Environ Res Public Health*. 2010;7:1540–1557.
367. Mende MA. Alcohol in the aging brain – the interplay between alcohol consumption, cognitive decline and the cardiovascular system. *Front Neurosci*. 2019;13.
368. Liu Y, Mitsuhashi T, Yamakawa M, et al. Alcohol consumption and incident dementia in older Japanese adults: the Okayama study. *Geriatr Gerontol Int*. 2019;19:740–746.
369. Gross AL, Rebok GW, Ford DE, et al. Alcohol consumption and domain-specific cognitive function in older adults: longitudinal data from the Johns Hopkins precursors study. *J Gerontol Psychol Sci*. 2010;66B(1):39–47. https://doi.org/10.1093/geronb/gbq062.
370. Panza F, Capurso C, D'Introno A, et al. Alcohol drinking, cognitive functions in older age, predementia, and dementia syndromes. *J Alzheimer's Dis*. 2009;17:7–31.
371. Rehm J, Hasan OSM, Black SE, Shield KD, Schwarzinger M. Alcohol use and dementia: a systematic scoping review. *Alzheimer's Res Ther*. 2019;11:1.
372. Thursz M, Kamath PS, Mathurin P, Szabo G, Shah VH. Alcohol-related liver disease: areas of consensus, unmet needs and opportunities for further study. *J Hepatol*. 2019;70:521–530.
373. Hydes T, Gilmore W, Sheron N, Gilmore I. Treating alcohol-related liver disease from a public health perspective. *J Hepatol*. 2019;70:223–236.
374. Ganne-Carrié N, Nahon P. Hepatocellular carcinoma in the setting of alcohol-related liver disease. *J Hepatol*. 2019;70:284–293.
375. Simpson RF, Hermon C, Liu B, et al. Alcohol drinking patterns and liver cirrhosis risk: analysis of the prospective UK Million Women Study. *Lancet Public Health*. 2019;4:e41–e48.
376. Britton A, Mehta G, O'Neill D, Bell S. Association of thirty-year alcohol consumption typologies and fatty liver: findings from a large population cohort study. *Drug Alcohol Depend*. 2019;194:225–229.

377. Mukherji A, Bailey SM, Staels B, Baumert TF. The circadian clock and liver function in health and disease. *J Hepatol*. 2019;71: 200–211.
378. Greuter T, Malhi H, Gores GJ, Shah VH. Therapeutic opportunities for alcoholic steatohepatitis and nonalcoholic steatohepatitis: exploiting similarities and differences in pathogenesis. *JCI Insight*. 2017;2:e95354.
379. Brar G, Tsukamoto H. Alcoholic and non-alcoholic steatohepatitis: global perspective and emerging science. *J Gastroenterol*. 2019;54:218–225.
380. Parker R, Kim S-J, Gao B. Alcohol, adipose tissue and liver disease: mechanistic links and clinical considerations. *Nat Rev Gastro Hepat*. 2017;15:50.
381. Louvet A, Mathurin P. Alcoholic liver disease: mechanisms of injury and targeted treatment. *Nat Rev Gastro Hepat*. 2015;12: 231.
382. Ohashi K, Pimienta M, Seki E. Alcoholic liver disease: a current molecular and clinical perspective. *Liver Res*. 2018;2:161–172.
383. Tolefree JA, Garcia AJ, Farrell J, et al. Alcoholic liver disease and mast cells: what's your gut got to do with it? *Liver Res*. 2019;3: 46–54.
384. Yang Z, Kusumanchi P, Ross RA, et al. Serum metabolomic profiling identifies key metabolic signatures associated with pathogenesis of alcoholic liver disease in humans. *Hepatol Commun*. 2019;3:542–557.
385. Seitz HK, Bataller R, Cortez-Pinto H, et al. Alcoholic liver disease. *Nat Rev Dis Primer*. 2018;4:16.
386. Aljomah G, Baker SS, Liu W, et al. Induction of CYP2E1 in nonalcoholic fatty liver diseases. *Exp Mol Pathol*. 2015;99:677–681.
387. Osna NA, Donohue Jr TM, Kharbanda KK. Alcoholic liver disease: pathogenesis and current management. *Alcohol Res*. 2017; 38:147–161.
388. Malhi H, Guicciardi ME, Gores GJ. Hepatocyte death: a clear and present danger. *Physiol Rev*. 2010;90:1165–1194.
389. Neuman GM, Maor Y, Nanau MR, et al. Alcoholic liver disease: role of cytokines. *Biomolecules*. 2015;5.
390. Diehl AM. Recent events in alcoholic liver disease V. Effects of ethanol on liver regeneration. *Am J Physiol Gastrointest Liver Physiol*. 2005;288:G1–G6.
391. O'Shea RS, Dasarathy S, McCullough AJ. Alcoholic liver disease. *Hepatology*. 2010;51:307–328.
392. Halsted CH. Nutrition and alcoholic liver disease. *Semin Liver Dis*. 2004;24:289–304.
393. Askgaard G, Grønbæk M, Kjær MS, Tjønneland A, Tolstrup JS. Alcohol drinking pattern and risk of alcoholic liver cirrhosis: a prospective cohort study. *J Hepatol*. 2015;62:1061–1067.
394. Sheron N. Alcohol and liver disease in Europe – simple measures have the potential to prevent tens of thousands of premature deaths. *J Hepatol*. 2016;64:957–967.
395. Joshi K, Kohli A, Manch R, Gish R. Alcoholic liver disease: high risk or low risk for developing hepatocellular carcinoma? *Clin Liver Dis*. 2016;20:563–580.
396. Ayubi E, Safiri S, Sani M, Khazaei S, Mansori K. Heavy daily alcohol intake at the population level predicts the weight of alcohol in cirrhosis burden worldwide: methodological issues of confounding and prediction models. *J Hepatol*. 2017;66:864–865.
397. Stein E, Cruz-Lemini M, Altamirano J, et al. Heavy daily alcohol intake at the population level predicts the weight of alcohol in cirrhosis burden worldwide. *J Hepatol*. 2016;65:998–1005.
398. Mendenhall C, Roselle GA, Gartside P, Moritz T. The veterans administration cooperative study G. Relationship of protein calorie malnutrition to alcoholic liver disease: a reexamination of data from two veterans administration cooperative studies. *Alcohol Clin Exp Res*. 1995;19:635–641.
399. Kallwitz ER. Sarcopenia and liver transplant: the relevance of too little muscle mass. *World J Gastroenterol*. 2015;21:10982–10993.
400. Ajmera VH, Terrault NA, Harrison SA. Is moderate alcohol use in nonalcoholic fatty liver disease good or bad? A critical review. *Hepatology*. 2017;65:2090–2099.
401. Carter AR, Borges M-C, Benn M, et al. Combined association of body mass index and alcohol consumption with biomarkers for liver injury and incidence of liver disease: a mendelian randomization study association of BMI and alcohol with biomarkers for liver injury and incidence of liver disease association of BMI and alcohol with biomarkers for liver injury and incidence of liver disease. *JAMA Netw Open*. 2019;2. e190305-(e).
402. World Cancer Research Fund/American Institute for Cancer Research. Continuous Update Project Expert Report 2018. Alcoholic drinks and the risk of cancer. Available at dietandcancerreport.org
403. Szabo G. Women and alcoholic liver disease — warning of a silent danger. *Nat Rev Gastro Hepat*. 2018;15:253.
404. Kawakita D, Matsuo K. Alcohol and head and neck cancer. *Cancer Metastasis Rev*. 2017;36:425–434.
405. McNabb S, Harrison TA, Albanes D, et al. Meta-analysis of 16 studies of the association of alcohol with colorectal cancer. *Int J Cancer*. 2019;0.
406. Seitz HK, Stickel F. Molecular mechanisms of alcohol-mediated carcinogenesis. *Nat Rev Cancer*. 2007;7:599–612.
407. Scoccianti C, Cecchini M, Anderson AS, et al. European code against cancer 4th edition: alcohol drinking and cancer. *Cancer Epidemiol*. 2015;39:S67–S74.
408. Ma K, Baloch Z, He T-T, Xia X. Alcohol consumption and gastric cancer risk: a meta-analysis. *Med Sci Monit*. 2017;23:238–246.
409. Ferro A, Morais S, Rota M, et al. Alcohol intake and gastric cancer: meta-analyses of published data versus individual participant data pooled analyses (StoP Project). *Cancer Epidemiol*. 2018;54: 125–132.
410. Bagnardi V, Rota M, Botteri E, et al. Alcohol consumption and site-specific cancer risk: a comprehensive dose–response meta-analysis. *Br J Canc*. 2014;112:580.
411. National Toxicology Program (NTP). Report on Carcinogens. 14th ed. Research Triangle Park, NC: U.S. Department of Health and Human Services, Public Health Service. https://ntp.niehs.nih.gov/go/roc14 2016.
412. Seitz HK, Stickel F. Acetaldehyde as an underestimated risk factor for cancer development: role of genetics in ethanol metabolism. *Genes Nutr*. 2010;5:121–128.
413. Nieminen MT, Salaspuro M. Local acetaldehyde—an essential role in alcohol-related upper gastrointestinal tract carcinogenesis. *Cancers*. 2018;10:11.
414. Bradbury KE, Murphy N, Key TJ. Diet and colorectal cancer in UK Biobank: a prospective study. *Int J Epidemiol*. 2019:1–13.
415. Cheng G, Xie L. Alcohol intake and risk of renal cell carcinoma: a meta-analysis of published case-control studies. *Arch Med Sci*. 2011;7:648–657.
416. Tramacere I, Pelucchi C, Bonifazi M, et al. Alcohol drinking and non-Hodgkin lymphoma risk: a systematic review and a meta-analysis. *Ann Oncol*. 2012;23:2791–2798.
417. Mizumoto A, Ohashi S, Hirohashi K, Amanuma Y, Matsuda T, Muto M. Molecular mechanisms of acetaldehyde-mediated carcinogenesis in squamous epithelium. *Int J Mol Sci*. 2017;18.
418. Yang S, Lee J, Park Y, et al. Interaction between alcohol consumption and methylenetetrahydrofolate reductase polymorphisms in thyroid cancer risk: national cancer center cohort in Korea. *Sci Rep*. 2018;8:4077.
419. Li CI, Chlebowski RT, Freiberg M, et al. Alcohol consumption and risk of postmenopausal breast cancer by subtype: the women's

health initiative observational study. *J Natl Cancer Inst*. 2010;102: 1422–1431.
420. Zhang SM, Lee IM, Manson JE, Cook NR, Willett WC, Buring JE. Alcohol consumption and breast cancer risk in the women's health study. *Am J Epidemiol*. 2007;165:667–676.
421. Jung S, Wang M, Anderson K, et al. Alcohol consumption and breast cancer risk by estrogen receptor status: in a pooled analysis of 20 studies. *Int J Epidemiol*. 2015;45:916–928.
422. Baglia ML, Cook LS, Mei-Tzu C, et al. Alcohol, smoking, and risk of Her2-overexpressing and triple-negative breast cancer relative to estrogen receptor-positive breast cancer. *Int J Cancer*. 2018;143: 1849–1857.
423. Kwan ML, Kushi LH, Weltzien E, et al. Alcohol consumption and breast cancer recurrence and survival among women with early-stage breast cancer: the life after cancer epidemiology study. *J Clin Oncol*. 2010;28:4410–4416.
424. Shield KD, Soerjomataram I, Rehm J. Alcohol use and breast cancer: a critical review. *Alcohol Clin Exp Res*. 2016;40:1166–1181.
425. Onland-Moret NC, Peeters PH, van der Schouw YT, Grobbee DE, van Gils CH. Alcohol and endogenous sex steroid levels in postmenopausal women: a cross-sectional study. *J Clin Endocrinol Metab*. 2005;90:1414–1419.
426. Scheideler JK, Klein WMP. Awareness of the link between alcohol consumption and cancer across the world: a review. *Cancer Epidem Biomar & Prev*. 2018;27:429.
427. Lizama N, Rogers P, Thomson A, et al. Women's beliefs about breast cancer causation in a breast cancer case–control study. *Psycho Oncol*. 2016;25:36–42.
428. Sinclair J, McCann M, Sheldon E, Gordon I, Brierley-Jones L, Copson E. The acceptability of addressing alcohol consumption as a modifiable risk factor for breast cancer: a mixed method study within breast screening services and symptomatic breast clinics. *BMJ Open*. 2019;9:e027371.
429. Petticrew M, Maani Hessari N, Knai C, Weiderpass E. How alcohol industry organisations mislead the public about alcohol and cancer. *Drug Alcohol Rev*. 2018;37:293–303.
430. Liu Y, Nguyen N, Colditz GA. Links between alcohol consumption and breast cancer: a look at the evidence. *Women's Health*. 2015;11:65–77.
431. Thibaut F. Alert out on tobacco and alcohol consumption in young European women. *Eur Arch Psychiatry Clin Neurosci*. 2018;268:317–319.
432. Hamajima N, Hirose K, Tajima K, et al. Alcohol, tobacco and breast cancer – collaborative reanalysis of individual data from 53 epidemiological studies, including 58 515 women with breast cancer and 95 067 women without the disease. *Br J Canc*. 2002; 87:1234–1245.
433. Hydes TJ, Burton R, Inskip H, Bellis MA, Sheron N. A comparison of gender-linked population cancer risks between alcohol and tobacco: how many cigarettes are there in a bottle of wine? *BMC Public Health*. 2019;19:316.
434. Pflaum T, Hausler T, Baumung C, et al. Carcinogenic compounds in alcoholic beverages: an update. *Arch Toxicol*. 2016;90:2349–2367.
435. Okaru AO, Rehm J, Sommerfeld K, Kuballa T, Walch SG, Lachenmeier DW. 1 – The threat to quality of alcoholic beverages by unrecorded consumption. In: Grumezescu AM, Holban AM, eds. *Alcoholic Beverages*. Woodhead Publishing; 2019:1–34.
436. Masaoka H, Ito H, Soga N, et al. Aldehyde dehydrogenase 2 (ALDH2) and alcohol dehydrogenase 1B (ADH1B) polymorphisms exacerbate bladder cancer risk associated with alcohol drinking: gene–environment interaction. *Carcinogenesis*. 2016;37: 583–588.
437. Ishioka K, Masaoka H, Ito H, et al. Association between ALDH2 and ADH1B polymorphisms, alcohol drinking and gastric cancer: a replication and mediation analysis. *Gastric Cancer*. 2018;21: 936–945.
438. Suo C, Yang Y, Yuan Z, et al. Alcohol intake interacts with functional genetic polymorphisms of aldehyde dehydrogenase (ALDH2) and alcohol dehydrogenase (ADH) to increase esophageal squamous cell cancer risk. *J Thorac Oncol*. 2019;14:712–725.
439. Zhuo X, Song J, Li D, Wu Y, Zhou Q. MTHFR C677T polymorphism interaction with heavy alcohol consumption increases head and neck carcinoma risk. *Sci Rep*. 2015;5:10671.
440. Kim HJ, Jung S, Eliassen AH, Chen WY, Willett WC, Cho E. Alcohol consumption and breast cancer risk in younger women according to family history of breast cancer and folate intake. *Am J Epidemiol*. 2017;186:524–531.
441. Simon L, Jolley SE, Molina PE. Alcoholic myopathy: pathophysiologic mechanisms and clinical implications. *Alcohol Res*. 2017;38: 207–217.
442. Sahni S, Mangano KM, McLean RR, Hannan MT, Kiel DP. Dietary approaches for bone health: lessons from the Framingham osteoporosis study. *Curr Osteoporos Rep*. 2015;13:245–255.
443. Fung TT, Mukamal KJ, Rimm EB, Meyer HE, Willett WC, Feskanich D. Alcohol intake, specific alcoholic beverages, and risk of hip fractures in postmenopausal women and men age 50 and older. *Am J Clin Nutr*. 2019;110(3):691–700.
444. Cheraghi Z, Doosti-Irani A, Almasi-Hashiani A, et al. The effect of alcohol on osteoporosis: a systematic review and meta-analysis. *Drug Alcohol Depend*. 2019;197:197–202.
445. Gaddini GW, Turner RT, Grant KA, Iwaniec UT. Alcohol: a simple nutrient with complex actions on bone in the adult skeleton. *Alcohol Clin Exp Res*. 2016;40:657–671.
446. Venkat KK, Arora MM, Singh P, Desai M, Khatkhatay I. Effect of alcohol consumption on bone mineral density and hormonal parameters in physically active male soldiers. *Bone*. 2009;45: 449–454.
447. L.H. Jin, S.J. Chang, S.B. Koh and et al., Association between Alcohol Consumption and Bone Strength in Korean Adults: The Korean Genomic Rural Cohort Study, Metabolism 60, 351–358
448. Feskanich D, Korrick SA, Greenspan SL, Rosen NH, Colditz GA. Moderate alcohol consumption and bone density among postmenopausal women. *J Women's Health*. 1999;8:65–73.
449. Tucker KL, Jugdaohsingh R, Powell JJ, et al. Effects of beer, wine, and liquor intakes on bone mineral density in older men and women. *Am J Clin Nutr*. 2009;89:1188–1196.
450. LaBrie JW, Boyle S, Earle A, Almstedt HC. Heavy episodic drinking is associated with poorer bone health in adolescent and young adult women. *J Stud Alcohol Drugs*. 2018;79:391–398.
451. Luo Z, Liu Y, Liu Y, Chen H, Shi S, Liu Y. Cellular and molecular mechanisms of alcohol-induced osteopenia. *Cell Mol Life Sci*. 2017; 74:4443–4453.
452. Noble N, Paul C, Turon H, Oldmeadow C. Which modifiable health risk behaviours are related? A systematic review of the clustering of Smoking, Nutrition, Alcohol and Physical activity ('SNAP') health risk factors. *Prev Med*. 2015;81:16–41.
453. Cruel M, Granke M, Bosser C, Audran M, Hoc T. Chronic alcohol abuse in men alters bone mechanical properties by affecting both tissue mechanical properties and microarchitectural parameters. *Morphologie*. 2017;101:88–96.
454. Maurel DB, Boisseau N, Benhamou CL, Jaffre C. Alcohol and bone: review of dose effects and mechanisms. *Osteoporos Int*. 2012;23:1–16.
455. Laitinen K, Valimaki M. Bone and the 'comforts of life'. *Ann Med*. 1993;25:413–425.
456. Jang H-D, Hong J-Y, Han K, et al. Relationship between bone mineral density and alcohol intake: a nationwide health survey analysis of postmenopausal women. *PLoS One*. 2017;12. e0180132-(e).
457. Ortolá R, García-Esquinas E, Galán I, et al. Patterns of alcohol consumption and risk of falls in older adults: a prospective cohort study. *Osteoporos Int*. 2017;28:3143–3152.

458. Chang VC, Do MT. Risk factors for falls among seniors: implications of gender. *Am J Epidemiol*. 2015;181:521–531.
459. Nakahara T, Hashimoto K, Hirano M, Koll M, Martin CR, Preedy VR. Acute and chronic effects of alcohol exposure on skeletal muscle c-myc, p53, and Bcl-2 mRNA expression. *Am J Physiol Endocrinol Metab*. 2003;285:E1273–E1281.
460. Preedy VR, Ohlendieck K, Adachi J, et al. The importance of alcohol-induced muscle disease. *J Muscle Res Motil*. 2003;24:55–63.
461. Steiner JL, Lang CH. Dysregulation of skeletal muscle protein metabolism by alcohol. *Am J Physiol Endocrinol Metab*. 2015;308: E699–E712.
462. Steiner JL, Kimball SR, Lang CH. Acute alcohol-induced decrease in muscle protein synthesis in female mice is REDD-1 and mTOR-independent. *Alcohol Alcohol*. 2016;51:242–250.
463. Vary TC, Frost RA, Lang CH. Acute alcohol intoxication increases atrogin-1 and MuRF1 mRNA without increasing proteolysis in skeletal muscle. *Am J Physiol Regul Integr Comp Physiol*. 2008;294: R1777–R1789.
464. Laonigro I, Correale M, Di Biase M, Altomare E. Alcohol abuse and heart failure. *Eur J Heart Fail*. 2009;11:453–462.
465. Piano MR. Alcoholic cardiomyopathy. *J Am Coll Cardiol*. 2018;71: 2303.
466. Steiner JL, Lang CH. Etiology of alcoholic cardiomyopathy: mitochondria, oxidative stress and apoptosis. *Int J Biochem Cell Biol*. 2017;89:125–135.
467. Dejong K, Olyaei A, Lo JO. Alcohol use in pregnancy. *Clin Obstet Gynecol*. 2019;62:142–155.
468. Denny L, Coles S, Blitz R. Fetal alcohol syndrome and fetal alcohol spectrum disorders. *Am Fam Physician*. 2017;96:515–522.
469. Calhoun F, Warren K. Fetal alcohol syndrome: historical perspectives. *Neurosci Biobehav Rev*. 2007;31:168–171.
470. Plant ML, Abel EL, Guerri C. Alcohol and pregnancy. In: Macdonald I, ed. *Health Issues Related to Alcohol Consumption*. Washington D.C: ILSI; 1999:182–213.
471. Georgieff MK, Tran PV, Carlson ES. Atypical fetal development: fetal alcohol syndrome, nutritional deprivation, teratogens, and risk for neurodevelopmental disorders and psychopathology. *Dev Psychopathol*. 2018;30:1063–1086.
472. Popova S, Lange S, Shield K, et al. Comorbidity of fetal alcohol spectrum disorder: a systematic review and meta-analysis. *Lancet*. 2016;387:978–987.
473. Popova S, Lange S, Probst C, Gmel G, Rehm J. Estimation of national, regional, and global prevalence of alcohol use during pregnancy and fetal alcohol syndrome: a systematic review and meta-analysis. *Lancet Global Health*. 2017;5:e290–e299.
474. Denny CH, Acero CS, Naimi TS, Kim SY. Consumption of alcohol beverages and binge drinking among pregnant women aged 18–44 years — United States, 2015–2017. *Morb Mortal Wkly Rep*. 2019;68:365–368.
475. Agrawal A, Rogers CE, Lessov-Schlaggar CN, Carter EB, Lenze SN, Grucza RA. Alcohol, cigarette, and cannabis use between 2002 and 2016 in pregnant women from a nationally representative sample evaluation of alcohol, cigarette, and cannabis use between 2002 and 2016 in pregnant women letters. *JAMA Pediatrics*. 2019;173:95–96.
476. Friedrich MJ. Subpopulations are vulnerable to fetal alcohol spectrum disorder subpopulations are vulnerable to fetal alcohol spectrum disorder global health. *J Am Med Assoc*. 2019; 321:2273.
477. Symons M, Pedruzzi RA, Bruce K, Milne E. A systematic review of prevention interventions to reduce prenatal alcohol exposure and fetal alcohol spectrum disorder in indigenous communities. *BMC Public Health*. 2018;18:1227.
478. O'Leary CM, Nassar N, Kurinczuk JJ, et al. Prenatal alcohol exposure and risk of birth defects. *Pediatrics*. 2010;126: e843–e850.
479. Hofer R, Burd L. Review of published studies of kidney, liver, and gastrointestinal birth defects in fetal alcohol spectrum disorders. *Birth Defects Res Part A Clin Mol Teratol*. 2009;85:179–183.
480. Petrelli B, Bendelac L, Hicks GG, Fainsod A. Insights into retinoic acid deficiency and the induction of craniofacial malformations and microcephaly in fetal alcohol spectrum disorder. *Genesis*. 2019;57:e23278.
481. Shukrun N, Shabtai Y, Pillemer G, Fainsod A. Retinoic acid signaling reduction recapitulates the effects of alcohol on embryo size. *Genesis*. 2019;57:e23284.
482. Zuccolo L, DeRoo LA, Wills AK, et al. Pre-conception and prenatal alcohol exposure from mothers and fathers drinking and head circumference: results from the Norwegian Mother-Child Study (MoBa). *Sci Rep*. 2016;6:39535.
483. Chang RC, Wang H, Bedi Y, Golding MC. Preconception paternal alcohol exposure exerts sex-specific effects on offspring growth and long-term metabolic programming. *Epigenet Chromatin*. 2019;12:9.
484. Rompala GR, Homanics GE. Intergenerational effects of alcohol: a review of paternal preconception ethanol exposure studies and epigenetic mechanisms in the male germline. *Alcohol Clin Exp Res*. 2019;43:1032–1045.
485. Maluenda F, Csendes A, De Aretxabala X, et al. Alcohol absorption modification after a laparoscopic sleeve gastrectomy due to obesity. *Obes Surg*. 2010;20:744–748.
486. Bal B, Koch TR, Finelli FC, Sarr MG. Managing medical and surgical disorders after divided Roux-en-Y gastric bypass surgery. *Nat Rev Gastro Hepat*. 2010;7(6):320–324 (advance online publication).
487. Mitchell JE, Lancaster KL, Burgard MA, et al. Long-term follow-up of patients' status after gastric bypass. *Obes Surg*. 2001;11:464–468.
488. Blackburn AN, Hajnal A, Leggio L. The gut in the brain: the effects of bariatric surgery on alcohol consumption. *Addict Biol*. 2017;22:1540–1553.
489. Ibrahim N, Alameddine M, Brennan J, Sessine M, Holliday C, Ghaferi AA. New onset alcohol use disorder following bariatric surgery. *Surg Endosc*. 2018;33:2521–2530.
490. Parikh M, Johnson JM, Ballem N. ASMBS position statement on alcohol use before and after bariatric surgery. *Surg Obes Relat Dis*. 2016;12:225–230.
491. Alizai PH, Akkerman MK, Kaemmer D, et al. Presurgical assessment of bariatric patients with the Patient Health Questionnaire (PHQ)—a screening of the prevalence of psychosocial comorbidity. *Health Qual Life Outcomes*. 2015;13:80.
492. Testino G, Fagoonee S. Alcohol use disorders and bariatric surgery. *Obes Surg*. 2018;28:3304–3305.
493. Mandal C, Halder D, Jung KH, Chai YG. In utero alcohol exposure and the alteration of histone marks in the developing fetus: an epigenetic phenomenon of maternal drinking. *Int J Biol Sci*. 2017;13:1100–1108.
494. Gilmore W, Chikritzhs T, Stockwell T, Jernigan D, Naimi T, Gilmore I. Alcohol: taking a population perspective. *Nat Rev Gastro Hepat*. 2016;13:426.
495. Suter PM, Häsler E, Vetter W. Effects of alcohol on energy metabolism and body weight regulation: is alcohol a risk factor for obesity? *Nutr Rev*. 1997;55:157–171.

CHAPTER

26

LIVER DISEASE

Craig James McClain[1,2,3,4], MD
Laura Smart[1], MD
Sarah Safadi[1], MD
Irina Kirpich[1,3], PhD

[1]Division of Gastroenterology, Hepatology and Nutrition, Department of Medicine, University of Louisville, Louisville, KY, United States
[2]Robley Rex VA Medical Center, Louisville, KY, United States
[3]University of Louisville Alcohol Research Center, Louisville, KY, United States
[4]Department of Pharmacology & Toxicology, University of Louisville, Louisville, KY, United States

SUMMARY

The liver is the largest and most complex metabolic organ of the body. It performs critical functions for anabolism, detoxification, immune regulation/tolerance, and protection from gut-derived toxins. Advanced liver disease is strongly associated with malnutrition, and the severity of malnutrition correlates with the development of complications of liver disease, as well as mortality and poor outcome following liver transplantation. Optimal nutritional support can improve malnutrition in patients with liver disease and may decrease infectious complications, improve cognitive function, and in some instances, even decrease mortality. Obesity with "insulin resistance" is also a wide-spread problem and frequently leads to nonalcoholic fatty liver disease (NAFLD), and in some instances, nonalcoholic steatohepatitis (NASH) and cirrhosis. Dietary modification and vitamin E supplementation, lifestyle modification, and bariatric surgery have all been shown to improve the hepatic steatosis/liver histology in NASH. In this chapter, we review important interactions between nutrition and various types/stages of liver disease.

Keywords: Liver disease; Malnutrition; Microbiome; Nutrition assessment.

I. NORMAL FUNCTION AND PHYSIOLOGY

The liver is the largest organ in the body, weighing approximately 1.5 kg in adults, and it is possibly the most complex organ in terms of metabolism. It has a unique dual blood supply, being perfused by both the portal vein and hepatic artery, and is comprised of multiple unique cell types having differing functions as described below.

Hepatocytes make up over 80% of total liver mass and 65% of the total number of cells in the liver. Hepatocytes perform multiple critical functions, including metabolism of amino acids and ammonia, biochemical oxidation reactions, detoxification of a variety of drugs, bile acid metabolism, storage of glycogen and certain vitamins (e.g., vitamin B12), and hormone production/metabolism, to name a few. Hepatocytes can be identified by their synthesis of certain proteins such as albumin and α-fetoprotein.

Kupffer cells represent the largest reservoir of fixed macrophages in the body. They comprise over 80% of the tissue macrophages in the body and about 15% of hepatic cells. They play a protective role against gut-derived

https://doi.org/10.1016/B978-0-12-818460-8.00026-5

toxins that have escaped into the portal circulation and in immune surveillance. They are also a major producer of cytokines, which can markedly influence nutritional status.

Stellate cells are major fat-storing cells and are a reservoir for vitamin A in the body. They play an important role in collagen formation during liver injury. When stellate cells are activated by various factors such as cytokines (e.g., transforming growth factor beta), they transform into myofibroblasts with loss of vitamin A and increased expression of genes responsible for collagen production and hepatic fibrosis.

Specialized liver endothelial cells line the hepatic sinusoids. These cells are fenestrated, and the fenestrations allow the passage of macromolecules such as lipoproteins. Subendothelial deposition of collagen and "capillarization of the sinusoids" may reduce nutrient transport across the sinusoids in advanced liver disease. Sinusoidal endothelial cells differ from continuous endothelial cells in the proteins they express, including higher levels of CD32, lipopolysaccharide-binding protein receptor (CD14), and CD36, to name only a few. These cells are also capable of endocytosis. The endothelial cell is highly susceptible to injury by factors such as endotoxemia and hypotension.

Cholangiocytes are epithelial cells that line the bile ducts, and they play an important role in solute transport and bile acid composition/metabolism. When activated, they secrete cytokines and participate in cross talk with the innate and adaptive immune system. Cholangiocytes can also participate in liver regeneration.

The liver is a central organ for nutrition and metabolism. The liver plays a vital role in protein, carbohydrate, and fat metabolism as well as micronutrient metabolism. It synthesizes plasma proteins, nonessential amino acids, urea (for ammonia excretion), glycogen, and critical hormones such as the anabolic molecule, insulin-like growth factor 1 (IGF-1). The liver is a major site for fatty acid metabolism, and bile synthesized in the liver is needed for fat absorption from the intestine. Thus, it is obvious that normal hepatic function is important for proper nutrition.

A strong association exists between advanced liver disease and malnutrition. However, malnutrition is not always recognized in patients with liver disease, at least in part because weight loss in these patients can be masked by fluid retention. The loss of glycogen stores predisposes patients with advanced liver disease to enter into a starvation state within a few hours of fasting that can lead to further protein catabolism and loss of function. Therefore, it is important to recognize malnutrition and initiate nutrition support early in these patients. Moreover, obesity and the metabolic syndrome are increasingly recognized as a major cause of abnormal liver enzymes and a spectrum of NAFLD. Thus, both undernutrition and obesity can play important roles in liver disease.

This chapter reviews the interactions between nutrition and liver disease and the role for nutritional intervention in liver disease. We begin with a discussion of the pathophysiology of liver disease (focusing on nutritional aspects). We present an overview of the prevalence, causes, and assessment of malnutrition in liver disease and the role of diet in the onset of liver disease. We then review primary treatment modalities with a focus on nutritional support, including specialized liver problems such as those related to obesity and liver transplantation. Lastly, we touch on selected drug/nutrient interactions and gaps in our knowledge.

II. PATHOPHYSIOLOGY

A. Abnormal Physiology and Function

Overview of liver disease

Liver disease is a growing problem in the United States and worldwide. Indeed, approximately 25% of the United States and world populations have NAFLD, and NAFLD is the greatest cause of abnormal liver enzymes in the United States. Alcoholic liver disease (ALD) also remains a major health problem and is increasing in the United States. Viral liver disease, a third major cause of liver disease, now has effective treatment. New direct-acting antiviral agents (DAAs) cure most cases of hepatitis C, and there are multiple agents that treat but generally do not cure hepatitis B. Importantly, large numbers of patients with cirrhosis due to hepatitis B/C are still at risk for liver failure and hepatocellular carcinoma (HCC). Some environmental exposures directly cause liver disease (can be histologically identical to NASH and alcoholic steatohepatitis) and can interact with the other above-noted forms of liver disease. Cirrhosis is the final stage of most chronic liver disease, and it is characterized by fibrosis and distortion of the hepatic architecture along with formation of regenerative nodules. It may be complicated by such resource-intensive and morbid problems as hepatic encephalopathy (HE), GI bleeding, renal failure, and infections. During the past approximate 15 years, annual deaths from cirrhosis have increased by 65% and deaths from HCC have doubled.[1] Below, we discuss prevalence, assessment and causes of malnutrition, and mechanisms of liver injury that have important links with nutrition.

Prevalence and assessment of malnutrition in liver disease

The most extensive studies of nutritional status in patients with liver disease are in those with ALD. Two early large studies in the Veterans Health Administration (VA) Cooperative Studies Program evaluated patients with alcoholic hepatitis (AH).[2–5] The first study demonstrated that virtually every patient with AH had some degree of malnutrition.[4] Patients (284 with complete nutritional assessments) were divided into groups with mild, moderate, or sAH based on clinical and biochemical parameters. Patients had a mean alcohol consumption of 228 g/d (almost 50% of energy intake from alcohol). The severity of liver disease was generally correlated with the severity of malnutrition. Similar data were generated in the 1993 follow-up VA study.[5]

In both of these studies, patients were given a balanced, 2500 kcal/d (10.5 MJ) hospital diet, monitored carefully by a dietitian, and encouraged to consume the study diet. In the second study, patients in the therapy arm of the protocol also received an enteral nutritional support product high in branched-chain amino acids (BCAAs), as well as the anabolic steroid oxandrolone (80 mg/d). Voluntary oral food intake during hospitalization correlated in a stepwise fashion with 6-month mortality data. Thus, patients who voluntarily consumed over 3000 kcal/d (12.6 MJ/d) had virtually no mortality, whereas those consuming under 1000 kcal/d (4.2 MJ/d) had more than an 80% 6-month mortality (Fig. 26.1).[2]

These VA studies evaluated hospitalized patients with severe acute AH. Nutritional status in patients with stable ALD without the severe inflammatory response that accompanies AH has also been determined. Patients with stable cirrhosis followed in an ascites clinic who were not actively drinking, were free of AH, and had bilirubin levels under 51 mmolL (3 mg/dL) were evaluated. They had indicators of malnutrition almost as severe as patients with AH (e.g., a creatinine height index of 71%).[6]

It can be argued that alcohol, rather than the underlying liver pathology, is the critical variable in malnutrition in liver disease. There have been several studies evaluating patients having both ALD and nonalcoholic (especially viral)-induced liver disease.[7–11] It is clear that non–alcohol-related liver disease also is complicated by malnutrition. However, patients with sAH and cirrhosis may have the most severe nutritional deficits.[12]

The assessment of malnutrition (in clinical care and clinical research settings) in patients with liver disease is often difficult. Some of the most commonly used assessment techniques are shown in Table 26.1 and are described in greater detail elsewhere in this book. Unfortunately, almost all of these tests can be influenced by either the underlying liver disease or the factors causing the liver disease, such as alcohol consumption or viral infection. Visceral proteins are commonly used by many clinicians; however, these proteins, such as albumin, prealbumin, and retinol-binding protein, are all produced in the liver and correlate better with severity

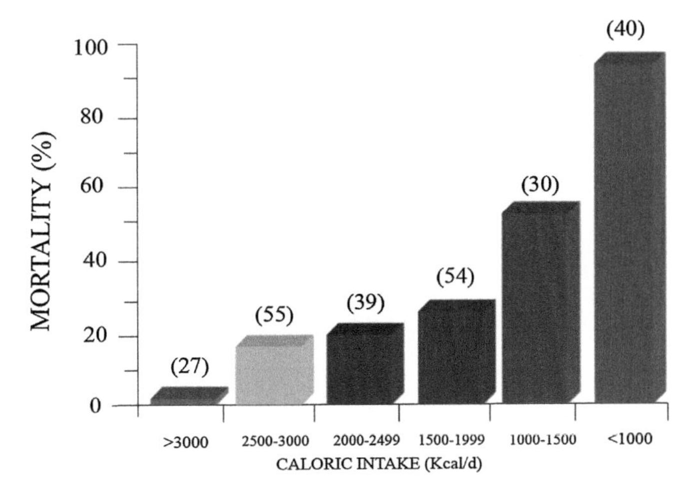

FIGURE 26.1 A direct relation was noted between mortality and voluntary caloric intake in Veterans Health Administration studies in patients with moderate and severe alcoholic hepatitis. It is not known whether providing enteral feeding to patients with inadequate caloric intake would have improved mortality. *From Mendenhall et al.*[2]

of the underlying liver disease than malnutrition in these patients. They are good predictors of risk for malnutrition but do not quantitatively evaluate nutritional status. Anthropometry is also frequently used but can be influenced by factors common in liver disease such as edema and ascites. We regularly use subjective global assessment.[13,14] Fig. 26.2 shows a patient with severe alcoholic cirrhosis and malnutrition diagnosed by subjective global assessment and markedly improved with 2 years of abstinence and appropriate nutritional support.

Multiple imaging modalities are increasingly used to assess muscle mass and body composition in cirr hosis.[15–17] A single cross-sectional computed tomography (CT) slice (most often at the third lumbar vertebra—L3) has been validated as an accurate method of assessing whole-body skeletal muscle and fat mass in healthy subjects and has been used in multiple patient populations.[17] Because patients with cirrhosis frequently have CT scans for clinical care including HCC surveillance, CT scans may be available for body composition analysis.

TABLE 26.1 Methods for assessing malnutrition.

- Anthropometry (triceps skinfold)
- Biological parameters (visceral proteins)
- Assessment of muscle strength
- Bioelectrical impedance
- Dual-energy X-ray absorptiometry, CT
- Subjective global assessment
- Energy balance
- 24-h urinary creatinine height index
- Metabolomics

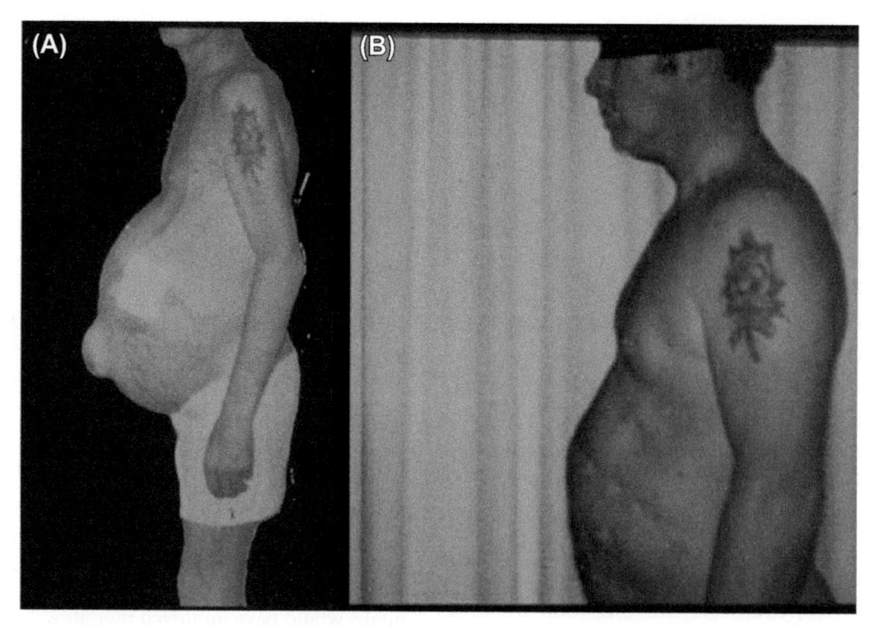

FIGURE 26.2 A patient in a VA Cooperative Study with decompensated cirrhosis with superimposed AH presented with severe ascites, muscle wasting, coagulopathy, and encephalopathy. The second panel shows the same patient after 2 years of abstinence with no ascites, a marked improvement in muscle strength, muscle mass, and functionality. This highlights the potential reversibility of even advanced ALD and the importance of abstinence and appropriate nutrition.

Bioelectrical impedance (BIA) is increasingly used as technology for body composition analysis. Early BIA technology was not very useful in patients with liver disease, especially those with edema or ascites. However, BIA is increasingly useful for patients with NASH, for posttransplant patients, for patients with cirrhosis and malnourished without ascites, and others. Indeed, in a study of 41 subjects, Pirlich and coworkers showed a strong correlation between BIA and the gold standard of body composition and total body potassium for assessing malnutrition.[18]

Causes of malnutrition in liver disease

The causes of malnutrition in liver disease, especially advanced liver disease, are multiple and often interrelated. We highlight below selected important causes of malnutrition in this population.

Food availability, diet quality, unpalatable diets; Patients with cirrhosis with fluid retention are usually prescribed a low-sodium diet that is often unpalatable.[19] Moreover, certain nutritional supplements also have palatability issues. Some patients with cirrhosis (with or without encephalopathy) are inappropriately prescribed a low-protein diet. Patients with alcohol- or NASH-related cirrhosis frequently have poor diets with a high intake of low nutrient-density foods and beverages, including alcoholic or sugar containing beverages. These cumulative effects can cause an overall decrease in energy or protein consumption and/or food quality leading to malnutrition.[20] For example, we recently reported that patients with early stages of ALD frequently consume ~50% of their calories as alcohol and are often deficient in serum zinc.[21]

Anorexia, altered taste, and smell; Anorexia is a major symptom associated with cirrhosis, which leads to decreased food intake. Over 60% of AH patients from VA hospitals had anorexia, and severity of liver disease was associated with the severity of the anorexia.[2–5,22] In an outpatient study of 200 patients from Eastern India, 100% of those with alcoholic cirrhosis reported anorexia.[23] A study from China reported that about 1/3 of patients with cirrhosis had anorexia, which correlated with the presence of depression.[24] Thus, anorexia was consistent across different liver diseases worldwide. Anorexia also is common with aging, and many malnourished patients with advanced liver disease are older. Lastly, decreased dietary intake and blood concentration of individual nutrients such as zinc may play a role in anorexia, anosmia, or dysgeusia observed in some patients with cirrhosis.

Nausea and gastroparesis; Nausea, vomiting, and abdominal bloating are frequent complaints in patients with advanced liver disease. In patients with sAH, about 50% had nausea.[5] In a large group of patients with cirrhosis who were not eligible for transplantation, 58% had nausea.[25] Autonomic dysfunction and gastroparesis are frequent in this patient population and often underdiagnosed.[26,27] Indeed, one report showed that

95% of patients with cirrhosis had gastroparesis, and this correlated with severity of autonomic dysfunction.[26]

Bacterial overgrowth and diarrhea; Small intestinal bacterial overgrowth (SIBO) is common in patients with cirrhosis[28] and may correlate with the degree of underlying liver disease.[29] SIBO can predispose to nausea, and bloating, which coupled with anorexia and gastric compression due to ascites, can deleteriously impact food intake in cirrhosis. Diarrhea also is common in patients with advanced liver disease.[5] Most of the time, this is iatrogenic and secondary to the use of nonabsorbable disaccharides (e.g., lactulose) in the treatment and prevention of HE. With advanced liver disease and further decline of hepatic synthetic function, hypoalbuminemia can cause small intestinal bowel wall edema that can serve as a mechanical barrier to nutrient absorption.

Hormones and cytokine effects; Proinflammatory cytokines, such as tumor necrosis factor (TNF), are frequently increased in liver disease and can mediate muscle wasting through increasing protein degradation and decreasing protein synthesis.[30] Catecholamines and sympathetic nervous system overactivity have been postulated to play a role in the sarcopenia in chronic liver disease.[30] Decreased levels of anabolic hormones also likely play a role in sarcopenia (loss of skeletal muscle mass) and malnutrition in liver disease. Testosterone levels are generally decreased in men with cirrhosis, and levels decrease as the severity of liver disease progresses.[31] IGF-1 is produced in the liver and mediates many of the effects of growth hormone. IGF-1 levels are low in chronic liver disease and decrease as severity of liver disease and sarcopenia increase.[32]

Complications of liver disease; Patients who have complications of liver disease, such as ascites or HE, are more likely to have sarcopenia and malnutrition. Patients with encephalopathy, even those with minimal encephalopathy, may be cognitively impaired and do not eat appropriately. Moreover, some dietitians and physicians inappropriately prescribe a low-protein diet for patients with encephalopathy. Patients with ascites may have abdominal fullness, anorexia, nausea, and increased energy expenditure, which improves with paracentesis to remove excess abdominal fluid.[33] Lastly, patients hospitalized for complications of liver disease often have meals interrupted due to fasting for medical and surgical procedures. Thus, nutrition support goals are frequently not met.

Nutritional mechanisms of liver disease

The mechanisms for liver disease (especially ALD and NASH) are highly complex, multifactorial, and often interactive. Patients with ALD or NASH initially develop fatty liver, and subsequent insults ("hits") then cause some patients to progress from fatty liver to steatohepatitis and/or cirrhosis (Fig. 26.3). Here, we review in detail the critical nutrition-related mechanisms of gut–barrier dysfunction and the gut:liver axis in liver disease development and progression. In a subsequent section, we discuss nutrition and metabolism in detail.

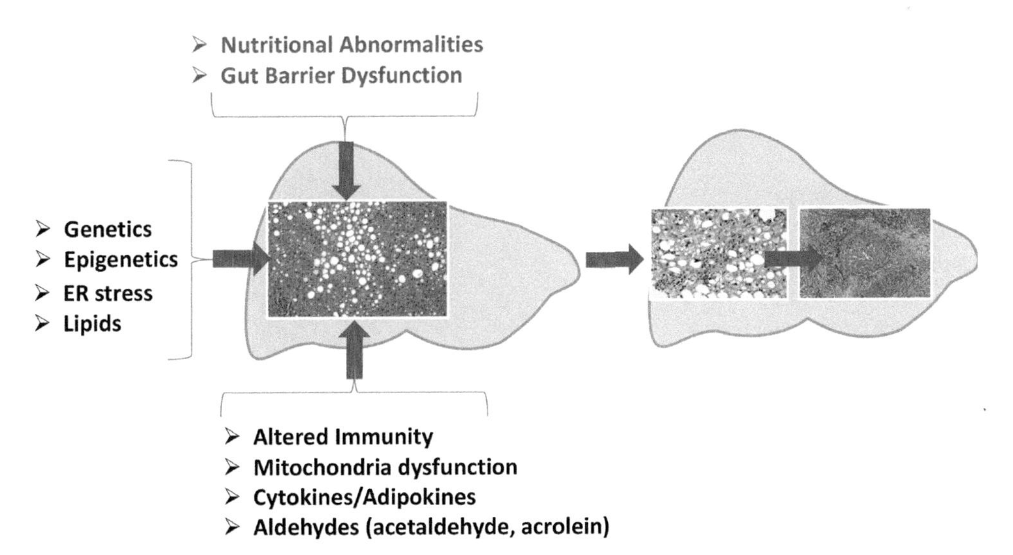

FIGURE 26.3 Fatty liver can develop due to many causes such as diet, alcohol, or environmental toxins and be adversely impacted by multiple factors ranging from nutrition to epigenetics or cytokines. These factors or second "hits" can cause progression from simple fatty liver disease to steatohepatitis and cirrhosis. These same metabolic factors are operational in most liver diseases ranging from viral liver disease to autoimmune liver injury. *ER*, endoplasmic reticulum.

Gut barrier dysfunction, lipopolysaccharides (LPS), and Gut: Liver axis

Nutrition and microbiome in liver disease The human intestinal tract harbors trillions of microbial cells and thousands of bacterial species known as the microbiota. Overall, the predominant bacterial groups in the gut microbiome are Gram-positive *Firmicutes* and Gram-negative *Bacteroidetes*.[34] Intestinal microbiota play an important role in the host health and have been implicated in the development of multiple pathologies, including liver disease. ALD and NAFLD in rodents and humans have been extensively studied, but other liver diseases, including viral and autoimmune, have also been evaluated in context of the microbiome. At the same time, compelling evidence supports the notion that diet plays a significant role in shaping the microbiome,[35–37] providing a rationale for a promising therapeutic strategy of the altering gut microbiota and preventing or treating liver disease through dietary intervention.

Dietary factors and microbial metabolites in liver disease Diet is a key component in the mutual relation between the host and the host resident microbial community. Moreover, diet is a major factor that modulates the gut microbiota composition, structure, and function. Nutritional factors, such as dietary carbohydrates, proteins, and fats, alter the gut microbiota, and these diet-induced changes, either beneficial or harmful for the host, influence the host physiology and pathology.

Gut microbes produce metabolites from dietary products that serve as signaling molecules between the gut and distal organs and play a role in host health and liver disease.[38] For instance, short-chain fatty acids, the primary end products of dietary fiber bacterial fermentation, play an important role in energy homeostasis, lipid, and carbohydrate metabolism and suppression of inflammatory signals.[39] Indolepropionic acid and indole-3-acetate, microbial metabolites of tryptophan, maintain intestinal homeostasis[40] and reduce hepatocyte and macrophage inflammation,[41] respectively. Trimethylamine, a microbial metabolite of choline, is oxidized to trimethylamine *N*-oxide (TMAO), is associated with cardiovascular risk,[42] and is implicated in the development of fatty liver disease.[43,44]

Dysbiosis and alcoholic liver disease Excessive alcohol consumption is one of the major risk factors for liver disease presenting as steatosis, steatohepatitis, acute AH, fibrosis, and cirrhosis. Both acute and chronic alcohol intake are associated with increased intestinal permeability and alterations in the gut microbiota community, metagenome, and metabolome, all of which may contribute to the abnormal gut–liver axis, thereby exacerbating alcohol-induced liver injury and inflammation. Patients with ALD develop dysbiosis and altered gut barrier function; allowing bacterial products such as LPS to enter the portal circulation and stimulate hepatic production of proinflammatory cytokines (e.g., TNF) with subsequent liver injury (Fig. 26.4). Our group was the first to demonstrate that chronic alcohol consumption altered the gut microbiota composition, and probiotic treatment improved moderate steatohepatitis in human alcoholics.[45] In mice, ethanol and a diet high in corn oil (~60% linoleic acid [LA], n6 PUFA) decreased both Bacteriodetes and Firmicutes phyla, with a proportional increase in the Gram-negative Proteobacteria and Gram-positive Actinobacteria phyla; these events were associated with disruption of the intestinal barrier, endotoxemia, liver steatosis, inflammation, and injury.[46] Chen et al., showed that dietary supplementation with saturated long-chain fatty acids corrected the bacterial dysbiosis, mainly by increasing

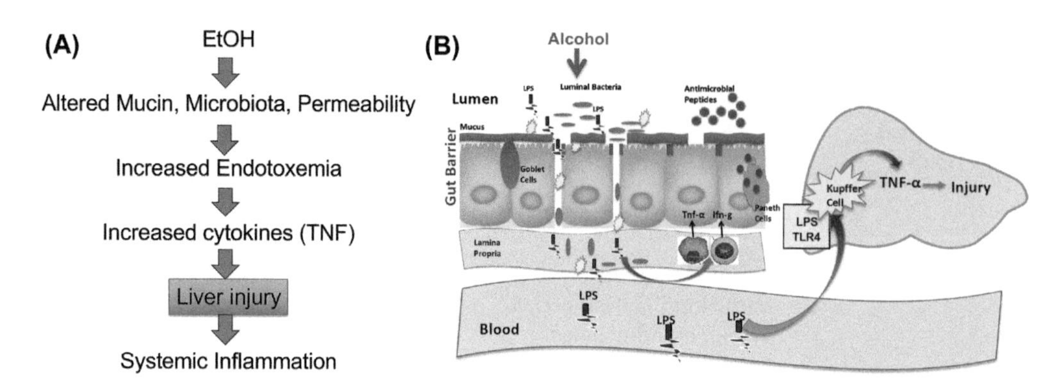

FIGURE 26.4 **Gut barrier dysfunction in alcoholic liver disease.** Alcohol consumption may cause dysbiosis and bacterial overgrowth. Intestinal bacteria alterations result in disruption of gut barrier integrity with the subsequent increase in gut permeability to bacteria-derived pathogens, including LPS. In the liver, LPS causes hepatocellular inflammation by stimulating hepatic Kupffer cells to release proinflammatory cytokines via TLR-4–mediated mechanisms leading to liver injury. High-fat or high-carbohydrate or fructose diet may act through very similar pathways. *EtOH*, ethyl alcohol; *IFN-γ*, interferon gamma; *LPS*, lipopolysaccharides; *TLR-4*, toll-like receptor 4.

the levels of *Lactobacilli* and reducing the ethanol-induced gut permeability and liver injury.[47]

The gut microbiota can influence the severity of AH. A study from France[48] reported distinct gut microbiota communities in patients with distinct degrees of severity of alcohol-induced liver injury. Thus, patients with sAH had elevated abundance of *Bifidobacteria* and *Streptococci*, and less *Atopobium* compared to patients with no AH (noAH). *Streptococci and Enterobacteria* were positively correlated with the AH severity. *Atopobium* and *Clostridium leptum,* known for antiinflammatory effects in the intestine, were negatively correlated with blood bilirubin and with liver fibrosis score, respectively. This study[48] also demonstrated that intestinal microbiota contribute to susceptibility to ALD, that the degree of susceptibility is transmissible from patients to mice, and that this susceptibility could be reversed with normalization of the gut microbiota. In this experiment, mice that received microbiota from a patient with sAH developed more severe alcohol-induced liver injury, inflammation, greater intestinal permeability, and higher translocation of bacteria than mice that received microbiota from an alcoholic patient without AH (noAH). Attenuated liver injury in noAH mice was associated with *Faecalibacterium* genus, a known antiinflammatory bacterium, and elevated levels of the primary bile acid, chenodeoxycholic acid, and the secondary bile acid, ursodeoxycholic acid with known hepatoprotective properties. The specific transferred bacteria associated with the sAH phenotype, the metabolites produced, or a combination of these factors may be transmissible factors contributing to ALD susceptibility. Fecal transplantation from "alcohol-resistant" mice or treatment with a prebiotic reversed intestinal dysbiosis and prevented steatosis and liver inflammation in alcohol-fed mice.[49]

Dysbiosis and nonalcoholic fatty liver disease Studies in animal models have shown a direct link between the gut microbiota and liver steatosis.[50] Using germ-free animal models, several research groups demonstrated that mice lacking gut microbiota are resistant to diet-induced obesity, liver steatosis, and insulin resistance.[51,52] Contribution of the gut bacteria to NAFLD is multifactorial and may occur via regulation of energy homeostasis[50]; modulation of choline[53] and bile acid metabolism[54]; production of the bacteria metabolites contributing to hepatic steatosis, e.g., TMAO[44]; and the ability to generate bacteria-derived toxins, e.g., LPS.[55] Small intestine bacterial overgrowth has also been linked to NASH pathogenesis.[56] Elevated representation of *Escherichia,* an alcohol-producing bacteria, was observed in parallel with increased blood alcohol concentration in patients with NASH, suggesting a novel mechanism for the pathogenesis of NASH: gut microbiota enriched in alcohol-producing bacteria (e.g., *Escherichia coli*) constantly produce more alcohol, which plays a role in the disruption of intestinal tight junctions, hepatic oxidative stress, and liver inflammation.[57]

Microbiota might be a factor in the progression of NAFLD to more severe forms of liver disease, e.g., NASH and fibrosis. Recent research in a well-character ized population of adult NAFLD patients revealed that two genera, *Bacteroides and Ruminococcus,* were significantly elevated, while the abundance of *Prevotella* was lower in patients with significant fibrosis compared to patients with no or mild fibrosis.[58] Increased abundance of *Bacteroides* was independently and positively associated with NASH, and the *Ruminococcus* genus was associated with fibrosis. A significant shift in metabolic function of the gut microbiota, specifically impacting metabolism of carbohydrates, lipids, and amino acids, was observed in NASH and in patients with significant fibrosis.[59]

An exciting advance in the field is the observation that gut microbiota transplantation from donor mice with NAFLD replicated the phenotype in wild-type recipients, demonstrating that NAFLD is a potentially transmissible process.[60] Gut microbiome transplantation has emerged as a novel intervention to manage obesity and related metabolic complications, including fatty liver disease.[61] The transplantation of fecal microbiota from mice with endogenous n3-PUFA enrichment improved metabolic alterations, including hepatic steatosis, and attenuated increased intestinal permeability caused by a high-fat/high-sucrose diet in mice.[62] This study provides evidence that modulation of the microbiota by n3 PUFAs may be beneficial for obese individuals and patients with NAFLD and supports the concept that the microbiome is a transmissible factor that can confer benefits to the host.

Novel therapeutic strategies: nutritional modulation of the gut microbiota The treatment of liver disease can be challenging. This is especially true for NAFLD and ALD where there is no FDA-approved therapy. Increasing data suggest beneficial effects of prebiotics (nondigestible food substances to promote growth of beneficial bacteria) and probiotics (live microorganisms that are favorable to the host) in NAFLD and ALD.[63] Given that diet modifies the microbiome, personalized dietary therapy may emerge as an approach in NAFLD and ALD. Listed in Table 26.2 are selected modalities that may be used to modulate the gut microbiome and treat various forms of liver disease.

TABLE 26.2 Modulation of microbiota to treat liver disease.

1. Diet/nutrition
2. Prebiotics
3. Probiotics
4. Fecal Transplant
5. Genetically engineered Bacteria
6. Antibiotics
7. Drugs

B. Role of Diet on Onset and Progression of Liver Disease

Protein

Protein malnutrition is common in cirrhosis. Multiple studies document that these patients consume inadequate amounts of protein. Early VA Cooperative studies indicated that 85 g of protein per day or more was required to maintain nitrogen balance, yet AH patients (both inpatient and outpatient) were consistently consuming about 20 gm/d less than this goal.[5] These same studies showed that protein-calorie malnutrition, assessed by a composite malnutrition score, was associated with significantly higher 30-day, 6-month, and 12-month mortality rates. In a more recent study, Moreno et al. performed a randomized trial comparing intense enteral nutrition (EN) with conventional nutrition support in hospitalized AH patients.[64] Patients receiving <21.5 kcal/kg per day had a significantly lower survival rate at 6 months than patients who consumed higher caloric intake. The decreased 6-month survival was also associated with <77.6 g/d of protein intake.[64] Thus, inadequate protein intake is frequently observed in patients with cirrhosis, especially those with superimposed AH.

Inadequate protein intake contributes to loss of muscle mass or sarcopenia.[65] Sarcopenia has been reported in ~40–60% of patients with cirrhosis. Patients can have both loss of muscle mass and impaired muscle strength. Decreased muscle mass is due to both increased breakdown of muscle tissue and impaired synthesis with liver cirrhosis. Sarcopenia has been associated with multiple poor outcomes in patients with cirrhosis, including fatigue, frailty, encephalopathy, and mortality.[58] Patients with cirrhosis are thought to be in a state of anabolic resistance with inadequate response to nutrient supplementation, and nutrition therapy is often not effective. Multiple factors appear to play a role in sarcopenia in cirrhosis, with elevated serum ammonia concentrations being a central mediator. Ammonia causes upregulation of myostatin, which inhibits muscle protein synthesis by impairing mTOR signaling.[65] Other factors include elevated blood endotoxin with catabolic cytokine effects and low levels of testosterone and IGF-1. Lastly, cirrhosis represents a state of accelerated starvation with an early shift from glucose to lipid utilization for energy during the postabsorptive state.[66] Thus, patients with cirrhosis literally go into a metabolic starvation mode with muscle breakdown during the overnight fast, and this pathologic state provides the rational for a late evening snack to block this overnight metabolic shift.

Fat

The amount and composition of dietary fat are known to contribute to human health and in many chronic diseases, including alcoholic[67,68] and non- ALD.[69] Evidence of a link between the dietary fat, alcohol consumption, and ALD came from the early epidemiologic studies demonstrating significant correlations between rates of alcoholic cirrhosis mortality and the products of dietary animal fat and alcohol consumption.[67,70] Subsequent experimental animal studies revealed that dietary saturated fat, specifically rich in medium-chain fatty acids, can attenuate liver damage; whereas, dietary unsaturated fat, specifically rich in corn oil and 56% LA, have shown to promote alcohol-induced liver damage.[71,72] Moreover, dietary LA, an omega-6 PUFA, was required for the development of experimental EtOH-induced liver injury, and the severity of ALD was correlated with the amount of LA in the diet.[73] This observation has an important public health implication given that LA is a major unsaturated fatty acid in the Western diet[74] and LA consumption has dramatically increased during the 20th century.[75] The deleterious effects of dietary USF in comparison to the protective effects of dietary SF are partially mediated through induction of lipid peroxidation and oxidative stress,[72,76–78] elevated blood endotoxin levels, disruption of intestinal barrier integrity, and the associated increased production of proinflammatory cytokines.[78–80] While the damaging effects of dietary omega-6 PUFAs, specifically LA, in ALD are well-documented (reviewed in[68]), studies examining effects of dietary omega-3 PUFAs are controversial. Protection,[81–83] exacerbation,[84,85] or no effects[86] of omega-3 PUFA supplementation on EtOH-induced hepatic steatosis and/or liver injury have been reported. The use of transgenic *fat-1* mice that endogenously convert omega-6 to omega-3 PUFAs is an innovative approach to study the role of omega-3 PUFAs in different pathologies. It has been shown that both endogenous omega-3 PUFA enrichment in *fat-1* mice as well as dietary DHA and EPA supplementation in wild-type mice alleviated EtOH-induced liver steatosis, liver injury, and inflammation.[87,88]

The hallmark of NAFLD is hepatic steatosis, which is a consequence of the alterations in liver lipid metabolism, i.e., the uptake of fatty acids and de novo lipogenesis surpassing rate of fatty acid oxidation and export. It is well documented that dietary fat plays an important role in NAFLD pathogenesis; dietary fatty acids are involved in hepatic lipogenesis and may prevent reverse or exacerbate hepatic fat accumulation.[89,90] Circulating fatty acids may also be toxic to hepatocytes via multiple molecular mechanisms (e.g., palmitic acid by inducing apoptosis).[91] The evidence from clinical and experimental studies demonstrates that different dietary fatty acids exert distinct effects on liver fat accumulation. Consumption of food rich in SF promotes hepatic and visceral fat storage. On the other hand, a combination of omega-6 PUFAs and cholesterol induced hepatic steatosis, inflam mation, and fibrosis accompanied by hepatic lipid peroxidation and oxidative stress in mice and closely resembles clinical features of NASH in patients with metabolic syndrome.[92] Consumption of the dietary monounsaturated fatty acid, oleate, compared to palmitate led to worse liver steatosis and adipose tissue inflammation mimicking the effects of the human Western diet in a preclinical animal study.[93] Studies investigating the dietary patterns of patients with NAFLD versus healthy individuals have reported that those with NAFLD have lower omega-3 PUFA intake and a higher omega-6/omega-3 PUFA intake ratio.[94] A metaanalysis conducted to assess the effect of omega-3 PUFA supplementation suggested that omega-3 PUFAs may decrease liver fat and blood gamma glutamyl transferase, TGs (triglycerides), and high-density lipoproteins in patients with NAFLD/NASH.[95]

Given the complexity and distinct effects of different dietary fatty acids on liver health and disease, further studies are warranted to elucidate the role of total dietary fat and specific fatty acids in nutritional strategies to prevent and treat patients with ALD and NAFLD.

Carbohydrate

Worldwide changes in dietary habits have led to increased consumption of processed foods rich in simple carbohydrates.[96] All carbohydrates consumed in excess can cause obesity and fatty liver, but fructose has received special attention. Increased fructose consumption in the United States parallels the increased prevalence of obesity and NAFLD. High fructose intake can induce a range of metabolic changes, including NAFLD, in both experimental animals and humans.[97–100] Fructose intake was reported to be significantly higher in patients with NAFLD than in those without hepatic steatosis or in healthy controls.[96,101] Moreover, increased fructose consumption is associated with more severe fibrosis in adult NAFLD patients.[102,103] Collectively, dietary fructose may be an important risk factor for the pathogenesis and disease progression of NAFLD.

The mechanisms of fructose-induced NAFLD are multifactorial. Gut fructose absorption is saturated at fairly low levels,[104,105] and excessive dietary intake can easily overwhelm the absorptive capacity leading to fructose malabsorption. The unabsorbed fructose may cause gut microbiota dysbiosis and gut barrier dysfunction.[97,106] Dietary fructose may lead to the development of NAFLD via at least two ways. The first is its unique metabolism contributing to the accelerated de novo lipogenesis.[107] The second occurs when unabsorbed fructose goes to the distal intestine leading to gut bacteria dysbiosis and gut barrier dysfunction. Increased intestinal permeability associated with high fructose consumption can lead to endotoxemia and Kupffer cell activation. This increases the secretion of inflammatory cytokines, subsequently causing insulin resistance and fatty liver.[97,106,108]

Studies in children offer unique opportunities for evaluating the role of excess dietary carbohydrates and fructose in the development of NAFLD. Children rarely have multiple other complicating metabolic diseases and are often consumers of sugary beverages. A recent clinical trial enrolled adolescent boys with histologically diagnosed NAFLD and randomized them to an intervention diet or typical diet.[109] The intervention diet consisted of individualized meal planning and provision of study meals to the entire household in order to restrict added sugar intake to less than 3% daily calories for 8 weeks. There was a significant decrease in hepatic steatosis, as well as a significant decrease in blood ALT in the low sugar intake group.[109] This type of well-controlled study documents the potential reversibility of NAFLD with dietary intervention.

Micronutrients

Chronic decreased dietary micronutrient intake and suboptimal status can cause a variety of complications in liver disease, and deficiencies may enhance liver disease development or progression. Table 26.3 lists micronutrient deficiencies seen in liver disease. Some deficiencies can accelerate liver disease or cause life-threatening complications.

Zinc regulates gene expression through metal-binding transcription factors and metal response elements in the promotor regions of regulated genes. The zinc-finger motifs are important to normal hepatic metabolism, such as hepatocyte nuclear factor 4 alpha and peroxisome proliferator-activated receptor-alpha.[110,111] Patients with cirrhosis, especially due to alcohol, are commonly zinc deficient. We recently showed that zinc deficiency occurs early in the development of ALD. Over the last two decades, a series of studies by Zhou and coworkers in experimental animals and in vitro

TABLE 26.3 Mineral and vitamin clinical signs and symptoms in patients with liver disease.

Mineral/Vitamin	Complications
Iron	Anemia, fatigue
Magnesium	Muscular cramps, weakness, insulin resistance, decreased bone density
Calcium	Decreased bone density, tetany
Zinc	Skin lesions, anorexia, growth retardation, decreased wound healing, hypogonadism, decreased immune function, diarrhea, depressed mental function
Copper	Anemia, neutropenia, neuropathy
Chromium	Glucose intolerance
Selenium	Myopathy, cardiomyopathy
Vitamin B12	Megaloblastic anemia, neuropathy
Folate	Macrocytic anemia, increased cancer risk, increased homocysteine
Thiamine	Ataxia, encephalopathy
Niacin	Dermatitis, diarrhea, dementia
Vitamin A	Decreased night vision, skin lesions
Vitamin D	Bone disease, immune and gut barrier dysfunction
Vitamin E	Oxidative stress
Vitamin K	Bruising, impaired clotting

has increased the understanding of mechanisms, whereby zinc deficiency exacerbate alcohol-induced liver injury and mechanisms of how zinc therapy may prevent or treat alcohol-induced liver injury. These include increased gut permeability, inflammation with increased cytokines and oxidative stress, mitochondrial dysfunction, and hepatocyte apoptosis.[110]

Copper is an essential trace element active in biological processes in the liver, including normal mitochondrial respiration, iron and lipid metabolism, detoxification of free radicals, and cross-linking of connective tissue. Dietary copper deficiency can induce hepatic steatosis and insulin resistance in rats (especially male rats), suggesting that copper availability may be involved in the development of NAFLD. Evidence suggests that hepatic copper concentrations are lower in patients with NAFLD, and steatosis correlates inversely with hepatic copper content. The Western diet is often low in copper. Dietary fructose and copper interact with high-fructose consumption enhancing copper deficiency–induced fatty liver disease. It is not uncommon to see NAFLD patients with high sugar-sweetened beverage consumption who have modestly low blood ceruloplasmin that normalizes with discontinuation of fructose intake. Severe copper deficiency can occur after gastric bypass surgery for obesity and present with microcystic anemia and peripheral neuropathy.[112] Excess copper intake with subsequent hepatotoxicity and fibrosis is well documented in Wilson disease and cholestatic liver diseases, including primary biliary cholangitis.[113] Copper toxicity occurs through multiple mechanisms, including oxidative stress.

Other minerals of particular relevance to liver disease include selenium (potential antioxidant function), chromium (glucose tolerance), magnesium (muscle cramps, insulin resistance), and manganese. Manganese is excreted via the biliary route and can be deposited in the brain with subsequent encephalopathy.[114]

End-stage chronic liver disease can result in thiamine deficiency caused primarily by depletion of liver thiamine stores. Thiamine deficiency is particular prevalent in patients with alcoholic cirrhosis, and there are direct effects of ethanol on dietary thiamine absorption from the gastrointestinal tract. Thiamine deficiency can cause Wernicke's encephalopathy, a metabolic encephalopathy that is characterized by ophthalmoplegia, ataxia, confusion, and memory loss. Importantly, neurologic complications can also occur after gastric bypass surgery, especially if patients develop nausea and vomiting. Wernicke's encephalopathy is a neurologic emergency and requires immediate IV thiamine administration.[115]

Malabsorption of the fat-soluble vitamins A, D, E, and K is well described in patients with advanced cholestatic liver disease.[116] Vitamin A plays a critical role in multiple metabolic pathways ranging from visual function to gene transcription. The liver is the major storage site for vitamin A (>90%), with most found in the liver stellate cells. Studies indicate that over 60% of patients with cirrhosis have low serum vitamin A levels, and 40% in one study had impaired dark adaptation that was not recognized by the patient.[117,118] Caution must be used in giving higher dose vitamin A supplements to patients with liver disease due to potential toxicity, including liver toxicity.[119] Vitamin E is a lipid-soluble antioxidant that prevents the propagation of free radicals. Low blood vitamin E has been found in patients with NASH as well as ALD, and in those with other forms of cirrhosis. Vitamin E is used as therapy in early NASH. Vitamin D is important for bone health and plays an important role in immune regulation and gut barrier function. Vitamin K plays an important role in blood clotting.

III. PRIMARY TREATMENT MODALITIES FOR LIVER DISEASE

A. Medical and Surgical Treatment

Of the three major forms of liver disease in the world (viral, alcohol, obesity-related), only viral-induced liver disease has FDA-approved therapies. The major types of chronic viral liver disease are hepatitis C and hepatitis B. Hepatitis C is diagnosed by an antibody test and confirmed by quantifying HCV RNA. Hepatitis C is a single-stranded RNA virus that does not have a latent host reservoir, and thus, patients are able to be cured of the virus. In 1991, alpha-interferon therapy was introduced, and in 2011, DAAs were introduced. Current DAA therapy provides >90% cure rate in most patient populations, and there has been a decrease in HCV deaths in the United States.[120] The diagnosis of hepatitis B is documented by the presence of a hepatitis B surface antigen. Patients are considered to have chronic hepatitis B if they have had the disease for at least 6 months. Hepatitis B can be spread by percutaneous and sexual exposure or by person-to-person contact.[121] Hepatitis B is different from most other forms of liver disease in that patients do not have to have cirrhosis to be at lifelong risk for HCC and requiring cancer surveillance. Hepatitis B is decreasing in many parts of the world due to the hepatitis B vaccine and effective nucleos(t)ide analogue therapies. These drugs are highly effective at suppressing the virus but do not cure the disease. While ALD and NASH have no FDA-approved therapies, it is projected that a NASH drug may be approved in the near future.

There are two therapies for certain forms of liver disease: bariatric surgery for NASH and liver transplantation. Bariatric surgery is indicated for rapid and permanent weight loss. It is currently indicated for severely obese individuals with a body mass index (BMI) $> 40\ kg/m^2$ or with a BMI $\geq 35\ kg/m^2$ and obesity-related comorbid conditions. It has the potential to improve metabolic syndrome, diabetes, and even liver histology in patients with NAFLD. It has the potential to reverse NAFLD risk factors, including insulin resistance, dyslipidemia, and inflammation.[122,123] The most commonly studied procedure for NAFLD is laparoscopic or open Roux-en-Y gastric bypass and other procedures like laparoscopic adjustable gastric banding, sleeve gastrectomy, gastroplasty, biliointestinal bypass, and biliopancreatic diversion. Similarly, endoscopic obesity treatment approaches such as gastric balloons have been evaluated. A metaanalysis of 15 cohort studies found an improvement or resolution in steatosis in 91.6% of patients, steatohepatitis in 81.3%, and fibrosis in 65.5% after bariatric surgery.[124] Similar results were also been shown is a prospective cohort study on 381 patients where improvement was documented in steatosis, ballooning, and overall NASH Activity Score, with a significant reduction in the percentage of patients who had NASH patients at five postsurgery years compared with before.[125] However, 5 years after surgery, 19.8% of patients had significant worsening of fibrosis for unknown reasons.

A metaanalysis that included 32 studies, 2649 biopsies, with a median follow-up period of 15 months showed a complete resolution of steatosis in 66% of patients, inflammation in 50% of patients, ballooning degeneration in 76%, and complete resolution of fibrosis in 40% of patients.[126] 12% of patients had worsening or development of fibrosis following bariatric surgery. These findings relate to the type of bariatric procedure or the malnutrition and malabsorption that can result from bariatric surgery for severe obesity.[127]

Mortality in obese patients with NAFLD has been studied following bariatric surgery. In one study, no increase in all-cause mortality after bariatric surgery was observed; however, there was an increased mortality rate ratio for gastrointestinal and liver diseases, including peritonitis and intestinal obstruction.[128] Overall, no significant increase of liver-related mortality after bariatric surgery is reported, but larger studies are needed.[129]

There were no randomized clinical trials included in the metaanalyses, as all studies were single-arm examining the effect of bariatric surgery on NAFLD before and after surgery, with no comparator groups. While randomized clinical trials are needed, the current literature supports improvement or resolution of fibrosis in obese NAFLD patients who undergo bariatric surgery, and it should be considered as a treatment option.

B. Nutritional Therapy

Outpatient

Interest in outpatient nutritional therapy for patients with cirrhosis was first stimulated when Patek et al.[130] demonstrated that a nutritious diet improved the 5-year outcome of patients with cirrhosis compared with a similar group of patients consuming their typical inadequate diet. Other studies further support the concept of improved outcomes with nutritional support in patients with cirrhosis. Hirsch et al.[131] demonstrated that a group of outpatients supplementing their diet with an enteral product (1000 kcal [4.2 MJ/d], 34 g protein) had significantly improved protein intake and fewer hospitalizations. These same investigators provided an enteral supplement to outpatients with alcoholic cirrhosis and observed an improvement in nutritional status and immune function.[132] A Japanese study evaluated over 200 patients with cirrhosis (of diverse etiology) who either received nutritional counseling from a dietitian following nutritional assessment or standard of care. Patients were followed for approximately 5 years, and those who had nutritional counseling had improved survival. Patients with Child's A cirrhosis showed the greatest benefits. The study highlights the importance of an initial nutritional assessment followed by dietary counseling and subsequent nutritional therapy and follow-up assessments.

When first evaluating an outpatient with cirrhosis, an initial assessment of fluid and electrolyte status is needed, as well as nutritional status using the subjective global assessment or other evaluation methods. Further nutritional evaluation and treatment can be implemented using more detailed assessment including body composition analysis and nutritional consultation to document current intake and plan for initial dietary management. The immediate evaluation of fluid and electrolyte status is critical because factors such as dehydration and renal dysfunction or hyperkalemia can lead to life-threatening consequences. Sodium is the primary electrolyte in body fluids (blood, serum, plasma) outside cells, with only 5% of total body sodium occurring intracellularly. Sodium, together with potassium, assists in maintaining the body's electrolyte and water balance. Hyponatremia (low serum sodium) is a frequent complication of liver disease[133] and usually occurs with typical or increased sodium intake being offset by increases in total body water volume. The increased water and sodium present as edema or ascites. Impaired free water clearance and the use of diuretics contribute to decreased sodium concentration. In patients with decompensated liver disease, the main way of treating hyponatremia is fluid restriction. Hypernatremia occurs less frequently in liver disease, and it is usually due to medical interventions with diuretics or lactulose therapy. Hypokalemia is frequently observed in liver disease.[133] Unlike sodium, potassium is predominantly an intracellular electrolyte. Hypokalemia may occur as a result of poor dietary intake; losses because of nausea, vomiting, or diarrhea; or use of diuretic medications to control edema or ascites. Various metabolic factors (e.g., increased insulin levels and respiratory alkalosis) may shift potassium from the extracellular fluid into cells, thus decreasing the serum potassium concentration. Hypokalemia can produce a spectrum of consequences ranging from muscular weakness to cardiac arrhythmias and even cardiac arrest. Hyperkalemia is much less commonly observed in liver disease and usually accompanies renal failure and use of potassium-sparing diuretics. It is vital that patients not be placed on potassium-containing salt substitutes while on potassium-sparing diuretics because severe hyperkalemia can occur. Hypophosphatemia may occur in very malnourished patients with liver disease and this can be exacerbated by refeeding. Thus, serum levels of these electrolytes need to be monitored, especially during refeeding of malnourished patients.

Dietary restrictions are necessary at times in the course of liver disease but are often detrimental in maintaining adequate nutritional intake. Sodium restriction is probably the most important change in the diet of patients with decompensated cirrhosis, and 1–2 g sodium diets are usually well-tolerated and can be followed by well-coached patients. Total fluid restriction is sometimes necessary to correct hyponatremia.[134]

Limiting protein intake was used in the past as part of the treatment for HE. Current evidence does not support protein restriction and will be explained throughout this chapter.[135,136] HE can be improved by interventions including optimizing adequate intestinal transit time; preventing small- and large-bowel bacterial overgrowth by decreasing portal hypertension and use of antibiotics, lactulose, and probiotics; maintaining electrolyte, vitamin, and mineral status; and possibly by supplementing casein or vegetable protein in the diet. HE occurs more often in patients with muscle mass depletion. Skeletal muscle is involved in ammonia detoxification due to the reduced capacity of urea synthesis in the cirrhotic liver. In malnourished patients with cirrhosis and HE, the improvement of nutritional status and muscle mass could be a potential treatment goal.[137] Early breakfast improves cognitive function in patients with minimal HE, and after food intake, alertness improves for a period of time, supporting the use of frequent small meals in advanced liver disease.[138]

A large body of evidence exists on the use and safety of BCAA preparations in the management of overt HE. BCAA has also been considered to treat malnourished patients with cirrhosis to improve nutritional status. However, a systematic review found the heterogeneity of studies due to variability in BCAA dose (total, relative proportions), duration, disease severity, and lack of uniformity in tools standardized for assessing patient outcomes limits overall strength of evidence and conclusions. Further studies of BCAA supplementation as a therapeutic treatment of malnutrition in chronic liver disease are warranted.[139]

Sarcopenia is a progressive and generalized loss of skeletal muscle mass, strength, and function and an important feature in malnourished patients with chronic liver disease. Optimizing bedtime nutrition intake can minimize and even reverse loss of muscle mass.[140] Late evening snacks are strongly encouraged for cirrhotic patients. When adequate oral intake cannot be maintained, nutritional intake should be supplemented with overnight enteral feedings via small-bore nasoenteric tubes. When the enteral support fails or is contraindicated, total parenteral nutrition (PN) should be considered. Lastly, physical inactivity contributes to sarcopenia. Modest exercise should be recommended in patients who can participate. Exercise can help maintain muscle mass and functionality, as well as improving quality of life and fatigue.[141–143]

Lifestyle modification is important for patients with liver disease, especially those with ALD or NASH. Patients with ALD should be referred to an alcohol treatment program for support to reduce alcohol intake. Current treatment recommendations for patients with NAFLD include both diet and physical activity for weight reduction and weight loss surgery for extreme obesity. One year of intensive lifestyle intervention in patients with type 2 diabetes was shown to reduce steatosis and incident NAFLD.[144] Studies examining the effects of dietary interventions reveal that caloric restriction can result in significant changes in both liver fat and volume within a few days.[145] The use of low-carbohydrate diets in NAFLD is an area of increasing interest. A low-carbohydrate, ketogenic diet in patients with NASH led to significant weight loss and histologic improvement of fatty liver disease at 6 months.[146] Dietary avoidance of lipogenic and simple sugars, especially fructose, is recommended.[147] A reduction in the consumption of sugar-sweetened beverages can lead to weight loss owing to a reduction in total calories consumed.[148] Regarding exercise, vigorous exercise may be most beneficial, as it appears that exercise intensity may be more important than duration or total volume in liver disease.[149] Weight loss by bariatric surgery attenuates both steatosis and steatohepatitis, but evidence supporting improvements in fibrosis are limited.[150] Coffee is the most popular beverage in the world, and it recently has been shown to have health benefits for patients with liver disease. Several studies from different parts of the world have shown that coffee consumption was associated with lower liver enzyme levels (AST, ALT, and gamma glutamyl transpeptidase).[151] Coffee consumption also significantly reduced the risk of hepatic fibrosis and cirrhosis.[152] A metaanalysis on coffee consumption in NAFLD patients showed an inverse association of coffee intake with fibrosis severity.[153] The relation between coffee consumption and HCC has been studied as well. A metaanalysis published in 2013 reported a 40% protective effect of coffee consumption on the development of HCC (RR −0.60).[154] The protection was higher in high consumption (≥3 cups/d, RR 0.44) versus low consumption (1–2 cups/d, RR 0.72). The exact mechanism of beneficial effects of coffee is not clear, but potential mechanisms include the effect of these bioactive compounds, in addition to the antioxidant properties of coffee.[155] Coffee also has antiinflammatory properties: a study showed significantly lower levels of inflammatory markers in coffee drinkers compared to nondrinkers.[156]

TABLE 26.4 Nutrition support goals for hospitalized patients with liver disease.

- Early nutrition assessment and evaluation of serum electrolytes
- Formulate water and electrolyte intake to individual needs, renal function, diuretic sensitivity
- Total energy intake goal: ~1.0–1.4× resting energy expenditure or ~25–40 kcal/kg body weight/day
- Protein: ~1.2–2.0 g/kg per day (upper range in hospital)
- Fat: ~30–40% of nonprotein energy
- Replace vitamins and minerals as indicated, and avoid excessive iron, copper, and vitamin A supplementation
- Supplement daily oral intake with enteral feedings (parental if enteral route otherwise contraindicated), if oral intake is insufficient
- Hypocaloric, high-protein diet for obese subjects
- Nutrition education with dietitian including implementation of nighttime snacks

There is no FDA-approved therapy for NAFLD. Pharmacologic therapies mostly target components of the metabolic syndrome or oxidative stress associated with the pathogenesis of NASH.[150] Vitamin E was initially reported to have beneficial effects in some but not all studies of patients with fatty liver (NASH).[157] The most important and compelling vitamin E data were from a large multicenter NIH-funded trial that assigned 247 adults with NASH (without diabetes) to receive pioglitazone at a dose of 30 mg daily (80 subjects), vitamin E at a dose of 800 IU daily, or placebo for 96 weeks.[158] Vitamin E therapy, as compared with placebo, was associated with a significantly higher rate of improvement in NASH (43% vs. 19%, $P = .001$). Serum alanine and aspartate aminotransferase were reduced with vitamin E and with pioglitazone, as compared to placebo ($P < .001$ for both comparisons). No treatment was associated with an improvement in fibrosis. Subjects who received pioglitazone gained more weight than did those who received vitamin E or placebo. In conclusion, vitamin E improved liver histology and liver enzymes and was not associated with the weight gain seen with pioglitazone. We consider 800 IU of vitamin E to be the preferred therapy for NASH without cirrhosis. AASLD guidelines recommend that patients should not have diabetes and should have biopsy-documented NASH.[157]

Inpatient care

Patients with liver disease, especially those with cirrhosis, are at high risk for malnutrition during hospitalization, especially when hospitalized in the intensive care unit (ICU). Thus, hospitalized patients should be monitored for malnutrition using tools described in Table 26.1. It is important to rapidly diagnose metabolic disturbances including alterations in sodium, potassium, and phosphorus. Monitor food consumption and utilize oral nutritional supplements, including a nighttime snack, in patients to ensure optimal protein/energy requirements by the oral route. A high-protein intake is critical, usually in the range of 1.2–2.0 g/kg BW/d (Table 26.4).

In patients with inadequate oral intake, early EN support is especially important because it has the potential to reduce complications and length of stay, and to positively impact patient outcomes. EN is favored over PN because of cost, risk of central line infection and sepsis with PN, and maintenance of the gut barrier function. Obese, very ill patients with liver disease represent a nutritional challenge. Current guidelines recommend the use of hypocaloric, high protein nutrition therapy in an attempt to preserve lean body mass, to mobilize fat stores, and to minimize overfeeding complications in these at-risk obese patients with liver disease.[159] Energy targets are low in patients with BMIs of 30–50, usually 65%–70% of requirements as measured by indirect calorimetry or approximately 11–14 kcal/kg of actual body weight per day. However, protein requirements are high, usually projected at 2.0–2.5 g/kg of ideal body weight per day.[159] It is a challenge to create and implement an appropriate diet plan that is high in protein, but restricted in calories and sodium.

The patient with acute liver failure is often not malnourished at presentation; however, the acuteness and severity of illness make the patient hypercatabolic prompting strong consideration for careful nutritional evaluation and support. A serious complication of acute liver failure is the development of hypoglycemia, which is seen in up to 45% of patients in the ICU. 1.5–4 gm/kg/d of intravenous glucose is recommended to prevent hypoglycemia and close monitoring of serum glucose every 2 h. In the patient who is receiving sufficient EN or PN, IV glucose may not be required. Because it is important to minimize the risk of brain edema, restriction of free water is often implemented. It is advisable to give the IV glucose in a 0.9% sodium solution and to choose an enteral formula with high caloric density to support fluid restrictions.

There is no consensus on nutrition support for patients with acute liver failure, and guidance is largely empirical. Calorie and protein requirements are considered to be similar to other critically ill patients. Early enteral feeding will maintain gut integrity, minimize muscle loss, and reduce the risk of gastrointestinal bleeding. Use of total PN based on baseline nutritional status and duration of low-calorie intake should be considered if EN is contraindicated.

Transplantation

Malnutrition is a risk factor for general postoperative morbidity (e.g., poor wound healing, infections) and mortality, and this holds true for liver transplantation. In one study, malnutrition was the only variable of six studied that significantly affected outcome, was potentially alterable, and was not completely dependent on underlying hepatic function.[160] Moderately to severely malnourished patients had prolonged ventilator times, ICU lengths of stay, total hospital lengths of stay, and increased hospitalization costs, and findings were similar to another study.[161] Mortality increased 3.2-fold when significant weight loss in body mass was present preoperatively.[162] Using a modified subjective global assessment of malnutrition, Pikul et al.[161] found a 79% incidence of malnutrition in 68 adult liver transplant recipients; in those with moderate and severe malnutrition, they found a significant increase in the number of days requiring ventilatory times, number of days in the ICU and in the hospital, and a higher incidence of tracheostomy. In this study, patients with moderate and severe malnutrition had a significantly higher mortality than did those with an adequate status or mild malnutrition. A universal component of chronic liver disease is the loss of muscle mass and strength, and these deficits are associated with impaired health-related quality of life, which persist to a lesser degree after liver transplantation.[163,164]

The pediatric literature presents similar information. Children awaiting a liver transplant are malnourished up to 60%–80% of the time, and malnourished patients have higher rates of morbidity and mortality, both before and after liver transplantation. Nutritional status should be assessed at every clinic including taking a detailed interval history, physical exam, laboratory testing, and anthropometric measurements. Nutritional needs vary among patients, but increasing caloric intake, supplementation with medium-chain TGs, and prevention of essential fatty acid and fat-soluble vitamin deficiencies are common dietary interventions in this population.[165]

Overweight and obesity can also complicate care for patients with chronic liver disease, especially if liver transplantation is indicated. An analysis of 18,172 liver transplant recipients showed that primary nonfunction and 1- and 2-year mortality rates were significantly higher in patients with morbid obesity (BMI >40 kg/m^2). The 5-year mortality rate was higher in patients with BMI >35 kg/m^2, largely due to cardiovascular events.[166] However, a similar study, which corrected BMI values for ascites, found no difference in survival across BMI categories.[167] In another study, liver transplant recipients with lower BMI (<18.5) were found to have higher 1-year graft loss and mortality rates while obese patients did not.[168]

Nutritional intake and status usually improve after liver transplant as the many metabolic alterations causing malnutrition in patients with cirrhosis are improved by a healthy, functioning liver. Dietary intake problems are expected to improve as patients improve postoperatively, but this is variable. After liver transplant, nutrition support should be initiated within 12–24 h. If patients are unable to tolerate sufficient oral intake, nutritional supplements are given though a nasoenteric tube, which is preferable to PN. Generally, nutrition goals include calories at 120%–130% of the estimated resting energy expenditure and 1.2–1.5 g/

kg/d of protein, since some hypermetabolism is present in the immediate postoperative phase and can persist for up to 6 months after liver transplant.[169] Additional posttransplant nutritional challenges include education regarding food–drug interactions with immunosuppressive medications (e.g., grapefruit products increase tacrolimus blood levels) and other potential risks such as raw and undercooked seafood that can transmit bacteria and cause infections in immunosuppressed individuals.

Weeks to months after transplantation, patients are prone to develop hyperglycemia, hypertension, and dyslipidemia as immunosuppressant drug-related side effects. Patients often have progressive weight gain, mostly as fat mass as opposed to lean mass, and continued skeletal muscle deficiency. A retrospective study of patients who underwent liver transplant found that 44% had some residual malnutrition 1 year after transplant.[170] In another study, only 6% of patients had reversal of sarcopenia after liver transplant, and 70% of those who were not sarcopenic before transplant developed sarcopenia posttransplant.[171] In several studies, patients evaluated 1–4 years after transplant found rates of obesity of 21%–31%, which increased over time.[170,172] This weight gain and increase in fat mass can lead to the metabolic syndrome, which is an increasing cause of long-term morbidity and mortality in patients after liver transplantation.

In the postliver transplant transition, there is a period of accelerated bone mineral density loss due to corticosteroid therapy and decreased patient mobility and physical activity. After this accelerated bone loss, there is a period of increase in bone mineral density that can continue for several years posttransplant.[173] Calcium supplementation is important during the period of increased bone formation. Bone mineral density monitoring is recommended for liver transplant recipients, especially in the first 5 years after transplant.[174]

IV. DRUG–NUTRIENT INTERACTIONS IN LIVER DISEASE

Food, nutritional supplements and drug–nutrient interactions, and potential hepatotoxicity are well established.[175] Dietary supplements are not regulated in the United States and can be contaminated with toxins or drugs. For example, supplements have been contaminated with small amounts of prescription drugs such as antibiotics or heavy metals, including lead or mercury. An example of a nutritional supplement–drug interaction is that of St. John's Wort.[175] This interaction was highlighted when postheart transplant patients developed rejection episodes after initiating St. John's Wort, likely due to the induction of cytochrome P4503A4 by St. John's Wort.[176] Grapefruit juice decreases the metabolism of over 80 drugs.[176] Thus, both increased and decreased metabolism can occur. The gut microbiome has an effect on metabolism, efficacy, and toxicity of some drugs used in liver disease. For example, certain bacterial species are present in the gut microbiome of patients who respond to PDE-1 checkpoint inhibitors used for cancer therapy compared to those who do not respond positively.[177] Transfer of these microbes into germ-free mice improved immunotherapy efficacy. In another example, urinary concentrations of the bacterial product p-cresol correlated with the rate of metabolism of acetaminophen. This is because p-cresol competes with the sulfonation step in acetaminophen metabolism, and thus in acetaminophen detoxification. There are also natural nutrient–nutrient interactions, such as zinc interacting with copper. Thus, zinc supplementation may impair copper absorption and can induce copper deficiency. Indeed, high doses of zinc are used therapeutically in Wilson's disease for this exact "side effect" of producing copper deficiency.[111]

RESEARCH GAPS

We need a better understanding of the interactions and cross talk between the liver and other organs and tissues (e.g., gut–liver axis and liver–adipose tissue axis). The role of the gut microbiome in liver disease onset and progression, as well as in obesity and systemic inflammation, is a likely target for therapeutic interventions. How liver disease alters the gut microbiome, and whether changing the gut microbiome with probiotics/prebiotics attenuates or prevents liver disease in humans are important areas of future investigation. Similarly, there are major gaps in our knowledge concerning drug–nutrient interactions in liver disease. Clinical trials, including dose-finding studies and finding appropriate biomarkers, are needed to study the efficacy of nutritional support and interventions on hepatic outcome. Major gaps exist in the understanding of sarcopenia, anabolic resistance, and nutritional interventions. Nutrients impact gene expression, and there are important gaps in knowledge of the role of nutrition-related epigenetics in liver disease. Research into the above areas will markedly expand our understanding of mechanisms of liver disease and potential nutritional interventions to prevent or treat liver disease.

Acknowledgments

This chapter is an update of the chapter titled "54. Liver Disease" by Craig J. McClain, Daniell B. Hill and Luis Marsano, in *Present Knowledge in Nutrition, 10th Edition*, edited by Erdman JW, Macdonald IA, and Zeisel SH and published by Wiley-Blackwell. © 2012 International Life Sciences Institute. Portions of this update are from the previously published chapter, and the contributions of previous authors are acknowledged.

V. REFERENCES

1. Tapper EB, Parikh ND. Mortality due to cirrhosis and liver cancer in the United States, 1999–2016: observational study. *BMJ*. 2018; 362. k2817.
2. Mendenhall C, Roselle GA, Gartside P, Moritz T. Relationship of protein calorie malnutrition to alcoholic liver disease: a reexamination of data from two Veterans Administration Cooperative Studies. *Alcohol Clin Exp Res*. 1995;19(3):635–641.
3. Mendenhall CL, Tosch T, Weesner RE, et al. VA cooperative study on alcoholic hepatitis. II: prognostic significance of protein-calorie malnutrition. *Am J Clin Nutr*. 1986;43(2):213–218.
4. Mendenhall CL, Anderson S, Weesner RE, Goldberg SJ, Crolic KA. Protein-calorie malnutrition associated with alcoholic hepatitis. Veterans administration cooperative study group on alcoholic hepatitis. *Am J Med*. 1984;76(2):211–222.
5. Mendenhall CL, Moritz TE, Roselle GA, et al. A study of oral nutritional support with oxandrolone in malnourished patients with alcoholic hepatitis: results of a Department of Veterans Affairs cooperative study. *Hepatology*. 1993;17(4):564–576.
6. Antonow DR, McClain C. Nutrition and alcoholism. In: Tarter RE, Van Thiel DH, eds. *Alcohol and the Brain: Chronic Effects*. New York: Plenum Publishing; 1985:81–120.
7. Sarin SK, Dhingra N, Bansal A, Malhotra S, Guptan RC. Dietary and nutritional abnormalities in alcoholic liver disease: a comparison with chronic alcoholics without liver disease. *Am J Gastroenterol*. 1997;92(5):777–783.
8. Caregaro L, Alberino F, Amodio P, et al. Malnutrition in alcoholic and virus-related cirrhosis. *Am J Clin Nutr*. 1996;63(4):602–609.
9. Lolli R, Marchesini G, Bianchi G, et al. Anthropometric assessment of the nutritional status of patients with liver cirrhosis in an Italian population. *Ital J Gastroenterol*. 1992;24(8):429–435.
10. Thuluvath PJ, Triger DR. Evaluation of nutritional status by using anthropometry in adults with alcoholic and nonalcoholic liver disease. *Am J Clin Nutr*. 1994;60(2):269–273.
11. DiCecco SR, Wieners EJ, Wiesner RH, Southorn PA, Plevak DJ, Krom RA. Assessment of nutritional status of patients with end-stage liver disease undergoing liver transplantation. *Mayo Clin Proc*. 1989;64(1):95–102.
12. Peng S, Plank LD, McCall JL, Gillanders LK, McIlroy K, Gane EJ. Body composition, muscle function, and energy expenditure in patients with liver cirrhosis: a comprehensive study. *Am J Clin Nutr*. 2007;85(5):1257–1266.
13. Makhija S, Baker J. The subjective global assessment: a review of its use in clinical practice. *Nutr Clin Pract*. 2008;23(4):405–409.
14. Zambrano DN, Xiao J, Prado CM, Gonzalez MC. Patient-generated subjective global assessment and computed tomography in the assessment of malnutrition and sarcopenia in patients with cirrhosis: is there any association? *Clin Nutr*. 2019;0(0). pii: S0261-5614(19)30274-2.
15. Durand F, Buyse S, Francoz C, et al. Prognostic value of muscle atrophy in cirrhosis using psoas muscle thickness on computed tomography. *J Hepatol*. 2014;60(6):1151–1157.
16. Mourtzakis M, Wischmeyer P. Bedside ultrasound measurement of skeletal muscle. *Curr Opin Clin Nutr Metab Care*. 2014;17(5): 389–395.
17. Paris M, Mourtzakis M. Assessment of skeletal muscle mass in critically ill patients: considerations for the utility of computed tomography imaging and ultrasonography. *Curr Opin Clin Nutr Metab Care*. 2016;19(2):125–130.
18. Pirlich M, Schutz T, Spachos T, et al. Bioelectrical impedance analysis is a useful bedside technique to assess malnutrition in cirrhotic patients with and without ascites. *Hepatology*. 2000; 32(6):1208–1215.
19. Moore KP, Aithal GP. Guidelines on the management of ascites in cirrhosis. *Gut*. 2006;55(suppl 6):vi1–12.
20. Ney M, Abraldes JG, Ma M, et al. Insufficient protein intake is associated with increased mortality in 630 patients with cirrhosis awaiting liver transplantation. *Nutr Clin Pract*. 2015;30(4): 530–536.
21. Vatsalya V, Kong M, Cave MC, et al. Association of serum zinc with markers of liver injury in very heavy drinking alcohol-dependent patients. *J Nutr Biochem*. 2018;59:49–55.
22. Mendenhall CL, Moritz TE, Roselle GA, et al. Protein energy malnutrition in severe alcoholic hepatitis: diagnosis and response to treatment. The VA Cooperative Study Group #275. *JPEN J Parenter Enteral Nutr*. 1995;19(4):258–265.
23. Ray S, Khanra D, Sonthalia N, et al. Clinico-biochemical correlation to histological findings in alcoholic liver disease: a single centre study from eastern India. *J Clin Diagn Res*. 2014;8(10): MC01–05.
24. Xu H, Zhou Y, Ko F, et al. Female gender and gastrointestinal symptoms, not brain-derived neurotrophic factor, are associated with depression and anxiety in cirrhosis. *Hepatol Res*. 2017;47(3): E64–E73.
25. Poonja Z, Brisebois A, van Zanten SV, Tandon P, Meeberg G, Karvellas CJ. Patients with cirrhosis and denied liver transplants rarely receive adequate palliative care or appropriate management. *Clin Gastroenterol Hepatol*. 2014;12(4):692–698.
26. Verne GN, Soldevia-Pico C, Robinson ME, Spicer KM, Reuben A. Autonomic dysfunction and gastroparesis in cirrhosis. *J Clin Gastroenterol*. 2004;38(1):72–76.
27. Aslam N, Kedar A, Nagarajarao HS, et al. Serum catecholamines and dysautonomia in diabetic gastroparesis and liver cirrhosis. *Am J Med Sci*. 2015;350(2):81–86.
28. Chesta J, Silva M, Thompson L, del Canto E, Defilippi C. Bacterial overgrowth in small intestine in patients with liver cirrhosis. *Rev Med Chile*. 1991;119(6):626–632.
29. Pande C, Kumar A, Sarin SK. Small-intestinal bacterial overgrowth in cirrhosis is related to the severity of liver disease. *Aliment Pharmacol Ther*. 2009;29(12):1273–1281.
30. Jeejeebhoy KN. Malnutrition, fatigue, frailty, vulnerability, sarcopenia and cachexia: overlap of clinical features. *Curr Opin Clin Nutr Metab Care*. 2012;15(3):213–219.
31. Sinclair M, Grossmann M, Gow PJ, Angus PW. Testosterone in men with advanced liver disease: abnormalities and implications. *J Gastroenterol Hepatol*. 2015;30(2):244–251.
32. Bonefeld K, Moller S. Insulin-like growth factor-I and the liver. *Liver Int*. 2011;31(7):911–919.
33. Knudsen AW, Krag A, Nordgaard-Lassen I, et al. Effect of paracentesis on metabolic activity in patients with advanced cirrhosis and ascites. *Scand J Gastroenterol*. 2016;51(5):601–609.

34. Ley RE, Turnbaugh PJ, Klein S, Gordon JI. Microbial ecology: human gut microbes associated with obesity. *Nature*. 2006;444(7122): 1022–1023.
35. Singh RK, Chang HW, Yan D, et al. Influence of diet on the gut microbiome and implications for human health. *J Transl Med*. 2017;15(1):73.
36. Willson K, Situ C. Systematic review on effects of diet on gut microbiota in relation to metabolic syndromes. *J Clin Nutr Metab*. 2017;1(2).
37. Gentile CL, Weir TL. The gut microbiota at the intersection of diet and human health. *Science*. 2018;362(6416):776–780.
38. Houghton D, Stewart CJ, Day CP, Trenell M. Gut microbiota and lifestyle interventions in NAFLD. *Int J Mol Sci*. 2016;17(4):447.
39. Tan J, McKenzie C, Potamitis M, Thorburn AN, Mackay CR, Macia L. The role of short-chain fatty acids in health and disease. *Adv Immunol*. 2014;121:91–119.
40. Alexeev EE, Lanis JM, Kao DJ, et al. Microbiota-derived Indole metabolites promote human and murine intestinal homeostasis through regulation of interleukin-10 receptor. *Am J Pathol*. 2018; 188(5):1183–1194.
41. Krishnan S, Ding Y, Saedi N, et al. Gut microbiota-derived tryptophan metabolites modulate inflammatory response in hepatocytes and macrophages. *Cell Rep*. 2018;23(4):1099–1111.
42. Heianza Y, Ma W, Manson JE, Rexrode KM, Qi L. Gut microbiota metabolites and risk of major adverse cardiovascular disease events and death: a systematic review and meta-analysis of prospective studies. *J Am Heart Assoc*. 2017;6(7).
43. Dumas ME, Barton RH, Toye A, et al. Metabolic profiling reveals a contribution of gut microbiota to fatty liver phenotype in insulin-resistant mice. *Proc Natl Acad Sci USA*. 2006;103(33):12511–12516.
44. Tan X, Liu Y, Long J, et al. Trimethylamine N-oxide aggravates liver steatosis through modulation of bile acid metabolism and inhibition of farnesoid X receptor signaling in nonalcoholic fatty liver disease. *Mol Nutr Food Res*. 2019:e1900257.
45. Kirpich IA, Solovieva NV, Leikhter SN, et al. Probiotics restore bowel flora and improve liver enzymes in human alcohol-induced liver injury: a pilot study. *Alcohol*. 2008;42(8):675–682.
46. Bull-Otterson L, Feng W, Kirpich I, et al. Metagenomic analyses of alcohol induced pathogenic alterations in the intestinal microbiome and the effect of *Lactobacillus rhamnosus* GG treatment. *PLoS One*. 2013;8(1):e53028.
47. Chen P, Torralba M, Tan J, et al. Supplementation of saturated long-chain fatty acids maintains intestinal eubiosis and reduces ethanol-induced liver injury in mice. *Gastroenterology*. 2015; 148(1), 203–214.e216.
48. Llopis M, Cassard AM, Wrzosek L, et al. Intestinal microbiota contributes to individual susceptibility to alcoholic liver disease. *Gut*. 2016;65(5):830–839.
49. Ferrere G, Wrzosek L, Cailleux F, et al. Fecal microbiota manipulation prevents dysbiosis and alcohol-induced liver injury in mice. *J Hepatol*. 2017;66(4):806–815.
50. Backhed F, Ding H, Wang T, et al. The gut microbiota as an environmental factor that regulates fat storage. *Proc Natl Acad Sci USA*. 2004;101(44):15718–15723.
51. Backhed F, Manchester JK, Semenkovich CF, Gordon JI. Mechanisms underlying the resistance to diet-induced obesity in germ-free mice. *Proc Natl Acad Sci USA*. 2007;104(3):979–984.
52. Rabot S, Membrez M, Bruneau A, et al. Germ-free C57BL/6J mice are resistant to high-fat-diet-induced insulin resistance and have altered cholesterol metabolism. *FASEB J*. 2010;24(12): 4948–4959.
53. Wang Z, Klipfell E, Bennett BJ, et al. Gut flora metabolism of phosphatidylcholine promotes cardiovascular disease. *Nature*. 2011; 472(7341):57–63.
54. Swann JR, Want EJ, Geier FM, et al. Systemic gut microbial modulation of bile acid metabolism in host tissue compartments. *Proc Natl Acad Sci USA*. 2011;108(Suppl 1):4523–4530.
55. Cani PD, Neyrinck AM, Fava F, et al. Selective increases of bifidobacteria in gut microflora improve high-fat-diet-induced diabetes in mice through a mechanism associated with endotoxaemia. *Diabetologia*. 2007;50(11):2374–2383.
56. Ferolla SM, Armiliato GN, Couto CA, Ferrari TC. The role of intestinal bacteria overgrowth in obesity-related nonalcoholic fatty liver disease. *Nutrients*. 2014;6(12):5583–5599.
57. Zhu L, Baker SS, Gill C, et al. Characterization of gut microbiomes in nonalcoholic steatohepatitis (NASH) patients: a connection between endogenous alcohol and NASH. *Hepatology*. 2013;57(2): 601–609.
58. Boursier J, Mueller O, Barret M, et al. The severity of nonalcoholic fatty liver disease is associated with gut dysbiosis and shift in the metabolic function of the gut microbiota. *Hepatology*. 2016;63(3): 764–775.
59. Miura K, Ohnishi H. Role of gut microbiota and Toll-like receptors in nonalcoholic fatty liver disease. *World J Gastroenterol*. 2014; 20(23):7381–7391.
60. Le Roy T, Llopis M, Lepage P, et al. Intestinal microbiota determines development of non-alcoholic fatty liver disease in mice. *Gut*. 2013;62(12):1787–1794.
61. Zhou Y, Zheng T, Chen H, et al. Microbial intervention as a novel target in treatment of non-alcoholic fatty liver disease progression. *Cell Physiol Biochem*. 2018;51(5):2123–2135.
62. Bidu C, Escoula Q, Bellenger S, et al. The transplantation of omega3 PUFA-altered gut microbiota of fat-1 mice to wild-type littermates prevents obesity and associated metabolic disorders. *Diabetes*. 2018;67(8):1512–1523.
63. Koopman N, Molinaro A, Nieuwdorp M, Holleboom AG. Review article: can bugs be drugs? The potential of probiotics and prebiotics as treatment for non-alcoholic fatty liver disease. *Aliment Pharmacol Ther*. 2019;50(6):628–639.
64. Moreno C, Deltenre P, Senterre C, et al. Intensive enteral nutrition is ineffective for patients with severe alcoholic hepatitis treated with corticosteroids. *Gastroenterology*. 2016;150(4), 903–910.e908.
65. Dasarathy S, Merli M. Sarcopenia from mechanism to diagnosis and treatment in liver disease. *J Hepatol*. 2016;65(6):1232–1244.
66. Owen OE, Reichle FA, Mozzoli MA, et al. Hepatic, gut, and renal substrate flux rates in patients with hepatic cirrhosis. *J Clin Investig*. 1981;68(1):240–252.
67. Nanji AA, French SW. Dietary factors and alcoholic cirrhosis. *Alcohol Clin Exp Res*. 1986;10(3):271–273.
68. Kirpich IA, Miller ME, Cave MC, Joshi-Barve S, McClain CJ. Alcoholic liver disease: update on the role of dietary fat. *Biomolecules*. 2016;6(1):1.
69. Hodson L, Rosqvist F, Parry SA. The influence of dietary fatty acids on liver fat content and metabolism. *Proc Nutr Soc*. 2019: 1–12.
70. Bridges FS. Relationship between dietary beef, fat, and pork and alcoholic cirrhosis. *Int J Environ Res Public Health*. 2009;6(9): 2417–2425.
71. Nanji AA, Mendenhall CL, French SW. Beef fat prevents alcoholic liver disease in the rat. *Alcohol Clin Exp Res*. 1989;13(1):15–19.
72. Nanji AA, Griniuviene B, Sadrzadeh SM, Levitsky S, McCully JD. Effect of type of dietary fat and ethanol on antioxidant enzyme mRNA induction in rat liver. *J Lipid Res*. 1995;36(4):736–744.
73. Nanji AA, French SW. Dietary linoleic acid is required for development of experimentally induced alcoholic liver injury. *Life Sci*. 1989;44(3):223–227.
74. *Dietary Reference Intakes for Energy, Carbohydrate, Fiber, Fat, Fatty Acids, Cholesterol, Protein, and Amino Acids*. Washington, DC: Institute of Medicine of the National Academy of Sciences. Standing Committee on the Scientific Evaluation of Dietary Reference Intakes, National Academy Press; 2005.
75. Blasbalg TL, Hibbeln JR, Ramsden CE, Majchrzak SF, Rawlings RR. Changes in consumption of omega-3 and omega-6

fatty acids in the United States during the 20th century. *Am J Clin Nutr*. 2011;93(5):950–962.
76. Nanji AA, Zhao S, Lamb RG, Dannenberg AJ, Sadrzadeh SM, Waxman DJ. Changes in cytochromes P-450, 2E1, 2B1, and 4A, and phospholipases A and C in the intragastric feeding rat model for alcoholic liver disease: relationship to dietary fats and pathologic liver injury. *Alcohol Clin Exp Res*. 1994;18(4):902–908.
77. Polavarapu R, Spitz DR, Sim JE, et al. Increased lipid peroxidation and impaired antioxidant enzyme function is associated with pathological liver injury in experimental alcoholic liver disease in rats fed diets high in corn oil and fish oil. *Hepatology*. 1998; 27(5):1317–1323.
78. Kono H, Enomoto N, Connor HD, et al. Medium-chain triglycerides inhibit free radical formation and TNF-alpha production in rats given enteral ethanol. *Am J Physiol Gastrointest Liver Physiol*. 2000;278(3):G467–G476.
79. Kirpich IA, Feng W, Wang Y, et al. The type of dietary fat modulates intestinal tight junction integrity, gut permeability, and hepatic toll-like receptor expression in a mouse model of alcoholic liver disease. *Alcohol Clin Exp Res*. 2012;36(5):835–846.
80. Zhong W, Li Q, Xie G, et al. Dietary fat sources differentially modulate intestinal barrier and hepatic inflammation in alcohol-induced liver injury in rats. *Am J Physiol Gastrointest Liver Physiol*. 2013;305(12). G919–932.
81. Song BJ, Moon KH, Olsson NU, Salem Jr N. Prevention of alcoholic fatty liver and mitochondrial dysfunction in the rat by long-chain polyunsaturated fatty acids. *J Hepatol*. 2008;49(2):262–273.
82. Wada S, Yamazaki T, Kawano Y, Miura S, Ezaki O. Fish oil fed prior to ethanol administration prevents acute ethanol-induced fatty liver in mice. *J Hepatol*. 2008;49(3):441–450.
83. Huang LL, Wan JB, Wang B, et al. Suppression of acute ethanol-induced hepatic steatosis by docosahexaenoic acid is associated with downregulation of stearoyl-CoA desaturase 1 and inflammatory cytokines. *Prostaglandins Leukot Essent Fatty Acids*. 2013;88(5): 347–353.
84. Nanji AA, Zhao S, Sadrzadeh SM, Dannenberg AJ, Tahan SR, Waxman DJ. Markedly enhanced cytochrome P450 2E1 induction and lipid peroxidation is associated with severe liver injury in fish oil-ethanol-fed rats. *Alcohol Clin Exp Res*. 1994;18(5): 1280–1285.
85. Morimoto M, Zern MA, Hagbjork AL, Ingelman-Sundberg M, French SW. Fish oil, alcohol, and liver pathology: role of cytochrome P450 2E1. *Proc Soc Exp Biol Med*. 1994;207(2):197–205.
86. Wang Y, Zhao Y, Li M, Wang Y, Yu S, Zeng T. Docosahexaenoic acid supplementation failed to attenuate chronic alcoholic fatty liver in mice. *Acta Biochim Biophys Sin (Shanghai)*. 2016;48(5): 482–484.
87. Wang M, Zhang X, Ma LJ, et al. Omega-3 polyunsaturated fatty acids ameliorate ethanol-induced adipose hyperlipolysis: a mechanism for hepatoprotective effect against alcoholic liver disease. *Biochim Biophys Acta Mol Basis Dis*. 2017;1863(12):3190–3201.
88. Huang W, Wang B, Li X, Kang JX. Endogenously elevated n-3 polyunsaturated fatty acids alleviate acute ethanol-induced liver steatosis. *Biofactors*. 2015;41(6):453–462.
89. Ferramosca A, Zara V. Modulation of hepatic steatosis by dietary fatty acids. *World J Gastroenterol*. 2014;20(7):1746–1755.
90. Juarez-Hernandez E, Chavez-Tapia NC, Uribe M, Barbero-Becerra VJ. Role of bioactive fatty acids in nonalcoholic fatty liver disease. *Nutr J*. 2016;15(1):72.
91. Malhi H, Gores GJ. Molecular mechanisms of lipotoxicity in nonalcoholic fatty liver disease. *Semin Liver Dis*. 2008;28(4): 360–369.
92. Henkel J, Coleman CD, Schraplau A, et al. Induction of steatohepatitis (NASH) with insulin resistance in wildtype B6 mice by a western-type diet containing soybean oil and cholesterol. *Mol Med*. 2017;23:70–82.
93. Duwaerts CC, Amin AM, Siao K, et al. Specific macronutrients exert unique influences on the adipose-liver Axis to promote hepatic steatosis in mice. *Cell Mol Gastroenterol Hepatol*. 2017;4(2): 223–236.
94. Araya J, Rodrigo R, Videla LA, et al. Increase in long-chain polyunsaturated fatty acid n - 6/n - 3 ratio in relation to hepatic steatosis in patients with non-alcoholic fatty liver disease. *Clin Sci (Lond)*. 2004;106(6):635–643.
95. Lu W, Li S, Li J, et al. Effects of omega-3 fatty acid in nonalcoholic fatty liver disease: a meta-analysis. *Gastroenterol Res Pract*. 2016; 2016:1459790.
96. Assy N, Nasser G, Kamayse I, et al. Soft drink consumption linked with fatty liver in the absence of traditional risk factors. *Can J Gastroenterol*. 2008;22(10):811–816.
97. Spruss A, Kanuri G, Wagnerberger S, Haub S, Bischoff SC, Bergheim I. Toll-like receptor 4 is involved in the development of fructose-induced hepatic steatosis in mice. *Hepatology*. 2009; 50(4):1094–1104.
98. Wada T, Kenmochi H, Miyashita Y, et al. Spironolactone improves glucose and lipid metabolism by ameliorating hepatic steatosis and inflammation and suppressing enhanced gluconeogenesis induced by high-fat and high-fructose diet. *Endocrinology*. 2010; 151(5):2040–2049.
99. Kelley GL, Allan G, Azhar S. High dietary fructose induces a hepatic stress response resulting in cholesterol and lipid dysregulation. *Endocrinology*. 2004;145(2):548–555.
100. Park OJ, Cesar D, Faix D, Wu K, Shackleton CH, Hellerstein MK. Mechanisms of fructose-induced hypertriglyceridaemia in the rat. Activation of hepatic pyruvate dehydrogenase through inhibition of pyruvate dehydrogenase kinase. *Biochem J*. 1992;282(Pt 3): 753–757.
101. Ouyang X, Cirillo P, Sautin Y, et al. Fructose consumption as a risk factor for non-alcoholic fatty liver disease. *J Hepatol*. 2008;48(6): 993–999.
102. Abdelmalek MF, Lazo M, Horska A, et al. Higher dietary fructose is associated with impaired hepatic adenosine triphosphate homeostasis in obese individuals with type 2 diabetes. *Hepatology*. 2012;56(3):952–960.
103. Abdelmalek MF, Suzuki A, Guy C, et al. Increased fructose consumption is associated with fibrosis severity in patients with nonalcoholic fatty liver disease. *Hepatology*. 2010;51(6): 1961–1971.
104. Fujisawa T, Riby J, Kretchmer N. Intestinal absorption of fructose in the rat. *Gastroenterology*. 1991;101(2):360–367.
105. Riby JE, Fujisawa T, Kretchmer N. Fructose absorption. *Am J Clin Nutr*. 1993;58(5 suppl):748S–753S.
106. Bergheim I, Weber S, Vos M, et al. Antibiotics protect against fructose-induced hepatic lipid accumulation in mice: role of endotoxin. *J Hepatol*. 2008;48(6):983–992.
107. Elliott SS, Keim NL, Stern JS, Teff K, Havel PJ. Fructose, weight gain, and the insulin resistance syndrome. *Am J Clin Nutr*. 2002; 76(5):911–922.
108. Spruss A, Bergheim I. Dietary fructose and intestinal barrier: potential risk factor in the pathogenesis of nonalcoholic fatty liver disease. *J Nutr Biochem*. 2009;20(9):657–662.
109. Schwimmer JB, Ugalde-Nicalo P, Welsh JA, et al. Effect of a low free sugar diet vs usual diet on nonalcoholic fatty liver disease in adolescent boys: a randomized clinical trial. *J Am Med Assoc*. 2019;321(3):256–265.
110. McClain C, Vatsalya V, Cave M. Role of zinc in the development/progression of alcoholic liver disease. *Curr Treat Options Gastroenterol*. 2017;15(2):285–295.
111. Mohammad MK, Zhou Z, Cave M, Barve A, McClain CJ. Zinc and liver disease. *Nutr Clin Pract*. 2012;27(1):8–20.
112. Coyle L, Entezaralmahdi M, Adeola M, De Hoyos P, Mehed A, Varon J. The perfect storm: copper deficiency presenting as

progressive peripheral neuropathy. *Am J Emerg Med*. 2016;34(2), 340.e345–346.
113. Song M, Schuschke DA, Zhou Z, et al. Modest fructose beverage intake causes liver injury and fat accumulation in marginal copper deficient rats. *Obesity (Silver Spring)*. 2013; 21(8):1669–1675.
114. McClain CJ, Marsano L, Burk RF, Bacon B. Trace metals in liver disease. *Semin Liver Dis*. 1991;11(4):321–339.
115. Butterworth RF. Thiamine deficiency-related brain dysfunction in chronic liver failure. *Metab Brain Dis*. 2009;24(1):189–196.
116. Sokol RJ. Fat-soluble vitamins and their importance in patients with cholestatic liver diseases. *Gastroenterol Clin N Am*. 1994; 23(4):673–705.
117. Chaves GV, Peres WA, Goncalves JC, Ramalho A. Vitamin A and retinol-binding protein deficiency among chronic liver disease patients. *Nutrition*. 2015;31(5):664–668.
118. Abbott-Johnson WJ, Kerlin P, Abiad G, Clague AE, Cuneo RC. Dark adaptation in vitamin A-deficient adults awaiting liver transplantation: improvement with intramuscular vitamin A treatment. *Br J Ophthalmol*. 2011;95(4):544–548.
119. Leo MA, Lieber CS. Alcohol, vitamin A, and beta-carotene: adverse interactions, including hepatotoxicity and carcinogenicity. *Am J Clin Nutr*. 1999;69(6):1071–1085.
120. Panel A-IHG. Hepatitis C guidance 2018 update: AASLD-IDSA recommendations for testing, managing, and treating hepatitis C virus infection. *Clin Infect Dis*. 2018;67(10):1477–1492.
121. Terrault NA, Lok ASF, McMahon BJ, et al. Update on prevention, diagnosis, and treatment of chronic hepatitis B: AASLD 2018 hepatitis B guidance. *Hepatology*. 2018;67(4):1560–1599.
122. Armstrong MJ, Gaunt P, Aithal GP, et al. Liraglutide safety and efficacy in patients with non-alcoholic steatohepatitis (LEAN): a multicentre, double-blind, randomised, placebo-controlled phase 2 study. *Lancet*. 2016;387(10019):679–690.
123. Mattar SG, Velcu LM, Rabinovitz M, et al. Surgically-induced weight loss significantly improves nonalcoholic fatty liver disease and the metabolic syndrome. *Ann Surg*. 2005;242(4):610–617. Discussion 618–620.
124. Mummadi RR, Kasturi KS, Chennareddygari S, Sood GK. Effect of bariatric surgery on nonalcoholic fatty liver disease: systematic review and meta-analysis. *Clin Gastroenterol Hepatol*. 2008;6(12): 1396–1402.
125. Mathurin P, Hollebecque A, Arnalsteen L, et al. Prospective study of the long-term effects of bariatric surgery on liver injury in patients without advanced disease. *Gastroenterology*. 2009;137(2): 532–540.
126. Lee Y, Doumouras AG, Yu J, et al. Complete resolution of nonalcoholic fatty liver disease after bariatric surgery: a systematic review and meta-analysis. *Clin Gastroenterol Hepatol*. 2019;17(6), 1040–1060.e1011.
127. Verna EC, Berk PD. Role of fatty acids in the pathogenesis of obesity and fatty liver: impact of bariatric surgery. *Semin Liver Dis*. 2008;28(04):407–426.
128. Gribsholt SB, Thomsen RW, Svensson E, Richelsen B. Overall and cause-specific mortality after Roux-en-Y gastric bypass surgery: a nationwide cohort study. *Surg Obes Relat Dis*. 2017;13(4):581–587.
129. Laursen TL, Hagemann CA, Wei C, et al. Bariatric surgery in patients with non-alcoholic fatty liver disease - from pathophysiology to clinical effects. *World J Hepatol*. 2019;11(2):138–149.
130. Patek Jr AJ, Post J, Ratnoff OD, et al. Dietary treatment of cirrhosis of the liver; results in 124 patients observed during a 10 year period, *J Am Med Assoc*. 138(8), 1948, 543-549
131. Hirsch S, Bunout D, de la Maza P, et al. Controlled trial on nutrition supplementation in outpatients with symptomatic alcoholic cirrhosis. *JPEN J Parenter Enteral Nutr*. 1993;17(2):119–124.
132. Hirsch S, de la Maza MP, Gattas V, et al. Nutritional support in alcoholic cirrhotic patients improves host defenses. *J Am Coll Nutr*. 1999;18(5):434–441.
133. Marsano LS, McClain C. Effects of alcohol on electrolytes and minerals. *Alcohol Health Res World*. 1989;13:255–260.
134. Lowell JA. Nutritional assessment and therapy in patients requiring liver transplantation. *Liver Transplant Surg*. 1996;2(5 suppl 1):79–88.
135. Cordoba J, Lopez-Hellin J, Planas M, et al. Normal protein diet for episodic hepatic encephalopathy: results of a randomized study. *J Hepatol*. 2004;41(1):38–43.
136. Gheorghe L, Iacob R, Vadan R, Iacob S, Gheorghe C. Improvement of hepatic encephalopathy using a modified high-calorie high-protein diet. *Rom J Gastroenterol*. 2005;14(3):231–238.
137. Nardelli S, Lattanzi B, Merli M, et al. Muscle alterations are associated with minimal and overt hepatic encephalopathy in patients with liver cirrhosis. *Hepatology*. 2019;70(5):1704–1713.
138. Vaisman N, Katzman H, Carmiel-Haggai M, Lusthaus M, Niv E. Breakfast improves cognitive function in cirrhotic patients with cognitive impairment. *Am J Clin Nutr*. 2010;92(1):137–140.
139. Ooi PH, Gilmour SM, Yap J, Mager DR. Effects of branched chain amino acid supplementation on patient care outcomes in adults and children with liver cirrhosis: a systematic review. *Clin Nutr ESPEN*. 2018;28:41–51.
140. Plank LD, Gane EJ, Peng S, et al. Nocturnal nutritional supplementation improves total body protein status of patients with liver cirrhosis: a randomized 12-month trial. *Hepatology*. 2008; 48(2):557–566.
141. Roman E, Garcia-Galceran C, Torrades T, et al. Effects of an exercise programme on functional capacity, body composition and risk of falls in patients with cirrhosis: a randomized clinical trial. *PLoS One*. 2016;11(3):e0151652.
142. Toshikuni N, Arisawa T, Tsutsumi M. Nutrition and exercise in the management of liver cirrhosis. *World J Gastroenterol*. 2014; 20(23):7286–7297.
143. Wu LJ, Wu MS, Lien GS, Chen FC, Tsai JC. Fatigue and physical activity levels in patients with liver cirrhosis. *J Clin Nurs*. 2012; 21(1–2):129–138.
144. Lazo M, Solga SF, Horska A, et al. Effect of a 12-month intensive lifestyle intervention on hepatic steatosis in adults with type 2 diabetes. *Diabetes Care*. 2010;33(10):2156–2163.
145. Yki-Jarvinen H. Nutritional modulation of nonalcoholic fatty liver disease and insulin resistance: human data. *Curr Opin Clin Nutr Metab Care*. 2010;13(6):709–714.
146. Tendler D, Lin S, Yancy Jr WS, et al. The effect of a low-carbohydrate, ketogenic diet on nonalcoholic fatty liver disease: a pilot study. *Dig Dis Sci*. 2007;52(2):589–593.
147. Lim JS, Mietus-Snyder M, Valente A, Schwarz JM, Lustig RH. The role of fructose in the pathogenesis of NAFLD and the metabolic syndrome. *Nat Rev Gastroenterol Hepatol*. 2010;7(5):251–264.
148. Zivkovic AM, German JB, Sanyal AJ. Comparative review of diets for the metabolic syndrome: implications for nonalcoholic fatty liver disease. *Am J Clin Nutr*. 2007;86(2):285–300.
149. Kistler KD, Brunt EM, Clark JM, et al. Physical activity recommendations, exercise intensity, and histological severity of nonalcoholic fatty liver disease. *Am J Gastroenterol*. 2011;106(3):460–468. Quiz 469.
150. Rafiq N, Younossi ZM. Effects of weight loss on nonalcoholic fatty liver disease. *Semin Liver Dis*. 2008;28(4):427–433.
151. Wadhawan M, Anand AC. Coffee and liver disease. *J Clin Exp Hepatol*. 2016;6(1):40–46.
152. Liu F, Wang X, Wu G, et al. Coffee consumption decreases risks for hepatic fibrosis and cirrhosis: a meta-analysis. *PLoS One*. 2015; 10(11):e0142457.

153. Marventano S, Salomone F, Godos J, et al. Coffee and tea consumption in relation with non-alcoholic fatty liver and metabolic syndrome: a systematic review and meta-analysis of observational studies. *Clin Nutr.* 2016;35(6):1269–1281.
154. Bravi F, Bosetti C, Tavani A, Gallus S, La Vecchia C. Coffee reduces risk for hepatocellular carcinoma: an updated meta-analysis. *Clin Gastroenterol Hepatol.* 2013;11(11), 1413–1421.e1411.
155. Inoue M, Tsugane S. Coffee drinking and reduced risk of liver cancer: update on epidemiological findings and potential mechanisms. *Curr Nutr Rep.* 2019;8(3):182–186.
156. Loftfield E, Shiels MS, Graubard BI, et al. Associations of coffee drinking with systemic immune and inflammatory markers. *Cancer Epidemiol Biomark Prev.* 2015;24(7):1052–1060.
157. Chalasani N, Younossi Z, Lavine JE, et al. The diagnosis and management of nonalcoholic fatty liver disease: practice guidance from the American Association for the Study of Liver Diseases. *Hepatology.* 2018;67(1):328–357.
158. Sanyal AJ, Chalasani N, Kowdley KV, et al. Pioglitazone, vitamin E, or placebo for nonalcoholic steatohepatitis. *N Engl J Med.* 2010; 362(18):1675–1685.
159. McClave SA, Taylor BE, Martindale RG, et al. Guidelines for the provision and assessment of nutrition support therapy in the adult critically ill patient: society of critical care medicine (SCCM) and American Society for parenteral and enteral nutrition (A.S.P.E.N.). *JPEN J Parenter Enteral Nutr.* 2016;40(2):159–211.
160. Shaw Jr BW, Wood RP, Gordon RD, Iwatsuki S, Gillquist WP, Starzl TE. Influence of selected patient variables and operative blood loss on six-month survival following liver transplantation. *Semin Liver Dis.* 1985;5(4):385–393.
161. Pikul J, Sharpe MD, Lowndes R, Ghent CN. Degree of preoperative malnutrition is predictive of postoperative morbidity and mortality in liver transplant recipients. *Transplantation.* 1994;57(3):469–472.
162. Muller MJ, Lautz HU, Plogmann B, Burger M, Korber J, Schmidt FW. Energy expenditure and substrate oxidation in patients with cirrhosis: the impact of cause, clinical staging and nutritional state. *Hepatology.* 1992;15(5):782–794.
163. Abbott WJ, Thomson A, Steadman C, et al. Child-Pugh class, nutritional indicators and early liver transplant outcomes. *Hepatogastroenterology.* 2001;48(39):823–827.
164. Pieber K, Crevenna R, Nuhr MJ, et al. Aerobic capacity, muscle strength and health-related quality of life before and after orthotopic liver transplantation: preliminary data of an Austrian transplantation centre. *J Rehabil Med.* 2006;38(5):322–328.
165. Normatov I, Kaplan S, Azzam RK. Nutrition in pediatric chronic liver disease. *Pediatr Ann.* 2018;47(11):e445–e451.
166. Nair S, Verma S, Thuluvath PJ. Obesity and its effect on survival in patients undergoing orthotopic liver transplantation in the United States. *Hepatology.* 2002;35(1):105–109.
167. Leonard J, Heimbach JK, Malinchoc M, Watt K, Charlton M. The impact of obesity on long-term outcomes in liver transplant recipients-results of the NIDDK liver transplant database. *Am J Transplant.* 2008;8(3):667–672.
168. Bambha KM, Dodge JL, Gralla J, Sprague D, Biggins SW. Low, rather than high, body mass index confers increased risk for post-liver transplant death and graft loss: risk modulated by model for end-stage liver disease. *Liver Transplant.* 2015;21(10): 1286–1294.
169. Plank LD, Metzger DJ, McCall JL, et al. Sequential changes in the metabolic response to orthotopic liver transplantation during the first year after surgery. *Ann Surg.* 2001;234(2):245–255.
170. de Carvalho L, Parise ER, Samuel D. Factors associated with nutritional status in liver transplant patients who survived the first year after transplantation. *J Gastroenterol Hepatol.* 2010;25(2): 391–396.
171. Tsien C, Garber A, Narayanan A, et al. Post-liver transplantation sarcopenia in cirrhosis: a prospective evaluation. *J Gastroenterol Hepatol.* 2014;29(6):1250–1257.
172. Ferreira LG, Santos LF, Anastacio LR, Lima AS, Correia MI. Resting energy expenditure, body composition, and dietary intake: a longitudinal study before and after liver transplantation. *Transplantation.* 2013;96(6):579–585.
173. Porayko MK, Wiesner RH, Hay JE, et al. Bone disease in liver transplant recipients: incidence, timing, and risk factors. *Transplant Proc.* 1991;23(1 Pt 2):1462–1465.
174. Lucey MR, Terrault N, Ojo L, et al. Long-term management of the successful adult liver transplant: 2012 practice guideline by the American Association for the Study of Liver Diseases and the American Society of Transplantation. *Liver Transplant.* 2013; 19(1):3–26.
175. Hanje AJ, Fortune B, Song M, Hill D, McClain C. The use of selected nutrition supplements and complementary and alternative medicine in liver disease. *Nutr Clin Pract.* 2006;21(3): 255–272.
176. Mouly S, Lloret-Linares C, Sellier PO, Sene D, Bergmann JF. Is the clinical relevance of drug-food and drug-herb interactions limited to grapefruit juice and Saint-John's Wort? *Pharmacol Res.* 2017;118: 82–92.
177. Williams S. How the microbiome influences drug action. In: *The Scientist. Ontario.* Canada: LabX Media Group; 2019:38–45.

CHAPTER

27

NUTRITIONAL ANEMIAS

Ajibola Ibraheem Abioye[1], *MD*
Wafaie W. Fawzi[1,2,3], *MBBS, MPH, MS, DrPH*
[1]Department of Nutrition, Harvard T.H. Chan School of Public Health, Boston, MA, United States
[2]Department of Global Health & Population, and Harvard T.H. Chan School of Public Health, Boston, MA, United States
[3]Department of Epidemiology, Harvard T.H. Chan School of Public Health, Boston MA, United States

SUMMARY

Anemia is the most prevalent nutritional problem globally, and poor nutrition is the foremost cause. Iron deficiency alone accounts for about half of all anemia cases, although deficiency of other nutrients may also occur. Anemia increases mortality risk especially in vulnerable groups, adverse pregnancy outcomes, poor cognitive development, increased health care costs, and lower productivity of workers.

Understanding iron metabolism will allow the design of anemia prevention and treatment programs. Dietary iron is absorbed in the duodenum, and the rate of absorption can be enhanced or inhibited by the coingestion of other food items. Transferrin and ferritin transport and store iron respectively. Hepcidin influences the rate iron is absorbed from intestines and released from the reticuloendothelial system into the blood.

Iron supplementation prevents anemia in pregnancy and thereby reduces the risk of adverse pregnancy outcomes. The World Health Organization recommends iron supplementation as part of standard care. Yet, fewer than 10% of pregnant women in many settings use them adequately. Food fortification with iron is cost-effective, and multiple countries have instituted fortification programs.

Other micronutrient deficiencies cause anemia too. Deficiencies of folate, vitamin B12, and vitamin A are reviewed in this chapter. Multiple micronutrient supplementation prevents anemia and reduces the risk of adverse pregnancy outcomes such as preterm births, small-for-gestational age, and low birth weight, compared to iron and folic acid alone. Anemia may also be prevented by delayed umbilical cord clamping at birth, control of infections, and most importantly, intake of high-quality, diverse diets.

Keywords: Anemia; Child; Fortification; Iron; Pregnancy; Supplementation.

I. NORMAL FUNCTION AND PHYSIOLOGY

A. Introduction

Anemia is the most prevalent nutritional problem globally. It refers to blood hemoglobin concentration below normal levels and a low oxygen-carrying capacity of the blood. People who are anemic may be pale, weak or easily tired. As anemia becomes severe, shortness of breath and palpitations occur when oxygen delivery to tissues is impaired. Anemia is a leading cause of death and disability worldwide. It accounted for 3.5% of the total years lived with disability from all conditions in 2017.[1] In 2012, the 65th World Health Assembly set a global nutrition target to halve the burden of anemia among women of reproductive age group by 2025.[2]

B. Epidemiology

Anemia disproportionately affects residents of low- and middle-income countries (LMICs), with the greatest burden in West Africa and South Asia.[3,4] Prevalence estimates vary by age, sex, socioeconomic status, and

https://doi.org/10.1016/B978-0-12-818460-8.00027-7

location. The public health significance of anemia in a country is classified mild if prevalence is >5%, moderate if 20%–40%, and severe if ≥ 40%.[5] The burden of anemia is greatest in children <5 years (43.6%) and pregnant women (38.2%).[2] The prevalence is >80% among children in Mali and Sierra Leone.[6,7] Anemia is more common in females than males, and the main causes of anemia differ by sex. Increased physiologic demands for maternal metabolism and fetal development during pregnancy is a major cause of anemia in females. The prevalence also differs by the burden of infections in the different countries. The average prevalence in high infection burden countries is 40%, and only about 12% and 7% in moderate and low infection burden countries, respectively.[8]

Anemia remains an important challenge in high-income countries. The burden is higher in certain demographic groups such as children, pregnant women, elderly persons, and racial minorities—especially non-Hispanic blacks and Hispanics.[9,10] The prevalence of anemia among pregnant women in high-income countries is about 22%. The prevalence of anemia in some of these countries is also on the rise, with >50% increase in the United States and Italy between 2002 and 2013.[9,10] Despite these distinctions by country income classification, anemia prevalence is only slightly influenced by national economic growth. For every 10% increase in income per capita, the prevalence of anemia among children <5 years reduces by 2.5%.[11] Even in the same country, it would take a fivefold increase in income to increase hemoglobin concentration by 1 g/dl.[12]

Iron deficiency (ID) is the most common cause of anemia globally—accounting for about half of all cases. Surveys using ferritin estimates corrected for inflammation suggest that the proportion of anemia due to ID range from 19%–38% in most countries.[3] Hookworm, malaria, and schistosomiasis (urinary and intestinal) infections, sickle cell anemia, thalassemia, chronic kidney disease, and cancers are also important causes.

Other common nutritional causes of anemia include deficiencies in vitamin A, folate, riboflavin (B2), and cyanocobalamin (B12). These often coexist with ID in resource-poor settings, making the attribution of etiology challenging.[8] Inadequate dietary iron intake during pregnancy and obstetric hemorrhage contribute to elevated risk of anemia in the immediate postpartum period.

The prevalence of anemia among children in many countries exceeds 60%. Age <2 years, low socioeconomic status, poor diet quality, malnutrition, and having been breastfed for <6 months are important predictors.[13–15] Anemia is also common in children with incomplete vaccination or who had a recent febrile illness.[16] Malaria is the most important cause of anemia in LMICs, and anemia is common among children who do not own a bednet. Children with repeated malaria episodes may have fourfold greater risk severe anemia compared to counterparts.[15] Anemia is also common in infants whose mothers were anemic during pregnancy—reflecting poor in utero iron transfer to the fetus, as well as poor quality of weaning diet and other environmental exposures.[13,17]

Adolescence is a critical period of increased nutritional demands for development, often coupled with behavioral challenges and reduced dietary intake and quality, and therefore warrants careful consideration.[18] Hormonal and reproductive peculiarities of adolescence, including menstrual abnormalities and inhibition of erythropoietin by estrogen, increase anemia risk among adolescent girls.[18] Adolescents who become pregnant have a greater risk of anemia compared to other adolescents and adult women.[19]

The burden of anemia among the elderly is considerable. In the United States, the prevalence was 4% among 50–59 year olds, 7% among 60–69 year olds, 12% among 70–79 year olds, and 19% among 80–85 year olds. Anemia is more common among elderly males than their female counterparts, and in non-Hispanic blacks compared to individuals belonging to other racial or ethnic groups.[9] Poor diet quality accounts for approximately one-third of anemia cases in the elderly. Of these, ID alone accounts for half. Anemia of inflammation (AI) accounts for >20%, often in association with kidney disease, cancers, and heart conditions. Anemia is negatively associated with quality of life, physical functioning, and muscle strength in the elderly.[20]

C. Consequences and Economic Burden

Mortality

Anemia can be so severe as to impair oxygen delivery to tissues considerably, leading to death. This is more likely to occur among the elderly,[20] children under the age of 5 years, pregnant women (especially if obstetric hemorrhage is excessive), and patients with advanced pulmonary tuberculosis or HIV.[21] Among pregnant women with anemia, modest amounts of obstetric hemorrhage may be associated with the occurrence of severe maternal outcomes, including mortality.[22] Among adults with HIV, studies examining the association of baseline anemia with all-cause mortality have consistently reported increased risk of mortality as anemia severity worsens.[23–25]

In the context of acute blood loss, severe anemia accompanies hypovolemic shock, hemodynamic instability, and organ damage leading to death.[26] If anemia is chronic and severe, impaired oxygen delivery to tissues can increase to compensatory increases in the workload of the heart, ultimately leading to heart failure and death. Anemia may also increase the risk of severe infections, leading to mortality.

Adverse pregnancy outcomes

The consequences of anemia in pregnancy stem from poor tissue oxygenation, reduced work capacity and exercise tolerance, blood pool expansion, disordered fetal and placental growth, and nutrient loss during childbirth. Anemia in pregnancy is associated with increased risk of critical pregnancy outcomes—preterm birth (by 63%), low birth weight (by 31%), perinatal mortality (by 51%), and neonatal mortality (by 2.72-fold).[4] In LMICs, 12% of low birth weight, 19% of preterm births, and 18% of perinatal mortality are attributable to maternal anemia.[4] These consequences are more likely if anemia occurs in the first and second trimester.[4]

Poor cognitive development

There is strong evidence that anemia is associated with depressed cognitive performance. The influence of anemia on cognitive function stems from reduced tissue oxygenation and diversion of critical iron from brain function to maintain erythropoiesis.[27] Iron is an important constituent of numerous metalloenzymes in the body. Iron is essential to maintain growth and differentiation in utero, especially in the first and second trimesters,[28,29] as well as during infancy.

Maternal iron status also influences infant neurocognitive development,[30] likely through iron status during infancy and early childhood.[31] Maternal micronutrient supplementation (MMS) prevents adverse consequences when provided early enough in pregnancy. It is critical that maternal ID be addressed before the third trimester because the impact of ID in the fetal brain may be irreversible afterward.[32] Children with iron depletion were 1.9- to 4.8-fold more likely to score poorly when their language, tractability, and fine motor skills were assessed.[33] The impact on cognitive development persists until late adolescence, and interventions after early childhood may not prevent long-term consequences.[34]

Iron serves multiple roles in brain development and function. During normal cognitive development, an adequate supply of iron is essential for neuronal and oligodendroglial cells to migrate to their final destination sites.[35] Iron is also critical for the myelination of nerve axons—essential for quick conduction of impulses across nerves.[36] Myelination begins at 12–14 weeks of pregnancy and continues through 2 years of age.[37] Iron depletion affects phosphorus utilization for ATP and lactate metabolism in the hippocampus, and iron is therefore critical in energy metabolism and regular functioning of nerves.[38,39] Iron is also important in the metabolism of neurotransmitters including dopamine, serotonin, and norepinephrine.[38,40] Finally, iron is important in the regulation of genes related to the function and production of myelin, synapses, and growth factors.[41,42]

Economic burden of nutritional anemia

The economic impact of nutritional anemia derives from increased mortality, higher cost of care for the complications of anemia, decreased productivity from exercise intolerance, decreased earnings potential from poor cognitive development, and possible intergenerational effects.[12] For instance, the annual health care costs for patients with anemia in the United States more than doubled the costs for nonanemic counterparts.[43] These costs were due to the increase in outpatient visits, emergency room visits, hospital days, laboratory tests, and therapies—including blood transfusion.[43]

The economic impact of poor cognitive development as a result of anemia during childhood is considerable. Infants with moderate ID anemia (IDA) tend to have test scores that are 0.5–1.5 standard deviations lower than their counterparts,[44] and a reduction in intelligence quotient by a half standard deviation results in 5%–12% lower wages, depending on country or how income was measured.[12]

National income is affected by the depressed productivity of anemic workers, due to excessive fatigue. The median loss in productivity was estimated to be approximately 0.9% in 1998,[44] and an updated understanding of the magnitude is necessary. The impact on lost productivity as a proportion of the gross domestic product was estimated to be greatest in South Asia due to the huge burden and the proportion of the population involved in manual work.[44] For instance, for every 1% decrease in hemoglobin concentration, the productivity of agricultural workers decreased by 1.5%.[45] Iron supplementation effectively improves labor productivity by 5%–17%,[12] and in labor-intensive economies, this can translate into improvements in earning ability.

Approaches to understand the economic burden of nutritional anemia have also examined the costs and benefits of interventions to address nutritional anemia.[45] These are discussed in the respective sections for the interventions.

II. PATHOPHYSIOLOGY

A. Nutritional Anemia: Iron Deficiency

As mentioned above, ID is by far the most important cause of anemia globally. The WHO estimates that 50% of anemia in women and 42% of anemia in children around the world could be effectively treated using iron supplementation.[2]

Iron metabolism

Iron is essential for life because it is a building block of (1) heme in hemoglobin and myoglobin and (2) iron-containing enzymes present in all cells. Like hemoglobin, myoglobin is an oxygen-carrying protein molecule. It is located in red muscle (cardiac and skeletal) and ensures the steady flow of oxygen to the mitochondria of muscle cells.[46] Iron requirements change during cell growth and therefore vary with the individual's age and sex—highest during pregnancy, childhood, and adolescence. The body obtains iron for metabolism from two sources: recycling of old red blood cells (RBCs)—22 mg/d—and from dietary intake (2–4 mg/d).[47]

Recycling from RBC contributes the greatest to plasma iron concentration. Senescent RBC and defective RBC precursors are catabolized by the macrophages in the reticuloendothelial system—especially spleen—as well as the liver and bone marrow. The degree to which iron is released from the reticuloendothelial system depends on the level of iron stores in the body and the presence of infection or inflammation.

Dietary sources of bioavailable iron include (1) heme iron: red meat, (2) nonheme iron: plant sources mostly such as beans, nuts, and green leafy vegetables, and (3) ferritin iron: mostly liver, but also from beans. Dietary iron absorption varies by dietary sources. Heme iron is consistently well absorbed (15%–35%). Nonheme iron absorption is more variable and could range from <1% to >90% depending on the coingestion of iron absorption inhibitors or enhancers, as well as the iron status of the individual. Examples of iron absorption inhibitors include tea and coffee. Examples of iron absorption enhancers include ascorbic acid in fruits and vegetables. Ferritin iron is also well absorbed—about as effectively absorbed as ferrous sulfate used for supplementation.[47]

Dietary iron is absorbed in the duodenum, predominantly, and in the jejunum. Systemic homeostasis ensures iron levels in plasma and extracellular fluid remain steady over a narrow range by regulating iron absorption. Factors affecting iron absorption in the gastrointestinal tract include the iron status of the individual, inflammation, and nature of food items in the individual's diet. Iron absorption is enhanced in response to iron depletion and depressed in the presence of inflammation, as part of a protective response to starve microbial invaders of essential iron.

Ferrous iron is first oxidized by enzymes, such as ferroxidase and ceruloplasmin, in macrophages, hepatocytes, duodenal enterocytes, and placental cells and then bound to ferroportin. Ferroportin is expressed on the surface of cells and is the only known cellular iron transport protein. Ferroportin transports iron across the membrane of duodenal enterocytes and macrophages in the reticuloendothelial system, to reach the systemic circulation. Thus, iron that is absorbed from the duodenum or recycled from the spleen, liver, or bone marrow is carried in the systemic circulation by transferrin. Transferrin is a glycoprotein in the plasma that transports iron to the cells, and transferrin saturation has a diurnal variation.[48] Iron that is absorbed into the enterocytes but is not transferred into the circulation is ultimately excreted in stool.

Iron uptake into cells occurs mainly via the transferrin receptor 1 (TfR1), by binding and internalizing transferrin. Iron is stored in cells as ferritin, and serum ferritin represents only a small fraction of the total ferritin. Total ferritin is in equilibrium with iron status—very low in ID. The divalent metal-ion transporter 1 (DMT1) is a transmembrane protein that facilitates iron entry into the cytoplasm but also transports nonheme iron across the apical membrane of duodenal enterocytes into the circulation.

Hepcidin is the master regulator of systemic iron homeostasis. It is produced by hepatocytes into blood and cleared by the kidney. It binds to ferroportin at numerous sites—including the surface of enterocytes in the gastrointestinal tract and macrophages in the reticuloendothelial system—to determine the degree to which ferroportin is available to transport iron across the plasma membrane for binding to transferrin.[49,50] The complex formed from hepcidin binding to ferroportin is degraded, thus limiting iron absorption. Hepcidin concentrations rises as total body iron increases, to prevent iron overload.[51]

Factors influencing hepcidin concentration include (1) erythropoietic rate—the greater the rate, the lower the hepcidin concentration, (2) iron stores in the liver—as iron stores increase, hepcidin levels increase to limit bioavailable iron, (3) hypoxia—reduces hepcidin synthesis via hypoxia-inducible factorll, (4) circulating iron, (5) inflammatory cytokines—interleukin 2 and 6, and (6) other pathways—related to nutrient metabolism, growth factors, and cellular proliferation. The erythropoietic rate is probably the greatest influence on hepcidin concentration as it overrides iron status.

Maternal iron stores are the main source of fetal iron for most of pregnancy. Placental iron transport is generally similar to the model described above for gastrointestinal iron absorption and uptake by macrophages with some peculiarities. Transferrin, ferrous iron, transferrin receptor (TfR), and ferroportin have the same roles as described above. Placental DMT1 and TfR facilitate the uptake of iron on the maternal side of the placenta.[52] Expression of placental TfR1 receptors is related to maternal iron status, and maternal ID upregulates its expression to facilitate transfer.[53] Here as well, ferric iron (Fe^{3+}) is oxidized to ferrous (Fe^{2+}) by a ferroxidase enzyme, permitting binding to ferroportin.

Iron transfer to the fetus is compromised when maternal stores are depleted. Neonatal and cord blood ferritin have been shown to be lower among neonates born to mothers with iron depletion, compared to iron-replete counterparts.[54,55] In a stable isotope study conducted among 41 Peruvian pregnant women, O'Brien et al. found a direct relationship between maternal iron absorption with ^{57}Fe and neonatal circulation.[56]

The role of maternal versus fetal hepcidin in facilitating iron transfer to the fetus is intriguing. Maternal circulating hepcidin concentrations decrease steadily during the course of pregnancy, to facilitate maternal iron absorption and thereby fetal iron uptake. The role of fetal hepcidin is less clear. Maternal iron depletion is associated with lower fetal hepcidin, to facilitate greater fetal iron uptake.[57,58] Fetal iron trafficking occurs as a result of a balance between maternal iron status determining placental iron uptake and fetal iron status determining placental iron efflux.[58–60] In fact, fetal iron needs are prioritized over maternal iron needs in the context of ID.[61]

Common causes of ID (Fig. 27.1)

- Inadequate intake—poor dietary diversity
- Iron malabsorption—from chronic intake of absorption inhibitors, celiac disease, chronic gastritis, iron refractory IDA
- Increased physiologic requirements unmet by dietary iron—during pregnancy, premature infants, early childhood, adolescent growth spurt. During pregnancy, for instance, iron status changes with the gestational age, reducing gradually from the first to third trimester as the fetal and placental needs for iron increase.
- Blood loss—menstruation, pathologic bleeding from gastrointestinal tract or urinary tract, helminth infections (hookworm, schistosomiasis)
- Intravascular hemolysis—accelerated breakdown of RBC within the blood vessels, faster than erythropoiesis to replace the cells (sickle cell anemia, celiac disease, thalassemia)

Stages of iron deficiency

Bothwell[62] proposed three stages of ID and these include (1) depletion of iron stores, (2) iron deficient erythropoiesis, and (3) IDA. Iron depletion is the first stage of ID and refers to the total exhaustion of body iron stores.[47] It is usually reflected as low serum ferritin concentration and the absence of stainable iron in the bone marrow. Anemia is unlikely to be present during this stage because erythropoiesis is not yet affected. Other iron status biomarkers are also normal.

If iron stores are not replenished, inadequate amounts of iron are incorporated into the hemoglobin during the formation of new RBC. This is known as iron deficient erythropoiesis and is the second stage of ID. Anemia is not present during this stage due to compensatory mechanisms that preserve hemoglobin synthesis. Specifically, zinc is incorporated into the hemoglobin molecule instead of iron. This stage can be identified by the elevated serum zinc protoporphyrin (ZPP). Soluble TfR levels also become elevated. Serum ferritin remains low, and the bone marrow still lacks stainable iron.

The third stage is IDA. Anemia results when the compensatory mechanisms to preserve hemoglobin and red cell production fail. The red cells tend to be microcytic (small size) and pale colored (hypochromic).

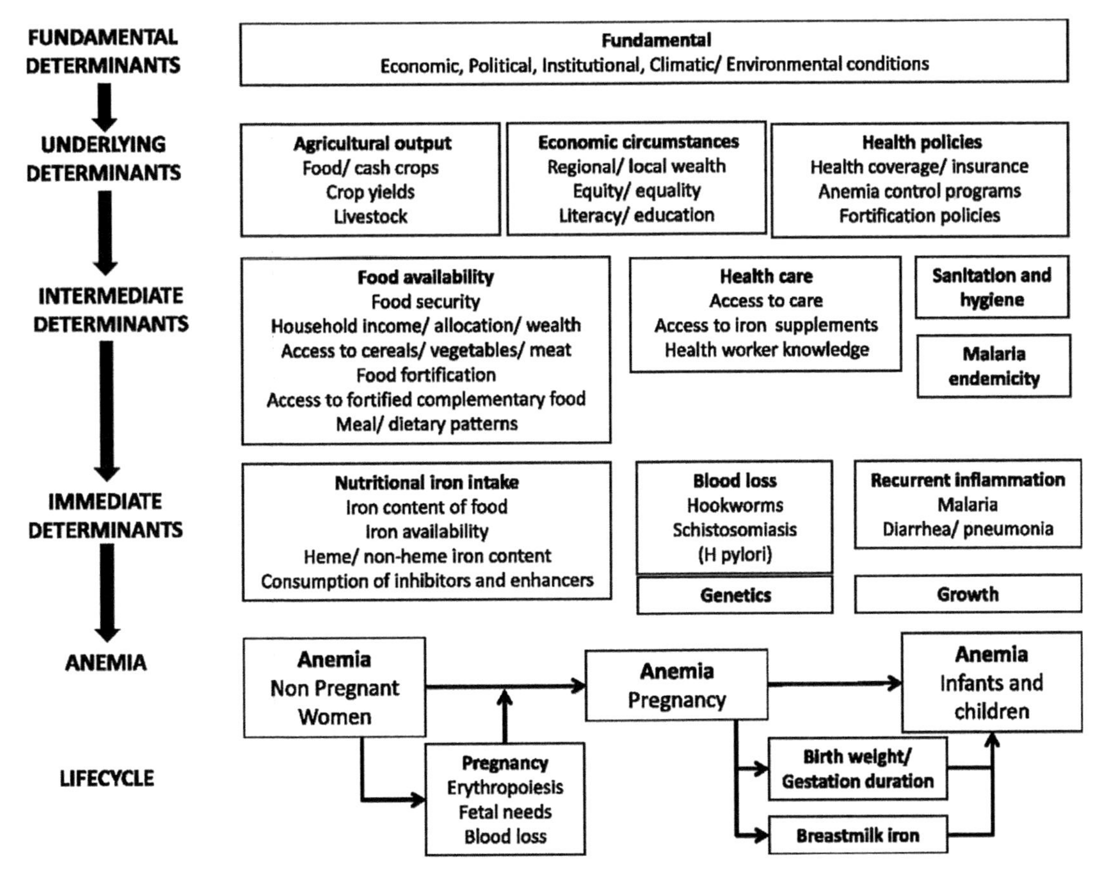

FIGURE 27.1 Causes of iron deficiency. *Source: Pasricha.*[162]

Iron and other micronutrients

As earlier mentioned, micronutrient deficiencies commonly cooccur, and studies have examined the impact of administering one other supplement with iron or coingesting iron with other micronutrients in diet (Table 27.1).

Iodine; Iron status and thyroid function are related, and ID predicts thyroid status during pregnancy.[63] Treatment of ID in individuals with goiter improves the effectiveness of thyroid treatment.[63,64] ID modifies thyroid function by altering the thyroid hormone feedback system and reducing levels of the active form of the thyroid hormone.[47] Integrating iron supplementation with measures to improve thyroid function such as promoting the intake of iodized salt may help.

Calcium; The WHO recommendations of routine iron and calcium supplementation are applicable to many of the same communities around the world. Both iron and calcium are divalent ions, and calcium intake likely inhibits iron absorption. It is possible that luminal calcium limits the uptake of iron by enterocytes because it leads to the internalization of DMT1 receptors, making them unavailable for iron absorption.[65] Population studies have yielded conflicting results.[66]

Calcium supplementation is important to prevent hypertension in pregnancy, and the risk that cosupplementation may worsen anemia risk among pregnant women is therefore concerning. As a precaution, the WHO recommends that calcium and iron supplements be taken at different times of the day. This makes it more likely that adherence to either supplement will be adversely affected. A recent metaanalysis of randomized trials and case-crossover studies suggests that calcium coingestion with iron is associated with impaired iron absorption and lower serum ferritin, with no impact on hemoglobin concentration.[67] Large randomized trials are also ongoing in Tanzania and India testing alternative dosing strategies that may allow safe delivery of calcium supplements in the context of routine iron supplementation in pregnant women.[68]

Zinc; The chemistry and metabolism of zinc is similar to that of iron, and zinc and iron compete for absorption when coadministered.[69] When iron stores are depleted, zinc replaces iron in the porphyrin ring of heme moiety of hemoglobin. Animal and human studies, including a large RCT of 2500 pregnant women, have reported reduced iron absorption due to high zinc intake leading to lower hemoglobin and ferritin concentration.[70,71]

The possible interaction of zinc with iron cosupplementation is important in the context of studies that have demonstrated that zinc supplementation may reduce the risk of placental malaria among pregnant women,[72] and the incidence of pneumonia, diarrhea, and diarrhea-specific mortality among children.[73] Clarifying this interaction is also important in the context of MMS. Further studies are warranted.

B. Nutritional Anemia: Other Micronutrients

Folate

Folate is essential throughout life. It is a cofactor for the de novo synthesis of purine and thymidine nucleotides. It is also a cofactor for the remethylation of homocysteine to

TABLE 27.1 Interaction of micronutrients with iron.

Micronutrient	Effect	Mechanism	Level of evidence
Vitamin A	Positive	Vitamin A enhances incorporation of iron into erythrocytes	
Iodine	Positive	Iron deficiency modifies thyroid function	
Calcium	Negative	Calcium intake reduces nonheme iron absorption and iron stores in the short term	Randomized trials and case-crossover studies
Zinc	Negative	Zinc and iron compete for incorporation into the porphyrin ring of the heme moiety during hemoglobin synthesis	Randomized trial
Copper	Negative	Copper and iron compete for absorption in the gastrointestinal tract	Observational studies

methionine, and homocysteine accumulation in folate deficiency is a basis for diagnosing the condition. Folate is important for cell growth and differentiation and is therefore required in greater amounts during pregnancy for the development of the fetus and the placenta.[74] The WHO recommends folate consumption of 400 μg/d for all women of reproductive age.[75] Deficiency of folate is well-known to increase the risk of neural tube and congenital heart defects, as well as fetal growth restriction, low birth weight, and preterm birth.[74] Folate deficiency may also result in the context of chronic alcoholism and use of phenytoin, metformin, sulfasalazine, and a few other common therapeutic drugs.[76]

Severe deficiency of folate and B_{12} is the cause of megaloblastic anemia—a form of macrocytic anemia (large size, few RBC) with hypersegmented neutrophils. Iron and folate deficiency may cooccur and may be unmasked when one deficiency is addressed. Folate deficiency results from intake of poor quality diets low in folate-rich sources (such as dark green leafy vegetables, beans, and nuts). Folate is the naturally occurring form in foods while folic acid is the synthetic form, used in supplements.

Mature RBCs accumulate folate during development and are therefore the optimal measure of long-term folate status. Too few national surveys and epidemiologic studies have used RBC folate biomarker and have opted for serum folate or homocysteine instead. RBC folate <400 μg/L is regarded as insufficient, per WHO guidelines.[75] In addition, serum folate <10 nmol/L or homocysteine ≥30 μmol/L. Folate fortification effectively increases serum folate concentrations.[77]

Vitamin B_{12}

Vitamin B_{12} is stored in the liver and takes a long time to be depleted. When this occurs, vitamin B12 deficiency causes megaloblastic anemia. If untreated, a demyelinating condition of the nervous system could result. Affected individuals present with neurologic and psychiatric features including paresthesia, peripheral neuropathy, irritability, depression, memory impairment, dementia, and psychosis. Vitamin B12 is an important cofactor in erythropoiesis. It is also involved in folate metabolism and the retention of folate in RBC.

Vitamin B12 deficiency occurs in individuals with chronic intake of limited quantities of animal source foods such as vegans and low-income individuals in developing countries. Less than 10% of individuals in Europe and the United States have inadequate intake.[78,79] Vitamin B12 deficiency may cooccur with ID in LMICs with 5%–10% of diet being from animal sources. Dietary sources of vitamin B12 include clams, liver and fortified breakfast cereal, meat, and dairy products.

Vitamin B12 is absorbed in the terminal ileum via endocytosis of a complex of vitamin B12 with intrinsic factor.[80] Therefore, vitamin B12 deficiency may also occur in the context of malabsorption syndromes or due to autoimmune atrophic gastritis, which impairs the production of intrinsic factor in the stomach.

Serum vitamin B12 < 200 pg/mL testing is useful for screening, and serum/plasma total homocysteine >21 μmol/L or serum methylmalonic acid may be used to confirm the diagnosis.[81] Age-specific cutoffs for these tests may be considered.[80,82] In clinical settings, additional tests to exclude pernicious anemia or atrophic gastritis may also be considered. Treatment with daily high-dose oral vitamin B12 (1000–2,000 mcg) and monthly intramuscular cyanocobalamin is similarly effective in resolution of B12 hematologic abnormalities within a few months.[83]

Vitamin A

Vitamin A deficiency is common in the context of low socioeconomic status and poor diet quality, especially in LMICs. Dietary sources of vitamin A are diverse. Animal sources of preformed vitamin A include liver, fish liver oils, dairy products, and egg yolk. Plant sources of carotenoid compounds include dark green leafy vegetables, yellow and orange vegetables, and fruits (such as carrots). Vitamin A–fortified foods in some developing countries such as sugar, cereal flours, edible oils, margarine, and noodles are also important sources of vitamin A.[76,84]

Vitamin A deficiency causes anemia by reducing the incorporation of iron into RBC during erythropoiesis[85] or as a result of depressed immunity and increased infection risk.[86] Other mechanisms have been suggested including altered RBC formation and differentiation, increased breakdown of malformed RBC, and impaired mobilization of iron from the reticuloendothelial system.[47] Rats fed with vitamin A–deficient diets over a long-term developed anemia and restoring vitamin A in the diet resolved the anemia.[85] Vitamin A supplementation trials among pregnant women and children <5 years have also demonstrated ≥14% lower risk of anemia.[87,88]

Vitamin A forms a soluble complex with iron in the intestinal lumen, enhancing its absorption and reducing the impact of inhibitors such as phytates and polyphenols. It is reasonable to expect vitamin A cosupplementation with iron to enhance the effectiveness of iron supplementation. While some studies have suggested that cosupplementing leads to a better hemoglobin and serum ferritin response than either micronutrient alone,[89,90] one RCT among pregnant women in Indonesia found no differences in either anemia and ID risk,[91] and a recent RCT among pregnant Tanzanian women found a better ferritin response, but an increased risk of severe anemia and no effect on the risk of mild to moderate anemia.[70] The Tanzanian trial specifically enrolled pregnant women in the first trimester, while the other studies enrolled women who were in the second or third trimester[89,91] or who were nonpregnant.[90] Clarifying this interaction is critical.

C. Anemia in Protein-Energy Malnutrition

Protein-energy malnutrition (PEM) deserves a distinct section when considering anemia because it is associated with an elevated mortality risk.[92] PEM may occur in the context of chronic poor quality diet or excess nutrient losses due to diseases such as severe diarrheal disease, kidney disease, or cancer. It results from disordered protein and/or total energy intake that does not match the physiologic requirements or increased needs in pathologic condition. Anemia is present in a substantial proportion of patients with PEM, regardless of the etiology of PEM, and may increase the risk of mortality and neurocognitive complications.[92,93]

PEM is accompanied by a lower overall production of visceral and blood proteins. Reduced serum transferrin production occurs as part of the global reduction in plasma proteins. As earlier mentioned, transferrin is essential for transport of iron in the systemic circulation, and low transferrin disrupts erythropoiesis, as well as other iron-dependent biological processes. ID, however, commonly occurs with PEM, often due to the poor-quality diet.[94] Iron depletion is usual in PEM, confirmed by the absence of stainable bone marrow iron in the majority of patients.[95] Deficiencies of folate, vitamin B12, and vitamin A are also possible, but less consistently seen.[94,95]

Production of blood cell progenitors is reduced in PEM.[96] This is due to bone marrow atrophy and inadequate nutrients essential for the proliferation, differentiation, and maturation of blood cells.[95–97] There is a decreased responsiveness to erythropoietin, a hormone that stimulates the production of RBC from stem cell progenitors.[95–97] Reticulocytopenia (low reticulocyte count) is therefore a fairly consistent feature of PEM. White blood cell counts are also low.

RBC membrane dysfunction results from depressed production of lipoproteins in the liver and disruption in the normal cholesterol–phospholipid balance of the plasma membrane.[98] This causes hemolysis and anemia.

Transfusion of packed RBC is associated with lower mortality risk, if anemia is severe.[99] Daily supplementation with micronutrients after the intensive phase of treatment is required.

D. Anemia in Chronic Inflammation and Infection

Anemia often occurs in the context of chronic inflammatory conditions and acute or chronic infections. It results from chronic blood loss, reduced dietary intake, poor-quality diet, hemolysis, inflammation, or a combination of these factors. Parasitic diseases such as hookworm and schistosomiasis are common causes of chronic gastrointestinal blood loss. Reduced dietary intake in the context of chronic infectious and noninfectious diseases is often due to anorexia and contributes to severe weight loss in these patients.

Inflammation in the context of chronic infectious and noninfectious diseases causes AI or anemia of chronic disease. AI refers to anemia, usually mild or moderate, in the presence of chronic inflammation that results in disordered gastrointestinal iron absorption and sequestration of iron in the duodenal enterocytes and in macrophages within the reticuloendothelial system.[51] It occurs as part of the immune response, which limits the amount of circulating iron. Ferritin concentrations increase inside macrophages, and overall iron available for biological processes is decreased. See Figs. 27.2 and 27.3. Anemia is present in approximately 50% of patients with HIV and 30% of patients with tuberculosis, and AI accounts for most cases.[21]

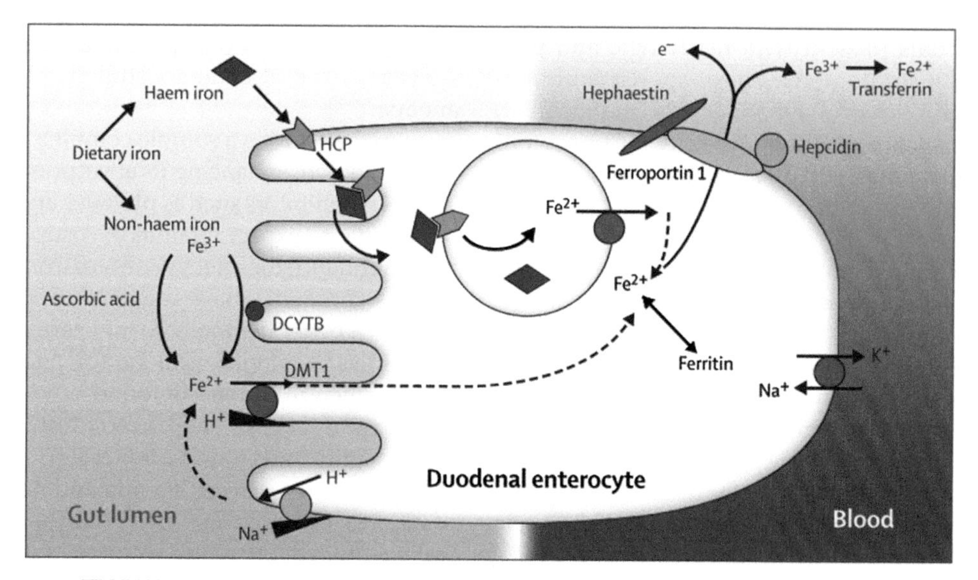

FIGURE 27.2 Regulation of intestinal iron uptake. *Source: Zimmerman and Hurrell.*[163]

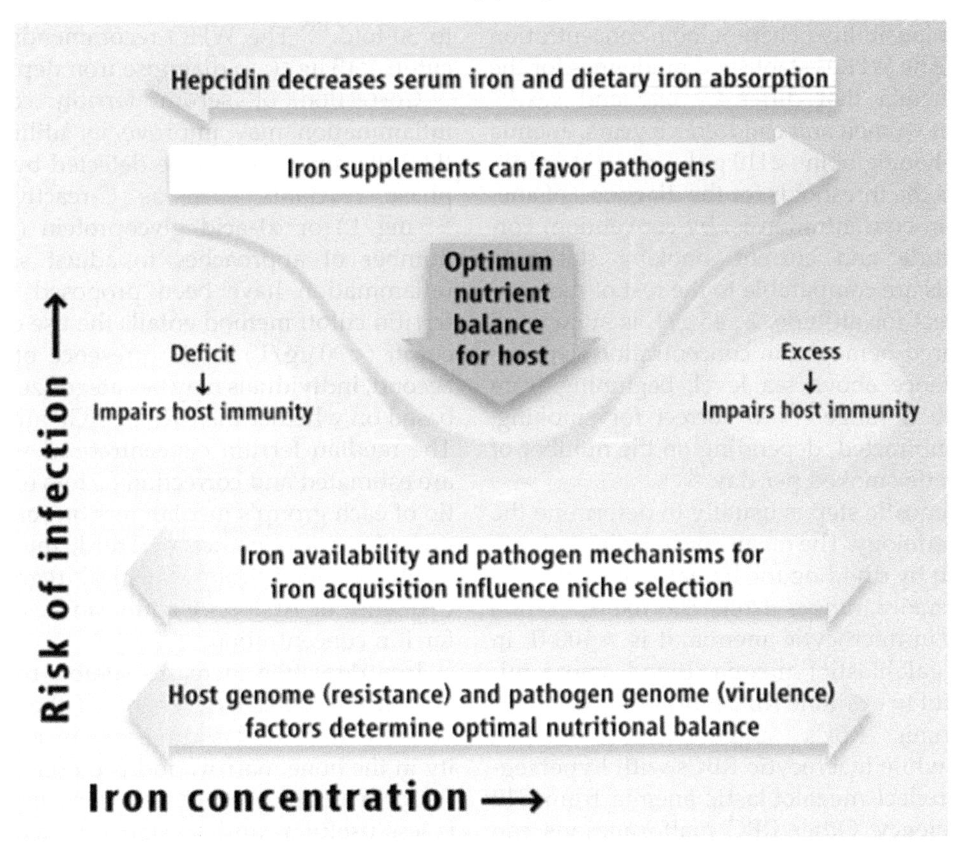

FIGURE 27.3 Risk of infection in relation to iron deficiency and iron excess. *Source: Drakesmith and Prentice.*[164]

Elevated hepcidin concentration is at the center of AI pathology. Hepcidin binds to ferroportin to determine how much iron is absorbed from the gastrointestinal tract or released from macrophages. Despite low serum iron, the total iron-binding capacity is low in AI. Red cell survival is also modestly decreased. Morphologically, affected RBC tend to be normocytic, with no increase in the red cell distribution width. Since AI reduces available iron for biological processes, it may cause some of the same consequences as IDA, and additional consequences due to the inflammation.

There is no standard definition for AI. Weiss and Goodnough suggested an approach based on the unique advantage of distinguishing individuals with AI from those with IDA and AI coexisting.[100] Briefly, in the presence of anemia, individuals with ferritin >100 μg/L or ferritin 30–100 μg/L and sTfR-ferritin ratio <1 are regarded as pure AI cases. If ferritin 30–100 μg/L and sTfR-ferritin >2, then AI and IDA are likely to be coexisting. If ferritin <30 μg/L, then IDA is likely. Hepcidin concentration may be further used to classify individuals with anemia, ferritin 30–100 μg/L and sTfR-ferritin of 1–2. Clearly, this approach is cumbersome, and simpler approaches to aid the diagnosis of AI are needed.

Some studies have instead considered noniron deficiency anemia (NIDA) as a proxy for AI, since AI accounts for the majority of anemia, which is not a result of ID. These studies have demonstrated that NIDA may be associated with an increased risk of all-cause mortality among adult HIV patients,[101] treatment failure among adults with tuberculosis,[21] and cognitive impairment among older children.[102]

The appropriate treatment for AI is unclear, although it is believed that treatment of the underlying infection or disease could ameliorate it. This question needs to be further examined, as limited available evidence does not necessarily support this hypothesis. For instance, while treatment with praziquantel for *Schistosoma japonicum* among Filipino pregnant women at 16 weeks' gestation did not modify the anemia type by 32 weeks' gestation,[59] antiretroviral therapy (ART) use was associated with a lower prevalence of AI after 18 months of follow-up among 400 Ugandan HIV-infected adults, compared to baseline.[103] Providing iron supplements alone to individuals with AI is unlikely to resolve the anemia.

E. Diagnosis—Clinical and Field

Anemia is diagnosed by assessing hemoglobin concentration, often as part of a complete or full blood count, or using point of care tests such as the hemoglobinometer (more commonly known by the brand name, HemoCue).

The range of plausibility of hemoglobin concentration is 25–200 g/L.[2] The WHO established guidelines for the diagnosis of anemia that differ by age and sex.[104] Among pregnant women and children <5 years, anemia is defined by hemoglobin <110 g/L (or <11 g/dl). Table 27.2 shows the thresholds for the diagnosis of anemia. Hemoglobin concentration is, by convention, corrected for altitude and current smoking status to ensure the results are comparable to the rest of the population. To correct for altitude, 2–45 g/L is subtracted from the measured hemoglobin concentration depending on the distance above sea level, beginning from 1,000 m to 4,500 m range.[104] To correct for smoking, 0.3–0.6 g/L is subtracted, depending on the number of packets of cigarette smoked per day.[104]

The next diagnostic step is usually to determine the anemia type or etiology. The mean corpuscular volume (MCV), obtained by dividing the hematocrit by the red cell count, normally ranges from 80–100 fL. While MCV is < 70 fL in microcytic anemia, it is > 100 fL in macrocytic (megaloblastic) anemia. Blood smear microscopy is useful to examine RBC morphology. Microcytic hypochromic RBCs suggest iron deficient erythropoiesis, while macrocytic RBCs with hypersegmented nuclei reflect megaloblastic anemia from B12 and folate deficiency. Other RBC malformations can be visualized to diagnose sickle cell anemia, hereditary spherocytosis, elliptocytosis, and myelodysplastic syndromes.

A number of methods are used to diagnose body iron status (Table 27.3). Bone marrow for stainable iron is the gold standard for diagnosing iron depletion. It is invasive and only rarely done in clinical practice. Iron status is most commonly assessed by measuring serum ferritin. Low serum ferritin (<10–12 μg/L) always reflects iron depletion. Higher ferritin concentrations may not necessarily exclude iron depletion or ID because ferritin can be increased with inflammation up to 30-fold.[105] The WHO recommends a serum ferritin cutoff <15 μg/L to diagnose iron depletion.[5]

Correction of serum ferritin concentrations for inflammation may improve its utility for diagnosing ID. Inflammation may be detected by measuring acute phase reactants such as C-reactive protein (CRP, >5 mg/L) or α1-acid glycoprotein (AGP, >1 g/L). A number of approaches to adjust serum ferritin for inflammation have been proposed. First, the higher ferritin cutoff method entails the use of a higher ferritin cutoff (<30 μg/L) in the presence of inflammation.[106] Second, individuals may be categorized into four groups based on whether the CRP or AGP are elevated or both. The median ferritin concentrations within each group are estimated and correction factors estimated as the ratio of each group's median ferritin relative to one of the group's as a reference[107]. Third, the regression coefficients obtained from statistical regression models of CRP and/or AGP on ferritin can be used to correct the ferritin concentration.[108]

Iron depletion increases soluble transferrin receptor (sTfR), the truncated version of the TfR with no iron bound to it.[109] sTfR is influenced by erythropoietic activity in the bone marrow and is therefore potentially useful for evaluating response to iron supplementation.[109] It is less useful as an iron status biomarker in conditions where altered erythropoiesis and ID coexist—such as pregnancy and hemolytic anemia.[109,110] sTfR is also influenced by inflammation, but to a lesser extent than serum ferritin. A ratio of sTfR to the $\log_{10}$ of ferritin, the sTfR-ferritin index, is often used an alternative to surmount some of these challenges. Results from the three commonly used assays often differ.[111,112] Therefore, sTfR tests need to be standardized.

As iron depletion progresses, levels become inadequate to maintain the production of the heme protein as part of erythropoiesis. Zinc may then be incorporated into the heme moiety, in place of iron, forming ZPP. ZPP

TABLE 27.2 Thresholds for diagnosis of anemia.

Children	Anemia	Mild anemia	Moderate anemia	Severe anemia
6–59 months	<110 g/L	100–109	70–99	<70
5–11 years	<115 g/L	110–114	80–109	<80
12–14 years	<120 g/L	110–119	80–109	<80
Adults				
Female, pregnant	<110 g/L	100–109	70–99	<70
Female, nonpregnant	<120 g/L	110–119	80–109	<80
Male	<130 g/L	110–129	80–109	<80

Source: World Health Organization (WHO). Haemoglobin concentration for the diagnosis of anaemia and assessment of severity. Vitamin and Mineral Nutrition Information System. *Geneva: WHO; 2011.*

TABLE 27.3 Iron status assessment.

Biomarker	Relevance	Method	Validity	Threshold/interpretation
Serum ferritin	Ferritin is the main store of intracellular iron	ELISA or using bedside rapid kits	Sensitive and specific, modified by inflammation	Levels are higher when iron stores are elevated and vice versa <15 μg/L is used to diagnose iron deficiency
Soluble transferrin receptor (sTfR)	An index of iron depletion or iron depleted erythropoiesis, refers to the level of soluble transferrin receptor with no bound iron	ELISA	Less influenced by inflammation. Levels may be elevated in hemolytic anemia, erythropoietin therapy, thalassemia major, or severe megaloblastic anemia	Levels are higher when iron stores are depleted. Elevated sTfR in the presence of anemia is more likely to be due to IDA than AI
sTfR-ferritin index or ratio	Helpful when sTfR (mg/L) and ferritin μg/L measures may have been altered by inflammation or infection	Estimated as a ratio of sTfR and $\log_{10}$ ferritin concentrations		Values are higher when iron stores are depleted. >1.5 is regarded as iron deficient
Zinc protoporphyrin	An excellent marker of iron-deficient erythropoiesis	Hematofluorometer	ZPP is however measured in whole blood, unlike ferritin and sTfR, and this greatly limits its utility in resource-limited settings	
Hepcidin	Is an antimicrobial peptide, produced from the liver, in response to the erythropoietic rate, elevated iron stores in the liver, circulating iron, hypoxia, and inflammation	ELISA		

is determined using hematofluorometer, in whole blood. ZPP testing is cheap and simple and less influenced by inflammation than the other iron status biomarkers. Concerns regarding training and supplies need to be addressed.[113] The concentration of ZPP may be elevated with thalassemia and sickle cell anemia, both highly prevalent in parts of Africa and Asia.[110]

Hepcidin is the primary regulator of iron homeostasis, and its concentration in serum is directly proportional to body iron stores, making it a suitable iron status biomarker. Recent studies among pregnant women in the Gambia and the Philippines have demonstrated its superior diagnostic accuracy for ID, compared to hemoglobin, sTfR, and ZPP.[59,114] Hepcidin levels are also modified by inflammation. While low hepcidin concentration ($\leq$1 μg/L) are more likely to reflect iron depletion, hepcidin levels tend to fall in pregnant women as the pregnancy advances. The erythropoietic drive is the most important determinant of hepcidin levels.[47] Hepcidin may distinguish between AI and IDA. Two common types of hepcidin ELISA assays are in use, and Wray and colleagues recently proposed a conversion factor between the tests.[115] Urinary hepcidin may be an alternative to blood testing, but it requires assessment of renal function by creatinine testing.

After establishing the diagnosis of anemia and characterizing the anemia type, it is often desirable to determine the etiology. Testing to determine the related pathology with HIV tests, blood smear for malaria, stool, and urine for occult blood loss may be indicated. Anemia may also be an early sign of undiagnosed conditions such as colorectal cancer or an indication of worsening disease such as in patients with chronic conditions such as kidney disease. Detailed clinical history and physical examination and additional tests may help characterize the clinical condition.

III. PRIMARY TREATMENT AND CONTROL MODALITIES

A. Dietary Diversification

Improved dietary diversity and access to healthful healthy iron-rich food options prevent anemia.[2] Intake of a diverse set of food groups ensures an adequate quantity and variety of calories, macronutrients, and micronutrients. Dietary diversity, therefore, reflects food security, nutrient adequacy, and diet quality.[116] Nutrition-sensitive programmes are required for successful dietary diversification. Agricultural and food security programmes increase the diversity of agricultural produce, nutrient diversity of crops, access to markets and farm productivity, and thereby, household and individual dietary diversity.[117,118] Women empowerment is also important to improve household dietary diversity since households where women can influence resource allocation spend more on fruit and vegetables and prioritize diet quality.[119]

Dietary diversity improves hematologic status, especially in children, the elderly, and the sick. In a cluster randomized trial in Burundi, providing food to children aged <2 years and their mothers improved hemoglobin concentration, partly through increased dietary diversity and consumption of iron-rich foods.[120] Among ART naïve patients with HIV in Uganda, intake of nutrient-rich foods was associated with lower risk of moderate anemia and mortality during follow-up.[121]

B. Iron Supplementation

Well-conducted systematic reviews and metaanalyses have demonstrated that daily iron supplementation (alone or as part of multivitamin supplements) prevents anemia in pregnant women,[122] menstruating women,[123] and school-age children.[124] The WHO has recommended iron supplementation as standard of care since the 1960s. Without iron supplementation during pregnancy, many pregnant women become iron depleted by third trimester though they may have been iron-replete in the first trimester.[125] Iron supplementation is cost-effective and costs \$2 − 5 for public health programs during the length of pregnancy and lactation costs.[12]

In one metaanalysis, pregnant women who used iron supplements any time during pregnancy had a higher mean hemoglobin concentration by 4.59 g/L, 50% lower risk of anemia, and 40% lower ID in the third trimester or at delivery.[122] Another metaanalysis found that supplementation was associated with a 41.2 g higher birth weight and a 19% lower risk of low birth weight, but no effect on preterm birth, SGA, length of gestation, or birth length.[122] Iron supplementation among infants is also associated with improved psychomotor development.[126] Infant iron supplementation, however, has not consistently been shown to be beneficial with regard to these nonhematologic clinical outcomes, making maternal iron supplementation more imperative.[127,128]

Multiple factors may influence the effectiveness of iron supplementation. Iron supplementation is more effective among pregnant women with poor hematologic status and if they use supplements for 90 days or more during pregnancy.[129] Only 10% of pregnant women in many sub-Saharan African countries use iron supplements adequately.[130] This is partly because pregnant women often commence antenatal care late. Other barriers to use of iron supplements in this setting include the inadequate or inconsistent supply, challenges to get patients to clinic regularly for refills, transport costs and convenience, and poor adherence once supplement is available. Iron supplementation is also less effective in malaria-endemic countries, likely due to inflammation.[122]

As an alternative to daily supplementation is intermittent supplementation—weekly or every 3 days. Intermittent iron supplementation is also effective to prevent anemia among pregnant women[131] and children <15 years.[132] Adherence, however, tends to be poorer among women on intermittent supplementation.

The WHO recommends the use of ferrous salts, due to their superior bioavailability, efficacy, and cost-effectiveness compared to ferric salts.[133] Ferrous sulfate is most commonly used, although ferrous gluconate and ferrous fumarate are alternatives. There are concerns that oral ferrous sulfate intake may be associated with adverse effects such as nausea, vomiting, and constipation due to mucosal irritation.[134]

The dose of supplementation affects how quickly anemia is treated or iron stores are restored. The WHO recommends 60 mg iron (which is 200 mg ferrous sulfate) daily during pregnancy in settings where anemia prevalence is >40%, and 30 mg if anemia prevalence is <40%. For every additional 10 mg iron/day among studies that provided ≤66 mg daily, iron supplementation was associated with 12% lower risk of maternal anemia. Supplementation is recommended to commence as early as possible, ideally before conception.[135]

Elevated iron status is potentially associated with adverse consequences in pregnancy and childhood. High hemoglobin concentration and iron status increase blood viscosity compromising placental blood flow, impairing systemic response to inflammation and infections, and increasing oxidative stress with elevated postprandial nontransferrin bound iron, lipid peroxidation, and DNA damage of placental cells, leading to adverse birth outcomes.[136] There is consistent evidence that elevated serum ferritin is associated with increased risk of gestational diabetes and preterm births.[137] Providing iron supplementation to iron-replete pregnant women and children in high-income countries could be associated with impaired fetal and child growth.[137,138] Evidence suggesting association with cognitive impairment, diarrhea, and changes in the gut microbiome are compelling but inconsistent.[137,139]

In malaria-endemic settings, there are unique concerns that providing routine iron supplementation to iron-replete pregnant women and children could be harmful. Iron supplementation trials among pregnant women and children in Tanzania and the Gambia found that iron supplementation may lead to increased risk of hospitalization for severe malaria and death.[140–142] The risk of adverse effects was greater in those who were iron-replete and in children <2 years.[142] In the absence of good malaria control, iron supplementation could also worsen hemolysis by increasing the parasite burden leading to no improvement in hemoglobin concentration on net.[142] However, malaria control has improved since these studies were conducted, and iron supplementation trials conducted among pregnant women and children more recently have not demonstrated any increased risk of harm.[143–145]

There are similar concerns that providing iron supplements to individuals with chronic infections such as HIV or tuberculosis may worsen disease outcomes, although the evidence is sparse. Among pregnant women with HIV, the WHO recommends universal supplementation with iron, in the absence of evidence of harm.[146] All individuals with HIV should aim for diverse diet.

C. Multiple Micronutrient Supplementation

In addition to iron, deficiency of other micronutrients, occurring singly or simultaneously, may contribute to anemia. Among pregnant women in Nepal, >50% had multiple micronutrient deficiencies during pregnancy.[147] Blood concentrations of most micronutrients decrease by 20%–50% between first and third trimesters of pregnancy.[148] MMS prevents and treats these deficiencies.

MMS typically include iron, folic acid, vitamin A, vitamin B12, and others (Table 27.4). These is evidence that MMS leads to greater reduction in the risk of adverse pregnancy outcomes such as preterm births, SGA, and low birth weight, compared to iron and folic acid alone.[149] MMS may be more effective to prevent stillbirth, low birth weight, SGA, and infant mortality at 6 months among anemic pregnant women than nonanemic counterparts.[150] MMS also provides 15% reduction in the risk of mortality through the first year of life for female infants.

There is no significant difference in the effect of MMS on maternal anemia risk, compared to standard iron and folic acid supplements alone.[149] Though the WHO recommends daily 60 mg iron supplementation, the commonly used multiple micronutrient supplements contain only 30 mg of iron. Compared to iron supplements, neonatal mortality is slightly higher in women who receive MMS, possibly due to the lower dose of iron in MMS.[151] Updated guidelines based on the use of MMS with 60 mg iron daily is warranted.

TABLE 27.4 Constituents of prototype multiple micronutrient supplement (UNIMMAP).

Nutrient	Dose
Vitamin A	800 μg
Vitamin D	5 μg
Vitamin E	10 mg
Vitamin C	70 mg
Vitamin B_1	1.4 mg
Vitamin B_2	1.4 mg
Niacin	18 mg
Vitamin B_6	1.9 mg
Vitamin B_{12}	2.6 μg
Folic acid	400 μg
Iron	30 mg
Zinc	15 mg
Copper	2 mg
Selenium	65 μg
Iodine	150 μg

UNIMMAP refers to the United Nations International Multiple Micronutrient Preparation.

D. Fortification

Eighty-seven countries worldwide have mandatory food fortification for at least one cereal grain—with varying success in implementation.[152] A recent metaanalysis of 19 studies among women and children showed that large-scale micronutrient fortification programs led to a 34% overall reduction in anemia.[153] The prevalence of ID decreased by 58% in some studies. In Costa Rica, fortifying wheat flour, maize flour, and milk for 7 years reduced anemia prevalence from 19% to 4%.[154] In China, iron fortification of soy sauce reduced anemia after 6 months, despite mean hemoglobin increasing by <10 g/L.[155] In Brazil, iron and ascorbic acid fortification of drinking water decreased the prevalence of anemia among preschool children attending daycare centers.[156]

A regularly consumed staple is required as the fortification vehicle.[76] Cereals/grains, such as wheat, maize, and rice, and staple seasoning cubes are frequently used. The fortificant compound should be a highly bioavailable source of the nutrient that does not alter the taste or smell of the food vehicle.[76] Iron compounds used to fortify include ferrous sulfate, ferrous fumarate, electrolytic iron/ferric pyrophosphate, sodium ferric ethylenediaminetetraacetic acid (EDTA), and iron amino acid chelates (e.g., iron glycinate chelate) in descending order of relative bioavailability and preference[47]. Unfortunately, poorly absorbed fortificants are more commonly used. Food processing—including milling, fermentation, and addition of ascorbic acid, phytase, or EDTA—may reduce the impact of iron absorption inhibitors and improve iron bioavailability.[157]

Food fortification cannot be well-targeted at individuals or groups, and there are concerns that iron fortification may be harmful to some or, at least, not beneficial. Large quantities of poorly absorbed iron fortificants may pass into the colon leading to gut inflammation and microbial dysbiosis.[158] For example, intake of iron-fortified biscuits increases the growth of potentially pathogenic gut microbes such as enterobacteria.[158]

Fortification costs $0.06–0.13 per person on average, being highest in Africa and lowest in Southeast Asia.[159] These costs are borne by customers in market-based fortification programs or by the government or other central funder. Economic models that account for the life-long impact, adherence, and geographic coverage have demonstrated that fortification is more cost-effective option at 95% coverage than iron supplementation.[159] The cost per DALY averted is lower for fortification than supplementation at 95% coverage but higher at 50% coverage. Iron supplementation is however more effective per capita due to its targeted nature. Fortification and supplementation are therefore best deployed together.

E. Delayed Umbilical Cord Clamping

By delaying the clamping of the umbilical cord for 1–5 min when a child is born, critical nutrients are transferred from the mother. This increases the newborn hematocrit and iron status immediately—demonstrable by 6 hours of life—and its impact lasts beyond the second month of age.[160,161] No harm occurs to the mother as a result of this procedure.[161] Unfortunately, the improvements in hematocrit do not protect the neonate from early mortality or birth asphyxia. The transfusion increases neonatal jaundice risk and birth weight by approximately 100 g.[161]

RESEARCH GAPS

Burden of disease

- Comprehensive and up-to-date estimates of the burden of the respective anemia types, especially among children, pregnant women, and individuals with HIV or TB infection
- Economic burden of anemia on health care utilization across high-, middle-, and low-income countries and regions
- Impact of anemia on national health care budgets by country income classification
- Impact of anemia on productivity of workers, given declines in participation in labor-intensive occupations and increased female employment

Normal function

- Identification of suitable functional biomarkers for the causes of nutritional anemia, not influenced by inflammation
- Interaction of the human microbiome and nutritional anemia, iron status, B12 metabolism

Pathophysiology

- Impact of vitamin A, calcium and zinc on iron absorption, erythropoiesis, hemoglobin concentration, and anemia risk in population studies
- Standardized definition of AI
- Consequences of AI on the risk of adverse pregnancy outcomes, maternal and infant survival, and clinical disease progression in HIV and TB
- Influence of pharmacologic agents on nutritional biomarkers

Prevention and treatment

- Barriers preventing optimal adherence to iron supplementation
- Role of maternal preconceptional iron and how best to deliver it
- Impact of treatment for chronic infections on anemia type
- Appropriate treatment modality for anemia of chronic disease, role of iron, and how it should be administered
- Role of iron supplementation in patients with HIV, TB, cancers, chronic kidney disease
- Feasibility and tolerability of intravenous iron among children, pregnant women, and HIV patients in developing countries
- Influence of dose of iron on the effectiveness of MMS
- Effectiveness and safety of iron fortification strategies in African countries
- Comprehensive and up-to-date evaluation of cost and cost-effectiveness of anemia treatment/prevention modalities

IV. REFERENCES

1. *GBD Results Tool*. University of Washington; 2017 [cited Aug 4, 2019].
2. World Health Organization (WHO). *The Global Prevalence of Anaemia in 2011*. 2015.
3. Petry N, Olofin I, Hurrell RF, et al. The proportion of anemia associated with iron deficiency in low, medium, and high human development index countries: a systematic analysis of national surveys. *Nutrients*. 2016;8(11).
4. Rahman MM, Abe SK, Rahman MS, et al. Maternal anemia and risk of adverse birth and health outcomes in low-and middle-income countries: systematic review and meta-analysis, 2. *Am J Clin Nutr*. 2016;103(2):495–504.
5. UNICEF/WHO. *Iron Deficiency Anaemia: Assessment, Prevention and Control, a Guide for Programme Managers*. 2001.
6. *Cellule de Planification et de Statistique - CPS/SSDSPF/Mali, Institut National de la Statistique - INSTAT/Mali, Centre d'Études et d'Information Statistiques - INFO-STAT/Mali, ICF International. Mali Enquête Démographique et de Santé (EDSM V) 2012–2013*. Rockville, Maryland, USA: CPS, INSTAT, INFO-STAT and ICF International; 2014.
7. Statistics Sierra Leone - SSL, ICF International. *Sierra Leone Demographic and Health Survey 2013*. Freetown, Sierra Leone: SSL and ICF International; 2014.
8. Wirth JP, Woodruff BA, Engle-Stone R, et al. Predictors of anemia in women of reproductive age: biomarkers reflecting inflammation and nutritional determinants of anemia (BRINDA) project. *Am J Clin Nutr*. 2017;106(suppl 1), 416s-27s.
9. Le CH. The prevalence of anemia and moderate-severe anemia in the US population (NHANES 2003-2012). *PLoS One*. 2016;11(11). e0166635.

10. Levi M, Rosselli M, Simonetti M, et al. Epidemiology of iron deficiency anaemia in four European countries: a population-based study in primary care. *Eur J Haematol*. 2016;97(6):583–593.
11. Mason J, Bailes A, Beda-Andourou M, et al. Recent trends in malnutrition in developing regions: vitamin A deficiency, anemia, iodine deficiency, and child underweight. *Food Nutr Bull*. 2005; 26(1):59–108.
12. Alderman H, Horton S. The economics of addressing nutritional anemia. *Nutritional anemia*. 2007;19:35.
13. Habib MA, Black K, Soofi SB, et al. Prevalence and predictors of iron deficiency anemia in children under five years of age in Pakistan, a secondary analysis of national nutrition survey data 2011–2012. *PLoS One*. 2016;11(5). e0155051.
14. Chandyo RK, Henjum S, Ulak M, et al. The prevalence of anemia and iron deficiency is more common in breastfed infants than their mothers in Bhaktapur, Nepal. *Eur J Clin Nutr*. 2016;70(4): 456–462.
15. Villamor E, Mbise R, Spiegelman D, Ndossi G, Fawzi WW. Vitamin A supplementation and other predictors of anemia among children from Dar Es Salaam, Tanzania. *Am J Trop Med Hyg*. 2000;62(5):590–597.
16. Ngnie-Teta I, Receveur O, Kuate-Defo B. Risk factors for moderate to severe anemia among children in Benin and Mali: insights from a multilevel analysis. *Food Nutr Bull*. 2007;28(1):76–89.
17. Abioye AI, McDonald EA, Park S, et al. Maternal anemia type during pregnancy is associated with anemia risk among offspring during infancy. *Pediatr Res*. 2019:1.
18. De Andrade Cairo RC, Rodrigues Silva L, Carneiro Bustani N, Ferreira Marques CD. Iron deficiency anemia in adolescents; a literature review. *Nutr Hosp*. 2014;29(6):1240–1249.
19. Weze K, Abioye AI, Obiajunwa C, Omotayo MO. *Spatial and Temporal Patterns and Determinants of Anemia Among Pregnant Women, Adolescents and Children in Sub-saharan Africa*. Unpublished. 2019.
20. Bianchi VE. Role of nutrition on anemia in elderly. *Clin Nutr ESPEN*. 2016;11:e1–e11.
21. Isanaka S, Mugusi F, Urassa W, et al. Iron deficiency and anemia predict mortality in patients with tuberculosis. *J Nutr*. 2012;142(2): 350–357.
22. Sheldon W, Blum J, Vogel J, et al. Postpartum haemorrhage management, risks, and maternal outcomes: findings from the World Health Organization multicountry survey on maternal and newborn health. *BJOG An Int J Obstet Gynaecol*. 2014;121:5–13.
23. McDermid JM, Jaye A, Schim van der Loeff MF, et al. Elevated iron status strongly predicts mortality in West African adults with HIV infection. *J Acquir Immune Defic Syndr*. 2007;46(4):498–507.
24. O'Brien ME, Kupka R, Msamanga GI, Saathoff E, Hunter DJ, Fawzi WW. Anemia is an independent predictor of mortality and immunologic progression of disease among women with HIV in Tanzania. *J Acquir Immune Defic Syndr*. 2005;40(2):219–225.
25. Haider BA, Spiegelman D, Hertzmark E, et al. Anemia, iron deficiency, and iron supplementation in relation 1 to mortality among HIV-infected patients receiving highly active antiretroviral therapy in Tanzania. *AJTM&H*. 2019;100(6):1512–1520.
26. Gutierrez G, Reines H, Wulf-Gutierrez ME. Clinical review: hemorrhagic shock. *Crit Care*. 2004;8(5):373.
27. Georgieff MK, Schmidt RL, Mills MM, Radmer WJ, Widness JA. Fetal iron and cytochrome c status after intrauterine hypoxemia and erythropoietin administration. *Am J Physiol*. 1992;262(3 Pt 2):R485–R491.
28. Anderson GJ, Frazer DM. Current understanding of iron homeostasis. *Am J Clin Nutr*. 2017;106(suppl 6):1559s–1566s.
29. Andersen HS, Gambling L, Holtrop G, McArdle HJ. Maternal iron deficiency identifies critical windows for growth and cardiovascular development in the rat postimplantation embryo. *J Nutr*. 2006;136(5):1171–1177.
30. Park S, Bellinger DC, Adamo M, et al. Mechanistic pathways from early gestation through infancy and neurodevelopment. *Pediatrics*. 2016;138(6). e20161843.
31. Abioye AI, McDonald EA, Park S, et al. Maternal anemia type during pregnancy is associated with anemia risk among offspring during infancy. *Pediatr Res*. 2019:1.
32. Burke R, Leon J, Suchdev P. Identification, prevention and treatment of iron deficiency during the first 1000 days. *Nutrients*. 2014;6(10):4093–4114.
33. Tamura T, Goldenberg RL, Hou J, et al. Cord serum ferritin concentrations and mental and psychomotor development of children at five years of age. *J Pediatr*. 2002;140(2):165–170.
34. Lozoff B, Beard J, Connor J, Barbara F, Georgieff M, Schallert T. Long-lasting neural and behavioral effects of iron deficiency in infancy. *Nutr Rev*. 2006;64(5 Pt 2):S34–S43. discussion S72-91.
35. Morath DJ, Mayer-Proschel M. Iron deficiency during embryogenesis and consequences for oligodendrocyte generation in vivo. *Dev Neurosci*. 2002;24(2–3):197–207.
36. Todorich B, Pasquini JM, Garcia CI, Paez PM, Connor JR. Oligodendrocytes and myelination: the role of iron. *Glia*. 2009;57(5): 467–478.
37. Prado EL, Dewey KG. Nutrition and brain development in early life. *Nutr Rev*. 2014;72(4):267–284.
38. Rao R, Tkac I, Townsend EL, Gruetter R, Georgieff MK. Perinatal iron deficiency alters the neurochemical profile of the developing rat hippocampus. *J Nutr*. 2003;133(10):3215–3221.
39. Dallman PR. Biochemical basis for the manifestations of iron deficiency. *Annu Rev Nutr*. 1986;6(1):13–40.
40. Rao R, Tkac I, Schmidt AT, Georgieff MK. Fetal and neonatal iron deficiency causes volume loss and alters the neurochemical profile of the adult rat hippocampus. *Nutr Neurosci*. 2011;14(2):59–65.
41. Clardy SL, Wang X, Zhao W, et al. Acute and chronic effects of developmental iron deficiency on mRNA expression patterns in the brain. *J Neural Transm Suppl*. 2006;(71):173–196.
42. Carlson ES, Stead JD, Neal CR, Petryk A, Georgieff MK. Perinatal iron deficiency results in altered developmental expression of genes mediating energy metabolism and neuronal morphogenesis in hippocampus. *Hippocampus*. 2007;17(8):679–691.
43. Nissenson AR, Wade S, Goodnough T, Knight K, Dubois RW. Economic burden of anemia in an insured population. *J Manag Care Pharm*. 2005;11(7):565–574.
44. Ross J, Horton S, Initiative M. *Economic Consequences of Iron Deficiency: Micronutrient Initiative*. Ottawa, ON, CA: IDRC; 1998.
45. Darnton-Hill I, Webb P, Harvey PW, et al. Micronutrient deficiencies and gender: social and economic costs. *Am J Clin Nutr*. 2005;81(5):1198S–1205S.
46. Wittenberg JB, Wittenberg BA. Myoglobin function reassessed. *J Exp Biol*. 2003;206(12):2011–2020.
47. Lynch S, Pfeiffer CM, Georgieff MK, et al. Biomarkers of nutrition for development (BOND)-Iron review. *J Nutr*. 2018;148(suppl l_1): 1001s–1067s.
48. Hamilton LD, Gubler CJ, Cartwright GE, Wintrobe MM. Diurnal variation in the plasma iron level of man. *Proc Soc Exp Biol Med*. 1950;75(1):65–68.
49. Kroot JJ, Tjalsma H, Fleming RE, Swinkels DW. Hepcidin in human iron disorders: diagnostic implications. *Clin Chem*. 2011; 57(12):1650–1669.
50. Nemeth E, Tuttle MS, Powelson J, et al. Hepcidin regulates cellular iron efflux by binding to ferroportin and inducing its internalization. *Science*. 2004;306(5704):2090–2093.
51. Nemeth E, Ganz T. Anemia of inflammation. *Hematol Oncol Clin N Am*. 2014;28(4):671–vi.
52. Young MF, Pressman E, Foehr ML, et al. Impact of maternal and neonatal iron status on placental transferrin receptor expression in pregnant adolescents. *Placenta*. 2010;31(11):1010–1014.

53. Best CM, Pressman EK, Cao C, et al. Maternal iron status during pregnancy compared with neonatal iron status better predicts placental iron transporter expression in humans. *FASEB J.* 2016; 30(10):3541–3550.
54. Lee S, Guillet R, Cooper EM, et al. Prevalence of anemia and associations between neonatal iron status, hepcidin, and maternal iron status among neonates born to pregnant adolescents. *Pediatr Res.* 2016;79(1–1):42–48.
55. Shao J, Lou J, Rao R, et al. Maternal serum ferritin concentration is positively associated with newborn iron stores in women with low ferritin status in late pregnancy. *J Nutr.* 2012;142(11): 2004–2009.
56. O'Brien KO, Zavaleta N, Abrams SA, Caulfield LE. Maternal iron status influences iron transfer to the fetus during the third trimester of pregnancy. *Am J Clin Nutr.* 2003;77(4):924–930.
57. Brickley EB, Spottiswoode N, Kabyemela E, et al. Cord blood hepcidin: cross-sectional correlates and associations with anemia, malaria, and mortality in a Tanzanian birth cohort study. *Am J Trop Med Hyg.* 2016:16–0218.
58. Gambling L, Czopek A, Andersen HS, et al. Fetal iron status regulates maternal iron metabolism during pregnancy in the rat. *Am J Physiol Regul Integr Comp Physiol.* 2009;296(4):R1063–R1070.
59. Abioye AI, Park S, Ripp K, et al. Anemia of inflammation during human pregnancy does not affect newborn iron endowment. *J Nutr.* 2018;148(3):427–436.
60. Finkelstein JL, O'Brien KO, Abrams SA, Zavaleta N. Infant iron status affects iron absorption in Peruvian breastfed infants at 2 and 5 mo of age. *Am J Clin Nutr.* 2013;98(6):1475–1484.
61. O'Brien KO, Zavaleta N, Abrams SA, Caulfield LE. Maternal iron status influences iron transfer to the fetus during the third trimester of pregnancy. *Am J Clin Nutr.* 2003;77(4):924–930.
62. Bothwell TH, Charlton R, Cook J, Finch CA. *Iron Metabolism in Man. Iron Metabolism in Man.* 1979.
63. Zimmermann M, Adou P, Torresani T, Zeder C, Hurrell R. Iron supplementation in goitrous, iron-deficient children improves their response to oral iodized oil. *Eur J Endocrinol.* 2000;142(3): 217–223.
64. Hess SY, Zimmermann MB, Adou P, Torresani T, Hurrell RF. Treatment of iron deficiency in goitrous children improves the efficacy of iodized salt in Cote d'Ivoire. *Am J Clin Nutr.* 2002;75(4): 743–748.
65. Shawki A, Mackenzie B. Interaction of calcium with the human divalent metal-ion transporter-1. *Biochem Biophys Res Commun.* 2010;393(3):471–475.
66. Omotayo M, Dickin K, Stolzfus R. Perinatal mortality due to preeclampsia in Africa: a comprehensive and integrated approach is needed. *Glob Health Sci Pract.* 2016.
67. Abioye AI, Okuneye TA, O AO, et al. *Effect of Calcium Intake on Iron Absorption and Hematologic Status: A Systematic Review and Dose-Response Meta-Analysis of Randomized Trials and Case-Cross-Over Studies.* 2019.
68. *Non-inferiority of Lower Dose Calcium Supplementation during Pregnancy.* US National Library of Medicine; 2017 [cited August 4, 2019]. Available from: https://clinicaltrials.gov/ct2/show/NCT03350516.
69. Solomons NW, Ruz M. Zinc and iron interaction: concepts and perspectives in the developing world. *Nutr Res.* 1997;17(1): 177–185.
70. Noor RA. *Effect of Prenatal Zinc, Vitamin A and Iron Supplementation on Maternal Hematological Outcomes at Delivery in Tanzania.* Boston, MA: Harvard University; 2019.
71. Olivares M, Pizarro F, Ruz M. Zinc inhibits nonheme iron bioavailability in humans. *Biol Trace Elem Res.* 2007;117(1–3):7–14.
72. Darling AM, Mugusi FM, Etheredge AJ, et al. Vitamin A and zinc supplementation among pregnant women to prevent placental malaria: a randomized, double-blind, placebo-controlled trial in Tanzania. *Am J Trop Med Hyg.* 2017;96(4):826–834.
73. Yakoob MY, Theodoratou E, Jabeen A, et al. Preventive zinc supplementation in developing countries: impact on mortality and morbidity due to diarrhea, pneumonia and malaria. *BMC Public Health.* 2011;11(3):S23.
74. Tamura T, Picciano MF, McGuire MK. Folate in pregnancy and lactation. In: Bailey LB, ed. *Folate in Health and Disease.* 2nd ed. Boca Raton (FL): CRC Press, Taylor and Francis Group; 2010:1–24.
75. Bailey LB, Stover PJ, McNulty H, et al. Biomarkers of nutrition for development—folate review. *J Nutr.* 2015;145(7):1636S–1680S.
76. Tanumihardjo SA, Russell RM, Stephensen CB, et al. Biomarkers of nutrition for development (BOND)-Vitamin A review. *J Nutr.* 2016;146(9):1816s–1848s.
77. Noor RA, Abioye AI, Ulenga N, et al. Large–scale wheat flour folic acid fortification program increases plasma folate levels among women of reproductive age in urban Tanzania. *PLoS One.* 2017;12(8):e0182099.
78. Bailey RL, Fulgoni 3rd VL, Keast DR, Dwyer JT. Examination of vitamin intakes among US adults by dietary supplement use. *J Acad Nutr Diet.* 2012;112(5):657–663. e4.
79. Roman Vinas B, Ribas Barba L, Ngo J, et al. Projected prevalence of inadequate nutrient intakes in Europe. *Ann Nutr Metab.* 2011; 59(2–4):84–95.
80. Allen LH, Miller JW, de Groot L, et al. Biomarkers of nutrition for development (BOND): vitamin B-12 review. *J Nutr.* 2018; 148(suppl_4):1995s–2027s.
81. Stabler SP. Vitamin B12 deficiency. *N Engl J Med.* 2013;368(2): 149–160.
82. Fedosov SN. Biochemical markers of vitamin B12 deficiency combined in one diagnostic parameter: the age-dependence and association with cognitive function and blood hemoglobin. *Clin Chim Acta.* 2013;422:47–53.
83. Vidal-Alaball J, Butler C, Cannings-John R, et al. Oral vitamin B12 versus intramuscular vitamin B12 for vitamin B12 deficiency. *Cochrane Database Syst Rev.* 2005;(3).
84. Joint FAO/WHO Expert Consultation. Vitamin A. In: *Vitamin and Mineral Requirements in Human Nutrition.* 2nd ed. 2004. Geneva, Switzerland.
85. Roodenburg A, West C, Beguin Y, et al. Indicators of erythrocyte formation and degradation in rats with either vitamin A or iron deficiency. *J Nutr Biochem.* 2000;11(4):223–230.
86. Thorne-Lyman AL, Fawzi WW. Vitamin A and carotenoids during pregnancy and maternal, neonatal and infant health outcomes: a systematic review and meta-analysis. *Paediatr Perinat Epidemiol.* 2012;26(Suppl 1):36–54.
87. da Cunha MSB, Campos Hankins NA, Arruda SF. Effect of vitamin A supplementation on iron status in humans: a systematic review and meta-analysis. *Crit Rev Food Sci Nutr.* 2018:1–15.
88. Fawzi WW, Villamor E, Msamanga GI, et al. Trial of zinc supplements in relation to pregnancy outcomes, hematologic indicators, and T cell counts among HIV-1-infected women in Tanzania. *Am J Clin Nutr.* 2005;81(1):161–167.
89. Suharno D, West CE, Muhilal, Karyadi D, Hautvast JG. Supplementation with vitamin A and iron for nutritional anaemia in pregnant women in West Java, Indonesia. *Lancet.* 1993;342(8883): 1325–1328.
90. Ahmed F, Khan MR, Jackson AA. Concomitant supplemental vitamin A enhances the response to weekly supplemental iron and folic acid in anemic teenagers in urban Bangladesh. *Am J Clin Nutr.* 2001;74(1):108–115.
91. Schmidt MK, Muslimatun S, West CE, Schultink W, Hautvast JG. Mental and psychomotor development in Indonesian infants of mothers supplemented with vitamin A in addition to iron during pregnancy. *Br J Nutr.* 2004;91(2):279–286.

92. Kovesdy CP, Kalantar-Zadeh K. Why is protein-energy wasting associated with mortality in chronic kidney disease? *Semin Nephrol*. 2009;29(1):3–14.
93. Kamel TB, Deraz TE, Elkabarity RH, Ahmed RK. Protein energy malnutrition associates with different types of hearing impairments in toddlers: anemia increases cochlear dysfunction. *Int J Pediatr Otorhinolaryngol*. 2016;85:27–31.
94. Thakur N, Chandra J, Pemde H, Singh V. Anemia in severe acute malnutrition. *Nutrition*. 2014;30(4):440–442.
95. Ozkale M, Sipahi T. Hematologic and bone marrow changes in children with protein-energy malnutrition. *Pediatr Hematol Oncol*. 2014;31(4):349–358.
96. Borelli P, Blatt S, Pereira J, et al. Reduction of erythroid progenitors in protein-energy malnutrition. *Br J Nutr*. 2007;97(2):307–314.
97. Cunha MC, Lima Fda S, Vinolo MA, et al. Protein malnutrition induces bone marrow mesenchymal stem cells commitment to adipogenic differentiation leading to hematopoietic failure. *PLoS One*. 2013;8(3). e58872.
98. Fondu P, Mozes N, Neve P, Sohet-Robazza L, Mandelbaum I. The erythrocyte membrane disturbances in protein-energy malnutrition: nature and mechanisms. *Br J Haematol*. 1980;44(4):605–618.
99. Schofield C, Ashworth A. Why have mortality rates for severe malnutrition remained so high? *Bull World Health Organ*. 1996; 74(2):223.
100. Weiss G, Goodnough LT. Anemia of chronic disease. *N Engl J Med*. 2005;352(10):1011–1023.
101. Isanaka S, Mugusi F, Hawkins C, et al. Effect of high-dose vs standard-dose multivitamin supplementation at the initiation of HAART on HIV disease progression and mortality in Tanzania: a randomized controlled trial. *Jama*. 2012;308(15):1535–1544.
102. Olson CL, Acosta LP, Hochberg NS, et al. Anemia of inflammation is related to cognitive impairment among children in leyte, the Philippines. *PLoS Neglected Trop Dis*. 2009;3(10):e533.
103. Ezeamama AE, Sikorskii A, Bajwa RK, et al. Evolution of anemia types during antiretroviral therapy-implications for treatment outcomes and quality of life among HIV-infected adults. *Nutrients*. 2019;11(4).
104. World Health Organization (WHO). *Haemoglobin Concentration for the Diagnosis of Anaemia and Assessment of Severity*. Geneva: WHO; 2011. Contract No.: WHO/NMH/NHD/MNM/11.1.
105. Thurnham DI, Northrop-Clewes CA. Inflammation and biomarkers of micronutrient status. *Curr Opin Clin Nutr Metab Care*. 2016;19(6):458–463.
106. Namaste SM, Rohner F, Huang J, et al. Adjusting ferritin concentrations for inflammation: biomarkers reflecting inflammation and nutritional determinants of anemia (BRINDA) project. *Am J Clin Nutr*. 2017;106(suppl l_1):359S–371S.
107. Thurnham DI, McCabe LD, Haldar S, Wieringa FT, Northrop-Clewes CA, McCabe GP. Adjusting plasma ferritin concentrations to remove the effects of subclinical inflammation in the assessment of iron deficiency: a meta-analysis. *Am J Clin Nutr*. 2010; 92(3):546–555.
108. Namaste SM, Rohner F, Huang J, et al. Adjusting ferritin concentrations for inflammation: biomarkers reflecting inflammation and nutritional determinants of anemia (BRINDA) project. *Am J Clin Nutr*. 2017;106(suppl 1):359s–371s.
109. Beguin Y. Soluble transferrin receptor for the evaluation of erythropoiesis and iron status. *Clin Chim Acta*. 2003;329(1):9–22.
110. Drakesmith H. Next-Generation biomarkers for iron status. In: Baetge EE, Dhawan A, Prentice A, eds. *Nestlé Nutr Inst Workshop Series*. 2016:59–69.
111. Wians FH, Urban JE, Kroft SH, Keffer JH. Soluble transferrin receptor (sTfR) concentration quantified using two sTfR kits: analytical and clinical performance characteristics. *Clin Chim Acta*. 2001; 303(1):75–81.
112. Pfeiffer CM, Cook JD, Mei Z, Cogswell ME, Looker AC, Lacher DA. Evaluation of an automated soluble transferrin receptor (sTfR) assay on the Roche Hitachi analyzer and its comparison to two ELISA assays. *Clin Chim Acta*. 2007;382(1):112–116.
113. Lamola AA, Yamane T. Zinc protoporphyrin (ZPP): a simple, sensitive, fluorometric screening test for lead poisioning. *Clin Chem*. 1975;21(1):93–97.
114. Bah A, Pasricha S-R, Jallow MW, et al. Serum hepcidin concentrations decline during pregnancy and may identify iron deficiency: analysis of a longitudinal pregnancy cohort in the Gambia. *J Nutr*. 2017;147(6):1131–1137.
115. Wray K, Allen A, Evans E, et al. Hepcidin detects iron deficiency in Sri Lankan adolescents with a high burden of hemoglobinopathy: a diagnostic test accuracy study. *Am J Hematol*. 2017;92(2): 196–203.
116. Kennedy G, Berardo A, Papavero C, et al. Proxy measures of household food consumption for food security assessment and surveillance: comparison of the household dietary diversity and food consumption scores. *Public Health Nutrition*. 2010;13(12).
117. Koppmair S, Kassie M, Qaim M. Farm production, market access and dietary diversity in Malawi. *Public Health Nutrition*. 2017; 20(2):325–335.
118. Bellon MR, Ntandou-Bouzitou GD, Caracciolo F. On-farm diversity and market participation are positively associated with dietary diversity of rural mothers in Southern Benin, West Africa. *PLoS One*. 2016;11(9). e0162535.
119. Ruel MT, Minot N, Smith L. *Patterns and Determinants of Fruit and Vegetable Consumption in Sub-saharan Africa: A Multicountry Comparison*. Geneva: WHO; 2005.
120. Leroy JL, Olney D, Ruel M. Tubaramure, a food-assisted integrated health and nutrition program in Burundi, increases maternal and child hemoglobin concentrations and reduces anemia: a theory-based cluster-randomized controlled intervention trial. *J Nutr*. 2016;146(8):1601–1608.
121. Rawat R, McCoy SI, Kadiyala S. Poor diet quality is associated with low CD4 count and anemia and predicts mortality among antiretroviral therapy-naive HIV-positive adults in Uganda. *J Acquir Immune Defic Syndr*. 2013;62(2):246–253.
122. Haider BA, Olofin I, Wang M, Spiegelman D, Ezzati M, Fawzi WW. Anaemia, prenatal iron use, and risk of adverse pregnancy outcomes: systematic review and meta-analysis. *Br Med J*. 2013;346:f3443.
123. Low MS, Speedy J, Styles CE, De-Regil LM, Pasricha SR. Daily iron supplementation for improving anaemia, iron status and health in menstruating women. *Cochrane Database Syst Rev*. 2016; 4. Cd009747.
124. Low M, Farrell A, Biggs BA, Pasricha SR. Effects of daily iron supplementation in primary-school-aged children: systematic review and meta-analysis of randomized controlled trials. *CMAJ*. 2013; 185(17):E791–E802.
125. Milman N, Paszkowski T, Cetin I, Castelo-Branco C. Supplementation during pregnancy: beliefs and science. *Gynecol Endocrinol*. 2016;32(7):509–516.
126. Szajewska H, Ruszczynski M, Chmielewska A. Effects of iron supplementation in nonanemic pregnant women, infants, and young children on the mental performance and psychomotor development of children: a systematic review of randomized controlled trials. *Am J Clin Nutr*. 2010;91(6):1684–1690.
127. Lozoff B, Georgieff MK. Iron deficiency and brain development. *Semin Pediatr Neurol*. 2006;13.
128. Vucic V, Berti C, Vollhardt C, et al. Effect of iron intervention on growth during gestation, infancy, childhood, and adolescence: a systematic review with meta-analysis. *Nutr Rev*. 2013;71(6): 386–401.
129. Abioye AI, Aboud S, Premji Z, et al. Iron supplementation affects hematologic biomarker concentrations and pregnancy outcomes

among iron-deficient Tanzanian women. *J Nutr.* 2016;146(6): 1162–1171.
130. Haddad L, Achadi E, Bendech MA, et al. The global nutrition report 2014: actions and accountability to accelerate the world's progress on nutrition–. *J Nutr.* 2015;145(4):663–671.
131. Pena-Rosas JP, De-Regil LM, Gomez Malave H, Flores-Urrutia MC, Dowswell T. Intermittent oral iron supplementation during pregnancy. *Cochrane Database Syst Rev.* 2015;(10):Cd009997.
132. De-Regil LM, Jefferds ME, Sylvetsky AC, Dowswell T. Intermittent iron supplementation for improving nutrition and development in children under 12 years of age. *Cochrane Database Syst Rev.* 2011;(12):Cd009085.
133. Cancelo-Hidalgo MJ, Castelo-Branco C, Palacios S, et al. Tolerability of different oral iron supplements: a systematic review. *Curr Med Res Opin.* 2013;29(4):291–303.
134. Ortiz R, Toblli JE, Romero JD, et al. Efficacy and safety of oral iron (III) polymaltose complex versus ferrous sulfate in pregnant women with iron-deficiency anemia: a multicenter, randomized, controlled study. *J Matern Fetal Neonatal Med.* 2011;24(11): 1347–1352.
135. Gunaratna NS, Masanja H, Mrema S, et al. Multivitamin and iron supplementation to prevent periconceptional anemia in rural Tanzanian women: a randomized, controlled trial. *PLoS One.* 2015;10(4):e0121552.
136. Dewey KG, Oaks BM. U-shaped curve for risk associated with maternal hemoglobin, iron status, or iron supplementation. *Am J Clin Nutr.* 2017;106(suppl l_6):1694S–1702S.
137. Brannon PM, Stover PJ, Taylor CL. Integrating themes, evidence gaps, and research needs identified by workshop on iron screening and supplementation in iron-replete pregnant women and young children. *Am J Clin Nutr.* 2017;106(suppl l_6): 1703S–1712S.
138. Lönnerdal B. Excess iron intake as a factor in growth, infections, and development of infants and young children. *Am J Clin Nutr.* 2017;106(suppl l_6):1681S–1687S.
139. Paganini D, Zimmermann MB. The effects of iron fortification and supplementation on the gut microbiome and diarrhea in infants and children: a review. *Am J Clin Nutr.* 2017;106(suppl l_6): 1688S–1693S.
140. Sazawal S, Black RE, Ramsan M, et al. Effects of routine prophylactic supplementation with iron and folic acid on admission to hospital and mortality in preschool children in a high malaria transmission setting: community-based, randomised, placebo-controlled trial. *Lancet.* 2006;367(9505):133–143.
141. Mwangi MN, Prentice AM, Verhoef H. Safety and benefits of antenatal oral iron supplementation in low-income countries: a review. *Br J Haematol.* 2017;177(6):884–895.
142. Veenemans J, Milligan P, Prentice AM, et al. Effect of supplementation with zinc and other micronutrients on malaria in Tanzanian children: a randomised trial. *PLoS Med.* 2011;8(11):e1001125.
143. Etheredge AJ, Premji Z, Gunaratna NS, et al. Iron supplementation in iron-replete and nonanemic pregnant women in Tanzania: a randomized clinical trial. *JAMA Pediatr.* 2015; 169(10):947–955.
144. Mwangi MN, Roth JM, Smit MR, et al. Effect of daily antenatal iron supplementation on Plasmodium infection in Kenyan women: a randomized clinical trial. *Jama.* 2015;314(10):1009–1020.
145. Neuberger A, Okebe J, Yahav D, Paul M. Oral iron supplements for children in malaria-endemic areas. *Cochrane Database Syst Rev.* 2016;(2).
146. World Health Organization. *Nutrient Requirements for People Living with HIV.* 2004.
147. Jiang T, Christian P, Khatry SK, Wu L, West Jr KP. Micronutrient deficiencies in early pregnancy are common, concurrent, and vary by season among rural Nepali pregnant women. *J Nutr.* 2005;135(5):1106–1112.
148. Christian P, Jiang T, Khatry SK, LeClerq SC, Shrestha SR, West Jr KP. Antenatal supplementation with micronutrients and biochemical indicators of status and subclinical infection in rural Nepal. *Am J Clin Nutr.* 2006;83(4):788–794.
149. Keats EC, Haider BA, Tam E, Bhutta ZA. Multiple-micronutrient supplementation for women during pregnancy. *Cochrane Database Syst Rev.* 2019;(3).
150. Smith ER, Shankar AH, Wu LS, et al. Modifiers of the effect of maternal multiple micronutrient supplementation on stillbirth, birth outcomes, and infant mortality: a meta-analysis of individual patient data from 17 randomised trials in low-income and middle-income countries. *The Lancet Global Health.* 2017;5(11):e1090–e1100.
151. Sudfeld CR, Smith ER. New evidence should inform WHO guidelines on multiple micronutrient supplementation in pregnancy. *J Nutr.* 2019;149(3):359–361.
152. Marks KJ, Luthringer CL, Ruth LJ, et al. Review of grain fortification legislation, standards, and monitoring documents. *Glob Health Sci Pract.* 2018;6(2):356–371.
153. Keats EC, Neufeld LM, Garrett GS, Mbuya MNN, Bhutta ZA. Improved micronutrient status and health outcomes in low- and middle-income countries following large-scale fortification: evidence from a systematic review and meta-analysis. *Am J Clin Nutr.* 2019;109(6):1696–1708.
154. Martorell R, Ascencio M, Tacsan L, et al. Effectiveness evaluation of the food fortification program of Costa Rica: impact on anemia prevalence and hemoglobin concentrations in women and children. *Am J Clin Nutr.* 2015;101(1):210–217.
155. Chen J, Zhao X, Zhang X, et al. Studies on the effectiveness of NaFeEDTA-fortified soy sauce in controlling iron deficiency: a population-based intervention trial. *Food Nutr Bull.* 2005;26(2): 177–186.
156. Rocha Dda S, Capanema FD, Netto MP, de Almeida CA, Franceschini Sdo C, Lamounier JA. Effectiveness of fortification of drinking water with iron and vitamin C in the reduction of anemia and improvement of nutritional status in children attending day-care centers in Belo Horizonte, Brazil. *Food Nutr Bull.* 2011;32(4): 340–346.
157. Hurrell R, Ranum P, de Pee S, et al. Revised recommendations for iron fortification of wheat flour and an evaluation of the expected impact of current national wheat flour fortification programs. *Food Nutr Bull.* 2010;31(1_suppl1):S7–S21.
158. Zimmermann MB, Chassard C, Rohner F, et al. The effects of iron fortification on the gut microbiota in African children: a randomized controlled trial in Cote d'Ivoire. *Am J Clin Nutr.* 2010;92(6): 1406–1415.
159. Baltussen R, Knai C, Sharan M. Iron fortification and iron supplementation are cost-effective interventions to reduce iron deficiency in four subregions of the world. *J Nutr.* 2004;134(10):2678–2684.
160. Hutton EK, Hassan ES. Late vs early clamping of the umbilical cord in full-term neonates: systematic review and meta-analysis of controlled trials. *JAMA.* 2007;297(11):1241–1252.
161. McDonald SJ, Middleton P, Dowswell T, Morris PS. Effect of timing of umbilical cord clamping of term infants on maternal and neonatal outcomes. *Evid Based Child Health Cochrane Rev J.* 2014;9(2):303–397.
162. Pasricha S-R, Drakesmith H, Black J, Hipgrave D, Biggs B-A. Control of iron deficiency anemia in low-and middle-income countries. *Blood.* 2013;121(14):2607–2617.
163. Zimmermann MB, Hurrell RF. Nutritional iron deficiency. *Lancet.* 2007;370(9586):511–520.
164. Drakesmith H, Prentice AM. Hepcidin and the iron-infection axis. *Science.* 2012;338(6108):768–772.

CHAPTER

28

NUTRITION AND BONE DISEASE

René Rizzoli, MD

Geneva University Hospitals and Faculty of Medicine, Geneva, Switzerland

SUMMARY

Osteoporosis increases the risk of fractures, which are associated with increased mortality and impaired quality of life. Patients with prevalent fracture are at high risk of sustaining another one. Optimal protein and calcium intakes, and vitamin D supply, together with regular weight bearing physical exercise, are the corner stones of fragility fracture prevention. Adherence to a Mediterranean diet or to a prudent diet pattern is associated with lower hip fracture risk. Inadequate dietary protein intakes may be a much more severe problem than protein excess in the oldest old population.

Keywords: Dietary calcium; Dietary protein; Fracture; IGF-I; Osteoporosis; Peak bone mass.

I. INTRODUCTION

Osteoporosis is defined as a systemic skeletal disease characterized by low bone mass and microarchitectural deterioration of bone tissue, with a consequent increase in bone fragility and in susceptibility to fracture risk.[1] The diagnosis of the disease relies on the quantitative assessment, using dual energy X-ray absorptiometry, of areal bone mineral density (aBMD) of the hip or spine. This represents an important determinant of bone strength and thereby of fracture risk. The operational definition of osteoporosis is based on aBMD lower than the lower limit of normal range of young healthy women, as defined in a WHO document.[2] An osteodensitometry-based diagnosis of osteoporosis together with a prevalent fragility fracture defines severe osteoporosis. Indications for treatment depend on the evaluation of fracture risk, which also integrates clinical risk factors in addition to densitometric osteoporosis diagnosis.[1]

II. BONE MASS ACCRUAL

At a given age, bone mass is determined by the amount of bone accumulated at the end of skeletal growth, the so-called peak bone mass, and by the amount of bone lost during the rest of the life[3] (Fig. 28.1). It is estimated that a 10% increase in peak bone mass could reduce the risk of osteoporotic fractures during adult life by 50%, or to be equivalent to a 13-year delay in the occurrence of menopause, after which bone loss accelerates.[4] Peak bone mass is achieved for most parts of the skeleton by the end of the second decade of life.[3] Body mineral mass nearly doubles during puberty, through an increase in the size of the skeleton, with little changes in volumetric bone density, i.e., the amount of bone in bone.[3] Then, a small percent of bone consolidation may occur during the third decade, particularly in males. Puberty is the period during which the sex difference in bone mass observed in adults becomes fully expressed. The important sex difference in bone mass that develops during pubertal maturation appears to result from a greater increase in bone size. There is no sex difference in the volumetric trabecular density at the end of the period of maturation, i.e., in young healthy adults in their third decade. The greater mean aBMD values observed in young healthy adult males as compared to females in the lumbar spine and at the level of the midfemoral or midradial diaphysis appear to be due to a more prolonged period of pubertal maturation rather than a greater maximal rate of bone accretion.[5]

III. BONE LOSS AND FRACTURE RISK

Bone mass decreases with age and with an accelerated bone loss after menopause, and the risk of osteoporotic

Present Knowledge in Nutrition, Volume 2
https://doi.org/10.1016/B978-0-12-818460-8.00028-9

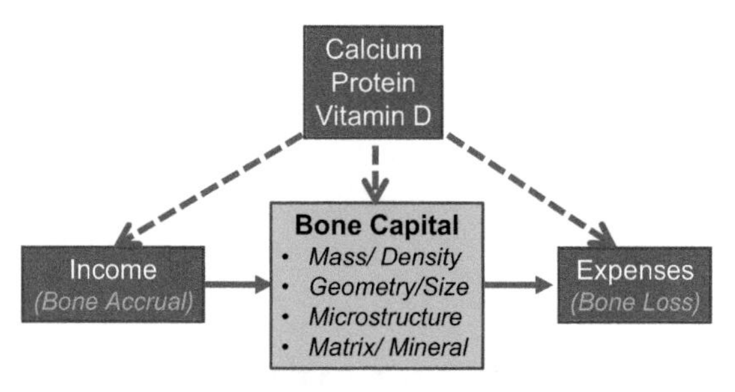

FIGURE 28.1 Roles of dietary intakes in the management of the "bone bank" through influences on bone accrual and bone loss.

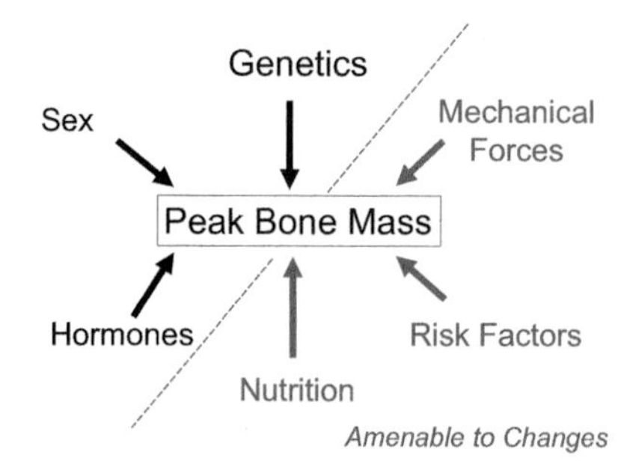

FIGURE 28.2 Factors influencing peak bone mass, i.e., the amount of bone accumulated at the end of skeletal growth. Some of these factors are amenable to modifications.

fracture increases. As the populations become older, the number of individuals who face the problem of bone fragility and increased fracture risk increases inexorably. At the age of 50, the lifetime risk of sustaining an osteoporotic fracture is around 50% for women and 20% for men.[1,6] Major osteoporotic fractures are those of the spine, hip, distal forearm, and proximal humerus.

A large majority of hip fractures associated with osteoporosis result from a fall from standing height, which defines fragility fractures. Around 2% of falls in the elderly lead to fractures. More than 50% of patients admitted to hospital with hip fracture are over 80 years old.[7] Only a limited number of X-ray–determined vertebral fractures comes to clinical attention and is diagnosed.[8] The incidence of osteoporotic fractures varies geographically. Up to 40% of hip fractures occur in people living in nursing homes.[9] This is probably related to advanced age, to a high prevalence of comorbidities requiring long-term institutional care, and to high risk of recurrent falls. All these factors are potentially related to malnutrition in the oldest old population.

Despite a rising number of older subjects and a forecasted increase of absolute number and incidence of hip fractures, a decrease in age-adjusted incidence has been observed in several countries and may indicate a reversal of a secular trend.[7] However, the incidence of nonhip osteoporotic fractures is continuing to increase, as is the total number of days of hospitalization in orthopedic and rehabilitation wards, for multiple fractures and comorbidities.[10]

There is a large body of evidences linking nutritional intakes, particularly calcium and protein, to bone growth and to bone loss later in life, both influencing fracture risk (Fig. 28.1).[11]

IV. NUTRITION AND BONE GROWTH (FIG. 28.2)

A. Calcium

Calcium plays major roles in the regulation of various cell functions, in the central and peripheral nervous systems, in muscle, and in exocrine/endocrine glands function.[12] In addition, this cation is implicated in the process of bone mineralization, by the formation of hydroxyapatite crystals.

Most of the studies carried out over a 1–3 year time period in children and adolescents have shown that supplementation with either calcium or dairy foods increases the rate of bone mineral acquisition, compared with unsupplemented (or placebo) control groups. A metaanalysis has reviewed 19 calcium intervention studies involving 2859 children,[13] with doses of calcium supplementation varying between 300 and 1200 mg per day, from calcium citrate malate, calcium carbonate, calcium phosphate, calcium lactate gluconate, calcium phosphate milk extract, or milk minerals. Calcium supplementation had a positive effect on whole body bone mineral content (BMC) and upper extremities bone mineral density (BMD), with standardized mean differences (effect size) of 0.14 for both. Changes at the upper extremities persisted up to 18 months after cessation of calcium supplementation. In the same analysis, calcium supplementation had no significant effect on weight, height, or body fat.

Among randomized, double-blind, placebo-controlled intervention trials, which have concluded that calcium supplementation increases bone mineral mass gain, the magnitude of the calcium effects appears to vary according to the skeletal sites examined, the stage of pubertal maturation at the time of the intervention, and the usual continuous dietary calcium intake.[13–16] Calcium supplementation effects have essentially been ascribed to a reduction in bone remodeling. Indeed, in one of the abovementioned studies, plasma concentration of osteocalcin, a biochemical marker of bone remodeling in adults, was significantly reduced in the calcium-supplemented children.[14] However, in a double-blind, placebo-controlled study on the effects of calcium supplementation in prepubertal girls, changes in projected scanned bone area and in standing height have suggested that calcium supplementation may influence bone modeling in addition to remodeling.[15] When BMD was measured 7.5 years after the end of calcium supplementation in adolescents, thus in young adult women, it appeared that menarche occurred earlier in the calcium-supplemented group and that persistent effects of calcium were mostly detectable in those subjects with an earlier puberty.[17]

B. Protein

In a prospective survey carried out in a cohort of female and male subjects aged 9–19 years, a positive correlation between lumbar and femoral bone mass yearly gain and protein intake was found.[18] This correlation was mainly detectable in prepubertal children, but not observed in those having reached a peri- or postpubertal stage. It remained statistically significant after adjustment for spontaneous calcium intakes. BMD/BMC at specific skeletal sites in prepubertal boys was positively associated with spontaneous protein intake.[19] In a prospective longitudinal study performed in healthy children and adolescents of both sexes, between the age of 6 and 18, dietary intakes were recorded over 4 years, using a yearly administered 3-day diary.[20] A positive association was detected between periosteal circumferences, cortical area, BMC, and a calculated strength strain index, and long-term protein intakes. In this cohort with a Western style diet, protein intakes were around 2 g/kg body weight x day in prepubertal children, whereas they were around 1.5 g/kg x day in post-pubertal individuals. There was no association between bone variables and intakes of nutrients with a high sulfur-containing amino acids, or intake of calcium. Overall, protein intakes accounted for 3% – 4% of the bone parameters variance.

Protein intake is to a large extent related to growth requirement during childhood and adolescence. Only intervention studies could reliably address this question. To our knowledge, there is no large randomized controlled trial having specifically tested the effects of dietary protein supplements on bone mineral mass accumulation, except those utilizing milk or dairy products, which provide protein, phosphorus, calories, and vitamins, in addition to calcium.[21] One liter of milk provides not only 32–35 g of protein, mostly casein, but also whey protein that contains numerous growth-promoting elements. In growing children, long-term milk avoidance is associated with smaller stature and lower bone mineral mass.[22] Low milk intake during childhood and/or adolescence increases the risk of fracture before puberty (a 2.6-fold higher risk has been reported).[23,24] In a 7 year observational study, there was a positive influence of dairy products consumption on BMD at the spine, hip, and forearm in adolescents, leading thereby to a higher peak bone mass.[25] In this study, calcium supplements did not affect spine BMD. But, higher dairy products intakes were associated with greater total and cortical proximal radius cross-sectional area. In agreement with this observation, milk consumption frequency and total daily milk intake at age 5 – 12 and 13 – 17 years were significant predictors of the height of 12- to 18-year-old adolescents, studied in the NHANES 1999–2002.[26]

Many intervention trials have demonstrated a favorable influence of dairy products on bone health during childhood and adolescence.[3,21,27,28] In an open randomized intervention controlled trial, 568 ml/day milk supplement for 18 months in 12-year-old girls[27] provided an additional 420 mg/day calcium and 14 g/day protein intakes at the end of the study. Compared to the control group, the intervention group had greater increases of whole body BMD and BMC. In the milk-supplemented group, serum insulin-like growth factor I (IGF-I) levels were 17% higher. In another study, cheese supplements appeared to be more beneficial for cortical bone accrual than a similar amount of calcium supplied as tablets.[28] The positive influence of milk on cortical bone thickness may be related to an effect on the modeling process, since metacarpal periosteal diameter was significantly increased in these Chinese children receiving milk supplements.

Based on these observations, it was suggested that while calcium supplements could influence volumetric BMD, thus the remodeling process, dairy products may have an additional effect on bone growth and periosteal bone expansion, i.e. an influence on modeling.[25]

V. PATHOPHYSIOLOGY OF BONE LOSS

After the age of 50 in women, bone loss accelerates through bone cortex thinning, increased cortical porosity, and trabeculae destruction by thinning and perforation.[29] Bone loss does not attenuate with age but continues throughout the whole life, at least in peripheral skeletal sites. Various factors contribute to age-related bone mass decrease and microstructural alterations.

A. Estrogens

Estrogen deficiency increases bone turnover with an imbalance between bone formation and resorption and appears to be a main cause of osteoporosis observed in women after the fifth decade.[30] Estrogen deficiency is associated with an increased production of a variety of cytokines released in the bone marrow environment, which stimulates bone resorption by raising the number and/or the activity of the bone-resorbing cells osteoclasts. Granulocyte-macrophage colony-stimulating factor (GM-CSF), tumor necrosis factor alpha, interleukin-1, interleukin-6, and receptor activator nuclear kappa-b ligand (RANKL) are cytokines implicated in hormones deficiency induced bone loss. GM-CSF and RANKL are necessary for osteoclast generation.[31]

B. Endocrine Disorders

Primary hyperparathyroidism increases bone turnover and is associated with some bone loss.[32] An excess of thyroid hormones also increases the rate of bone remodeling. Thus, bone loss can occur in hyperthyroidism and in patients under long-term thyroid hormone therapy at doses that suppress TSH. The main net effect of excess glucocorticoid is the reduction of bone formation, early bone loss, and increased fracture risk.[33] In addition, excess glucocorticoids cause muscle wasting.

C. Nutrition

Nutritional insufficiency and malnutrition are frequent in older people and are particularly prevalent in patients with a recent hip fracture. Nutritional deficiencies play a significant role in osteoporosis in elderly[11] (Fig. 28.3). With aging, there is a decrease in calcium intake, the intestinal absorption of calcium, the absorptive capacity of the intestinal epithelium to adapt to a low calcium intake, the exposure to sunlight, and the capacity of the skin to produce vitamin D. Vitamin D plays an essential role in the maintenance of bone strength and muscle function.[34] This nutrient/cofactor is involved in the absorption of calcium and phosphorus from the intestine, in the mineralization of bone, and maintenance of muscle quality as well as potentially in a variety of beneficial effects on other organ systems. Vitamin D is synthesized in skin during sun exposure or ingested as part of a balanced diet. Many older people suffer from hypovitaminosis D. This is particularly true in patients with hip fracture.[35] A state of chronic secondary hyperparathyroidism resulting from calcium and vitamin D deficiencies increases bone turnover and favors a negative bone balance, hence osteoporosis.

The prevalence of protein-energy malnutrition is as high as 4% – 10% in elderly persons living at home, 15% – 38% in those in institutional care, and 30% – 70% in hospitalized older patients.[36] A state of undernutrition at admission can adversely influence the clinical outcome (Fig. 28.4). Intervention studies using supplements, or even an oral one that normalizes protein intake, may improve the clinical outcome after hip fracture by lowering the rate of complications, such as bedsore, severe anemia, intercurrent lung or renal infections,[11] and shorten the length of stay in rehabilitation wards. Malnutrition and particularly protein-energy malnutrition is a risk factor for osteoporosis, sarcopenia, and frailty.[11,37] Various studies have found a relationship between protein intakes and calcium phosphate or bone metabolism and have come to the conclusion that either a deficient or an excessive protein supply could negatively affect the balance of calcium.[38] However, a deficient intake is a much higher risk than excess intake in the oldest old. A sufficient protein intake is a major contributor to for bone health, particularly in elderly.[11,38,39]

Protein intakes influence the production of IGF-I, which is an important trophic hormone, having growth-promoting effects on almost every cell in the body, especially skeletal muscle, cartilage, and bone (Fig. 28.5). In addition, it regulates phosphate reabsorption in the kid-

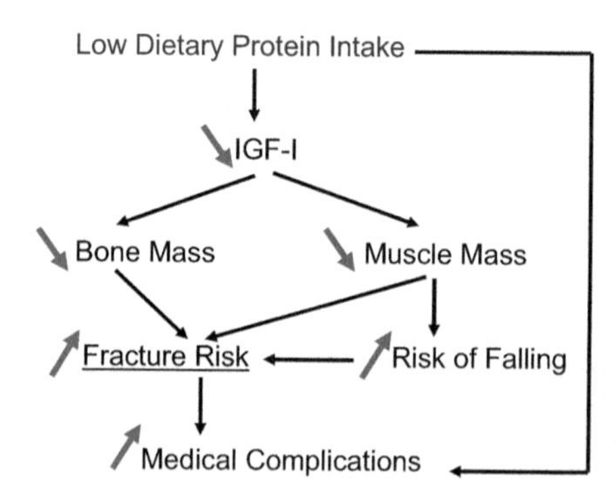

FIGURE 28.4 Consequences on musculoskeletal health of a low-protein diet. IGF-I: insulin-like growth factor I; red arrows: increase or decrease.

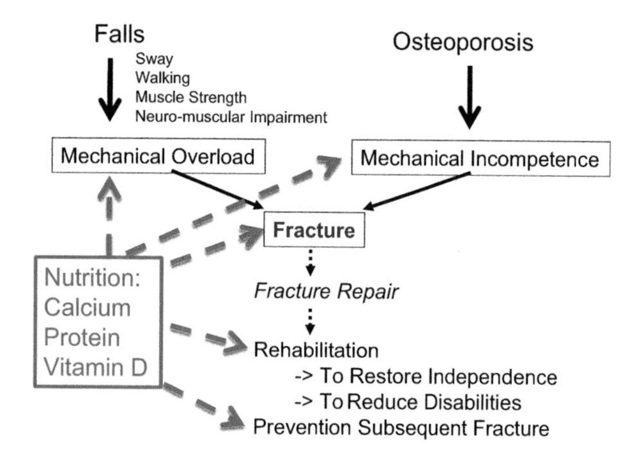

FIGURE 28.3 Multiple sites of action of nutrition in the pathogenesis of fragility fractures.

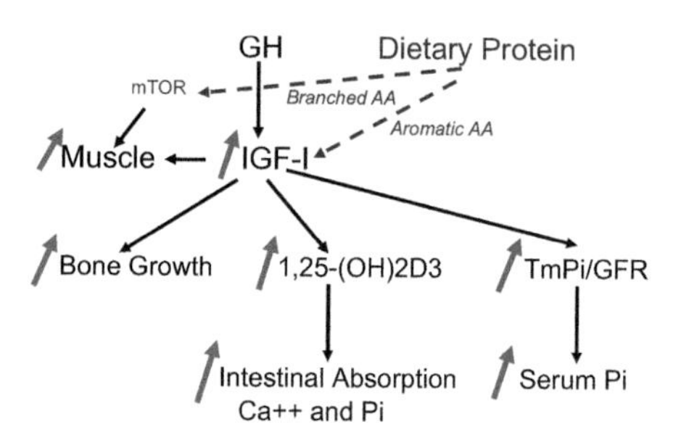

FIGURE 28.5 Modulation of the growth hormone–IGF-I axis by dietary protein. AA: amino acids; Ca++: calcium; GH: growth hormone; IGF-I: insulin-like growth factor I; mTOR: mammalian target of rapamycin; 1,25(OH)2D3: calcitriol; Pi: inorganic phosphate; red arrows: increase; TmPi/GFR: maximal renal tubular reabsorption of phosphate.

ney and has a stimulatory effect on the active uptake of calcium and phosphate from the intestine via the renal synthesis of calcitriol.[12,40] The determination of plasma IGF-I concentration has utility as a nutritional biomarker. Questionnaires such as the Mini Nutritional Assessment or the SNAQ65+, which have been validated in older persons, are useful in this respect to assess nutritional status.[36]

VI. STRATEGIES TO PREVENT FALLS

Although a number of risk factors for falling are not modifiable, such as age, others are amenable to changes, like decreased visual acuity, medications that can diminish awareness and/or balance, home environment (slippery floors and mats, poor lighting), and undernutrition.[41] In a comparative metaanalysis, the lowest relative risk of injurious falls was observed when calcium and vitamin D supplementations were combined with quality improvement strategies and multifactorial assessment and treatment. Exercise programs focusing on gait, coordination, and functional tasks, as well as muscle strengthening exercises other than just walking, seem to improve clinical balance outcomes in older people.[42] A multitask music-based training like Jacques-Dalcroze eurhythmic exercise has been shown to reduce gait and balance variability and lower fall risk.[43,44] Reducing falls were associated with a lower fracture risk.[42,45]

Trials of protein or selective amino acids supplementation on muscle mass and function have provided inconsistent results,[46,47] with even a prevention of falls in one study.[48] However, a recent trial in elderly men with 1.3 g/kg body weight dietary protein versus 0.8 (Recommended Daily Allowance [RDA] in adults) failed to detect any difference in muscle function and performance.[49] Protein supplements seem to magnify the effects of resistance training on muscle mass and function.[50,51] A pattern of even distribution of protein intake over the daily meals and some temporal link to physical activity are important factors for optimal muscle protein synthesis.[52]

VII. NUTRITIONAL SUPPLEMENTATIONS AND BONE HEALTH

A. Vitamin D

The associations between rickets in children or osteomalacia in adults with vitamin D deficiency and their effective treatment with vitamin D have been recognized for centuries.[53] Many clinical studies have tested the effects of vitamin D supplementation (often in combination with calcium) on fracture risk in participants who were older and/or osteoporotic. Metaanalyses of several of these trials have returned equivocal results.[54] For example, in a pooled analysis of 11 trials ($N = 31,000$), a lower fracture risk was associated with subjects having a plasma concentration of 25-hydroxy vitamin D (25-(OH)D) of at least 60 nmol/L at baseline as compared with those having concentrations below 30 nmol/L.[55] In contrast, fracture risk did not appear to be influenced by vitamin D alone in other studies.[54] Vitamin D supplementation has beneficial effects beyond bone health. Raising the levels of 25-(OH)D may decrease the incidence of falls in older persons, particularly in vitamin D insufficient subjects. Other studies and metaanalyses on vitamin D supplementation given with calcium have concluded that it is associated with a reduction in all-cause mortality.[56]

Sufficient concentrations of vitamin D are a prerequisite for the efficacy of antiosteoporosis medications, as all studies with these agents have been conducted in calcium and vitamin D–supplemented patients. Vitamin D supplementation should thus precede any antiosteoporosis therapy. The recommendation of a dose of 800 IU/day (20 μg/day) in older adults (>70 years) has been adopted by most European guidelines, as well as the International Osteoporosis Foundation, the Institute of Medicine, and in a European Society of Clinical and Economic Aspects of Osteoporosis, Osteoarthritis and Musculoskeletal Disease consensus paper.[34,57,58] There is no strong indication to systematically measure circulating 25-(OH)D in older patients with suspected high fracture risk since the price of testing far exceeds the cost of supplementation. The adverse effects of hypercalcemia/hypercalciuria and nephrolithiasis are more frequently associated with high serum 25-(OH)D (>125 nmol/L), which has been set as the potential upper limit of safety. Studies with large annual doses of vitamin D have reported an increased risk of falls and hip fracture.[59] Thus, a yearly high-dose regimen rather than a daily or weekly low-dose supplementation should be avoided.

B. Calcium

It is important to ensure a sufficient calcium intake through a balanced diet. Calcium and vitamin D supplements decrease secondary hyperparathyroidism and reduce the risk of proximal femur fracture, particularly in the elderly living in nursing homes.[60] Intakes of at least 800–1000 mg/day of calcium in addition to 800 IU of vitamin D can be recommended in the general management of patients with osteoporosis.[1,58]

A metaanalysis has concluded that calcium supplements without coadministered vitamin D may be associated with an increased risk of myocardial infarction.[61] There was no increased risk when calcium was of dietary origin. Large long-term observational studies have not confirmed this hypothesis.[62,63] Overall, it can be concluded that (1) calcium and vitamin D supplementation may lead to a modest reduction in fracture risk; (2) supplementation with calcium alone does not reduce fracture risk; (3) side effects of calcium supplementation may include renal stones and gastrointestinal symptoms; (4) vitamin D supplementation, rather than calcium, may reduce falls risk; (5) increased cardiovascular risk consequent to calcium supplementation is not convincingly supported by current evidence; and (6) calcium and vitamin D supplementation is recommended for patients at higher risk of calcium and vitamin D insufficiency, and in those who are receiving medications for osteoporosis.[64]

VIII. DIETARY PROTEIN

Correction of protein insufficiency can lead to a rapid normalization of IGF-I levels in frail older adults and in patients with a recent hip fracture.[65] In view of the impaired protein assimilation of older individuals, RDA (0.8 g/kg body weight) has been suggested to be increased to 1.0−1.2 g/kg per day in the older age group or even higher in case of severe diseases.[39,65] For additional review, see reference 38.

A. Dietary Protein and Bone Mineral Density

The association between BMD and dietary protein intakes has been investigated in four recent systematic reviews and metaanalyses.[66–69] Variations in protein intakes between approximately 0.8 and 1.2 g/kg body weight/day, thus above the RDA, accounted for 2% − 4% of BMD variance in adults.[66] In a metaanalysis of five RCT with lumbar spine BMD as an outcome, higher protein intake was associated with +0.52% change difference (95% CI: 0.06 − 0.97).[67]

Regarding intervention trials with protein above the current RDA, three studies assessed protein supplements on lumbar spine, with one showing an improvement in BMD with protein intakes at 163% of RDA for 26 weeks. For femoral neck, 1 out of 2 trials having assessed BMD changes showed an improvement with protein at 150% of RDA after 104 weeks.[68]

In a randomized placebo-controlled trial, conducted in vitamin D and calcium-replete subjects with a recent hip fracture, a protein supplement of 20 g per day for 6 months led to a 50% reduction in proximal BMD decrease at 1 year[70] and to a shorter length of stay in rehabilitation unit. An estimation of bone strength of peripheral skeleton sites, using finite element analysis, showed a positive association between predicted failure load and total animal and dairy protein intakes.[71]

B. Dietary Protein and Fracture Risk

No randomized controlled trial has examined the effect of dietary protein on fracture risk.[38] Five systematic reviews and metaanalyses have assessed this issue since 2009. Darling et al. found no significant reduction in hip fracture risk comparing the highest to the lowest quartile/quintile of dietary protein intakes in four cohort studies (RR: 0.75; 95% CI: 0.47 − 1.20).[66] Wu et al. pooled five cohorts with data on hip fracture risk and found a relative risk of 0.89 (0.82 − 0.97) comparing the highest to the lowest quartile/quintile of dietary protein intakes.[72] In a 2017 systematic review and metaanalysis, the conclusion was that higher protein intakes had no adverse effects on the bone.[67] In another systematic review and metaanalysis, high versus low dietary protein intakes were associated with a 16% reduction of hip fracture risk, with a relative risk of 0.84 (0.73 − 0.95).[68] The conclusion was that dietary protein at or above the current RDA could be beneficial for reducing hip fracture risk. In their metaanalysis update, Darling et al. concluded that there is little benefit of increasing protein intake for bone health in healthy adults, but there is no clear indication of any detrimental effect.[69]

C. Dietary Protein−Calcium Interaction

The slight discrepancy in the metaanalyses conclusions may reside in different included studies.[38] Furthermore, some studies have detected higher fracture risk in relation with dietary protein, when calcium intakes were low, suggesting some interaction between protein and calcium. A significant interaction was found in a calcium−vitamin D intervention trial.[73] Only in the calcium−vitamin D supplemented group, higher protein intake was associated with greater femoral neck and whole body BMD outcomes. Conversely, the positive effects of calcium−vitamin D supplementation on femoral neck BMD were more evident in the higher dietary protein tertile.[73]

Dairy products are a source of both protein and calcium, since 1 liter of milk provides 32 g of protein and 1200 mg of calcium. In some countries, yogurts are enriched in milk powder, leading to an up to 50% increased content of these nutrients as compared with yogurt prepared from plain milk. For Swiss cheese, protein and calcium contents are 26 g/100 g and 89 0mg/100 g, respectively.[21]

Numerous studies have tested the influence of both protein and calcium supplementation on bone health variables, through administration of dairy products, in randomized controlled trials (for review, see 21,38). These trials were relatively small, including between 11 and 408 subjects, precluding thus the assessment of fracture risk. The length of follow-up was between 1 week and 2.5 years, with a large variety of studied populations and outcomes. Altogether, dairy products, some being fortified with calcium or vitamin D, were consistently associated with a decrease in circulating PTH, an increase in IGF-I, and a decrease in bone resorption markers. In 10 out of 13 studies, a blunted decrease and even an increase in BMD were observed in response to dairy products, depending on the age of the subjects.[21] Dairy products are associated with higher estimated bone strength.[71]

With metaanalyses of cohort and case–control studies, Bian et al. have shown a lower risk of hip fracture in dairy products consumers.[74] This is in agreement with a recent report in older US men and women, where higher milk consumption was associated with a lower hip fracture risk.[75] Probiotics contained in fermented dairy products may provide additional benefits. In a prospective cohort of healthy postmenopausal women, age-related cortical bone loss was attenuated at nonbearing bone sites in yoghurt consumers, not in milk or ripened cheese consumers, independently of total energy, calcium, or protein intakes.[76] The effects of dairy products specifically attributable to fermented compounds have been recently reviewed[77] and are in agreement with those of other dairy intake-related studies. In contrast, a diet devoid of dairy foods, such as a vegan diet, is associated with lower BMD and higher fracture risk as demonstrated in a recent metaanalysis.[78] The cardiovascular safety of dairy products has been shown in metaanalysis combining data from 29 prospective cohort studies that concluded to neutral associations between dairy products and cardiovascular and all-cause mortality.[79] Even, specific analyses of fermented dairy like cheese and yogurt showed diets with cheese to have a 2% lower risk of CVD (RR 0.98, 95% CI 0.95 – 1.00) per 10 g/day intake. In a large multinational cohort study of individuals aged 35–70 years enrolled from 21 countries in 5 continents, dairy consumption was associated with lower risk of mortality and major cardiovascular disease events.[80] Interestingly, following a Mediterranean diet with additional dairy foods to meet the calcium intakes recommendations improved markers of cardiovascular risk over 8 weeks as compared with a low-fat diet.[81] Indeed, saturated fat irrespective of the fatty acids type and food sources may not be as harmful on the cardiovascular system as previously considered, and recommendation to avoid these foods may distract from intake of nutrient-dense foods that decrease the risk of malnutrition and various chronic disease including osteoporosis.[82]

From a health economics point of view, increasing dairy products intake with an impact on osteoporotic fracture and health costs may be a cost-effective measure.[83,84] Indeed, vitamin D–fortified dairy products have the potential to lower the burden of osteoporotic fractures, particularly in the general population aged more than 70 years.

IX. DIETARY PATTERN

In several cohort studies, adherence to Mediterranean diet was associated with a lower hip fracture risk.[85–87] In a metaanalysis of these data, the reduction of fracture risk amounted to 21% with adherence to Mediterranean diet.[88] For one unit increase in the Mediterranean diet score, a 5% reduction in the risk of hip fracture (RR 0.95, 95% CI 0.92 – 0.98) was found. Similarly, a lower risk of fracture was detected in a metaanalysis when intakes in the highest categories were compared with the lowest categories of prudent/healthy dietary pattern (OR = 0.81; 95% CI: 0.69, 0.95) 89 and was confirmed in another metaanalysis.[90]

X. DIETARY MODULATION OF GUT MICROBIOTA COMPOSITION AND/OR METABOLISM

The gut microbiota has been implicated in the pathogenesis of a large series of disorders, including bone diseases.[91] Diet is a major factor to determine the types and proportion of the microorganisms present in gut microbiota. Conversely, microbiota contributes to influence food nutritional value. Bone mass accrual, bone homeostasis, and prevention of sex hormone deficiency–induced bone loss may benefit from pre- or probiotics ingestion, which modifies gut microbiota composition and metabolism.[91] The fiber content of the diet markedly influences gut microbiota composition, by its prebiotic properties,[92] as does the ingestion of foods containing probiotics.[93] Gut microbiota is able to modulate and stimulate IGF-I synthesis by the host. Changes in gut microbiota have been reported with the Mediterranean diet, which provides fiber, fermented dairy products, and bioactive food compounds such as polyphenols.[94,95]

Genetic background, sex, immune status, age, dietary intakes, living conditions, geography, and medications are likely important confounding factors necessary to consider in evaluating the effects of gut microbiota on bone health. However, well-conducted long-term randomized controlled trials, with nutritional interventions changing gut microbiota composition[96] and/or function, and able of preventing bone loss and/or reducing fracture risk, are not yet available.

XI. CONCLUSIONS

The risk of osteoporotic fractures is a major health care concern. The impact of a major fracture on patients' lives is large. The costs borne by society are also significant, both in terms of immediate care and rehabilitation and loss of independence and quality of life. Many older people are undernourished and vitamin D deficient. These are clinical issues that should be identified and treated, by adequate dietary intakes of vitamin D, calcium, protein, and calories. Inadequate dietary protein intake in the oldest old members of the population is likely a much more severe problem than protein excess.

Practice points for nutritional approach of fracture prevention

- Correct or prevent vitamin D insufficiency ($\geq$ 800 IU/d)
- Ensure dietary calcium intake $\geq$ 1000 mg/d
- Ensure adequate dietary protein intake $\geq$ 1 g/kg body weight x d
- Promote weight-bearing physical exercise
- Treat any disease that might be causing bone loss
- Reduce the risk of falls
- Follow-up patients to encourage adherence to fracture prevention recommendations

RESEARCH GAPS

- To validate management models to optimize nutritional approaches as preventive strategies of bone disorders
- To demonstrate antifracture efficacy of nutritional intervention and determine its effect size
- To evaluate whether diet-mediated changes in gut microbiota are associated with reduction in fracture risk
- To further estimate the benefit–risk ratio and the cost-effectiveness of nutritional interventions in fracture prevention
- To identify intervention thresholds in nutritional status for fracture prevention
- To further estimate the benefit–risk ratio of foods for bone health instead of single nutrient intakes
- To explore new pathways of biological response to dietary intake change
- To revisit potential adverse effects such as cardiovascular system precluding adequate use of foods favorable to bone health

XII. REFERENCES

1. Kanis JA, Cooper C, Rizzoli R, Reginster JY. European guidance for the diagnosis and management of osteoporosis in postmenopausal women. *Osteoporos Int*. 2019;30:3–44.
2. Assessment of fracture risk and its application to screening for postmenopausal osteoporosis: report of a WHO Study Group. *World Health Organ Tech Rep Ser*. 1994;843:1–129.
3. Rizzoli R, Bianchi ML, Garabedian M, McKay HA, Moreno LA. Maximizing bone mineral mass gain during growth for the prevention of fractures in the adolescents and the elderly. *Bone*. 2010;46: 294–305.
4. Hernandez CJ, Beaupre GS, Carter DR. A theoretical analysis of the relative influences of peak BMD, age-related bone loss and menopause on the development of osteoporosis. *Osteoporos Int*. 2003;14: 843–847.
5. Theintz G, Buchs B, Rizzoli R, et al. Longitudinal monitoring of bone mass accumulation in healthy adolescents: evidence for a marked reduction after 16 years of age at the levels of lumbar spine and femoral neck in female subjects. *J Clin Endocrinol Metab*. 1992;75:1060–1065.
6. Lippuner K, Johansson H, Kanis JA, Rizzoli R. Remaining lifetime and absolute 10-year probabilities of osteoporotic fracture in Swiss men and women. *Osteoporos Int*. 2009;20:1131–1140.
7. Chevalley T, Guilley E, Herrmann FR, Hoffmeyer P, Rapin CH, Rizzoli R. Incidence of hip fracture over a 10-year period (1991–2000): reversal of a secular trend. *Bone*. 2007;40: 1284–1289.
8. Casez P, Uebelhart B, Gaspoz JM, Ferrari S, Louis-Simonet M, Rizzoli R. Targeted education improves the very low recognition of vertebral fractures and osteoporosis management by general internists. *Osteoporos Int*. 2006;17:965–970.
9. Schurch MA, Rizzoli R, Mermillod B, Vasey H, Michel JP, Bonjour JP. A prospective study on socioeconomic aspects of fracture of the proximal femur. *J Bone Miner Res*. 1996;11: 1935–1942.
10. Lippuner K, Popp AW, Schwab P, et al. Fracture hospitalizations between years 2000 and 2007 in Switzerland: a trend analysis. *Osteoporos Int*. 2011;22:2487–2497.
11. Rizzoli R. Nutritional aspects of bone health. *Best Pract Res Clin Endocrinol Metabol*. 2014;28:795–808.
12. Rizzoli R, Bonjour JP. Physiology of calcium and phosphate homeostases. In: Seibel MJ, Robins SP, Bilezikian JP, eds. *Dynamics of Bone and Cartilage Metabolism*. 2nd ed. San Diego: Academic Press; 2006:345–360.
13. Winzenberg T, Shaw K, Fryer J, Jones G. Effects of calcium supplementation on bone density in healthy children: meta-analysis of randomised controlled trials. *Br Med J*. 2006;333:775–778.

14. Johnston CC, Miller JZ, Slemenda CW, et al. Calcium supplementation and increases in bone mineral density in children. *N Engl J Med*. 1992;327:82–87.
15. Bonjour JP, Carrie AL, Ferrari S, et al. Calcium-enriched foods and bone mass growth in prepubertal girls: a randomized, double-blind, placebo-controlled trial. *J Clin Investig*. 1997;99:1287–1294.
16. Chevalley T, Bonjour JP, Ferrari S, Hans D, Rizzoli R. Skeletal site selectivity in the effects of calcium supplementation on areal bone mineral density gain: a randomized, double-blind, placebo-controlled trial in prepubertal boys. *J Clin Endocrinol Metab*. 2005; 90:3342–3349.
17. Chevalley T, Rizzoli R, Hans D, Ferrari S, Bonjour JP. Interaction between calcium intake and menarcheal age on bone mass gain: an eight-year follow-up study from prepuberty to postmenarche. *J Clin Endocrinol Metab*. 2005;90:44–51.
18. Bonjour JP, Ammann P, Chevalley T, Rizzoli R. Protein intake and bone growth. *Can J Appl Physiol*. 2001;26(Suppl):S153–S166.
19. Chevalley T, Bonjour JP, Ferrari S, Rizzoli R. High-protein intake enhances the positive impact of physical activity on BMC in prepubertal boys. *J Bone Miner Res*. 2008;23:131–142.
20. Alexy U, Remer T, Manz F, Neu CM, Schoenau E. Long-term protein intake and dietary potential renal acid load are associated with bone modeling and remodeling at the proximal radius in healthy children. *Am J Clin Nutr*. 2005;82:1107–1114.
21. Rizzoli R. Dairy products, yogurts, and bone health. *Am J Clin Nutr*. 2014;99:1256s–1262s.
22. Opotowsky AR, Bilezikian JP. Racial differences in the effect of early milk consumption on peak and postmenopausal bone mineral density. *J Bone Miner Res*. 2003;18:1978–1988.
23. Goulding A, Rockell JE, Black RE, Grant AM, Jones IE, Williams SM. Children who avoid drinking cow's milk are at increased risk for prepubertal bone fractures. *J Am Diet Assoc*. 2004;104:250–253.
24. Konstantynowicz J, Nguyen TV, Kaczmarski M, Jamiolkowski J, Piotrowska-Jastrzebska J, Seeman E. Fractures during growth: potential role of a milk-free diet. *Osteoporos Int*. 2007;18:1601–1607.
25. Matkovic V, Landoll JD, Badenhop-Stevens NE, et al. Nutrition influences skeletal development from childhood to adulthood: a study of hip, spine, and forearm in adolescent females. *J Nutr*. 2004;134:701S–705S.
26. Wiley AS. Does milk make children grow? Relationships between milk consumption and height in NHANES 1999–2002. *Am J Hum Biol*. 2005;17:425–441.
27. Cadogan J, Eastell R, Jones N, Barker ME. Milk intake and bone mineral acquisition in adolescent girls: randomised, controlled intervention trial. *Br Med J*. 1997;315:1255–1260.
28. Cheng S, Lyytikainen A, Kroger H, et al. Effects of calcium, dairy product, and vitamin D supplementation on bone mass accrual and body composition in 10-12-y-old girls: a 2-y randomized trial. *Am J Clin Nutr*. 2005;82:1115–1126. quiz 1147-1118.
29. Seeman E. Age- and menopause-related bone loss compromise cortical and trabecular microstructure. *J Gerontol A Biol Sci Med Sci*. 2013;68:1218–1225.
30. Almeida M, Laurent MR, Dubois V, et al. Estrogens and androgens in skeletal physiology and pathophysiology. *Physiol Rev*. 2017;97: 135–187.
31. Rao S, Cronin SJF, Sigl V, Penninger JM. RANKL and RANK: from mammalian physiology to cancer treatment. *Trends Cell Biol*. 2018; 28:213–223.
32. Khan AA, Hanley DA, Rizzoli R, et al. Primary hyperparathyroidism: review and recommendations on evaluation, diagnosis, and management. A Canadian and international consensus. *Osteoporos Int*. 2017;28:1–19.
33. Rizzoli R, Biver E. Glucocorticoid-induced osteoporosis: who to treat with what agent? *Nat Rev Rheumatol*. 2015;11:98–109.
34. Rizzoli R, Boonen S, Brandi ML, et al. Vitamin D supplementation in elderly or postmenopausal women: a 2013 update of the 2008 recommendations from the European Society for Clinical and Economic Aspects of Osteoporosis and Osteoarthritis (ESCEO). *Curr Med Res Opin*. 2013;29:305–313.
35. Bischoff-Ferrari HA, Can U, Staehelin HB, et al. Severe vitamin D deficiency in Swiss hip fracture patients. *Bone*. 2008;42:597–602.
36. Trombetti A, Cheseaux J, Herrmann FR, Rizzoli R. A critical pathway for the management of elderly inpatients with malnutrition: effects on serum insulin-like growth factor-I. *Eur J Clin Nutr*. 2013;67:1175–1181.
37. Gaffney-Stomberg E, Insogna KL, Rodriguez NR, Kerstetter JE. Increasing dietary protein requirements in elderly people for optimal muscle and bone health. *J Am Geriatr Soc*. 2009;57: 1073–1079.
38. Rizzoli R, Biver E, Bonjour JP, et al. Benefits and safety of dietary protein for bone health-an expert consensus paper endorsed by the European Society for Clinical and Economical Aspects of Osteopororosis, Osteoarthritis, and Musculoskeletal Diseases and by the International Osteoporosis Foundation. *Osteoporos Int*. 2018;29:1933–1948.
39. Bauer J, Biolo G, Cederholm T, et al. Evidence-based recommendations for optimal dietary protein intake in older people: a position paper from the PROT-AGE Study Group. *J Am Med Dir Assoc*. 2013; 14:542–559.
40. Dawson-Hughes B, Harris SS, Rasmussen HM, Dallal GE. Comparative effects of oral aromatic and branched-chain amino acids on urine calcium excretion in humans. *Osteoporos Int*. 2007;18: 955–961.
41. Tricco AC, Thomas SM, Veroniki AA, et al. Comparisons of interventions for preventing falls in older adults: a systematic review and meta-analysis. *J Am Med Assoc*. 2017;318:1687–1699.
42. de Souto Barreto P, Rolland Y, Vellas B, Maltais M. Association of long-term exercise training with risk of falls, fractures, hospitalizations, and mortality in older adults: a systematic review and meta-analysis. *JAMA Intern Med*. 2018;179(9).
43. Trombetti A, Hars M, Herrmann FR, Kressig RW, Ferrari S, Rizzoli R. Effect of music-based multitask training on gait, balance, and fall risk in elderly people: a randomized controlled trial. *Arch Intern Med*. 2011;171:525–533.
44. Hars M, Herrmann FR, Fielding RA, Reid KF, Rizzoli R, Trombetti A. Long-term exercise in older adults: 4-year outcomes of music-based multitask training. *Calcif Tissue Int*. 2014;95: 393–404.
45. El-Khoury F, Cassou B, Charles MA, Dargent-Molina P. The effect of fall prevention exercise programmes on fall induced injuries in community dwelling older adults: systematic review and meta-analysis of randomised controlled trials. *Br Med J*. 2013;347:f6234.
46. Bauer JM, Verlaan S, Bautmans I, et al. Effects of a vitamin D and leucine-enriched whey protein nutritional supplement on measures of sarcopenia in older adults, the PROVIDE study: a randomized, double-blind, placebo-controlled trial. *J Am Med Dir Assoc*. 2015;16:740–747.
47. Tieland M, Franssen R, Dullemeijer C, et al. The impact of dietary protein or amino acid supplementation on muscle mass and strength in elderly people: individual participant data and meta-analysis of RCT's. *J Nutr Health Aging*. 2017;21:994–1001.
48. Neelemaat F, Lips P, Bosmans JE, Thijs A, Seidell JC, van Bokhorst-de van der Schueren MA. Short-term oral nutritional intervention with protein and vitamin D decreases falls in malnourished older adults. *J Am Geriatr Soc*. 2012;60:691–699.
49. Bhasin S, Apovian CM, Travison TG, et al. Effect of protein intake on lean body mass in functionally limited older men: a randomized clinical trial. *JAMA Intern Med*. 2018;178:530–541.

50. Fiatarone MA, O'Neill EF, Ryan ND, et al. Exercise training and nutritional supplementation for physical frailty in very elderly people. *N Engl J Med.* 1994;330:1769–1775.
51. Cermak NM, Res PT, de Groot LC, Saris WH, van Loon LJ. Protein supplementation augments the adaptive response of skeletal muscle to resistance-type exercise training: a meta-analysis. *Am J Clin Nutr.* 2012;96:1454–1464.
52. Paddon-Jones D, Campbell WW, Jacques PF, et al. Protein and healthy aging. *Am J Clin Nutr.* 2015;101:1339s–1345s.
53. Ebeling PR, Adler RA, Jones G, et al. Management of endocrine disease: therapeutics of vitamin D. *Eur J Endocrinol.* 2018;179: R239–r259.
54. Bolland MJ, Grey A, Avenell A. Effects of vitamin D supplementation on musculoskeletal health: a systematic review, meta-analysis, and trial sequential analysis. *Lancet Diabetes Endocrinol.* 2018;6: 847–858.
55. Bischoff-Ferrari HA, Willett WC, Orav EJ, et al. A pooled analysis of vitamin D dose requirements for fracture prevention. *N Engl J Med.* 2012;367:40–49.
56. Rejnmark L, Avenell A, Masud T, et al. Vitamin D with calcium reduces mortality: patient level pooled analysis of 70,528 patients from eight major vitamin D trials. *J Clin Endocrinol Metab.* 2012; 97:2670–2681.
57. Dawson-Hughes B, Mithal A, Bonjour JP, et al. IOF position statement: vitamin D recommendations for older adults. *Osteoporos Int.* 2010;21:1151–1154.
58. Ross AC, Manson JE, Abrams SA, et al. The 2011 report on dietary reference intakes for calcium and vitamin D from the Institute of Medicine: what clinicians need to know. *J Clin Endocrinol Metab.* 2011;96:53–58.
59. Sanders KM, Stuart AL, Williamson EJ, et al. Annual high-dose oral vitamin D and falls and fractures in older women: a randomized controlled trial. *J Am Med Assoc.* 2010;303:1815–1822.
60. Tang BM, Eslick GD, Nowson C, Smith C, Bensoussan A. Use of calcium or calcium in combination with vitamin D supplementation to prevent fractures and bone loss in people aged 50 years and older: a meta-analysis. *Lancet.* 2007;370:657–666.
61. Bolland MJ, Avenell A, Baron JA, et al. Effect of calcium supplements on risk of myocardial infarction and cardiovascular events: meta-analysis. *Br Med J.* 2010;341:c3691.
62. Prentice RL, Pettinger MB, Jackson RD, et al. Health risks and benefits from calcium and vitamin D supplementation: women's Health Initiative clinical trial and cohort study. *Osteoporos Int.* 2013;24:567–580.
63. Paik JM, Curhan GC, Sun Q, et al. Calcium supplement intake and risk of cardiovascular disease in women. *Osteoporos Int.* 2014;25: 2047–2056.
64. Harvey NC, Biver E, Kaufman JM, et al. The role of calcium supplementation in healthy musculoskeletal ageing : an expert consensus meeting of the European Society for Clinical and Economic Aspects of Osteoporosis, Osteoarthritis and Musculoskeletal Diseases (ESCEO) and the International Foundation for Osteoporosis (IOF). *Osteoporos Int.* 2017;28:447–462.
65. Rizzoli R, Stevenson JC, Bauer JM, et al. The role of dietary protein and vitamin D in maintaining musculoskeletal health in postmenopausal women: a consensus statement from the European Society for Clinical and Economic Aspects of Osteoporosis and Osteoarthritis (ESCEO). *Maturitas.* 2014;79:122–132.
66. Darling AL, Millward DJ, Torgerson DJ, Hewitt CE, Lanham-New SA. Dietary protein and bone health: a systematic review and meta-analysis. *Am J Clin Nutr.* 2009;90:1674–1692.
67. Shams-White MM, Chung M, Du M, et al. Dietary protein and bone health: a systematic review and meta-analysis from the National Osteoporosis Foundation. *Am J Clin Nutr.* 2017;105: 1528–1543.
68. Wallace TC, Frankenfeld CL. Dietary protein intake above the current RDA and bone health: a systematic review and meta-analysis. *J Am Coll Nutr.* 2017;36:481–496.
69. Darling AL, Manders RJF, Sahni S, et al. Dietary protein and bone health across the life-course: an updated systematic review and meta-analysis over 40 years. *Osteoporos Int.* 2019;30:741–761.
70. Schurch MA, Rizzoli R, Slosman D, Vadas L, Vergnaud P, Bonjour JP. Protein supplements increase serum insulin-like growth factor-I levels and attenuate proximal femur bone loss in patients with recent hip fracture. A randomized, double-blind, placebo-controlled trial. *Ann Intern Med.* 1998;128:801–809.
71. Durosier-Izart C, Biver E, Merminod F, et al. Peripheral skeleton bone strength is positively correlated with total and dairy protein intakes in healthy postmenopausal women. *Am J Clin Nutr.* 2017; 105:513–525.
72. Wu AM, Sun XL, Lv QB, et al. The relationship between dietary protein consumption and risk of fracture: a subgroup and dose-response meta-analysis of prospective cohort studies. *Sci Rep.* 2015;5:9151.
73. Dawson-Hughes B, Harris SS. Calcium intake influences the association of protein intake with rates of bone loss in elderly men and women. *Am J Clin Nutr.* 2002;75:773–779.
74. Bian S, Hu J, Zhang K, Wang Y, Yu M, Ma J. Dairy product consumption and risk of hip fracture: a systematic review and meta-analysis. *BMC Public Health.* 2018;18:165.
75. Feskanich D, Meyer HE, Fung TT, Bischoff-Ferrari HA, Willett WC. Milk and other dairy foods and risk of hip fracture in men and women. *Osteoporos Int.* 2018;29:385–396.
76. Biver E, Durosier-Izart C, Merminod F, et al. Fermented dairy products consumption is associated with attenuated cortical bone loss independently of total calcium, protein, and energy intakes in healthy postmenopausal women. *Osteoporos Int.* 2018;29:1771–1782.
77. Rizzoli R, Biver E. Effects of fermented milk products on bone. *Calcif Tissue Int.* 2018;102:489–500.
78. Iguacel I, Miguel-Berges ML, Gomez-Bruton A, Moreno LA, Julian C. Veganism, vegetarianism, bone mineral density, and fracture risk: a systematic review and meta-analysis. *Nutr Rev.* 2019;77:1–18.
79. Guo J, Astrup A, Lovegrove JA, Gijsbers L, Givens DI, Soedamah-Muthu SS. Milk and dairy consumption and risk of cardiovascular diseases and all-cause mortality: dose-response meta-analysis of prospective cohort studies. *Eur J Epidemiol.* 2017;32:269–287.
80. Dehghan M, Mente A, Rangarajan S, et al. Association of dairy intake with cardiovascular disease and mortality in 21 countries from five continents (PURE): a prospective cohort study. *Lancet.* 2018;392:2288–2297.
81. Wade AT, Davis CR, Dyer KA, Hodgson JM, Woodman RJ, Murphy KJ. A Mediterranean diet supplemented with dairy foods improves markers of cardiovascular risk: results from the MedDairy randomized controlled trial. *Am J Clin Nutr.* 2018;108: 1166–1182.
82. Astrup A, Bertram HC, Bonjour JP, et al. WHO draft guidelines on dietary saturated and trans fatty acids: time for a new approach? *Br Med J.* 2019;366:l4137.
83. Lotters FJ, Lenoir-Wijnkoop I, Fardellone P, Rizzoli R, Rocher E, Poley MJ. Dairy foods and osteoporosis: an example of assessing the health-economic impact of food products. *Osteoporos Int.* 2013;24:139–150.

84. Hiligsmann M, Burlet N, Fardellone P, Al-Daghri N, Reginster JY. Public health impact and economic evaluation of vitamin D-fortified dairy products for fracture prevention in France. *Osteoporos Int*. 2017;28:833–840.
85. Byberg L, Bellavia A, Larsson SC, Orsini N, Wolk A, Michaelsson K. Mediterranean diet and hip fracture in Swedish men and women. *J Bone Miner Res*. 2016;31:2098–2105.
86. Haring B, Crandall CJ, Wu C, et al. Dietary patterns and fractures in postmenopausal women: results from the women's health initiative. *JAMA Intern Med*. 2016;176:645–652.
87. Benetou V, Orfanos P, Feskanich D, et al. Mediterranean diet and hip fracture incidence among older adults: the CHANCES project. *Osteoporos Int*. 2018;29:1591–1599.
88. Malmir H, Saneei P, Larijani B, Esmaillzadeh A. Adherence to Mediterranean diet in relation to bone mineral density and risk of fracture: a systematic review and meta-analysis of observational studies. *Eur J Nutr*. 2018;57:2147–2160.
89. Denova-Gutierrez E, Mendez-Sanchez L, Munoz-Aguirre P, Tucker KL, Clark P. Dietary patterns, bone mineral density, and risk of fractures: a systematic review and meta-analysis. *Nutrients*. 2018;10.
90. Fabiani R, Naldini G, Chiavarini M. Dietary patterns in relation to low bone mineral density and fracture risk: a systematic review and meta-analysis. *Adv Nutr*. 2019;10:219–236.
91. Rizzoli R. Nutritional influence on bone: role of gut microbiota. *Aging Clin Exp Res*. 2019;31:743–751.
92. Whisner CM, Weaver CM. Prebiotics and bone. *Adv Exp Med Biol*. 2017;1033:201–224.
93. Druart C, Alligier M, Salazar N, Neyrinck AM, Delzenne NM. Modulation of the gut microbiota by nutrients with prebiotic and probiotic properties. *Adv Nutr*. 2014;5:624s–633s.
94. Mitsou EK, Kakali A, Antonopoulou S, et al. Adherence to the Mediterranean diet is associated with the gut microbiota pattern and gastrointestinal characteristics in an adult population. *Br J Nutr*. 2017;117:1645–1655.
95. Tosti V, Bertozzi B, Fontana L. Health benefits of the Mediterranean diet: metabolic and molecular mechanisms. *J Gerontol A Biol Sci Med Sci*. 2018;73:318–326.
96. Nilsson AG, Sundh D, Backhed F, Lorentzon M. Lactobacillus reuteri reduces bone loss in older women with low bone mineral density: a randomized, placebo-controlled, double-blind, clinical trial. *J Intern Med*. 2018;284:307–317.

CHAPTER

29

FOOD ALLERGIES, SENSITIVITIES, AND INTOLERANCES

Steve L. Taylor, PhD
Joseph L. Baumert, MS, PhD
University of Nebraska-Lincoln, Food Allergy Research & Resource Program, Department of Food Science & Technology, Lincoln, NE, United States

SUMMARY

Food allergies, sensitivities, and intolerances affect a small but significant portion of the population. Symptoms can range from mildly annoying to severe and life-threatening. The true food allergies present the biggest risk because symptoms can occasionally be quite severe and the threshold dose for the offending food needed to provoke a reaction is quite low. The prevalence of true food allergies is growing and dietary management in infancy may be a preventive strategy. In general, food sensitivities are poorly defined and difficult to diagnose. Food intolerances generally present with moderate symptoms and affected individuals can often tolerate small doses of the offending food. Individuals affected with food allergies, sensitivities, and intolerances must avoid the causative food. Construction of safe and effective avoidance diets can be quite difficult for individuals with true food allergies in part due to the low threshold doses.

Keywords: Avoidance diet; Celiac disease; Eosinophilic esophagitis; Food allergy; Food intolerance; Food protein-induced enterocolitis; Gluten; Lactose intolerance; IgE; Sulfite.

I. NORMAL FUNCTION AND PHYSIOLOGY

Centuries ago, Lucretius stated "What is food to one is bitter poison to another." Food allergies, sensitivities, and intolerances can be collectively referred to as "*individualistic* adverse reactions to foods" because these illnesses affected only certain individuals within the population. In unaffected individuals, food components are digested, absorbed, and/or metabolized by normally functioning mechanisms. Unaffected individuals can eat all foods in the diet without harm. With true food allergies where naturally occurring dietary proteins elicit abnormal immune responses, the unaffected individuals safely digest these proteins and utilize the amino acids in the same manner as for all dietary proteins (see Chapter 2). With food sensitivities and intolerances, altered metabolic processes are known to be involved in some conditions, but the mechanisms involved in other conditions remain obscure.

II. DISEASES

Although these food allergies, sensitivities, and intolerances are often grouped together under the general heading of "food allergy", a variety of different types of illnesses are involved. The existence of several different types of adverse reactions to foods with varied symptoms, severity, prevalence, and causative factors is not recognized by some physicians or nutrition professionals. Consumers are even more likely to be confused regarding the definition and classification of adverse reactions to foods. Consumers perceive that "food allergies"

Present Knowledge in Nutrition, Volume 2
https://doi.org/10.1016/B978-0-12-818460-8.00029-0

are quite common,[1] but many self-diagnosed cases of "food allergy" incorrectly associate foods with a particular malady or ascribe various mild forms of postprandial eating discomfort to this category of illness. In this chapter, we will describe each of these conditions separately in an attempt to add clarity.

III. ABNORMAL PHYSIOLOGY OR FUNCTION

Table 29.1 provides a classification scheme for the different types of illnesses that are known to occur in association with food ingestion that only involve certain individuals in the population. Three major groups of individualistic adverse reactions to foods are known: true food allergies, food sensitivities, and food intolerances. The true food allergies involve abnormal immunological mechanisms, whereas the food sensitivities and intolerances do not. Knowing and recognizing the difference between immunological food allergies and nonimmunological food sensitivities and intolerances is crucial. True food allergies can be provoked in some cases by very low doses of the offending foods while those with sensitivities and intolerances can often tolerate larger doses of the offending food before symptoms are experienced.

A food allergy is an abnormal immunological response to a food or food component, usually a naturally occurring protein.[2] Two different types of abnormal immunological responses are known to occur. Immediate hypersensitivity reactions are antibody-mediated, while delayed hypersensitivity reactions are cell-mediated. Additionally, mixed responses involving both antibodies and immune cells occur in several conditions. Finally, other illnesses appear to be food allergies but have obscure mechanisms.

In contrast, food sensitivities and intolerances do not involve abnormal responses of the immune system.[2] Food intolerances are also known as metabolic food disorders because they are caused by abnormalities in metabolic functions that are only physiologically evident when certain foods are consumed. Food sensitivities are idiosyncratic with observed heightened sensitivities to certain food components that occur through unknown mechanisms.

IV. IGE-MEDIATED FOOD ALLERGY

Immediate hypersensitivity reactions are mediated by allergen-specific IgE antibodies (Fig. 29.1). In IgE-mediated food allergies, allergen-specific IgE antibodies are produced by B cells in response to the immunological stimulus created by exposure of the immune system to the allergen.[3] Food allergens are usually naturally occurring proteins present in the food.[4] The allergen-specific IgE antibodies bind to the surfaces of mast cells in the tissues and basophils in the blood, which is the sensitization phase of the allergic response. The sensitization phase is asymptomatic. On subsequent exposure to the specific allergenic food, the allergens cross-link two or more of the IgE antibodies affixed to the surfaces of mast cells or basophils. This interaction triggers the degranulation of the mast cell or basophil and the release of a variety of potent physiologically active mediators into the bloodstream and tissues. The granules within mast cells and basophils contain many of the important mediators of the allergic reaction. These potent mediators are actually responsible for the symptoms of immediate hypersensitivity reactions. Histamine is perhaps the most important of the mediators released from mast cells and basophils in an allergic reaction. Histamine can elicit inflammation, pruritis, and contraction of the smooth muscles in the blood vessels, gastrointestinal tract, and respiratory tract.[2] Other important mediators include various leukotrienes and prostaglandins. The leukotrienes are associated with some of the symptoms that develop more slowly in IgE-mediated food allergies, such as late-phase asthmatic reactions. This same type of IgE-mediated reaction is also responsible for allergic reactions to other environmental substances such as pollens, mold

TABLE 29.1 Classification of individualistic adverse reactions to foods.

Classification
True Food Allergies
Antibody-Mediated Food Allergies
IgE-mediated food allergies (peanut, cows' milk, etc.)
Exercise-associated food allergies
Cell-Mediated Food Allergies
Celiac disease
Other types of delayed hypersensitivity
Food Intolerances
Anaphylactoid Reactions
Metabolic Food Disorders
Lactose intolerance
Idiosyncratic Reactions
Sulfite-induced asthma

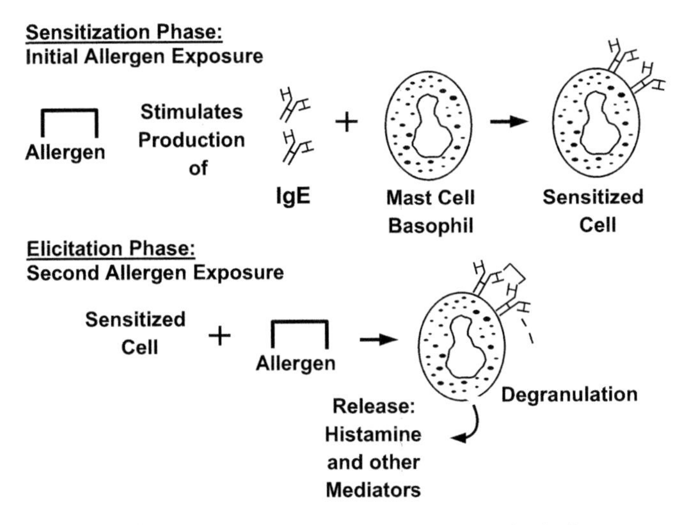

FIGURE 29.1 Mechanism of IgE-mediated food allergy.

TABLE 29.2 Symptoms associated with IgE-mediated food allergy.

Gastrointestinal:	Nausea
	Vomiting
	Diarrhea
	Abdominal cramping
Cutaneous:	Urticaria
	Dermatitis or eczema
	Angioedema
	Pruritis
Respiratory:	Rhinitis
	Asthma
	Laryngeal edema
Generalized:	Anaphylactic shock

spores, animal danders, and bee venoms; only the source of the allergen is different.

During the sensitization phase, an individual forms allergen-specific IgE antibodies after exposure to a specific food protein. However, even among individuals predisposed to allergies, exposure to food proteins usually does not result in the formation of IgE antibodies. Normally even among individuals predisposed to food allergies, exposure to a food protein in the gastrointestinal tract results in oral tolerance through either the formation of protein-specific IgG, IgM, or IgA antibodies or other mechanisms including clonal anergy (no immunological response whatsoever), apoptosis of antigen-specific T cells, active immune suppression, or bystander suppression.[5] Heredity and other physiological factors are important in predisposing individuals to the development of IgE-mediated allergies including food allergies.[6] Studies with monozygotic and dizygotic twins demonstrate that genetics is an extremely important parameter and that identical twins may even inherit the likelihood of responding to the same allergenic food, e.g., peanuts.[7] Approximately 65% of patients with clinically documented allergy have first degree relatives with allergic disease.[8] Conditions that increase the permeability of the small intestinal mucosa to proteins have been considered to possibly increase the risk of development of food allergy. An increased risk is seen in cystic fibrosis patients perhaps due to increased gut permeability,[9] but no increased risk for food allergy is encountered in premature infants who manifest with increased gut permeability.[10]

The onset time for IgE-mediated food allergy reactions ranges from a few minutes to several hours after the consumption of the offending food. IgE-mediated food allergies involve numerous symptoms ranging from mild and annoying to severe and life-threatening (Table 29.2). No individual with IgE-mediated food allergy suffers from all of the symptoms noted in Table 29.2. Furthermore, the symptoms are not necessarily consistent from one episode to another for an individual. The nature and severity of symptoms can also vary as a result of the amount of the offending food that has been ingested and the length of time since the previous exposure. An individual who experiences only mild symptoms on ingestion of a specific food, e.g., oral pruritis, may develop more serious manifestations on subsequent occasions especially if avoidance of the offending food is not routinely practiced.

Gastrointestinal symptoms and cutaneous symptoms are among the more common manifestations of IgE-mediated food allergies. Respiratory symptoms are less commonly encountered but can be severe and life-threatening. Mild respiratory symptoms such as rhinitis and rhinoconjunctivitis are more likely to be encountered with exposure to environmental allergens such as directly inhaled airborne pollens or animal danders. However, respiratory reactions associated with food allergies can occasionally be severe (asthma and laryngeal edema). Those few food-allergic individuals who experience severe respiratory reactions in connection with the inadvertent ingestion of the offending food are most likely to be at risk for life-threatening episodes.[11] Of the many symptoms involved in IgE-mediated food allergies, systemic anaphylaxis is the most severe manifestation.[12] Systemic anaphylaxis, also sometimes referred to as anaphylactic shock, involves multiple organ systems and numerous symptoms. The symptoms can involve the gastrointestinal tract, respiratory tract, skin, and cardiovascular system. Death can occur from severe hypotension coupled with respiratory and cardiovascular complications. Anaphylactic shock is the most common cause of death in the occasional fatalities associated with IgE-mediated food allergies.[11,13–16] The number of deaths occurring from IgE-mediated food allergies is not recorded in most countries. Fatal food allergy reactions may be underreported in the United States; estimates vary widely from 10 to 100 deaths per year.[16,17]

Food allergies are not often severe. In fact, the most common manifestation of IgE-mediated food allergies is oral allergy syndrome, which typically elicits rather mild oropharyngeal symptoms: pruritis, urticaria, and angioedema associated with the ingestion of the offending foods—often fresh fruits and vegetables.[18] Fresh fruits and vegetables contain comparatively low quantities of the protein allergens, but oral allergy syndrome is an IgE-mediated response involving reactions to certain specific proteins.[18] Apparently, the allergens in these fresh fruits and vegetables are rapidly digested by the proteases of the gastrointestinal tract,[19] and systemic reactions are rarely encountered. The allergens are also apparently heat labile[19] because heat processing eliminates their effects. Individuals with oral allergy syndrome are initially sensitized to one or more environmental pollens, frequently birch pollen, or mugwort pollen.[18] Once sensitized to the pollen allergens, these individuals are reactive to proteins that exist in foods that cross-react with these allergens.

Several environmental factors can exacerbate IgE-mediated food allergies. The best studied of these conditions is food-dependent, exercise-induced anaphylaxis. Exercise-induced food allergies are a subset of the immediate hypersensitivity reactions to foods. They involve allergen-specific IgE antibodies but occur only when the food is eaten in conjunction with exercise.[20] Numerous foods have been implicated, including shellfish, wheat, celery, and peach. The symptoms are as individualistic and variable as those for other food allergies. Exercise-induced allergies can also exist without any role for food intake.[20] The mechanism of this illness is not well understood except the involvement of IgE antibodies is clear. With the recent national emphasis on increased physical activity, reports of this condition could increase.

The overall prevalence of IgE-mediated food allergies for all age groups may be as high as 8%–10% for the United States.[21,22] However, an epidemiologic analysis of the data on prevalence of food allergies revealed that the evidence basis was remarkably weak.[23] For example, few investigations involving clinical confirmation of IgE-mediated food allergies have been conducted using representative groups of the population; the largest studies in the United States relied upon surveys.[21,22] Selection biases also plague the prevalence data because many clinical prevalence investigations have involved groups of patients seen at allergy clinics. Such selected groups are unlikely to represent the entire population, and the prevalence rates for these groups are likely to be higher than for the general population. A large-scale epidemiological investigation of the prevalence of IgE-mediated food allergy was conducted in the Netherlands.[24] This study revealed that although >10% of Dutch adults believed that they had adverse reactions to foods, the prevalence of these reactions was ~2% when clinical histories were confirmed by blinded food challenges.[24] The prevalence rate for IgE-mediated food allergies among infants and young children is better defined than for adults.[25] Clinical trials among groups of unselected infants suggest that the prevalence of IgE-mediated food allergies is in the range of 4%–8%.[26,27] Surveys conducted in the United States, Canada, and England indicate that the self-perceived prevalence of peanut allergy alone is 0.5%–0.8% among all age groups,[28–30] although the survey by Gupta et al.[21] in the United States suggested a prevalence of peanut allergy of 2.0% among children and 1.8% among adults in the United States. A survey in the United States of the self-perceived prevalence of tree nut, fish, and crustacean shellfish allergies indicated that 0.5%, 0.4%, and 1.9%, respectively, believes that they have these particular food allergies.[30,31] Higher prevalence levels among US adults were indicated in a more recent survey[22] of 1.2% for tree nuts, 0.9% for fish, and 2.9% for crustacean shellfish. None of these surveys included clinical investigations to confirm that peanut, tree nut, fish, or crustacean shellfish allergies truly existed in these individuals.

Many food-allergic infants outgrow their food allergies within a few months to several years after the onset of the sensitivity.[32] Allergies to certain foods, such as cows' milk, are more commonly outgrown than are allergies to certain other foods such as peanut. Allergies to peanuts were considered to be a lifelong affliction until clinical researchers demonstrated that peanut allergy, especially when acquired very early in life, can be outgrown,[33] although that does not seem to be a frequent occurrence. While milk and egg allergy is more frequently outgrown than peanut allergy, several studies have documented that these allergies are increasingly persistent in a subgroup of patients with milk and egg allergy.[34,35] Tolerance to baked milk and egg products seems to precede tolerance to less-heated forms of these foods.[36,37] The mechanisms involved in the loss of sensitivity to specific foods are not precisely known, but the development of immunological tolerance is definitely involved.[5] More heat-stable allergen epitopes may result in greater persistence.[38]

Eight foods or food groups—milk, eggs, fish, crustacea (shrimp, crab, lobster, etc.), peanuts, soybeans, tree nuts (walnuts, almonds, hazelnuts, etc.), and wheat—are responsible for the vast majority of IgE-mediated food allergies worldwide,[39] but regional differences exist. Examples of food allergies that occur more frequently in certain parts of the world than in others would include celery allergy in Europe,[40] sesame seed allergy in Israel,[41] and buckwheat allergy in Japan.[42] These regional differences are likely related to food preferences in those areas and sometimes to coexistent pollen allergies (e.g., celery allergy in individuals sensitized to mugwort pollen). Beyond the eight major foods or food groups, >160 other foods have been documented to cause IgE-mediated food allergies.[43] Because food allergens are proteins, any food that contains protein is likely to elicit allergic sensitization on at least rare occasions. The eight most commonly allergenic foods or food groups contain comparatively high amounts of protein and are commonly consumed in the diet. However, several other commonly consumed foods with high protein contents, such as beef, pork, chicken, and turkey, are rarely allergenic.

Food allergens are almost always naturally occurring proteins.[4] Foods contain hundreds of thousands of different proteins, and only a small percentage is known allergens. The major allergens have been identified, purified, and characterized for most of the commonly allergenic foods.[4] Multiple allergenic proteins exist in some commonly allergenic foods. Foods may contain both major and minor allergens. Major allergens are defined as proteins that bind to serum IgE antibodies from >50% of patients with a specific food allergy. For example, milk contains three major allergens: casein, β-lactoglobulin, and α-lactalbumin.[44] These also happen to be the major milk proteins. Milk may also contain several minor allergens, e.g., bovine serum albumin and lactoferrin, although the level of evidence for clinical relevance is less convincing for these minor allergens.[45] Peanuts contain multiple allergens including four major allergens, named *Ara h* 1, *Ara h* 2, *Ara h* 3, and *Ara h* 6,[46] although it is doubtful that all of the minor IgE-binding proteins from peanut are clinically significant. In contrast, codfish (*Gad c* 1) and Brazil nut (*Ber e* 1) contain primarily one major allergenic protein.[4]

For some foods, cross-reactions occur with closely related foods. For example, shrimp-allergic individuals will also typically be sensitive to other crustaceans including crab and lobster.[47] Similarly, cross-reactions commonly occur between different species of fish,[47] different species of avian eggs,[48] and milk from cows and goats.[49] In contrast, some peanut-allergic individuals are allergic to other legumes such as soybean,[50] but this is not common. Clinical hypersensitivity to one legume, such as peanuts or soybeans, does not warrant exclusion of the entire legume family from the diet unless allergy to each individual legume is confirmed by clinical challenge trials.[51] However, there are a few instances with legumes where cross-reactions become a more serious concern. The best example would be cross-reactions between lupine seed flour and peanut.[52,53]

Cross-reactions are also known to occur between certain types of pollens and foods. These reactions are often involved with oral allergy syndrome that was described earlier. Examples would include ragweed pollen and melons, mugwort pollen and celery, mugwort pollen and hazelnut, and birch pollen and various foods including carrots, apples, hazelnuts, and potatoes.[54]

Cross-reactions are also known to occur between allergies to natural rubber latex and banana, chestnut, avocado, and kiwi among others.[55]

V. DELAYED IGE-MEDIATED HYPERSENSITIVITIES

As noted, IgE-mediated reactions typically involve immediate onset. But one type of delayed hypersensitivity reaction mediated by IgE antibodies has been identified—the so-called alpha-gal syndrome.[56] This condition is triggered by ingestion of mammalian meats with symptoms appearing 3–6 h after meat ingestion. Diagnosis is established by presence of elevated levels of IgE antibodies directed against an oligosaccharide, galactose-α-1,3-galactose (alpha-gal). Sensitization occurs from the bite of several species of ticks.[57] Subsequently affected individuals have adverse reactions from the ingestion of meat products that apparently contain glycoproteins with alpha-gal moieties. IgE-mediated food allergies usually involve immediate onset of symptoms, and the explanation for the delayed basis of the alpha-gal syndrome is not known. Also most allergens are proteins, but in this unique situation, the antibodies are directed at carbohydrate structures.

VI. CELL-MEDIATED HYPERSENSITIVITIES

Some forms of delayed hypersensitivities are mediated by immune cells involving tissue-bound T lymphocytes that are sensitized to a specific foodborne substance that triggers the reaction.[2] These reactions often result in localized tissue inflammation. In such reactions, symptoms begin to appear 6–24 h after consumption of the offending food.

The principal example of this type of delayed hypersensitivity reaction is celiac disease (also known as celiac sprue, nontropical sprue, or gluten-sensitive enteropathy), a malabsorption syndrome occurring in sensitive individuals upon the consumption of wheat, rye, barley, triticale, spelt, kamut, and other grains containing prolamin proteins.[2,58] Celiac disease is a chronic, immune-mediated, enteropathy resulting from consumption of the offending grains or protein-containing products derived from those grains.[58,59] Histologic examination reveals characteristic villous atrophy, crypt hyperplasia, and intraepithelial lymphocytosis.[59] Although the inflammatory process specifically targets the small intestine, both intestinal and extraintestinal symptoms may occur.[60] The mucosal damage, especially the villous atrophy, leads to nutrient malabsorption. Some symptoms such as weight loss, anemia, and bone pain are associated with nutrient deficiencies associated with active celiac disease. Intestinal T cells reactive to gliadin, the prolamin from wheat, are found in celiac patients including infants predisposed to development of the disease.[61] Celiac disease is an inherited trait, occurring in ~5% of first degree relatives of celiac patients and ~75% of monozygotic twin pairs.[62] Histocompatibility locus antigen (HLA) class II genes (DQ8 and DQ2) are the major genes associated with celiac disease, but concordance for celiac disease is only 25%–40% in siblings who are identical for one or both HLA haplotypes.[63] Thus, genes outside of the HLA locus likely have some as-yet undefined role in disease susceptibility.

The prevalence of celiac disease is between 0.5% and 1.0% in the United States.[64,65] Prevalence estimates from different parts of the world are somewhat variable[60] perhaps complicated by the use of different diagnostic approaches. Celiac disease appears to be latent or asymptomatic in some individuals whose symptoms only appear occasionally.[58] The prevalence of celiac disease in the United States has increased over the past few decades for unexplained reasons.[66]

Celiac disease is associated with the ingestion of gliadin from wheat and related prolamin proteins from other grains.[2] The prolamin fraction of wheat is known as gliadin. Gliadin together with a more insoluble protein called glutenin forms the gluten complex in wheat. Hence, celiac disease is sometimes called gluten-sensitive enteropathy. A defect in mucosal processing of gliadin in patients with celiac disease provokes the generation of toxic peptides that contribute to the abnormal T-cell response and the subsequent inflammatory reaction.[61] The risk of death as a direct result of celiac disease is low,[67] but individuals suffering from celiac disease for prolonged periods are at increased risk for development of T-cell lymphoma.[68] Patients also appear more likely to have various other autoimmune diseases including dermatitis herpetiformis, thyroid diseases, Addison's disease, pernicious anemia, autoimmune thrombocytopenia, sarcoidosis, insulin-dependent diabetes mellitus, and IgA nephropathy.[58,69]

VII. MIXED IGE- AND CELL-MEDIATED HYPERSENSITIVITIES

Eosinophilic esophagitis (EoE) is the most common illness that fits into this category of immune-mediated illness. EoE has rapidly emerged as an illness of increasing importance over the past 10 years. EoE is typically characterized by symptoms of esophageal dysfunction.[70] Esophageal rings and strictures can develop leading to food impaction and dysphagia.[71] Vomiting can also occur. Food allergies are often involved with milk, wheat, egg, beef, soy, and chicken most commonly implicated.[72] The prevalence of EoE is increasing and may be as high as 1 in 1000 among adults and children.[73]

Several other eosinophilic disorders of the gastrointestinal tract also appear to fit within this category including eosinophilic colitis (EC), eosinophilic gastritis (EG), and eosinophilic gastroenteritis (EGE).[72] These illnesses are rather rare compared to EoE. EC affects primarily infants, and causative foods seem restricted to milk and soy. EG is more common in adults than children and can involve wheat, soy, egg, and tree nuts. EGE is encountered almost exclusively in adults, and seafoods and meats are implicated.

VIII. OTHER NONIGE-MEDIATED FOOD ALLERGIES

Several illnesses should be discussed in this section including food protein–induced enterocolitis syndrome (FPIES), food protein–induced allergic proctocolitis (FPIP), and food protein enteropathy (FPE).[72] All of these illnesses are considered as food allergies even though the direct involvement of the immune system in these disorders requires further elucidation. FPIES has recently been recognized clinically as an important disorder among infants and young children.[74] FPIES presents with repeated, profuse vomiting, pallor, lethargy, and often with diarrhea leading to acute dehydration.[74,75] Chronically, FPIES can lead to weight loss and failure to thrive in infants.[75] The acute dehydration can lead to severe hypotension in some cases.[74] FPIES most commonly is associated with cows' milk but can also be triggered by soy, rice, oats, and egg.[72] In a large study involving more than 13,000 Israeli infants, 0.34% developed FPIES to milk, but 90% of the cases had resolved by the age of 3 years.[76] FPIES rarely occurs in exclusively breastfed infants.[75] In contrast, FPIP is a benign condition occurring in otherwise healthy young infants who produce bloody stools.[75] FPIP most often develops with breastfed infants and resolves when the lactating mothers remove milk and soy from their diets.[75] FPIP typically resolves by the end of the first year of life.[75] FPE usually presents in infancy with recurrent abdominal pain and chronic malabsorptive diarrhea.[77] Celiac disease is an example of an FPE. However, cases have been described on children who have similar reactions to foods other than gluten-containing grains, particularly milk.[77] Even some patients with celiac disease have been described who are also reactive to a second food, usually milk.[77]

IX. FOOD SENSITIVITIES

Some individuals have heightened sensitivities to certain food components that have unknown mechanisms. Since the components are typically not proteins, the immune system is unlikely to be involved. While such complaints are numerous and involve many food components, especially additives, the cause–effect relationships have not been clearly established in many cases. Psychosomatic illnesses are included in this category. In this section, we will discuss two illnesses where the cause–effect relationship is reasonably clear, but the mechanism of action remains unknown. The first will be nonceliac gluten sensitivity which is likely related to gluten, a protein component of certain grains. The second will be sulfite-induced asthma where the food component is an additive.

Nonceliac gluten sensitivity is diagnosed by exclusion. Patients do not have celiac disease or wheat allergy (negative diagnostic tests) but yet experience intestinal or extraintestinal symptoms or both upon ingestion of gluten-containing grains such as wheat, barley, or rye.[60] The symptoms are similar to celiac disease so the diagnosis cannot be made by symptomatic history alone. The condition does improve upon the removal of gluten-containing grains and ingredients from the diet and that becomes part of the diagnostic criteria. Because no biomarkers are available and the diagnosis is difficult, no estimates exist regarding the prevalence of nonceliac gluten sensitivity. Because the condition is associated with gluten-containing grains, it is often thought to be associated with gluten or other proteins from wheat and related grains,[63] but definitive proof of that association is lacking. While the mechanism of nonceliac gluten sensitivity has not been elucidated, the exposure of peripheral blood mononuclear cells from patients with this condition included an overactivation of the proinflammatory chemokine, CXCL10.[78]

Sulfites are common food additives that also occur naturally in certain foods, especially fermented foods, usually in small amounts.[79] Although asthma is the only well-established symptom associated with sulfite sensitivity, only a small percentage of asthmatics are sulfite sensitive.[79] Individuals with severe asthma who require steroids for control of symptoms are the primary risk group for sulfite sensitivity, but only ~5% of these are sulfite sensitive.[79] Sulfite-induced asthma can be quite severe, and deaths have been documented.[79] The mechanism of sulfite-induced asthma remains unclear although several hypotheses have been put forward.[79] Immunological mechanisms are not likely to be involved.

X. FOOD INTOLERANCES

Food intolerances also known as metabolic food disorders occur as the result of genetically determined metabolic deficiencies that either affect the ability to metabolize a specific substance in foods or heighten sensitivity to a particular foodborne chemical.[2] Lactose intolerance is an example of a metabolic food disorder.[2] Inborn errors of metabolism such as phenylketonuria could be discussed within this context as some of them do respond to dietary restrictions. Conditions such as phenylketonuria are much more serious than lactose intolerance and involve special clinical oversight. They will not be discussed further in this chapter.

Lactose intolerance is associated with a deficiency of the enzyme, β-galactosidase (lactase), in the intestinal tract that leads to an inability to metabolize lactose from milk and other dairy products.[80] The symptoms of lactose intolerance are mild, confined to the gastrointestinal tract, and include abdominal discomfort, flatulence, and frothy diarrhea.[80] Lactose intolerance affects a large number of people worldwide with a frequency as high as 60%–90% among people with African, Native American, Hispanic, Asian, Jewish, and Arab ancestry.[2] In contrast, the prevalence among North American Caucasians is ~6–12%.[2]

XI. ROLE OF DIET IN THE ONSET OF THE CONDITION

Dietary components clearly trigger food allergies, sensitivities, and intolerances, but in most of these conditions, diet is not known to play any role in the onset of the condition. Dietary factors could play some role in certain conditions, but more research will be needed to understand those relationships. The exceptions are IgE-mediated food allergies and celiac disease where the diet and epigenetic factors related to diet appear to play a key role in the onset of the condition.

With IgE-mediated food allergies, genetics is clearly important because IgE-mediated food allergies are most likely to develop in high-risk infants—those born to parents with histories of allergic disease of any type (pollens, mold spores, animal danders, bee venoms, food, etc.). Preventing the development of food allergies in such infants has been a subject of great interest but limited progress until recently. The restriction of the diet of the mother during pregnancy (excluding commonly allergenic foods such as peanuts) does not appear to help prevent allergy in the infant[81] suggesting that sensitization does not occur in utero. Breastfeeding for extended periods of time appears to delay but may not prevent the development of IgE-mediated food allergies.[82] The exclusion of certain commonly allergenic foods, such as peanuts, from the maternal diet during the lactation period has often been recommended. The use of probiotics during lactation may also help to lessen the likelihood of allergic sensitization.[83] Hypoallergenic infant formula may also prevent the development of food allergies in high-risk infants,[84] although these formulas are more often used to prevent reactions after sensitization has already occurred. The use of partial whey hydrolyzate formula has been advocated because the partial hydrolyzate is more likely to prevent sensitization than a formula based on whole milk.[85] High-risk infants may still develop food allergies once solid foods are introduced into the diet.[82]

As the prevalence of IgE-mediated food allergies continued to increase rather rapidly in recent decades, researchers continued to probe for more effective preventive measures. Multiple factors are likely involved to one degree or another,[86] but weaning practices appear to play a significant role. The Learning Early About Peanut (LEAP) trial demonstrated that the introduction of peanut to high-risk infants (with a history of egg allergy and dermatitis) beginning at 4–6 months of age resulted in a dramatically lower prevalence of peanut allergy at age of 5 years.[87] This finding confirmed an initial observation that Jewish children in Tel Aviv had a much lower prevalence of peanut allergy than genetically similar Jewish children in London attributed to the consumption of a popular extruded peanut snack in Israel.[88] Before the LEAP trial, pediatric societies had recommended delaying the introduction of peanuts during the weaning period until 3 years of age or longer. These recommendations have now been changed.[89] The early introduction of other commonly allergenic foods during the early weaning period may also be beneficial,[90] but continued research is needed to explore this approach more fully. Breastfeeding remains highly recommended, but the early introduction of commonly allergenic foods may serve to prevent the development of food allergies.

Epigenetic factors beyond weaning practices are increasingly considered as contributors to the development of food allergies.[86] Dietary factors may be involved including vitamin A, vitamin D, long-chain n-3 fatty acids, and antioxidants. Vitamin A is known to stimulate an antiinflammatory microenvironment within mucosal tissues through boosting of the production of Treg cells.[5] As a result, vitamin A appears to stimulate the development of oral tolerance. However, the specific role of vitamin A in the development of food allergy remains to be determined.[91] The role of vitamin D in prevention of food allergies is also not clearly defined.[92] Vitamin D definitely exerts potentially beneficial effects at the immunological level.[86] However, a case–control study showed that vitamin D insufficiency during the first 6 months was not associated with an increased risk of challenge-proven egg allergy in infants at age of 1 year.[93] Evidence does suggest that the positive effect of vitamin D on food sensitization is associated with certain genetic variants.[86] The effects of vitamin D supplementation during pregnancy have not been studied. The intake of long-chain n-3 polyunsaturated fatty acids appears to have a preventive effect on the development of IgE-mediated allergies.[94] These n-3 PUFAs may exert the preventive effect by inducing a favorable balance of prostaglandins and cytokines affecting T-cell classes.[86] The roles of other dietary antioxidants such as vitamin E, vitamin C, and β-carotene on the development of food allergy are less clear and not as well investigated.[86]

The gastrointestinal microbiome likely influences the development of food allergy,[95] but the extent of the effect remains unclear. Infants born by Cesarean section have a sterile intestinal tract at birth and do not inherit their mother's protective microbiome. Infants born by Cesarean are at increased risk of the development of food allergies.[96,97] Prebiotics such as oligosaccharides and especially the human milk oligosaccharides can alter the intestinal microbiome in a manner that seems to protect against the development of food allergy.[98] The addition of prebiotic oligosaccharides to infant formula is being explored as one potential strategy to prevent food allergies in early life.[98]

With celiac disease, the main driver appears to be genetic. Because not all individuals with the genetic predisposition get celiac disease, the possibility exists that other factors may be involved. Two randomized control trials have demonstrated that neither the delayed introduction of gluten or breastfeeding of genetically predisposed infants affected the risk of development of celiac disease.[59] Host–microbe interactions may also play a role in prevention of celiac disease in infants.[59] The addition of probiotics into the infant diet is being explored.

XII. MEDICAL TREATMENT

Medical treatment primarily exists only for IgE-mediated food allergies, although novel therapies are also being explored for celiac disease. Medical treatments have not been developed for alpha-gal syndrome, mixed IgE- and cell-mediated hypersensitivities, non–IgE-mediated food allergies, food sensitivities, or food intolerances.

Pharmacological approaches (epinephrine and antihistamines) are available for treating the symptoms of IgE-mediated allergic reactions.[99] Antihistamines are often used to treat the symptoms of mild to moderate food allergy reactions. However, epinephrine is the drug of choice to treat severe anaphylactic reactions to foods.

Several immunotherapeutic approaches have been developed for the treatment of IgE-mediated food allergies. The first of the immunotherapeutic approaches involved administration of antiIgE antibodies.[100] While this approach has not gained approval, it does appear to be effective in increasing the level of tolerance to the offending food.[101] Subsequently, oral, sublingual, and epicutaneous immunotherapies have shown promise.[102] These approaches do not lead to sustained unresponsiveness or tolerance to the offending food but do increase the individual's threshold dose thereby decreasing the risk of unexpected reactions occurring in the community.[103] Individuals who have achieved some degree of desensitization through immunotherapy must continue to consume a maintenance dose of the food or risk reverting to a lower threshold dose. Other novel therapies are under active development with the hope to achieve sustained oral tolerance.[104]

Several novel therapies are in the development stages for celiac disease including both pharmacological and tolerogenic approaches. Pharmacological approaches, all in the early stages of development, include the oral administration of endopeptidases, tight junction modulators, transglutaminase inhibitors, inflammatory protease inhibitors, HLA-DQ2 blockers, and gluten-binding agents.[59] Tolerogenic approaches include a peptide-based vaccine, parasitic immunoregulation, and nanoparticle therapy but none are yet approved by FDA for clinical use.[59] Additionally, plant breeding and agricultural biotechnology approaches to develop wheat varieties with low gliadin content are being pursued.[105]

XIII. DIETARY MANAGEMENT

At present, avoidance diets remain as the mainstay approach for preventing food allergies, sensitivities, and intolerances.[63,106,107] For example, if allergic to peanuts, simply avoid peanuts in all forms. A competent diagnosis with identification of the causative food or food ingredient is a necessary preamble to any advice on a suitable avoidance diet for any of these conditions.

In the case of IgE-mediated food allergies, a careful history of the individual's reactions of various foods and oral challenges are typically sufficient to identify the causative foods.[108] The presence of food-specific IgE antibodies as determined by serum testing or skin prick tests is insufficient to establish clinical reactivity.[108] Consultation with knowledgeable dietitians is then critical to the construction of a safe and nutritionally adequate avoidance diet for children and adults. More individuals are being diagnosed with multiple food allergies,[21] which increases the criticality of nutritional consultation. Nutritionally inadequate avoidance diets can lead to micronutrient deficiencies.[109]

In IgE-mediated food allergies, individual minimal provoking doses (thresholds) are highly variable. In some affected individuals, exposure to trace levels of the offending food can elicit adverse reactions. Anecdotal reports suggest that reactions could occur from exposure to the small quantities via using shared utensils or containers, kissing the lips of someone who has eaten the offending food, opening packages of the offending food, or inhalation of vapors from the offending food. Although these situations are not well documented, the amount of the offending food that would be ingested from such occurrences would be quite low. The anecdotes and reports of reactions to "hidden" allergens in foods (not always trivial doses)[110] have led to the widespread belief that very small doses of the offending food can elicit severe allergic reactions. Thus complete avoidance is the most frequently recommended approach for IgE-mediated food allergies. In reality, threshold doses do exist, below which allergic individuals will not experience adverse reactions.[111] Threshold doses do not appear to be the same for all allergenic foods.[111] Since most food-allergic individuals do not know their personal threshold dose, caution remains necessary for safe and effective avoidance diets. With packaged foods, food-allergic consumers rely upon the ingredient labels to identify the allergens that must be avoided; the enactment of labeling legislation in several countries including the United States has simplified this effort.[39] Food-allergic consumers are advised to avoid all ingredients derived from foods that provoke their allergies.[106] However, the levels of allergenic protein from the source food in various ingredients can vary from trivial to substantial thus complicating avoidance diets.[112] Allergic consumers frequently worry about cross contamination in food processing operations resulting from shared equipment and shared facilities. Since public health agencies have not established threshold levels for allergenic foods, the significance of such concerns is difficult to assess. Accordingly, precautionary allergen labeling (e.g. "may contain X" and similar) abounds on packaged foods and additionally places stress on consumers following avoidance diets.[113,114] Avoidance diets are a practical approach for individuals with IgE-mediated food allergies, but this management approach has become increasingly complex in recent years.

Alpha-gal syndrome is also treated with avoidance diets. All types of red meat must be avoided.[56] No information is available on threshold doses for this condition.

An avoidance diet, in this case gluten avoidance, is also the mainstay for management of celiac disease.[63] The usual recommendation is complete avoidance of gluten, which comes with many of the same challenges outlined above for IgE-mediated food allergies. A concentration of <20 ppm gluten has been defined as the consensus level for gluten-free foods globally.[115] The tolerance for gluten is likely to be variable among celiac sufferers. Clinical studies have indicated the daily gluten consumption of 10 mg is safe[116] and supports the establishment of the gluten-free definition. Patients with celiac disease avoid all gluten-containing grains including wheat, barley, rye, spelt, and kamut. Most celiac sufferers have also historically avoided oats, although the role of oats in the elicitation of celiac disease was refuted.[117] Because oats are often contaminated with wheat and/or barley in commerce, some caution may still be necessary. However, gluten-free oat products, grown or processed to remove wheat or barley contamination, are now available in the marketplace. Gluten-free oats and many other gluten-free foods have become quite popular in the United States. Thus, the maintenance of a gluten-free diet has become easier.

With EoE, avoidance diets are implemented in management although it can be more difficult to clinically determine the identity of the specific causative foods.[118,119] While the threshold dose for elicitation of EoE is unknown, some evidence suggests that low-dose exposures can be problematic for some affected persons.[118] Avoidance diets are also employed in the management of other eosinophilic disorders[72] but typically involve a limited number of foods.

With the other non–IgE-mediated food allergies (FPIES, FPIP, and FPE), only short-term avoidance diets are needed in most cases because the illnesses affect infants and spontaneously resolves as the child gets older.[72] Although no studies have been conducted on threshold doses for these conditions, strict avoidance of low doses is likely not necessary in the case of FPIES.[118]

Food sensitivities are treated with specific avoidance diets. In the case of nonceliac gluten sensitivity, affected individuals are advised to follow the same gluten-free diet as with celiac disease.[60] However, nonceliac gluten sensitivity is thought to be a transient condition, so avoidance periods of 12–24 months are often employed.

Sulfites added to foods must be declared on product labels so avoidance diets are reasonably easy to develop.[79] Sulfite-sensitive individuals with asthma can tolerate the ingestion of small quantities of sulfite, especially when the sulfites are incorporated in certain types of foods where the sulfite is bound to other food components such as shrimp or dehydrated potatoes.[120] Although sulfite-induced asthma poses a considerable risk to sensitive individuals, this condition is manageable once it is recognized.

The usual treatment for lactose intolerance is the avoidance of dairy products containing lactose, but lactose-intolerant individuals can tolerate some lactose in their diets[2] and most have virtually no symptoms on consumption of the amount of lactose in 235 mL (1 cup) of milk.[2] Additionally, some dairy products (e.g., yogurt, acidophilus milk) are better tolerated than others, apparently because they contain bacteria with β-galactosidase.[2] Lactase (β-galactosidase) tablets are available commercially and assist affected individuals in tolerating modest doses of lactose. Thus, lactose intolerance is a manageable condition.

XIV. CONCLUSION

Knowledge about some of the more important clinical conditions involved with food allergies, sensitivities, and intolerances including IgE-mediated food allergies, celiac disease, and EoE has increased substantially in recent years. Meanwhile other conditions are only recently being recognized including nonceliac gluten sensitivity and FPIES. Knowledge surrounding food sensitivities and intolerances is limited and primarily associated with lactose intolerance and sulfite sensitivity. Nutrition professionals have long played an important role in providing individuals with advice on the construction of safe and effective avoidance diets. However recently, attention has also focused on the role of nutrition in prevention of the development of food allergies, sensitivities, and intolerance. Research box includes a short-term list of key nutritional research studies. Table 29.3 (box) provides emerging areas where many nutrition professionals need to gain knowledge to provide the best advice to their clients.

TABLE 29.3 Emerging areas of knowledge important to nutrition professionals.

- Early introduction of commonly allergenic foods for the prevention of food allergy development and the benefits to families of high risk and all infants
- Food allergen immunotherapy (oral and epicutaneous) for desensitization to allergenic foods and the need to ongoing maintenance doses
- Dietary avoidance advice to children with multiple food allergies
- The persistence or natural history of various food allergies
- Role of food processing on the allergenicity of certain foods, e.g., baked milk or egg
- Threshold doses for commonly allergenic foods
- Dose versus severity for IgE-mediated food allergy
- Understanding of the role of diet in emerging conditions such as eosinophilic disorders, food protein–induced enterocolitis, and others

RESEARCH GAPS

Nutritional research gaps on food allergies, sensitivities, and intolerances

- Determine if early introduction of peanuts into the diets of infants who are NOT high risk for development of food allergies has any benefit
- Determine if early introduction of other allergenic foods into the diets of infants, both high risk and not high risk, has any benefit for the prevention of food allergy development
- Further assess the potential nutritional epigenetic factors on the prevention of the development of food allergies
- Determine if breastfeeding, with or without early supplementation with allergenic foods, has any effect on the prevention of food allergy development
- Assess the dietary behavior of patients who have achieved partial desensitization through food allergen immunotherapy
- Explore the relationship between the gut microbiome on food allergy prevention and persistence
- Determine if early introduction of gluten has any impact of the prevention of celiac disease
- Explore the relationship of the gut microbiome on celiac disease and other cell-mediated or non-IgE-mediated food allergy
- Assess the potential impact of nutritional epigenetic factors on the prevention of the development of celiac disease and other cell-mediated or non-IgE-mediated food allergy
- Determine the persistence of nonceliac gluten sensitivity

XV. REFERENCES

1. Sloan AE, Powers ME. A perspective on popular perceptions of adverse reactions to foods. *J Allergy Clin Immunol.* 1986;78: 127–133.
2. Taylor SL, Hefle SL. Food allergies and other food sensitivities. *Food Technol.* 2001;55(9):68–83.
3. Sampath V, Tupa D, Graham MT, et al. Deciphering the black box of food allergy mechanisms. *Ann Allerg Asthma Immunol.* 2017;118: 21–27.
4. Breiteneder H, Mills ENC. Food allergens: molecular and immunological characteristics. In: Metcalfe DD, Sampson HA, Simon RA, eds. *Food Allergy: Adverse Reactions to Foods and Food Additives.* 4th ed. Malden MA: Blackwell Publishing; 2008: 43–61.
5. Sricharunrat T, Pumirat P, Leaungwutiwong. Oral tolerance: recent advances on mechanisms and potential applications. *Asian Pac J Allergy Immunol.* 2018;36:207–216.
6. Tsai H-J, Kumar R, Pongracic J, et al. Familial aggregation of food allergy and sensitization to food allergens: a family-based study. *Clin Exp Allergy.* 2009;39:101–109.
7. Sicherer SH, Furlong TJ, Maes HH, et al. Genetics of peanut allergy: twin study. *J Allergy Clin Immunol.* 2000;106:53–56.
8. Hourihane JO'B, Dean TP, Warner JO. Peanut allergy in relation to heredity, maternal diet, and other atopic diseases: results of a questionnaire survey, skin prick testing, and food challenge. *Br Med J.* 1996;313:518–521.
9. Lucarelli S, Quattrucci S, Zingoni AM, et al. Food allergy in cystic fibrosis. *Minerva Pediatr.* 1994;46:543–548.
10. Liem JJ, Kozyrskyj AL, Hug SI, et al. The risk of developing food allergy in premature or low-birth-weight children. *J Allergy Clin Immunol.* 2007;119:1203–1209.
11. Sampson HA, Mendelson L, Rosen J. Fatal and near-fatal anaphylactic reactions to foods in children and adolescents. *N Engl J Med.* 1992;327:380–384.
12. Greenhawt M, Gupta RS, Meadows JA, et al. Guiding principles for the recognition, diagnosis, and management of infants with anaphylaxis: an expert panel consensus. *J Allergy Clin Immunol Pract.* 2019;7:1148–1156.
13. Yunginger JW, Sweeney KG, Sturner WQ, et al. Fatal food-induced anaphylaxis. *J Am Med Assoc.* 1988;260:1450–1452.
14. Bock SA, Munoz-Furlong A, Sampson HA. Further fatalities caused by anaphylactic shock, 2001-2006. *J Allergy Clin Immunol.* 2007;119:1016–1018.
15. Pumphrey RSH, Gowland H. Further fatal allergic reactions to foods in the United Kingdom, 1999–2006. *J Allergy Clin Immunol.* 2007;119:1018–1019.
16. Turner PJ, Jerschow E, Umasunthar T, et al. Fatal anaphylaxis: mortality and risk factors. *J Allergy Clin Immunol Pract.* 2017;5: 1169–1175.
17. Sampson HA. Anaphylaxis and emergency treatment. *Pediatrics.* 2003;111:1601–1608.
18. Wang J. Oral allergy syndrome. In: Metcalfe DD, Sampson HA, Simon RA, eds. *Food Allergy: Adverse Reactions to Foods and Food Additives.* 4th ed. Malden MA: Blackwell Publishing; 2008: 133–143.
19. Taylor SL, Lehrer SB. Principles and characteristics of food allergens. *Crit Rev Food Sci Nutr.* 1996;36:S91–S118.
20. Foong R-X, Giovannini M, du Toit G. Food-dependent exercise-induced anaphylaxis. *Curr Opin Allergy Clin Immunol.* 2019;19: 224–228.
21. Gupta RS, Springston EE, Warrier MR, et al. The prevalence, severity, and distribution of childhood food allergy in the United States. *Pediatrics.* 2011;128:e9–e16.
22. Gupta RS, Warren CM, Smith BM, et al. Prevalence and severity of food allergy among U.S. adults. *JAMA Netw Open.* 2019;2. e185630, 14 pp.
23. Rona RJ, Keil T, Summers C, et al. The prevalence of food allergy: a meta analysis. *J Allergy Clin Immunol.* 2007;120:638–646.
24. Neistijl Jansen JJ, Kardinaal AFM, Huijbers G, et al. Prevalence of food allergy and intolerance in the adult Dutch population. *J Allergy Clin Immunol.* 1994;93:446–456.
25. Sampson HA. Food allergy. *Curr Opin Immunol.* 1990;2:542–547.
26. Bock SA, Lee WY, Remigio LK, May CD. Studies of hypersensitivity reactions to foods in infants and children. *J Allergy Clin Immunol.* 1978;62:327–334.
27. Sampson HA. Update on food allergy. *J Allergy Clin Immunol.* 2004;113:805–819.

28. Emmett SE, Angus FJ, Fry JS, et al. Perceived prevalence of peanut allergy in Great Britain and its association with other atopic conditions and with peanut allergy in other household members. *Allergy.* 1999;54:380–385.
29. Ben-Shoshan M, Harrington DW, Soller L, et al. A population-based study on peanut, tree nut, fish, shellfish, and sesame allergy prevalence in Canada. *J Allergy Clin Immunol.* 2010;125:1327–1335.
30. Sicherer SH, Munoz-Furlong A, Godbold JH, et al. US prevalence of self- reported peant, tree nut, and sesame allergy: 11-year follow-up. *J Allergy Clin Immunol.* 2010;125:1322–1326.
31. Sicherer SH, Munoz-Furlong A, Sampson HA. Prevalence of seafood allergy in the United States by a random telephone survey. *J Allergy Clin Immunol.* 2004;114:159–165.
32. Savage J, Sicherer S, Wood R. The natural history of food allergy. *J Allergy Clin Immunol Pract.* 20, 1916;4:196–203.
33. Skolnick H, Conover Walker MK, Barnes-Koerner C, et al. The natural history of peanut allergy. *J Allergy Clin Immunol.* 2001; 107:367–374.
34. Savage JH, Matsui EC, Skripak JM, et al. The natural history of egg allergy. *J Allergy Clin Immunol.* 2007;120:1413–1417.
35. Skripak JM, Matsui EC, Mudd K, et al. The natural history of IgE-mediated cow's milk allergy. *J Allergy Clin Immunol.* 2007;120: 1172–1177.
36. Leonard SA, Caubet J-C, Kim JS, et al. Baked milk- and egg-containing diet in the management of milk and egg allergy. *J Allergy Clin Immunol Pract.* 2015;1:131–23.
37. Nowak-Wegrzyn A, Lawson K, Musilamani M, et al. Heat-denatured (baked) milk products in milk-allergicv children. *J Allergy Clin Immunol Pract.* 2018;6:486–495.
38. Bloom KA, Huang FR, Bencharitiwong R, et al. Effect of heat treatment on milk and egg proteins allergenicity. *Pediatr Allergy Immunol.* 2015;25:740–746.
39. Taylor SL, Baumert JL. Worldwide food allergy labeling and detection of allergens in processed foods. In: Ebisawa M, Ballmer-Weber B, Vieths S, Wood R, Karger S, eds. *Food Allergy: Molecular Basis and Clinical Practice, Chemical Immunology & Allergy Series.* Vol. 101. 2015:227–234. Basel, Switzerland.
40. Woods RK, Abramson M, Bailey M, et al. International prevalence of reported food allergies and intolerances. Comparisons arising from the European Community Respiratory Health Survey (ECRHS) 1991–1994. *Eur J Clin Nutr.* 2001;55:298–304.
41. Dalal I, Goldberg M, Katz Y. Sesame seed food allergy. *Curr Allergy Asthma Rep.* 2012;12:339–345.
42. Ebisawa M, Nishima S, Ohnishi H, et al. Pediatric allergy and immunology in Japan. *Pediatr Allergy Immunol.* 2013;24:704–714.
43. Hefle SL, Nordlee JA, Taylor SL. Allergenic foods. *Crit Rev Food Sci Nutr.* 1996;36:S69–S89.
44. Tsabouri S, Douras K, Priftis KN. Cow's milk allergenicity. *Endocr Metab Immune Disord Drug Targets.* 2014;14:16–26.
45. Hochwallner H, Schulmeister U, Swoboda I, et al. Cow's milk allergy: from allergens to new forms of diagnosis, therapy, and prevention. *Methods.* 2014;66:22–33.
46. Palladino C, Breiteneder H. Peanut allergens. *Mol Immunol.* 2018; 100:58–70.
47. Leung NYH, Wai CYY, Shu S, et al. Current immunological and molecular biological perspectives on seafood allergy: a comprehensive review. *Clin Rev Allergy Immunol.* 2014;46:180–197.
48. Langeland T. A clinical and immunological study of allergy to hen's egg white. VI. Occurrence of proteins cross-reacting with allergens in hen's egg white as studied in egg white from Turkey, duck,goose, seagull, and in hen egg yolk, and hen and chicken sera and flesh. *Allergy.* 1983;39:339–412.
49. Pham MN, Wang J. Mammalian milk allergy: a case presentation and review of prevalence, diagnosis, and treatment. *Ann Allerg Asthma Immunol.* 2017;118:406–410.
50. Herian AM, Taylor SL, Bush RK. Identification of soybean allergens by immunoblotting with sera from soy-allergic adults. *Int Arch Allergy Appl Immunol.* 1990;92:193–198.
51. Bernhisel-Broadbent J, Sampson HA. Cross-allergenicity in the legume botanical family in children with food hypersensitivity. *J Allergy Clin Immunol.* 1989;83:435–440.
52. Moneret-Vautrin DA, Guerin L, Kanny G, et al. Cross-allergenicity of peanut and lupine: the risk of lupine allergy in patients allergic to peanut. *J Allergy Clin Immunol.* 1999;104:883–888.
53. Bingemann TA, Santos CB, Russell AF, et al. Lupin – an emerging food allergen in the United States. *Ann Allerg Asthma Immunol.* 2019;122:8–10.
54. Van Ree R. Clinical importance of cross-reactivity in food allergy. *Curr Opin Allergy Clin Immunol.* 2004;4:235–240.
55. Blanco C. Latex – fruit syndrome. *Curr Allergy Asthma Rep.* 2003;3: 47–53.
56. Commins SP, Platts-Mills TA. Delayed anaphylaxis to red meat in patients with IgE specific to galactoseo-alpha-1,3-galactose (alpha-gal). *Curr Allergy Asthma Rep.* 2013;13:72–77.
57. Crispell G, Commins SP, Archer-Hartman SA, et al. Discovery of alpha-gal-containing antigens in North American tick species believed to induce red meat allergy. *Front Immunol.* 2019;10. Article 1056, 16 pp.
58. Rubio-Tapia A, Murray JA. Gluten-sensitive enteropathy. In: Metcalfe DD, Sampson HA, Simon RA, eds. *Food Allergy: Adverse Reactions To Foods And Food Additives.* 4th ed. Malden MA: Blackwell Publishing; 2008:211–222.
59. Tye-Din JA, Galipeau HJ, Agardh D. Celiac disease: a review of current concepts in pathogenesis, prevention, and movel therapies. *Front Pediatr.* 2018;6(350), 19 pp.
60. Leonard MM, Sapone A, Catassi C, et al. Celiac disease and non-celiac gluten sensitivity – a review. *J Am Med Assoc.* 2017;318: 647–658.
61. Camarca A, Auricchio R, Picascia S, et al. Gliadin-reactive T cells in Italian children from preventCD cohort at high risk of celiac disease. *Pediatr Allergy Immunol.* 2017;28:362–369.
62. Holtmeier W, Rowell DL, Nyberg A, et al. Distinct δ T cell receptor repertoires in monozygotic twins concordant for coeliac disease. *Clin Exp Immunol.* 1997;107:148–157.
63. Green PHR, Lebwohl B, Greywoode R. Celiac disease. *J Allergy Clin Immunol.* 2015;135:1099–1106.
64. Fasano A, Berti I, Gerarduzzi T, et al. Prevalence of celiac disease in at-risk and not-at-risk groups in the United States. *Arch Intern Med.* 2001;163:286–292.
65. Rubio-Tapia A, Ludvigsson JF, Branter T, et al. The prevalence of celiac disease in the United States. *Am J Gastroenterol.* 2012;107: 1538–1544.
66. Ludvigsson JF, Murray JA. Epidemiology of celiac disease. *Gastroenterol Clin N Am.* 2019;48:11–18.
67. Biagi F, Corazzo GR. Mortality in celiac disease. *Nat Rev Gastroenterol Hepatol.* 2010;7:158–162.
68. Meijer JW, Mulder CJ, Goerres MG, et al. Coeliac disease and (extra)intestinal T-cell lymphomas: definition, diagnosis, and treatment. *Scand J Gastroenterol Suppl.* 2004;241:78–84.
69. McGough N, Cummings JH. Coeliac disease: a diverse clinical syndrome caused by intolerance to wheat, barley, and rye. *Proc Nutr Soc.* 2005;64:434–450.
70. Bochner BS, Book W, Busse WW, et al. Workshop report from the National Institute of Health Task Force on the research needs of eosinophil-associated diseases (TREAD). *J Allergy Clin Immunol.* 2012;130:587–596.
71. Chehade M, Jones SM, Pesek RD, et al. Phenotypic characterization of eosinophilic esophagitis in a large multicenter patient population from the Consortium for Food Allergy Research. *J Allergy Clin Immunol Pract.* 2018;6:1534–1544.

72. Yu W, Freedland DM, Nadeau KC. Food allergy: immune mechanisms, diagnosis and immunotherapy. *Nat Rev Immunol.* 2016;16:751–765.
73. Dellon ES. Epidemiology of eosinophilic esophagitis. *Gastroenterol Clin N Am.* 2014;43:201–218.
74. Sopo SM, Green M, Monaco S, et al. Food protein-induced enterocolitis syndrome, from practice to theory. *Expert Rev Clin Immunol.* 2013;9:707–715.
75. Nowak-Wegrzyn A. Food protein-induced enterocolitis syndrome and allergic proctocolitis. *Allergy Asthma Proc.* 2015;3:172–184.
76. Katz Y, Goldberg MR, Rajuan N, et al. The prevalence and natural course of food protein-induced enterocolitis syndrome to cow's milk: a large-scale, prospective population study. *J Allergy Clin Immunol.* 2011;127:647–653.
77. Ruffner MA, Spergel JM. Non-IgE-mediated food allergy syndromes. *Ann Allerg Asthma Immunol.* 2016;117:452–454.
78. Valerii MC, Ricci C, Spisni E, et al. Responses of peripheral blood mononucleated cells from non-celiac gluten sensitivity patients to various cereal sources. *Food Chem.* 2015;176:167–174.
79. Taylor SL, Bush RK, Nordlee JA. Sulfites. In: Metcalfe DD, Sampson HA, Simon RA, eds. *Food Allergy: Adverse Reactions to Foods and Food Additives.* 4th ed. Malden MA: Blackwell Publishing; 2008:353–368.
80. Suarez FL, Savaiano DA. Diet, genetics, and lactose intolerance. *Food Technol.* 1997;51(3):74–76.
81. Lack G, Du Toit G. Prevention of food allergy. In: Metcalfe DD, Sampson HA, Simon RA, eds. *Food Allergy: Adverse Reactions to Foods and Food Additives.* 4th ed. Malden MA: Blackwell Publishing; 2008:470–481.
82. Zeiger RS, Heller S. The development and prediction of atopy in high-risk children: follow-up at seven years in a prospective randomized study of combined maternal and infant food allergy avoidance. *J Allergy Clin Immunol.* 1995;95:1179–1190.
83. Kirjavainen PV, Apostolou E, Salminen SJ, et al. New aspects of probiotics – a novel approach in the management of food allergy. *Allergy.* 1999;54:909–915.
84. Businco L, Dreborg S, Einarsson R, et al. Hydrolysed cow's milk formulae. Allergenicity and use in treatment and prevention. An ESPACI position paper. *Pediatr Allergy Immunol.* 1993;4:101–111.
85. Vandenplas Y, Hauser B, Van den Borre C, et al. The long-term effect of a partial whey hydrolysate formula on the prophylaxis of atopic disease. *Eur J Pediatr.* 1995;154:488–494.
86. Hong X, Wang X. Early life precursors, epigenetics, and the development of food allergy. *Semin Immunopathol.* 2012;34:655–669.
87. Du Toit G, Roberts G, Sayre PH, et al. Randomized trial of peanut consumption in infants at risk for peanut allergy. *N Engl J Med.* 2015;372:803–813.
88. Du Toit G, Katz Y, Sasieni P, et al. Early consumption of peanuts in infancy is associated with a low prevalence of peanut allergy. *J Allergy Clin Immunol.* 2008;122:984–991.
89. Fleischer DM, Sicherer S, Greenhawt M, et al. Consensus communication on early peanut introduction and the prevention of peanut allergy in high-risk infants. *J Allergy Clin Immunol.* 2015;136:258–261.
90. Fisher HR, Du Toit G, Bahnson HT, et al. The challenges of preventing food allergy. Lessons from LEAP and EAT. *Ann Allerg Asthma Immunol.* 2018;121:313–319.
91. Berin MC, Sampson HA. Food allergy: an enigmatic epidemic. *Trends Immunol.* 2013;34:390–397.
92. Koplin JJ, Allen KJ, Tang MLK. Important risk factors for the development of food allergy and potential options for prevention. *Expert Rev Clin Immunol.* 2019;15:147–152.
93. Molloy J, Koplin JJ, Allen KJ, et al. Vitamin D insufficiency in the first 6 months of infancy and challenge-proven IgE-mediated food allergy at 1 year of age: a case-control study. *Allergy.* 2017;72:1222–1231.
94. Venter C, Brown KR, Maslin K, et al. Maternal dietary intake in pregnancy and lactation and allergic disease outcomes in offspring. *Pediatr Allergy Immunol.* 2017;28:135–143.
95. Zhao W, Ho H, Bunyavanich S. The gut microbiome in food allergy. *Ann Allerg Asthma Immunol.* 2019;122:276–282.
96. Papathoma E, Triga M, Fouzas S, et al. Cesarean section delivery and development of food allergy and atopic dermatitis in early childhood. *Pediatr Allergy Immunol.* 2016;27:419–424.
97. Mitselou N, Hallberg J, Stephansson O, et al. Cesarean delivery, preterm birth, and risk of food allergy: a nationwide Swedish cohort study of more than 1 million children. *J Allergy Clin Immunol.* 2018;142:1510–1514.
98. Jeurink PV, van Esch BCAM, Rijnierse A, et al. Mechanisms underlying immune effects of dietary oligosaccharides. *Am J Clin Nutr.* 2013;98:572S–577S.
99. Wang J, Sampson HA. Food anaphylaxis. *Clin Exp Allergy.* 2007;37:651–660.
100. Leung DYM, Sampson HA, Yunginger JW, et al. Effect of anti-IgE therapy in patients with peanut allergy. *N Engl J Med.* 2003;348:986–993.
101. Fiocchi A, Artesani MC, Riccardi C, et al. Impact of omalizumab on food allergy in patients treated for asthma: a real-life study. *J Aller Cl Imm-Pract.* 2019;7:1901–1909.
102. Nurmatov U, Dhami S, Arasi S, et al. Allergen immunotherapies for IgE-mediated food allergy: a systematic review and meta-analysis. *Allergy.* 2017;72:1133–1147.
103. Baumert JL, Taylor SL, Koppelman SJ. Quantitative assessment of the safety benefits associated with increasing clinical peanut thresholds through immunotherapy. *J Allergy Clin Immunol Pract.* 2018;6:457–465.
104. Keet CA, Wood RA. Emerging therapies for food allergy. *J Clin Investig.* 2014;124:1880–1886.
105. Garcia-Molina MD, Gimenez MJ, Sanchez-Leon S, et al. Gluten-free wheat: are we there? *Nutrients.* 2019;11:487, 13 pp.
106. Taylor SL, Hefle SL, Munoz-Furlong A. Food allergies and avoidance diets. *Nutr Today.* 1999;34:15–22.
107. Stear GIJ, Horsburgh K, Steinman HA. Lactose intolerance: a review. *Curr Opin Allergy Clin Immunol.* 2005;18:114–119.
108. Stukus DR, Mikhail I. Pearls and pitfalls in diagnosing IgE-mediated food allergy. *Curr Allergy Asthma Rep.* 2016;16(34), 10 pp.
109. Meyer R, De Koker C, Dzubiak R, et al. Malnutrition in children with food allergies in the U.K. *J Hum Nutr Diet.* 2014;27:227–235.
110. Crevel RWR, Taylor SL, Pfaff S, et al. Managing food allergens: case histories and how they are handled. In: Madsen CB, Crevel RWR, Mills C, Taylor SL, eds. *Risk Management of Food Allergy.* Oxford, U.K: Elsevier; 2014:167–187.
111. Taylor SL, Baumert JL, Kruizinga AG, et al. Establishment of reference doses for residues of allergenic foods: report of the VITAL expert panel. *Food Chem Toxicol.* 2014;63:7–17.
112. Taylor SL, Hefle SL. Ingredient and labeling issues associated with allergenic foods. *Allergy.* 2001;56(Suppl. 67):64–69.
113. Allen KJ, Taylor SL. The consequences of precautionary allergen labeling: safe haven or unjustifiable burden? *J Allergy Clin Immunol Pract.* 2018;6:400–407.
114. DunnGalvin A, Chan CH, Crevel R, et al. Precautionary allergen labeling: perspectives from key stakeholder groups. *Allergy.* 2015;70:1039–1051.
115. Thompson T. The gluten-free labeling rule: what registered dietitian professionals need to know to help clients with gluten-related disorders. *J Acad Nutr Diet.* 2015;115:13–16.
116. Catassi C, Fabiani E, Iacono G, et al. A prospective, double-blind, placebo-controlled trial to establish a safe gluten threshold for patients with celiac disease. *Am J Clin Nutr.* 2007;85:160–166.

117. Janatuinen EK, Pikkarainen PH, Kemppainen TA, et al. A comparison of diets with and without oats in adults with celiac disease. *N Engl J Med*. 1995;333:1033–1037.
118. Venter C, Fleischer DM. Diets for diagnosis and management of food allergy. The role of the dietitian in eosinophilic esophagitis in adults and children. *Ann Allerg Asthma Immunol*. 2013;117:468–471.
119. Molina-Infante J, Lucendo AT. Dietary therapy for eosinophilic esophagitis. *J Allergy Clin Immunol*. 2018;142:42–47.
120. Taylor SL, Bush RK, Selner JC, et al. Sensitivity to sulfited foods among sulfite-sensitive asthmatics. *J Allergy Clin Immunol*. 1988; 81:1159–1167.

CHAPTER

30

NUTRITION AND AUTOIMMUNE DISEASES

Simin Nikbin Meydani[1,*], *DVM, PhD*
Weimin Guo[1], *PhD*
Sung Nim Han[2], *PhD, RD*
Dayong Wu[1,*], *MD, PhD*

[1]Nutritional Immunology Laboratory, Jean Mayer USDA Human Nutrition Research Center on Aging at Tufts University, Boston, MA, United States
[2]Department of Food and Nutrition, College of Human Ecology, Seoul National University, Seoul, Korea

SUMMARY

Autoimmune diseases are a host of diseases characterized by abnormal immune response against normal tissues of the body. There are about 100 autoimmune diseases, and they are estimated to affect at least 3% –5% of population. While the etiology is still unclear, both genetic and environmental factors are recognized to play key roles in the disease development. Pharmaceutical therapies have substantially improved the disease control and prognosis. However, the adverse effects and high cost of the drugs limit their use. There has been an increasing interest in alternative and complementary means to improve the outcomes of conventional therapies in many autoimmune diseases. Diet as a modifiable factor has the potential to improve clinical outcomes for several major autoimmune diseases. This chapter provides a summary and analysis of both observational and experimental studies as well as perspectives on the role of nutrition in prevention and treatment of some of the most prominent autoimmune diseases.

Keywords: Autoimmune diseases; Inflammatory bowel disease; Inflammatory cytokines; Multiple sclerosis; Nutrition; Phytochemicals; Polyunsaturated fatty acids; Rheumatoid arthritis; Vitamins.

I. INTRODUCTION

Food not only provides nutrients to maintain an individual's normal development, growth, and physiological functions but also significantly impacts risk and prognosis of various diseases, including both infectious and noninfectious diseases. In this chapter, we will discuss the role of diet as a modifiable environmental factor in etiology and management of autoimmune diseases.

It has long been known that certain diet components including both nutrients and nonnutrient phytochemicals can modulate a variety of immune and inflammatory events, many of which are key players in pathogenesis of autoimmune diseases. Thus nutritional intervention may be a promising approach to prevent and mitigate autoimmune diseases. Although there are many autoimmune diseases, most are rare and/or we have limited knowledge about their immunopathology. Only three of

*SNM and DW share senior authorship.

Present Knowledge in Nutrition, Volume 2
https://doi.org/10.1016/B978-0-12-818460-8.00030-7

the most common, prototypic autoimmune diseases, namely, inflammatory bowel disease (IBD), rheumatoid arthritis (RA), and multiple sclerosis (MS), will be reviewed in this chapter, for prevalence, etiology, pathogenesis, evidence for the impact of dietary factors on disease development, and treatment. We have not included discussion of other common autoimmune diseases, such as Graves' disease, type-1 diabetes, systemic lupus erythematosus, and Sjogren's disease, because of the limited information available regarding the impact of nutritional factors on these diseases. Fig. 30.1 provides an overview of the autoimmune diseases.

II. AUTOIMMUNE DISEASE

A. Definition

The immune system serves to protect the body against infection from invading pathological microorganisms, clear damaged tissues, and monitor for malignant cells. Coordinated activities of various immune cells in both the innate and adaptive immune systems are required for the optimal function of immune system. A functioning immune system can distinguish "foreign" from "self" because of the "self-tolerance" mechanism of the immune system. When this self-tolerance mechanism fails, immune system can be activated in response to self-antigens in the absence of external assaults or internal threats. This immune response to self is called autoimmunity, which can cause damage and dysfunction in various tissues and organs leading to the corresponding clinical manifestations collectively called autoimmune diseases. It is worth pointing out that autoimmune diseases are commonly defined as diseases in which self-reactive T cells or B cells (antibodies) are the causal factors or the primary drivers of pathogenesis and do not include those characterized by excess inflammatory response of activated innate immune cells without a clear autoantigen target.

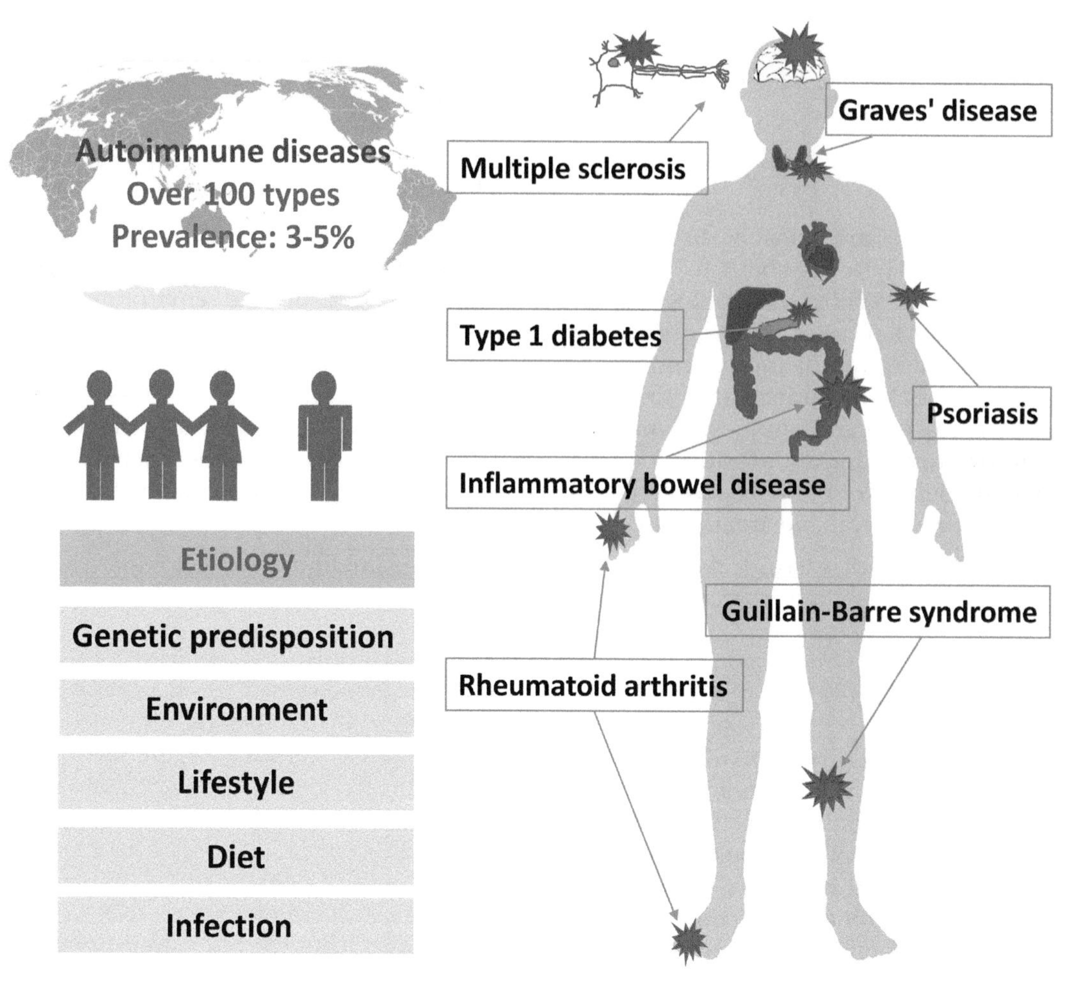

FIGURE 30.1 Overview of autoimmune diseases. There are about 100 autoimmune diseases and they are estimated to affect at least 3%–5% of population. Women are at 2.7 times greater risk than men in acquiring autoimmune diseases The etiology is still unclear, and both genetic and environmental factors are recognized to play key roles in the disease development. The most common autoimmune diseases include inflammatory bowel disease (IBD), rheumatoid arthritis (RA), multiple sclerosis (MS).

B. Type and Prevalence

There is no widely accepted and/or standard classification for autoimmune diseases, which is mainly due to lack of clear characterization of pathogenesis. Nevertheless, clinically, it is helpful to divide them into two major categories: organ-specific and systemic autoimmune diseases, based on whether autoimmunity targets a specific organ/tissue or multiple organs/tissues. However, this classification is mainly based on clinical manifestations rather than in which tissue autoantigens are expressed. In fact, some autoantigens may be widely expressed across the body but clinical impact may be seen in only one organ. Thus not all autoimmune diseases can be unequivocally classified by this categorizing system.

Incidence of autoimmune diseases is relatively low. However, they often result in disability and morbidity. Further, they are one of the leading causes of morbidity and mortality in young and middle-aged women and thus have a significant health and economic impact. There are no reliable estimates to date for the total number of autoimmune diseases or the incidence and prevalence of all or individual diseases. A generally accepted estimate is that there are more than 80,[1] or nearly 100,[2] distinct autoimmune diseases. The prevalence of total diseases is estimated to be 3%–5%, which is primarily based on the results from two large epidemiological surveys: one in the United States that included 24 autoimmune diseases[3] and the other in Denmark that included 31 autoimmune diseases.[4] This estimate was later supported by an updated comprehensive review.[1] The prevalence of individual diseases varies greatly ranging from rare to common. Given the lack of information for many of the less common conditions, this estimate is believed to be conservative. There is a clear sex bias in the disease burden, and overall, for majority of autoimmune diseases, women are at 2.7 times greater risk than men in acquiring autoimmune diseases.[1,3,5,6]

C. Etiology

The exact causes of autoimmune diseases are unknown. The current view is that development involves multiple factors including genetic predisposition and environmental impact (Fig. 30.1). The evidence for the role of genetic factor is from epidemiological studies showing that in contrast to the low frequency of most autoimmune diseases in the general population (0.0%–1.0%), the first-degree relatives of the patients exhibit about five times higher prevalence, and the concordance of an autoimmune disease in monozygotic twins can be as high as 20%–30%.[7] While some rare monogenic hereditary autoimmune diseases do exist, multiple genetic factors contribute to development of the majority of autoimmune diseases,[2] including polymorphisms, single-nucleotide polymorphisms, and epigenetic modifications.[7] Despite the key role of genetic predisposition, the fact that even identical twins exhibit only partial concordance highlights the importance of external factors such as environment, lifestyle, diet, and infection. These modifiable external factors have thus become targets for developing preventive and therapeutic strategies against autoimmune diseases. In this chapter, we will discuss the role of nutritional interventions including use of nutrients, nonnutrient phytochemicals, and other dietary components in prevention and treatment of autoimmune diseases.

D. Immunopathology

Autoimmune diseases are clinical manifestations of autoimmunity; however, autoimmunity may not necessarily develop into autoimmune disease. Despite the rapid development and significant progress, the complex immunopathology involved in initiation and progression of autoimmune diseases is not completely understood. While there is heterogeneity in autoimmune mechanisms among different diseases, in general, they are primarily attributed to disorders of the adaptive immune responses. A brief description of the current view regarding immunopathogenesis of autoimmune diseases is provided to help the readers to better understand the results of nutritional intervention studies and underlying mechanisms. Several previous publications provide a comprehensive review of the topic.[7–10]

From the immunological perspective, the fundamental cause of autoimmune diseases is loss of self-tolerance. For this to happen, autoreactive lymphocytes must escape elimination by the body's central tolerance mechanisms (mainly in thymus) and travel to the periphery where these cells encounter specific autoantigens. Further, the peripheral tolerance mechanisms (in secondary lymphoid organs and/or sites of inflammation) also fail in stopping activation of autoreactive lymphocytes and their mounting of specific response against autoantigen-bearing cells, leading to tissue damage.

Clinical symptoms of most autoimmune diseases are due to the responses of autoantibodies and autoreactive effector T cells against autoantigens. Activated effector T cells release proinflammatory cytokines, which can in turn activate innate immune cells (such as macrophages and neutrophils) as well as nonhematopoietic cells (such as endothelial cells and fibroblasts) to induce the production of more cytokines. Autoreactive CD4+ cells, or helper T (Th) cells, also help autoreactive B cells in autoantibody production. In addition, these Th cells can activate autoreactive CD8+ cytotoxic T (Tc) cells. Both autoantibodies and autoreactive effector T cells as well as the released cytokines attack cells that express autoantigens leading to inflammation and damage of the target as well as the surrounding cells. Antigen-specific lymphocyte activation occurs only when T cells form an immune synapse with antigen-presenting cells (APCs, mainly dendritic cells [DCs]) through antigens expressed on the surface of APCs. Thus, reactivity of APC also plays an important role in autoimmunity development.

CD4+ T cells are the primary player in initiation and progression of autoimmune diseases. In particular, several distinct Th cell subpopulations are recognized to play specific roles in autoimmunity (Fig. 30.2). These CD4+ T cells are critical for host defense against diverse pathogens (both intracellular and extracellular) mainly via activation of B cells and also cells in the innate immune system. However, CD4+ T cells can also drive development of major T cell–mediated autoimmune diseases. Th1 (producing interferon-γ [IFN-γ], tumor necrosis factor-α [TNF-α], interleukin [IL]-2) and Th17 (producing IL-17, IL-21, IL-22) cells are prominent proinflammatory CD4+ T cells and considered main drivers for major autoimmune diseases. Th9 cells (producing IL-9) may also play a similar role. On the other hand, a distinct Th subset called regulatory T cells (Tregs) help maintain self-tolerance and control autoimmune responses. Tregs are identified as CD4+CD25+ T cells expressing transcription factor Foxp3 and producing antiinflammatory cytokines IL-10 and transforming growth factor-β (TGF-β). While the role of Th2 in autoimmunity is not well characterized, they are shown to antagonize Th1 differentiation and to ameliorate some autoimmune diseases. As will be discussed later in this chapter, nutritional intervention can improve autoimmune diseases by modulating differentiation and effector functions of these T cell subsets. Fig. 30.2 illustrates the primary subtypes of CD4 T cells, regulatory proteins, and transcription factors that drive their differentiation, the key cytokines produced by them, and their main roles in immunity. Major functions of cytokines involved in autoimmunity are summarized in Table 30.1.

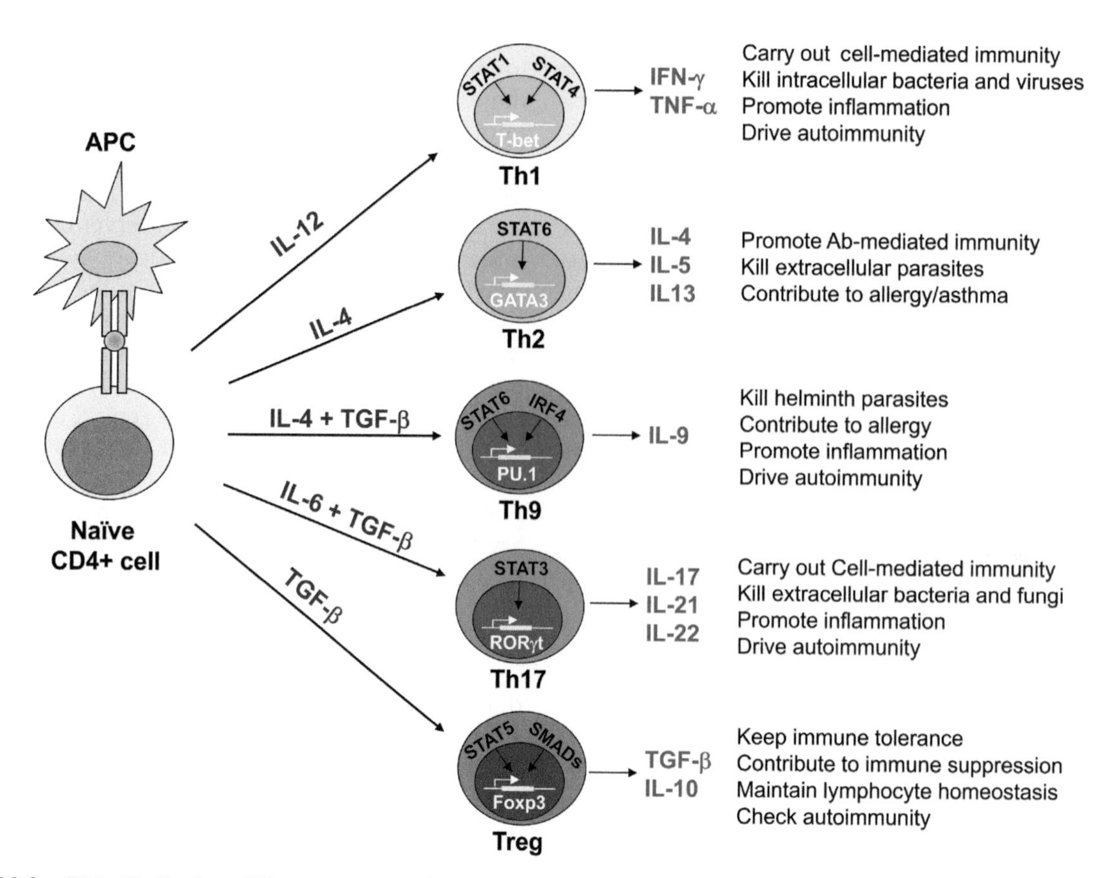

FIGURE 30.2 CD4+ T cell subset differentiation and effector function. After engaging with specific antigens presented by antigen presenting cells (APCs), naive CD4+ T cells are activated and differentiate into subsets including Th1, Th2, Th9, Th17, and Treg cells under appropriate cytokine milieu (shown in blue print). The differentiation process is controlled by the corresponding regulatory network mainly composed of specific signal transducers (shown in black print inside cells) and downstream transcription factors (shown in white print in cell nuclei). These CD4+ T cell subsets produce distinct sets of cytokines (shown in red print) that contribute to adaptive immunity including the clearance of pathogens, development of inflammation, regulation of autoimmunity, maintenance of immune homeostasis, and immune responses again tumors. CD4+ T cell subsets interact with each other at their differentiation stage as well as in their functional stage. *Foxp3*, forkhead box protein 3; *IFN*, interferon; *IL*, interleukin; *IRF4*, interferon regulatory factor 4; *PU.1*, transcription factor PU.1; *RORγt*, retinoic acid receptor-–related orphan receptor gamma t; *STAT*, signal transducers and activators of transcription; *T-bet*, T-box protein expressed in T cells; *TGF*, transforming growth factor beta; *Th*, helper T cell; *TNF*, tumor necrosis factor; *Treg*, regulatory T cell.

TABLE 30.1 Major functions of cytokines involved in autoimmunity.

Cytokines	Major functions
IL-1β	Promotes progression of autoimmune diseases by inducing proinflammatory molecules and promoting expansion of Th1/Th17 cells.
IL-2	Prevents autoimmune diseases partially by inhibiting naïve CD4+ T cell differentiation into Th17 lymphocytes and promoting differentiation of certain immature T cells into Treg cells.
IL-4	Induces Th2 differentiation; suppresses IL-1 and TNF production.
IL-5	Stimulates B cell growth and increases immunoglobulin secretion (primarily IgA); activates eosinophil.
IL-6	Stimulates inflammatory and autoimmune processes; inhibits TGF-β-induced Treg differentiation and promotes Th17 cell differentiation; stimulates differentiation of activated B cells into immunoglobulin (Ig)-producing plasma cells.
IL-8	Recruits neutrophils, NK cells, T cells, basophils, and eosinophils to lesion site; stimulates neutrophil to a higher activation state.
IL-9	Stimulates proliferation of CD8+ T cells and mast cells; promotes Th2 cell differentiation and enhances Th17 cell survival.
IL-10	Induces tolerance and maintenance of immunological homeostasis; inhibits IFN-γ secretion and monocytes/macrophages activation.
IL-12	Promotes Th1 cell differentiation; activates NK cells; supports DC maturation; stimulates IFN-γ and TNF-α production.
IL-17	Induces proinflammatory cytokines, chemokines, and metalloproteases.
IL-18	Induces IFN-γ in presence of IL-12; enhances NK cell cytotoxicity.
IL-21	Promotes Th2 and Th17 cell differentiation and inhibits Th1 and Treg cell development; induces maturation and enhances cytotoxicity of CD8+ T cells and NK cells; stimulates B cell differentiation into plasma cells and production of immunoglobulins.
IL-22	Promotes inflammatory tissue pathology; regulates cell regeneration, tissue remodeling, and wound healing.
IL-23	Stimulates IL-17 production; enhances T cell proliferation; activates NK cells.
TGF-β	Suppresses immune response and Treg differentiation.
IFN-γ	Activates macrophages; promotes inflammation; induces Th1 differentiation.
TNF-α	Promotes inflammatory tissue pathology; induces other proinflammatory cytokines, metalloproteinases, and free radicals.

Note: *IL*, interleukin; *TGF-β*, transforming growth factor-β; *IFN-γ*, interferon-γ; *TNF-α*, tumor necrosis factor-α; *Treg*, regulatory T cell.

III. NUTRITIONAL INTERVENTION IN MAJOR AUTOIMMUNE DISEASES

Development in pharmaceutical therapies against autoimmune diseases has provided specific immunosuppressive synthetic drugs or biologicals resulting in improved disease prognosis. However, the adverse effects and high cost of these drugs make them beyond the reach of many patients. Thus, there has been an increasing interest in alternative and complementary means in conjunction with conventional therapies. Diet as a modifiable factor has received attention based on the findings from both observational and experimental studies. Epidemiologic studies on the relationship between diet pattern/nutrient intake and prevalence of certain autoimmune diseases have revealed some interesting associations. Experimental studies have demonstrated that a variety of diet components favorably modulate the immune and inflammatory responses involved in the pathogenesis of autoimmune diseases (the effects of nutrition intervention on MS, RA, and IBD are summarized on Table 30.2). Furthermore, some of these nutritional agents are found to improve disease symptoms and tissue pathology in various animal models and to a limited extent in clinical trials. These results, discussed in detail below, suggest that dietary intervention might be helpful in both prevention and treatment of autoimmune disease.

A. Multiple Sclerosis

General information about MS

MS is a chronic, autoimmune neuroinflammatory disease of the central nervous system (CNS). Estimated prevalence of MS is more than 400,000 in the United States[11] and more than 2.5 millions worldwide, and the incidence is anticipated to continue to increase.[12] MS is more common in Europe, North America, Australia, and New Zealand than the other countries and is rare in Asia.[13] MS mainly affects people aged 20–40 years with higher prevalence in women,[14] and it is one of the leading causes of disability in young adults.[15] Clinical presentations of MS vary widely, but commonly include fatigue, depression and anxiety, spasticity and incoordination, chronic pain, cognitive impairment, bladder and bowel dysfunction, visual and speech impairments, sensory disturbance, sexual dysfunction, and impaired mobility. The hallmark pathophysiological characters of MS are demyelination, axonal/neuronal damage, and gliosis in the brain and spinal cord.[16–18] Clinical symptoms and course of MS are heterogeneous and are believed to correlate with the site lesion pathology.[19] About 85% of patients initially show a relapsing-remitting pattern, but eventually 80% of them go on to

TABLE 30.2 Effects of nutrition intervention on multiple sclerosis, rheumatoid arthritis, and inflammatory bowel disease.

		MS		RA		IBD	
		Human	Animal	Human	Animal	Human	Animal
Diet	Mediterranean diet	Limited data	N/A	Reduced disease activity	N/A	No data available	N/A
	Green tea	No data available	Delayed disease onset Improved symptoms	Limited data	Limited data	Limited data	Limited data
	n-3 PUFA	Insufficient evidence	Delayed disease onset Reduced disease scores	Improved symptoms	Limited data	Insufficient evidence	Ameliorated IBD symptoms
Vitamins	Vitamin D	Not consistent results	Improved symptoms	Reduced disease activity	Improved clinical indexes	Insufficient evidence	Ameliorated IBD symptoms
	Vitamin E	Limited data	Limited data	Improved symptoms	Prevented joint destruction	No data available	No data available
	Vitamin K	No data available	No data available	Reduced disease activity	Limited data	No data available	No data available
Minerals	Calcium	Limited data	Limited data	Limited data	Limited data	No data available	Limited data
	Zinc	No data available	No data available	Insufficient evidence	No data available	Limited data	No data available
	Selenium	No data available	No data available	Limited data	Limited data	No data available	No data available
Phytochemicals	Catechins	No data available	Delayed disease onset Improved symptoms	No data available	No data available	Limited data	Ameliorated IBD symptoms
	Curcumin	Limited data	Ameliorated EAE symptoms	Not consistent results	Limited data	Insufficient evidence	Limited data
	Resveratrol	No data available	Delayed disease onset	Improved symptoms	Limited data	Limited data	Limited data
	Hesperidin Hesperetin	No data available	Reduced the incidence Delayed disease onset Improved symptoms	No data available	Improved clinical indexes	No data available	No data available
	Tannins	No data available	No data available	No data available	Delayed RA development	No data available	No data available
	Quercetin	No data available	No data available	Improved symptoms	Limited data	No data available	Ameliorated IBD symptoms

Note: *MS*, multiple sclerosis; *RA*, rheumatoid arthritis; *IBD*, inflammatory bowel disease; *N/A*, not applicable.

develop secondary progressive MS; a minority of patients are diagnosed as primary progressive MS.[14]

The etiology of MS remains elusive. As with many other autoimmune diseases, it is believed to be multifactorial. It may involve dysregulated immune responses influenced by and interacted with genetic, environmental, and behavioral factors. MS cases appear to cluster within families, and MS risk among the first-degree relatives of MS patients is 10–50 times higher than the general population.[20] A genome-wide association analysis in MS patients versus healthy controls has identified 48 MS risk variants,[21] and genes coding for molecules of immunological relevance, or controlling neurobiological pathways are shown to be related to MS incidence.[22] However, genetic factor alone is estimated to account for only 25% of the lifetime risk of developing MS,[12] and epidemiological studies have suggested that various environmental factors have great contribution to the disease susceptibility. For example, viral infection including Epstein–Barr virus, human endogenous retroviruses, measles and the related canine distemper virus, and human herpesvirus,[23] cigarette smoking,[24] and nutritional factors including vitamin D deficit,[25,26] increased salt intake,[27] and obesity[28] are all shown to be associated with MS prevalence.

Interaction of genetic and environmental factors is also important in impacting susceptibility to MS. Environmental signals may affect gene expression by inducing epigenetic changes[29]; modification in DNA methylation is associated with pathogenesis of MS[30] and T cell profile.[31] Studies also showed involvement of microRNA in MS pathogenesis.[32] For example, miR-141 and miR-200a were upregulated in relapsing phase of MS patients compared to remitting and control groups.[33] The brain of active MS patients had upregulated miR-34a, miR-155, and miR-326, which might mediate macrophage activation leading to active lesions.[34]

The pathogenesis of MS involves autoreactive myelin-specific T cells orchestrating with B cells and innate immune cells to cause demyelination and consequent neurodegeneration in the CNS. Our knowledge regarding the immunopathological mechanisms of MS is mostly established through studies in animal models, in particular the experimental autoimmune encephalomyelitis (EAE), the best defined and highly reproducible rodent model for human MS. EAE is typically induced by immunizing animals with emulsified CNS antigens (myelin components). Antigen-specific T cells (mainly Th1 and Th17) generated in the draining lymph nodes enter circulation and eventually cross the blood–brain barrier to cause inflammatory damage in the CNS. Th1 and Th17 cells are the main drivers, while Treg cells provide control; macrophages, neutrophils, and microglia are primary innate immune cells involved; many cytokines serve as regulators or effectors. Although there are differences between EAE and MS, many of the CNS pathologies observed in EAE mice are similar to those found in the CNS of MS patients.[35,36]

MS cannot be cured and the disease management mainly depends on immunomodulatory drug therapies that are developed largely based on studies in animal models. These therapies are usually designed to either broadly suppress immune response or selectively target single molecules or pathways in the immune system. Although the pharmaceutical therapies have improved the disease control, they have limited efficacy, in particular during the progressive phase, and often introduce significant side effects.

Role of nutrition and dietary factors and underlying mechanisms

Evidence from observational studies; Early epidemiological studies indicated diet as a modifiable environmental factor for MS prevention and management.[37] Diet-related MS risk factors proposed include low vitamin D, high fat/saturated fatty acids, childhood obesity, and diet-related dysbiosis.

Since the link between vitamin D and MS was first proposed about 45 years ago,[38] low vitamin D intake and low exposure to sunlight (major source of vitamin D synthesis) have been shown to be associated with high MS risk and disease activity.[39] Serum vitamin D levels are typically lower in MS patients than in the healthy controls,[40,41] and seasonal variation of serum vitamin D levels are inversely associated with clinical disease activity in MS patients.[42] In addition, early exposure to low vitamin D status during childhood[43] or even in utero[44,45] may increase MS risk in later life.

Intake of total fat and fat types have long been known to be a factor influencing MS development. Early studies by Swank et al. revealed that MS incidence may be related to consumption of saturated fats of animal sources such as those from dairy and meat.[37,46] Similar observation was reported by Arganoff and Goldberg who reported that vegetables, nuts, and fish intakes were associated with reduced risk of MS.[47] High energy intake from fat, in particular saturated fat, increased MS risk while fruit and vegetable intake is protective in both adult[48] and pediatric patients.[49] Impact of polyunsaturated fatty acids (PUFAs) intake on MS incidence is not very clear. The Nurses' Health Study I (92,422 women, 1980–94) and the Nurses' Health Study II (95,389 women, 1991–95) that documented 195 new cases of MS found no significant relations between intakes of total fat or specific types of fat and MS risk, except for a trend toward inverse correlation between α-linolenic acid (ALA) intake and MS risk.[50] Extended follow-up of these studies (1980–2004 for Study I and 1991–2009 for Study II) that identified 479 incident MS cases found that MS risk had inverse relationship with total PUFA and ALA intake, but not other specific types of PUFA.[51]

Dietary pattern analysis in relationship to MS has also been conducted, including evaluation of Mediterranean,[52] Paleolithic (no dairy and grains),[53] and McDougall diets (low fat vegetarian),[54] as well as various diet indices based on diet quality defined by researchers as "prudent," such as the Alternative Healthy Eating Index-2010, Alternate Mediterranean Diet, and Dietary Approaches to Stop Hypertension, relative to "Western" style diets.[55–57] However, the information in this regard is limited and inconsistent with no particular diet pattern confirmed to have clear benefit for preventing or improving MS.

Evidence from intervention studies; Based on epidemiologic results, and to a larger extent based on the information about the nutrients and food components that are known to have immunomodulatory, antiinflammatory, neuroprotective, and antioxidant properties, nutritional intervention trials have been conducted using a variety of nutrients in both animal models and MS patients.

Given the inverse association between vitamin D status and MS risk reported in epidemiologic studies, together with vitamin D's immunomodulatory function, in particular the suppressive effect on adaptive immune responses and antigen-presenting process, vitamin D supplementation in MS patients has been strongly recommended. Indeed, a number of studies using the EAE, a rodent model for MS, have reported that dietary vitamin D improves disease symptoms and tissue pathology, and this protective effect is associated with reduced development of pathogenic Th1[58,59] and Th17[60,61] cells, and suppressed Tregs differentiation,[60] as well as appropriate changes in cytokines and transcription factors that regulate T cell activation and differentiation. Modulatory effect of vitamin D on effector CD4+ T cells, leading to protection against EAE, may be in part mediated by its effect on DCs.[62] However, translational value of these results is questionable. Clinical trials in humans with vitamin D alone or together with other agents thus far have not provided consistent evidence to support the findings from animal models.[63,64] This uncertainty calls for further studies with better design taking particular consideration of range of doses used, baseline conditions such as nutrition and vitamin D status, and genetic and epigenetic heterogeneity. It is worth adding that caution should be taken in using higher doses of vitamin D because a recent case report showed worse outcomes in an MS patient who had taken 50,000 IU/day vitamin D for several months (<6) and had serum 25-hydroxy vitamin D3 above the upper limit of detection with routine laboratory tests (>160 ng/mL or 400 nmol/L).[65]

High saturated fat and n-6/n-3 PUFA ratio intakes, typically found in the Western diets, are considered risk factors for MS, which may partly explain the higher MS prevalence in Western countries. N-3 PUFA (ALA, eicosapentaenoic acid [EPA], docosahexaenoic acid [DHA]) and some n-6 PUFA (γ-linolenic acid, dihomo-γ-linolenic acid) have antiinflammatory effect and thus, theoretically, may play a protective role in MS. Moderate improvement of MS symptoms was reported in the patients receiving 1 year of low-fat diet together with increased fish intake or olive oil alone.[66] An animal study showed that mice fed DHA for 4 weeks before EAE induction had delayed EAE onset and reduced disease scores.[67] However, overall results from clinical trials thus far are insufficient to suggest a significant impact of changing the intake of n-3 or n-6 PUFA on MS patients.[68]

A variety of nonnutrient bioactive dietary components of plant origin (phytochemicals) with favorable effects on the immune and inflammatory responses of MS pathogenesis have been studied. Oral administration (diet or drinking water) of green tea and its catechins, in particular epigallocatechin-3-gallate (EGCG), has been shown to be protective in EAE mouse model as indicated by delayed disease onset, improved symptoms, and attenuated pathology in brain and spinal cord. These effects were accompanied by suppressed responses of pathological T cells and production of proinflammatory cytokines.[69–71] Mechanistic investigation revealed that the EGCG effect on EAE mainly involves its immunomodulating and antiinflammatory effects such as inhibiting differentiation of naive CD4+ T cells into Th1, Th9, and Th17 subsets via respective regulatory network, enhancing Treg development and switching Th17/Treg balance toward favoring Treg by inhibiting IL-6 signaling, and production of inflammatory cytokines.[71,72]

Information for use of EGCG in MS patients is limited (two studies identified). In a randomized-controlled trial (RCT) with crossover design, 18 patients with relapsing-remitting MS received EGCG (600 mg/d) and placebo for 12 week with a 4 week washout in between. The authors reported that EGCG improved muscle metabolism during moderate exercise but did not report neurological and immunological outcomes.[73] Another study was a combined phase I (single group) and phase II (randomized, placebo-controlled) trials to determine safety and neuroprotective effect of a green tea extract containing 50% EGCG.[74] In this study, MS patients received 800 mg EGCG/d for 6 mo. In the phase I study, 10 participants were enrolled and completed all assessments with no serious side effects; the phase II study using a new batch but the same source of EGCG supplement in 12 patients was halted due to high frequency (5/7) of elevated serum liver enzyme concentrations for unknown reason. The outcomes from these two human studies cannot validate or dispute the findings reported in animal studies using EAE models, and thus, the benefit of using EGCG in MS patients is yet to be determined. However, future trials should pay particular attention to possible side effects.

Curcumin, a principal component of the dietary spice turmeric, is suggested to have a protective effect for several autoimmune diseases including MS. Studies have shown the efficacy of curcumin in EAE treatment, which is thought to be mediated through its modulation of both innate and adaptive immune cell functions as well as the APC function that bridges innate and adaptive immunity.[75–78] As with EGCG, few human clinical trials have been conducted. In a placebo-controlled trial, MS patients who received nanoparticulated curcumin for 6 months had lower peripheral blood mononuclear cell (PBMC) mRNA expression for inflammatory cytokines and chemokines, transcription factors (nuclear factor-κB [NF-κB], activator protein 1 [AP-1], STAT1, STAT5), inflammatory miRNAs (miR-145, miR-132, miR-16), and an improved clinical status as determined with the Expanded Disability Status Scale.[79] Reduced frequency of Th17 cells and expression levels of IL-17 were also observed in these curcumin-treated patients.[80]

Resveratrol is a polyphenolic compound found in at least more than 70 plant species; it is particularly enriched in fresh grape skin. The first evidence implying the potential protective effect of resveratrol came from an animal study using EAE model that showed that oral gavage of resveratrol decreased clinical symptoms and inflammation in spinal cord, decreased serum levels of proinflammatory cytokines and chemokines.[81] In a study using the remitting-relapsing EAE model, oral gavage of SRT501, a pharmaceutical-grade formulation of resveratrol, from day 8 or 10 postimmunization (1 day prior to or after disease onset) to day 14 (peak of disease) attenuated neuronal damage in spinal cords but had no effect on EAE onset and symptom up to day 14; SRT501 reduced symptom during later remission (days 20–25) but did not prevent subsequent onset of remission (day 30).[82] Using the progressive EAE model, the same group found that both resveratrol and SRT501 delayed the onset of EAE by several days, prevented neuronal loss, and delayed visual decline in EAE mice but did not affect spinal cord inflammation, T cells number in the periphery and CNS, and % CD4+ and CD8+ T cells in the spinal cord and spleen.[83] In contrast, using the same EAE model, Imler and Petro showed that dietary resveratrol improved EAE symptom and also differentially affected production of IL-17, IFN-γ, and TNF-α by spleen cells.[84] These conflicting results may be related to different experimental protocols used in the two studies. Compared to the study by Fonseca-Kelly et al., Imler and Pedro used the purified form of resveratrol in diet, started the feeding earlier (right after immunization), and lasted longer (to day 56 postimmunization). In addition to immunomodulating and neuroprotective effects that may be involved in the resveratrol effect on EAE, resveratrol intraperitoneally injected to EAE mice has been shown to attenuate disease by protecting blood–brain barrier integrity, which in turn was associated with maintained expression of tight junction proteins and reduced expression of adhesion molecules.[85] Using a less common, copper chelator cuprizone–induced EAE mouse model, Ghaiad et al. found that resveratrol attenuated the impairment in balance and locomotor coordination, reversed cuprizone-induced demyelination, improved brain mitochondrial function, and reduced cuprizone-induced oxidative stress and inflammation.[86] Thus far, there are no reports from human studies using resveratrol alone.

Several citrus-derived flavonoids (naringin/naringenin, hesperidin/hesperitin, apigenin, diosmetin, nobiletin, auraptene) have been shown to have beneficial effect against inflammation and inflammatory diseases.[87–90] Oral or subcutaneous administration of hesperidin in mice inhibited EAE development and inflammation in CNS, increased IL-10 and TGF-β, decreased IL-1β, IL-6, TNF-α, and IL-17 production, and reduced Th17 cells, but increased Treg cells in the spleen and lymph nodes.[91,92] Dietary naringenin reduced the incidence, delayed the onset, and attenuated the symptoms of EAE, together with reduced immune cell infiltration and demyelination in the spinal cord. Proinflammatory Th1, Th9, and Th17 cells as well as their respective transcription factors were reduced in both CNS and lymph nodes of EAE mice.[93] A further mechanistic study reported that naringenin inhibited CD4+ T cell proliferation and differentiation to Th1 and Th17 via altering expression of their respective regulatory proteins.[94]

Studies reviewed above suggest that EGCG, resveratrol, curcumin, and naranginin have efficacy in ameliorating EAE symptoms and pathology. This is consistent with, and explained by, their favorable modulatory effects on immune and inflammatory processes involved in EAE development. Additional benefit of these phytochemicals is their neuroprotective effect, which is important because current MS drugs target immune and inflammatory dysregulations, but does little to prevent permanent neurological damages. The findings from animal studies, however, have not been reproduced in humans. There are several reasons that contribute to this discrepancy. First, animals and humans have different genetic backgrounds. Furthermore, bioavailability, metabolism, and dose–response pattern of these phytochemicals are not the same in animals and humans. More importantly, although several EAE models mimic individual aspects and immunologic mechanisms in MS pathogenesis, none completely exhibit the spectrum of pathological and clinical features of MS seen in humans. This may explain while several drugs have shown efficacy in animals, few have been developed for human use. Phytochemicals are relatively safe, easy to obtain, and inexpensive and thus should be further studied for their use in humans on their own or as a complement to conventional therapies.

B. Rheumatoid Arthritis

General information about RA

RA is one of the most prevalent chronic autoimmune diseases with an estimated prevalence of 0.5%–1% in the general population, more commonly occurring in women than in men (2–3:1).[95,96] Although RA primarily involves the joints, it is in fact considered a systemic autoimmune disease, or a syndrome, because it has extraarticular manifestations in various tissues and organ systems such as the skin, eyes, lungs, heart, blood vessels, and kidneys.[96,97] RA is a debilitating disease that severely impairs quality of life and is burden to both individuals and those who care for them.[98]

RA is believed to develop in the individuals possessing high-risk genetic background in combination with exposure to certain environmental factors resulting in epigenomic modifications favorable to RA pathogenesis. 12%–15% monozygotic twins share RA, and first-degree relatives of RA patients have several folds higher risk relative to general population.[99] The most important genetic factor for RA risk is the shared susceptibility epitopes coded by specific class II human leukocyte antigen (also known as MHC-II) loci.[100] Genome-wide association studies have identified more than 100 loci associated with RA risk and most of them involve immune mechanisms.[101] Several epigenetic mechanisms are implicated in RA including DNA methylation, histone modification, and microRNA expression.[102] Environmental factors for RA risk include smoking, dust inhalation, mucosal microbes, high salt intake, low serum vitamin D concentrations, and obesity.[95,103] Increasing evidence has also pointed to the involvement of altered gut microbiota, or dysbiosis, in RA pathogenesis and development.[104,105]

Consistent with the findings mentioned above, pathogenesis is mainly driven by immune dysregulation. RA is characterized by persistent inflammation of the synovial membrane (synovitis), which involves activation of macrophage-like synovial fibroblasts (synoviocytes), and infiltration of T cells, B cells, macrophages, neutrophils, and mast cells into synovial compartments. These cells produce soluble mediator/effector molecules such as cytokines, chemokines, matrix metalloproteinases, eicosanoids, and autoantibodies. Antibodies against Fc portion of IgG (rheumatoid factors), and citrullinated peptides (ACPAs), the hallmarks of RA, are found in blood of 80%–90% RA patients.[102] The presence of these autoantibodies in blood (serapositivity) is associated with severity in symptoms, joint damage, and mortality, and their concentrations decrease with effective therapy.[96] These findings highlight the key role of autoantibody-producing B cells in RA pathogenesis. In contrast, the role of T cells in RA has long been debated. The differentiation state of CD4+ T cells in RA is not well defined. The role of Th17 cells is strongly supported in animal RA models but not consistently confirmed in human studies, which may explain why IL-17–targetting therapy has been disappointing.

As with many other autoimmune diseases, currently RA is not curable; however, development in diagnostic and therapeutic strategies in the past two decades, achieving the goal of remission or low disease activity to avoid joint damage, has become possible in many patients. The current treatment of RA primarily involves use of general immunosuppressants, inhibitors for cytokines and their receptors (particularly IL-6 and TNF-α), and inhibitors for specific signaling pathways (such as Janus kinase). These drugs have significant side effects and are expensive, which limits their broad utilization by RA patients.

Role of nutrition and dietary factors and underlying mechanisms

Evidence from observational studies; Diet and nutrition have long been known to impact RA initiation and progression. Studies have shown that severity of RA process adversely affects nutritional status. The nutritional status of the patients also impacts disease severity. For instances, malnourished RA patients had more active disease than those without malnutrition.[106] Earlier observational studies reported that RA patients have low serum concentrations of albumin, prealbumin, transferrin, zinc, and folic acid.[107–109] Trace minerals such as zinc and selenium may be protective in RA as the mean hair zinc content,[110] and serum selenium levels[111,112] were significantly lower in RA patients compared to the healthy controls.[111,112] Furthermore, both cross-sectional and longitudinal studies showed that lower selenium levels in RA patients were associated with the clinical disease activity.[113] RA patients are recommended to receive dietary education and consume adequate amount of calcium, folic acid, vitamin E, zinc, and selenium.[114]

Dietary pattern and certain foods are suggested to affect RA. Consumption of fruits, vegetables, olive oil, and oil-rich fish is shown to be associated with reduced risk of RA onset.[115] A large population-based case-control study reported an inverse correlation between the Mediterranean diet and RA risk among men,[116] but this correlation was not observed in women.[117] In patients with established disease, there was no association between severity of disease and high dietary quality, i.e., high intake of fish, shellfish, whole grains, fruits, and vegetables, and low intake of sausages and sweets. However, high dietary quality was significantly related to reduction in plasma levels of inflammation biomarker C-reactive protein (CRP).[118] A systematic review of prospective human studies[119] indicated beneficial effect of Mediterranean diet including reduced pain and increased physical function in RA patient. Monounsaturated fatty acids in the Mediterranean diet are suggested to be the key factor contributing to reduced disease activity in RA patients.[120] Overall, the evidence for a role of dietary pattern in RA development is limited and supported with only a small number of observational studies.

N-3 PUFAs have antiinflammatory and immunomodulating properties, which may underlie their suggested beneficial effects in RA.[121–123] EPA levels in both serum and erythrocytes of RA patients were found to be significantly lower compared to healthy controls.[124,125] Consumption of oily fish, the main source of n-3 long-chain PUFAs in human diet, was associated with a modest decrease in risk of developing RA.[126] Daily consumption of more than 0.21 g n-3 PUFAs was found to be associated with a 35% reduction in risk of developing RA in middle-aged and older women from the Swedish Mammography Cohort, a population-based prospective study.[127] A cross-sectional analysis showed that compared to those who never ate fish or had fish less than once a month, the RA patients consuming fish $\geq$2 times/week had a significantly lower disease activity score.[128] In a prospective study in 727 patients with early RA, higher intake of dietary vitamin D and n-3 PUFAs during the year preceding initiation of conventional drug therapy was associated with better treatment results,[129] and dietary intake of n-3 PUFAs was inversely associated with unacceptable pain among methotrexate-treated early RA patients.[130]

Accumulating evidence indicates that vitamin D, a fat-soluble vitamin able to regulate calcium/phosphate metabolism and immune function, may affect RA pathogenesis. Lower serum vitamin D levels in 50 Indian RA patients relative to the healthy controls were shown to correlate with disease activity.[131] Low vitamin D levels in newly diagnosed RA patients not receiving any RA drugs were associated with reduced response to treatment and increased disease activity.[132] Several meta-analysis studies consistently reported low serum vitamin D level in RA patients and its inverse association with disease activity.[133–135] A study evaluating vitamin D status in 1413 RA patients from 15 countries showed that low blood vitamin D level was common in RA patients in different countries and at different latitudes.[136] Low vitamin D intake–associated elevation in RA risk is supported by a meta-analysis involving three cohort studies with 215,757 participants, 874 cases of RA, and follow-up period of 11, 12, and 22 years, respectively.[134] However, it should be pointed out that it is not clear at this time whether the low serum vitamin D status seen in RA patients is a cause or consequence of RA. Thus, further investigation, in particular, clinical trials of adequate size is needed before benefit of additional vitamin D intake for RA patients is confirmed.

Other vitamins are suggested to impact RA risk. For example, a prospective cohort study in 29,368 women aged 55–69 years old found that higher intake of vitamin C, vitamin E, and zinc was inversely correlated with RA development.[137] Together, these studies suggest that intake of antioxidant micronutrients may be protective against RA development.

Evidence from intervention studies; Prospective studies have been conducted to determine the role of nutrients, food, food components, and dietary patterns in RA prevention and management. Studies have shown that dietary intervention may be effective in relieving symptoms and mitigating disease progression in RA patients.[138–141] In a small Swedish cohort study, stable or modestly active RA patients who consumed Mediterranean diet for 3 months showed significant reduction in disease activity and serum CRP levels compared to patients who continued their regular diet.[142]

Beneficial effect of n-3 PUFAs on RA disease activity has been investigated in several clinical trials. For example, in an RCT, patients with active RA who received daily fish oil containing 1000 mg EPA and 1500 mg DHA for 12 week showed reduction in disease symptoms and blood CRP levels.[143] In a cross-over RCT with 10 week intervention/10 week washout period, RA patients who received daily 2.1 g DHA supplementation had a significant decline in number of tender and swollen joints.[144] In another RCT, patients with recent onset RA who received fish oil containing 5.5 g EPA + DHA/day for 1 year exhibited decrease in failure rate of conventional therapy (combination of antirheumatic drugs) as well as increased disease remission.[145]

Fruits and vegetables contain high levels of phytochemicals that have antiinflammatory properties.[146] A recent RCT reported that female RA patients who consumed daily 500 mL of low-calorie cranberry juice containing 150 mg vitamin C, 131.92 mg proanthocyanidins, 258.75 mg total phenolics, and 0.30 mg folic acid for 90 days had reduced disease activity compared to those who did not.[147] In an animal study, oral administration of tannins prepared from apples delayed RA development in a mouse RA model.[148]

Dietary polyphenols, which have antiinflammatory and antioxidant properties, have been shown to have anti-RA activity via reduced production of cytokines, chemokines, and osteoclastogenic factors and inhibition of activation of transcription factors such as MAP kinase, c-Fos, and NFκB in the in vitro cell culture and animal models.[149]

Fibroblast-like synoviocytes (FLSs) are the predominant cell type comprising the structure of the synovial intima in healthy human synovium. In inflamed rheumatoid synovium, activated FLS plays a key role in RA pathogenesis by producing cytokines that perpetuate inflammation and proteases that degrade the cartilage matrix promoting joint destruction. Synovial hyperplasia is a consequence of an increased proliferation and impaired apoptosis of FLS in RA. In vitro studies have shown that resveratrol may have beneficial effects on RA because it has been shown to induce apoptosis of FLS isolated from RA patients as well as MH7A cells, a human RA synovial cell line.[150,151] A recent RCT reported that RA patients who consumed daily 1 g resveratrol with conventional treatment for 3 months had significantly reduced disease activity and improved biochemical markers compared to those who received conventional treatment alone[152]

IL-17, a predominant cytokine of Th17 cells with osteoclastogenic activity, induces production of destructive cytokines (such as MIF, TNF-α, and RANKL). In the pathogenesis of RA, TNF-α promotes synovitis and stimulates cartilage and bone breakdown by stimulating production of proinflammatory mediators like prostaglandin E_2 (PGE_2) and IL-1β. Quercetin, a dietary polyphenol found in vegetables and fruits such as onions, kale, apples, and berries, inhibited LPS-induced TNF-α secretion from macrophage cell line, RAW 264.7 cells.[153] Quercetin also suppressed Th17 differentiation and IL-17 production in cultured PBMCs and inhibited IL-17–induced RANKL mRNA and protein expression in cultured FLS from RA patients.[154] In an RCT conducted in female RA patients, quercetin supplementation (500 mg/day) for 8 weeks significantly alleviated clinical symptoms including early morning stiffness, morning pain, and after-activity pain.[155]

Since vitamin D deficiency (defined as plasma 25-hydroxy vitamin D < 75 nmol/L) is common in RA patients, studies have investigated if correction of deficiency would improve RA. A study showed that administration of a single oral high dose (300,000 IU) of vitamin D3, followed by daily dose of 800–1000 IU for 6 months, could effectively correct low vitamin D status in RA patients.[156] In a randomized open-label trial, administration of 60,000 IU vitamin D for 6 weeks followed by 3 months of 60,000 IU vitamin D once a month significantly increased serum vitamin D levels and decreased disease activity.[157] It is worth noting that vitamin D supplementation may not always prevent vitamin D deficiency, and vitamin D deficiency may still be found in RA patients who regularly take vitamin D supplementation. A study reported that among 318 patients who consumed daily supplements ≥800 IU of vitamin D, 28% patients did not reach adequate levels of vitamin D. Furthermore, vitamin D supplementation is often ineffective in RA patients with more severe disease.[158] A study in 1,191 RA patients and 1,019 control subjects (not on vitamin D supplement) from 22 Italian rheumatology centers showed that one-third of total 557 RA patients who received vitamin D supplements were still vitamin D deficient.[159] These studies suggest that in addition to optimizing vitamin D supplement dosage, other factors, such as sun exposure and BMI, which are well-established risk factors for vitamin D deficiency, should be considered when correcting deficient vitamin D status in RA patients.

Although several studies demonstrated beneficial effects of vitamin D on RA, the potential role of vitamin D supplementation in preventing RA or as a component of RA treatment is controversial. Daily supplementation for 5.1 years with 1,000 mg calcium plus daily low dose vitamin D3 was not effective in reducing the risk of developing RA in an RCT that included 32,435 postmenopausal women. Further, both solar irradiance and dietary vitamin D intake may be associated with increased RA incidence.[160] These results underscore the necessity of further studies for characterizing the role of vitamin D in RA as well as optimizing and personalizing supplementation strategies.

Pain is a common symptom experienced by RA patients, which is caused by inflammatory or noninflammatory factors. In an open-labeled randomized trial, supplementation with 1,25-$(OH)_2D_3$ for 8 weeks in recently diagnosed RA patient receiving conventional therapy drugs produced additional pain relief.[161] In another study, this pain-relieving effect of vitamin D was only observed in the RA patients who had low serum vitamin D levels before supplementation[162]; similarly, significant reduction of Health Assessment Questionnaire score was only observed in the RA patients who had low before supplementation serum vitamin D levels (<20 ng/mL).[163]

Vitamin E, a potent antioxidant with antiinflammatory properties, has been suggested to have anti-RA potential. Rats with experimental RA treated with vitamin E for 6 weeks had significantly lower serum levels of PGE_2 and nitric oxide[164] compared to those that were untreated. Further, supplementation with glucosamine plus vitamin E had a synergistic effect against RA symptoms in rats.[165] Vitamin E treatment in transgenic mouse model of RA, which spontaneously develops polyarthritis that is similar to the human RA, prevented joint destruction.[166] Supplementation with vitamin E plus fish oil in a mouse model of RA significantly decreased the levels of IL-6, IL-10, IL-12, and TNF-α compared to fish oil alone.[167] RA patients receiving 600 mg vitamin E twice a day for 12 weeks had a pain reduction.[168] In addition, lower inflammation was observed in patients with active RA after combined supplementation with linoleic acid and vitamin E.[169,170]

Vitamin K has been suggested to have antiinflammatory activity and its potential benefit in RA has been tested. Vitamin K1 (phylloquinone) treatment is not effective in improving clinical symptoms and biochemical indices of RA patients.[171–173] However, vitamin K2 (menaquinone-4, MK-4) was reported to inhibit FLS proliferation and also induce apoptosis,[174] indicating that vitamin K2 could be potentially used for RA treatment. In a cross-sectional study, RA patients treated with MK-7, an MK with greater bioavailability than MK-4, exhibited a significant decrease in serum inflammatory markers and disease activity score.[175] These studies suggest that therapeutic potential of vitamin K worths further investigation.

C. Inflammatory Bowel Diseases

General information about IBD

IBD, primarily Crohn's disease (CD) and ulcerative colitis (UC), is a chronic and relapsing inflammatory disorder that affects gastrointestinal tract. The prevalence of IBD is highest in developed Western countries including North America, Europe, and Australia. There are approximately 1.6 million US residents with IBD, including 785,000 with CD and 910,000 with UC.[176] Mean hospitalization rates for IBD from 2010 to 2015 in the United States, Europe, and Australia were 33.9, 72.9, and 31.5 per 100,000 individuals, respectively.[177] The incidence of IBD is increasing in Asia. Annual incidence of CD was 0.05 cases per 100,000 person-years in 1986–1990 and increased to 1.34 per 100,000 person-years in 2001–2005 in a population-based study from South Korea. In the ACCESS cohort, the highest incidence of IBD was in India at 9.3 cases per 100,000 person-years and the incidence of IBD within China ranged from 0.05 to 3.14 per 100,000 person-years.[178]

CD and UC share some similarities and also have distinct clinical and pathological features. In CD, inflammation is discontinuous and affects all layers of the bowel wall while UC involves the large intestine beginning in the rectum and affects first two layers of the intestinal wall.[179] Although IBD is not only an autoimmune disease, some autoantibodies were common in IBD patients and all autoimmune diseases except for thyroiditis were more prevalent among IBD patients compared with the non-IBD controls in Israel. Possible explanations suggested for association between IBD and autoimmune diseases were underlying genetic factors predisposing patients for both IBD and autoimmune diseases, autoimmunity triggered by IBD-related inflammation and increased permeability, and use of immunomodulatory medications.[180]

Etiologies of IBD are not clear, but both genetic susceptibility and environmental factors play a role in development and pathogenesis of the disease. IBD seems to result from an inappropriate immune response to the host gut microbiome in a genetically susceptible individuals. Therefore, a balance between the effector and regulatory cells, composition of the microbiome, integrity of the intestinal barrier, and environmental factors that affect microbiome and immune responses play important roles in IBD pathogenesis.[181] Genetic factors implicated in susceptibility to CD are those related to innate immune system pattern recognition receptors, differentiation of Th17 cells, autophagy, maintenance of epithelial barrier integrity, and the orchestration of the secondary immune responses.[182]

Environmental factors are believed to have a significant influence on the development of IBD. Cigarette smoking increases the risk of developing CD possibly by affecting intestinal microbiota. Dietary factors are associated with IBD, and a diet high in animal fat and low in fruits and vegetables is the dietary pattern associated with an increased risk of IBD. Low serum vitamin D level appears to be a risk factor for IBD. Use of medications such as antibiotics, oral contraceptives, and nonsteroidal antiinflammatory drugs is associated with increased IBD risk.[178,183]

Both innate and acquired immune systems play important roles in IBD. Defects in innate immune system, overly aggressive activity of effector lymphocytes and proinflammatory cytokines, and failure of regulatory mechanisms could contribute to the pathogenesis of IBD. Inability to recognize bacterial products results in defective intestinal innate immune response and could lead to increased risk of CD development. Mutations in the *NOD2* gene are a risk factor for CD; the risk for CD increases by 2- to 4-fold with one pathologic allele and by 15- to 40-fold with two pathologic allele. NOD2 recognizes the lysosomal breakdown product of bacteria peptidoglycan and activates innate immune system and induces autophagy.[179,184] Exaggerated T cell response is seen in both CD and UC; however, the two show differences in T cell response pattern. In CD, excessive Th1 and Th17 responses due to the production of IL-12, IL-18, IL-23, and TGF-β by APC and macrophages are observed. In fact, animals deficient in IL-12 p40 subunit and IL-23 are resistant to the induction of colitis. In UC, inflammation is secondary to Th2 cytokine profile and increased production of IL-5 is observed. Tregs can suppress the inflammation driven by Th17 cells and control innate inflammatory mechanisms.[181]

Role of nutrition and dietary factors in IBD and underlying mechanisms

Evidence from observational studies; Vitamin D status shows strong association with IBD risk and disease activity. In the Nurses' Health Study, 72,719 women were followed from 1986 through 2008 during which 122 cases of CD and 123 cases of UC were diagnosed. Higher vitamin D prediction score, which was developed from diet and lifestyle assessment and validated against circulating 25(OH)D, was associated with reduced risk of CD. The median predicted 25(OH)D level was 22.3 ng/mL in the lowest and 32.2 ng/mL in the highest quartiles, and the multivariate-adjusted hazard ratio associated with the highest quartile of vitamin D for

CD was 0.54 (95% confidence interval [CI], 0.30–0.99) compared with the lowest quartile.[185] In a retrospective study that included 504 IBD patients (403 CD and 101 UC patients), 49.8% of patients were vitamin D deficient and deficiency was associated with greater disease activity and lower health-related quality of life.[186]

In a meta-analysis by Mozaffari et al.,[187] association of fish consumption and dietary intake of n-3 PUFAs with the risk of IBD was investigated using ten observational studies (four prospective and six case–control). Total sample size of 282,610 participants with 2002 cases of IBD (1061 CD and 937 UC) were included. A negative association between fish consumption and the risk of CD (pooled effect size: 0.54, 95% CI: 0.31–0.96, $P = .03$) was found. A significant inverse association between dietary long-chain n-3 PUFAs and the risk of UC (pooled effect size: 0.75, 95% CI: 0.57–0.98, $P = .03$) was observed. However, no association was found between total dietary n-3 PUFAs or ALA intake with IBD.

Evidence from intervention studies; Dietary interventions to reduce relapse and disease activity in IBD patients have used different strategies/targets including promotion of favorable gut microbiota, decrease in intestinal permeability and intestinal epithelial injury, and reduction of inflammation. Dietary interventions tested for their efficacy against IBD include specific carbohydrate diet, low-FODMAP (fermentable oligosaccharides, disaccharides, monosaccharides, and polyols) diet, gluten-free diet, antiinflammatory diet, immunoglobulin-G4-guided exclusion diet, high-fiber diet, low-residue diet, semivegetarian diet, Mediterranean diet, and paleolithic diet. Dietary supplements investigated for benefits in IBD patients are curcumin, glutamine, n-3 fatty acids, vitamin D, prebiotics, and probiotics. The effects of these dietary interventions and nutrition supplementations on pathogenesis and treatment of IBD have been reviewed in several recent articles.[183,188–190]

Vitamin D exerts diverse effects on immune system. Vitamin D activates innate immune system by inducing monocyte proliferation and the expression of IL-1 and cathelicidin by macrophages. Vitamin D decreases DC maturation and IL-12 production while inducing the production of IL-10. Further, vitamin D decreases the production of IL-2, IL-17, and IFN-γ, attenuates proliferation of CD4+ and CD8+ T cells, and promotes the development of Treg cells and IL-10–producing type 1 Treg cells.[191] All these vitamin D–induced changes have the potential to impact IBD development and pathogenesis. In human monocytes and epithelial cells, vitamin D stimulated the expression of NOD2/CARD15/IBD1 genes and proteins, providing the molecular basis for the role of vitamin D deficiency in pathogenesis of CD.[192] In a mouse model, proper vitamin D receptor (VDR) signaling was critical for the innate immune response during experimental IBD and vitamin supplementation improved colitis.[193,194] When IL-10 knockout mice were fed vitamin D–deficient diet, they rapidly developed diarrhea and a wasting disease and exhibited 58% mortality. On the other hand, those fed the vitamin D–sufficient diet or provided with $1,25(OH)_2D_3$ supplementation showed significantly ameliorated IBD symptoms and no mortality was observed.[193] In dextran sulfate sodium–induced IBD model, VDR knockout mice showed shorter colon length, greater weight loss, and higher histology scores and mortality compared with the wild-type mice.[194] VDR seemed to play a critical role in mucosal barrier homeostasis by preserving the integrity of intercellular junctions and healing capacity of colonic epithelium.[195] Proper balance between Tregs and Th17 cells is important for the control of inflammation in IBD. Impaired delivery of IL-15 to CD4+ T cells in the colon downmodulated Foxp3 expression and enhanced RORγt expression, which resulted in rapid triggering of IBD characterized by enhanced production of proinfiammatory cytokines (IFN-γ and IL-6) and accumulation of Th1/Th17 cells in mice.[196] Foxp3 gene expression was promoted by vitamin D in CD4+ T cells isolated from human PBMCs through direct VDR binding to the vitamin D response element within Foxp3 gene and the enhancement of the Foxp3 promoter activity.[197]

However, there are few RCTs in which clinical benefits of vitamin D have been demonstrated. In a randomized controlled study, 94 CD patients received either daily placebo or 1,200 IU vitamin D for 12 months. Serum vitamin D levels increased significantly with supplementation, and the relapse rate tended to be lower ($P = .06$) among patients treated with vitamin D3 (6/46 or 13%) compared with patients treated with placebo.[198] In a small study with 18 mild-to-moderate CD patients, 24 weeks of supplementation with up to 5,000 IU/d vitamin D3 effectively raised serum $25(OH)D_3$ levels and reduced the unadjusted mean CD activity index scores. Quality-of-life scores also improved following vitamin D supplementation.[199]

N-3 fatty acids can exert antiinflammatory actions by various mechanisms including inhibition of leukocyte chemotaxis, production of lipid mediators with less biological potency, inhibition of inflammatory cytokine production, alteration in activation of transcription factors (activation of PPAR-γ and reduced activation of NF-κB), and decrease in T cell reactivity (inhibition of T cell proliferation and decreased IL-2 production).[200] Despite strong mechanistic associations including antiinflammatory properties and epidemiological data, clinical trials of n-3 fatty acids in IBD patients have produced mixed results, showing some beneficial effects, but failing to demonstrate a protective effect in preventing clinical relapse. These trials have been reviewed by several investigators.[201,202] Cabré et al.[202] evaluated omega-3 PUFA as therapeutic agents in IBD patients from the total of 19 RCTs. They concluded that available data do not allow recommendation to use omega-3 PUFA supplementation for treatment of either active or inactive IBD. However, authors pointed out several issues that might have influenced the outcomes of the RCTs: (1) doses of omega-3 PUFA used were too low to elicit therapeutic effects, (2) dietary n-6 to n-3 ratio, or plasma, red blood cell, or gut mucosal fatty acid profiles were not monitored, (3) different n-3 formulations had different pharmacokinetic characteristics, and (4) the choice of placebo was not optimal. Olive oil, oleic acid, or medium chain triglyceride were used in some studies, and these were reported to attenuate intestinal inflammation.

IV. CONCLUSIONS AND PERSPECTIVES

A normally functioning immune system can distinguish "foreign" from "self." "Self-tolerance" prohibits an individual's immune system from attacking normal tissues of the body. When this self-tolerance mechanism fails, immune system can be activated in response to self-antigens in the absence of external assaults or internal threats. This host-directed immune response is called autoimmunity, which can cause damage and dysfunction in various tissues and organs leading to the corresponding clinical manifestations collectively called autoimmune diseases.

Incidence of autoimmune diseases is relatively low. However, they often result in disability and morbidity. Further, they are one of the leading causes of mortality in young and middle-aged women and thus have a significant health and economic impact. About 100 different types of autoimmune diseases have been identified, although not all may fit all of the criteria set for autoimmune disorders.

Nutrition can impact regulation of the immune system and thus prevalence and pathogenesis of autoimmune diseases. Information related to impact of nutrition on autoimmune diseases is somewhat limited. Nutrition intervention experiments, whether preclinical or clinical, have focused on few of the 100 different autoimmune diseases. The results, thus far, are encouraging and show efficacy of specific nutrients or dietary patterns on reducing pathogenesis and clinical symptoms of some of the autoimmune diseases, e.g., vitamin D and IBD, green tea catechins and MS, or n-3 PUFA and RA. Majority of evidence, thus far, has been obtained using experimental animal models. Further investigation including clinical trials of adequate size and duration are needed to firmly establish the value of nutritional intervention in reducing the risk and pathogenesis of these autoimmune diseases. In addition, the role of nutrition in pathogenesis of other autoimmune diseases needs to be explored. A hindrance to this effort is lack of a complete understanding of etiology and underlying mechanism of pathogenesis of several of these autoimmune disorders, which makes selection of appropriate nutritional intervention difficult. Thus, more investigation is needed to better understand etiology and pathogenesis of several autoimmune diseases before nutrition intervention can be attempted. Finally, understanding the mechanism of those nutritional interventions that have been successful is needed. This information will help determine the most efficient preventive and therapeutic nutritional approach for specific autoimmune diseases.

V. REFERENCES

1. Hayter SM, Cook MC. Updated assessment of the prevalence, spectrum and case definition of autoimmune disease. *Autoimmun Rev.* 2012;11(10):754–765.
2. Wang L, Wang FS, Gershwin ME. Human autoimmune diseases: a comprehensive update. *J Intern Med.* 2015;278(4):369–395.
3. Jacobson DL, Gange SJ, Rose NR, Graham NM. Epidemiology and estimated population burden of selected autoimmune diseases in the United States. *Clin Immunol Immunopathol.* 1997;84(3):223–243.
4. Eaton WW, Rose NR, Kalaydjian A, Pedersen MG, Mortensen PB. Epidemiology of autoimmune diseases in Denmark. *J Autoimmun.* 2007;29(1):1–9.
5. Youinou P, Pers JO, Gershwin ME, Shoenfeld Y. Geo-epidemiology and autoimmunity. *J Autoimmun.* 2010;34(3):J163–J167.
6. Cooper GS, Stroehla BC. The epidemiology of autoimmune diseases. *Autoimmun Rev.* 2003;2(3):119–125.
7. Wahren-Herlenius M, Dorner T. Immunopathogenic mechanisms of systemic autoimmune disease. *Lancet.* 2013;382(9894):819–831.
8. Cho JH, Gregersen PK. Genomics and the multifactorial nature of human autoimmune disease. *N Engl J Med.* 2011;365(17):1612–1623.
9. Davidson A, Diamond B. Autoimmune diseases. *N Engl J Med.* 2001;345(5):340–350.
10. Goodnow CC. Multistep pathogenesis of autoimmune disease. *Cell.* 2007;130(1):25–35.
11. Dilokthornsakul P, Valuck RJ, Nair KV, Corboy JR, Allen RR, Campbell JD. Multiple sclerosis prevalence in the United States commercially insured population. *Neurology.* 2016;86(11):1014–1021.
12. Hemmer B, Kerschensteiner M, Korn T. Role of the innate and adaptive immune responses in the course of multiple sclerosis. *Lancet Neurol.* 2015;14(4):406–419.
13. Ascherio A, Munger KL. Epidemiology of multiple sclerosis: from risk factors to prevention-an update. *Semin Neurol.* 2016;36(2):103–114.
14. Filippi M, Bar-Or A, Piehl F, et al. Multiple sclerosis. *Nat Rev Dis Primers.* 2018;4(1):43.
15. Kister I, Chamot E, Salter AR, Cutter GR, Bacon TE, Herbert J. Disability in multiple sclerosis: a reference for patients and clinicians. *Neurology.* 2013;80(11):1018–1024.
16. Compston A, Coles A. Multiple sclerosis. *Lancet.* 2002;359(9313):1221–1231.
17. Sospedra M, Martin R. Immunology of multiple sclerosis. *Annu Rev Immunol.* 2005;23:683–747.

18. Ciccarelli O, Barkhof F, Bodini B, et al. Pathogenesis of multiple sclerosis: insights from molecular and metabolic imaging. *Lancet Neurol*. 2014;13(8):807–822.
19. Dendrou CA, Fugger L, Friese MA. Immunopathology of multiple sclerosis. *Nat Rev Immunol*. 2015;15(9):545–558.
20. Garg N, Smith TW. An update on immunopathogenesis, diagnosis, and treatment of multiple sclerosis. *Brain Behav*. 2015;5(9): e00362.
21. International Multiple Sclerosis Genetics C, Beecham AH, Patsopoulos NA, et al. Analysis of immune-related loci identifies 48 new susceptibility variants for multiple sclerosis. *Nat Genet*. 2013;45(11):1353–1360.
22. Mechelli R, Annibali V, Ristori G, Vittori D, Coarelli G, Salvetti M. Multiple sclerosis etiology: beyond genes and environment. *Expert Rev Clin Immunol*. 2010;6(3):481–490.
23. Ascherio A, Munger KL. Environmental risk factors for multiple sclerosis. Part I: the role of infection. *Ann Neurol*. 2007;61(4): 288–299.
24. Wingerchuk DM. Smoking: effects on multiple sclerosis susceptibility and disease progression. *Ther Adv Neurol Disord*. 2012;5(1): 13–22.
25. Ascherio A, Munger KL, Simon KC. Vitamin D and multiple sclerosis. *Lancet Neurol*. 2010;9(6):599–612.
26. Correale J, Ysrraelit MC, Gaitan MI. Immunomodulatory effects of Vitamin D in multiple sclerosis. *Brain*. 2009;132(Pt 5): 1146–1160.
27. Kleinewietfeld M, Manzel A, Titze J, et al. Sodium chloride drives autoimmune disease by the induction of pathogenic TH17 cells. *Nature*. 2013;496(7446):518–522.
28. Hedstrom AK, Olsson T, Alfredsson L. High body mass index before age 20 is associated with increased risk for multiple sclerosis in both men and women. *Mult Scler*. 2012;18(9):1334–1336.
29. Aslani S, Jafari N, Javan MR, Karami J, Ahmadi M, Jafarnejad M. Epigenetic modifications and therapy in multiple sclerosis. *Neuromolecular Med*. 2017;19(1):11–23.
30. Li X, Xiao B, Chen XS. DNA methylation: a new player in multiple sclerosis. *Mol Neurobiol*. 2017;54(6):4049–4059.
31. Maltby VE, Graves MC, Lea RA, et al. Genome-wide DNA methylation profiling of CD8+ T cells shows a distinct epigenetic signature to CD4+ T cells in multiple sclerosis patients. *Clin Epigenet*. 2015;7:118.
32. Huang Q, Xiao B, Ma X, et al. MicroRNAs associated with the pathogenesis of multiple sclerosis. *J Neuroimmunol*. 2016; 295–296:148–161.
33. Naghavian R, Ghaedi K, Kiani-Esfahani A, Ganjalikhani-Hakemi M, Etemadifar M, Nasr-Esfahani MH. miR-141 and miR-200a, revelation of new possible players in modulation of Th17/treg differentiation and pathogenesis of multiple sclerosis. *PLoS One*. 2015;10(5):e0124555.
34. Junker A, Krumbholz M, Eisele S, et al. MicroRNA profiling of multiple sclerosis lesions identifies modulators of the regulatory protein CD47. *Brain*. 2009;132(Pt 12):3342–3352.
35. Procaccini C, De Rosa V, Pucino V, Formisano L, Matarese G. Animal models of multiple sclerosis. *Eur J Pharmacol*. 2015;759: 182–191.
36. Robinson AP, Harp CT, Noronha A, Miller SD. The experimental autoimmune encephalomyelitis (EAE) model of MS: utility for understanding disease pathophysiology and treatment. *Handb Clin Neurol*. 2014;122:173–189.
37. Swank RL, Lerstad O, Strom A, Backer J. Multiple sclerosis in rural Norway its geographic and occupational incidence in relation to nutrition. *N Engl J Med*. 1952;246(19):722–728.
38. Goldberg P. Multiple sclerosis: vitamin D and calcium as environmental determinants of prevalence (A viewpoint) part 1: sunlight, dietary factors and epidemiology. *Int J Environ Stud*. 1974;6(1): 19–27.
39. Lucas RM, Byrne SN, Correale J, Ilschner S, Hart PH. Ultraviolet radiation, vitamin D and multiple sclerosis. *Neurodegener Dis Manag*. 2015;5(5):413–424.
40. Mazdeh M, Seifirad S, Kazemi N, Seifrabie MA, Dehghan A, Abbasi H. Comparison of vitamin D3 serum levels in new diagnosed patients with multiple sclerosis versus their healthy relatives. *Acta Med Iran*. 2013;51(5):289–292.
41. Munger KL, Levin LI, Hollis BW, Howard NS, Ascherio A. Serum 25-hydroxyvitamin D levels and risk of multiple sclerosis. *J Am Med Assoc*. 2006;296(23):2832–2838.
42. Hartl C, Obermeier V, Gerdes LA, Brugel M, von Kries R, Kumpfel T. Seasonal variations of 25-OH vitamin D serum levels are associated with clinical disease activity in multiple sclerosis patients. *J Neurol Sci*. 2017;375:160–164.
43. Munger KL, Chitnis T, Frazier AL, Giovannucci E, Spiegelman D, Ascherio A. Dietary intake of vitamin D during adolescence and risk of multiple sclerosis. *J Neurol*. 2011;258(3):479–485.
44. Mirzaei F, Michels KB, Munger K, et al. Gestational vitamin D and the risk of multiple sclerosis in offspring. *Ann Neurol*. 2011;70(1): 30–40.
45. Munger KL, Aivo J, Hongell K, Soilu-Hanninen M, Surcel HM, Ascherio A. Vitamin D status during pregnancy and risk of multiple sclerosis in offspring of women in the finnish maternity cohort. *JAMA Neurol*. 2016;73(5):515–519.
46. Swank RL. Multiple sclerosis; a correlation of its incidence with dietary fat. *Am J Med Sci*. 1950;220(4):421–430.
47. Agranoff BW, Goldberg D. Diet and the geographical distribution of multiple sclerosis. *Lancet*. 1974;2(7888):1061–1066.
48. Bagheri M, Maghsoudi Z, Fayazi S, Elahi N, Tabesh H, Majdinasab N. Several food items and multiple sclerosis: a case-control study in Ahvaz (Iran). *Iran J Nurs Midwifery Res*. 2014; 19(6):659–665.
49. Azary S, Schreiner T, Graves J, et al. Contribution of dietary intake to relapse rate in early paediatric multiple sclerosis. *J Neurol Neurosurg Psychiatry*. 2018;89(1):28–33.
50. Zhang SM, Willett WC, Hernan MA, Olek MJ, Ascherio A. Dietary fat in relation to risk of multiple sclerosis among two large cohorts of women. *Am J Epidemiol*. 2000;152(11):1056–1064.
51. Bjornevik K, Chitnis T, Ascherio A, Munger KL. Polyunsaturated fatty acids and the risk of multiple sclerosis. *Mult Scler*. 2017; 23(14):1830–1838.
52. Katz Sand I, Benn EKT, Fabian M, et al. Randomized-controlled trial of a modified Mediterranean dietary program for multiple sclerosis: a pilot study. *Mult Scler Relat Disord*. 2019;36:101403.
53. Wahls TL, Chenard CA, Snetselaar LG. Review of two popular eating plans within the multiple sclerosis community: low saturated fat and modified paleolithic. *Nutrients*. 2019;11(2).
54. Yadav V, Marracci G, Kim E, et al. Low-fat, plant-based diet in multiple sclerosis: a randomized controlled trial. *Mult Scler Relat Disord*. 2016;9:80–90.
55. Black LJ, Rowley C, Sherriff J, et al. A healthy dietary pattern associates with a lower risk of a first clinical diagnosis of central nervous system demyelination. *Mult Scler*. 2019;25(11):1514–1525.
56. Katz Sand I. The role of diet in multiple sclerosis: mechanistic connections and current evidence. *Curr Nutr Rep*. 2018;7(3):150–160.
57. Rotstein DL, Cortese M, Fung TT, Chitnis T, Ascherio A, Munger KL. Diet quality and risk of multiple sclerosis in two cohorts of US women. *Mult Scler*. 2019;25(13):1773–1780.
58. Muthian G, Raikwar HP, Rajasingh J, Bright JJ. 1,25 Dihydroxyvitamin-D3 modulates JAK-STAT pathway in IL-12/IFNgamma axis leading to Th1 response in experimental allergic encephalomyelitis. *J Neurosci Res*. 2006;83(7):1299–1309.
59. Nashold FE, Hoag KA, Goverman J, Hayes CE. Rag-1-dependent cells are necessary for 1,25-dihydroxyvitamin D(3) prevention of experimental autoimmune encephalomyelitis. *J Neuroimmunol*. 2001;119(1):16–29.

60. Chang JH, Cha HR, Lee DS, Seo KY, Kweon MN. 1,25-Dihydroxyvitamin D3 inhibits the differentiation and migration of T(H)17 cells to protect against experimental autoimmune encephalomyelitis. *PLoS One*. 2010;5(9):e12925.
61. Joshi S, Pantalena LC, Liu XK, et al. 1,25-dihydroxyvitamin D(3) ameliorates Th17 autoimmunity via transcriptional modulation of interleukin-17A. *Mol Cell Biol*. 2011;31(17):3653–3669.
62. Xie Z, Chen J, Zheng C, et al. 1,25-dihydroxyvitamin D3 -induced dendritic cells suppress experimental autoimmune encephalomyelitis by increasing proportions of the regulatory lymphocytes and reducing T helper type 1 and type 17 cells. *Immunology*. 2017; 152(3):414–424.
63. McLaughlin L, Clarke L, Khalilidehkordi E, Butzkueven H, Taylor B, Broadley SA. Vitamin D for the treatment of multiple sclerosis: a meta-analysis. *J Neurol*. 2018;265(12):2893–2905.
64. Sintzel MB, Rametta M, Reder AT. Vitamin D and multiple sclerosis: a comprehensive review. *Neurol Ther*. 2018;7(1):59–85.
65. Feige J, Salmhofer H, Hecker C, et al. Life-threatening vitamin D intoxication due to intake of ultra-high doses in multiple sclerosis: a note of caution. *Mult Scler*. 2019;25(9):1326–1328.
66. Weinstock-Guttman B, Baier M, Park Y, et al. Low fat dietary intervention with omega-3 fatty acid supplementation in multiple sclerosis patients. *Prostaglandins Leukot Essent Fatty Acids*. 2005;73(5): 397–404.
67. Adkins Y, Soulika AM, Mackey B, Kelley DS. Docosahexaenoic acid (22:6n-3) ameliorated the onset and severity of experimental autoimmune encephalomyelitis in mice. *Lipids*. 2019; 54(1):13–23.
68. Farinotti M, Vacchi L, Simi S, Di Pietrantonj C, Brait L, Filippini G. Dietary interventions for multiple sclerosis. *Cochrane Database Syst Rev*. 2012;12:CD004192.
69. Aktas O, Prozorovski T, Smorodchenko A, et al. Green tea epigallocatechin-3-gallate mediates T cellular NF-kappa B inhibition and exerts neuroprotection in autoimmune encephalomyelitis. *J Immunol*. 2004;173(9):5794–5800.
70. Herges K, Millward JM, Hentschel N, Infante-Duarte C, Aktas O, Zipp F. Neuroprotective effect of combination therapy of glatiramer acetate and epigallocatechin-3-gallate in neuroin flammation. *PLoS One*. 2011;6(10):e25456.
71. Wang J, Ren Z, Xu Y, Xiao S, Meydani SN, Wu D. Epigallocatechin-3-gallate ameliorates experimental autoimmune encephalomyelitis by altering balance among CD4+ T-cell subsets. *Am J Pathol*. 2012;180(1):221–234.
72. Wang J, Pae M, Meydani SN, Wu D. Green tea epigallocatechin-3-gallate modulates differentiation of naive CD4(+) T cells into specific lineage effector cells. *J Mol Med*. 2013;91(4): 485–495.
73. Mahler A, Steiniger J, Bock M, et al. Metabolic response to epigallocatechin-3-gallate in relapsing-remitting multiple sclerosis: a randomized clinical trial. *Am J Clin Nutr*. 2015;101(3): 487–495.
74. Lovera J, Ramos A, Devier D, et al. Polyphenon E, non-futile at neuroprotection in multiple sclerosis but unpredictably hepatotoxic: phase I single group and phase II randomized placebo-controlled studies. *J Neurol Sci*. 2015;358(1–2):46–52.
75. Bruck J, Holstein J, Glocova I, et al. Nutritional control of IL-23/Th17-mediated autoimmune disease through HO-1/STAT3 activation. *Sci Rep*. 2017;7:44482.
76. Chearwae W, Bright JJ. 15-deoxy-Delta(12,14)-prostaglandin J(2) and curcumin modulate the expression of toll-like receptors 4 and 9 in autoimmune T lymphocyte. *J Clin Immunol*. 2008;28(5): 558–570.
77. Kanakasabai S, Casalini E, Walline CC, Mo C, Chearwae W, Bright JJ. Differential regulation of CD4(+) T helper cell responses by curcumin in experimental autoimmune encephalomyelitis. *J Nutr Biochem*. 2012;23(11):1498–1507.
78. Xie L, Li XK, Funeshima-Fuji N, et al. Amelioration of experimental autoimmune encephalomyelitis by curcumin treatment through inhibition of IL-17 production. *Int Immunopharmacol*. 2009;9(5):575–581.
79. Dolati S, Ahmadi M, Aghebti-Maleki L, et al. Nanocurcumin is a potential novel therapy for multiple sclerosis by influencing inflammatory mediators. *Pharmacol Rep*. 2018;70(6):1158–1167.
80. Dolati S, Ahmadi M, Rikhtegar R, et al. Changes in Th17 cells function after nanocurcumin use to treat multiple sclerosis. *Int Immunopharmacol*. 2018;61:74–81.
81. Singh NP, Hegde VL, Hofseth LJ, Nagarkatti M, Nagarkatti P. Resveratrol (trans-3,5,4′-trihydroxystilbene) ameliorates experimental allergic encephalomyelitis, primarily via induction of apoptosis in T cells involving activation of aryl hydrocarbon receptor and estrogen receptor. *Mol Pharmacol*. 2007;72(6): 1508–1521.
82. Shindler KS, Ventura E, Dutt M, Elliott P, Fitzgerald DC, Rostami A. Oral resveratrol reduces neuronal damage in a model of multiple sclerosis. *J Neuro Ophthalmol*. 2010;30(4):328–339.
83. Fonseca-Kelly Z, Nassrallah M, Uribe J, et al. Resveratrol neuroprotection in a chronic mouse model of multiple sclerosis. *Front Neurol*. 2012;3:84.
84. Imler Jr TJ, Petro TM. Decreased severity of experimental autoimmune encephalomyelitis during resveratrol administration is associated with increased IL-17+IL-10+ T cells, CD4(-) IFN-gamma+ cells, and decreased macrophage IL-6 expression. *Int Immunopharmacol*. 2009;9(1):134–143.
85. Wang D, Li SP, Fu JS, Zhang S, Bai L, Guo L. Resveratrol defends blood-brain barrier integrity in experimental autoimmune encephalomyelitis mice. *J Neurophysiol*. 2016;116(5):2173–2179.
86. Ghaiad HR, Nooh MM, El-Sawalhi MM, Shaheen AA. Resveratrol promotes remyelination in cuprizone model of multiple sclerosis: biochemical and histological study. *Mol Neurobiol*. 2017;54(5): 3219–3229.
87. Ahmad SF, Zoheir KM, Abdel-Hamied HE, et al. Amelioration of autoimmune arthritis by naringin through modulation of T regulatory cells and Th1/Th2 cytokines. *Cell Immunol*. 2014;287(2):112–120.
88. Azuma T, Shigeshiro M, Kodama M, Tanabe S, Suzuki T. Supplemental naringenin prevents intestinal barrier defects and inflammation in colitic mice. *J Nutr*. 2013;143(6):827–834.
89. Cui Y, Wu J, Jung SC, et al. Anti-neuroinflammatory activity of nobiletin on suppression of microglial activation. *Biol Pharm Bull*. 2010;33(11):1814–1821.
90. Okuyama S, Minami S, Shimada N, Makihata N, Nakajima M, Furukawa Y. Anti-inflammatory and neuroprotective effects of auraptene, a citrus coumarin, following cerebral global ischemia in mice. *Eur J Pharmacol*. 2013;699(1–3):118–123.
91. Ciftci O, Ozcan C, Kamisli O, Cetin A, Basak N, Aytac B. Hesperidin, a citrus flavonoid, has the ameliorative effects against experimental autoimmune encephalomyelitis (EAE) in a C57BL/J6 mouse model. *Neurochem Res*. 2015;40(6):1111–1120.
92. Haghmorad D, Mahmoudi MB, Salehipour Z, et al. Hesperidin ameliorates immunological outcome and reduces neuroinflammation in the mouse model of multiple sclerosis. *J Neuroimmunol*. 2017;302:23–33.
93. Wang J, Qi Y, Niu X, Tang H, Meydani SN, Wu D. Dietary naringenin supplementation attenuates experimental autoimmune encephalomyelitis by modulating autoimmune inflammatory responses in mice. *J Nutr Biochem*. 2018;54:130–139.
94. Wang J, Niu X, Wu C, Wu D. Naringenin modifies the development of lineage-specific effector CD4(+) T cells. *Front Immunol*. 2018;9:2267.
95. Smolen JS, Aletaha D, Barton A, et al. Rheumatoid arthritis. *Nat Rev Dis Primers*. 2018;4:18001.
96. Smolen JS, Aletaha D, McInnes IB. Rheumatoid arthritis. *Lancet*. 2016;388(10055):2023–2038.

97. Prete M, Racanelli V, Digiglio L, Vacca A, Dammacco F, Perosa F. Extra-articular manifestations of rheumatoid arthritis: an update. *Autoimmun Rev.* 2011;11(2):123–131.
98. Cross M, Smith E, Hoy D, et al. The global burden of rheumatoid arthritis: estimates from the global burden of disease 2010 study. *Ann Rheum Dis.* 2014;73(7):1316–1322.
99. Frisell T, Saevarsdottir S, Askling J. Family history of rheumatoid arthritis: an old concept with new developments. *Nat Rev Rheumatol.* 2016;12(6):335–343.
100. Gregersen PK, Silver J, Winchester RJ. The shared epitope hypothesis. An approach to understanding the molecular genetics of susceptibility to rheumatoid arthritis. *Arthritis Rheum.* 1987;30(11): 1205–1213.
101. Okada Y, Wu D, Trynka G, et al. Genetics of rheumatoid arthritis contributes to biology and drug discovery. *Nature.* 2014;506(7488): 376–381.
102. Firestein GS, McInnes IB. Immunopathogenesis of rheumatoid arthritis. *Immunity.* 2017;46(2):183–196.
103. Deane KD, Demoruelle MK, Kelmenson LB, Kuhn KA, Norris JM, Holers VM. Genetic and environmental risk factors for rheumatoid arthritis. *Best Pract Res Clin Rheumatol.* 2017;31(1):3–18.
104. Maeda Y, Takeda K. Role of gut microbiota in rheumatoid arthritis. *J Clin Med.* 2017;6(6).
105. Zhong D, Wu C, Zeng X, Wang Q. The role of gut microbiota in the pathogenesis of rheumatic diseases. *Clin Rheumatol.* 2018;37(1): 25–34.
106. Helliwell M, Coombes EJ, Moody BJ, Batstone GF, Robertson JC. Nutritional status in patients with rheumatoid arthritis. *Ann Rheum Dis.* 1984;43(3):386–390.
107. Helliwell M, Batstone GF, Coombes EJ, Moody BJ. Nutritional status in rheumatoid arthritis. *Arthritis Rheum.* 1983;26(12): 1532–1533.
108. Burnham R, Russell AS. Nutritional status in patients with rheumatoid arthritis. *Ann Rheum Dis.* 1986;45(9):788–789.
109. Gomez-Vaquero C, Nolla JM, Fiter J, et al. Nutritional status in patients with rheumatoid arthritis. *Jt Bone Spine.* 2001;68(5):403–409.
110. Mierzecki A, Strecker D, Radomska K. A pilot study on zinc levels in patients with rheumatoid arthritis. *Biol Trace Elem Res.* 2011; 143(2):854–862.
111. Yu N, Han F, Lin X, Tang C, Ye J, Cai X. The association between serum selenium levels with rheumatoid arthritis. *Biol Trace Elem Res.* 2016;172(1):46–52.
112. Xin L, Yang X, Cai G, et al. Serum levels of copper and zinc in patients with rheumatoid arthritis: a meta-analysis. *Biol Trace Elem Res.* 2015;168(1):1–10.
113. Tarp U. Selenium and the selenium-dependent glutathione peroxidase in rheumatoid arthritis. *Dan Med Bull.* 1994;41(3):264–274.
114. Stone J, Doube A, Dudson D, Wallace J. Inadequate calcium, folic acid, vitamin E, zinc, and selenium intake in rheumatoid arthritis patients: results of a dietary survey. *Semin Arthritis Rheum.* 1997; 27(3):180–185.
115. Pattison DJ, Harrison RA, Symmons DP. The role of diet in susceptibility to rheumatoid arthritis: a systematic review. *J Rheumatol.* 2004;31(7):1310–1319.
116. Johansson K, Askling J, Alfredsson L, Di Giuseppe D, group Es. Mediterranean diet and risk of rheumatoid arthritis: a population-based case-control study. *Arthritis Res Ther.* 2018; 20(1):175.
117. Hu Y, Costenbader KH, Gao X, Hu FB, Karlson EW, Lu B. Mediterranean diet and incidence of rheumatoid arthritis in women. *Arthritis Care Res.* 2015;67(5):597–606.
118. Barebring L, Winkvist A, Gjertsson I, Lindqvist HM. Poor dietary quality is associated with increased inflammation in Swedish patients with rheumatoid arthritis. *Nutrients.* 2018;10(10).
119. Forsyth C, Kouvari M, D'Cunha NM, et al. The effects of the Mediterranean diet on rheumatoid arthritis prevention and treatment: a systematic review of human prospective studies. *Rheumatol Int.* 2018;38(5):737–747.
120. Matsumoto Y, Sugioka Y, Tada M, et al. Monounsaturated fatty acids might be key factors in the Mediterranean diet that suppress rheumatoid arthritis disease activity: the TOMORROW study. *Clin Nutr.* 2018;37(2):675–680.
121. Miles EA, Calder PC. Influence of marine n-3 polyunsaturated fatty acids on immune function and a systematic review of their effects on clinical outcomes in rheumatoid arthritis. *Br J Nutr.* 2012;107(Suppl 2):S171–S184.
122. Calder PC. n-3 fatty acids, inflammation and immunity: new mechanisms to explain old actions. *Proc Nutr Soc.* 2013;72(3): 326–336.
123. Abdulrazaq M, Innes JK, Calder PC. Effect of omega-3 polyunsaturated fatty acids on arthritic pain: a systematic review. *Nutrition.* 2017;39–40:57–66.
124. Rodriguez-Carrio J, Alperi-Lopez M, Lopez P, Ballina-Garcia FJ, Suarez A. Non-esterified fatty acids profiling in rheumatoid arthritis: associations with clinical features and Th1 response. *PLoS One.* 2016;11(8):e0159573.
125. Lee AL, Park Y. The association between n-3 polyunsaturated fatty acid levels in erythrocytes and the risk of rheumatoid arthritis in Korean women. *Ann Nutr Metab.* 2013;63(1–2): 88–95.
126. Rosell M, Wesley AM, Rydin K, Klareskog L, Alfredsson L, group Es. Dietary fish and fish oil and the risk of rheumatoid arthritis. *Epidemiology.* 2009;20(6):896–901.
127. Di Giuseppe D, Wallin A, Bottai M, Askling J, Wolk A. Long-term intake of dietary long-chain n-3 polyunsaturated fatty acids and risk of rheumatoid arthritis: a prospective cohort study of women. *Ann Rheum Dis.* 2014;73(11):1949–1953.
128. Tedeschi SK, Bathon JM, Giles JT, Lin TC, Yoshida K, Solomon DH. Relationship between fish consumption and disease activity in rheumatoid arthritis. *Arthritis Care Res.* 2018;70(3):327–332.
129. Lourdudoss C, Wolk A, Nise L, Alfredsson L, Vollenhoven RV. Are dietary vitamin D, omega-3 fatty acids and folate associated with treatment results in patients with early rheumatoid arthritis? data from a Swedish population-based prospective study. *BMJ Open.* 2017;7(6):e016154.
130. Lourdudoss C, Di Giuseppe D, Wolk A, et al. Dietary intake of polyunsaturated fatty acids and pain in spite of inflammatory control among methotrexate-treated early rheumatoid arthritis patients. *Arthritis Care Res.* 2018;70(2):205–212.
131. Meena N, Singh Chawla SP, Garg R, Batta A, Kaur S. Assessment of vitamin D in rheumatoid arthritis and its correlation with disease activity. *J Nat Sci Biol Med.* 2018;9(1):54–58.
132. Di Franco M, Barchetta I, Iannuccelli C, et al. Hypovitaminosis D in recent onset rheumatoid arthritis is predictive of reduced response to treatment and increased disease activity: a 12 month follow-up study. *BMC Muscoskelet Disord.* 2015;16:53.
133. Lee YH, Bae SC. Vitamin D level in rheumatoid arthritis and its correlation with the disease activity: a meta-analysis. *Clin Exp Rheumatol.* 2016;34(5):827–833.
134. Song GG, Bae SC, Lee YH. Association between vitamin D intake and the risk of rheumatoid arthritis: a meta-analysis. *Clin Rheumatol.* 2012;31(12):1733–1739.
135. Lin J, Liu J, Davies ML, Chen W. Serum vitamin D level and rheumatoid arthritis disease activity: review and meta-analysis. *PLoS One.* 2016;11(1):e0146351.
136. Hajjaj-Hassouni N, Mawani N, Allali F, et al. Evaluation of vitamin D status in rheumatoid arthritis and its association with disease activity across 15 countries: "the COMORA study. *Internet J Rheumatol.* 2017;2017:5491676.
137. Cerhan JR, Saag KG, Merlino LA, Mikuls TR, Criswell LA. Antioxidant micronutrients and risk of rheumatoid arthritis in a cohort of older women. *Am J Epidemiol.* 2003;157(4):345–354.

138. Khanna S, Jaiswal KS, Gupta B. Managing rheumatoid arthritis with dietary interventions. *Front Nutr.* 2017;4:52.
139. Stamp LK, James MJ, Cleland LG. Diet and rheumatoid arthritis: a review of the literature. *Semin Arthritis Rheum.* 2005;35(2):77–94.
140. Li S, Micheletti R. Role of diet in rheumatic disease. *Rheum Dis Clin N Am.* 2011;37(1):119–133.
141. Badsha H. Role of diet in influencing rheumatoid arthritis disease activity. *Open Rheumatol J.* 2018;12:19–28.
142. Skoldstam L, Hagfors L, Johansson G. An experimental study of a Mediterranean diet intervention for patients with rheumatoid arthritis. *Ann Rheum Dis.* 2003;62(3):208–214.
143. Veselinovic M, Vasiljevic D, Vucic V, et al. Clinical benefits of n-3 PUFA and -linolenic acid in patients with rheumatoid arthritis. *Nutrients.* 2017;9(4).
144. Dawczynski C, Dittrich M, Neumann T, et al. Docosahexaenoic acid in the treatment of rheumatoid arthritis: a double-blind, placebo-controlled, randomized cross-over study with microalgae vs. sunflower oil. *Clin Nutr.* 2018;37(2):494–504.
145. Proudman SM, James MJ, Spargo LD, et al. Fish oil in recent onset rheumatoid arthritis: a randomised, double-blind controlled trial within algorithm-based drug use. *Ann Rheum Dis.* 2015;74(1): 89–95.
146. Zhu F, Du B, Xu B. Anti-inflammatory effects of phytochemicals from fruits, vegetables, and food legumes: a review. *Crit Rev Food Sci Nutr.* 2018;58(8):1260–1270.
147. Thimoteo NSB, Iryioda TMV, Alfieri DF, et al. Cranberry juice decreases disease activity in women with rheumatoid arthritis. *Nutrition.* 2019;60:112–117.
148. Nakamura K, Matsuoka H, Nakashima S, Kanda T, Nishimaki-Mogami T, Akiyama H. Oral administration of apple condensed tannins delays rheumatoid arthritis development in mice via downregulation of T helper 17 (Th17) cell responses. *Mol Nutr Food Res.* 2015;59(7):1406–1410.
149. Sung S, Kwon D, Um E, Kim B. Could polyphenols help in the control of rheumatoid arthritis? *Molecules.* 2019;24(8).
150. Nakayama H, Yaguchi T, Yoshiya S, Nishizaki T. Resveratrol induces apoptosis MH7A human rheumatoid arthritis synovial cells in a sirtuin 1-dependent manner. *Rheumatol Int.* 2012;32(1): 151–157.
151. Byun HS, Song JK, Kim YR, et al. Caspase-8 has an essential role in resveratrol-induced apoptosis of rheumatoid fibroblast-like synoviocytes. *Rheumatology.* 2008;47(3):301–308.
152. Khojah HM, Ahmed S, Abdel-Rahman MS, Elhakeim EH. Resveratrol as an effective adjuvant therapy in the management of rheumatoid arthritis: a clinical study. *Clin Rheumatol.* 2018;37(8):2035–2042.
153. Gokhale JP, Mahajan HS, Surana SJ. Quercetin loaded nanoemulsion-based gel for rheumatoid arthritis: in vivo and in vitro studies. *Biomed Pharmacother.* 2019;112:108622.
154. Kim HR, Kim BM, Won JY, et al. Quercetin, a plant polyphenol, has potential for the prevention of bone destruction in rheumatoid arthritis. *J Med Food.* 2019;22(2):152–161.
155. Javadi F, Ahmadzadeh A, Eghtesadi S, et al. The effect of quercetin on inflammatory factors and clinical symptoms in women with rheumatoid arthritis: a double-blind, randomized controlled trial. *J Am Coll Nutr.* 2017;36(1):9–15.
156. Sainaghi PP, Bellan M, Nerviani A, et al. Superiority of a high loading dose of cholecalciferol to correct hypovitaminosis d in patients with inflammatory/autoimmune rheumatic diseases. *J Rheumatol.* 2013;40(2):166–172.
157. Chandrashekara S, Patted A. Role of vitamin D supplementation in improving disease activity in rheumatoid arthritis: an exploratory study. *Int J Rheum Dis.* 2017;20(7):825–831.
158. Varenna M, Manara M, Cantatore FP, et al. Determinants and effects of vitamin D supplementation on serum 25-hydroxy-vitamin D levels in patients with rheumatoid arthritis. *Clin Exp Rheumatol.* 2012;30(5):714–719.
159. Rossini M, Maddali Bongi S, La Montagna G, et al. Vitamin D deficiency in rheumatoid arthritis: prevalence, determinants and associations with disease activity and disability. *Arthritis Res Ther.* 2010;12(6):R216.
160. Racovan M, Walitt B, Collins CE, et al. Calcium and vitamin D supplementation and incident rheumatoid arthritis: the women's health initiative calcium plus vitamin D trial. *Rheumatol Int.* 2012; 32(12):3823–3830.
161. Mukherjee D, Lahiry S, Thakur S, Chakraborty DS. Effect of 1,25 dihydroxy vitamin D3 supplementation on pain relief in early rheumatoid arthritis. *J Fam Med Prim Care.* 2019;8(2):517–522.
162. Adami G, Rossini M, Bogliolo L, et al. An exploratory study on the role of vitamin D supplementation in improving pain and disease activity in rheumatoid arthritis. *Mod Rheumatol.* 2018:1–8.
163. Soubrier M, Lambert C, Combe B, et al. A randomised, double-blind, placebo-controlled study assessing the efficacy of high doses of vitamin D on functional disability in patients with rheumatoid arthritis. *Clin Exp Rheumatol.* 2018;36(6):1056–1060.
164. Alorainy M. Effect of allopurinol and vitamin e on rat model of rheumatoid arthritis. *Int J Health Sci.* 2008;2(1):59–67.
165. Dai W, Qi C, Wang S. Synergistic effect of glucosamine and vitamin E against experimental rheumatoid arthritis in neonatal rats. *Biomed Pharmacother.* 2018;105:835–840.
166. De Bandt M, Grossin M, Driss F, Pincemail J, Babin-Chevaye C, Pasquier C. Vitamin E uncouples joint destruction and clinical inflammation in a transgenic mouse model of rheumatoid arthritis. *Arthritis Rheum.* 2002;46(2):522–532.
167. Venkatraman JT, Chu WC. Effects of dietary omega-3 and omega-6 lipids and vitamin E on serum cytokines, lipid mediators and anti-DNA antibodies in a mouse model for rheumatoid arthritis. *J Am Coll Nutr.* 1999;18(6):602–613.
168. Edmonds SE, Winyard PG, Guo R, et al. Putative analgesic activity of repeated oral doses of vitamin E in the treatment of rheumatoid arthritis. Results of a prospective placebo controlled double blind trial. *Ann Rheum Dis.* 1997;56(11):649–655.
169. Aryaeian N, Djalali M, Shahram F, Djazayery A, Eshragian MR. Effect of conjugated linoleic Acid, vitamin e, alone or combined on immunity and inflammatory parameters in adults with active rheumatoid arthritis: a randomized controlled trial. *Int J Prev Med.* 2014;5(12):1567–1577.
170. Aryaeian N, Shahram F, Djalali M, et al. Effect of conjugated linoleic acid, vitamin E and their combination on lipid profiles and blood pressure of Iranian adults with active rheumatoid arthritis. *Vasc Health Risk Manag.* 2008;4(6):1423–1432.
171. Shishavan NG, Gargari BP, Kolahi S, Hajialilo M, Jafarabadi MA, Javadzadeh Y. Effects of vitamin K on matrix metalloproteinase-3 and rheumatoid factor in women with rheumatoid arthritis: a randomized, double-blind, placebo-controlled trial. *J Am Coll Nutr.* 2016;35(5):392–398.
172. Kolahi S, Pourghassem Gargari B, Mesgari Abbasi M, Asghari Jafarabadi M, Ghamarzad Shishavan N. Effects of phylloquinone supplementation on lipid profile in women with rheumatoid arthritis: a double blind placebo controlled study. *Nutr Res Pract.* 2015;9(2):186–191.
173. Ghamarzad Shishavan N, Pourghassem Gargari B, Asghari Jafarabadi M, Kolahi S, Haggifar S, Noroozi S. Vitamin K1 supplementation did not alter inflammatory markers and clinical status in patients with rheumatoid arthritis. *Int J Vitam Nutr Res.* 2019: 1–7.
174. Okamoto H, Shidara K, Hoshi D, Kamatani N. Anti-arthritis effects of vitamin K(2) (menaquinone-4)—a new potential therapeutic strategy for rheumatoid arthritis. *FEBS J.* 2007;274(17): 4588–4594.
175. Abdel-Rahman MS, Alkady EA, Ahmed S. Menaquinone-7 as a novel pharmacological therapy in the treatment of rheumatoid arthritis: a clinical study. *Eur J Pharmacol.* 2015;761:273–278.

176. Shivashankar R, Tremaine WJ, Harmsen WS, Loftus Jr EV. Incidence and prevalence of Crohn's disease and ulcerative colitis in Olmsted county, Minnesota from 1970 through 2010. *Clin Gastroenterol Hepatol*. 2017;15(6):857–863.
177. King JA, Underwood FE, Panaccione N, et al. Trends in hospitalisation rates for inflammatory bowel disease in western versus newly industrialised countries: a population-based study of countries in the Organisation for Economic Co-operation and Development. *Lancet Gastroenterol Hepatol*. 2019;4(4):287–295.
178. Aniwan S, Park SH, Loftus Jr EV. Epidemiology, natural history, and risk stratification of Crohn's disease. *Gastroenterol Clin N Am*. 2017;46(3):463–480.
179. Bamias G, Nyce MR, De La Rue SA, Cominelli F, American College of P, American Physiological S. New concepts in the pathophysiology of inflammatory bowel disease. *Ann Intern Med*. 2005;143(12):895–904.
180. Bar Yehuda S, Axlerod R, Toker O, et al. The association of inflammatory bowel diseases with autoimmune disorders: a report from the epi-IIRN. *J Crohns Colitis*. 2019;13(3):324–329.
181. Ramos GP, Papadakis KA. Mechanisms of disease: inflammatory bowel diseases. *Mayo Clin Proc*. 2019;94(1):155–165.
182. Van Limbergen J, Wilson DC, Satsangi J. The genetics of Crohn's disease. *Annu Rev Genom Hum Genet*. 2009;10:89–116.
183. Lewis JD, Abreu MT. Diet as a trigger or therapy for inflammatory bowel diseases. *Gastroenterology*. 2017;152(2), 398–414 e396.
184. Verway M, Behr MA, White JH. Vitamin D, NOD2, autophagy and Crohn's disease. *Expert Rev Clin Immunol*. 2010;6(4):505–508.
185. Ananthakrishnan AN, Khalili H, Higuchi LM, et al. Higher predicted vitamin D status is associated with reduced risk of Crohn's disease. *Gastroenterology*. 2012;142(3):482–489.
186. Ulitsky A, Ananthakrishnan AN, Naik A, et al. Vitamin D deficiency in patients with inflammatory bowel disease: association with disease activity and quality of life. *J Parenter Enter Nutr*. 2011;35(3):308–316.
187. Mozaffari H, Daneshzad E, Larijani B, Bellissimo N, Azadbakht L. Dietary intake of fish, n-3 polyunsaturated fatty acids, and risk of inflammatory bowel disease: a systematic review and meta-analysis of observational studies. *Eur J Nutr*. 2020;59(1):1–17.
188. Limketkai BN, Wolf A, Parian AM. Nutritional interventions in the patient with inflammatory bowel disease. *Gastroenterol Clin N Am*. 2018;47(1):155–177.
189. Levine A, Sigall Boneh R, Wine E. Evolving role of diet in the pathogenesis and treatment of inflammatory bowel diseases. *Gut*. 2018;67(9):1726–1738.
190. Fletcher J, Cooper SC, Ghosh S, Hewison M. The role of vitamin D in inflammatory bowel disease: mechanism to management. *Nutrients*. 2019;11(5).
191. Mora JR, Iwata M, von Andrian UH. Vitamin effects on the immune system: vitamins A and D take centre stage. *Nat Rev Immunol*. 2008;8(9):685–698.
192. Wang TT, Dabbas B, Laperriere D, et al. Direct and indirect induction by 1,25-dihydroxyvitamin D3 of the NOD2/CARD15-defensin beta2 innate immune pathway defective in Crohn disease. *J Biol Chem*. 2010;285(4):2227–2231.
193. Cantorna MT, Munsick C, Bemiss C, Mahon BD. 1,25-Dihydroxycholecalciferol prevents and ameliorates symptoms of experimental murine inflammatory bowel disease. *J Nutr*. 2000;130(11):2648–2652.
194. Froicu M, Cantorna MT. Vitamin D and the vitamin D receptor are critical for control of the innate immune response to colonic injury. *BMC Immunol*. 2007;8:5.
195. Kong J, Zhang Z, Musch MW, et al. Novel role of the vitamin D receptor in maintaining the integrity of the intestinal mucosal barrier. *Am J Physiol Gastrointest Liver Physiol*. 2008;294(1): G208–G216.
196. Tosiek MJ, Fiette L, El Daker S, Eberl G, Freitas AA. IL-15-dependent balance between Foxp3 and RORgammat expression impacts inflammatory bowel disease. *Nat Commun*. 2016;7:10888.
197. Kang SW, Kim SH, Lee N, et al. 1,25-Dihyroxyvitamin D3 promotes FOXP3 expression via binding to vitamin D response elements in its conserved noncoding sequence region. *J Immunol*. 2012;188(11):5276–5282.
198. Jorgensen SP, Agnholt J, Glerup H, et al. Clinical trial: vitamin D3 treatment in Crohn's disease – a randomized double-blind placebo-controlled study. *Aliment Pharmacol Ther*. 2010;32(3): 377–383.
199. Yang L, Weaver V, Smith JP, Bingaman S, Hartman TJ, Cantorna MT. Therapeutic effect of vitamin d supplementation in a pilot study of Crohn's patients. *Clin Transl Gastroenterol*. 2013;4:e33.
200. Calder PC. Marine omega-3 fatty acids and inflammatory processes: effects, mechanisms and clinical relevance. *Biochim Biophys Acta*. 2015;1851(4):469–484.
201. Scaioli E, Liverani E, Belluzzi A. The imbalance between n-6/n-3 polyunsaturated fatty acids and inflammatory bowel disease: a comprehensive review and future therapeutic perspectives. *Int J Mol Sci*. 2017;18(12).
202. Cabre E, Manosa M, Gassull MA. Omega-3 fatty acids and inflammatory bowel diseases - a systematic review. *Br J Nutr*. 2012; 107(Suppl 2):S240–S252.

CHAPTER

31

SPECIALIZED NUTRITION SUPPORT

Vivian M. Zhao[1], *PharmD*
Thomas R. Ziegler[1,2], *MD*

[1]Emory University Hospital Nutrition and Metabolic Support Service, Atlanta, GA, United State
[2]Division of Endocrinology, Metabolism and Lipids, Department of Medicine, Emory University School of Medicine, Atlanta, GA, United States

SUMMARY

Malnutrition is common in hospitalized patients and is associated with adverse clinical outcomes. A variety of factors commonly present in hospital patients contribute to protein–energy malnutrition and loss of essential vitamins, minerals, and electrolytes. Assessment of nutritional status requires comprehensive evaluation and integration of medical and surgical history, current clinical and fluid status, dietary intake patterns, body weight changes, gastrointestinal (GI) symptoms, physical examination, and selected biochemical tests. Current guidelines suggest that goals for caloric intake between 20 and 25 kcal/kg/day and protein/amino acids between 1.2 and 2.0 g/kg/day are appropriate for most adult hospital patients. Adequate vitamins, minerals, electrolytes, essential amino acids, and essential fatty acids must be provided based on recommended allowances for healthy individuals; however, true requirements in subtypes of hospital patients are unknown. The GI (enteral) route should be the first choice for specialized feeding in the hospital setting, with parenteral nutrition modalities, via peripheral or central vein, reserved for those patients in whom adequate enteral nutrition is not possible. Metabolic, infectious, and mechanical complications can occur with both enteral and parenteral feeding modalities and can be prevented or reduced with careful monitoring and adherence to current standards of practice. Relatively few rigorous, randomized controlled clinical trials have been conducted within the field of specialized feeding in the hospital setting, and many areas of uncertainty remain.

Keywords: Enteral nutrition; Malnutrition; Nutritional assessment; Parenteral nutrition.

I. INTRODUCTION

The incidence and prevalence of malnutrition, which includes significant loss of lean body mass and/or depletion of essential vitamins and minerals, are quite high in hospitalized patients.[1–7] Based on various observational studies of total hospital admissions and in intensive care unit (ICU) settings, malnutrition (depletion of essential micronutrients and/or loss of significant lean body mass or body weight) may occur in 20% to as high as 60% of patients.[4,8–12] Further, the incidence of malnutrition worsens over time in patients requiring prolonged hospitalization, in part due to inadequate ad libitum food intake and repeated catabolic insults.[9,13–15] Protein–energy malnutrition prior to and inadequate nutritional intake during hospitalization are each associated with higher rates of morbidity and mortality.[12,15–18] The importance of adequate macronutrient and micronutrient intake for optimal cellular, immune, and organ function is outlined elsewhere in this book. In highly catabolic ICU patients, protein–energy depletion has been associated with higher rates of hospital-acquired infection, poor wound healing, and skeletal muscle weakness.[3,6,12,16,18] Multiple pathophysiologic factors common in hospital patients put these individuals at risk for generalized protein–energy malnu-trition and/or micronutrient depletion[19] (see Box 31.1). The specialized enteral and parenteral nutrition

https://doi.org/10.1016/B978-0-12-818460-8.00031-9

BOX 31.1

Major pathophysiologic factors that contribute to malnutrition in hospital patients

- Decreased spontaneous food intake prior to or during hospitalization (e.g., due to anorexia, fatigue, gastrointestinal (GI) symptoms, NPO status).
- Increased concentrations of catabolic hormones and cytokines (e.g., cortisol, catecholamines, tumor necrosis factor-α, interleukins).
- Decreased blood concentrations of anabolic hormones (e.g., insulin-like growth factor I, testosterone).
- Resistance to anabolic hormones with consequent decreased substrate utilization (e.g., insulin resistance).
- Abnormal nutrient losses (e.g., wounds, drainage tubes, renal replacement therapy, diarrhea, emesis, polyuria).
- Decreased protein synthesis due to physical inactivity (e.g., bed rest, pharmacological paralysis).
- Drug–nutrient interactions (e.g., diuretics, pressor effects, corticosteroids).
- Increased energy, protein, and/or specific micronutrient requirements (e.g., with infection, trauma, oxidative stress).
- Iatrogenic factors related to prolonged periods of inadequate enteral or parenteral nutrient provision in relation to metabolic requirements.

NPO, nil per os (enteral food restriction due to diagnostic tests or therapeutic procedures).

(PN) support modalities that are currently available and that are the subject of this chapter have been developed to support vital cell and organ functions, muscle capacity, and wound healing. Both enteral nutrition (EN) and PN formulations provide fluid, calories (as various carbohydrate, protein/amino acid, and fat sources), essential amino acids and fats, electrolytes, vitamins, and minerals, as outlined below.

II. NUTRITIONAL ASSESSMENT

Important aspects of comprehensive nutritional assessment, which involves integration of multiple factors, are outlined in Box 31.2.[19] There is currently no "gold standard" for nutritional assessment in hospital patients. For example, blood concentrations of albumin and prealbumin, which may be useful in outpatient or epidemiologic settings, may be markedly decreased by inflammation, infection, decreased hepatic synthesis, and/or increased clearance from blood in hospital settings. Levels of these proteins in plasma may also be increased during fluid depletion or decreased with fluid overload. Blood concentrations of specific vitamins and minerals, as with blood electrolytes, are useful to follow in certain at-risk patients, but the possibility of changes due to fluid status and interorgan shifts necessitate serial monitoring to guide repletion strategies. Body weight often changes dramatically due to fluid status alterations.

A method to assess nutritional status, termed "Subjective Global Assessment" (SGA), has been validated as a way to assess nutritional status and to predict clinical outcomes in stable patients without marked fluid shifts.[20,21] The SGA incorporates patient history regarding body weight loss, usual dietary intake, functional capacity, GI symptoms, and physical-examination evidence of malnutrition (loss of muscle or fat mass, presence of edema) to classify patients as well nourished, moderately or suspected of being malnourished, or severely malnourished.[20,21] In Europe, a method of nutritional risk screening (NRS) is commonly utilized in hospital settings, which involves scoring risk based on body mass index (BMI), decrease in percent of usual food intake, body weight changes, age, and whether or not the patient is severely ill.[22,23] However, NRS is not yet validated for its use for ICU patients.[3] The NUTRIC (Nutrition Risk in Critically Ill) and modified NUTRIC scores are nutritional risk assessment tools developed and validated specifically for ICU patients; patients with high scores may benefit the most from advanced nutritional supplementation, based on data to date.[24–26] The NUTRIC score and modified NUTRIC score rapidly assess nutritional state based on illness severity, age, and comorbidities, with or without interleukin-6 concentrations in blood as a score parameter.[24,25] The American Society for Parenteral and Enteral Nutrition (ASPEN) and the Academy of Nutrition and Dietetics have also recommended a standardized, etiological set of diagnostic criteria be used to identify and document adult malnutrition in routine clinical practice.[26] Patient are diagnosed as malnourished when at least two of the following six criteria are met: inadequate dietary intake; recent weight loss; muscle loss; subcutaneous fat loss; present of localized or generalized edema; and weaken hand grip strength.

BOX 31.2

Important steps in nutritional assessment of hospitalized patients

- Review past medical and surgical history, tempo of current illness, and expected hospital course.
- Determine dietary intake pattern and history of use of specialized nutrition support.
- Obtain body weight history.
- Perform physical examination with attention to fluid status, organ functions, and evidence of protein–energy malnutrition or lesions consistent with vitamin and/or mineral deficiency.
- Evaluate GI tract function to evaluate ability to tolerate enteral feeding.
- Determine ambulatory capacity and mental status.
- Measure or evaluate standard blood tests (organ function indices, electrolytes, pH, triglycerides, and selected vitamins and minerals if at risk for depletion).
- Estimate current calorie and protein requirements.
- Evaluate options for enteral and parenteral access for nutrient delivery.

Patients with involuntary body weight loss of >5%–10% of usual body weight in the previous several weeks or months, patients weighing less than 90% of their ideal body weight, or those with a BMI less than 18.5 kg/m^2 should be carefully evaluated for malnutrition.

In recent years, various new technologies have been available and utilized to assess body composition to potentially provide unique methods to characterize ongoing nutrition status by providing real-time information on the adequacy of nutrition interventions.[26–28] The most commonly available clinical technologies for assessment of body composition include bioelectrical impedance analysis, computed tomography, dual-energy X-ray absorptiometry, and musculoskeletal ultrasound. Unfortunately, the utilization of these tools is limited by cost and accessibility, as well as standardized approaches to interpret results. With constant development of technologies, more clinical studies are needed to validate use in hospitalized patients. More details regarding methods of hospital-based comprehensive nutritional assessment are available.[19]

III. NUTRIENT INTAKE GOALS

Guidelines for energy and protein/amino acid intake in adult hospital patients have been outlined by nutrition-related professional societies.[3,6,27–29] Specific approaches for pediatric patients are beyond the scope of this chapter but have been recently published.[30,31] It is important to note that energy (calorie) needs in hospitalized patients, especially those who are critically ill, may vary considerably due to serial changes in clinical conditions.[3,6,29–31] Optimal caloric and protein/amino acid requirements in hospital patients are unknown due to a relative lack of rigorous, randomized, controlled clinical trials, necessitating the use of clinical judgment and clinical practice guidelines.[3,6,30–32]

Resting energy expenditure (REE) can be estimated using bedside metabolic cart measurements (indirect calorimetry), but technical issues can cause inaccuracies.[6,33] REE can be estimated using standard predictive equations, most commonly the Harris–Benedict equation, which incorporates the patient age, sex, weight, and height.[6,19,33,34] Unfortunately, this method may over- or underestimate REE in certain patients when clinical conditions are changing and/or with body weight changes due to changes in fluid status.[19,33] Recently published European and American Clinical Practice Guidelines suggest that an adequate energy goal for most patients can be estimated at 20–25 kcal/kg/day (using the most recent prehospital clinic body weight), which is approximately equivalent to measured or estimated REE × 1.0–1.2. Ongoing randomized controlled trials (RCTs) are designed to better define caloric dosing guidelines in ICU patients, as data are particularly conflicting in this clinical care setting. Prehospital and preoperative body weight should be used in energy intake estimates because measured body weight in the hospital (especially in the ICU) may reflect fluid status and is typically much higher than recent "dry" weight. An alternative is to use ideal body weight derived from routine tables or equations if recent dry weight is unavailable. In obese subjects, adjusted body weight should be used in the Harris–Benedict equation.[19] Published ASPEN guidelines recommend that in obese patients, caloric goals should start with hypocaloric feeds at 50%–70% of estimated REE (or <14 kcal/kg actual weight), and the recommended protein/amino acid dose may be started with 1.2 g/kg actual weight or 2–2.5 g/kg ideal body weight.[31]

Studies conducted in the 1980s in ICU patients indicate that protein intake of more than 2.0 g/kg/day are not efficiently utilized for protein synthesis and the excess is oxidized and contributes to azotemia.[35,36] The commonly recommended protein/amino acid dose range is 1.2–1.5 g/kg/day for most individuals with normal renal and hepatic function (50%–100% above the RDA of 0.8 g/kg/day); although, some guidelines recommend higher doses (up to 2.0–2.5 g/kg/day) in specific conditions such as burns and in patients requiring renal replacement therapy.[3,6,19,30] The administered protein/amino acid dose should be adjusted downward depending on the degree and tempo of azotemia (in the absence of renal replacement therapy). Patients with evidence of acute liver failure and encephalopathy are at risk for amino acid–induced increases in arterial blood ammonia concentrations. In such patients, it may be prudent to provide lower doses of EN/PN protein/amino acids (0.6–1.2 g/kg/day), based on the degree of liver dysfunction. Dietary protein restriction is not currently recommended in stable patients with chronic liver failure.

IV. ENTERAL NUTRITION SUPPORT

Whenever possible, EN in hospital patients should consist of oral diets with regular foods as tolerated, supplemented as indicated with the wide variety of commercially available flavored oral liquid formulations or solid nutrient–rich products. Most hospital patients should also receive a complete multivitamin–mineral product to cover needs, although this recommendation is not evidence-based. Enteral tube feeding is the preferred route of nutritional delivery for patients who have a functional GI tract but are unable to maintain adequate nutrient intake with voluntary oral intake. The current Society for Critical Care Medicine (SCCM) and ASPEN guideline recommends starting early EN (within 24–48 h) in ICU patients who cannot tolerate adequate oral intake.[6]

EN is more physiologic, associated with less severe infectious, metabolic, and mechanical complications, and less costly than PN.[6,15,37] Specific indications for EN in adults and children are described in clinical practice guidelines.[15,19,26–30] Although not evidence-based, common contraindications to EN include inability to gain access to the GI tract, intestinal obstruction, intractable vomiting, severe diarrhea, diffuse peritonitis, paralytic ileus, bowel ischemia, and hemodynamic instability requiring mid- to high-dose vasopressors.[3,15,16,19]

EN administration must be individualized to each patient's specific needs. In order to determine the appropriate EN delivery method, GI tract integrity and functional capacity, presence and degree of malnutrition, underlying disease states, and patient tolerance must be assessed prior to and following the initiation of tube feeding. GI, mechanical, and metabolic complications, as well as pulmonary aspiration of feeds, can occur with enteral tube feeding. It is therefore essential to monitor enterally fed patients closely in order to identify complications.[38]

A. Routes for Enteral Tube Feeding

Successful enteral tube feeding is in part dependent upon selection of the appropriate enteral access device and placement technique. Understanding the indications, contraindications, advantages, and disadvantages of each different access device for enteral feedings will allow clinicians to select the best delivery method for patients. Commercially available feeding tubes vary in materials and diameters (5–24 French). Small-bore tubes (5–12 French) are usually made of polyurethane, silicone, or a mixture of the two, whereas large-bore tubes (≥14 French) are usually made of polyvinyl, which is a stiffer material.[39,40] Compared with small-bore tubes, the large-bore tubes are more uncomfortable for patients, but they are less prone to clog.[41] In addition, large-bore tubes are easier to use for aspirating gastric contents than small-bore tubes due to their larger diameters. The tubes are typically classified according to insertion site (nasal, oral, percutaneous) and location of the terminal end of the enteral device (stomach, duodenum, proximal small bowel) (Table 31.1). Orogastric and nasogastric tubes are large-bore tubes, which are commonly placed at bedside. Oroenteral and nasoenteral tubes may be inserted blindly at the bedside by experienced personnel or with the assistance of endoscopy, fluoroscopy, radiology, or with bedside devices such as ultrasound, carbon dioxide sensor, and electromagnetic devices.[40] Gastrostomy and jejunostomy tubes can be placed endoscopically, fluoroscopically, laparoscopically, and percutaneously. Surgeons may also place the feeding tube intraoperatively when patients have preexisting moderate or severe malnutrition and/or are anticipated to require prolonged support after operation.[39] Radiographic verification of correct placement of a blindly inserted small- or large-bore feeding tube is mandatory before administering feeding and medications.[39,41–43] Nasal or oral tubes are usually placed for short-term (<4–6 weeks) use, whereas tube enterostomies are typically placed for long-term (≥4 weeks) EN support.[27,39–43]

The selection of an enteral access route depends on patient-specific factors, including comorbidities, GI anatomy with consideration of prior surgery, gastric and intestinal motility and function, risk of aspiration, and the anticipated duration of therapy.[27,39–44] Although some studies suggested postpyloric feeding is associated with

TABLE 31.1 Advantages and disadvantages of different enteral nutrition access routes.

Route	Indications	Advantages	Disadvantages
Nasoenteric (NE) tube feeding (short term, <4 weeks)			
Orogastric (OG)	Intubated and sedated; Chemically paralyzed	Easy to place tube	Patient discomfort
Nasogastric (NG)	Normal gastric emptying No esophageal reflux Gastric decompression Medication administration	Easy to place tube Larger reservoir capacity in stomach	Highest aspiration risk Tube displacement
Nasoduodenal (ND)	Gastroparesis Impaired gastric emptying Esophageal reflux (see NJ below)	Lower aspiration risk than NG	May require endoscopic placement Tube displacement Potential aspiration
Nasojejunal (NJ)	Gastric dysfunction	May initiate feedings immediately after injury or operation	Potential GI intolerance (bloating, cramping, diarrhea)
	Pancreatitis	Possible lower aspiration risk than NG in some patients	Potential aspiration
Tube enterostomy (long-term feeding required)			
Gastrostomy	See NG	Can be placed during GI surgery	Surgery is needed for surgical gastrostomies Tube dislodgement
Percutaneous[a] gastrostomy (PEG)	No NE route available Persistent dysphasia	No surgery needed for PEG PEG less costly than surgical gastrostomy	Requires stoma care
Operative laparoscopic[b] gastrostomy	Patient already in operating room for another surgical procedure	Lower tube occlusion risk with large-bore tube	Potential complications: • Aspiration risk • Stoma site skin infection • Skin excoriation at stoma site • Fistula following tube removal
Jejunostomy	See NJ	Lower aspiration risk	Requires stoma care
Percutaneous[a] endoscopic jejunostomy (PEJ)	High aspiration risk Esophageal reflux Intolerance of gastric feeding	Can be placed during GI surgery No surgery needed for PEJ	Tube occlusion with small-bore tube or needle catheter
Needle catheter jejunostomy (NCJ)	Inability to access upper GI tract (esophagus, stomach, duodenum)	PEJ less costly than surgical jejunostomy	Surgery required for jejunostomy placement
Operative laparoscopic jejunostomy		May initiate feeding immediately after operation	Potential complications: • GI intolerance • Stoma site infection • Skin excoriation at stoma site • Fistula following tube removal

[a]*Percutanously placed tubes avoid risks of surgery and general anesthesia; however, these may require endoscopy, abdominal ultrasound, or radiologic procedure with contrast media. Endoscopy may be difficult in the presence of a tumor or stricture, altered anatomy, or severe obesity.*
[b]*Laparoscopically or operatively placed tubes require general anesthesia; however, patients may be able to return home on the same day after the procedure.*

lower risk of pneumonia and increased nutrition delivery than gastric feeding, most studies showed no significant difference in clinical outcomes, including mortality, ICU length of stay, incidence of pneumonia, and/or ventilator days.[6] The current guidelines do not provide a consensus recommendation for the preferred routes of gastric versus postpyloric, hence the selection of feeding tubes is based on clinician and practice preference.[3,6]. Gastric feedings generally require a functional stomach without delayed gastric emptying, obstruction, or fistula. Small-bowel feedings are most appropriate for patients with gastroparesis, gastric outlet obstruction, prior pancreatitis, known esophageal reflux, and high aspiration risk. Although nasojejunal feedings are not required unless patients have gastric feeding intolerance, small-bowel feedings have been associated with a significant reduction in ventilator-associated pneumonia in some, but not all, studies.[38] Combined gastrojejunal tubes are indicated when gastric decompression is needed, but jejunal feeding is possible, as occurs in patients who have impaired gastric motility but normal small-bowel motility and absorption.[38,44]

B. Tube Feeding Formula Selection

Once an enteral route has been established for the initiation of tube feeding, an appropriate formula must be selected. There are numerous commercially available products, which fall into one of the following categories: standardized or polymeric, hydrolyzed, caloric-dense, fiber-enriched, fat-modified, disease-specific, immune-modulated, and powdered formulas, to meet the various needs of most patients (Table 31.2).[45] EN formulas vary in terms of caloric density, composition of macronutrients, macronutrient digestibility, viscosity, osmolarity, and cost. The polymeric formulas contain intact protein, complex carbohydrates, long- and medium-chain triglycerides, vitamins, minerals, and trace elements. All formulations are lactose- and gluten-free, and most are low residue as well as isotonic or slightly hypertonic, with a caloric content ranging from 1 to 2 kcal/mL.

Because of the variations between enteral formulas, a systematic comparison of the patient-specific variables and nutrient needs with the specific characteristics of the available formulas can be used to select an appropriate formula that will most approximate the individual's estimated requirements. Patient-specific variables include clinical status, nutritional status and requirements, metabolic abnormalities, digestive and absorptive capacity of the GI tract, disease state, expected outcomes, and possible routes available for administration. The simple consideration of a medical diagnosis with a specifically marketed formula can result in the administration of inappropriate nutrition support product and an increased cost of nutrient provision.

Most hospital patients can be safely fed with standard, inexpensive, polymeric, enteral formulas (Table 31.2). The more calorically dense mixtures are useful for patients requiring fluid restriction. The addition of soluble fiber in enteral products is increasingly common in commercial formulas and may prevent constipation or control diarrhea. Available research in the role of fiber-enriched formulas in the management of diarrhea, however, has not demonstrated consistent benefit, possibly because a myriad of factors can cause diarrhea in hospital patients (e.g., antibiotics).[46] The polymeric formulas are usually tolerated as well as, or better than, much more expensive hydrolyzed formulas.[47,48] Hydrolyzed formulas, which contain hydrolyzed casein or whey as the protein source (also known as oligomeric, semi-elemental, or peptide-based), are designed for patients with malabsorption and pancreatic insufficiency. Clinical data documenting the advantages of routine use of peptide-based formulas are limited; however, their use in patients with acute pancreatitis in one study showed a significantly shorter hospital length of stay when compared with polymeric formulas.[49]

Commercial enteral formulas have been developed for use in disease-specific conditions such as diabetes, renal failure, and pulmonary disease,. Diabetes-specific formulas are developed with lower amounts of carbohydrate and higher amounts of fat as energy sources to improve glycemic control; some studies show that their use in hospitalized diabetic patients resulted in improved blood glucose control and decreased insulin requirements.[50–52] Renal-specific products are available for patients with different degrees of renal failure (presence or absence of renal replacement therapy) (Table 31.2). Several RCTs suggest that formulas containing increased amounts of antioxidant nutrients (e.g., vitamins C and E) and anti-inflammatory lipids (e.g., eicosapentanoic acid, gammalinolenic acid) result in improved clinical outcomes compared with standard EN formulations in patients with adult respiratory distress syndrome (ARDS),[30,53] although results of a recent Phase II trial of omega-3 fatty acid enriched EN showed no benefit.[54] A variety of so-called "immune-modulating" EN formulations are commercially available and are supplemented with, typically, a combination of glutamine, arginine, omega-3 fatty acids, probiotics, and or/antioxidants.[38,45] Most recently, plant-based enteral formulas, which contain soluble fiber without dairy, soy, gluten, corn, nuts, artificial sweetener or additives, have become available and are gaining interest, however, there are limited data available to evaluate benefits.[55,56] Individuals with allergies to specific constituents in the standard EN formulations may benefit from these newer plant-based EN formulations. Routine use of EN "immune-modulating" formulations remains controversial because of inconsistent results (especially in ICU patients) and lack of effects on mortality.[57,58]

TABLE 31.2 Examples of commercially available enteral nutrition formulas in the United States.

Categories	Potential indications	kcal (per mL)	Protein (g/L)	Fat (g/L)	Carbohydrate (g/L)	% Water	Osmolality (mOsm/kg H_2O)
Polymeric							
Standard (e.g., Osmolite; Isosource)	Most patients	1.0	44	35	144	84	300
		1.2	56	39	158	82	360
		1.5	63	49	204	76	525
Caloric dense (e.g., TwoCal HN)	Fluid-restricted	2.0	84	90	218	70	725
Fiber-enriched (e.g., Jevity; Fibersource HN)	Diarrhea	1.0	44	35	155	84	300
		1.2	56	39	169	82	450
		1.5	63	49	216	76	525
Hydrolyzed							
Semielemental/peptide-based (e.g., Crucial; Peptamen)	Pancreatitis, malabsorption	1.0	40–51	28–39	127–138	83–85	300–585
Disease-specific							
Immune-modulating (e.g., Impact with Glutamine)	Immunosuppressed, critical illness	1.3	78	43	150	81	630
Oxepa	Adult respiratory distress syndrome	1.5	63	94	105	79	535
Nepro	Renal failure, on dialysis	1.8	81	96	167	73	600
Suplena	Renal failure, predialysis	1.8	45	96	202	73	600
Glucerna	Diabetes	1.0	42	54	95.6	85	355
		1.2	60	60	114.5	81	720
		1.5	82	75	133.1	76	875
Promote	Wound healing	1.0	62	26–28	130.0–138	84	340–380

This table does not constitute an all-inclusive list. Information provided by manufacturers.

However, metaanalyses in GI surgery patients suggest that use of some of these "immune-modulating" formulations results in lower rates of hospital total complications and infections and decreased length of hospital stay compared with standard EN products.[59]

C. Methods of Tube Feeding Administration

In the initial administration of tube feeding, diluting enteral formulas is not necessary. The practice of diluting formulas is more likely to promote microbial growth than full-strength formulations and increases the risk of intolerance due to diarrhea secondary to microbial contamination.[38] There are limited data to form recommendations for the best starting rate for enteral feeding at initiation and should be based on clinician judgment and clinical conditions. EN can be administered as rate-based (cc/hr) continuous 24 h feeds, as bolus feeds, or, in clinically stable patients as "cycled" feeds over 12–16 h (Table 31.3).

Continuous feedings are delivered over 24 h via gravity drip or with the assistance of an enteral infusion device (electronic feeding pump). A feeding pump is more advantageous than gravity drip because it can enhance safety and accuracy in delivery by sustaining a constant infusion rate and accidental bolus delivery unlikely to occur. Most commercially available formulas are well tolerated at full strength when delivered into the stomach or small intestine at 10–30 mL/h. The infusion rate can generally be advanced in increments of 10–20 mL/h every 8–12 h as tolerated until goal rate is reached.[38] Medically stable patients can tolerate a fairly rapid progression of infusion rate and achieve the goal rate within 24–48 h of initiation. There is also evidence to support starting EN at goal rates in stable adult patients.[60,61] Continuous administration is usually better tolerated, with lower incidence of GI intolerance and risk of aspiration than bolus tube feeds in hospital settings. Continuous infusion may be necessary for postpyloric feedings because the small bowel cannot act as a reservoir for large feeding volumes over a short period of time. Hospitalized patients may initially benefit from a continuous infusion to establish tolerance and later transition to an intermittent bolus or cyclic infusion schedule.

Bolus and cycled feedings are the most physiologic feeding techniques because they mimic normal dietary habits, take advantage of physiologic gastric emptying, and allow bowel rest in between feedings[38] (Table 31.3). These are the easiest to deliver and can be administered over a short period of time via syringe bolus or a feeding container by gravity drip or with an enteral feeding pump.[62] Bolus feedings generally deliver the formula in less than 15 min, whereas intermittent feedings deliver it over 30–45 min. The feeding is initiated with full-strength formula three to eight times daily with increases of 60–120 mL every 8–12 h as tolerated up to the goal volume of 250–500 mL per feeding, four to six times daily. Bolus and intermittent methods are primarily reserved for medically stable patients with gastric feeding tubes because the stomach acts as a reservoir to handle relatively large volumes within a short time. Feedings provided by this method may result in adverse GI effects (pain, diarrhea) due to the sudden delivery of a large, hyperosmolar formula.[38,62]

TABLE 31.3 Methods of administration of enteral tube feeding.

Method	Indications	Advantages	Disadvantages
Continuous	Initiation of feeding Critically ill patient Small-bowel feeding Intermittent or bolus feeding intolerance	Pump-assisted Enhances tolerance Minimizes risk due to • high gastric residual • aspiration • metabolic abnormalities	Restricts ambulation Increased cost due to equipment and supplies
Bolus—intermittent	Noncritically ill patient Home TF Rehabilitation patient Gastric feeding	Ease of administration No pump required Short feeding time Most physiological	Highest aspiration risk Potential GI intolerance (nausea, vomiting, abdominal pain, diarrhea)
Cyclic—intermittent	Noncritically ill patient Home TF Rehabilitation patient Small-bowel feeding	Physical and psychological freedom from pump Beneficial for transitioning TF to oral diet	Requires high infusion rate over short time (8–16 h) May require formula with higher calorie and protein density to meet needs Potential GI intolerance
Volume-based	Critically ill patient	Mitigates feeding deficits Reaches nutrition goal quickly	Requires a well-written nurse-driven protocol/algorithm

GI, gastrointestinal; *TF*, tube feeding.

Cyclic feedings are defined as continuous infusion in an intermittent fashion, for which the formula is infused continuously over a set number of hours (i.e., 8–16 h). Tube feedings can be cycled for patients with duodenal or jejunal feeding tubes, patients who are transitioning from tube to oral feeding (in which cycled feeding may stimulate appetite), or for those requiring eventual home EN. A cyclic feeding schedule allows bowel rest, free time off the pump, and flexibility to administer EN overnight and discontinue during the day to afford the patient greater mobility and an opportunity to eat oral food.

Underfeeding is common with EN using the traditional rate-based delivery method due to frequent interruptions for various reasons, such as holding EN for diagnostic testing, procedures, medication administrations, etc. Volume-based feeding (VBF) in one recent delivery method developed to improve nutrition deficits. VBF orders are written with a total volume for a 24-hour period (e.g., 1000 mL/day) with a maximum compensatory rate 150 mL/h with or without an end-of-day bolus given to replace remaining deficits. The usual rate and volumes are individualized to meet patient's nutrition needs, and the nurses follow an algorithm/protocol to adjust the delivery rate to make for interruptions. In recent years, several studies have compared and evaluated the effectiveness and clinical outcome between the widely used rate-based feeding versus VBF.[6,62,63] VBF has shown to be safe as well as improved delivery to better energy needs without increasing complications, such as feeding intolerance, mortality, ICU length of stay, ventilation days, or hyperglycemia.[63,64] However, large, multicenter randomized controlled studies are needed to determine evidence-based outcomes related to improved nutrition delivery.

Of note, a recent study in 46 Australian and New Zealand ICUs compared clinical outcomes in patients receiving energy-dense (1.5 kcal/mL) EN, which provided 1863 ± 478 kcal per day of EN versus routine EN (1.0 kcal/mL) that provided 1262 ± 313 kcal/day.[64] Results showed no difference in the primary end point (90-day survival) or any other predefined clinical outcomes between the two groups.[64] Also, a recent randomized study of 894 clinically similar critically ill adults with medical or surgical issues at seven academic centers assigned patients to permissive underfeeding (40%–60% of calculated energy needs) versus standard EN (70%–100% of calculated energy needs), with similar daily protein intake (approximately 60 g/day).[65] During intervention, the permissive underfed group received 835 ± 297 kcal/day versus 1299 ± 467 kcal/day in the standard group; no difference in mortality or other clinical outcomes occurred.[65]

Regardless of the delivery technique, most patients on EN will require additional fluid to meet minimum fluid requirements (typically 30–40 mL/kg body weight). Supplemental fluid (i.e., sterile water or normal saline) is administered intermittently as flushes throughout the day (i.e., flush tube with at least 30 mL every 8 h). To calculate additional fluid requirements, begin by determining the patient's total fluid needs. Then, determine that amount of free water provided by the tube feeding formula by multiplying the percent free water content by the total volume of enteral formula to be administered daily (Table 31.2). Subtraction of the free water supplied by the formula from the calculated total free water requirement equals the remaining volume of free water required. The remaining volume is divided into three or four boluses per day.[66–69]

D. Complications of Enteral Tube Feeding

While the administration of EN may appear less complex compared with PN, it is not without potential complications. Serious harm and death can result due to issues occurring throughout the process of ordering, administering, and monitoring. Complications include GI intolerance, mechanical tube complications, bronchopulmonary aspiration, enteral access device misplacement and displacement, metabolic abnormalities, and drug–nutrient interactions.[38,70,71] The acceptable ranges for gastric residual volumes (GRVs) at which to decrease tube feeding rates have been reevaluated in recent years, and higher amounts than previous routine have been advocated based on available data.[72] Many clinicians feel that if the GRV is ≥ 250 mL after two consecutive gastric residual checks, a promotility agent should be considered in adult patients. However, no adequately powered studies have to date demonstrated that elevated GRVs are reliable markers for increased risk of aspiration pneumonia.[72] The current SCCM/ASPEN guidelines for nutrition support in critical illness do not recommend checking GRV as a sign of GI intolerance.[6] Nonetheless, in clinical practice, gastric residuals are checked more frequently (i.e., every 4–6 h for the first 48 h) when gastric feedings are first initiated and clinical judgment coupled with residual volume dictates EN tube feeding rate changes (typically made by the primary nurses). After the desired gastric feeding rate is established, gastric residual monitoring may be decreased to every 6–12 h in the noncritically ill patients.[72] Patient positioning, use of postpyloric continuous feeding, and judicious use of prokinetic agents (e.g., metoclopramide or erythromycin) have been advocated as important to prevent pulmonary aspiration of tube feeding in patients demonstrating intolerance (e.g., emesis, gastric distention).[44,73] Patients should be monitored frequently for evidence of

TABLE 31.4 Complications of tube feeding.

Complications	Possible causes	Possible management
Gastrointestinal		
Diarrhea (>4 bowel movements per day or large loose stool)	Medications (e.g., antibiotics) Formula intolerance Bacterial overgrowth Osmotic overload Decreased bulk *Clostridium difficile*	Medication modifications: • Eliminate antibiotics, antacids, liquid formulations containing sorbitol. • Further dilute hypertonic medications. • Administer medications by intravenous route. • Administer bulking agents (e.g., psyllium). • Administer probiotics. • Administer antidiarrheal agents.[a] Stool culture for pathogens. Feeding modifications: • Change to a low-fat, high-fiber, or isotonic formula. • Decrease concentration of formula or rate.
Nausea or vomiting	Patient position Volume overload Delayed gastric emptying Nutrient intolerances GI tract obstruction Hyperglycemia	Elevate head of bed to 35–45 degrees. Position patient on right side to facilitate passage of gastric contents through pylorus. Medication modifications: • Consider reducing narcotic use. • Administer prokinetic agents (i.e., metoclopramide). • Consider antiemetic. Feeding modification: • Decrease total volume or delivery rate. • Advance delivery rate slowly over 12–24 h. • Stop feeding for 2 h and check residuals. • Change to lactose-free or low-fat formula.
Constipation	Dehydration Decreased fiber GI obstruction	Change to fiber formula. Administer bulking agents. Tube flush with water. Stop feeding temporarily.
Mechanical		
Pulmonary aspiration	Supine position Impaired gag reflex Reflux Tube malposition or displacement Abnormal mental status	Elevate head of bed 30–45 degrees. Infuse feedings into the duodenum or jejunum Change to smaller bore tube. Radiographic confirmation for proper placement after insertion and after severe coughing, vomiting, or a seizure. Tape tube in place and mark with indelible ink at exit point for reference. Reconfirm placement prior to each feeding by checking residuals, ink mark.
Tube obstruction	Acid precipitation of formula Insufficient tube irrigation Medications	Flush tube before and after each medication, residual check, bolus feeding, and every 8 h during continuous feeding, or whenever feeding is stopped. Infuse feedings into the duodenum or jejunum. Do not mix medications with enteral formula. Adequately crush meds and mix powder with water. Use liquid meds where possible or administer via alternative route. Avoid administering bulk-forming agents via small-bore tube.

[a]*Begin antidiarrheal agent only when infectious and inflammatory etiologies and fecal impaction have been ruled out and causal hypertonic medications (e.g., acetaminophen elixir) have been changed or discontinued.*

complications from EN support. Table 31.4 lists common potential complications of tube feedings and suggested inter-ventions.

Feeding tubes are prone to clogging for a variety of reasons, including use of small-bore feeding tubes, improper medication administration, and formula sediment accumulation in the lower segment of the tube, especially during slow administration rates of caloric-dense or fiber-enriched formulas.[43,62] Most clogging can be prevented by use of a clean technique to minimize formula contamination, and adherence to protocols for proper flushing of tubes before and after each medication administration. Water is the preferred flush solution (e.g., every 4 h) during continuous feeding, before and after intermittent feedings, or after residual volume measurements in an adult patient.[43,62] Use of sterile water for tube flushes in immunocompromised or critically ill patients, especially when the safety of tap water cannot be reasonably assumed, is recommended.[62] The recommended first-line method to unclog an EN tube is to instill warm water using slight manual pressure. Flushing with a combination of pancrelipase and sodium bicarbonate solution or with carbonated soda drink may dissolve the clog.[62]

Metabolic complications of EN are similar to those that occur during PN, although the incidence and severity may be less. As with PN, outlined below, prevention of refeeding syndrome and monitoring patient tolerance of EN are essential for the safe delivery of EN.[74] Monitoring metabolic parameters prior to the initiation of enteral feedings and periodically during enteral therapy should be based on protocols and patient underlying disease state and length of therapy. Patients at risk of developing refeeding syndrome should be identified, and severe electrolyte abnormalities should be corrected prior to the initiation of nutrition support.

V. PARENTERAL NUTRITION SUPPORT

As with EN support, relatively few well-designed, adequately powered RCTs on PN efficacy in hospital settings have been published.[75–80] Thus, practices of PN use in hospital patients are largely based on guidelines from professional societies, which in turn are largely derived from observational studies, small clinical trials, and expert opinion.[3,6,15,28–30] A caveat regarding efficacy of PN is that no rigorous RCT has featured an unfed or minimally fed control group. Such studies would be difficult to perform, particularly as the clinical effect of various durations of minimal or no feeding is unknown in the modern ICU and other hospital settings.[80] Also, many of the earlier RCTs in nutrition support provided excessive PN caloric doses and less stringent blood glucose control strategies compared with current practice. Nonetheless, available data suggest that patients with moderate to severe generalized malnutrition benefit from PN in terms of overall morbidity and possibly mortality when EN is not possible.[19]

A. Indications for Parenteral Nutrition

Although not evidence-based, commonly accepted indications for PN in hospital patients when EN is not appropriate or not tolerated (especially in already malnourished patients) are as follows: (1) following massive small bowel $\pm$ colonic resection; (2) with perforated small bowel or a proximal high-output fistula; and (3) in other conditions associated with prolonged intolerance to EN (e.g., severe diarrhea or emesis, significant abdominal distention, partial or complete bowel obstruction, or acute GI bleeding, severe hemodynamic instability) precluding adequate EN for >3–7 days.[3,6,19] There are no data to support withholding of PN in patients with preexisting protein–energy malnutrition who cannot tolerate EN. However, a large RCT from Belgium (4640 patients) explored the impact of timing of PN initiation in adult ICU patients receiving inadequate amounts of early enteral feeding.[79] In the early initiation group, supplemental PN to meet the caloric goal of 25–30 kcal/kg/day was started on ICU day 2, according to 2009 European clinical practice guidelines.[3] In the late-initiation group, supplemental PN to meet the caloric goal of 25–30 kcal/kg/day was started on ICU day 7, according to 2009 American clinical practice guidelines.[6] The early initiation of PN was associated with modestly increased ICU and hospital length of stay, infectious complications, indices of organ dysfunction, and total hospital costs.[79,80]

In a more recent study in critically ill children by the same Belgian group, early initiation of PN (within 24 h after admission to the ICU) was associated with higher hospital morbidity rates than the group in which PN was initiated on the eighth day after ICU admission.[81] Of interest, a study in 2388 critically ill adults admitted to 1 of 33 English ICUs with functional GI tracts randomly assigned patients to either EN or PN in a pragmatic randomized trial.[82] Results showed that there were no differences between the EN and PN groups in terms of caloric intake or in clinical outcomes; this study suggests that, when properly administered, PN administration is safe in ICU patients.[82]

Contraindications for PN (largely not evidence-based) include (1) when the GI tract is functional and access for enteral feeding is available; (2) if the patient cannot tolerate the intravenous fluid load required for PN, or has severe hyperglycemia or severe electrolyte abnormalities on the planned day of PN initiation; (3) when PN is unlikely to be required for >5–7 days; and (4) if new placement of an intravenous line solely for PN poses undue risks (Singer et al., 2009,[3,6,19]).

B. Parenteral Nutrition Administration

PN can be delivered as complete solutions given by either peripheral or central vein. A comparison of typical fluid, macronutrient and micronutrient content, and characteristics of peripheral and central vein PN is

TABLE 31.5 Composition of typical parenteral nutrition formulations.

Component	Peripheral vein PN	Central vein PN
Volume (L/day)	2–3	1–1.5
Dextrose (%)	5	10–25
Amino acids (%)	2.5–3.5	3–8
Lipid (%)	3.5–5.0	2.5–5.0
Sodium (meq/L)	50–150	50–150
Potassium (meq/L)	20–35	30–50
Phosphorus (mmol/L)	5–10	10–30
Magnesium (meq/L)	8–10	10–20
Calcium (meq/L)	2.5–5	2.5–5
Vitamins[a]		
Trace elements/minerals[b]		

[a]*Vitamins typically added on a daily basis to peripheral vein and central vein PN are comprised of commercial mixtures of vitamins A, B1 (thiamin), B2 (riboflavin), B3 (niacinamide), B6 (pyridoxine), B12, C, D, and E, biotin, folate, and pantothenic acid. Vitamin K is added on an individual basis (e.g., in patients with cirrhosis). Specific vitamins can also be supplemented individually.*
[b]*Trace elements/minerals typically added on a daily basis to the peripheral vein and central vein PN are comprised of commercial mixtures of chromium, copper, manganese, selenium, and zinc. Minerals can also be supplemented individually.*

shown in Table 31.5. Because of the risk of phlebitis, peripheral vein PN provides lower amounts of dextrose (5%; dextrose = 3.4 kcal/g) and amino acids (≤3.5%; 4 kcal/g), and a large proportion of the caloric content is given as fat emulsion (50%–60% of total calories).[15] Fluid restriction due to cardiac, hepatic, and/or renal dysfunction may be a contraindication to the use of larger fluid volumes for PN; thus, peripheral vein PN is generally not indicated in ICU patients as larger volumes are required to meet energy and amino acid goals. Central venous PN allows concentrated dextrose and amino acid delivery via the superior vena cava. Adequate energy and amino acid intake in the vast majority of adults can thus be achieved with central venous volumes of 1–1.5 L/day (Table 31.5). Depending on fluid status, non-PN hydration fluid rate should be proportionally decreased when PN is infused.[6,15]

PN electrolytes are adjusted as indicated to maintain serially measured serum levels within the normal range. With elevated blood concentrations, lower doses (or elimination) of specific electrolytes, as compared with the typical ranges outlined in Table 31.5, may be indicated until blood values are within the normal range. Higher dextrose concentrations in central vein PN may increase potassium, magnesium, and phosphorus requirements. The relative percentage of sodium and potassium salts as chloride is increased to correct metabolic alkalosis, and the percentage of these salts as acetate is increased to correct metabolic acidosis. Tighter blood glucose control in ICU and other hospital patients is now the standard of care (<180 mg/dL).[83–85] To achieve these goals, regular insulin can be added to PN and/or the dextrose load can be reduced as needed (separate intravenous insulin infusions are commonly required with hyperglycemia in ICU settings).[19,86]

Conventional PN provide nine essentials amino acids and several nonessential amino acids, depending on the commercial amino acid formulation used.[32,87] Although controversial, some authors recommend addition of glutamine as a conditionally essential amino acid in some ICU patients, given the evidence that this amino acid may become conditionally essential in certain catabolic patients.[3,32,87,88] The dose of amino acids is adjusted downward or upward in relation to goal amounts as a function of the degree of azotemia or hyperbilirubinemia in patients with acute renal and hepatic failure, respectively. For patients with renal failure, specialized amino acid formulations containing mainly or only essential amino acid are available for use. For patients with hepatic failure, clinicians can use the specialized amino acid mixtures with increased amounts of branched-chain amino acids and decreased amounts of methionine, phenylalanine, and tryptophan.[87]

Complete PN provides intravenous lipid emulsions (IVFs) as a source of both energy and essential linoleic and linolenic fatty acids. In the United States, historically, the commercially available lipid emulsion is soybean oil (SO)–based; now, an intravenous SO/olive oil emulsion, an intravenous SO/medium-chain triglyceride mixture, a fish oil/medium-chain triglyceride/olive oil/SO emulsion, and a fish oil–based emulsion have been approved for use in PN. The different formulations vary in the fatty acid content, composition of the emulsion, and dosing.[89] The use of SO-based emulsions have been associated with elevated serum bilirubin levels, intestinal failure associated liver disease, and cholestasis in some patients, particularly at chronic doses exceeding 1.0 g/kg/day.[89] It is thought that the amount of polyunsaturated fatty acids, alpha-tocopherol, and phytosterol amounts in alternative products may alleviate or reduce the impact on the liver.[89–91] Recent reviews of fish oil–containing IVF lowered inflammatory markers, improved triglyceride levels and liver enzymes, and reduced infectious complications, morbidity, and mortality in ICU patients.[92–94] When compared with SO-based IVF, olive oil–based IVFs are a safe alternative, but clinical and metabolic differences between these two IVF were not statistically significant.[92,93,95]

Lipid is typically mixed with dextrose and amino acids in the same PN infusion bag ("all-in-one" solution) and given with PN over 16–24 h. Lipid emulsion may also be infused separately from the main PN bag over 10–12 h. The maximal recommended dose of lipid emulsion infusion in adults is 1.0–1.3 g/kg/day, with monitoring of blood triglyceride levels at baseline and then approximately weekly and as indicated to assess clearance of intravenous fat.[15,19,28] Triglyceride levels should be maintained below 400–500 mg/dL by decreasing the amount of lipid infused to decrease risk of pancreatitis and diminished pulmonary diffusion capacity in patients with severe chronic obstructive lung disease (Box 31.3). In central venous PN, a reasonable initial guideline is to provide 60%–70% of non–amino acid calories as dextrose and 30%–40% of non–amino acid calories as fat emulsion.[6,15,19,28]

Specific requirements for intravenous vitamins and minerals have not been rigorously defined in hospital patients.[3,6,14,19,80] Therapy is therefore guided at meeting published recommended doses that maintain blood concentrations in the normal range in most patients using commercially available intravenous preparations of combined vitamins and minerals (Table 31.5). However, several studies show that a significant proportion of ICU patients receiving conventional PN or EN nutrition support variously exhibit low blood zinc, copper, selenium, vitamin C, vitamin E, and vitamin D concentrations.[1,2,7] This may be due to pre-ICU admission nutrient depletion, increased ICU requirements (possibly secondary to oxidative stress), increased excretion, and/or tissue redistribution. Essential nutrient depletion may impair antioxidant capacity, immunity, wound healing, and other important nutrient-related body functions. Thus, as with electrolytes, therapy is directed at maintaining normal blood status, with serial monitoring in blood as clinically and biochemically indicated.

PN formulations can be prepared under a sterile hood by trained hospital pharmacists, but commercially prepared formulations are also available. PN is administered by infusion pump to control delivery rates, and the infusion catheters incorporate an in-line filter to prevent microbial contamination.

C. Clinical Monitoring of Parenteral Nutrition

Monitoring of PN therapy in the hospital setting requires daily assessment of the multiple factors outlined in Boxes 31.1 and 31.2. Blood glucose should be monitored several times daily, and blood electrolytes and renal function tests should generally be determined daily. Blood triglyceride levels should be measured at baseline and then weekly until stable. Although guidelines are few, some centers routinely monitor periodic blood levels of copper, selenium, zinc, whole blood thiamin (vitamin B_1), vitamin B6, vitamin C, retinol, and 25-hydroxyvitamin D.[7,19] Liver function tests should be measured at least a few times weekly. pH should be monitored generally daily in ventilated patients when arterial blood gas pH measurements are available; blood carbon dioxide ($C0_2$) concentrations are a surrogate marker for acid–base status (low $C0_2$ levels = acidosis; high $C0_2$ levels = alkalosis).[19] Frequent monitoring of blood glucose, electrolytes, and organ function is routine in the ICU setting.

D. Adverse Effects of Parenteral Nutrition

Metabolic, infectious, and mechanical complications may occur with PN.[19,28,96–101] Mechanical complications, particularly with central venous catheters, include pneumothorax, hemothorax, thrombosis, and bleeding

BOX 31.3

Characteristics of overfeeding and the refeeding syndrome in patients receiving PN

- Extracellular to intracellular shift of magnesium, phosphorus, and/or potassium due to excess dextrose infusion and refeeding hyperinsulinemia.
- Immune cell dysfunction and infection (hyperglycemia).
- Cardiac failure or arrhythmias (excess fluid, excess sodium and other electrolytes, refeeding-induced electrolyte shifts).
- Neuromuscular dysfunction (thiamin depletion, refeeding-induced electrolyte shifts).
- Azotemia (excess amino acid, inadequate PN total energy supplied in relation to amino acid dose).
- Fluid retention (excess fluid, sodium, refeeding hyperinsulinemia).
- Elevated liver function tests and/or hepatic steatosis (excess kilocalories, dextrose or fat).
- Increased blood ammonia levels (excess amino acids with liver failure).
- Hypercapnia (excess total kilocalories).
- Respiratory insufficiency (refeeding-induced hypophosphatemia, excess fluid, kilocalories, carbohydrate or fat).
- Hypertriglyceridemia (excess carbohydrate or fat).

with insertion. Catheter-related bloodstream infections can occur in PN patients and are not uncommon in these individuals, who typically have other risk factors for infection. For example, in a recent study of 1325 patients receiving PN in a tertiary-care hospital over a 12-year period, the catheter-related bloodstream infection rate was 10–13 per 1000 central venous catheter days, depending on the criteria used.[99] Proper and safe administration of both peripheral and central vein PN requires strict catheter care and nursing care protocols, including use of dedicated catheter ports for PN administration and subclavian vein insertion sites for central venous PN.[15,19,28]

Potential metabolic and clinical consequences of overfeeding and refeeding syndrome during central venous PN in critically ill patients are shown in Box 31.3. High calorie, dextrose, amino acid, and fat doses ("hyperalimentation") are readily administered via a central vein. While not the standard of care based upon current guidelines, administration of excess dextrose, fat, and total calorie remains a common practice in some centers.[15,28] Risk factors for PN-associated hyperglycemia include (1) use in obese, diabetic, and/or septic patients; (2) poorly controlled blood glucose at PN initiation; (3) initial use of high dextrose concentrations (>10%) or dextrose load (>150 g/day); (4) insufficient insulin administration and/or inadequate monitoring of blood glucose; and (5) concomitant administration of corticosteroids and pressor agents.[6,28]

Electrolyte administration requires careful monitoring and general day-to-day adjustment in PN to maintain normal blood levels. Overfeeding can induce several metabolic complications of varying degrees of severity affecting several organ systems (Box 31.3). A large study found that PN use per se, overfeeding, and sepsis were the major risk factors for liver dysfunction in critically ill patients.[97] Elevated transaminases and eventual PN-induced liver dysfunction that may lead to hepatic failure occur with PN administration, especially in individuals receiving chronic PN therapy.[28] The mechanisms for PN-induced liver dysfunction remain unclear but are probably multifactorial.[28] Of interest, some studies suggest that switching from conventional soybean oil–based lipid emulsion to fish oil–based lipid emulsion was associated with decreased PN-associated liver failure in children receiving chronic PN, but mechanisms remain obscure.[98] PN should be advanced carefully to goal rates and the composition adjusted as appropriate based on the results of close daily metabolic and clinical monitoring performed daily. The calories provided by dextrose present in non-PN intravenous fluids, the SO lipid emulsion carrier of propofol, a commonly used intravenous ICU sedative, and clevidipine, an intravenous calcium-channel blocker, as well as the nutrients provided in any administered EN, must be taken into account in the PN prescription to avoid caloric or electrolyte overfeeding.

Refeeding syndrome is relatively common in at-risk patients (alcoholic dependency, preexisting malnutrition or electrolyte depletion, recent significant body weight loss, prolonged periods of intravenous hydration therapy alone, or administration of insulin or diuretics prior to refeeding).[96,100–103] In a study of at-risk hospital patients given EN, PN, or both, 25% of 92 patients developed refeeding-induced hypophosphatemia.[101] In a recent systemic review, involving a total of 6608 patients, the incidence of refeeding syndrome was reported as high as 80% based on various definitions.[102] Refeeding syndrome is mediated by administration of excessive intravenous dextrose (>150–250 g or 1 L of PN with 15%–25% dextrose). This markedly stimulates insulin release, which may rapidly decrease blood potassium, magnesium, and especially phosphorus concentrations due to intracellular shift and utilization in metabolic pathways.[96,100–103] High doses of carbohydrate increase thiamin utilization and can precipitate symptoms of thiamin deficiency. Hyperinsulinemia may cause sodium and fluid retention by the kidney. This, together with decreased blood electrolyte concentrations (which can cause cardiac arrhythmias), can result in heart failure, especially in patients with preexisting heart disease.[96,100–103] Prevention of refeeding syndrome requires identification of at-risk patients, use of initially low PN dextrose (e.g., 1 L.d of PN with 10% dextrose), empiric provision of higher PN doses of potassium, magnesium, and phosphorus, based on blood levels and renal function, and supplemental PN thiamin (e.g., 100 mg/day for 3–5 days),[19,74,101].

Consultation with an experienced multidisciplinary nutrition support team for recommendations regarding the PN prescription is ideal when such personnel are available. Nutrition support team daily monitoring has been shown to reduce complications and costs and to decrease inappropriate use of PN.[104–106]

VI. FUTURE DIRECTIONS

Numerous areas of uncertainty remain with regard to administration of specialized EN and PN, despite routine use in hospitals and other settings. For example, the optimal timing for EN and PN initiation in hospital patients remains areas of uncertainty. Few prospective data are available on the clinical effects of minimal or no feeding over time (e.g., >7 days), and such data are unlikely to be forthcoming. Rigorous RCTs are needed to define optimal caloric and protein/amino acid dose regimens in subgroups of ICU and non-ICU patients. Some studies show that larger doses of standard soybean oil–based intravenous fat emulsions induce proinflammatory and prooxidative effects and possibly immune suppression. However, conflicting results of small RCTs comparing soybean oil–based lipid emulsion with other types of lipid emulsion have not clarified optimal use. Available data suggest that glutamine may become a conditionally essential amino acid in ICU patients. Glutamine serves as an important fuel for immune and gut mucosal cells and has cytoprotective properties among other potentially beneficial functions. Several clinical trials have shown that glutamine-supplemented PN (0.2–0.5 g/kg/day as the L-amino acid or as glutamine dipeptides) has protein-anabolic effects, enhances indices of immunity, and decreases hospital infections. Thus, some expert panels recommend that glutamine be routinely added to PN in ICU patients, if available. However, a large RCT in adults with severe critical illness showed that very high doses of supplemental glutamine, given concomitantly via enteral and parenteral routes worsened clinical outcomes.[107] Phase III level, double-blind, intent-to-treat RCTs are needed in specific ICU patient subgroups to define clinically optimal calorie, protein/amino acid, and specific vitamin and mineral requirements, as well as to determine the efficacy of supplemental PN combined with EN to achieve caloric and protein/amino acid goals. In addition, rigorous trials to verify proposed "pharmaconutrition" strategies (e.g., use of high doses of supplemental parenteral and enteral glutamine, vitamin C and other antioxidants, selenium, and/or zinc, etc.) are also needed.[108]

Additional sources of information are available in the published literature.[109]

V. REFERENCES

1. Nathens AB, Neff MJ, Jurkovich GJ, et al. Randomized, prospective trial of antioxidant supplementation in critically ill surgical patients. *Ann Surg*. 2002;236:814–822.
2. Luo M, Fernandez-Estivariz C, Jones DP, et al. Depletion of plasma antioxidants in surgical intensive care unit patients requiring parenteral feeding: effects of parenteral nutrition with or without alanyl-glutamine dipeptide supplementation. *Nutrition*. 2008;24:37–44.
3. Singer P, Blaser AR, Berger MM, et al. ESPEN guidelines on clinical nutrition in the intensive care unit. *Clin Nutr*. 2019;38:48–79.
4. Barker LA, Gout BS, Crowe TC. Hospital malnutrition: prevalence, identification and impact on patients and the healthcare system. *Int J Environ Res Public Health*. 2011;8:514–527.
5. De Luis DA, López Mongil R, Gonzalez Sagrado M, et al. Nutritional status in a multicenter study among institutionalized patients in Spain. *Eur Rev Med Pharmacol Sci*. 2011;15:259–265.
6. McClave SA, Taylor BE, Martindale RG, et al. Guidelines for the provision and assessment of nutrition support therapy in the adult critically ill patient: Society of Critical Care Medicine (SCCM) and American Society for Parenteral and Enteral Nutrition (A.S.P.E.N.). *JPEN J Parenter Enter Nutr*. 2016;40: 159–211.
7. Blaauw R, Osland E, Sriram K, et al. Parenteral provision of micronutrients to adult patients: an expert consensus paper. *JPEN J Parenter Enter Nutr*. 2019;43(1 suppl):S5–S23.
8. Giner M, Laviano A, Meguid MM, et al. In 1995 a correlation between malnutrition and poor outcome in critically ill patients still exists. *Nutrition*. 1996;12:23–29.
9. Pirlich M, Schütz T, Norman K, et al. The German hospital malnutrition study. *Clin Nutr*. 2006;25:563–572.
10. Konturek PC, Herrmann HJ, Schink K, et al. Malnutrition in hospitals: it was, is now, and must not remain a problem!. *Med Sci Monit*. 2015;21:2969–2975.
11. Allard JP, Keller H, Jeejeebhoy KN, et al. Decline in nutritional status is associated with prolonged length of stay in hospitalized patients admitted for 7 days or more: a prospective cohort study. *Clin Nutr*. 2016;35(1):144–152.
12. Kang MC, Kim JH, Ryu SW, et al. Prevalence of malnutrition in hospitalized patients: a multicenter cross-sectional study. *J Korean Med Sci*. 2018;33(2):e10.
13. Rinninella E, Ruggiero A, Maurizi P, Triarico S, Cintoni M, et al. Clinical tools to assess nutritional risk and malnutrition in hospitalized children and adolescents. *Eur Rev Med Pharmacol Sci*. 2017; 21:2690–2701.
14. Patel MD, Martin FC. Why don't elderly hospital inpatients eat adequately? *J Nutr Health Aging*. 2008;12:227–231.
15. Druyan ME, Compher C, Boullata JL, et al. Clinical guidelines for the use of parenteral and enteral nutrition in adult and pediatric patients: applying the GRADE system to development of ASPEN clinical guidelines. *JPEN J Parenter Enter Nutr*. 2012; 36(1):77–80.
16. Schneider SM, Veyres P, Pivot X, et al. Malnutrition is an independent factor associated with nosocomial infections. *Br J Nutr*. 2004; 92:105–111.
17. O'Brien Jr JM, Phillips GS, Ali NA. Body mass index is independently associated with hospital mortality in mechanically ventilated adults with acute lung injury. *Crit Care Med*. 2006;34: 738–744.
18. Zaloga GP. Parenteral nutrition in adult inpatients with functioning gastrointestinal tracts: assessment of outcomes. *Lancet*. 2006;367:1101–1111.
19. Ziegler TR. Parenteral nutrition in the critically ill patient. *N Engl J Med*. 2009;361:1088–1097.
20. Detsky AS, McLaughlin JR, Baker JP, et al. What is subjective global assessment of nutritional status? *JPEN J Parenter Enter Nutr*. 1987;11:8–13.
21. Norman K, Schütz T, Kemps M, et al. The Subjective Global Assessment reliably identifies malnutrition-related muscle dysfunction. *Clin Nutr*. 2005;24:143–150.
22. Kondrup J, Allison SP, Elia M, et al. ESPEN guidelines for nutrition screening 2002. *Clin Nutr*. 2002;22:415–421.
23. Rasmussen HH, Holst M, Kondrup J. Measuring nutritional risk in hospitals. *Clin Epidemiol*. 2010;2:209–216.
24. Heyland DK, Dhaliwal R, Jiang X, et al. Identifying critically ill patients who benefit the most from nutrition therapy: the development and initial validation of a novel risk assessment tool. *Crit Care*. 2011;15:R268.
25. de Vries MC, Koekkoek WK, Opdam MH, et al. Nutritional assessment of critically ill patients: validation of the modified NUTRIC score. *Eur J Clin Nutr*. 2018;72:428–435.
26. Jeong DH, Hong SB, Lim CM, et al. Comparison of accuracy of NUTRIC and modified NUTRIC scores in predicting 28-days mortality in patients with sepsis: a single center retrospective study. *Nutrients*. 2018;10:911.
27. Heyland DK, Drover JW, Dhaliwal R, et al. Optimizing the benefits and minimizing the risks of enteral nutrition in the critically ill: role of small bowel feeding. *JPEN J Parenter Enter Nutr*. 2002; 26(6 Suppl):S51–S57.
28. Sheean P, Gonzalez MC, Prado CM, et al. American Society for Parenteral and Enteral Nutritional Clinical Guidelines: the validity of body composition assessment in clinical populations. *JPEN J Parenter Enter Nutr*. 2019. https://doi.org/10.1002/jpen.1669.

29. Kreymann KG, Berger MM, Deutz NE, et al. ESPEN guidelines on enteral nutrition: intensive care. *Clin Nutr.* 2006;25:210–223.
30. Mehta NM, Skillman HE, Irving SY, et al. Guidelines for the provision and assessment of nutrition support therapy in the pediatric critically ill patient: Society of Critical Care Medicine and American Society for Parenteral and Enteral Nutrition. *JPEN J Parenter Enter Nutr.* 2017;41:706–742.
31. Choban P, Dickerson R, Malone A, et al. A.S.P.E.N. Clinical guidelines: nutrition support for hospitalized adult patients with obesity. *JPEN J Parenter Enter Nutr.* 2013;37:714–744.
32. Yarandi SS, Zhao VM, Hebbar G, et al. Amino acid composition in parenteral nutrition: what is the evidence? *Curr Opin Clin Nutr Metab Care.* 2011;14:75–78.
33. Anderegg BA, Worrall C, Barbour E, et al. Comparison of resting energy expenditure prediction methods with measured resting energy expenditure in obese, hospitalized adults. *JPEN J Parenter Enter Nutr.* 2009;33:168–175.
34. Parker EA, Feinberg TM, Wappel S, et al. Considerations when using predictive equations to estimate energy needs among older, hospitalized patients: a narrative review. *Curr Nutr Rep.* 2017;6: 102–110.
35. Shaw JH, Wildbore M, Wolfe RR. Whole body protein kinetics in severely septic patients. The response to glucose infusion and total parenteral nutrition. *Ann Surg.* 1987;205:288–294.
36. Streat SJ, Beddoe AH, Hill GL. Aggressive nutritional support does not prevent protein loss despite fat gain in septic intensive care patients. *J Trauma.* 1987;27:262–266.
37. Allen K, Hoffman L. Enteral nutrition in the mechanically ventilated patient. *Nutr Clin Pract.* 2019;34:540–557.
38. Boullata J, Carrera A, Harvey L, et al. ASPEN safe practices for enteral nutrition therapy. *JPEN J Parenter Enter Nutr.* 2017;41:36–46.
39. Minard G. Enteral access. *Nutr Clin Pract.* 1994;9:172–182.
40. Pash E. Enteral nutrition: options for short-term access. *Nutr Clin Pract.* 2018;33:170–176.
41. Kozeniecki M, Fritzshall R. Enteral nutrition for adults in the hospital setting. *Nutr Clin Pract.* 2015;30:634–651.
42. Baskin WN. Acute complications associated with bedside placement of feeding tubes. *Nutr Clin Pract.* 2006;21:40–55.
43. DeLegge MH. Enteral access and associated complications. *Gastroenterol Clin N Am.* 2018;47:23–37.
44. Metheny NA, Clouse RE, Chang YH, et al. Tracheobronchial aspiration of gastric contents in critically ill tube-fed patients: frequency, outcomes, and risk factors. *Crit Care Med.* 2006;34:1–9.
45. Brown B, Roehl K, Betz M. Enteral nutrition formula selection: current evidence and implications for practice. *Nutr Clin Pract.* 2015;30:72–85.
46. Yang G, Wu XT, Zhou Y, et al. Application of dietary fiber in clinical enteral nutrition: a meta-analysis of randomized controlled trials. *World J Gastroenterol.* 2005;11:3935–3938.
47. Ford E, Hull S, Jenning L, et al. Clinical comparison of tolerance to elemental or polymeric enteral feedings in the postoperative patient. *J Am Coll Nutr.* 1992;11:11–16.
48. Mowatt-Larssen C, Brown R, Wojtysial S, et al. Comparison of tolerance and nutritional outcome between a peptide and a standard formula in critically ill, hypoalbuminemic patients. *JPEN J Parenter Enter Nutr.* 1992;16:20–24.
49. Tiengou LE, Gloro R, Pouzoulet J, et al. Semi-elemental formula or polymeric formula: is there a better choice for enteral nutrition in acute pancreatitis? Randomized comparative study. *JPEN J Parenter Enter Nutr.* 2006;30:1–5.
50. Leon-Sanz M, Garcia-Luna PP, Planas M, et al. Glycemic and lipid control in hospitalized type 2 diabetic patients: evaluation of 2 enteral nutrition formulas (low carbohydrate-high monosaturated fat vs. high carbohydrate). *JPEN J Parenter Enter Nutr.* 2005;29:21–29.
51. Pohl M, Mayr P, Mertl-Roetzer M, et al. Glycaemic control in type II diabetic tube-fed patients with a new enteral formula low in carbohydrates and high in monosaturated fatty acids: a randomized controlled trial. *Eur J Clin Nutr.* 2005;59:1121–1132.
52. Alish CJ, Garvey WT, Maki KC, et al. A diabetes-specific enteral formula improves glycemic variability in patients with type 2 diabetes. *Diabetes Technol Ther.* 2010;12:419–425.
53. Gadek JE, DeMichele SJ, Karlstad MD, et al. Effect of enteral feeding with eicosapentaenoic acid, gamma-linolenic acid and antioxidants in patients with acute respiratory distress syndrome. Enteral nutrition in ARDS study group. *Crit Care Med.* 1999;27: 1409–1420.
54. Stapleton RD, Martin TR, Weiss NS, et al. A phase II randomized placebo-controlled trial of omega-3 fatty acids for the treatment of acute lung injury. *Crit Care Med.* 2011;39:1655–1662.
55. Yeh A, Conners EM, Ramos-Jimenez RG, et al. Plant-based enteral nutrition modifies the gut microbiota and improves outcomes in murine models of colitis. *Cell Mol Gastroenterol Hepatol.* 2019;7:872–874.
56. McClanahan D, Yeh A, Firek E, et al. Pilot study of the effect on plant-based enteral nutrition on the gut microbiota in chronically ill tube-fed children. *JPEN J Parenter Enter Nutr.* 2019;43:899–911.
57. Marik PE, Zaloga GP. Immunonutrition in critically ill patients: a systematic review and analysis of the literature. *Intensive Care Med.* 2008;34:1980–1990.
58. Dupertuis YM, Meguid MM, Pichard C. Advancing from immunonutrition to pharmaconutrition: a gigantic challenge. *Curr Opin Clin Nutr Metab Care.* 2009;12:398–403.
59. Cerantola Y, Hübner M, Grass F, et al. Immunonutrition in gastrointestinal surgery. *Br J Surg.* 2011;98:37–48.
60. Rees RG, Keohane PP, Grimble GK, et al. Tolerance of elemental diet administered without starter regimen. *Br Med J.* 1985;290: 1869–1870.
61. Mentec H, Dupont H, Bocchetti M, et al. Upper digestive intolerance during enteral nutrition in critically ill patients: frequency, risk, factors, and complications. *Crit Care Med.* 2001;29:1922–1961.
62. Lord LM. Restoring and maintaining patency of enteral feeding tubes. *Nutr Clin Pract.* 2003;18:422–426.
63. Roberts S, Brody R, Rawal S, et al. Volume-based vs rate-based enteral nutrition in the intensive care unit: impact on nutrition delivery and glycemic control. *Nutr Clin Pract.* 2018;33:170–176.
64. TARGET Investigators for the ANZICS Clinical Trials Group, Chapman M, Peake SL, Bellomo R, et al. Energy-dense versus routine enteral nutrition in the critically ill. *N Engl J Med.* 2018; 379:1823–1834.
65. Arabi VM, Aldawood AS, Haddad SH, et al. Permissive underfeeding or standard enteral feeding in critically ill adults. *N Engl J Med.* 2015;372:2398–2408.
66. Hirai F, Takeda T, Takada Y, et al. Efficacy of enteral nutrition in patients with Crohn's disease on maintenance anti-TNF-alpha antibody therapy: a meta-analysis. *J Gastroenterol.* 2019. https://doi.org/10.1007/s00535-019-01634-1.
67. Fetterplace K, Gill BMT, Chapple LS, Presneill JJ, MacIsaac C, Deane AM. Systematic review with meta-analysis of patient-centered outcomes, comparing international guideline-recommended enteral protein delivery with usual care. *JPEN J Parenter Enter Nutr.* 2019. https://doi.org/10.1002/jpen.1725 [Epub ahead of print].
68. Brown BD, Hoffman SR, Johnson SJ, Nielsen WR, Greenwaldt HJ. Developing and maintaining an RDN-led bedside feeding tube placement program. *Nutr Clin Pract.* 2019. https://doi.org/10.1002/ncp.10411 [Epub ahead of print].
69. Di Caro S, Fragkos KC, Keetarut K, et al. Enteral nutrition in adult crohn's disease: toward a paradigm shift. *Nutrients.* 2019;(9):11. https://doi.org/10.3390/nu11092222. pii:E2222.
70. Malone AM, Seres DS, Lord L. Complications of enteral nutrition. In: Gottschlich MM, ed. *The ASPEN Nutrition Support Core Curriculum: A Case-Based Approach – the Adult Patient.* Silver Spring, MD: American Society of Parenteral and Enteral Nutrition; 2007: 246–263.

71. Guenter P, Hicks RW, Simmons D, et al. Enteral feeding misconnections: a consortium position statement. *Jt Comm J Qual Patient Saf.* 2008;34:285–292.
72. Hurt RT, McClave SA. Gastric residual volumes in critical illness: what do they really mean? *Crit Care Clin.* 2010;26:481–490.
73. Torres A, Serra-Batlles J, Ros E, et al. Pulmonary aspiration of gastric contents in patients receiving mechanical ventilation: the effect of the body position. *Ann Intern Med.* 1992;116: 540–543.
74. Stanga Z, Brunner A, Leuenberger M, et al. Nutrition in clinical practice—the refeeding syndrome: illustrative cases and guidelines for prevention and treatment. *Eur J Clin Nutr.* 2008;62:687–694.
75. Doig GS, Simpson F, Delaney A. A review of the true methodological quality of nutritional support trials conducted in the critically ill: time for improvement. *Anesth Analg.* 2005;100:527–533.
76. Doig GS, Simpson F, Sweetman EA. Evidence-based nutrition support in the intensive care unit: an update on reported trial quality. *Curr Opin Clin Nutr Metab Care.* 2009;12:201–206.
77. Koretz RL. Parenteral nutrition and urban legends. *Curr Opin Gastroenterol.* 2008;24:210–214.
78. Koretz RL. Enteral nutrition: a hard look at some soft evidence. *Nutr Clin Pract.* 2009;24:316–324.
79. Loss SH, Franzosi OS, Nunes DSL, Teixeira C, Viana LV. Seven deadly sins of nutrition therapy in critically ill patients. *Nutr Clin Pract.* 2019. https://doi.org/10.1002/ncp.10430 [Epub ahead of print].
80. Ziegler TR. Nutrition support in critical illness – bridging the evidence gap. *N Engl J Med.* 2011;365:562–564.
81. Fivez T, Kerklaan D, Mesotten D, et al. Early versus late parenteral nutrition in critically ill children. *N Engl J Med.* 2016;374: 1111–1122.
82. Harvey SE, Parrott F, Harrison DA, et al. Trial of the route of early nutritional support in critically ill adults. *N Engl J Med.* 2014;371: 1673–1684.
83. NICE–SUGAR Study Investigators, Finfer S, Chittock DR, et al. Intensive versus conventional glucose control in critically ill patients. *N Engl J Med.* 2009;360:1283–1297.
84. Kavanagh BP, McCowen KC. Clinical practice. Glycemic control in the ICU. *N Engl J Med.* 2010;363:2540–2546.
85. McMahon MM, Nystrom E, Braunschweig C, et al. A.S.P.E,N. Clinical guidelines: nutrition support of adult patients with hyperglycemia. *JPEN J Parenter Enter Nutr.* 2013;37:23–36.
86. McCulloch A, Bansiya V, Woodward JM. Addition of insulin to parenteral nutrition for control of hyperglycemia. *JPEN J Parenter Enter Nutr.* 2018;42:846–854.
87. Hoffer LJ. Parenteral nutrition: amino acids. *Nutrients.* 2017;9: 257–266.
88. van Zanten AR, Hofman Z, Heyland DK. Consequences of the REDOXS and METAPLUS trials: the end of an era of glutamine and antioxidant supplementation for critically ill patients? *JPEN J Parenter Enter Nutr.* 2015;39:890–892.
89. Gabe SM. Lipids and liver dysfunction in patients receiving parenteral nutrition. *Curr Opin Clin Nutr Metab Care 16.* 2013: 150–155.
90. Anez-bustillos L, Dao DT, Baker MA, et al. Intravenous fat emulsion formulations for the adult and pediatric patient: understanding the differences. *Nutr Clin Pract.* 2016;31:596–609.
91. Jones CJ, Calder PC. Influence of different intravenous lipid emulsions on fatty acid status and laboratory and clinical outcomes in adult patients receiving home parenteral nutrition: a systematic review. *Clin Nutr.* 2018;37:285–291.
92. Edmunds CE, Brody RA, Parrott JS, et al. The effects of different IV fat emulsions on clinical outcomes in critically ill patients. *Crit Care Med.* 2014;42:1168–1177.
93. Manzanares W, Langlois PL, Hardy G. Intravenous lipid emulsions in the crucially ill: an update. *Curr Opin Crit Care.* 2016;22: 308–315.
94. Honeywell S, Zelig R, Radler DR. Impact of intravenous lipid emulsions containing fish oil on clinical outcomes in critically ill surgical patients: a literature review. *JPEN J Parenter Enter Nutr.* 2019;26:112–122.
95. Umpierrez GE, Spiegelman R, Zhao V, et al. A double-blind, randomized clinical trial comparing soybean oil-based versus olive oil-based lipid emulsions in adult medical-surgical intensive care unit patients requiring parenteral nutrition. *Crit Care Med.* 2012;40:1792–1798.
96. Solomon SM, Kirby DF. The refeeding syndrome: a review. *JPEN J Parenter Enter Nutr.* 1990;14:90–97.
97. Grau T, Bonet A, Rubio M, et al. Liver dysfunction associated with artificial nutrition in critically ill patients. *Crit Care.* 2007;11:R10.
98. Biesboer AN, Stoehr NA. A product review of alternative oil-based intravenous fat emulsions. *Nutr Clin Pract.* 2016;31: 610–618.
99. Madnawat H, Welu AL, Gilbert EJ, Taylor DB, Jain S, et al. Mechanisms of parenteral nutrition-associated liver and gut injury. *Nutr Clin Pract.* 2020;35:63–71.
100. Byrnes MC, Stangenes J. Refeeding in the ICU: an adult and pediatric problem. *Curr Opin Clin Nutr Metab Care.* 2011;14:186–192.
101. Zeki S, Culkin A, Gabe SM, et al. Refeeding hypophosphataemia is more common in enteral than parenteral feeding in adult in patients. *Clin Nutr.* 2011;30:365–368.
102. Friedli E, Stanga Z, Sobotka L, et al. Revisiting the refeeding syndrome: results of a systemic review. *Nutrition.* 2017;35: 151–160.
103. Friedli N, Stanga Z, Culkin A, et al. Management and prevention of refeeding syndrome in medical inpatients: an evidence-based and consensus-supported algorithm. *Nutrition.* 2018;47:13–20.
104. Trujillo EB, Young LS, Chertow GM, et al. Metabolic and monetary costs of avoidable parenteral nutrition use. *JPEN J Parenter Enter Nutr.* 1999;23:109–113.
105. Kennedy JF, Nightingale JM. Cost savings of an adult hospital nutrition support team. *Nutrition.* 2005;21:1127–1133.
106. Cong MH, Li SL, Cheng GW, et al. An interdisciplinary nutrition support team improves clinical and hospitalized outcomes of esophageal cancer patients with concurrent chemoradiotherapy. *Chin Med J (Engl).* 2015;128:3003–3307.
107. Heyland D, Muscedere J, Wischmeyer PE, et al. A randomized trial of glutamine and antioxidants in critically ill patients. *N Engl J Med.* 2013;368:1489–1497.
108. Wischmeyer PE, Heyland DK. The future of critical care nutrition therapy. *Crit Care Clin.* 2010;26:433–441.
109. ASPEN Board of Directors and Enteral Nutrition Practice Recommendations Task Force. Enteral nutrition practice recommendations. *JPEN J Parenter Enter Nutr.* 2009;33:122–167.

CHAPTER

32

NUTRITION SUPPORT IN CRITICALLY ILL ADULTS AND CHILDREN

Sharon Y. Irving[1], PhD, CRNP, FCCM, FAAN
Liam McKeever[2], PhD, RDN, LDN
Vijay Srinivasan[3], MBBS, MD, FAAP, FCCM
Charlene Compher[4], PhD, RD, CNSC, LDN, FADA, FASPEN

[1]University of Pennsylvania School of Nursing, Nurse Practitioner, Department of Critical Care Nursing, Children's Hospital of Philadelphia, Philadelphia, PA, United States
[2]Department of Biostatistics, Epidemiology, & Informatics, Perelman School of Medicine, University of Pennsylvania, Philadelphia, PA, United States
[3]Department of Anesthesiology, Critical Care and Pediatrics, Perelman School of Medicine, University of Pennsylvania, Philadelphia, PA, United States
[4]University of Pennsylvania School of Nursing and Clinical Nutrition Support Service at the Hospital of the University of Pennsylvania, Philadelphia, PA, United States

SUMMARY

Gastrointestinal physiology involves an intricate network of mechanical, hormonal, and motility functions, including enzymatic secretions, and acid production that work in concert to ensure the breakdown of ingested food for utilization by the body. In critical illness, this delicate interplay is disrupted with marked alterations in absorptive physiology and energy metabolism. This combination of changes necessitates a careful and nuanced approach to nutritional therapy for critically ill patients. The preillness nutrition status of the patient determines their ability to withstand and survive the critical illness state. Nutrition assessment is essential to characterize and define the nutrition status of the patient, determine appropriate nutrient intake goals, and identify the best mode for nutrient delivery. This chapter describes the current state of knowledge and evidence for the provision of nutritional therapy in the ICU patient and explains the nutritional relevance of selected diseases common to adult and pediatric ICU patients.

Keywords: Adult; Critical care nutrition; Critical illness; Energy expenditure; ICU adult nutrition; ICU pediatric nutrition; Nutrition assessment; Nutrition support; Pediatric.

I. CHANGES IN FUNCTION AND PHYSIOLOGY DURING CRITICAL ILLNESS

A. Introduction

Changes in gastrointestinal (GI) physiology and metabolism of critically ill patients may lead to intolerance of enteral formulas and nutritional deficits. During health, GI physiology involves an intricate network of mechanical, hormonal, and motility functions involving enzymatic secretions and acid production that work in concert to ensure the breakdown of ingested food for utilization by the body and promotion of homeostasis in healthy individuals. During critical illness, key

https://doi.org/10.1016/B978-0-12-818460-8.00032-0

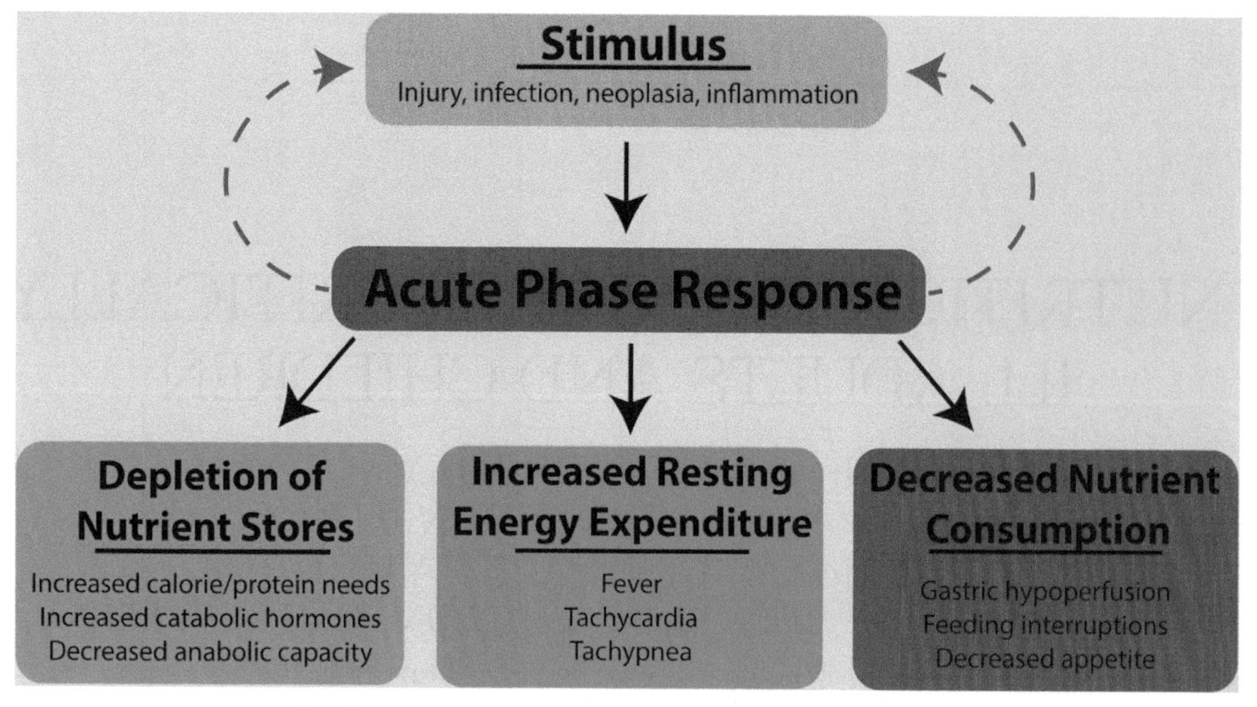

FIGURE 32.1 Nutritional considerations in the acute phase response.

components of this network become disrupted, with inflammatory changes causing acute metabolic stress. In turn, this results in disordered carbohydrate, lipid, and protein metabolism with alterations in the innate hormonal environment.[1] Disease or injury processes alter absorptive physiology and energy metabolism—both key factors that need to be accounted for with a nuanced approach to nutritional support.

Manifestation of these alterations vary with the preillness nutritional condition of the patient. Therefore, these disruptive processes can have disparate presentations in patients depending on their overall health and nutrition status at the onset of illness and subsequent evolution of disease in the intensive care unit (ICU). Nutrition assessment of the critically ill patient is necessary to characterize and define nutrition status, determine appropriate nutrient intake goals, identify the best mode for nutrient delivery, monitor for tolerance, and determine associations with patient outcomes.

The objectives of this chapter are to present the current state of knowledge regarding the provision of nutrition therapy in the ICU patient and describe the nutritional relevance of selected diseases common to the adult and pediatric ICU patients. It is beyond the scope of this chapter to address physiologic changes that occur in the still developing GI tract in premature infants who are critically ill.

B. The Acute Phase Response

Critical illness is characterized by an increase in catabolism mediated by counterregulatory catabolic hormones, which is termed the acute phase response (Fig. 32.1). While catabolic states induced by starvation have muscle-preserving mechanisms to protect lean mass in advanced stages, the acute phase response overrides these protections creating a relentless catabolic state. The catabolic state begins with an "ebb phase" lasting 12–24 h during which oxygen utilization and body temperature decrease. The ebb phase is followed by the catabolic "flow phase," which can last one to 3 weeks, during which time increased catecholamines induce the breakdown of endogenous macronutrient stores through pathways of lipolysis and gluconeogenesis.[1] These changes coupled with the immobilization associated with critical illness can result in severe muscle wasting in the critically ill patient. In the first few days of ICU admission, lean mass loss can be as high as 17.7% in adults[2] and greater than 10% in children.[3] The catabolic activity of the acute phase response to injury or illness is likely not resolved by provision of energy and protein. Instead, excess energy provided during this catabolic state is converted to fat and glucose and can lead to hyperglycemia and hypertriglyceridemia.[4–6] Whether increased protein intake can ameliorate the losses of lean mass is not yet clear.

Cytokines released during the acute phase response result in profound alterations in hepatic protein synthesis. Synthesis of positive acute phase proteins such as C-reactive protein (CRP), fibrinogen, haptoglobin, ceruloplasmin, complement, alpha-1 glycoprotein, and serum amyloid is stimulated, with resulting increase in serum concentrations. Concurrently, suppression of negative acute phase proteins such as albumin, transferrin, transthyretin, and retinol-binding protein occurs, with resulting decrease in serum concentrations of these proteins. Additionally, serum concentrations also decline due to decreases in oncotic pressure within the vasculature leading to capillary leak with accumulation of protein-rich interstitial fluid in tissues and from dilution with fluid resuscitation. These changes in protein synthesis and concentration during critical illness render measurements of albumin, prealbumin, and retinol-binding protein less reliable as biomarkers of nutrition status during the acute phase of critical illness. These nutritional biomarkers are more reflective of the acute phase response than they are of nutritional status of the patient.

Changes in blood micronutrient concentrations may also occur during critical illness (Fig. 32.2). During the acute phase response, many vitamins (A, B6, C, D, and E) and minerals (copper, iron, selenium, and zinc) are impacted by inflammation and best interpreted in light of the CRP concentration. Renal failure requiring dialysis therapy may result in excess losses of copper, selenium, zinc, thiamin, and vitamin B6.[7] Oxidative stress related to the production of oxygen free radicals may require greater use of antiinflammatory vitamins.[8] Thus, it can be difficult to interpret blood concentrations of micronutrients during critical illness.[1]

Studies of supplementation of selenium (Se) and vitamin C in critical illness are promising. Selenium supplementation may improve renal function and decrease

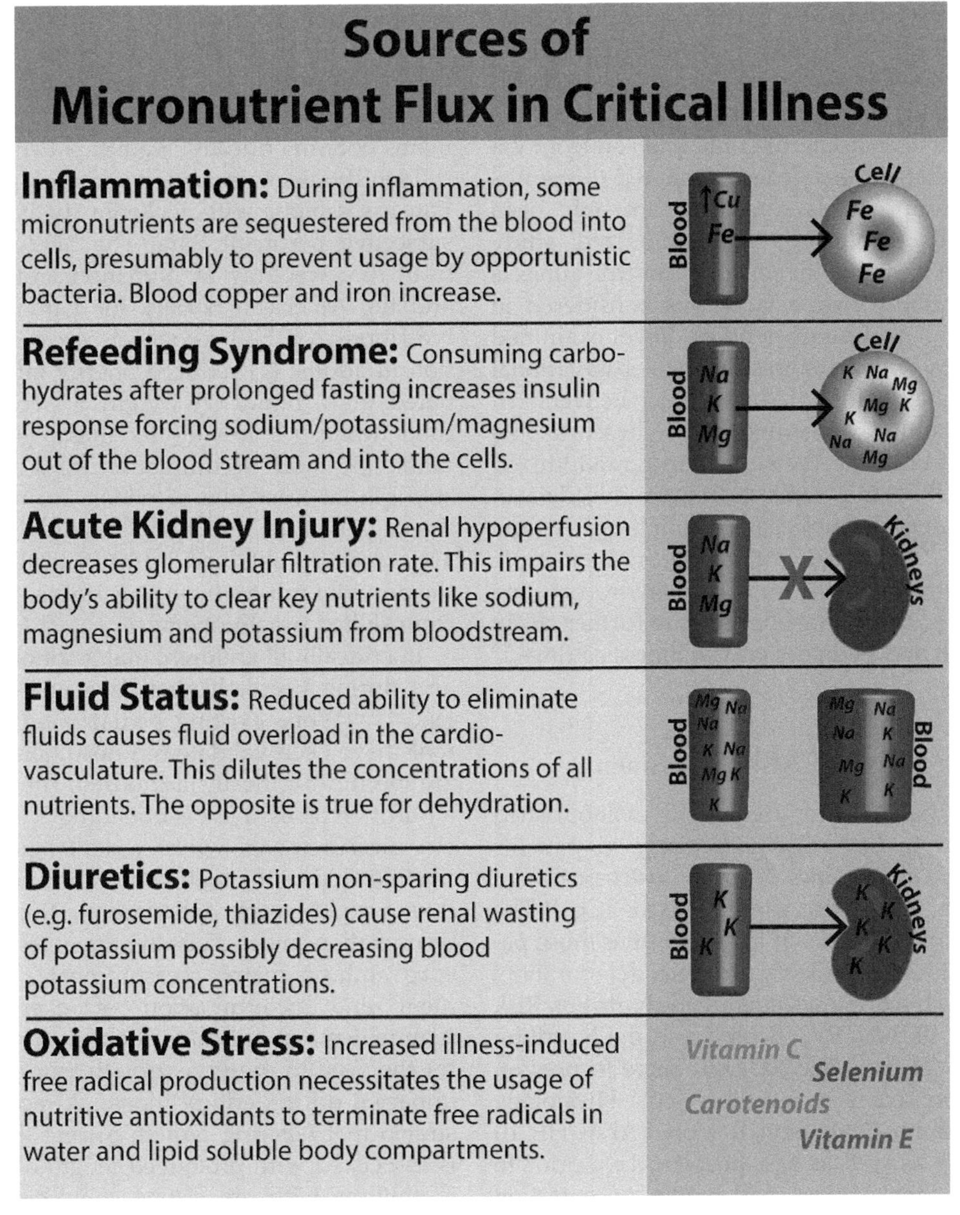

FIGURE 32.2 Causes of micronutrient shifts in critical illness, Cu = copper, Fe = iron, Na = sodium, K = potassium, and Mg = magnesium.

infectious complications.[9] Vitamin C administration, particularly in combination with thiamine and hydrocortisone, may be important in sepsis.[10] Demand for vitamin C increases during sepsis due to the adaptive processes in the body to reduce plasma-free iron and free radicals, but concentrations may also be decreased due to inflammation and fluid resuscitation. Vitamin C administration has also been shown to preserve cardiovascular integrity and responsiveness to vasopressors in animal models of sepsis.[11,12] A randomized placebo-controlled trial in 26 adult ICU subjects demonstrated a more rapid decline in sequential organ failure assessment (SOFA) scores (indicating improvement in organ dysfunction) over 96 h in patients receiving intravenous (IV) vitamin C doses of 200 mg/kg body weight per 24 h.[13] In an open-label study of 47 adult subjects with severe sepsis compared to historic controls that tested IV administrations of vitamin C (1.5 g every 6 h), thiamine (200 mg every 12 h), and hydrocortisone (50 mg every 6 h), mortality in the treatment group was 8.5% versus 40.4% in the control group. Additionally, there was a significant decrease in the time to wean from vasopressors in the treatment group compared to the historic control group.[10] This study has not only been criticized for its unblinded, nonrandomized study design but also because the historic control subjects had greater mortality risk, a factor not considered in the comparison. Additional studies have examined this triple therapy with mixed results. One observational study (n = 94 subjects) found no association between triple therapy (vitamin C, thiamine, and hydrocortisone) and any clinical outcome.[14] One pediatric randomized controlled trial (RCT) in 24 subjects found reduced vasopressor requirements in subjects receiving triple therapy versus controls.[15] Although vitamin C and/or triple therapy with vitamin C, thiamine, and hydrocortisone maybe promising, these strategies require further study in both the adult and pediatric critical illness settings.[16]

C. Nutrition Status and Risk Assessment

Critically ill patients are frequently malnourished upon admission to the ICU, particularly in patients with preexisting comorbidities. Nutrition risk assessment should occur for each patient admitted to the ICU.[17] The use of nutrition risk assessment tools identifies those patients who are at highest risk of nutritional deterioration. In adults, two such scoring systems are the Nutrition Risk in the Critically Ill (NUTRIC) Score[18] and the Nutrition Risk Score 2002 (NRS).[19] The NUTRIC Score focuses on severity of illness scores such as the Acute Physiology and Chronic Health Evaluation II score (APACHE II) and SOFA score, as well as age, hospital days prior to ICU admission, comorbidities, and serum concentration of interleukin-6 (IL-6), a proinflammatory cytokine. A modified version of the NUTRIC score without IL-6 is also available.[20] While the NUTRIC score has been shown to predict mortality[21,22] and identify patients who benefit most from nutrition support with lower mortality in observational studies,[20,23–25] one prospective trial[26] did not convincingly demonstrate its ability to predict the impact of nutrition therapy on clinically relevant outcomes. However, this trial was relatively small (n = 245 subjects), and survivors consistently received greater intake of protein and energy after day 6, though still only about 70% of goal requirements. The nonsurvivor group had significantly more patients with high NUTRIC score (82% vs. 41%) and with malnutrition (23% vs. 33%). The NRS score has been validated to predict the impact of nutrition support on clinical outcomes in two prospective randomized control trials.[27,28] Limitations of the NRS score include the need for APACHE II calculated score greater than 10, which is achieved by age alone (greater than 45 years), and ICU admission.[29] Thus, the ability to assess nutrition status and identify nutrition risk remains poor in critically ill adult patients.

Identifying malnutrition requires a complete nutrition assessment with inclusion of both objective and subjective pertinent data. The 2012 consensus report from the Academy of Nutrition and Dietetics (AND) and the American Society for Parenteral and Enteral Nutrition (ASPEN) recognizes six criteria of malnutrition in adults: (1) reduced energy intake over a designated time frame, (2) weight loss over a designated time frame, (3) loss of fat mass, (4) loss of muscle mass, (5) fluid accumulation, and (6) reduced grip strength, at least two of which are needed to classify the degree of malnutrition.[30] Many of these parameters are not easily obtained in the critically ill patient, and the provider must rely on physical assessment and input from skilled practitioners.[31]

In critically ill children, malnutrition upon admission and during hospitalization is a well-established problem.[32–35] While existing pediatric nutrition assessment tools have been validated in hospitalized patients, none are specific to critically ill children. The key to performing a nutrition assessment is obtaining accurate anthropometry measurements, which is challenging in the critically ill child due to fluctuations in fluid volume status, and thus weight, from dehydration, fluid overload from resuscitation, and various treatment modalities that influence anthropometry measurements. Nutrition assessment and determination of energy and protein requirements in critically ill children must also account for the need to preserve growth that is often negatively impacted during critical illness. A recent study demonstrated that faltering growth during the ICU admission is associated with prolonged length of stay, particularly in children with preexisting comorbidities.[36] Similar to the adult consensus statement, a pediatric consensus statement by AND and ASPEN recommends the use of standard diagnostic indicators to identify and document pediatric malnutrition. These include (1) weight-for-height/length z-score, (2) body mass index (BMI)–for-age z-score, (3) length/height-for-age z-score, and/or (4) mid-upper arm circumference. If more than one anthropometric data point is available, the recommendations include the use of (1) weight gain velocity in < 2-year-olds, (2) weight loss in 2- to 20-year-olds, (3) deceleration in weight-for-length/height z-score, and (4) inadequate nutrient intake to assess malnutrition. Current standards encourage assessment of nutrition status with accurate documentation upon hospital admission as the basis to direct nutrition therapy. Systematic nutrition assessment is vital for both adult and pediatric critically ill patients to identify those patients at risk for nutritional deterioration and to prescribe and appropriately adapt nutrition therapy to thwart nutrition-related complications during critical illness.

D. Determining Nutritional Needs in the Critically Ill Patient

The determination of nutritional requirements in the critically ill patient is best assessed by measurement of individual patient needs for energy and protein. Current guidelines for nutrition support in critically ill adult[17] and pediatric patients[37] recommend use of indirect calorimetry (IC) to determine energy needs whenever possible. In the absence of IC, use of a predictive or weight-based equation (25–30 kcal/kg (kg)/d) is recommended in nonobese adults (BMI<30) (Table 32.1).[6]

Current guidelines for the pediatric critically ill patient recommend use of the Schofield equation[39] or the World Health Organization (WHO) predictive equation based on kg body weight without the addition of a stress factor to estimate energy requirements (when IC is not available) (Table 32.2).[37,40,41] The adult guidelines recommend that critically ill patients receive protein at 1.2–2 g/kg body weight[17] (Table 32.1), though recommendations are based on limited strength of evidence. The clinical registry–based EFFORT trial in adult ICU patients is underway to answer whether protein delivery at 2.2 g/kg/day is associated with lower mortality and shorter time to hospital discharge than usual intake of 1.2 g/kg/day.[42] By contrast, in critically ill children, a minimum of 1.5 g/kg/day of protein is recommended to avoid protein deficit and attain a positive nitrogen balance. These thresholds appear to correlate with improved outcomes.[37] The evidence for protein requirements in critically ill children accounts for increased protein breakdown and exceeds recommendations of the WHO and the Dietary Reference Intake values.[37] Tables 32.3 and 32.4 provide pediatric recommendations for protein and fat allowances. Further study is necessary in both adult and pediatric populations to determine more precise protein requirements during critical illness.

E. Obesity in the Critically Ill Patient

It is important for providers to recognize that malnutrition often accompanies obesity and has an impact on nutritional support. The increased rate of obesity seen globally in the general population is also encountered in adult and

TABLE 32.1 Guidelines for feeding nonobese and obese ICU patients.

Summary of 2016 ASPEN/SCCM General guideline recommendations for energy and protein provision in critically ill adult patients			
Nonobese patients	BMI[a]: 18–30 kg/m²	Calories[b]	25–30 kcal/kg ***actual*** body weight
	BMI: 18–30 kg/m²	Protein	1.2–1.5 g/kg ***actual*** body weight
Obese patients	BMI: 30-50 kg/m²	Calories[b]	11–14 kcal/kg ***actual*** body weight
	BMI > 50 kg/m²	Calories[b]	22–25 kcal/kg ***ideal*** body weight[c]
	BMI: 30–40 kg/m²	Protein	2 g/kg ***ideal*** body weight
	BMI > 40 kg/m²	Protein	2.5 g/kg ***ideal*** body weight

[a]*BMI is body mass index represented as weight (kg) divided by height (m²).*
[b]*This or other predictive equations to be used when indirect calorimetry is contraindicated or unavailable.*
[c]*Ideal body weight in lbs (for men) = 106 + 6 X (Ht − 60 in). Ideal body weight in lbs (for women) = 105 + 5 X (Ht − 60 in).[38] ASPEN: American Society of Parenteral and Enteral Nutrition; SCCM: Society of Critical Care Medicine.*

TABLE 32.2 Energy equations to estimate energy for critically ill children.

Equation	Sex	Age (years)	Resting energy requirements estimate
Schofield[44]	Female	0–3 3–10 10–18	[16.252 × Wt + 1023.2 x Ht] – 413.5 [16.969 × Wt + 161.8 x Ht] + 371.2 [8.365 × Wt + 465 x Ht] + 200
	Male	0–3 3–10 10–18	[0.167 × Wt + 1517.4 x Ht] – 617.6 [19.59 × Wt + 130.3 x Ht] + 414.9 [16.25 × Wt + 137.2 x Ht] + 515.5
FAO/WHO/UNU[40]	Female	0–3 3–10 10–18	[61 × Wt] – 51 [22.5 × Wt] + 499 [12.2 × Wt] + 746
	Male	0–3 3–10 10–18	[60.9 × Wt] – 54 [22.7 × Wt] + 495 [17.5 × Wt] + 651

Wt, weight, kg; *Ht*, height, m.
FAO, *Food and Agriculture Organization*; UNU, *United Nations University*, WHO, *World Health Organization*.

TABLE 32.3 Pediatric recommendations for dietary protein allowance.

Recommended pediatric dietary allowance for protein			
Age group	**ASPEN g/kg/day**	**WHO g/kg/day**	**IOM g/kg/day**
0–6 months	2.0–3.0	1.5	1.52[a]
7–12 months	1.5–3.0	1.5	1.1[b]
1–2 years	2.0–3.0	1.2	0.88
3–12 years	1.5–2.0	0.9–1.0	0.76
14–18 years	1.5	0.85–1.0	0.76

ASPEN: American Society of Parenteral and Enteral Nutrition; WHO: World Health Organization; IOM: Institute of Medicine.
[a]*Adequate Intake: recommended average daily nutrient intake based on a group of healthy individuals.*
[b]*Estimated Average Requirement: average nutrient intake level at which the needs of 50% of population will be met.*
Adapted from Kleinman RE, Greer FR, eds, American Academy of Pediatrics, Committee on Nutrition. Pediatric Nutrition Handbook seventh edition. *Elk Grove Village, IL: Academy of Pediatrics; 2014; Mehta NM, Compher C, ASPEN Board of Directors. ASPEN clinical guidelines: nutrition support of the critically ill child.* JPEN J Parenter Enter Nutr, 33*(3): 260–276; 2009. Institute of Medicine.* Dietary Reference Intakes for Energy, Carbohydrates, Fiber, Fat, Fatty Acids, Cholesterol, Protein and Amino Acids. *Washington, DC: National Academies Press; 2002/2005.*

TABLE 32.4 Pediatric recommendations for fat intake as percent of total calories.

Age group	Total fat intake recommendations
2–3 years	30%–40% of total calories
> 4 years	25%–35% of total calories

Adapted from: Dietary Recommendations for Healthy Children. https://www.heart.org/en/healthy-living/healthy-eating/eat-smart/nutrition-basics/dietary-recommendations-for-healthy-children

pediatric ICU patient populations. In the United States in 2015–16, the prevalence of obesity in adults was about 40%.[43] Excess adiposity in adults can mask loss of muscle mass that has accrued due to chronic, low-grade inflammation. The hypercatabolic state that occurs in the acute phase of critical illness accelerates the rate of loss of lean mass with a risk of worsening muscle mass and function after ICU discharge.[1] No high-quality data based on strength of evidence exist to guide energy requirements in ICU patients with obesity. However expert consensus guidelines from ASPEN[17] recommend a hypocaloric, high-protein strategy in adults. It is suggested that obese adult patients receive 65%–70% of calorie goals as determined through IC. If IC is not available, the guidelines suggest 11–14 kcal/kg/day of *actual* body weight for an adult patient with a BMI between 30 and 50 kg/m^2 and 22–25 kcal/kg/day of *ideal* body weight (IBW) for patients with a BMI >50 kg/m^2.[6] Protein recommendations in adult obese patients are 2 g/kg/day of IBW for those patients with a BMI between 30 and 40 kg/m^2 and 2.5 g/kg/day of IBW for those patients with a BMI >40 kg/m^2. These suggestions for intake of energy and protein are based on low strength of evidence.

Similarly, obesity increasingly affects large numbers of children in the United States. The National Health and Nutrition Examination Survey 2015–16 found the prevalence of obesity in children ages 2–5 years to be 14%, ages 6–11 years to be 18%, and ages 12–19 years to be 21%.[43] Critically ill children with obesity are at increased nutrition risk, and there are no standards to define IBW in children with obesity. IC will more accurately assess energy requirements in this population but may not be available. Accuracy of IC is a concern if ventilator settings are high or if the child requires supplemental oxygen therapy, both of which are common interventions in the ICU setting.

Use of standard predictive equations or BMI may over or underestimate energy needs. Predictive equations should be used with caution and combined with close monitoring of the patient's weight pattern in response to nutrition therapy, often adjusting as necessary to achieve appropriate energy and weight goals.[45] Specific protein intake recommendations are not available for pediatric patients with obesity. The ASPEN guidelines for all hospitalized children suggest caution when using recommendations for nonobese pediatric patients as they may over- or underestimate needs by as much as 20% depending on patient age, nutritional status, clinical presentation, and severity of illness.[37,45,46]

In general, nutrition guidelines are not designed to recognize the nuanced illness states associated with an ICU admission or the changing nutritional needs of the patient during the course of critical illness. Therefore, it is important that providers view current guidelines as a starting point to initiate nutrition care and monitor patient response to nutritional therapy. Real-time monitoring of clinical and laboratory determinants such as serum electrolytes, blood urea nitrogen (BUN), serum proteins, inflammatory markers, micronutrient concentrations, and serial anthropometry patterns is essential and may be the best indicators of successful nutrition therapy in the critically ill patient with obesity.

F. Provision of Nutrition Support

Enteral nutrition

Numerous factors contribute to the inability of ICU patients to participate in volitional feeding by mouth. When critically ill patients with a functioning GI tract are unable to consume nutrients orally, enteral nutrition (EN) is the preferred mode of nutrition therapy. EN is defined as the delivery of nutrients distal to the oral cavity through tube, catheter, or stoma. The joint ASPEN and Society of Critical Care Medicine (SCCM) guidelines for nutrition support in critically ill adults[17] and children[37] recommend that EN be initiated within 48 h of ICU admission. Early EN for critically ill patients is associated with a decrease in the hypercatabolic response, preservation of GI mucosal integrity and motility, and increased caloric and protein intake stimulating insulin secretion and protein preservation.[47,48] Providing a flow of nutrients through the GI tract is believed to maintain the structural integrity of intestinal cells and the gut-associated lymph tissues that participate in overall immune function.[49] Enteral feeding stimulates cholecystokinin release, which may protect against cholelithiasis. Providing EN is associated with significant cost savings. Doig and colleagues demonstrated hospital cost reduction of more than $14,000 per patient attributable to the use of early EN during the course of ICU stay.[50]

For most adult and pediatric patients, a tube delivering bolus feedings directly into the stomach (gastric feeding) is appropriate and similar to normal gastric physiology with meal ingestion. In situations where the GI motility of the patient is slowed, or where gastric feeds are contraindicated, postpyloric feeding (distal to the stomach) may be appropriate. Continuous feeding directly into the duodenum or jejunum may improve EN tolerance and secondarily increase attainment of goal nutrient intake.

In patients who do not tolerate EN well, nutritional deficits can easily accumulate. Practices such as delayed feeding initiation, feeding interruptions with less than optimal resumption, along with issues of tube dislodgement or obstruction, provider discomfort with feeding practice, and lack of necessary equipment (replacement feeding tubes, formula infusion pump, etc.) can cause shortfalls in the planned volume of nutrition delivery and worsen nutritional deficits during the phase where nutrition is needed most for recovery. The ASPEN/SCCM adult and pediatric Critical Care Nutrition Support Guidelines recommend the use of EN feeding protocols as a strategy to increase the delivery of EN.[17,29]

Adult patients

The choice of feeding tube may be based on the estimated duration of EN provision. In general, if the duration of EN is expected to be less than 6 weeks, a feeding tube is inserted through the nose to the gastric cavity, the duodenum, or the proximal portion of the jejunum. However, if the anticipated duration of EN is greater than 6 weeks, a more permanent GI tract access device is necessary, and the patient requires placement of a gastrostomy, jejunostomy or gastrojejunostomy tube. The type of tube used is dependent on patient needs, safety, and comfort.

Once the appropriate EN feeding tube is in place, and the energy and caloric needs of the patient are determined, a suitable formula is prescribed with appropriate dosing to meet the patient's needs. Formula selection is best performed by a registered dietitian experienced in working with ICU patients, in collaboration with the clinical team to meet patient-specific nutritional needs. Specialty formulas are available for specific disease states such as renal or pulmonary disease, as well as immune-enhanced formulas. However, data on the association of immune-enhanced formulas with improved patient outcomes are limited.[17]

Pediatric patients

In critically ill children with an intact and functioning GI tract, EN is the preferred method of nutrient delivery.

Results from a pilot study observed that bolus gastric feeding improved EN delivery more than continuous EN in mechanically ventilated, critically ill children.[51] Studies of early EN in children with thermal injuries have demonstrated reduced caloric deficits and improved protein retention.[52] In general, EN in critically ill children is associated with improved feeding tolerance and early attainment of energy and protein goals. EN should be initiated within 48 h of ICU admission unless contraindicated.[37] Similar to adult patients, formula prescription for critically ill children is selected to meet the needs of the patient. In addition, patient age must be considered as well as the protein source. For example, whey protein based formulas are thought to accelerate gastric emptying, which may decrease the risk of reflux of gastric contents.[53]

G. Parenteral Nutrition

Parenteral nutrition (PN) is the IV formulation of nutrients consisting of carbohydrates delivered as dextrose, protein as amino acids, fat as lipid emulsion, and micronutrients as indicated for those patients who are unable to meet nutritional needs solely via the GI tract or where use of the GI tract is contraindicated. For the adult ICU patient of low nutritional risk, the recommendation is to withhold PN for the initial week of illness. However, in adults with high nutrition risk, when EN is not feasible, exclusive PN should be initiated as soon as possible after ICU admission.[6] In both adult and pediatric patients, initiation of PN after a week of ICU admission is associated with decreased infection risk, increased number of ventilator free days, and reduced duration of hospitalization.[54,55] However, the adult trial that observed these outcomes has been criticized because the subjects were low-risk (3 days of ventilation), largely postcardiac surgery patients who would not be fed in many clinical settings. Large multicenter RCTs in adults have shown that PN did not result in greater mortality[56,57] or increased infectious complications over EN.[57] The earlier recommendations for EN over PN due to lower infectious risk were based on data for provision of PN before the understanding of the negative impact of excess energy provision and those due to hyperglycemia were fully appreciated. By contrast, modern practice includes avoidance of overfeeding, glycemic control, and careful IV catheter care.

As PN is a hyperosmolar solution that relies on cardiovascular circulation for dilution, PN administration requires central venous access for safe delivery. While PN can be given peripherally, the osmolality should be diluted to less than 900 mOsm/L to decrease the risk of phlebitis in peripheral veins. In addition, peripheral PN often does not deliver full nutrient requirements for critically ill patients. These patients may also have challenging peripheral IV access due to edema. For these reasons, the use of peripheral PN is not recommended.

H. Refeeding Syndrome

Refeeding syndrome constitutes a constellation of symptoms related to the reintroduction of calories after an extended period with limited energy intake. As a metabolic adaptation to starvation, insulin secretion is reduced while glucagon and growth hormone secretion is increased. Endogenous fats and proteins are the primary source of energy, while lean mass with its associated mineral components is reduced with weight loss. The rapid introduction of carbohydrates to the system during refeeding leads to an abrupt shift from glucagon-driven oxidation of endogenous fuel sources to insulin-driven utilization of exogenous glucose for fuel. This sharp increase in insulin response leads to a shift of glucose into the cells and concurrently drives the migration of electrolytes such as potassium, phosphorus, and magnesium into the cell. The combination of depleted body stores of potassium, phosphorus, and magnesium, together with the rapid intracellular migration of these electrolytes, induces hypokalemia, hypophosphatemia, and hypomagnesemia, with the most prominent being low phosphorus concentrations (Table 32.2). Potential complications related to refeeding syndrome include heart failure with dysrhythmias, hyperglycemia, respiratory failure/fatigue, anemia, red blood cell lysis, and immune suppression.[58] Recovering ICU patients are at increased risk for refeeding syndrome, and reintroduction of EN or PN must be implemented with caution and with close monitoring of fluid and electrolyte status with repletion as indicated.

II. PATHOPHYSIOLOGY AND NUTRITION MANAGEMENT OF SPECIFIC CRITICAL ILLNESS STATES

A. Sepsis and Multiple Organ Dysfunction Syndrome

Annually approximately 270,000 people in the United Status die from sepsis, which is an extreme, life-threatening response to infection characterized by inflammation, capillary leak, and fluid shifts with organ dysfunction. Patients with sepsis are often malnourished at ICU admission and frequently do not receive nutrition support during the first days of illness due to unstable clinical status. Even previously healthy patients are at risk for developing malnutrition due to an increase in metabolic rate and the inflammatory response that are characteristic of sepsis. A variety of metabolic derangements, including changes in carbohydrate, protein, and fat metabolism, are driven by the acute phase response mediated by counterregulatory hormones and inflammatory cytokines. The most noticeable changes include increases in gluconeogenesis and glycogenolysis (early), proteolysis and lipolysis with resulting stress hyperglycemia and insulin resistance, hypertriglyceridemia, and negative nitrogen balance. Energy expenditure is highly variable in sepsis and multiple organ dysfunction states and is influenced by variable lean body mass, severity of illness, and ICU interventions (including sedation, mechanical ventilation, and steroid and vasoactive medications).

The early phases of sepsis are frequently accompanied by organ hypoperfusion. Tolerance to oral feeding or EN drastically decreases with hypoperfusion to the gut. In the kidneys, the consequence of hypoperfusion is acute kidney injury (AKI), which results in an accumulation of nitrogenous compounds, imbalances of electrolytes and minerals, development of metabolic acidosis, and fluid retention. Decreased glomerular filtration rate (GFR) leads to hyperkalemia, hyperphosphatemia, and hypermagnesemia, while increased fluid retention leads to hyponatremia, hypochloremia, and hypocalcemia (Table 32.2). Monitoring of electrolyte status in AKI is crucial.[59]

Adult patients

Both the 2016 Surviving Sepsis Campaign[60] and the 2016 ASPEN Guidelines for Nutrition Support in the adult critically ill patient[17] recommend early EN, once resuscitation is complete and the patient has attained hemodynamic stability. Early EN is associated with better clinical outcomes, possibly by preventing gut mucosal atrophy and bacterial translocation. If the patient is unable to attain full EN, then small volume trophic/hypocaloric feeds are acceptable. Even trophic/hypocaloric feeds preserve gut integrity, potentially decrease inflammation, and to a lesser degree, abate the caloric deficit that accumulates early in the course of illness. Neither guideline recommends administering PN within the first few days of illness when EN is not possible.[6,19] However, an Australian RCT employing current strategies of catheter care, glycemic control, and avoidance of overfeeding energy confirmed that early PN was not associated with worse outcomes when early EN was relatively contraindicated.[56]

Pediatric patients

Data from a recent global study of pediatric severe sepsis reported that severe undernutrition status was associated with higher all-cause ICU mortality while severe overnutrition/obesity status was associated with greater ICU length of stay.[61] Studies of critically ill children with severe sepsis using measured energy expenditure have observed that these children often have persistently negative energy and nitrogen balances during the first week of illness.[62–64] However, these findings were confounded by timing and frequency of measurements, as well as challenges with providing consistent nutrition support.

The 2012 Surviving Sepsis Campaign pediatric guidelines recommend EN in children whenever possible and PN in those who are unable to tolerate EN once hemodynamically stable. Limited studies have demonstrated that early EN is associated with lower mortality in general populations of critically ill children. The multicenter pediatric version of the effect of early parenteral nutrition to complete insufficient enteral nutrition in ICU patients (PEPaNIC) trial observed that initiation of PN within 24 h of ICU admission was associated with worse clinical outcomes compared to delayed initiation in critically ill children at medium to high risk of malnutrition.[55] Children with sepsis frequently require increased glucose delivery and consequently increased fluids. To manage fluid imbalances during sepsis, renal dialysis therapies may be required with corresponding adjustments in nutrition therapy. While studies of immune-enhancing diets have not demonstrated improved outcomes in critically ill children, preexisting immune status may influence outcomes. Recent data[65,66] suggest that diets with whey-based protein may be associated with a decrease in acquired sepsis in critically ill immune-competent children without lymphopenia, while increased supplementation of Zn, Se, and glutamine appeared to be protective for critically ill immunocompromised children.

B. Acute Respiratory Failure, Acute Lung Injury, and Acute Respiratory Distress Syndrome

Acute respiratory failure (ARF) occurs when respiratory muscle demand for metabolic substrate and oxygen delivery exceeds supply. The energy cost of breathing, duration of contraction per breath, velocity of contraction, operational length of muscle fibers, energy supply, efficiency of muscles, and state of muscle training can all influence respiratory failure.[67] Prolonged malnutrition can affect diaphragmatic structure and function, impairing the ability of the diaphragm to generate force. ARF due to acute neuromuscular weakness is often associated with hypermetabolism, with consequent muscle wasting and negative nitrogen balance. Prolonged mechanical ventilation particularly with sedation and neuromuscular blockade reduces metabolic expenditure and also predisposes the patient to respiratory muscle atrophy with potentially deleterious consequences for survivors.

Under normal conditions, inspiration accounts for almost all the work of the breathing cycle. Nearly half of the work of breathing during inspiration dissipates as heat to overcome frictional resistance to chest wall deformation. The remaining inspiratory work is stored as potential energy to perform the work of expiration. Increased airway resistance and decreased respiratory compliance impose a greater workload on the respiratory muscles and increase the oxygen cost of breathing. Eventually, respiratory failure may ensue due to muscle fatigue.

Macronutrient metabolism uses oxygen to create ATP and produces carbon dioxide (CO_2) as a by-product through aerobic respiration, while anaerobic respiration creates lactate. These waste products enter the bicarbonate/carbonic acid buffering system in the blood stream for transport to the lungs for exhalation in the form of CO_2. This process requires a functional respiratory system. Any condition that impairs this vital gas exchange in the lungs increases circulating CO_2 thereby disturbing acid−base balance. Excessive or overfeeding disrupts CO_2 and oxygen exchange, placing an increased burden on the lungs, and can worsen ARF. Patients who are unable to adequately clear CO_2 from blood require mechanical ventilation to remove CO_2 and preserve acid−base balance.

Gut dysfunction also plays an important role in the pathogenesis of ARF, acute lung injury, and acute respiratory distress syndrome (ARDS). As per the "gut lymph" hypothesis, the injured gut allows translocation of bacteria and bacterial products together with cytokines and toxins across damaged intestinal barriers into the lymphatic system; this activates alveolar macrophages and the inflammatory cascade that causes ARDS. In the "intestinal crosstalk" theory, disruptions of the intestinal microbiota, immune system, and intestinal epithelial barrier result in systemic inflammation and development of ARDS.[68]

In ARDS, the goals of optimal nutrition are to modulate cytokine responses, improve antioxidant defenses, preserve gut integrity, and support the patient during the hypermetabolic phase by minimizing catabolism and reducing the risk of malnutrition. Avoidance of overfeeding and/or underfeeding the patient with ARDS is critical to avoid complications and further decline in respiratory status. Overfeeding is associated with delayed ventilator weaning, lipogenesis, hepatic dysfunction, hyperglycemia, increased mortality, and prolonged hospitalization.[68,69] Complications associated with underfeeding include delayed ventilator weaning, impaired protein synthesis, organ failure, and an increased risk of hospital associated infections, particularly sepsis.[68,69]

While measured energy expenditure by IC maybe superior to predictive equations to determine energy expenditure, IC is not accurate for any mechanically ventilated patient requiring high inspired oxygen concentrations ($FiO2 \geq 60\%$) and high mean airway pressures. Energy expenditure is quite variable in ARF and is often influenced by severity of illness, and ICU interventions (including sedation, mechanical ventilation, and steroid and vasoactive medications). Thus, IC is unusable for the early stages of many ICU patients requiring mechanical ventilation.

Nutritional deficits can easily accumulate in critically ill patients with ARDS and other causes of respiratory failure. Competing priorities of ICU care may require interruptions in delivery of feedings. Various tests and procedures in the ICU often require that EN be stopped for concerns of patient safety. Preparation for extubation from mechanical ventilation can interrupt EN for several hours. Once extubated, the patient is often observed for an extended period (hours to days) prior to resumption of EN to ensure that a stable respiratory status is achieved and maintained. Additionally, it is not uncommon for EN to be resumed at a lower infusion rate than prior to the interruption, further extending the risk for nutrition deficit. Dysphasia can occur following a prolonged intubation, necessitating a swallow evaluation which can delay the resumption of oral feeds or EN, and put the patient at risk for further caloric, protein, and micronutrient deficits.

Adult patients

The current recommendations for nutrition support in ARF and ARDS are the same as those generally used for critical illness. In the absence of IC, initiation of nutrition support at 25−30 kcal/kg/day of dosing weight and 1.5−2 g/kg/day of protein in the nonobese adult is recommended.[17] To decrease burden on the lungs in those patients with persistently high pCO_2 despite adjustments in mechanical ventilation, reduction in carbohydrate load may be considered. If the patient is also in a volume-overloaded state with fluid retention, the use of a more concentrated formula providing up to 2 kcal/mL may be appropriate. Since hypophosphatemia is common in critically ill patients with risk for further respiratory muscle weakness, serum phosphorus concentration should be monitored, and phosphorus repleted as needed.[17]

Pediatric patients

A retrospective study demonstrated that adequate energy and nutrient delivery in children with ARDS was associated with improved clinical outcomes.[52] Protein delivery may be even more important than energy delivered. There is no current evidence to guide initiation, advancement, or withholding of EN for patients with ARDS. EN intolerance is common in more than 50% of patients with ARDS making it an important cause for inability to attain target energy and protein goals. Many studies report that only 40%–75% of median goal calories are delivered over the first 7 days in children with ARDS. While EN is preferred over PN, if target EN is not achieved within 72 h of onset of ARDS, initiation of PN should be considered to supplement or replace EN and prevent worsening malnutrition.[68,70] Immune-enhancing formulas containing omega-3 fatty acids and antioxidants are associated with improvements in the biochemical inflammatory profile,[71] but these changes have not translated to clinical benefits (compared to standard enteral formulas) in children with ARDS.

C. Acute Kidney Injury

AKI is characterized by an abrupt decline of renal function causing decreased GFR and diminished renal tubular function. Clinical manifestations of AKI include fluid overload, decreased urine output with an associated rise in serum creatinine, BUN concentration, and electrolyte imbalances. As the GFR declines, electrolyte abnormalities such as hyperkalemia, hyperphosphatemia, and hypermagnesemia ensue (Table 32.2). Additional complications include glucose intolerance, azotemia, and acidosis. Restricting potassium and phosphorus intake along with careful fluid management is an essential aspect for optimal management of AKI. Current clinical consensus favors early initiation of renal dialysis to prevent complications and support initiation of adequate nutrition provision.[59] In patients with AKI, baseline and ongoing weight assessment is essential to assess fluid management, direct other aspects of therapy, and prescribe nutrition. Patients with AKI often become hypercatabolic and have altered metabolism. Nutrition requirements are generally unchanged when AKI accompanies sepsis. Fluid management, usually in the form of restriction, often predicts nutrition delivery and places the patient at risk for nutrient deficits due to decreased nutrition therapy.[59,70,72–74]

Adult patients

Nutrition management is an important component to deliver optimal care in patients with AKI. Return of renal function with a decrease in protein catabolism and improved nitrogen balance may be favorably influenced by provision of adequate nutrition therapy.[59] Priority is given to attainment of positive energy balance and neutral nitrogen balance along with restoration of electrolyte and appropriate fluid balance. Ongoing inflammation can prolong renal dysfunction. Therefore, it is imperative that the underlying disease be treated. Reasonable targets for sodium, potassium, and phosphorus administration are 2–3 g/day (87–130 mmol), 2–3 g/k/day (50–80 mmol), and 8–15 mg/kg (0.25–0.48 mmol/kg) per day, respectively.[59] However, it is essential to monitor these serum electrolyte concentrations frequently and adjust intake as indicated.

Pediatric patients

No standards exist for estimating requirements or provision of adequate nutrition therapy for critically ill children with AKI. Nutrition requirements in AKI are unchanged from standard age-based recommendations. Recognizing that hypercatabolism, metabolic, and fluid shifts are common in this population, a primary goal of nutrition therapy is to prevent or abate catabolism. A recent study demonstrated that less than 68% of energy and less than 35% of protein needs were delivered by day 5 of illness to critically ill children with AKI.[73] To facilitate optimal nutrition delivery, consideration should be given to early initiation of renal dialysis with close monitoring of fluid status and electrolyte balance. Following guidelines for patients with chronic kidney disease, use of nutrient-dense, low-solute and low-volume formulas is recommended to meet nutritional requirements.[75]

D. Cardiovascular Disease States

Cardiovascular disease is the leading cause of mortality in adults accounting for one in every three deaths, with heart failure occurring in 20% of all Americans over the age of 40.[67] In general, heart failure (which can involve either the left, right, or both sides of the heart) results in an inability to adequately circulate blood in the systemic circulation. Left-sided heart failure causes fluid congestion in the pulmonary circulation, while right-sided failure results in fluid congestion in the systemic circulation with both types constituting congestive heart failure (CHF). The hallmark symptoms of CHF are dyspnea, fatigue, and fluid retention. Medical therapies center on relief of the vascular congestion and are accomplished through vasodilation, diuresis, and in severe cases, use of inotropic agents.

The normal myocardium uses fatty acids, lactate, and glucose to meet energy needs. The failing myocardium preferentially uses glucose via glycolytic pathways as an adaptive mechanism to conserve energy and reduce oxygen losses. The glucose transporter protein GLUT-4 facilitates myocardial glucose uptake and is upregulated during the early stages of cardiac failure. If cardiac failure progresses, continuous activation of the sympathetic nervous system results in lipolysis with elevated plasma free fatty acids that predispose to insulin resistance. Insulin resistance results in impaired glucose oxidation and worsening of myocardial energetics.

Adult cardiovascular disease

Malnutrition is common in CHF and is related to a combination of fluid restriction and increased energy expenditure from increased metabolic demands. CHF can predispose patients to anorexia and disturbances in GI function including malabsorption, hepatic congestion, intestinal edema, and gastroesophageal reflux. Additionally, these patients are at risk for micronutrient deficiencies. The micronutrients of greater concern are magnesium and thiamine as these deficiencies can exacerbate symptoms of CHF. Magnesium deficiency can also alter renal handling of sodium and potassium leading to a positive sodium balance with renal potassium wasting resulting in increased fluid retention. Thiamine is a key coenzyme in metabolism of macronutrients to ATP; therefore, thiamine deficiency leads to decreased energy availability for cardiac function.[76] In patients with CHF, nutrition status and assessment of metabolic state are often unpredictable in critical illness states. In 10%–15% of patients with CHF, cardiac cachexia will ensue causing a 6% drop in nonfluid body weight that is refractory to increased nutrition therapy, accompanied by a rapid drop in lean muscle mass. In patients with cardiac cachexia, 18-month mortality is approximately 50%.[76]

Pediatric cardiovascular disease

Nearly 40,000 infants are born annually in the United Status with congenital heart disease (CHD).[77] Children with CHD are at increased risk for malnutrition, ranging between 15% and 65%.[78] Malnutrition in children with CHD is due to multifactorial causes and results from increased energy needs concurrent with inadequate nutrition intake resulting in an energy imbalance. Nutrition delivery is often impeded due to ongoing needs for vasopressor support and fluid intake restrictions. Also, these children have a high incidence of EN intolerance related to intestinal edema, oral aversion, and inadequate feeding skills. CHD is often part of a spectrum of genetic abnormalities that may have a role in energy balance and malnutrition in this population of infants.[79] Preoperatively, children with CHD, particularly those with cyanotic disease, have higher resting energy expenditure (REE) compared to healthy children.[80,81] Following surgical palliation or complete repair, some studies have observed that differences in REE dissipate.[82,83] Other studies have observed no differences in REE before and after surgery or between those infants with cyanotic and noncyanotic disease.[84] Additionally, studies have shown no differences in EE between infants with palliative intervention, completely repaired infants, and healthy infants following surgical intervention.[85,86] Due to the variable results from numerous studies in this population, the question of energy expenditure and its relationship to malnutrition in children with CHD remains essentially unanswered. Negative nitrogen balance is common in this population due to increased protein metabolism and turnover, and this may be indicative of skeletal muscle wasting. However, due to limited evidence, protein needs in children with CHD remain largely unknown. Postoperative risk factors for malnutrition in these children include frequent feeding interruptions, vocal cord dysfunction, and protein-losing enteropathy, especially in those with single ventricle physiology. Children who require staged palliative repair for CHD are at particularly high risk for malnutrition. Overall, malnutrition in infants and children with CHD is associated with suboptimal clinical outcomes (greater ICU length of stay, prolonged mechanical ventilation, and increased risk of hospital acquired infections), growth failure, and neurodevelopmental impairment.[87]

Adult patients

Energy and protein recommendations in CHF are identical to those for sepsis and respiratory failure with an added emphasis on preventing further fluid retention. Concentrated formulas that provide 1.5–2 kcal/mL may be more appropriate for providing adequate nutrition while restricting fluid intake. However, the hyperosmolarity of these formulas may draw water into the GI tract, increasing the risk of osmotic diarrhea and electrolyte imbalances.

Pediatric patients

Early postoperative EN has demonstrated decreased intestinal complications, improved anthropometric measurements, and better outcomes in children with CHD.[88] While human milk is the preferred form of nutrition, it often needs fortification with additional calories to provide optimal energy intake in infants with CHD. Infants with CHD, especially those with single ventricle physiology, often require an enteral feeding tube to attain adequate energy, protein, and fluid intake to meet nutritional requirements. These infants may benefit from early PN in both the preoperative and early postoperative periods in conjunction with enteral feeds (as tolerated) to optimize nutrient intake. Consultation with a registered dietitian to prescribe nutrition in these infants coupled with use of a feeding protocol can achieve enhanced nutrient delivery.[78,89,90] It is also important to recognize behavioral and neurodevelopmental aspects of care that are necessary for the growing infant, including attention to cues for feeding readiness. No specific recommendations exist for energy and protein intake to support recovery from cardiac surgery and optimize postoperative growth in infants and children with CHD. Though target energy intake between 120–150 kcal/kg/day in infants is believed to be necessary to facilitate daily weight gain up to 30 g/day, data suggest that only two-thirds of both well-nourished and malnourished children (including infants) met their protein and energy requirements by day 7 following corrective cardiac surgery.[78] A systematic approach to feeding that includes ICU care bundles, while optimizing energy and protein intake is essential to support nutrient intake in children with CHD. Monitoring anthropometry measurements and the overall clinical status of the infant and child are the best approaches to nutritional care for children with CHD to improve short- and long-term patient outcomes.

E. Traumatic Brain Injury

Traumatic brain injury (TBI) results from blunt or penetrating trauma to the head and is responsible for 50,000 deaths per year in the United States.[91] The severity of TBI is staged according to degree of consciousness measured through the Glasgow Coma Scale and ranges from mild to severe TBI. Following the primary injury, the brain experiences altered regulation of cerebral blood flow and nutrient metabolism. Nutrient oxidation in the brain switches from favoring oxidative phosphorylation to anaerobic respiration, likely due to depleted oxygenation, causing an increase in lactic acid levels with resultant edema and a decrease in ATP production. This drop in available energy leads to a decrease in the activity of energy-dependent ion pumps, further dysregulating the ability to maintain normal cellular gradients, leading to a series of events driven by excessive glutamate release that triggers catabolic processes within the cell and increase oxidative stress.[92] The timing of initiation of nutrition therapy has been shown to impact outcomes in patients with TBI, and specific nutrients have been theorized to impact some of the secondary effects of cerebral edema, oxidative stress, and inflammation in TBI.[93]

The developing healthy brain almost exclusively uses glucose as a metabolic fuel for energy needs and biosynthesis. In addition to using glucose, activated neurons use lactate as an energy substrate. When glucose supplies are limited, the brain uses ketone bodies, free fatty acids, and amino acids as alternative fuels for metabolism. The metabolic stress response of critical illness affects cerebral metabolism in many ways. Prolonged or recurrent severe hypoglycemia can result in neurologic injury, especially in the setting of hypoxia and ischemia. Insulin-induced hypoglycemia may be more injurious to the developing brain than spontaneous hypoglycemia due to the lack of available alternative fuels, ketones, and fatty acids. The resulting energy failure mediates neuronal damage via glutamate-induced excitotoxicity, accumulation of oxygen free radicals, and activation of cellular apoptosis. Glucose overload results in increased production of reactive oxygen species, impaired vasodilatation, cellular apoptosis, and neuronal failure. Alterations in protein metabolism result in glutamate-induced neurotoxicity and alterations in lipid metabolism which predispose the patient to memory loss and cognitive deficits.

Adult patients

The 2016 ASPEN Guidelines for Nutrition Support in critically ill adult patients recommend initiation of EN in the hemodynamically stable patient with TBI within 24–48 h of injury but do not provide specific guidelines for energy and protein delivery. This recommendation is largely based on observational data that noted association of decreased mortality with early EN.[94,95] An RCT that enrolled 82 head injured subjects requiring mechanical ventilation found that those randomized to meet goal energy requirements on day 1 had fewer infections and overall complications compared to standard care.[96] Supplements such as Zn, magnesium, and nicotinamide are associated with decreased secondary effects of TBI such as decreased oxidative stress, inflammation, and apoptosis in animal models.[93]

Pediatric patients

TBI in children is associated with hypermetabolic states ranging from 130% to 170% higher than predicted energy expenditure for age, sex, and size.[97] Seizures and elevated temperatures are common derangements that occur following TBI and potentially increase energy expenditure. Additionally, elevated muscle tone may account for a significant component of increased energy expenditure.[98] After an initial transient increase in glucose metabolism, the patient may experience a prolonged period of apparent age-dependent, reduced glucose metabolism. In a retrospective multicenter study,[99] children with severe TBI were more likely to have delayed initiation of EN, which was an independent risk factor for worse functional status at ICU discharge. Contemporary care with guideline-based therapies such as antiepileptic medications, antipyretic therapies, and mechanical ventilation using sedation with neuromuscular blockade can significantly reduce mean energy expenditure. While adult guidelines for TBI recommend early EN, the 2019 guidelines for management of severe TBI in pediatric patients loosely endorse early EN in the absence of strong evidence to support such an approach. The 2017 ASPEN/SCCM guidelines for Nutrition Support in critically ill children recommend early EN if appropriate and tolerated by critically ill children.[100]

TABLE 32.5 Gaps in the current adult ICU nutrition literature.

Research domain topic	Topic
Protein dose	• Comparison of different levels of protein dosage at different levels of passive and active limb mobilization in postacute illness and recovery • explore the impact of high- versus low protein dosage in context of permissive underfeeding
Energy dose	• Comparison of different levels of calorie exposure at different levels of passive and active limb mobilization in acute and postacute illness as well as in recovery
Nutrition assessment	• Randomized control trials are needed to validate specific nutrition assessment tools for the exploration of group-specific nuances of benefits/harms of specific nutritional therapies • explore bedside methods for determining skeletal muscle mass and for charting/predicting improved function
EN infusion method	• explore impact of continuous versus intermittent enteral nutrition on markers of muscle preservation as well as mortality and functional status
Parenteral micronutrient supplementation	• Pragmatic trials to explore effect of parenteral supplementation of 100% of micronutrient needs until full enteral nutrition is possible on functional recovery/mortality
EN tolerance	• Examine usage of prokinetic agents when patient is intolerant to EN

TABLE 32.6 Gaps in the current pediatric ICU nutrition literature.

Research domain topic	Topic
Malnutrition in pediatric critical illness	• Define malnutrition as it related to pediatric critical illness • Describe and define phases of critical illness • Impact of critical illness on body composition (muscle mass)
Nutrition assessment	• Nutrition assessment tool for critically ill children • Impact of nutrition status at PICU admission on delivery of care and outcomes • ID changing nutrition status • Measures of muscle wasting
Energy requirements in critical illness	• Timing for assessment of energy requirements • Variables that impact energy expenditure • Develop and validate a physiology-based predictive equation for energy needs in critical illness
Protein intake	• Determination of protein goals • Impact of early protein delivery on preservation of muscle mass • Combined protein delivery and early mobilization on mobility function • Optimal approach for protein delivery
Pharmaconutrition	• Role of micronutrients in critical illness • Impact of pharmaconutrition on outcomes

TABLE 32.6 Gaps in the current pediatric ICU nutrition literature.—cont'd

Research domain topic	Topic
Enteral nutrition	• Site for EN • Impact of EN on gut (microbiome, motility, integrity) • Impact of nurse-driven feeding protocols on outcomes • Define permissive underfeeding and its impact on outcomes
Feeding intolerance	• Define EN feeding intolerance • Develop a tool to ID feeding intolerance • Indications for small bowel feeding • Use of probiotics
Parenteral nutrition	• Optimal timing of initiation of PN • Role of PN supplementation
Nutrition therapy	• Impact of combined targeted nutrition strategy on early mobilization/rehabilitation • Impact of catch-up feeding regimes • Nutrition status at discharge and long-term outcomes
Nutrition therapy in special population	• Identify "readiness to feed" for high-risk groups • Nutrition requirements in AKI or CKD • Nutrition needs and optimal feeding in noninvasive ventilation • Optimal EN on vasoactive medications; "safe dose"

III. CONCLUSION

Optimal nutrition is essential to improving outcomes in critically ill patients. Lack of careful attention to nutrition therapy while administering additional treatments during critical illness can result in development of nutrient deficits or excesses (if overfeeding) in both adults and children. Accurate nutrition assessment, obtaining anthropometric measurements, determining nutritional requirements, and the prescription and delivery of nutrients all present challenges when caring for critically ill patients. However, lack of attention to the nutritional needs of patients puts them at risk for nutritional deficits, which can delay recovery and healing. There is an urgent need for robust nutrition research and refinement of evidence-based guidelines for nutrition therapy in critically ill patients. A comprehensive, interdisciplinary approach to development of disease-specific best practices in nutrition therapy for critically ill adult and pediatric patients is necessary to diminish barriers and improve the delivery of nutrition care and optimize clinical outcomes.

RESEARCH GAPS

Adults

In 2017, an international panel of renowned nutrition researchers collaborated to identify areas of uncertainty and gaps in the adult critical care nutrition literature. Their literature review[101] revealed a dearth of knowledge in protein/calorie dosage during rehabilitative therapies, nuanced feeding therapies to address the individualized patient needs, impact of different enteral feeding methods, and more (Table 32.5).

Pediatrics

Using a 3-round Delphi process, an interdisciplinary group of experts devised a 10-point domain for research topics in nutrition support for Pediatric Critical Care, an abbreviated presentation of the topics identified in each domain is presented in Table 32.6.[102]

Acknowledgments

This chapter is an update of the chapter titled "57. Specialized Nutrition Support" by Vivian M. Zhao and Thomas R. Ziegler in Present Knowledge in Nutrition, 10th Edition, edited by Erdman JW, Macdonald IA, and Zeisel SH and published by Wiley-Blackwell. © 2012 International Life Sciences Institute. Portions of this update are from the previously published chapter and the contributions of previous authors are acknowledged.

IV. REFERENCES

1. Mehta NM, Duggan CP. Nutritional deficiencies during critical illness. *Pediatr Clin N Am.* 2009;56(5):1143–1160.
2. Puthucheary ZA, Rawal J, McPhail M, et al. Acute skeletal muscle wasting in critical illness. *J Am Med Assoc.* 2013;310(15):1591–1600.
3. Johnson RW, Ng KWP, Dietz AR, et al. Muscle atrophy in mechanically-ventilated critically ill children. *PLoS One.* 2018; 13(12):e0207720.
4. Streat SJ, Beddoe AH, Hill GL. Aggressive nutritional support does not prevent protein loss despite fat gain in septic intensive care patients. *J Trauma.* 1987;27(3):262–266.
5. Wilmore DW. Catabolic illness. Strategies for enhancing recovery. *N Engl J Med.* 1991;325(10):695–702.
6. Ziegler TR, Gatzen C, Wilmore DW. Strategies for attenuating protein-catabolic responses in the critically ill. *Annu Rev Med.* 1994;45:459–480.
7. Blaauw R, Osland E, Sriram K, et al. Parenteral provision of micronutrients to adult patients: an expert consensus paper. *J Parenter Enter Nutr.* 2019;43(Suppl 1):S5–S23.
8. Halliwell B, Gutteridge JMC. In: Oxford, ed. *Free Radicals in Biology and Medicine.* 5th ed. United Kingdom: Oxford University Press; 2015.
9. Geoghegan M, McAuley D, Eaton S, Powell-Tuck J. Selenium in critical illness. *Curr Opin Crit Care.* 2006;12(2):136–141.
10. Marik PE, Khangoora V, Rivera R, Hooper MH, Catravas J. Hydrocortisone, vitamin C, and thiamine for the treatment of severe sepsis and septic shock: a retrospective before-after study. *Chest.* 2017;151(6):1229–1238.
11. Armour J, Tyml K, Lidington D, Wilson JX. Ascorbate prevents microvascular dysfunction in the skeletal muscle of the septic rat. *J Appl Physiol.* 2001;90(3):795–803.
12. Wu F, Wilson JX, Tyml K. Ascorbate protects against impaired arteriolar constriction in sepsis by inhibiting inducible nitric oxide synthase expression. *Free Radic Biol Med.* 2004;37(8): 1282–1289.
13. Fowler 3rd AA, Syed AA, Knowlson S, et al. Phase I safety trial of intravenous ascorbic acid in patients with severe sepsis. *J Transl Med.* 2014;12:32.
14. Litwak JJ, Cho N, Nguyen HB, Moussavi K, Bushell T. Vitamin C, hydrocortisone, and thiamine for the treatment of severe sepsis and septic shock: a retrospective analysis of real-world application. *J Clin Med.* 2019;8(4).
15. Balakrishnan M, Gandhi H, Shah K, et al. Hydrocortisone, vitamin C and thiamine for the treatment of sepsis and septic shock following cardiac surgery. *Indian J Anaesth.* 2018;62(12): 934–939.
16. Kalil AC, Johnson DW, Cawcutt KA. Vitamin C is not ready for prime time in sepsis but a solution is close. *Chest.* 2017; 152(3):676.
17. McClave SA, Taylor BE, Martindale RG, et al. Guidelines for the provision and assessment of nutrition support therapy in the adult critically ill patient: Society of Critical Care Medicine (SCCM) and American Society for Parenteral and Enteral Nutrition (A.S.P.E.N.). *J Parenter Enter Nutr.* 2016;40(2): 159–211.

18. Heyland DK, Dhaliwal R, Jiang X, Day AG. Identifying critically ill patients who benefit the most from nutrition therapy: the development and initial validation of a novel risk assessment tool. *Crit Care*. 2011;15(6):R268.
19. Kondrup J, Rasmussen HH, Hamberg O, Stanga Z, Ad Hoc EWG. Nutritional risk screening (NRS 2002): a new method based on an analysis of controlled clinical trials. *Clin Nutr*. 2003; 22(3):321–336.
20. Rahman A, Hasan RM, Agarwala R, Martin C, Day AG, Heyland DK. Identifying critically-ill patients who will benefit most from nutritional therapy: further validation of the "modified NUTRIC" nutritional risk assessment tool. *Clin Nutr*. 2016;35(1): 158–162.
21. Kalaiselvan MS, Renuka MK, Arunkumar AS. Use of nutrition risk in critically ill (NUTRIC) score to assess nutritional risk in mechanically ventilated patients: a prospective observational study. *Indian J Crit Care Med*. 2017;21(5):253–256.
22. Ata Ur-Rehman HM, Ishtiaq W, Yousaf M, Bano S, Mujahid AM, Akhtar A. Modified nutrition risk in critically ill (mNUTRIC) score to assess nutritional risk in mechanically ventilated patients: a prospective observational study from the Pakistani population. *Cureus*. 2018;10(12):e3786.
23. Compher C, Chittams J, Sammarco T, Higashibeppu N, Higashiguchi T, Heyland DK. Greater nutrient intake is associated with lower mortality in western and eastern critically ill patients with low BMI: a multicenter, multinational observational study. *J Parenter Enter Nutr*. 2019;43(1):63–69.
24. Compher C, Chittams J, Sammarco T, Nicolo M, Heyland DK. Greater protein and energy intake may be associated with improved mortality in higher risk critically ill patients: a multicenter, multinational observational study. *Crit Care Med*. 2017; 45(2):156–163.
25. Nicolo M, Heyland DK, Chittams J, Sammarco T, Compher C. Clinical outcomes related to protein delivery in a critically ill population: a multicenter, multinational observation study. *J Parenter Enter Nutr*. 2016;40(1):45–51.
26. Lew CCH, Wong GJY, Cheung KP, et al. When timing and dose of nutrition support were examined, the modified nutrition risk in critically ill (mNUTRIC) score did not differentiate high-risk patients who would derive the most benefit from nutrition support: a prospective cohort study. *Ann Intensive Care*. 2018; 8(1):98.
27. Johansen N, Kondrup J, Plum LM, et al. Effect of nutritional support on clinical outcome in patients at nutritional risk. *Clin Nutr*. 2004;23(4):539–550.
28. Starke J, Schneider H, Alteheld B, Stehle P, Meier R. Short-term individual nutritional care as part of routine clinical setting improves outcome and quality of life in malnourished medical patients. *Clin Nutr*. 2011;30(2):194–201.
29. Kondrup J. Nutritional-risk scoring systems in the intensive care unit. *Curr Opin Clin Nutr Metab Care*. 2014;17(2):177–182.
30. White JV, Guenter P, Jensen G, et al. Consensus statement of the Academy of Nutrition and Dietetics/American Society for Parenteral and Enteral Nutrition: characteristics recommended for the identification and documentation of adult malnutrition (undernutrition). *J Acad Nutr Diet*. 2012;112(5):730–738.
31. Sheean PM, Peterson SJ, Gomez Perez S, et al. The prevalence of sarcopenia in patients with respiratory failure classified as normally nourished using computed tomography and subjective global assessment. *J Parenter Enter Nutr*. 2014;38(7):873–879.
32. Pollack MM, Wiley JS, Holbrook PR. Early nutritional depletion in critically ill children. *Crit Care Med*. 1981;9(8):580–583.
33. Pollack MM, Wiley JS, Kanter R, Holbrook PR. Malnutrition in critically ill infants and children. *J Parenter Enter Nutr*. 1982;6(1): 20–24.
34. Hulst J, Joosten K, Zimmermann L, et al. Malnutrition in critically ill children: from admission to 6 months after discharge. *Clin Nutr*. 2004;23(2):223–232.
35. Pawellek I, Dokoupil K, Koletzko B. Prevalence of malnutrition in paediatric hospital patients. *Clin Nutr*. 2008;27(1):72–76.
36. Valla FV, Berthiller J, Gaillard-Le-Roux B, et al. Faltering growth in the critically ill child: prevalence, risk factors, and impaired outcome. *Eur J Pediatr*. 2018;177(3):345–353.
37. Mehta NM, Skillman HE, Irving SY, et al. Guidelines for the provision and assessment of nutrition support therapy in the pediatric critically ill patient: Society of Critical Care Medicine and American Society for Parenteral and Enteral Nutrition. *Pediatr Crit Care Med*. 2017;18(7):675–715.
38. Peterson CM, Thomas DM, Blackburn GL, Heymsfield SB. Universal equation for estimating ideal body weight and body weight at any BMI. *Am J Clin Nutr*. 2016;103(5):1197–1203.
39. Schofield WN. Predicting basal metabolic rate, new standards and review of previous work. *Hum Nutr Clin Nutr*. 1985;39(Suppl 1): 5–41.
40. World Health Organization. *FAO/WHO/UNU Expert Consultation. Energy and Protein Requirements: Technical Report Series #724*. 1985: 71–112. Geneva.
41. Carpenter A, Pencharz P, Mouzaki M. Accurate estimation of energy requirements of young patients. *J Pediatr Gastroenterol Nutr*. 2015;60(1):4–10.
42. Heyland DK, Patel J, Bear D, et al. The effect of higher protein dosing in critically ill patients: a multicenter registry-based randomized trial: the EFFORT trial. *J Parenter Enter Nutr*. 2019;43(3): 326–334.
43. Hales CMCM, Fryar CD, Ogden CL. *Prevalence of Obesity Among Adults and Youth: United States, 2015–2016.NCHS Data Brief No. 288*. October 2017.
44. Schofield WN. Predicting basal metabolic rate, new standards and review of previous work. *Hum Nutr Clin Nutr*. 1985;39C(Suppl 1): 5–41.
45. Jesuit C, Dillon C, Compher C, American Society for P, Enteral Nutrition Board of Directors, Lenders CM. A.S.P.E.N. clinical guidelines: nutrition support of hospitalized pediatric patients with obesity. *J Parenter Enteral Nutr*. 2010;34(1):13–20.
46. Bechard LJ, Rothpletz-Puglia P, Touger-Decker R, Duggan C, Mehta NM. Influence of obesity on clinical outcomes in hospitalized children: a systematic review. *JAMA Pediatr*. 2013;167(5):476–482.
47. Mehta NM, Bechard LJ, Cahill N, et al. Nutritional practices and their relationship to clinical outcomes in critically ill children—an international multicenter cohort study. *Crit Care Med*. 2012;40(7): 2204–2211.
48. Mikhailov TA, Kuhn EM, Manzi J, et al. Early enteral nutrition is associated with lower mortality in critically ill children. *J Parenter Enter Nutr*. 2014;38(4):459–466.
49. Turner JR. Intestinal mucosal barrier function in health and disease. *Nat Rev Immunol*. 2009;9(11):799–809.
50. Doig GS, Chevrou-Severac H, Simpson F. Early enteral nutrition in critical illness: a full economic analysis using US costs. *Clinicoecon Outcomes Res*. 2013;5:429–436.
51. Brown AM, Fisher E, Forbes ML. Bolus vs continuous nasogastric feeds in mechanically ventilated pediatric patients: a pilot study. *J Parenter Enter Nutr*. 2019;43(6):750–758.
52. Gottschlich MM, Jenkins ME, Mayes T, Khoury J, Kagan RJ, Warden GD. The 2002 Clinical Research Award. An evaluation of the safety of early vs delayed enteral support and effects on clinical, nutritional, and endocrine outcomes after severe burns. *J Burn Care Rehabil*. 2002;23(6):401–415.
53. Tolia V, Lin CH, Kuhns LR. Gastric emptying using three different formulas in infants with gastroesophageal reflux. *J Pediatr Gastroenterol Nutr*. 1992;15(3):297–301.

54. Casaer MP, Mesotten D, Hermans G, et al. Early versus late parenteral nutrition in critically ill adults. *N Engl J Med*. 2011;365(6):506–517.
55. Fivez T, Kerklaan D, Mesotten D, et al. Early versus late parenteral nutrition in critically ill children. *N Engl J Med*. 2016;374(12):1111–1122.
56. Doig GS, Simpson F, Sweetman EA, et al. Early parenteral nutrition in critically ill patients with short-term relative contraindications to early enteral nutrition: a randomized controlled trial. *J Am Med Assoc*. 2013;309(20):2130–2138.
57. Harvey SE, Parrott F, Harrison DA, et al. Trial of the route of early nutritional support in critically ill adults. *N Engl J Med*. 2014; 371(18):1673–1684.
58. Byrnes MC, Stangenes J. Refeeding in the ICU: an adult and pediatric problem. *Curr Opin Clin Nutr Metab Care*. 2011;14(2):186–192.
59. Byham-Gray LS J, Weisen K. *A Clinical Guide to Nutrition Care in Kidney Disease*. 2nd ed. 2013.
60. Rhodes A, Evans LE, Alhazzani W, et al. Surviving sepsis campaign: international guidelines for management of sepsis and septic shock: 2016. *Intensive Care Med*. 2017;43(3):304–377.
61. Irving SY, Daly B, Verger J, et al. The association of nutrition status expressed as body mass index z score with outcomes in children with severe sepsis: a secondary analysis from the Sepsis Prevalence, Outcomes, and Therapies (SPROUT) study. *Crit Care Med*. 2018;46(11):e1029–e1039.
62. Briassoulis G, Venkataraman S, Thompson AE. Energy expenditure in critically ill children. *Crit Care Med*. 2000;28(4):1166–1172.
63. Ismail J, Bansal A, Jayashree M, Nallasamy K, Attri SV. Energy balance in critically ill children with severe sepsis using indirect calorimetry: a prospective cohort study. *J Pediatr Gastroenterol Nutr*. 2019;68(6):868–873.
64. Spanaki AM, Tavladaki T, Dimitriou H, et al. Longitudinal profiles of metabolism and bioenergetics associated with innate immune hormonal inflammatory responses and amino-acid kinetics in severe sepsis and systemic inflammatory response syndrome in children. *J Parenter Enter Nutr*. 2018;42(6):1061–1074.
65. Carcillo JA, Dean JM, Holubkov R, et al. The randomized comparative pediatric critical illness stress-induced immune suppression (CRISIS) prevention trial. *Pediatr Crit Care Med*. 2012;13(2):165–173.
66. Carcillo JA, Dean JM, Holubkov R, et al. Interaction between 2 nutraceutical treatments and host immune status in the pediatric critical illness stress-induced immune suppression comparative effectiveness trial. *J Parenter Enter Nutr*. 2017;41(8):1325–1335.
67. Kasper DL, Fauci AS, Hauser SL, Longo DL, Jameson JL, Loscalzo J. *Harrison's Principles of Internal Medicine*. 19th ed. New York: McGraw Hill Education Medical; 2015.
68. Wilson B, Typpo K. Nutrition: a primary therapy in pediatric acute respiratory distress syndrome. *Front Pediatr*. 2016;4:108.
69. Krzak A, Pleva M, Napolitano LM. Nutrition therapy for ALI and ARDS. *Crit Care Clin*. 2011;27(3):647–659.
70. Wong JJ, Han WM, Sultana R, Loh TF, Lee JH. Nutrition delivery affects outcomes in pediatric acute respiratory distress syndrome. *J Parenter Enter Nutr*. 2017;41(6):1007–1013.
71. Jacobs BR, Nadkarni V, Goldstein B, et al. Nutritional immunomodulation in critically ill children with acute lung injury: feasibility and impact on circulating biomarkers. *Pediatr Crit Care Med*. 2013; 14(1):e45–56.
72. Wei Q, Xiao X, Fogle P, Dong Z. Changes in metabolic profiles during acute kidney injury and recovery following ischemia/reperfusion. *PLoS One*. 2014;9(9):e106647.
73. Kyle UG, Akcan-Arikan A, Orellana RA, Coss-Bu JA. Nutrition support among critically ill children with AKI. *Clin J Am Soc Nephrol*. 2013;8(4):568–574.
74. Sethi SK, Maxvold N, Bunchman T, Jha P, Kher V, Raina R. Nutritional management in the critically ill child with acute kidney injury: a review. *Pediatr Nephrol*. 2017;32(4):589–601.
75. Nelms CLJM, Warady BA. *Renal Disease. A.S.P.E.N. Pediatric Nutrition Support Core Curriculum*. 2nd ed. Silver Spring, MD: American Society of Parenteral and Enteral Nutrition; 2015.
76. Raymond JLaC SC. Medical nutrition therapy for cardiovascular disease. In: Mahan KaR JL, ed. *Krause's Food & the Nutrition Care Process*. 14th ed. Saint Louis, MO: Elsevier; 2017.
77. Hoffman JI, Kaplan S. The incidence of congenital heart disease. *J Am Coll Cardiol*. 2002;39(12):1890–1900.
78. Medoff-Cooper B, Ravishankar C. Nutrition and growth in congenital heart disease: a challenge in children. *Curr Opin Cardiol*. 2013;28(2):122–129.
79. Burnham N, Ittenbach RF, Stallings VA, et al. Genetic factors are important determinants of impaired growth after infant cardiac surgery. *J Thorac Cardiovasc Surg*. 2010;140(1):144–149.
80. Leitch CA, Karn CA, Peppard RJ, et al. Increased energy expenditure in infants with cyanotic congenital heart disease. *J Pediatr*. 1998;133(6):755–760.
81. Farrell AG, Schamberger MS, Olson IL, Leitch CA. Large left-to-right shunts and congestive heart failure increase total energy expenditure in infants with ventricular septal defect. *Am J Cardiol*. 2001;87(9):1128–1131. A1110.
82. Mitchell IM, Davies PS, Day JM, Pollock JC, Jamieson MP. Energy expenditure in children with congenital heart disease, before and after cardiac surgery. *J Thorac Cardiovasc Surg*. 1994;107(2):374–380.
83. Leitch CA, Karn CA, Ensing GJ, Denne SC. Energy expenditure after surgical repair in children with cyanotic congenital heart disease. *J Pediatr*. 2000;137(3):381–385.
84. Barton JS, Hindmarsh PC, Scrimgeour CM, Rennie MJ, Preece MA. Energy expenditure in congenital heart disease. *Arch Dis Child*. 1994;70(1):5–9.
85. Irving SY, Medoff-Cooper B, Stouffer NO, et al. Resting energy expenditure at 3 months of age following neonatal surgery for congenital heart disease. *Congenit Heart Dis*. 2013;8(4):343–351.
86. Trabulsi JC, Irving SY, Papas MA, et al. Total energy expenditure of infants with congenital heart disease who have undergone surgical intervention. *Pediatr Cardiol*. 2015;36(8):1670–1679.
87. Medoff-Cooper B, Irving SY, Hanlon AL, et al. The association among feeding mode, growth, and developmental outcomes in infants with complex congenital heart disease at 6 and 12 Months of age. *J Pediatr*. 2016;169, 154–159 e151.
88. Kaufman J, Vichayavilas P, Rannie M, et al. Improved nutrition delivery and nutrition status in critically ill children with heart disease. *Pediatrics*. 2015;135(3):e717–725.
89. Tsintoni A, Dimitriou G, Karatza AA. Nutrition of neonates with congenital heart disease: existing evidence, conflicts and concerns. *J Matern Fetal Neonatal Med*. 2019:1–6.
90. Sables-Baus S, Kaufman J, Cook P, da Cruz EM. Oral feeding outcomes in neonates with congenital cardiac disease undergoing cardiac surgery. *Cardiol Young*. 2012;22(1):42–48.
91. Vella MA, Crandall ML, Patel MB. Acute management of traumatic brain injury. *Surg Clin N Am*. 2017;97(5):1015–1030.
92. Werner C, Engelhard K. Pathophysiology of traumatic brain injury. *Br J Anaesth*. 2007;99(1):4–9.
93. Lucke-Wold BP, Logsdon AF, Nguyen L, et al. Supplements, nutrition, and alternative therapies for the treatment of traumatic brain injury. *Nutr Neurosci*. 2018;21(2):79–91.
94. Chiang YH, Chao DP, Chu SF, et al. Early enteral nutrition and clinical outcomes of severe traumatic brain injury patients in acute stage: a multi-center cohort study. *J Neurotrauma*. 2012;29(1):75–80.
95. Hartl R, Gerber LM, Ni Q, Ghajar J. Effect of early nutrition on deaths due to severe traumatic brain injury. *J Neurosurg*. 2008; 109(1):50–56.
96. Taylor SJ, Fettes SB, Jewkes C, Nelson RJ. Prospective, randomized, controlled trial to determine the effect of early enhanced enteral nutrition on clinical outcome in mechanically ventilated

patients suffering head injury. *Crit Care Med.* 1999;27(11):2525–2531.

97. Redmond C, Lipp J. Traumatic brain injury in the pediatric population. *Nutr Clin Pract.* 2006;21(5):450–461.
98. Phillips R, Ott L, Young B, Walsh J. Nutritional support and measured energy expenditure of the child and adolescent with head injury. *J Neurosurg.* 1987;67(6):846–851.
99. Balakrishnan B, Flynn-O'Brien KT, Simpson PM, Dasgupta M, Hanson SJ. Enteral nutrition initiation in children admitted to pediatric intensive care units after traumatic brain injury. *Neurocritical Care.* 2019;30(1):193–200.
100. Kochanek PM, Tasker RC, Carney N, et al. Guidelines for the management of pediatric severe traumatic brain injury, third edition: update of the brain trauma foundation guidelines. *Pediatr Crit Care Med.* 2019;20(3S Suppl 1):S1–S82.
101. Arabi YM, Casaer MP, Chapman M, et al. The intensive care medicine research agenda in nutrition and metabolism. *Intensive Care Med.* 2017;43(9):1239–1256.
102. Tume LN, Valla FV, Floh AA, et al. Priorities for nutrition research in pediatric critical care. *J Parenter Enteral Nutr.* 2019;43(7):853–862.

CHAPTER

33

CLINICAL NUTRITION IN PATIENTS WITH CANCER

Asta Bye[1,2,3], *RD, PhD*
Ellisiv Lærum-Onsager[4], *RN, PhD*

[1]Department of Nursing and Health Promotion, Faculty of Health Sciences, OsloMet - Oslo Metropolitan University, Oslo, Norway
[2]Regional Advisory Unit for Palliative Care, Department of Oncology, Oslo University Hospital, Oslo, Norway
[3]European Palliative Care Research Centre (PRC), Department of Oncology, Oslo University Hospital, Oslo, Norway
[4]Lovisenberg Diaconal University College, Oslo, Norway

SUMMARY

In this chapter, we aim to describe the important features of malnutrition and cachexia in patients with cancer, in addition to assessment of nutritional status and symptoms affecting nutritional status in this group of patients. Furthermore, nutritional interventions will be described in accordance to relevant clinical guidelines both for patients currently receiving anticancer treatment and patients receiving palliative care. We have particularly emphasized the role symptoms and side effects of anticancer treatment in the development of malnutrition in patients. Systematic symptom assessment is strongly recommended in addition to nutritional risk screening. Furthermore, we advocate that evaluation of physical performance status should be included when goals for nutritional treatment are set. Nutrition support for patients with cancer is described with focus on enteral and parenteral nutrition. The chapter concerns cancer diagnosis in general, and different types of cancer are mentioned as examples, but not described in detailed.

Keywords: Cancer cachexia; Malnutrition; Nutritional assessment; Nutritional treatment; Patients.

I. NUTRITION IN CANCER

According to the European Society of Clinical Nutrition and Metabolism (ESPEN) Guidelines for nutrition in patients with cancer, there are no diets known to cure cancer or prevent cancer recurrence.[1] However, the international organization World Cancer Research Fund (WCRF) that regularly analyses the evidence on cancer prevention and survival recommend cancer survivors (people diagnosed with cancer, including those who have recovered) to follow the recommendations for cancer prevention if they can.[2] Following the recommendations are likely to promote nutritional adequacy and a healthful body composition. The recommendations are therefore also applicable for patients living with cancer who want to follow a healthful diet, unless they struggle with weight loss or are advised otherwise by their physician or other health professionals. Table 33.1 summarizes the cancer prevention recommendations and comments on the evidence base associated with each recommendation. The main points are that people should maintain a healthy weight, be physically active, and eat whole grains, vegetables, fruits, and beans. The consumption of processed foods high in fat, starches or sugar, red and processed meat, and sugar sweetened drinks and alcohol should be limited. In addition, it is recommended to meet these nutritional needs through foods alone, rather than not through dietary supplements,

Present Knowledge in Nutrition, Volume 2
https://doi.org/10.1016/B978-0-12-818460-8.00033-2

TABLE 33.1 The World Cancer Research Fund cancer prevention recommendations with comments.

Recommendation	Comments
1. Recommendation: Be a healthy weight	**Comments**
Keep a weight within the healthy range (BMI of 18.5–24.9) and avoid weight gain in adult life.	*Convincing evidence that a healthy weight protects against* cancers of the esophagus (adenocarcinoma), pancreas, liver, colorectum, breast (menopausal) and kidney. *Overweight and obesity is probably a cause of* cancers of the mouth, pharynx and larynx, stomach (cardia), gallbladder, ovary, and prostate (advanced).
2. Recommendation: Be physically active	**Comments**
Be at least moderately physically active and follow or exceed national guidelines and limit sedentary habits	*Convincing* evidence that physical activity[a] protects against colon cancer. *Physical activity[a] probably protect against the following:* Postmenopausal breast cancer and endometrial cancer. Physical activity of *vigorous intensity probably* protects against premenopausal breast cancer. In addition, physical activity protects against weight gain, overweight, and obesity and therefore against those cancers for which these conditions are a cause (see recommendation 1).
3. Recommendation: Eat whole grains, vegetables, fruit, and beans	**Comments**
Make whole grains, vegetables, fruits, and pulses (legumes) such as beans and lentils a major part of your daily diet	*Strong* evidence that eating whole grains and food containing dietary fiber protects against colorectal cancer.
4. Recommendation: Limit "fast food"	**Comments**
Limit processed foods high in fat, starches, or sugars——including fast foods	*Strong* evidence that glycemia load is a cause of endometrial cancer. In addition, a high consumption of fast food can cause weight gain, overweight, and obesity and therefore increase the risk of cancers for which these conditions are a cause (see recommendation 1).
5. Recommendation: Limit red and processed meat	**Comments**
Eat no more than moderate amounts[b] of red meat and little, if any, processed meat	*Strong* evidence that consumption of either red or processed meat are causes of colorectal cancer.
6. Recommendation: Limit sugar-sweetened drinks	**Comments**
Drink mostly water and unsweetened drinks	Consumption of sugar-sweetened drinks can cause weight gain, overweight, and obesity and therefore increase the risk of those cancers for which these conditions are a cause (see recommendation 1).
7. Recommendation: Limit alcohol consumption	**Comments**
For cancer prevention, it is best not to drink alcohol.	*Strong evidence that consumption of alcohol is a cause of* cancers of the mouth, pharynx and larynx, esophagus (squamous cell carcinoma), liver, colorectum, breast (pre- and postmenopause), and stomach.
8. Recommendation: Do not use supplements for cancer prevention	**Comments**
High-dose dietary supplements are not recommended for cancer prevention. Aim to meet nutritional needs through diet alone.	*Strong* evidence that consumption of high-dose beta-carotene supplements may increase risk of lung cancer in some people. No strong evidence that dietary supplements, apart from calcium for colorectal cancer, can reduce cancer risk.
9. Recommendation: Mothers should be recommended to breastfeed their infants if possible	**Comments**
Evidence on cancer and other diseases shows that sustained, exclusive breastfeeding is protective for the mother and the child	***Strong* evidence that breastfeeding protects against the following:** Breast cancer in the mother and promotes healthy growth in the infant. Breastfeeding protects children against overweight and obesity and therefore against those cancers for which these conditions are a cause.

TABLE 33.1 The World Cancer Research Fund cancer prevention recommendations with comments.—cont'd

10. Recommendation: After a cancer diagnosis, follow WCRFs recommendation if possible	**Comments**
Unless otherwise advised from health personnel, all cancer survivors, if they can, are advised to follow the Cancer Prevention Recommendations as far as possible after the acute stage of treatment. There may be specific situations where the Cancer Prevention Recommendations may not apply and guidance from health professionals may be needed.	There is currently a lack of high-quality randomized controlled trials (RCTs) regarding nutrition, diet, and physical activity effect on risk of cancer in cancer survivors. Due to this, WCRF has only reviewed the evidence for the effects of these lifestyle factors on survival and future risk in breast cancer. The evidence is persuasive that nutritional factors, such as body fatness, and physical activity predict important outcomes from breast cancer.

[a]*of moderate or vigorous intensity, for example, walking, cycling, gardening (moderate-intensity) and running, fast swimming, and aerobics (vigorous intensity).*
[b]*no more than three (350–500 g/12–18 oz) portions per week.*

unless medically recommended. Finally, WCRF underscores and recommends breastfeeding, if possible, since it protects against breast cancer in the mother and promotes typical growth patterns in the infant.[2]

Patients with cancer with unintentional weight loss and food intake are complicated by symptoms induced by physical responses to tumor growth and side effects of antineoplastic regimes. A primary focus is to ensure sufficient energy intake to prevent decline in nutritional status.[1] Patients with cancer have one of the highest prevalences of malnutrition,[3] yet the prevalence tends to vary depending on factors such as malnutrition assessment techniques, setting, and heterogeneity within in the population of oncological patients. Without treatment, malnutrition contributes to a downward trajectory [4] and has consequences not only for the individual but also for the society. Malnutrition in patients with cancer is associated with adverse outcomes such as lower survival rates and may be related to increased treatment toxicity, reduced immune competence, psychosocial stress, longer hospital stays, poorer quality of life, and frailty.[5] Societal consequences of malnutrition include longer hospital stay, which increase hospital costs.[6]

It has been suggested that approximately 25%–30% of patients with cancer die as a consequence of emaciation rather than tumor growth in vital organ systems.[7] Despite this, it has not been well demonstrated that nutritional therapy in patients with cancer who are malnourished or at risk of malnutrition improves survival.[1] On the other side, there is good evidence that nutrition interventions lead to increased food intake, weight gain, and improvement in some aspects of quality of life. Thus, nutritional interventions are an important part of the medical treatment of patients with cancer, especially with significant malnourished patients.

II. CANCER-ASSOCIATED WEIGHT LOSS AND MALNUTRITION

A. Etiology and Pathophysiology

About 50% of all newly diagnosed patients with cancer experience unintentional (involuntary) weight loss.[8] However, there is great variation in this rate between diagnoses. In patients with gastric and intestinal tract cancers, more than 80% have weight loss at the time of diagnosis.[8,9] In patients with colorectal cancer and lung carcinoma, the estimated prevalence is 50%–60%.[8–11] Weight loss is less frequent in lymphoma, leukemia, and breast cancer where the prevalence is reported to be below 50%.[8] The prevalence of weight loss increases during treatment and disease progression regardless of diagnosis, and more than 80% of patients with advanced and incurable cancer experience weight loss.[12] If the weight loss is more than 5% of usual body weight over a period of 6 to 12 months, it is defined as clinically relevant.[13]

The etiology of weight loss in patients with cancer is complex, but generally, it is attributed to two key components: reduced dietary intake and increased energy expenditure.[1] Reduced intake is normally related to poor appetite, poor uptake of nutrients due to pathological changes in the intestinal tract, and/or eating problems due to symptoms associated with the disease and the anticancer treatment.[14] The body thus breaks down its own energy reserves, primarily fat, and also protein (muscle), and results in weight loss. In cancer and specifically in patients with incurable disease, weight loss may occur as a result of metabolic changes including increased energy expenditure.[1,15] This occurs through a variety of mechanisms related to the tumor growth and metabolism and the host response to the tumor (such as hormones and inflammatory cytokines). This condition is referred to as cancer cachexia and is closely connected to the underlying disease (see section "Cancer Cachexia").[1,16] Patients with cachexia usually have insufficient food intake in addition to increased resting energy expenditure.[15] The combination of these factors causes the patient to lose weight faster than one might expect from the metabolic changes alone.[16] The possibility of cachexia must be taken into consideration when assessing nutritional status and making therapeutic decisions for the care of patients with cancer.

Inadequate food intake over longer periods of time leads to changes in the nutritional status and result in malnutrition. There is currently no universal agreement on the definition of malnutrition. In the 2017 guideline from ESPEN, malnutrition is defined as "a state resulting from lack of uptake or intake of nutrition leading to altered body composition (decreased fat free mass) and body cell mass leading to diminished physical and mental function." [17] One recent study reported prevalence of malnutrition in hospitalized patients with cancer measured with the Subjective Global Assessment (SGA) method at two time points (2012, n = 1677 participants and 2014, n = 1913 participants) from a population that was representative of all treatment settings, tumor types, and stages of disease.[18] The overall prevalence of malnutrition was 31% in 2012 and 26% in 2014. At both time points, patients with tumors in the upper gastrointestinal tract, in addition to endocrine and thyroid tumors, had the highest prevalence of malnutrition (2012: 61%, 2014: 48%), followed by head and neck cancer (2012:40%, 2014: 36%) and lung cancer (2012: 37%, 2014: 33%). The lowest prevalence of malnutrition was reported for breast cancer (2012:14%, 2014: 13%). It is important to underscore that in patients with advanced cancer with metastases, the prevalence of weight loss and malnutrition tends to be higher.[19]

The pathophysiology of cancer-associated malnutrition is complex due to underlying mechanisms and cannot be explained by one singular factor.[14] Consequently, the development of malnutrition in patients with cancer is a multimodal process due to the factors that collude to decrease food intake, increase energy and protein needs, decrease anabolic stimuli such as physical activity, and alter metabolism in different organs or tissues.[1] Cancer-related factors that cause appetite loss and eating difficulties include pain or mechanical obstructions and treatment toxicity. Cancer-related inflammation may lead to higher resting energy expenditure and increased muscle catabolism, and metabolic changes affect appetite regulation and lead to decreased appetite.[9,20] Poor appetite is considered of great importance in the development of cancer-related malnutrition, and the effect is enhanced by the many symptoms that potentially affect food intake during the disease course.[21] Several studies have demonstrated strong associations between cancer, symptom burden, and food intake. It is unclear which nutritional treatment will reverse weight loss or if some groups of patients will benefit more than others from specific nutritional treatments.[1]

B. Role of Symptoms and Treatment-Related Side Effects

A symptom is defined as any subjective evidence of disease. In cancer, symptoms rarely occur in isolation but coexist with others. It is reported that the cancer patient experience an average of 11–13 symptoms.[22] Appetite loss is probably the most common nutrition-related symptom in cancer, and it is independently linked to survival.[23] As mentioned, it may be caused by the cancer itself and also by a number of other medical symptoms leading to decreased appetite. Appetite loss is found to coexist with symptoms such as nausea, vomiting, taste changes, dry mouth, and fatigue.[24]

The symptoms associated with appetite loss and compromised dietary intake are often referred to as nutrition impact symptoms (NIS).[10,25] NIS may occur early in the disease course, for instance in patients with pancreatic cancer, or NIS may emerge at an advanced stage of the disease, such as in breast cancer and lymphoma. It is also important to be aware that NIS may continue after the end of treatment, which may raise concern in patients of a permanent inability to eat and enjoy food.[26] Systematic symptom assessment and management is therefore mandatory and of great importance during the entire disease trajectory.[27]

Appetite loss

The regulation of appetite and satiety in the human body is a complex process including peripheral endocrine and neuronal signals as well as cognition, perception, and learned behavior.[28] Normally, nervous signals provide information about energy consumption and availability from recently ingested food as well as energy stores, and the body uses this to maintain energy homeostasis and body weight. In cancer and specifically in cancer cachexia may several hormones and signaling molecules be involved in the appetite regulation. This includes insulin, leptin, ghrelin, corticosteroids, and cytokines such as interleukin 1.[29] It is also suggested that inflammatory reactions caused by cytokines initiate both appetite loss and mobilization of body energy and protein reserves. These responses are thought to reflect adaptive reactions intended to enact immune reactions and tissue repair, independent of food supply.

Disease and treatment-related symptoms

Tumors in the oral cavity, pharynx, esophagus, or stomach can cause obstructions, making food difficult to pass.[30] The prevalence of swallowing problems among patients with cancer varies with diagnosis, stage, and treatment,[31] but in general, these are associated with cancer of the ear, nose, throat, and esophagus. Swallowing dysfunction can also occur in brain metastases or central nervous system tumors.[32] In addition to dysphagia, the patient may experience pain when eating which may cause avoidance of food or meals and changes in eating habits. Similar eating problems occur if a tumor is obstructing the intestine, inhibits passage of food, and impacts digestion and absorption. Abdominal pain, nausea, vomiting, and early satiety may result. Suppressed appetite due to sensory changes occurs frequently. Changes in the ability to perceive the basic flavors (sweet, salty, sour, bitter, and umami) are common due to both increased and decreased taste detection.[33] Elevated salt thresholds have for example been documented during and following chemotherapy for advanced cancer. Bitter, chemical, or metallic tastes also seem to be common after chemotherapy.[30] However, these changes seem to be reversible if the tumor responds to treatment.[34] Oral dryness due to salivary gland hypofunction and specific drugs (antiemetics and opioids) may cause sensory dysfunction and dysphagia. This may predispose to bacterial or fungal infections in the oral mucosa.[30] Such infections make the mucosa sore and painful and cause discomfort or swallowing difficulties, thus resulting in a reduced food intake. In addition to the discomfort, soreness in the oral mucosa may result in difficulty to perform good oral hygiene and to oral or dental complications.

Cancer-related surgery can affect the gastrointestinal tract and interfere with digestion and absorption of nutrients.[30] A typical example is gastrectomy, where anatomical changes make it impossible to eat as much food per meal as before and therefore results in energy deficits. In the case of radiotherapy to the upper part, gastrointestinal tract (oral cavity, pharynx, esophagus), soreness, mucositis, and edema often occur and cause swallowing problems.[1] The radiation side effects usually persist for a few weeks after treatment, but for some patients, these are irreversible.[30] In the case of radiotherapy to the stomach and intestines, patients may experience problems such as nausea, vomiting, and diarrhea. These side effects usually disappear a few weeks after discontinuation of treatment. Some may experience late side effects that appear months to years after discontinuation of treatment. Chemotherapy usually produces side effects such as taste and smell changes, nausea and vomiting, diarrhea, stomatitis, and esophagitis.[1,30] Some chemotherapeutic regimens affect the intestinal muscle and mucosal activity and cause constipation and ileus. The effect on appetite and physical ability to eat depends on which chemotherapy agents are used and target tissue.[30] Generally, it is difficult to maintain the nutritional status during ongoing more toxic chemotherapy regimens because of the side effects. This implies that patients receiving chemotherapy treatment are regularly exposed to periods of hunger and weight loss. New treatment approaches, such as immunotherapy, are generally less toxic and more comfortable to the patient than traditional chemotherapy, but they may cause side effects that may influence food intake.[35] Immune-related adverse events include colitis, diarrhea, and gastrointestinal bleeding.

Finally, psychosocial conditions such as isolation, anxiety, or depression can lead to poor appetite and reduced food intake. However, there is no strong evidence of a causal relationship between food intake or nutritional status and mental stress in patients with advanced cancer. Table 33.2 provides an overview of the abovementioned symptoms that can cause eating problems and reduced appetite in patients with cancer, regardless of diagnosis and treatment modality.

TABLE 33.2 Overview of symptoms (defined as any subjective evidence of disease) that can affect food intake and nutritional status in cancer patients.

Organ	Symptoms
Oral cavity and throat	Altered taste sense Dry mouth Sore mucosa Swallow pain
Gastrointestinal tract	Nausea Vomiting Diarrhea Constipation Obstruction
Other disease and/or treatment-related symptoms	Pain Dyspnea Fatigue Depression Delirium Problems with cooking and preparing food Loneliness Physical impermeant

C. Cancer Cachexia

The word cachexia stems from the Greek words *kakos* and *hexis*, meaning "bad condition." [36] It is generally agreed upon that cancer cachexia emerges from a complex interaction between cancer growth and host response. This results in progressive weight loss that is a consequence of a negative protein and energy balance, often associated with signs of systemic inflammation.[37] Cachexia is referred to as a syndrome, i.e., a combination of symptoms and signs that together represent a disease process. The symptoms and signs of cancer cachexia include anorexia, fatigue, involuntary weight loss, and loss of skeletal muscle mass, with or without the loss of fat mass.[37–39] Cachexia is associated with poor tolerability of cancer treatment, decline in performance status, and reduced quality of life and survival.[40–42]

Based on different consensus definitions of cachexia from three expert groups, an international consensus definition of cachexia was proposed in 2011:[43] "*Cancer cachexia is a multifactorial syndrome characterized by an ongoing loss of skeletal muscle mass (with or without the loss of fat mass) that cannot be fully reversed by conventional nutritional support and leads to progressive functional impairment. The pathophysiology is characterized by negative protein and energy balance driven by a variable combination*

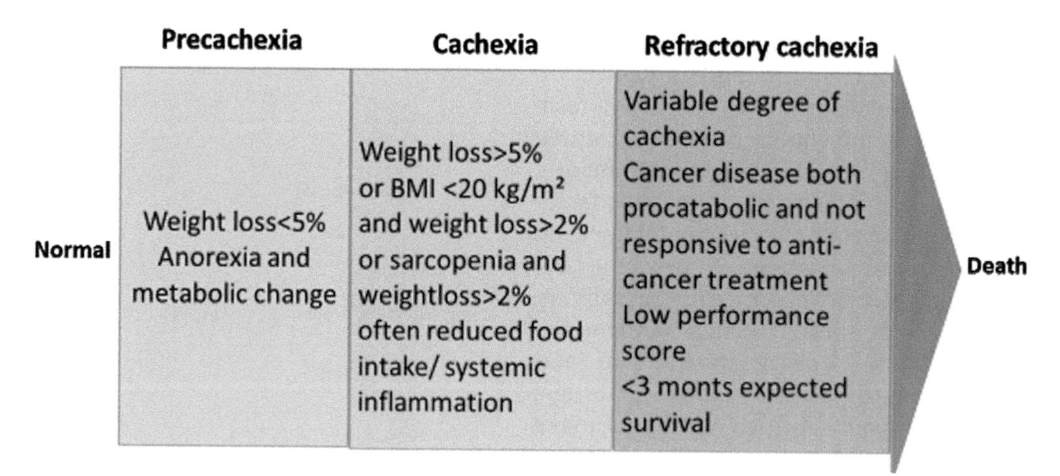

FIGURE 33.1 Stages of cancer cachexia. *Adapted from Fearon et al., 2011 Ref.* [43]*{Fearon, 2011 #2114}.*

of reduced food intake and abnormal metabolism." It is important to be aware of that the present definition of cancer cachexia states that opposed to malnutrition, weight loss in cachexia cannot be compensated by optimal energy intake alone.[40,43] In addition, metabolic alterations in cachexia cause greater loss of muscle mass than in malnutrition.[30,37] The muscle wasting seem to be accelerated by a combination of metabolic changes (i.e., increased resting energy expenditure and increased turnover of protein, lipids, and glucose), hormonal changes (i.e., insulin resistance), systemic inflammation (i.e., cytokine release), and tumor-inducing factors (i.e., proteolysis-inducing factor).[37,38]

Classification of cancer cachexia

Although several factors involved in the development of cachexia are described, the underlying mechanisms remain unclear.[44,45] Because of this and the fact that cachexia is associated with a wide range of clinical manifestations, it is difficult to precisely define this condition and establish criteria for diagnosis. This also makes it difficult to give an exact estimate of the prevalence of cancer cachexia.[46,47] The prevalence rates between 12% and 82% have been reported depending on definitions, study designs, and cancer diagnosis.[16,48,49] Even with the same tumor type and stage of disease, one patient may develop cachexia whereas another may not. Such variation may relate, at least in part, to the patient genotype. In order to identify, treat, and/or prevent this condition and to develop potential therapeutic interventions, a definition that is accepted by both clinicians and researchers is needed.[15,39]

Weight loss alone is not enough to capture the complexity of cachexia.[50] Based on the 2011 cachexia definition,[43] a set of criteria for a classification was defined of which one of the following had to be present: weight loss more than 5% of usual body weight over a period of 6 months (in absence of simple starvation); BMI <20 kg/m^2 and any degree of weight loss >2% of usual body weight, or appendicular skeletal muscle index consistent with sarcopenia and any degree of weight loss >2% of usual body weight. It was emphasized that cachexia can develop progressively through various stages (Fig. 33.1). The spectrum starts with precachexia and then progresses to cachexia and finally to refractory cachexia. The progression can be modulated by factors like cancer type and stage, systemic inflammation, reduced food intake, and response to anticancer therapy. Not all patients progress through each stage. Cancer cachexia has traditionally been associated with advanced disease;[47] however, it is now recognized that it may occur early in the disease course.[30] The international consensus definition is considered a framework that can be modified over time.[43] Thus, efforts to validate the definition and the classification system in clinical studies are important and ongoing.[36,43]

Wallengren et al.[48] compared the consensus definition and the classifications by Fearon et al.[16] and Evans et al.[39] in 405 patients with different cancer diagnoses in advanced stages. The conclusion was that weight loss, fatigue, and markers of systemic inflammation were most strongly associated with adverse outcomes like reduced QoL, functional decline, more symptoms, and shorter survival. Based on the results, an alternative three-factor classification was developed: weight loss >2% since before onset of disease; fatigue of >3 points (on a 1–10 scale); and C-reactive protein (CRP) >10 mg/l. Blum et al. [51] also validated the consensus definition in a heterogeneous sample of patients with advanced cancer. They concluded that the combination of weight loss (>5% of usual weight) and low BMI (<20 kg/m^2) showed the strongest association with short survival. A recent review from ESPEN expert group recommends that assessment of inflammatory biomarkers

TABLE 33.3 Summary of ESPEN expert group recommendations for improved nutritional care for patients with cancer (Arends, Baracos, et al., 2017[5]), p.1194.

- Perform nutritional risk screen in all cancer patients and regularly rescreen the patient, regardless of present body mass index and weight history. Screening should be performed early in the course of care and rescreen regularly.
- Nutritional assessment should include anorexia, body composition, resting energy expenditure, physical function, and inflammatory biomarkers.
- Develop individualized nutritional intervention plans with focus on increasing nutritional intake and physical activity and lowering hypermetabolic stress and inflammation.

be added, for example, Glasgow prognostic score based on serum concentrations of albumin and CRP, in the process to identify cachexia[5] (see Table 33.3).

Considering the limited specific treatment options for cancer cachexia, emphasis is placed on the precachexia phase, in which multimodal interventions may slow down weight loss.[52] Discrepancy in the prevalence of precachexia was found in two studies in patients with advanced cancer, and no significant difference in survival was found between precachexia and cachexia.[53,54] Moreover the clinical relevance of a precachexia diagnosis has been questioned in a study by Blauwhoff-Buskermolen et al.[55] and showed that the use of the present framework depicted in Fig. 33.1 identified very few patients i.e., 0.5%–2%.

Although the multifactorial pathophysiology of cachexia is now better understood, there is no standard of care or approved drug treatment, and it remains an unmet medical need. This lack of progress is paradoxical given the role cachexia plays in cancer and the way it contributes to excess morbidity and mortality. The specific elements (systemic inflammation, muscle wasting, reduced physical activity, negative energy, and protein balance) lend themselves to therapeutic reversal through multimodal approaches and emerging treatments. Large trials are lacking, but a feasibility study investigating a 6-week intervention combining nonsteroidal antiinflammatory drugs such as celecoxib, nutritional advice, and oral supplements including eicosapentaenoic fatty acid and exercise in patients with advanced lung or pancreatic cancer commencing chemotherapy showed promising effects on weight and muscle mass.[56]

III. NUTRITIONAL TREATMENT IN PATIENTS WITH CANCER

All patients with cancer should be observed continuously for weight loss, decreased appetite, and food intake.[1] The following practices are recommended to prevent and treat weight loss and malnutrition caused by disease and/or treatment (see Table 33.3)

- Identify patients who are at risk of becoming malnourished
- Assess symptoms and food intake in all patients who are at risk of becoming malnourished
- Take action – start individualized nutritional treatment

A. Risk Screening and Nutritional Assessment

In order to achieve effective of nutritional treatment, it is important to detect the deterioration of nutritional status early and prevent further weight loss through dietary advice adapted to the individual patient's specific situation. This includes not only identification of obvious malnourished individuals but also those at risk of developing malnutrition. Diagnosing malnutrition is a two-step process.[17] First, a patient must be screened with a validated screening tool and be identified "at nutritional risk." Further assessment of those who are at risk is then conducted. The nutritional diagnosis is dependent on criteria or definition selected by the care team or investigator as no standardized method for identification of malnutrition has reached full consensus.

Several guidelines emphasized risk screening as an important measure to detect nutritional disturbances at an early stage.[1,5,57] It is recommended to evaluate nutritional risk in all patients with cancer with validated nutrition screening instruments that include weight assessment and information about weight development.

If the patient is at risk of malnutrition, a more thorough assessment is done to determine likely causes of weight loss so that targeted treatment can be implemented. Current methods and standards to assess nutritional status are not designed for use in patients with cancer. Biochemical variables are for example affected by the cancer and the values can therefore be difficult to interpret.[58] Especially serum proteins such as albumin and transthyretin (i.e., prealbumin) have been employed to determine nutritional status. Albumin is a hepatic protein and is characterized as negative acute phase protein with a half-life of 14–20 days.[59] Albumin is known to decline after prolonged poor nutrition, i.e., insufficient food intake (calories and protein), but in patients with cancer, low albumin values also may be due to infections and/or catabolic conditions. Thus, albumin is an unreliable serum marker for malnutrition in patients with ongoing disease processes as in cancer. Transthyretin has a shorter half-life than albumin, 2–3 days, and therefore regarded more reliable to detect acute changes in nutritional status than albumin, but it is affected in the same way as albumin from inflammatory states.[59] In general, it is difficult to obtain reliable nutrition status information from laboratory findings alone in patients with cancer.[59] This is specifically relevant in connection with incurable disease where weight loss also may a result of cachexia.

In the absence of trustworthy biochemical variables, the Patient-Generated Subjective Global Assessment (PG-SGA) can be used to detect malnutrition in patients with cancer.[59,60] Ottery et al.[61] adapted PG-SGA from the SGA, earlier developed and described by Detsky et al.[62] PG-SGA was developed for use in patients with cancer and covers all domains of the malnutrition definition by ESPEN.[63] The tool has been validated as a nutritional assessment instrument in the cancer population[60,64] and classified patients as well-nourished, moderately/suspected malnourished, or severely malnourished.

When treating weight loss in patients with cancer, it is important to distinguish between malnutrition and cachexia, in order to set treatment goals. Unfortunately, simple methods that distinguish between malnutrition and cachexia are lacking.[57] The patient's baseline clinical condition is used when interpreting nutritional status including evaluation of performance status that measures functional capabilities. Physical performance status is a strong predictor of survival in cancer and is considered in treatment decisions.[65] The performance status is determined using one of two scoring systems, either the Karnofsky Performance Status score or the Eastern Cooperative Oncology Group Performance Status score.[66,67] When diagnosing malnutrition and nutritional treatment in patients with advanced cancer, it is important to consider physical performance status, identify weight loss that can be reversed or stopped, and avoid intervention for weight loss that does not respond to nutritional management.

B. Symptom Assessment

The patients are the best sources of information about the symptoms they are experiencing. Several studies show systematic underestimation of patient's frequency and severity of symptoms by health care providers.[68,69] The use of patient reported outcomes (PROs) is recommended in both clinical practice and research.[27] Symptom relief is a prerequisite for the patient to benefit from any nutritional therapy or intervention. Thus, a thorough assessment of disease and treatment-related symptoms in relation to nutritional status is an important part of the nutrition care.[27] Systematic symptom assessment indicates which physiological abnormalities are contributing to the symptoms, for example, a tumor that obstructs intestinal passage and leads to a high risk for developing constipation or ileus.

In relation to nutrition in cancer, PROs are used to provide information about weight change and symptoms that may cause reduced food intake such as anorexia and nausea.[70] However, exploring patient symptoms requires thoroughness and persistence, and it is a vital aspect of patient-centered care.[71] Multiple assessment tools are available to assess symptoms in individual patients, for example, Rotterdam Symptom Checklist[72] and the revised Edmonton Symptom Assessment System (ESAS-r).[73] These assessment tools provide information regarding treatment effect, response to specific symptomatic interventions, for example, nutritional therapy, and recognition of unreported symptoms.[71] In palliative care of patients with cancer ESAS-r is frequently employed, with nine core symptoms that are pain, tiredness, nausea, depression, anxious, drowsiness, appetite, feeling of well-being, shortness of breath, and an optional 10th symptom provided by the patient. Each symptom is scored on an 11-point numeric rating scale ranging from 0 (no symptom) to 10 (worst possible).[73]

C. Nutritional Treatment

Nutritional problems leading to malnutrition in cancer are complex and multifactorial. Thus treatment requires a multifactorial and holistic treatment approach, coordinated across different health care disciplines that include dialog with the patient about his or her concerns, symptoms, and preferences.[74] Patients who are malnourished or at risk of malnutrition require a nutritional plan with dietary advice tailored to the patient's clinical condition, preferences, and needs.[1,75] It is essential that prior to initiating any dietary interventions, underlying factors to poor appetite such as nausea, constipation, dysphagia, and pain are satisfactorily treated.[75] It is also important that both the patient and their relatives are allowed to participate in the development of the nutritional plan and realistic goals for the treatment. The nutritional plan and the effect of the intervention must be continuously assessed to be able to modify it if the patient's clinical condition changes or the treatment is ineffective. The fact that the patient is unable to eat as planned can be stressful and can result in concerns of starving to death.

The dietary goals for malnourished or at risk patients is primarily to ensure adequate energy (calories) and nutrients to retain or maintain weight.[75] The expected effects of setting such goals are improved general health condition and strengthened immune system. If the patient is overweight, initially guidance is needed to preserve body weight during the treatment period and to be aware that dieting and weight loss is not recommended during cancer treatment. It is assumed that the total energy expenditure in patients with cancer is similar to healthy subjects ranging between 25 and 30 kcal/kg/day.[1] Furthermore, it is recommended that protein intake should be above 1.0 g/kg/day and, if possible, up to 1.5 g/kg/day during treatment.[1]

In general, patients with poor appetite are encouraged to eat small meals but more often and to eat when they feel hungry. The food should be energy-dense, i.e., contains high levels of energy or calories per 100 g food.[76] All beverages should contain energy and evening and night snacks or small meals can be beneficial. Wine or other alcoholic beverages can stimulate appetite as well as containing some calories. Oral nutritional supplements may help to improve the dietary intake of those who are unable to meet nutritional requirements with foods and beverages despite counseling.[75] The success of supplementation depends on the acceptability and routine use of the product by the patient.

Nutritional treatment in cachexia

Cancer patients with cachexia respond differently to nutritional treatment than malnourished patients without cachexia.[77] This is attributed to the metabolic changes previously described (see the section *Cancer cachexia*). Still, in patients with advanced cancer, cachexia and malnutrition tend to occur simultaneously and insufficient dietary intake is the common etiology. Nutritional treatment in these patients should not be ignored.[15] However, the goal of the nutritional treatment for cachexia will be different from patients without cachexia. Dietary interventions are individualized, and both symptoms and physical performance are considered as described above. The treatment goals will also vary across the different stages of cachexia. It is important that the patients and their relatives are aware of the treatment goals and that the treatment does not increase the psychological burden the patients already experience.

In precachexia, the goal may maintain or increase the patient's weight and physical function, and the patient is advised to consume frequent meals and use high energy density foods and oral nutritional supplements.[78] In refractory cachexia, the most important goal is symptom relief that includes modification of foods.

Pharmacologic treatment of cachexia

Several pharmacologic agents have been investigated for use in cancer cachexia to improve appetite and to preserve muscle mass. Systematic reviews and metaanalyzes have summarized the effects of megestrol acetate (Megase).[79,80] The evidence suggests this agent has a positive effect on appetite and weight, but not on muscle mass preservation and quality of life. However, the evaluations are short term (8–12 weeks), and side effects such as fluid retention, risk of thromboembolism, and a potential excess mortality are reported.[79] Megestrol acetate is considered in patients where poor appetite affects the patient's quality of life when the life expectancy is longer than 2–3 months. The optimal is not well established but 160–800 mg daily is commonly used.

Glucocorticosteroids also increase appetite, well-being, and physical function.[81] Weight is often not significantly affected. Corticosteroids have serious side effects such as proximal myopathy, immunosuppression, and insulin resistance. The effect of corticosteroids on appetite often ceases after a few weeks. The treatment is therefore more suitable for patients with short life span and with other symptoms where steroids may be useful (e.g., liver disorder, nausea, and brain edema). Corticosteroids are used in connection with important social and life events where better appetite is of importance to the patient.

Anamorelin[82] is a ghrelin receptor agonist, i.e., a compound that acts by mimicking the hormone ghrelin that stimulates appetite and positive energy balance.[83] The drug has shown positive effects on appetite and muscle mass preservation in clinical trials with no impact on physical function.[82]

Nutrition at the end of life

When the patient approaches end of life, the focus of all care is to facilitate the best possible symptom relief and quality of life.[84] Weight development and nutritional needs are no longer of relevance, and the patient should be offered the food he or she wants. Most patients will not experience hunger at this stage, but both patient and relatives need information and support on how to manage plans and expectations for food and meals.

Using intravenous fluid treatment in the terminal phase is debated, but mostly not indicated.[85] If there is an indication for maintaining basic hydration, typical 500–1000 ml of fluid per day is sufficient. Mouth dryness symptoms should be treated primarily with oral products and not systemic treatment, as this is not necessarily alleviated by parenteral fluids.

Physical activity as part of nutritional treatment

Many patients with cancer experience fatigue as a result of disease and treatment. Fatigue is a very troublesome symptom that adversely affects quality of life. Fatigue often leads the patients into a vicious circle, with the reduction of daily physical activity which in turn leads to reduction of muscle mass, muscle strength, aerobic capacity, and physical function. However, there is good evidence to recommend physical activity and exercise in patients with cancer who have a good prognosis.[86] Physical activity can reduce muscle catabolism and increase anabolism as well the potential to reduce systemic inflammation and may have a positive impact on nutritional status.

Also patients with advanced disease should be advised to increase activity if possible since muscle catabolism and inflammation are important elements in the pathophysiology of cancer-related cachexia. A few studies have considered the effect of physical activity and exercise in patients with advanced cancer and demonstrated that patients are both capable and willing to participate in physical activity despite advanced disease.[87,88] A recent systematic summary of physical activity in patients with advanced disease shows good effect on physical function, reduction of fatigue, and maintenance of quality of life.[89] The patient is counseled to maintain daily activity and to find a balance between rest and activity.[1] Exercise under supervision shows the best effect on quality of life and physical fitness,[90] and individualization based on previous patient experiences of physical activity, motivation, and performance status is necessary.

D. Special Nutritional Support

Special nutritional support (also referred to as artificial or therapeutic nutritional support) includes oral nutrition supplements (ONS), enteral nutrition, and parenteral nutrition.[91] When possible, food is preferred compared to therapeutic products for the treatment of patients with cancer.[1] However, in accordance to the ESPEN guidelines on nutrition in patients with cancer '*artificial nutrition is indicated if patients are unable to eat adequately*, e.g., *no food for more than 1 week or less than 60% of requirement for more than 1–2 week*'.[1] As with all medical interventions, special nutrition requires an indication for treatment, a definition of a therapeutic goal to be achieved through the treatment, and the agreement of the patient and his or her informed consent.[92] Before initiating artificial nutritional support, health care personnel must assess the pros and cons, including the ethical aspects of the treatment. In patients with advanced cancer, it is important to consider whether artificial nutrition will improve the patient's nutritional status and quality of life by providing increased physical strength and better resistance to infections and other complications related to poor nutritional status. In addition, it should be discussed whether artificial nutrition will provide emotional well-being, reduce anxiety about the disease, and increase self-esteem by making the patients feel more satisfied with his or her body.

When considering whether initiating special nutrition therapy is appropriate, it is important to consider the patient's wishes and include the patient and, if relevant, relatives and family in the discussion.[74] Poor food intake may be of concern to the patient and family and that the patient wants this form of intervention. The patients and relatives should be included in the discussion, but it is important to empathize that the decision of initiating or terminating the treatment is the responsibility of the treating physician in close cooperation with the patient and his or hers wishes.[92]

When a decision has been made to feed a patient, ESPEN Guidelines recommend '*enteral nutrition if oral nutrition remains inadequate despite nutritional interventions* (e.g., *counselling and oral nutrition supplement), and parenteral nutrition if enteral nutrition is not sufficient or feasible*.'[1] The impact of special nutrition support tends to vary depending on the underlying causes of the patient's poor nutritional status, for example, malnutrition or cachexia.[93] Finally, in patients with advanced cancer and shorter expected survival, the decision to continue or withdraw special nutrition support should be intermediately reevaluated.

Enteral nutrition

Enteral nutrition is the science, technique, and practical implementation of nutritionally completed food provided through a stoma or a tube into the intestinal tract distal to oral cavity.[91] This form of nutritional treatment can be given to all patients who have a functioning gastrointestinal tract.[1] Enteral nutrition can also be initiated if there is a problem with gastric motility, by administering nutrition postpylorically, for example, through a jejunostomy, nasoduodenal or nasojejunal tube.[94] Enteral nutrition should be considered if there are swallowing problems, for instance, if it is tumor growth in the oral cavity, pharynx, or esophagus, as well as with insufficient voluntary food intake.

Some clinicians consider enteral nutrition as a burden for the patient, thus react negatively when this treatment option is considered. If health professionals do not regard enteral nutrition as a good alternative, the patient will probably react negatively. In such contexts, we should consider that some patients will be relived to get nutrition through a tube or stoma and avoid the constant hassle of eating sufficient volumes of food despite pain, dysphagia, or other symptoms.

It is also a common misconception that patients receiving enteral nutrition cannot eat regular food. On the contrary, patients should be encouraged continuously to eat and drink when capable if there are no contradictions. If the patient can eat some regular food, enteral nutrition may act as a supplement and help maintain the energy intake and weight.

Parenteral nutrition

Parenteral nutrition is considered when the patient does not have a functioning gastrointestinal tract or has fistulas.[1] Parenteral nutrition is most frequently initiated in patients with tumors in the gastrointestinal tract, for example, gastric carcinoma, colorectal carcinoma and pancreatic carcinoma,[95] and gynecological cancer diagnosis.[93] Sometimes parenteral nutrition is used as the sole source of nutrition, but it is more common that it is an adjunct to food or enteral nutrition. It is beneficial for the patient to eat some food orally or administrate small doses of enteral nutrition daily, so that the function of the gastrointestinal tract is stimulated. Some oral or enteral nutrition facilitates the transition to regular food later and ensures optimal intestinal function.

In patients with advanced cancer and short life expectancy (under 2–3 months), enteral and parenteral nutrition is usually not indicated unless these nutritional treatments are expected to provide clear relief and improvement of symptoms.[1] Other exceptions include use to support the patient through an infection, surgery, or other tumor-related treatment. Parenteral nutrition is also used in complicated gastrointestinal conditions where there is uncertainty about the prognosis. Risk of organ failure and infection makes it difficult to initiate intensive nutrition treatment when life expectancy is short. If the patient accumulates fluid or experiences other side effects, the volume of nutritional support fluids is reduced or terminated to support overall care. Parenteral nutrition might be preferred over enteral nutrition, as patients receiving parenteral nutrition receive more calories compared to those patients who are feed enterally.[96,97] Due to a higher calorie intake, parenteral nutrition may be more efficient for patients with cancer suffering from malnutrition and/or weight loss, compared to enteral nutrition. However, in a recent metaanalysis and systematic review,[95] outcomes of parenteral nutrition and enteral nutrition in patients with cancer were compared and the results indicated that neither parenteral nor enteral nutrition was superior with respect to major complications (e.g., morbidity), nutrition support complications (nausea, vomiting), or survival in patients with cancer. The only difference reported between parenteral nutrition and enteral nutrition was an increased incidence of infections in patients receiving parenteral nutrition.[95]

RESEARCH GAPS

The authors suggest that more research should be conducted regarding:

- Nutritional treatment and the ability to reverse weight loss and malnutrition
- Which diagnostic groups that will benefit from nutritional treatment more than others
- Development and validation of objective cancer cachexia diagnostic criteria
- Well-designed randomized controlled trials to assess the efficacy of nutritional interventions on outcomes such as survival, physical function, and quality of life in malnourished patients with cancer and patients with cancer with cachexia

In addition, we highlight the six areas where more research on diet, nutrition, physical activity, and cancer is needed according to the Expert Panel of World Cancer Research Fund Continuous Update Project[2]:

- Biological mechanisms by which diet, nutrition, and physical activity affect cancer processes
- The impact of diet, nutrition, and physical activity throughout the life course on cancer risk
- Better characterization of diet, nutrition, body composition, and physical activity exposures
- Better characterization of cancer-related outcomes
- Stronger evidence for the impact of diet, nutrition, and physical activity on outcomes in cancer survivors
- Globally representative research on specific exposures and cancer

Acknowledgments

This chapter is an update of the chapter titled "51. Cancer" by Holly Nicastro and John A. Milner, in Present Knowledge in Nutrition, 10th Edition, edited by Erdman JW, Macdonald IA, and Zeisel SH and published by Wiley-Blackwell. © 2012 International Life Sciences Institute. The previously published chapter was an inspiration and the authors are acknowledged. We also want to acknowledge Nima Wesseltoft-Rao who contributed with her knowledge to the part about cancer cachexia.

IV. REFERENCES

1. Arends J, Bachmann P, Baracos V, et al. ESPEN guidelines on nutrition in cancer patients. *Clin Nutr.* 2017;36(1):11–48.
2. World Cancer Research Fund, American Institute for Cancer Research, Continuous Update Project. *Diet, Nutrition, Physical Activity and Cancer: A Global Perspective.* 2018.
3. Agarwal E, Ferguson M, Banks M, Bauer J, Capra S, Isenring E. Nutritional status and dietary intake of acute care patients: results from the Nutrition Care Day Survey 2010. *Clin Nutr.* 2011;31(1): 41–47.
4. Chen CC-H, Schilling LS, Lyder CH. A concept analysis of malnutrition in the elderly. *J Adv Nurs.* 2001;36(1):131–142.
5. Arends J, Baracos V, Bertz H, et al. ESPEN expert group recommendations for action against cancer-related malnutrition. *Clin Nutr.* 2017;36(5):1187–1196.
6. Isabel TD, Correia M, Waitzberg DL. The impact of malnutrition on morbidity, mortality, length of hospital stay and costs evaluated through a multivariate model analysis. *Clin Nutr.* 2003;22(3): 235–239.

7. Muscaritoli M, Bossola M, Aversa Z, Bellantone R, Rossi Fanelli F. Prevention and treatment of cancer cachexia: new insights into an old problem. *Eur J Cancer.* 2006;42(1):31–41.
8. Dewys WD, Begg C, Lavin PT, et al. Prognostic effect of weight loss prior to chemotherapy in cancer patients. Eastern Cooperative Oncology Group. *Am J Med.* 1980;69(4):491–497.
9. Muscaritoli M, Lucia S, Farcomeni A, et al. Prevalence of malnutrition in patients at first medical oncology visit: the PreMiO study. *Oncotarget.* 2017;8(45):79884.
10. Khalid U, Spiro A, Baldwin C, et al. Symptoms and weight loss in patients with gastrointestinal and lung cancer at presentation. *Support Care Canc.* 2007;15(1):39–46.
11. Burden ST, Hill J, Shaffer JL, Todd C. Nutritional status of preoperative colorectal cancer patients. *J Hum Nutr Diet.* 2010;23(4): 402–407.
12. Tan BH, Fearon KC. Cachexia: prevalence and impact in medicine. *Curr Opin Clin Nutr Metab Care.* 2008;11(4):400–407.
13. Wong CJ. Involuntary weight loss. *Med Clin.* 2014;98(3):625–643.
14. Rock CL, Doyle C, Demark-Wahnefried W, et al. Nutrition and physical activity guidelines for cancer survivors. *Cancer J Clin.* 2012;62(4):242–274.
15. Sadeghi M, Keshavarz-Fathi M, Baracos V, Arends J, Mahmoudi M, Rezaei NJC. Cancer cachexia: diagnosis, assessment, and treatment. *Crit Rev Oncol Hematol.* 2018;127:91–104.
16. Fearon KC, Voss AC, Hustead DS, Cancer Cachexia Study Group. Definition of cancer cachexia: effect of weight loss, reduced food intake, and systemic inflammation on functional status and prognosis. *Am J Clin Nutr.* 2006;83(6):1345–1350.
17. Cederholm T, Barazzoni R, Austin P, et al. ESPEN guidelines on definitions and terminology of clinical nutrition. *Clin Nutr.* 2017; 36(1):49–64.
18. Marshall KM, Loeliger J, Nolte L, Kelaart A, Kiss NK. Prevalence of malnutrition and impact on clinical outcomes in cancer services: a comparison of two time points. *Clin Nutr.* 2019;38(2):644–651.
19. Teunissen SC, Wesker W, Kruitwagen C, de Haes HC, Voest EE, de Graeff A. Symptom prevalence in patients with incurable cancer: a systematic review. *J Pain Symptom Manag.* 2007;34(1):94–104.
20. Kaysen GA. Association between inflammation and malnutrition as risk factors of cardiovascular disease. *Blood Purif.* 2006;24(1): 51–55.
21. Yavuzsen T, Walsh D, Davis MP, et al. Components of the anorexia–cachexia syndrome: gastrointestinal symptom correlates of cancer anorexia. *Support Care Cancer.* 2009;17(12):1531.
22. Chow E, Fan G, Hadi S, Wong J, Kirou-Mauro A, Filipczak LJCO. Symptom clusters in cancer patients with brain metastases. *Clin Oncol.* 2008;20(1):76–82.
23. Shragge JE, Wismer WV, Olson KL, Baracos VE. The management of anorexia by patients with advanced cancer: a critical review of the literature. *Palliat Med.* 2006;20(6):623–629.
24. Barsevick A. Defining the symptom cluster: how far have we come?. In: *Paper Presented at: Seminars in Oncology Nursing.* 2016.
25. Bye A, Jordhoy MS, Skjegstad G, Ledsaak O, Iversen PO, Hjermstad MJ. Symptoms in advanced pancreatic cancer are of importance for energy intake. *Support Care Cancer.* 2013;21(1): 219–227.
26. Bressan V, Bagnasco A, Aleo G, et al. The life experience of nutrition impact symptoms during treatment for head and neck cancer patients: a systematic review and meta-synthesis. *Support Care Cancer.* 2017;25(5):1699–1712.
27. Kaasa S, Loge JH, Aapro M, et al. Integration of oncology and palliative care: a lancet oncology commission. *Lancet Oncol.* 2018;19(11): e588–e653.
28. Pilgrim A, Robinson S, Sayer AA, Roberts HJN. An overview of appetite decline in older people. *Nurs Older People.* 2015; 27(5):29.
29. Ezeoke CC, Morley JE. Pathophysiology of anorexia in the cancer cachexia syndrome. *J Cachexia Sarcopenia Muscle.* 2015;6(4): 287–302.
30. Nicolini A, Ferrari P, Masoni MC, et al. Malnutrition, anorexia and cachexia in cancer patients: a mini-review on pathogenesis and treatment. *Biomed Pharmacothe.* 2013;67(8):807–817.
31. Schindler A, Denaro N, Russi EG, et al. Dysphagia in head and neck cancer patients treated with radiotherapy and systemic therapies: literature review and consensus. *Crit Rev Oncol Hematol.* 2015;96(2):372–384.
32. Lister R. Oropharyngeal dysphagia and nutritional management. *Curr Opin Gastroenterol.* 2006;22(4):341–346.
33. Spotten L, Corish CA, Lorton C, et al. Subjective and objective taste and smell changes in cancer. *Ann Oncol.* 2017;28(5):969–984.
34. Bernhardson B-M, Tishelman C, Rutqvist LE. Self-reported taste and smell changes during cancer chemotherapy. *Support Care Cancer.* 2008;16(3):275–283.
35. Kroschinsky F, Stölzel F, von Bonin S, et al. New drugs, new toxicities: severe side effects of modern targeted and immunotherapy of cancer and their management. *Crit Care.* 2017;21(1):89.
36. Argiles JM, Anker SD, Evans WJ, et al. Consensus on cachexia definitions. *J Am Med Dir Assoc.* 2010;11(4):229–230.
37. Ronga I, Gallucci F, Riccardi F, Uomo G. Anorexia-cachexia syndrome in pancreatic cancer: recent advances and new pharmacological approach. *Adv Med Sci.* 2014;59(1):1–6.
38. Tan CR, Yaffee PM, Jamil LH, et al. Pancreatic cancer cachexia: a review of mechanisms and therapeutics. *Front Physiol.* 2014;5:88.
39. Evans WJ, Morley JE, Argiles J, et al. Cachexia: a new definition. *Clin Nutr.* 2008;27(6):793–799.
40. de Luca C, Olefsky JM. Inflammation and insulin resistance. *FEBS Lett.* 2008;582(1):97–105.
41. Tisdale MJ. Mechanisms of cancer cachexia. *Physiol Rev.* 2009;89(2): 381–410.
42. Tuca A, Jimenez-Fonseca P, Gascon P. Clinical evaluation and optimal management of cancer cachexia. *Crit Rev Oncol-Hematol.* 2013;88(3):625–636.
43. Fearon K, Strasser F, Anker SD, et al. Definition and classification of cancer cachexia: an international consensus. *Lancet Oncol.* 2011; 12(5):489–495.
44. Bozzetti F, Mariani L. Defining and classifying cancer cachexia: a proposal by the SCRINIO Working Group. *J Parenter Enter Nutr.* 2009;33(4):361–367.
45. Baracos VE, Martin L, Korc M, Guttridge DC, Fearon KC. Cancer-associated cachexia. *Nat Rev Dis Primers.* 2018;4:17105.
46. Hahne F, LeMeur N, Brinkman RR, et al. FlowCore: a bioconductor package for high throughput flow cytometry. *BMC Bioinformatics.* 2009;10:106.
47. Seelaender M, Batista Jr M, Lira F, Silverio R, Rossi-Fanelli F. Inflammation in cancer cachexia: to resolve or not to resolve (is that the question?). *Clin Nutr.* 2012;31(4):562–566.
48. Wallengren O, Lundholm K, Bosaeus I. Diagnostic criteria of cancer cachexia: relation to quality of life, exercise capacity and survival in unselected palliative care patients. *Support Care Cancer.* 2013;21(6):1569–1577.
49. Thoresen L, Frykholm G, Lydersen S, et al. Nutritional status, cachexia and survival in patients with advanced colorectal carcinoma. Different assessment criteria for nutritional status provide unequal results. *Clin Nutr.* 2013;32(1):65–72.
50. Prado CM, Heymsfield SB. Lean tissue imaging: a new era for nutritional assessment and intervention. *J Parenter Enter Nutr.* 2014;38(8):940–953.
51. Blum D, Stene GB, Solheim TS, et al. Validation of the consensus-definition for cancer cachexia and evaluation of a classification model—a study based on data from an international multicentre project (EPCRC-CSA). *Ann Oncol.* 2014;25(8):1635–1642.

52. Reneman MF, Kleen M, Trompetter HR, et al. Measuring avoidance of pain: validation of the acceptance and action questionnaire II-pain version. *Int J Rehabil Res*. 2014;37(2):125–129.
53. Namazi S, Baba MB, Halaliah Mokhtar H, Ghani Hamzah MS. Validation of the Iranian version of the University of California at Los Angeles posttraumatic stress disorder index for DSM-IV-R. *Trauma Mon*. 2013;18(3):122–125.
54. Rostami M, Noorian N, Mansournia MA, Sharafi E, Babaki AE, Kordi R. Validation of the Persian version of the fear avoidance belief questionnaire in patients with low back pain. *J Back Musculoskelet Rehabil*. 2014;27(2):213–221.
55. Blauwhoff-Buskermolen S, de van der Schueren MA, Verheul HM, Langius JA. 'Pre-cachexia': a non-existing phenomenon in cancer? *Ann Oncol*. 2014;25(8):1668–1669.
56. Solheim TS, Laird BJ, Balstad TR, et al. A randomized phase II feasibility trial of a multimodal intervention for the management of cachexia in lung and pancreatic cancer. *J Cachexia Sarcopenia Muscle*. 2017;8(5):778–788.
57. Cederholm T, Jensen G, Correia M, et al. GLIM criteria for the diagnosis of malnutrition–A consensus report from the global clinical nutrition community. *Clin Nutr*. 2019;10(1):207–217.
58. Barbosa-Silva MCG. Subjective and objective nutritional assessment methods: what do they really assess? *Curr Opin Clin Nutr Metab Care*. 2008;11(3):248–254.
59. Bharadwaj S, Ginoya S, Tandon P, et al. Malnutrition: laboratory markers vs nutritional assessment. *Gastroenterol Rep*. 2016;4(4): 272–280.
60. Bauer J, Capra S, Ferguson M. Use of the scored Patient-Generated Subjective Global Assessment (PG-SGA) as a nutrition assessment tool in patients with cancer. *Eur J Clin Nutr*. 2002; 56(8):779–785.
61. Ottery FD. Definition of standardized nutritional assessment and interventional pathways in oncology. *Nutrition*. 1996;12(1 Suppl): S15–S19.
62. Detsky AS, Baker J, Johnston N, Whittaker S, Mendelson R, Jeejeebhoy K. What is subjective global assessment of nutritional status? *J Parenter Enteral Nutr*. 1987;11(1):8–13.
63. Cederholm T, Bosaeus I, Barazzoni R, et al. Diagnostic criteria for malnutrition–an ESPEN consensus statement. *Clin Nutr*. 2015; 34(3):335–340.
64. Thoresen L, Fjeldstad I, Krogstad K, Kaasa S, Falkmer UG. Nutritional status of patients with advanced cancer: the value of using the subjective global assessment of nutritional status as a screening tool. *Palliat Med*. 2002;16(1):33–42.
65. Leal AD, Allmer C, Maurer MJ, et al. Variability of performance status assessment between patients with hematologic malignancies and their physicians. *Leuk Lymphoma*. 2018;59(3):695–701.
66. Oken MM, Creech RH, Tormey DC, et al. Toxicity and response criteria of the Eastern cooperative oncology group. *Am J Clin Oncol*. 1982;5(6):649–656.
67. Mor V, Laliberte L, Morris JN, Wiemann MJC. The Karnofsky performance status scale: an examination of its reliability and validity in a research setting. *Cancer*. 1984;53(9):2002–2007.
68. Gravis G, Marino P, Joly F, et al. Patients' self-assessment versus investigators' evaluation in a phase III trial in non-castrate metastatic prostate cancer (GETUG-AFU 15). *Eur J Cancer*. 2014;50(5): 953–962.
69. Laugsand EA, Sprangers MA, Bjordal K, Skorpen F, Kaasa S, Klepstad P. Health care providers underestimate symptom intensities of cancer patients: a multicenter European study. *Health Qual Life Outcome*. 2010;8:104.
70. Bosaeus I, Daneryd P, Svanberg E, Lundholm K. Dietary intake and resting energy expenditure in relation to weight loss in unselected cancer patients. *Int J Canc*. 2001;93(3):380–383.
71. Chang VT. *Approach to Symptom Assessment in Palliative Care*. 2017:4.
72. De Haes J, Van Knippenberg F, Neijt J. Measuring psychological and physical distress in cancer patients: structure and application of the Rotterdam symptom checklist. *Br J Cancer*. 1990;62(6):1034.
73. Watanabe SM, Nekolaichuk C, Beaumont C, et al. A multicenter study comparing two numerical versions of the Edmonton symptom assessment system in palliative care patients. *J Pain Symptom Manage*. 2011;41(2):456–468.
74. Sladdin I, Ball L, Bull C, Chaboyer W. Patient-centered care to improve dietetic practice: an integrative review. *J Hum Nutr Diet*. 2017;30(4):453–470.
75. Ravasco P. Nutritional approaches in cancer: relevance of individualized counseling and supplementation. *J Nephrol*. 2015;31(4): 603–604.
76. Wallengren O, Bosaeus I, Lundholm K. Dietary energy density, inflammation and energy balance in palliative care cancer patients. *Clin Nutr*. 2013;32(1):88–92.
77. Balstad TR, Solheim TS, Strasser F, Kaasa S, Bye A. Dietary treatment of weight loss in patients with advanced cancer and cachexia: a systematic literature review. *Crit Rev Oncol-Hematol*. 2014;91(2):210–221.
78. Radbruch L, Elsner F, Trottenberg P, Strasser F, Baracos V, Fearon K. *Clinical Practice Guidelines on Cancer Cachexia in Advanced Cancer Patients*. Aachen: Department of Palliative Medicin/European Palliative Care Research Collaborative; 2010.
79. Ruiz Garcia V, Lopez-Briz E, Carbonell Sanchis R, Gonzalvez Perales JL, Bort-Marti S. Megestrol acetate for treatment of anorexia-cachexia syndrome. *Cochrane Database Syst Rev*. 2013; 3(3):CD004310.
80. Yavuzsen T, Davis MP, Walsh D, LeGrand S, Lagman R. Systematic review of the treatment of cancer-associated anorexia and weight loss. *J Clin Oncol*. 2005;23(33):8500–8511.
81. Holtan A, Aass N, Nordoy T, et al. Prevalence of pain in hospitalised cancer patients in Norway: a national survey. *Palliat Med*. 2007; 21(1):7–13.
82. Temel JS, Abernethy AP, Currow DC, et al. Anamorelin in patients with non-small-cell lung cancer and cachexia (ROMANA 1 and ROMANA 2): results from two randomized, double-blind, phase 3 trials. *Lancet Oncol*. 2016;17(4):519–531.
83. DeBoer MD. The use of ghrelin and ghrelin receptor agonists as a treatment for animal models of disease: efficacy and mechanism. *Curr Pharm Des*. 2012;18(31):4779–4799.
84. Dy SM, Apostol CC. Evidence-based approaches to other symptoms in advanced cancer. *Cancer J*. 2010;16(5):507–513.
85. Dev R, Dalal S, Bruera E. Is there a role for parenteral nutrition or hydration at the end of life? *Curr Opin Support Palliat Care*. 2012; 6(3):365–370.
86. Segal R, Zwaal C, Green E, Tomasone J, Loblaw A, Petrella T. Exercise for people with cancer: a systematic review. *Curr Oncol*. 2017; 24(4):e290.
87. Oldervoll LM. Physical exercise for cancer patients with advanced disease: a randomized controlled trial. *Oncol*. 2011;16:1649–1657.
88. Oldervoll LM, Loge JH, Paltiel H, et al. Are palliative cancer patients willing and able to participate in a physical exercise program? *Palliat Support Care*. 2005;3(4):281–287.
89. Dittus KL, Gramling RE, Ades PA. Exercise interventions for individuals with advanced cancer: a systematic review. *Prev Med*. 2017; 104:124–132.
90. Fong DY, Ho JW, Hui BP, et al. Physical activity for cancer survivors: meta-analysis of randomized controlled trials. *Br Med J*. 2012;344:e70.
91. Valentini L, Volkert D, Schütz T, et al. Suggestions for terminology in clinical nutrition. *E-SPEN J*. 2014;9(2):e97–e108.
92. Druml C, Ballmer PE, Druml W, et al. ESPEN guideline on ethical aspects of artificial nutrition and hydration. *Clin Nutr*. 2016;35(3): 545–556.

93. Orrevall Y, Tishelman C, Permert J, Lundström S. A national observational study of the prevalence and use of enteral tube feeding, parenteral nutrition and intravenous glucose in cancer patients enrolled in specialized palliative care. *Nutrients.* 2013;5(1):267–282.
94. Pearce CB, Duncan HD. Enteral feeding. Nasogastric, nasojejunal, percutaneous endoscopic gastrostomy, or jejunostomy: its indications and limitations. *Postgrad Med J.* 2002;78(918):198–204.
95. Chow R, Bruera E, Chiu L, et al. Enteral and parenteral nutrition in cancer patients: a systematic review and meta-analysis. *Ann Palliat Med.* 2016;5(1):30–41.
96. Bozzetti F, Braga M, Gianotti L, Gavazzi C, Mariani L. Postoperative enteral versus parenteral nutrition in malnourished patients with gastrointestinal cancer: a randomised multicentre trial. *Lancet.* 2001;358(9292):1487–1492.
97. Hamaoui E, Lefkowitz R, Olender L, et al. Enteral nutrition in the early postoperative period: a new semi-elemental formula versus total parenteral nutrition. *J Parenter Enteral Nutr.* 1990;14(5):501–507.

CHAPTER

34

SPECIALIZED NUTRITION SUPPORT IN BURNS, WASTING, DECONDITIONING, AND HYPERMETABOLIC CONDITIONS

Juquan Song[1], MD

Steven E. Wolf[1], MD

Charles E. Wade[2], PhD

Thomas R. Ziegler[3], MD

[1]University of Texas Medical Branch, Galveston, TX, United States

[2]University of Texas Health Science Center at Houston, Houston, TX, United States

[3]Emory University, Atlanta, GA, United States

SUMMARY

Severe burn caused hypermetabolism-sustained muscle wasting and other comorbidities. The goal of nutrition support and other care management is to maintain energy homeostasis in burn patients. Due to dramatic changes and other factors that influence over the time course after burn, the plan of nutrition support has to be adjusted continuously with monitoring patient conditions. Inappropriate management of nutrition support adverses patients' status and progress. The current principal of care management has been encouraged in severe burn patients, which includes earlier enteral feeding, 1.5–2 g/kg of protein intake, and others. However, the detail of each territory in nutrition care is still under investigation. Further, nutrition support is more specialized for certain population as the time being.

Keywords: Energy requirement; Hypermetabolism; Nutrition composition; Nutrition delivery route; Nutrition monitoring; Nutrition support; Severe burn.

I. NORMAL FUNCTION AND PHYSIOLOGY

Metabolism is essential and critical to maintain the biological homeostasis. The World Health Organization (WHO) recommends 2100 kcal/day requirement for normal healthy adults, with increases as needed for any additional medical stress.[1,2] Energy metabolism includes resource materials, such as macronutrient and micronutrient, energy production cycles, and energy production location (mitochondrial).

The skin and other accessory structures make a protective barrier to define each individual biological system. The skin is not only a barrier; it is more than a path to connect the environment with signal exchanges. In general, the skin plays important roles in protection, sensing, thermoregulation, and vitamin D synthesis.

II. SEVERE BURN AND CARE MANAGEMENT

A. Introduction

Nutritional support is fundamental for clinically ill patients. With critical illness, surgery, and severe injury,

Present Knowledge in Nutrition, Volume 2
https://doi.org/10.1016/B978-0-12-818460-8.00034-4

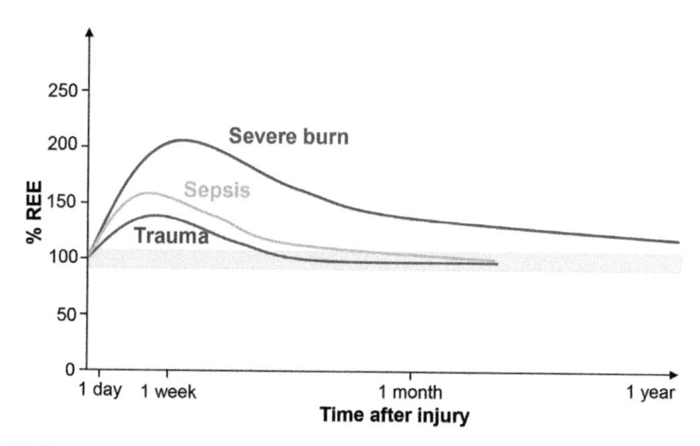

FIGURE 34.1 Hypermetabolic response after severe burn, sepsis, and trauma. *Adapted from Jan BV, Lowry SF. Systemic response to injury and metabolic support. In: Brunicardi FC, Andersen DK, Billiar TR, Dunn DL, Hunter JG, Matthews JB, Pollock RE, eds.* Schwartz's Principles of Surgery. *9th ed. 2010:15–50.*

there is a hypermetabolic response that occurs. Burns represent the extreme of this response with almost a doubling of resting energy expenditure (REE). Trauma and sepsis also result in increased REE with a lesser amplitude and duration (Fig. 34.1).[3] For this reason, the present treatment of burns has been used as an extreme example of nutritional support of the severely injured patients. This chapter will discuss the nutritional care in severe burns, which also gains knowledge to all injury states.

B. Characteristics of Burns

Burn description

Burn is the type of trauma to the skin or other tissues. Most burn injuries are heat related from hot liquids. Other physical and chemical factors also can be the cause. By the depth of injury, burns are categorized to superficial (I), partial thickness (superficial and deep II), full thickness (III), and even deeper to the underlying other tissue, such as muscle and bone (IV). Superficial burns involve only the epidermis and can self-heal within 3–4 days. Partial thickness burns involve the whole epidermis and partial dermis layers, papillary dermis to reticulum dermis. Burns over the deep superficial layer require excision and grafting, while partial thickness burns is treated with bacitracin and petroleum-based dressing application. Burns with greater than 20% total body surface area (TBSA) are considered severe and result in a dramatic systemic metabolic response.[4] Though the globe trend of burn incidence has declined,[5] it is still recognized as a major contributor to morbidity and mortality, in part, due to the dynamic postinjury systemic hypermetabolic response.[6] This chapter focused on the discussion of nutritional care in severe burns.

Hypermetabolism after severe burn

The metabolic status is characterized into the "ebb" acute stress phase and the later "flow" hypermetabolism stage following the injury. After surviving the acute ischemic shock phase, there is a pronounced increase in metabolism that persist for 7–10 days, followed by the flow phase in which a hypermetabolic state persists for years.[7] The catabolic status dominates to provide energy consumption for function maintenance in essential organs. Patients with greater than 40% TBSA burn increased REE up to 40%–100%.[8] The substrate cycling of fatty acids and glucose is greatly enhanced in response to burns. The total fatty acid cycling can increase fivefold, and the glycolytic/gluconeogenic cycle can double.[9] Compared to other types of trauma and sepsis, this hypermetabolic status also lasts longer in burn patients.[10] This persistent hypermetabolic response is further exacerbated with lean body mass loss, immune function compromise, delayed wound healing, etc.[11]

Energy metabolism and mitochondrial dysfunction after severe burn

The efficiency of energy production is damped after severe burns. In normal adults, about 80% of mitochondrial respiration is coupled to ADP phosphorylation with the rest attributing to proton leaks (such as heat production).[12] Adenosine triphosphate (ATP)–consuming reactions in adults with burns contribute to 57% of the increased total energy expenditure for protein synthesis, the substrate cycling of glucose and fatty acids.[13] Increased heating production could be due to uncoupling of mitochondrial respiration from ADP phosphorylation.[14] At the cellular level, oxygen consumption and ATP production turnover increase resulting in the hypermetabolism status after severe burn.

The underlying mechanisms of hypermetabolism after burns are complicated. Mitochondria are the cellular organelle to produce ATP for energy. Mitochondrial structure and functional impairment has been observed in response to severe burns.[15–18] These alterations in mitochondria could explain why attempts to maintain the normal proportion of macronutrients could not be helpful or if not at times harmful in burns. In addition, the use of nonnutritional agents that restore mitochondrial function may therefore improve the metabolic statue. A clinical trial (NCT number: NCT01812941) is ongoing to evaluate mitochondrial functional damage, by analyzing plasma levels of mtDNA damage-associated molecular patterns associated with multiorgan dysfunction syndrome to gain a better understating of mitochondrial changes in the hypermetabolic response to burns.

C. Nutrition Disarrangement in Burns

Malnutrition

Malnutrition, in the presence of acute injury and chronic disease, has serious consequences and increased risk of mortality. Malnutrition was defined at the guidelines and clinical resources in the American Society for Parenteral and Enteral Nutrition (ASPEN), including adults[19] and pediatric patients.[20,21] In adults, body mass involuntary changes (including loss and gain) are 5% in a month or 10% within 6 months and are considered malnutrition with body mass index (BMI) alterations ($18.5\,kg/m^2 < BMI > 25\,kg/m^2$). In children, the malnutrition threshold of BMI (for age or gender) is less than 5% or greater than 85%.

Overnutrition/hyperalimentation

Overnutrition/hyperalimentation is relatively rare but risky. In the 1970s, burn patients received 5000 kcal/day as the standard care, which led to hyperalimentation development.[22] Overnutrition, with overcalory input, causes hyperglycemia, overload of the respiratory system, and fat restoration. Overfeeding carbohydrates increases fatty acid synthesis in the liver and whole body. Three weeks of overfeeding carbohydrates increased 27% of liver fat accumulation but just 2% of body weight in human subjects.[23] Overfeeding caused fatty liver infiltration, which has been associated with increases in infection rate.[24] In rats overfed after burns, there was a threefold higher mortality rate.[25]

Refeeding syndrome

Refeeding syndrome is rare and defined as potentially fatal shifts in fluids and electrolytes with typical hypophosphatemia, hypokalemia, and hypomagnesemia.[26] In a small retrospective study, hypophosphatemia blood levels of less than 2.5 mg/dL (0.8 mmol/L) were observed at 2–6 days and the phosphate blood levels were back to the baseline at 18–20 days after burns.[27] Refeeding syndrome is due to endogenous insulin secretion in response to hyperglycemia after refeeding.

Undernutrition

Patients are more fragile to resistant severe insult when undernutrition support is either before or after injury. Demographic factors are also associated to nutritional disarrangement after injury, including aging, chronic disease, and even social, psychiatric, economic, and religious (i.e., vegetarian) factors. Malnourishment occurred in burn pediatric patients with delayed admission, which also increased length of stay.[28] Patients with undernutrition suffer from malnutrition and worse subsequences, such as immunosuppression, prolonged dependency on mechanical ventilation, delay in the healing processes, and increased risk of morbidity and mortality.[29]

Nutrition support is vital for the maintenance and recovery of burn patients. An inappropriate nutrition supply could lead malnutrition in patients. Either a lack of nutritional supplement or overnutrition makes detrimental effects in patients with worse progress. Many factors affect inappropriate nutritional supplements during the injury. The postburn hypermetabolic dynamic changes are the major challenges, and in addition, they are related to other inappropriate nutritional management. Using a single static energy expenditure formula might not fully reflect a patient's dynamic metabolic status. Periodic monitoring of nutrition management is critical to meet a patient's energy consumption. The nutrition disarrangement covers the affective range from preinjury till postadmission in patients. The hypermetabolic status persists years after burn, which is far from when patients are discharged. Nutritional support for patients should extend even after they are discharged.

D. Nutrition Support in Burn Care Management Overview

General guideline of nutritional management

The principle of burn critical care nutrition is to attenuate the magnitude of burn-induced hypermetabolism and meet the patient energy demands. To date, general rules are in agreement with nutritional management in burn critical care, including energy consumption measurement, the prioritized route and time of feeding, and proportion of nutrition supplement, etc. The European Society for Clinical Nutrition and Metabolism (ESPEN) endorsed eight recommendations of nutritional support in major burns in 2013, including earlier enteral feeding, adjustment of nutrient intake, appropriate energy expenditure assessment, and nonnutritional strategies (Table 34.1).[30] The International Society for Burn Injuries (ISBI) in 2016 also provides recommendation criteria in the similar range.[31]

Though most clinicians agree in the principles of nutritional support guidelines, there are no uniformed standard procedures for critical burn care. The differences of nutritional management after burns are inconsistent from local to worldwide regions and are affected by many practical factors, such as economics and social factors.

Clinical management of nutrition support

Nutritional support in the care of the patient with burns requires a multidisciplinary approach. Integration

TABLE 34.1 Malnutrition criteria ASPEN.

1. Early enteral feeding
2. Protein intake (1.5–2 g/kg in adults, 3 g/kg in children)
3. Glucose delivery (55% of energy requirement, 5 mg/kg/hours)
4. Trace element and vitamin substitution
5. Nonnutritional strategies (pharmacological agents and physical tools)
6. Indirect calorimetry for energy requirement determination
7. Toronto equation in adults and Schoffield equation in children
8. Fat administration ≤30% of total energy delivery

First five are strongly recommended and rest three are suggested.
Adapted from 2013 ESPEN recommendations. (Cited from Rousseau A-F, Losser M-R, Ichai C, et al. ESPEN endorsed recommendations: nutritional therapy in major burns. Clin Nutr. *2013;32(4):499–502).*

of the dietitian, with burn surgeons and other health care team members, to personalize the nutritional care of the patient is essential. In addition, they should educate the patient and family as to their long-term metabolic requirements. The nutrition plan needs to be adjusted and compatible with treatment requirements and during all phases of recovery. For example, loss of skin after excision and grafting, as well as wound healing, will increase metabolic requirements due to heat loss as well and increase energy expenditure associated with wound healing. The optimal efficiency of nutritional support can be achieved in harmony of teamwork. We outline the nutrition support management in burn care as an example. The practical procedure development from each hospital is encouraged.

III. CLINICAL NUTRITION MANAGEMENT IN BURN

A. Resting Energy Expenditure Requirement and Measurement

The goal of energy measurement

Nutritional support is to compensate the increase in caloric needs from burn patients who are hypermetabolic. Calculating energy (calorie) is fundamental for nutritional support and is also challenging due to metabolic dynamic changes in burn patients.

Energy expenditure typically increased within a week after earlier stressed at the earlier acute phase. Many factors affect this general dynamic energy expenditure curve, including surgical treatment, nutrition support, comorbidity, complications, medication, physical therapy, and ambient temperature. The Society of Critical Care Medicine and ASPEN recommend providing a minimum of 50%–60% of caloric goal during the first week after injury.[32,33]

Indirect calorimetry

Indirect calorimetry (IC) is the gold standard for REE measurement in critical care.[34] IC has been developed for 200 years following the Dynamic Energy Budget theory and applied to clinical nutrition management in past decades.[35] IC is a respiratory test to measure the exchange gas of oxygen and carbon dioxide in lungs and thus calculate actual REE. REE is calculated based on the Weir formula[36] compensated with practical fed state. The formula used is below:[37]

Metabolic rate (kcal per day) $= 1.44 \times (3.94 \times VO_2 + 1.11 \times VCO_2)$,
VO_2 is oxygen consumption, VCO_2 is carbon dioxide production, and the unit is mL/min.

The ratio of carbon dioxide production to oxygen consumption is defined as respiratory quotient (RQ), which also could be the monitor or evaluator of nutrition status. Under a normal feeding status, body stored fat is the main resource for energy consumption (RQ ranges from 0.75 to 0.90). RQ is greater than 1.0 when overfeeding occurs. Glucose/protein will be an energy resource, and the metabolic pathway shifts toward fat synthesis. RQ is thus useful to interpret the results of the REE.

Mathematical equations

IC is not always available based on reality concerns of its financial cost and users' training experience.[38] Thus, mathematical equations have been developed to estimate energy expenditure and applied widely. Mathematical calculations cost less and are more readily available compared to IC. However, when employing these formulas, the user should be aware of the consequences of misfeeding, as these static formulas do not account for the highly variable energy expenditure in burn patients.[39]

Among those mathematical equations, the Curreri formula is the oldest with the most important factors of age, body weight, and burn size. The formula is based on limited data from nine patients and tends to overestimate energy expenditure when compared to IC.[40] The equation by Davies and Liljedahl is the easiest and can be quickly calculated, but it also has a tendency of overestimation.[4] The Harris Benedict equation determines the basal energy expenditure (BEE), which is then multiplied by 1.5 to estimate the energy requirement for burns. The Toronto formula based on BEE is more accurate and is justified with injury progression to adjust for wound healing. Multiple regression analysis of an important number of calorimetric studies showed that the Toronto equation is a well-validated alternative when IC is not available.[41,42] Some other

TABLE 34.2 Mathematical equation for energy requirement in burns adults.

Formula name	Calculation equation	Estimated daily energy consumption (kcal)	Comments
Harris benedict	BEE for Men: 665 + (13.8 × W) + (5 × H) − (6.76 × A); Women: 655 + (9.6 × W) + (1.85 × H) − (4.68 × A). Multiplying by factor 1.2–2.0 for stress adjusting	BEE = 1915 For burn, 1915 × 1.5 = 2872	Basal energy expenditure (BEE) estimation, multiply by 1 for common burn stress adjustment
Curreri	Age 16–59: (25 × W) + (40 × TBSA); Age >60: (20 × W) + (65 × TBSA)	4400	Overestimation tendency, aging factor considered
Davies and Lilijedahl	(20 × W) + (70 × TBSA)	5800	Overestimation tendency, gross estimation for large injury
Toronto	−4343 + (10.5 × TBSA) + (0.23 × Cl) + (0.84 × BEE) + (114 × T) − (4.5 × PBD)	2782	Complicated, continuous data collection
Ireton-Jones	Ventilated patient: 1784 − (11 × A) + (5 × W) + (244 × S) + × (239 × T) + (804 × B) Nonventilated patient: 629 − (11 × A) + (25 × W) − (609 × O)	2957 2384	Considered injury type and obesity

For all equations, *A*, age in years; *B*, burn (present = 1, absent = 0); *BEE*, Basal energy expenditure; *Cl*, calorie intake the previous day; *H*, height in centimeters; *HBE*, Harris–Benedict estimates; *O*, obesity (present = 1, absent = 0); *PBD*, postburn day; *S*, sex (male = 1, female = 0); *T*, temperature (C°); *T*, trauma (present=1, absent=0); *TBSA*, burn size (percent total body surface area); *W*, weight in kilograms; Estimated Daily Energy Consumption based on an example subject: 25 A, 80kg, BSA 2m^2, TBSA 60%.

Adapted from Saffle JR, Graves C. Nutritional support of the burned patient. In: Herndon DN, ed. Total Burn Care, *3rd edition. Edinburgh: Saunders Elsevier, 2007: 398–419.*

equations are also developed to meet special needs, such as ventilation. The current popular equations are listed in Table 34.2. Pediatric formula is discussed separately in special populations.

B. Nutrition Component

Nutritional support includes macronutrients and micronutrients. Macronutrients include protein, carbohydrates, and fat to provide body with energy. Micronutrients include vitamins and minerals to maintain the body metabolic process. Dieticians can arrange the food menu for patients based on their calorie requirement. The amount and proportion of nutritional supplements are both adjusted. The earliest formulas for burn patients consisted of milk and eggs. Commercial products were then developed with different proportions of nutrients via different delivery routes. Specialized nutritional formulas are convenient and designed with differing amounts of carbohydrates, proteins, fats, and micronutrients. Numerous commercially prepared enteral formulas have been developed and listed partially. Diets having higher proportions of fat, such as Glucerna or Pulmocare, are not suitable for burns. Nepro can be applied when supplemented with protein for burn patients.

In 2007, ASPEN endeavored to standardize the PN production process to improve patient safety and clinical efficiency.[43] Premixed commercial products are also available for parenteral nutrition (PN).[44] PN products are grouped based on the component mixture with the fat emulsion systemic (Pro), PN solution systemic, PN solution systemic with electrolytes systemic, and trace elements systemic.[45] PN products are generally costly and can serve to supplement enteral nutrition (EN) in critically ill patients with severe nutritional needs.

When commercial formulas are not available under emergency situations, or in the area of developing countries, the alternative or replacement has to be considered and local nutrition supplements could have benefits as well. The disaster plans should be installed with nutritional options in local hospitals, which can be guided under the institutions of medicine.[46] WHO provides detailed information about local foods and nutrient contents.[47]

Macronutrients (proteins, carbohydrates, lipids)

Proteins; Under the hypermetabolic status, proteolysis dominates after severe burns. Protein is degraded into peptides and amino acids, which are redistributed to support function maintenance in other important organs, such as the heart and brain. Amino acids are ready to convert energy when calories are limited. Either one further degrades to carbon skeleton for the intermediates into citric acid cycle, or EAA coverts to acetyl-CoA. In addition, glutamine, alanine, and arginine are released from the skeletal muscle and transaminated to alpha-keto acid in the liver, a crossover to further convert to energy production, fat, glucose, and new amino acid production.

Burn injury increases urea production resulting in increased nitrogen excretion. In addition, protein loss can occur as it exudates directly through damaged skin and as the result of increased permeability of the blood vascular system. Nitrogen loss in burn patients is about 0.2 g/kg/day, leading to 10% body weight loss during the first week. The acute protein depletion is associated with immune dysfunction and infection incidence.[8] Thus, a protein supplement is needed.

Current ASPEN recommendation is 1.5–2 g protein intake per kilogram of body weight per day in the critically ill adult patient.[33] ISBI recommended that nonprotein calories to nitrogen ratios should be maintained between 150:1 for smaller burns and 100:1 for larger burns.[31] Excess protein intake has not been demonstrated to correlate with protein synthesis or to show a significant clinical benefit. An isotope study in pediatric patients with burns showed that 2.92 g/kg body weight/day of a high-protein diet only enhanced skin protein synthesis, without altering whole-body protein breakdown and synthesis.[48]

Special amino acid managements are under investigation. Glutamine is a conditional essential amino acid that is depleted quickly in serum and muscle after burn.[49] As an antioxidant, glutamine supplementation improves immune function and clinical outcomes in burns.[50–52] However, the effect of glutamine is not always consistent. Administration (0.3 g/kg/day) of glutamine during less than 3 days has no benefits in burned children.[53] In a multiple center trial, 1123 patients showed that patients supplemented with glutamine (0.35 g/kg/day) are associated with higher mortality after 28 days.[54] Currently, a double-blind, multicenter randomized trial is ongoing, which expects 2700 critically ill burned patients to be enrolled in over 60 burn centers worldwide. Patients are treated with enteral glutamine (0.5 g/kg/day) to assess hospital survival (RE-ENERGIZE study, NCT number: NCT00985205).[55]

The supplementation of arginine in burn patients was shown to improve wound healing and immune function,[56,57] but data from critically ill nonburn patients suggest that arginine could be detrimental due to over nitric oxide production.[58] Though current formula of immune enteral diet includes those amino acids, the conclusion is still dependent on more studies.

Carbohydrates; Carbohydrate metabolism is the central energy metabolism pathway. Once food is digested, it is mechanically and biochemically transformed to monomer monosaccharides such as glucose, fructose, and galactose. Eighty percent of food breaks down to glucose. Aerobic respiration results in 36 ATP from a molecular of glucose after the stages of glycolysis (2 ATPs), the citric acid circle (2 ATPs), and the electron transport system (32 ATPs). Carbohydrates provide the primary energy source for burn patients.

High-carbohydrate diets have been demonstrated to facilitate wound healing and to convey a protein-sparing effect. Awareness of excessive intake of carbohydrates is considered especially when treatment is via parenteral route. The maximum intravenous carbohydrate infusion rate for adults is 5–7 mg/kg/min. Exceeding this range increases the risk of shock in liver and hyperglycemia.[39] In contrast, insufficient carbohydrate supplementation leads to hypoglycemia. Van den Berghe and Jeschke,[59,60] respectively, reported 5% and 26% incidence rates of hypoglycemia in critically ill and burn patients. Hypoglycemia was associated with increased morbidity and mortality in pediatric burn patients.[61] Under tight glucose control, carbohydrate intake should be sufficient with 55%–60% of total energy requirements. In other words, carbohydrate intake should be about 5 g/kg/day with a daily limit of 1400–1500 kcal. A maximum of 7 g/kg/day is the glucose rate in severely burned patients, which glucose can be oxidized.[62,63]

Lipids; Lipids break down to triglycerides and further split to fatty acids and cholesterol in the small intestine. Transported with lipoprotein, triglycerides break down to glycerol and fatty acids and arrive to cells to biofunction of metabolic processing. Glycerol alters glycolysis and oxidation and fatty acids beta-oxidation in mitochondria. One molecule of fatty acids creates over three times the amount of energy than glucose.

The basal rate of lipolysis increases after burn,[64] and elevated beta-oxidation of fatty acids provides more fuel. However, only 30% of the free fatty acids are degraded, and the rest go through reesterification and accumulate in the liver.[65] Thus, a restriction of a low-fat diet is recommended for burn patients. Diets contain less than 15% of total calories from lipids and are beneficial in burn patients.[66] Patients with total lipid intakes reaching 35% of energy requirements have greater infection rates and increased lengths of stay.[67] Nutritional supplements containing fat are required to prevent essential fatty acid deficiency. Current commercial dietary formulas provide 30%–50% of total energy as fat, thus limitation of fat intake should be considered. Total lipid intake from all sources should be accounted as well to avoid overfeeding of fats. For instance, propofol

(DIPRIVAN Injectable Emulsion), as a sedation or anesthetic, is often applied by 15–30 g/day in adult burn patients. The present formulation contains soybean oil (100 mg/mL), glycerol (22.5 mg/mL), and egg lecithin (12 mg/mL), therefore, contributing to lipid intake. When calculating lipid intake daily, nonnutritional lipid intake such as propofol infusion needs to be counted in the total daily lipid calculation.

The composition of administered fatty acids also should be considered. The common dietary formula contains *omega*-6 fatty acids, such as linoleic acid, which converts to arachidonic acid, a precursor of proinflammatory cytokines (e.g., prostaglandin E2). On the other hand, supplementations with *omega*-3 fatty acids are observed to improve immune function.[68] In a study of 92 patients served a low-fat enteral diet with fish oil, *omega*-3 fatty acids had clinical benefits in sepsis control with reductions of nonseptic complications, such as mechanical ventilation requirements and gastric residual volumes. However, the mortality was not altered.[69] The ideal composition and amount of fat in nutritional support for burn patients remains to be clearly defined.

Micronutrients (minerals, vitamins)

Vitamins; Vitamin A and C improve wound healing via epithelial growth and protection,[70] and other vitamins such as vitamins B and E provide antioxidant protection as well in clinical benefits.[71] Vitamin B1 thiamine deficiency has been noted acutely with the potential threat of beriberi and Gayet-Wernicke encephalopathy. Local injection of thiamine reduces pain in the burn animal model.[72] Recently, the guidance on vitamin therapy in critically ill patients has been updated, recommending 300 mg of thiamine IV daily in at-risk patients and 100 mg iv for other patients.[73] Vitamin C is an electron donor and has pleiotropic effects during burn. Vitamin C reduced epithelial damage and capillary leakage in burn rats.[74] Normal healthy adults require 100 mg of vitamin C per day while burn and critically ill patients should receive up to 3 g/day.[75] Vitamin D (usually defined as 25(OH) D<= 20 ng/mL) and its binding protein are reduced in serum after burn.[76] Besides the depletion under oxidative stress, vitamin D3 production is obstructed due to skin damage. Pediatric burn patients extremely suffered calcium and vitamin D deficiency.[77] Vitamin D can be given from a standard range of 600–800 IU up to 10, 000 IU daily.[78] Vitamin E was depleted in fat tissue from pediatric burn patients.[79] Vitamin E applications prevent fibroblast from a heat-stressed environment.[80]

Minerals; Trace elements contribute to many biosynthesis processes and are often decreased from burn. The loss of minerals including zinc, copper, selenium, and others occurs through urination and cutaneous losses through burned skin.[81] The need of supplemental minerals increased, and the administration of minerals is based on the wound closing time after burn.[82] Minerals are an essential component of PN, deficiencies in and toxicity of certain trace elements necessitate vigilance of clinical symptoms in patients with burns, and appropriate and prompt corrections are made.[83]

Copper is an essential enzymatic cofactor involving iron metabolism, hematopoiesis, connective tissue formation, and nervous system function.[84] Clinical manifestations of copper deficiency are pancytopenia, skeletal, and neurologic abnormalities.[85] The recommendation of ASPEN is copper with a supplement of 0.3–0.5 mg/day.[86]

Zinc is important for DNA replication and protein synthesis in wound healing and lymphocyte activities.[87] 86% of total body zinc is stored in skeletal muscle and bone, and only 0.1% is found in plasma with a concentration of 12–18 μmol/L.[84] The clinical features of zinc deficiency are nonspecific. ASPEN-recommended supplementation in PN for zinc is 2.5–5 mg/day.[86] Patients with sepsis and burns require additional supplementation.[33] Up to 36 mg/day of supplementation has shown the benefits of infection reduction in burn patients without toxicity.[88] Oral doses of more than 200 mg/day may lead to acute zinc toxicity with associated gastrointestinal symptoms.

Selenium has multiple functions. It is served as an antiinflammatory by inhibiting of NF-κB, antioxidant via selenoproteins, such as glutathione peroxidase (GSH-Px),[89] and regulates thyroid hormone metabolism.[90] Selenium deficiency was first recognized as Keshan cardiomyopathy disease.[91] Selenium (Se) loss occurs from skin and urine both in adults and pediatric patients with burns resulting in an acute reduction in serum levels.[92] Selenium deficiency is also caused by continuous clinical manipulations, including continuous renal replacement therapy, high urine output, diarrhea/fistula output, multiple drains, and medications, such as corticosteroids and statins.[93] Therefore, selenium levels should be monitored and supplementation considered if necessary.

Trivalent chromium is a component of metalloenzymes, influencing glucose levels and insulin resistance.[84] Chromium deficiency can result in glucose intolerance refractory to insulin and subsequently hyperglycemia and neuropathy.[94] Trivalent chromium competes with iron for transport with transferrin and albumin. Overdose of chromium may disturb iron metabolism.[95] The current ASPEN guidelines recommend 10–15 μg/day of chromium in PN.[86]

Manganese is a component of metalloenzymes that are involved in immune function, reproduction, and neurological functions.[96] Excessive manganese deposit in the basal ganglia of the brain results where patients develop Parkinson-like signs and other neuropsychiatric symptoms.[97] Due to the risk of hypermanganesemia in patients with home parental nutrition, the current recommended dose of manganese drops from 60 to 100 mcg/day to a lower dose of 55 μg/day.[86]

Ferrous acts as a cofactor for oxygen-carrying proteins. The British National Diet estimated dietary iron daily intake in healthy individuals to be 13.2 mg for men and 10.0 mg for women.[98] However, the ASPEN guidelines indicate that iron is "not routinely added." Anemia is the most familiar clinical means by which iron deficiency is recognized. Serum ferritin and transferrin can be measured to access the need for iron supplementation.

Aluminum is rarely studied. Klein et al.[99] observed that elevated aluminum concentrations were associated with bone disease after burn in pediatric patients. The elevation could be from use of antacids and albumin administration, partial immobilization, and increased production of endogenous glucocorticoids.

Micronutrients include vitamins and minerals, which are required more in burn patients than in healthy individuals as a result of consumption due to hypermetabolism and wound healing, as well as losses from the injured skin or in urine. Severe burns caused hyperinflammation and intensive oxidative stress that result in depletion of endogenous antioxidants. Decreased levels of vitamins and minerals negatively impact immune function and body homeostasis.[81] ASPEN in 2014 released the guidelines of micronutrients for the use of PN and EN.[99]

C. Nutrition Delivery Route

Oral

The oral route is usually employed in patients with smaller burns. Patients with less than 10% TBSA burns do not significantly increase their energy requirement and can readily meet alterations in metabolism with their regular diet. Patients with 10%–20% TBSA burns generally are able to meet caloric needs by increasing the amount and quality of a high-protein/calorie diet.[100] This is facilitated by consultation with a dietitian.

In patients with severe burns, oral/facial burns, or requiring mechanical ventilation, the oral route is insufficient to meet energy requirements.[101] EN and/or PN need to be implemented when oral delivery is less than 60% of the daily energy requirement. Under certain extreme conditions when these routes are not available, the oral route with high-protein foods and small frequent feeding is encouraged. Patients might be allowed to eat and drink whenever possible based on triage treatment plans and individual patient tolerance. Monitoring a patient's nutritional status is always necessary.[102]

Enteral

EN is the first choice for severe burn patients. The presence of nutrients maintains the integrity of digestive physiologic function by stimulating blood supply, preserving gut mucosa integrity, and decreasing bacterial translocation.[103,104] In addition to its biological benefits, EN is a clinically safe and effective feeding route.

Early enteral nutrition (EEN) is more amenable for patients' recovery and survival. EN prior to surgical procedures provides more benefits, including fewer complications, a reduction in length of stay, and reduced financial cost compared to PN.[105] Animal studies with enteral feedings initialized 2 h after burns demonstrated metabolic improvements in pigs.[106] Early enteral feeding even initiated within the first 6–12 h after injury improves immune and metabolic function and reduces complications.[107] EEN was also accessed to be effective and safe.[108] A reduction in mortality was reported with early (3–6 h) vs. delayed (>48 h) EN in a randomized clinical trial with 688 children.[109] However, EEN benefit is not always reported to be significant. A British study of about 2400 patients showed that the route of delivery of early nutritional support enteral vs. parenteral did not affect the 30-day mortality in critically ill patients, but the enteral route attenuated the incidence of hypoglycemia and vomiting.[110] Another study found EEN did not affect the hypermetabolism in burns.[111] The clinical practice guidelines (CPGs) from the European Society of Intensive Care Medicine sites 17 recommendations of EEN within 48 h in critically ill patients. Seven were sited of delaying enteral nutrition in those with uncontrolled shock and GI symptoms.[112] At the present, the consensus is to initiate enteral feeding early.

Small-bore (5–12 French) or large-bore (≥14 French) feeding tubes are typically selected dependent on the insertion site (nasal, oral, percutaneous) and location of the terminal end of the enteral device (stomach, duodenum, proximal small bowel).[113] Gastric feeding has the advantages of large-bore tubes to give bolus feeds; however, the ileus often develops following burn injury. Smaller postpyloric tubes are more prone to clogging and malposition, but they are more comfortable and postpyloric feedings can be initiated safely. Nasal/oral tubes are usually placed for short-term (<4–6 weeks) use, while tube enterostomies are employed for long-term (≥4 weeks) EN support.[114] In the most severely burned patients, the gastric route should be attempted first, keeping the postpyloric access option or even percutaneous endoscopic gastrostomy as backup in case of pyloric dysfunction.[115] Radiographic verification of blindly tube insertion is advocated before initiating feeding.[116]

EN products are commercially available and discussed above. Continuous feeds are more favorable with less chance of aspiration, infection rate, and moralities.[117–119] Burn patients usually take a lower residue containing 1 kcal/mL product with protein supplement. Routine water flushes are recommended to maintain tube cleanness without block. ASPEN Safe Practices for Enteral Nutrition Therapy updated in 2018[117] described general EN use procedures, which include the following steps: patient assessment; prescribe EN regimen; EN order review-procedure material preparation; EN regimen administration; monitor and reassess; and feedback to justification of the first step of patient assessment.

The common complications with EN are gastrointestinal tract symptoms including nausea, vomiting, abdominal distention, diarrhea, constipation, and aspiration. Clinical management to avoid these complications should include chlorhexidine mouthwash in orally intubated patients,[33] inclined bed,[119] and prokinetic agents.[120]

Other rare enteral feeding complications are refeeding syndrome and nonobstructive bowel necrosis. Burn patients with preexisted malnutrition are at greater risk for these complications. Aggressive enteral feeding can cause nonobstructive bowel necrosis. Thus, initial fiber-free enteral feeding should be undertaken cautiously, especially in patients with critical conditions, such as shock, on mechanical ventilation, or being administered anesthetic and analgesic medications, etc.

Parenteral

PN can quickly deliver energy and nutrients into the body system for those patients who are not able to meet nutrition requirements when other routes are not available or insufficient. PN was routinely used back to 1970s; however, now PN is the alternative after EN consideration for burn patients because of purported EN biological benefits.[121] Intravenous route of PN increases the tendency of infection mechanical and infectious complications of catheters, and PN solutions are also costive compared to EN formulas. Van Den Berg's group reported that initiation of PN after 8 days has a better recovery effect with less complications compared to earlier PN initiated within 48 h in 2312 adults in the intensive care unit (ICU).[122]

The commercial formula for PN consist all essential nine amino acids.[123] PN is recommended to provide 60%–70% of nonamino acid calories as dextrose and 30%–40% of nonamino acid calories as fat emulsion in ICU patient. The maximal dose of lipid emulsion infusion is 1.0–1.3 g/kg/day.[124–127] The composition of PN, infusion rate, and delivery line care are considered when providing this form of nutrition. PN can be delivered as complete solutions given by either a peripheral or central vein. The use of a central vein allows more volume of concentrated dextrose and amino acid to be delivered to meet the nutrition requirements in ICU critical patients (Table 34.3). The ESPEN recommendation of PN in critically ill patients[126] supported the use of 6–8 mmol/L (100–150 mg/dL) of glucose, which has also been advocated for use in major burns.[30]

Previously, PN was suggested to result in overfeeding, especially when calculation of energy requirements was not accurate. In the late 80's, overfeeding/hyperalimentation was observed in patients with PN specifically due to the lack of glucose control.[24] PN formulations can cause increases in proinflammatory mediators,[128] which are associated with steatosis,[129] immunosuppression,[24] and elevated mortality.[130] Patients with PN should be monitored closely for tight glucose control with administration regulated in response to the changing energy requirements over the course of recovery.

PN complications are associated with technical line placement. Inappropriate line placement can cause pneumothorax, hemothorax, and pericardial tamponade. Indwelling central venous line may lead hemorrhage or air embolism. A long-term use of central lines for PN delivery is also suggested to increase the risk of infections. PN solutions have been reported to result in metabolic complications, which may be severe to moderate or common to rare.

EN and PN are given based on clinical judgment. Table 34.4 presented three examples to demonstrate nutrition derangements during the delivery route changes: a typical maintenance regimen for severe burns containing a high-protein formula; enteral feeding decreasing to reduce glucose intolerance; and using a high-fat diet resulting in fewer carbohydrate calories, which is especially for patients with diabetes or insulin resistance as a result of burns.

D. Nutrition Monitoring and Evaluation

Nutrition risk screening and monitor procedure

Though there is no defined clinical procedure of nutritional evaluation in burn and trauma, the guidelines should be in place to monitor the patient nutrition status. Monitoring has been defined as "the chance of a better or worse outcome from disease or surgery according to actual or potential nutritional and metabolic status," and nutritional risk scaled by ESPEN and Nutritional Risk Screening 2002.[131] The procedure of nutrition assessment covers several administrative steps for different levels of health care personals. A predesigned format of survey or procedure should include

TABLE 34.3 Parenteral nutrition components.

Component	Peripheral vein PN	Central vein PN
Volume (L/day)	2–3	1–1.5
Dextrose (%)	5	10–25
Amino acids (%)	2.5–3.5	3–8
Lipid (%)	3.5–5.0	2.5–5.0
Sodium (meq/L)	50–150	50–150
Potassium (meq/L)	20–35	30–50
Phosphorus (mmol/L)	5–10	10–30
Magnesium (meq/L)	8–10	10–20
Calcium (meq/L)	2.5–5	2.5–5
Vitamins	*	
Trace elements/minerals	**	

**Vitamins typically added on a daily basis to peripheral vein and central vein PN comprise commercial mixtures of vitamins A, B1 (thiamin), B2 (riboflavin), B3 (niacinamide), B6 (pyridoxine), B12, C, D, and E, biotin, folate, and pantothenic acid. Vitamin K is added on an individual basis (e.g., in patients with cirrhosis). Specific vitamins can also be supplemented individually.*
***Trace elements/minerals typically added on a daily basis to peripheral vein and central vein PN comprise commercial mixtures of chromium, copper, manganese, selenium, and zinc. Minerals can also be supplemented individually.*
Adapted from Zhao VM, Ziegler TR. Specialized nutrition support. In: Erdman Jr, JW, Macdonald IA, Zeisel SH, eds. Present Knowledge in Nutrition, *10th edition. Oxford: Wiley-Blackwell, 2012:982–999.*

TABLE 34.4 Nutrition change with delivery route.

	Feedings	IV dextrose	Total
	Example 1: Maintenance feeding and IV		
mL/h	100	200	300
Kcal/d	2400	680	3080
Protein g/d	150	0	150
Carbs g/d	271	240	511
Fat g/d	82	0	82
	Example 2: Decreasing feeding and increasing IV		
mL/h	50	250	300
Kcal/d	1200	1020	2220
Protein g/d	75	0	75
Carbs g/d	136	300	436
Fat g/d	41	0	41
	Example 3: Changing formula to glucerna		
mL/h	100	200	300
Kcal/d	2400	680	3080
Protein g/d	100	0	100
Carbs g/d	229	240	169
Fat g/d	131	0	131

Adapted from Saffle JR, Graves C. Nutritional support of the burned patient. In: Herndon DN, ed. Total Burn Care, *3rd edition. Edinburgh: Saunders Elsevier, 2007: 398–419.*

standardized data collection procedures and periodic monitoring throughout a patient's hospitalization.

Nutrition assessment of the burned patient begun at admission as it depends on a complete review of the history and physical exam. Patients' demographic information as to preexist diseases affects the nutrition plan. Hypermetabolism changes fluxes the nutritional need in the patient, certain comorbidities, and manipulation such as infections, ventilator support, and hypoproteinemia, further varying nutrition requirements. The hypermetabolic state persists for over years after burn, and the continuous nutrition support and assessment are also important for patients even after discharge from the hospital. Considering environmental limitations, such as it is practical for patients to regularly weigh and feed themselves in order to maintain body weight as instructed by the physician and dietician need to be considered. An increased caloric intake with a high-protein component is usually recommended for about a year after discharge.

Nutrition assessment methods

Clinical examination and additional laboratory measurements are recommended not only for the initial assessment but also for the continued monitoring postburn. Serum proteins, nitrogen balance, anthropometric measurements, intake and output of fluids, IC, and tests of immune function are methods that provide a fair overview of the metabolic alterations in the postburn period. A survey from 65 burn care resources in North America summarized the order of parameters used to assess the adequacy of nutritional support: prealbumin (86% of centers), body weight (75%), calorie count (69%), and nitrogen balance (54%).[132] In addition, measurement of BMI is easy to acquire. However, body weight value could be affected during resuscitation at the early stage. The body weight increases as great as 10% have been reported during the acute phase. Though eventually via diuresis this weight gain is lost, the time course of the loss depends on clinical needs, thus body weight is unpredictable during this period. Dual X-ray absorptiometry medical imaging of lean body mass and bone density can also assist nutrition monitoring of patients.

Nitrogen is a fundamental component of amino acids metabolism. Nitrogen balance is the parameter to assess the efficiency of protein metabolism, and a negative nitrogen balance often occurs with burns, trauma, and periods of fasting, while measurement requires accurate urine collection for determination of urea nitrogen (UUN) as well as documentation of dietary nitrogen intake.[133] Nitrogen balance is calculated between the daily amount of nitrogen intake and nitrogen excreted: Nitrogen balance $=$ [Daily protein intake/6.25]$-$[$1.25 \times (\text{UUN} + 4)$]. Nonurinary nitrogen losses (4 g) and 1.25 multiply correction are for excessive loss in burns, mostly protein-enriched exudate from skin wound.[134]

Lab examination of serum hepatic protein levels has been used with limitations noted. Albumin was depressed after burns even with proper nutrition and appears to be more closely correlated with the inflammatory response than nutritional status.[135] Prealbumin is theoretically sensitive for nutrition monitoring; however, its half-life is over 2 days, tempering its association with nutritional status especially in the dynamic phase immediately postburn.[136] Protein markers, if used, should be interpreted in context with the patient's clinical status.

Monitoring hyperglycemia

Hyperglycemia is extremely common in burn patients. With the hypermetabolic state, patients develop insulin resistance. Persistent hyperglycemia has been associated with an increased risk of infection and other poor outcomes. Intensive glucose control with glucose levels of 80–110 mg/dL has been attributed to beneficiary effects, such as less multiple organ failure, a decreased rate of infection, shorter length of stay, and decreased mortality when compared to tradition control, which show glucose levels in a 180–200 mg/dL range.[137] Since tight blood glucose controls have been recognized, comprehensive protocols were adopted in many burn ICUs. Because of the nature of insulin resistance, effective glucose controls require glucose monitoring, nurse time, and substantial insulin doses.

IV. NONNUTRITIONAL SUPPORT AGENTS AND MANIPULATIONS

Pharmacological and nonnutritional clinical management strategies have been developed during past decades to improve nutritional care. Clinical manipulation, such as increasing the ambient environmental temperature, anabolic agents, pain relievers, and physical rehabilitation, is to attenuate stress and reduce catabolism in critically ill burned patients.[30] The primary target of these applications is to maintain metabolism in burn patients; therefore, they are closely correlated to clinical nutrition care management.

A. Medications

Oxandrolone is an anabolic steroid and synthetic androgen. It has been shown to significantly increase lean body mass retention, bone mineral content, and density and decrease length of hospital stay.[138] The dose of 0.1 mg/kg bid from 6 to 12 months postburn in children has been demonstrated to have beneficial effects.[139] Oxandrolone is often continued in the outpatient setting. Elevated aminotransferase (ALT over 200 U/L) levels are a reported side effect, thus liver function tests should be considered.

Propranolol is a nonselective beta-adrenergic receptor blocker and previously shown to lower heart rate by 20% in patients with burns who have an increased rate due to their hypermetabolic state. Recent studies, by the Galveston group, showed its benefit on the skeletomuscular system as long-term usage of propranolol (4 mg/kg/d) improved lean body mass and decreased bone loss.[140] A systemic review from 10 clinical trials also showed the benefit of propranolol with additional effects of reducing BEE and central fat deposition.[141] The studies were in consensus by the American Burn Association in 2013.[142] The awareness of side effects is bradycardia and hypotension.

Insulin affects both anabolism and decrease proteolysis. Insulin can decrease hyperglycemia and is associated with improved wound healing resulting in a short length of hospital stay when applied with a high-carbohydrate, high-protein diet.[143,144] However, the side effect of insulin is hypoglycemia, subsequently leading to worse outcome of infection risk.[145] Current critical care nutrition guidelines recommend blood sugar control at a target range of 140–180 mg/dL. Patients must be monitored closely with a tight blood sugar control as there is an increased risk of hypoglycemia.

Metformin decreases blood sugar with other potential benefits. Several small clinical trials demonstrate the benefit of glucose control in burn patients with 850 mg qid for 7 days[146] and a lower incidence of hypoglycemia compared to insulin treatment.[147] The side effect note in burns is lactate acidosis.

Other medications have been evaluated in burns. The effect of recombinant human growth hormone is controversial. It improved LBM accretion after burns in pediatric patients,[148] but in studies of critically ill adults, an increase in mortality has been reported.[149] Insulin-like growth factor 1 (IGF-1) is 3–4 times lower than normal in burn patients, and several studies showed that exogenous infusion of IGF-1 maintains metabolic status.[150] More research is needed regarding the efficacy and safety of these anabolic agents in patients.

B. Probiotics and Synbiotics

The development of probiotics treatment, to restore normal bacteria flora (microbiome) of the gut, has been investigated in other types of critically ill patients (*Lactobacillus* and *Bifidobacterium*). However, the progress of clinical application is slow in burns. El-Ghazely et al.[151] suggested clinical benefits in children with burns on probiotic treatment, with improved wound healing and a reduced length of stay, without changes in the rate of infections. Mayes[152] reported the nonclinical benefit in burn pediatric patients with probiotic administration. Additional research as to the clinical efficacy of probiotic treatment appears to be warranted.

C. Fluid Resuscitation

Though it is not a direct nutritional support, fluid resuscitation influences nutrition delivery and absorption. Composition and volume of the fluids are related to nutritional support. Some colloids and albumin serve dual roles in regulating osmolarity and metabolism. Fluid supplements are affected by the calorie nutrition calculation as well as the concentrations of various macro- and micronutrients.

Burns less than 15%–20% TBSA can be cared for by oral hydration, while burns greater than 20% TBSA often require intravenous resuscitation. The increase in fluid requirements in the patient with severe burns is due to increases in vascular permeability and increased fluid loss from damaged skin. Sufficient fluid resuscitation is thus important to maintain the body function. The most commonly used formulas to direct fluid resuscitation are the Parkland, modified Parkland, Brooke, modified Brooke, and Evans and Monafo's formulas.[153] The Parkland formula is 4 mL lactated Ringers/kg per % TBSA burned, with half of total volume given over the first 8 h and the remaining half of total volume given over the next 16 h, titrated to maintain adequate urine output. The use of lactate solutions in burns up to 40% TBSA without inhalation injury is safe. Be aware, the volume of colloid solution used in resuscitation needs to be lower in patients with preexisted heart disease, larger burns (>40%), or inhalation injury.[154]

V. SPECIAL POPULATIONS IN BURN NUTRITION MANAGEMENT

A. Pediatrics

Pathophysiological responses to burns are differed from children to adults due to differences in the body mass to body surface relationship. As a result regarding nutritional support, pediatric patients require special care as they have an increased risk of hypothermia after burn. In addition, following the general rule of nutrition management after burn of determining energy expenditure, when gold standard of IC is not available, the Schofield equation is suitable for children (Table 34.5).[155]

TABLE 34.5 Schofield equation of pediatric energy requirement.

Age	Sex	Requirements
3–10 years	Male	(19.6 × weight) + (1033 × height) + 200
	Female	(16.97 × weight) + (1618 × height) + 371.2
10–18 years	Male	(16.25 × weight) + (1372 × height) + 515.5
	Female	(8365 × weight) + (4.65 × height) + 200

Weight (kg), height (cm).
Adapted from Rousseau A-F, Losser M-R, Ichai C, et al. ESPEN endorsed recommendations: nutritional therapy in major burns. Clin Nutr *2013;32(4):499–502.*

The disadvantage of the Schofield equation, a fixed equation, is not integrating changes over time. The Galveston group developed a formula that can be used in children down to 1 year of age (Table 34.6).

Additionally, for consideration in the nutritional management for children, they have a smaller energy reserve and higher energy and protein requirements than adults. There are commercially available products that are designed especially for pediatric patients. Based on the additional need of growth development, protein could increase to 2.5–4.0 g/kg/day for burned children. Nutrition delivery with postpyloric tube feeding is easier in children than in adults.

B. Obesity

The rate of obesity has increased, in the past decades, worldwide. In obesity patients, chronic inflammation triggered intracellular signals[156] that have an impact on physiological responses, especially metabolic homeostasis.[157] Obesity can interfere with initial nutritional assessment, when body weight is the primary parameter. Though hypocaloric feeding with a low calorie and high protein diet is suggested to maintain lean body mass for obesity patients, there is currently limited data to endorse care guidelines for patients who are obese.

C. Military

Military-based burn care has its specialty. The adversity of burns in the military field is that burns often combined with multisystem traumatic injuries, limited medical supplies, equipment and care on the battlefield, and multiple-treatment levels. Among combat casualties, 2%–10% involved burn-related injuries.[158] About 20% of combat burns are greater than 30% TBSA.[159] Burn CPGs were created in 2006 to guide medical care of the combat casualty with burns.[160] The Milner equation was applied to determine REE in the military field with ≥20% TBSA burns.[161] Nutritional care on the battlefield follows the general guideline promulgated by consensus of military and civilian providers. Earlier enteral nutrition within 24 h is the recommended. The EN rate starts at 20 mL/h and increased by 2 0 mL/h every 4 h to reach the goal of calorie requirements (100 ± 20%) on day 3 after admission.[33] As military casualties are often transported over long distances, EN can be started 96 h after injury and later when patients settled down and in the flow phase of metabolism.[158] Later EN is also delayed to limit the potential risk of aspiration during the transportation.[162] While a taxing environment in which to care for the casualty in combat, the outcomes are similar to those attained in civilian populations.[163]

Humane catastrophe scenario possibly generates a large number of combined or multiple trauma injury types with the inclusion of severe burn in a short time

TABLE 34.6 Galveston pediatric energy calculation.

Formula name		Calculation equation by age							
Age (years)		0–0.5	0.5–1	1–3	3–10	10–11	11–14	14–15	15–18
BSA (m^2)		0.5	–	0.6	1.1	–	1.6	–	–
BEE (WHO)	Female Male		(61 × W) − 51 (60.9 × W) − 54		(22.5 × W) + 499 (22.7 × W) + 495			(12.2 × W) + 746 (17.5 × W) + 651	
Recommended dietary intake (RDI)[3,28]		108 × W	98 × W	102 × W	90 × W	55 × W	55 × W	47 × W	47 × W
Galveston		2100 × BSA + 1000 × BSA × TBSA		1800 × BSA + 1300 × BSA × TBSA			1500 × BSA + 1500 × BSA × TBSA		
Curreri junior		RDA + (15 × TBSA)		RDA + (25 × TBSA)		RDA + (40 × TBSA)			–

BEE, basal energy expenditure; *CI*, calorie intake the previous day; *RDA*, Recommended dietary allowance; *RDI*, Recommended dietary intake; *TBSA*, burn size (percent total body surface area); *W*, weight in kilograms.
*** BSA average 0.5 m², 10 kg, 1 month old; 0.6 m², 12 kg, 3 years; 1.1 m², 30 kg, 10 years; 1.6 m², 10 years; 60 kg, 14 years.*
Adapted from Saffle JR, Graves C. Nutritional support of the burned patient. In: Herndon DN, ed. Total Burn Care, *third edition. Edinburgh: Saunders Elsevier, 2007; p. 398–419.*

period. In emergency situations with limited resources, nutritional management is compromised and alternative procedures employed. In 2016, ABA summarized the recommendation of burn nutrition guidelines under austere conditions.[102] The recommendations simplified the medical professional criteria with a general preparation plan and care principles for the public. However, there are limited data as to nutritional care under a crisis, such as a mass casualty, and investigations should be continued.

RESEARCH GAPS

Burn injury belongs to trauma, and it represents the extreme in nutritional support requirements. Burns produce the greatest alteration metabolism, with a hypermetabolic state that persists for years after the injury. General guidelines have been developed to address each aspect of nutritional management, taking into account the unique requirements of the patient with burns. This chapter presents the mechanistic and "material" aspect of nutrition care. The varied "human" side of health care, including a network of education, management, coordination, and procedure implantation, needs to be established. A fully developed protocol involved all team members who provide optimal nutritional care to burn patients. Mainly due to the characterization of severe burn, the treatment procedure is difficult and standardized. Furthermore, nutritional support should be specialized as the current population change. A feasible and broad applicable procedure of burn care management for austere scenario should be considered for preparation in the future.

Nowadays, high technology related to health care has been developed including a cloud database, an artificial intelligence (AI) program, a telemedicine diagnosis of home nutrition support, and robotic surgery, all new techniques could help to manage nutrition at every aspect, will change the current nutrition support setting. Recently, Dr. McMahon, the president of the ASPEN, has created an AI program called FEED (Feeding Effectively Using Electronic Data) Mayo Clinic. The program is to focus on the safety and quality of patients receiving nutritional support. Technology such as this will greatly improve compliance with guidelines resulting in better outcomes and function of the patient with severe injuries.

VI. REFERENCES

1. World Health Organization. *The Management of Nutrition in Major Emergencies*. Geneva: World Health Organization; 2000. Available at: http://search.ebscohost.com/login.aspx?direct=true&scope=site&db=nlebk&db=nlabk&AN=91370.
2. Hanfling D, Hick J. *Committee on Crisis Standards of Care: A Toolkit for Indicators and Triggers, Board on Health Sciences Policy.* Institute of Medicine; 2013. Available at: http://www.acphd.org/media/330265/crisis%20standards%20of%20care%20toolkit.pdf.
3. Brunicardi FC, Schwartz SI. *Schwartz's Principles of Surgery.* New York, NY: McGraw-Hill Education LLC.; 2010. Available at: https://login.proxy.bib.uottawa.ca/login?url=https://accessmedicine.mhmedical.com/book.aspx?bookid=352.
4. Herndon DN. *Total Burn Care*. 5th ed. Philadelphia: Elsevier; 2017.
5. Smolle C, Cambiaso-Daniel J, Forbes AA, et al. Recent trends in burn epidemiology worldwide: a systematic review. *Burns*. 2017; 43:249–257.
6. Zavlin D, Chegireddy V, Boukovalas S, et al. Multi-institutional analysis of independent predictors for burn mortality in the United States. *Burns Trauma*. 2018;6:24.
7. Cuthbertson DP, Angeles Valero Zanuy MA, Leon Sanz ML. Post-shock metabolic response. 1942. *Nutr Hosp*. 2001;16:176–182. discussion 175–176.
8. Hart DW, Wolf SE, Mlcak R, et al. Persistence of muscle catabolism after severe burn. *Surgery.* 2000;128:312–319.
9. Wolfe RR, Herndon DN, Jahoor F, et al. Effect of severe burn injury on substrate cycling by glucose and fatty acids. *N Engl J Med*. 1987; 317:403–408.
10. Clark A, Imran J, Madni T, Wolf SE. Nutrition and metabolism in burn patients. *Burns Trauma*. 2017;5:11.
11. Williams FN, Herndon DN, Jeschke MG. The hypermetabolic response to burn injury and interventions to modify this response. *Clin Plast Surg*. 2009;36:583–596.
12. Rolfe DF, Brown GC. Cellular energy utilization and molecular origin of standard metabolic rate in mammals. *Physiol Rev.* 1997; 77:731–758.
13. Yu YM, Tompkins RG, Ryan CM, Young VR. The metabolic basis of the increase of the increase in energy expenditure in severely burned patients. *JPEN J Parenter Enteral Nutr.* 1999;23:160–168.
14. Porter C, Tompkins RG, Finnerty CC, et al. The metabolic stress response to burn trauma: current understanding and therapies. *Lancet*. 2016;388:1417–1426.
15. Padfield KE, Astrakas LG, Zhang Q, et al. Burn injury causes mitochondrial dysfunction in skeletal muscle. *Proc Natl Acad Sci USA*. 2005;102:5368–5373.
16. Porter C, Herndon DN, Sidossis LS, Borsheim E. The impact of severe burns on skeletal muscle mitochondrial function. *Burns.* 2013;39:1039–1047.
17. Szczesny B, Brunyanszki A, Ahmad A, et al. Time-dependent and organ-specific changes in mitochondrial function, mitochondrial DNA integrity, oxidative stress and mononuclear cell infiltration in a mouse model of burn injury. *PLoS One.* 2015;10:e0143730.
18. Berger MM, Pantet O. Nutrition in burn injury: any recent changes? *Curr Opin Crit Care.* 2016;22:285–291.
19. White JV, Guenter P, Jensen G, et al. Consensus statement: Academy of Nutrition and Dietetics and American Society for Parenteral and Enteral Nutrition: characteristics recommended for the identification and documentation of adult malnutrition (undernutrition). *JPEN J Parenter Enter Nutr.* 2012;36:275–283.
20. Mehta NM, Corkins MR, Lyman B, et al. Defining pediatric malnutrition: a paradigm shift toward etiology-related definitions. *JPEN J Parenter Enter Nutr.* 2013;37:460–481.

21. Becker P, Carney LN, Corkins MR, et al. Consensus statement of the Academy of Nutrition and Dietetics/American Society for Parenteral and Enteral Nutrition: indicators recommended for the identification and documentation of pediatric malnutrition (undernutrition). *Nutr Clin Pract*. 2015;30:147–161.
22. Rodriguez NA, Jeschke MG, Williams FN, et al. Nutrition in burns: Galveston contributions. *JPEN J Parenter Enter Nutr*. 2011; 35:704–714.
23. Sevastianova K, Santos A, Kotronen A, et al. Effect of short-term carbohydrate overfeeding and long-term weight loss on liver fat in overweight humans. *Am J Clin Nutr*. 2012;96:727–734.
24. Herndon DN, Barrow RE, Stein M, et al. Increased mortality with intravenous supplemental feeding in severely burned patients. *J Burn Care Rehabil*. 1989;10:309–313.
25. Mittendorfer B, Jeschke MG, Wolf SE, Sidossis LS. Nutritional hepatic steatosis and mortality after burn injury in rats. *Clin Nutr*. 1998;17:293–299.
26. Mehanna HM, Moledina J, Travis J. Refeeding syndrome: what it is, and how to prevent and treat it. *BMJ*. 2008;336: 1495–1498.
27. Castana O, Rempelos G, Faflia C, et al. Hypophosphataemia in burns. *Ann Burns Fire Disasters*. 2009;22:59–61.
28. Dylewski ML, Prelack K, Weber JM, et al. Malnutrition among pediatric burn patients: a consequence of delayed admissions. *Burns*. 2010;36:1185–1189.
29. Schulman CI, Ivascu FA. Nutritional and metabolic consequences in the pediatric burn patient. *J Craniofac Surg*. 2008;19: 891–894.
30. Rousseau AF, Losser MR, Ichai C, Berger MM. ESPEN endorsed recommendations: nutritional therapy in major burns. *Clin Nutr*. 2013;32:497–502.
31. ISBI Practice Guidelines Committee, Steering Subcommittee, Advisory Subcommittee. ISBI practice guidelines for burn care. *Burns*. 2016;42:953–1021.
32. Taylor BE, McClave SA, Martindale RG, et al. Guidelines for the provision and assessment of nutrition support therapy in the adult critically ill patient: society of critical care medicine (SCCM) and American society for parenteral and enteral nutrition (A.S.P.E.N.). *Crit Care Med*. 2016;44:390–438.
33. McClave SA, Taylor BE, Martindale RG, et al. Guidelines for the provision and assessment of nutrition support therapy in the adult critically ill patient: society of critical care medicine (SCCM) and American society for parenteral and enteral nutrition (A.S.P.E.N.). *JPEN J Parenter Enter Nutr*. 2016;40: 159–211.
34. Turza KC, Krenitsky J, Sawyer RG. Enteral feeding and vasoactive agents: suggested guidelines for clinicians. *Pract Gastroenterol*. 2009;33, 11–12, 15–7, 21–22.
35. McClave SA, Snider HL. Use of indirect calorimetry in clinical nutrition. *Nutr Clin Pract*. 1992;7:207–221.
36. Weir JB. New methods for calculating metabolic rate with special reference to protein metabolism. *J Physiol*. 1949;109:1–9.
37. Ferrannini E. The theoretical bases of indirect calorimetry: a review. *Metabolism*. 1988;37:287–301.
38. Davis KA, Kinn T, Esposito TJ, et al. Nutritional gain versus financial gain: the role of metabolic carts in the surgical ICU. *J Trauma*. 2006;61:1436–1440.
39. Gottschlich MM, American Society for Parenteral Enteral Nutrition. *The A.S.P.E.N. Nutrition Support Core Curriculum: A Case-Based Approach - the Adult Patient*. Silver Spring, MD: American Society for Parenteral and Enteral Nutrition (A.S.P.E.N.); 2007.
40. Curreri PW. Assessing nutritional needs for the burned patient. *J Trauma*. 1990;30:S20–S23.
41. Allard JP, Pichard C, Hoshino E, et al. Validation of a new formula for calculating the energy requirements of burn patients. *JPEN J Parenter Enter Nutr*. 1990;14:115–118.
42. Royall D, Fairholm L, Peters WJ, et al. Continuous measurement of energy expenditure in ventilated burn patients: an analysis. *Crit Care Med*. 1994;22:399–406.
43. Kochevar M, Guenter P, Holcombe B, et al. ASPEN statement on parenteral nutrition standardization. *JPEN J Parenter Enter Nutr*. 2007;31:441–448.
44. Gervasio J. Compounding vs standardized commercial parenteral nutrition product: pros and cons. *JPEN J Parenter Enter Nutr*. 2012; 36:40S–41S.
45. Total Parenteral Nutrition. Drugs.com; 2019; Available at: https://www.drugs.com/cdi/total-parenteral-nutrition.html. Accessed June 3, 2019.
46. Stroud C. Institute of Medicine Forum on Medical Public Health Preparedness for Castastrophic Events. In: *Crisis Standards of Care: Summary of a Workshop Series*. Washington, D.C: National Academies Press; 2010.
47. World Health Organization, United Nations, High Commissioner for Refugees. *Food and Nutrition Needs in Emergencies*. Geneva: World Health Organization; 2004. Available at: https://apps.who.int/iris/handle/10665/68660.
48. Patterson BW, Nguyen T, Pierre E, et al. Urea and protein metabolism in burned children: effect of dietary protein intake. *Metabolism*. 1997;46:573–578.
49. Gore DC, Jahoor F. Glutamine kinetics in burn patients. Comparison with hormonally induced stress in volunteers. *Arch Surg*. 1994;129:1318–1323.
50. Souba WW. Glutamine: a key substrate for the splanchnic bed. *Annu Rev Nutr*. 1991;11:285–308.
51. Peng X, Yan H, You Z, et al. Glutamine granule-supplemented enteral nutrition maintains immunological function in severely burned patients. *Burns*. 2006;32:589–593.
52. Garrel D, Patenaude J, Nedelec B, et al. Decreased mortality and infectious morbidity in adult burn patients given enteral glutamine supplements: a prospective, controlled, randomized clinical trial. *Crit Care Med*. 2003;31:2444–2449.
53. Sheridan RL, Prelack K, Yu YM, et al. Short-term enteral glutamine does not enhance protein accretion in burned children: a stable isotope study. *Surgery*. 2004;135:671–678.
54. Heyland D, Muscedere J, Wischmeyer PE, et al. A randomized trial of glutamine and antioxidants in critically ill patients. *N Engl J Med*. 2013;368:1489–1497.
55. Heyland DK, Wischmeyer P, Jeschke MG, et al. A randomized trial of enteral glutamine to minimize thermal injury (The RE-ENERGIZE Trial): a clinical trial protocol. *Scars Burn Heal*. 2017;3.
56. Marin VB, Rodriguez-Osiac L, Schlessinger L, et al. Controlled study of enteral arginine supplementation in burned children: impact on immunologic and metabolic status. *Nutrition*. 2006;22: 705–712.
57. Wibbenmeyer LA, Mitchell MA, Newel IM, et al. Effect of a fish oil and arginine-fortified diet in thermally injured patients. *J Burn Care Res*. 2006;27:694–702.
58. Heyland DK, Samis A. Does immunonutrition in patients with sepsis do more harm than good? *Intensive Care Med*. 2003;29: 669–671.
59. Van den Berghe G, Wouters PJ, Kesteloot K, Hilleman DE. Analysis of healthcare resource utilization with intensive insulin therapy in critically ill patients. *Crit Care Med*. 2006;34:612–616.
60. Jeschke MG, Kulp GA, Kraft R, et al. Intensive insulin therapy in severely burned pediatric patients: a prospective randomized trial. *Am J Respir Crit Care Med*. 2010;182:351–359.
61. Jeschke MG, Pinto R, Herndon DN, et al. Hypoglycemia is associated with increased postburn morbidity and mortality in pediatric patients. *Crit Care Med*. 2014;42:1221–1231.
62. Sheridan RL, Yu YM, Prelack K, et al. Maximal parenteral glucose oxidation in hypermetabolic young children: a stable isotope study. *JPEN J Parenter Enter Nutr*. 1998;22:212–216.

63. Wolfe RR. Maximal parenteral glucose oxidation in hypermetabolic young children. *JPEN J Parenter Enter Nutr.* 1998;22:190.
64. Wolfe RR, Herndon DN, Peters EJ, et al. Regulation of lipolysis in severely burned children. *Ann Surg.* 1987;206:214–221.
65. Mochizuki H, Trocki O, Dominioni L, et al. Optimal lipid content for enteral diets following thermal injury. *JPEN J Parenter Enter Nutr.* 1984;8:638–646.
66. Demling RH, Seigne P. Metabolic management of patients with severe burns. *World J Surg.* 2000;24:673–680.
67. Garrel DR, Razi M, Lariviere F, et al. Improved clinical status and length of care with low-fat nutrition support in burn patients. *JPEN J Parenter Enter Nutr.* 1995;19:482–491.
68. Alexander JW, Gottschlich MM. Nutritional immunomodulation in burn patients. *Crit Care Med.* 1990;18:S149–S153.
69. Tihista S, Echavarria E. Effect of omega 3 polyunsaturated fatty acids derived from fish oil in major burn patients: a prospective randomized controlled pilot trial. *Clin Nutr.* 2018;37:107–112.
70. Rock CL, Dechert RE, Khilnani R, et al. Carotenoids and antioxidant vitamins in patients after burn injury. *J Burn Care Rehabil.* 1997;18:269–278. discussion 268.
71. Al-Jawad FH, Sahib AS, Al-Kaisy AA. Role of antioxidants in the treatment of burn lesions. *Ann Burns Fire Disasters.* 2008;21: 186–191.
72. Zhang K, Pei Y, Gan Z, et al. Local administration of thiamine ameliorates ongoing pain in a rat model of second-degree burn. *J Burn Care Res.* 2017;38:e842–e850.
73. Amrein K, Oudemans-van Straaten HM, Berger MM. Vitamin therapy in critically ill patients: focus on thiamine, vitamin C, and vitamin D. *Intensive Care Med.* 2018;44:1940–1944.
74. Kremer T, Harenberg P, Hernekamp F, et al. High-dose vitamin C treatment reduces capillary leakage after burn plasma transfer in rats. *J Burn Care Res.* 2010;31:470–479.
75. Anand T, Skinner R. Vitamin C in burns, sepsis, and trauma. *J Trauma Acute Care Surg.* 2018;85:782–787.
76. Klein GL, Chen TC, Holick MF, et al. Synthesis of vitamin D in skin after burns. *Lancet.* 2004;363:291–292.
77. Gottschlich MM, Mayes T, Khoury J, Warden GD. Hypovitaminosis D in acutely injured pediatric burn patients. *J Am Diet Assoc.* 2004;104:931–941. quiz 1031.
78. Klein GL, Rodriguez NA, Branski LK, Herndon DN. Vitamin and trace element homeostasis following severe burn injury. In: Herndon DN, ed. *Total Burn Care.* 4th ed. London: Saunders Elsevier; 2012, 321–324. e322.
79. Traber MG, Leonard SW, Traber DL, et al. alpha-Tocopherol adipose tissue stores are depleted after burn injury in pediatric patients. *Am J Clin Nutr.* 2010;92:1378–1384.
80. Butt H, Mehmood A, Ali M, et al. Protective role of vitamin E preconditioning of human dermal fibroblasts against thermal stress in vitro. *Life Sci.* 2017;184:1–9.
81. Berger MM, Shenkin A. Trace element requirements in critically ill burned patients. *J Trace Elem Med Biol.* 2007;21(Suppl 1):44–48.
82. Berger MM, Cavadini C, Bart A, et al. Cutaneous copper and zinc losses in burns. *Burns.* 1992;18:373–380.
83. Jin J, Mulesa L, Carrilero Rouillet M. Trace elements in parenteral nutrition: considerations for the prescribing clinician. *Nutrients.* 2017;9:440.
84. Shils ME, Shike M, Ross AC, et al. *Modern Nutrition in Health and Disease.* 10th ed. Lippincott Williams & Wilkins; 2015.
85. Danks DM. Copper deficiency in humans. *Annu Rev Nutr.* 1988;8: 235–257.
86. Vanek VW, Borum P, Buchman A, et al. A.S.P.E.N. position paper: recommendations for changes in commercially available parenteral multivitamin and multi-trace element products. *Nutr Clin Pract.* 2012;27:440–491.
87. Selmanpakoglu AN, Cetin C, Sayal A, Isimer A. Trace element (Al, Se, Zn, Cu) levels in serum, urine and tissues of burn patients. *Burns.* 1994;20:99–103.
88. Jeejeebhoy K. Zinc: an essential trace element for parenteral nutrition. *Gastroenterology.* 2009;137:S7–S12.
89. Fessler TA. Trace elements in parenteral nutrition: a practical guide for dosage and monitoring for adult patients. *Nutr Clin Pract.* 2013;28:722–729.
90. Boosalis MG. The role of selenium in chronic disease. *Nutr Clin Pract.* 2008;23:152–160.
91. Shenkin A. Selenium in intravenous nutrition. *Gastroenterology.* 2009;137:S61–S69.
92. Dylewski ML, Bender JC, Smith AM, et al. The selenium status of pediatric patients with burn injuries. *J Trauma.* 2010;69:584–588. discussion 588.
93. Hardy G, Hardy I, Manzanares W. Selenium supplementation in the critically ill. *Nutr Clin Pract.* 2012;27:21–33.
94. Plogsted S, Adams SC, Allen K, et al. Parenteral nutrition trace element product shortage considerations. *Nutr Clin Pract.* 2016; 31:843–847.
95. Moukarzel A. Chromium in parenteral nutrition: too little or too much? *Gastroenterology.* 2009;137:S18–S28.
96. Santos D, Batoreu C, Mateus L, et al. Manganese in human parenteral nutrition: considerations for toxicity and biomonitoring. *Neurotoxicology.* 2014;43:36–45.
97. Dickerson RN. Manganese intoxication and parenteral nutrition. *Nutrition.* 2001;17:689–693.
98. Gibson S, Ashwell M. The association between red and processed meat consumption and iron intakes and status among British adults. *Public Health Nutr.* 2003;6:341–350.
99. A.S.P.E.N. Clinical Practice Committee Shortage Subcomittee. A.S.P.E.N. parenteral nutrition trace element product shortage considerations. *Nutr Clin Pract.* 2014;29:249–251.
100. Saffle JR, Gibran N, Jordan M. Defining the ratio of outcomes to resources for triage of burn patients in mass casualties. *J Burn Care Rehabil.* 2005;26:478–482.
101. Herndon DN. *Total Burn Care.* 4th ed. London: Saunders Elsevier; 2012.
102. Young AW, Graves C, Kowalske KJ, et al. Guideline for burn care under austere conditions: special care topics. *J Burn Care Res.* 2017; 38:e497–e509.
103. Magnotti LJ, Deitch EA. Burns, bacterial translocation, gut barrier function, and failure. *J Burn Care Rehabil.* 2005;26:383–391.
104. Andel D, Kamolz LP, Donner A, et al. Impact of intraoperative duodenal feeding on the oxygen balance of the splanchnic region in severely burned patients. *Burns.* 2005;31:302–305.
105. Abunnaja S, Cuviello A, Sanchez JA. Enteral and parenteral nutrition in the perioperative period: state of the art. *Nutrients.* 2013;5: 608–623.
106. Mochizuki H, Trocki O, Dominioni L, et al. Mechanism of prevention of postburn hypermetabolism and catabolism by early enteral feeding. *Ann Surg.* 1984;200:297–310.
107. Lam NN, Tien NG, Khoa CM. Early enteral feeding for burned patients–an effective method which should be encouraged in developing countries. *Burns.* 2008;34:192–196.
108. Venter M, Rode H, Sive A, Visser M. Enteral resuscitation and early enteral feeding in children with major burns–effect on McFarlane response to stress. *Burns.* 2007;33:464–471.
109. Khorasani EN, Mansouri F. Effect of early enteral nutrition on morbidity and mortality in children with burns. *Burns.* 2010;36: 1067–1071.
110. Harvey SE, Parrott F, Harrison DA, et al. Trial of the route of early nutritional support in critically ill adults. *N Engl J Med.* 2014;371: 1673–1684.

111. Peck MD, Kessler M, Cairns BA, et al. Early enteral nutrition does not decrease hypermetabolism associated with burn injury. *J Trauma*. 2004;57:1143–1148. discussion 1148–1149.
112. Reintam Blaser A, Starkopf J, Alhazzani W, et al. Early enteral nutrition in critically ill patients: ESICM clinical practice guidelines. *Intensive Care Med*. 2017;43:380–398.
113. Minard G. Enteral access. *Nutr Clin Pract*. 1994;9:172–182.
114. Baskin WN. Acute complications associated with bedside placement of feeding tubes. *Nutr Clin Pract*. 2006;21:40–55.
115. Kreis BE, Middelkoop E, Vloemans AF, Kreis RW. The use of a PEG tube in a burn centre. *Burns*. 2002;28:191–197.
116. Metheny NA, Meert KL, Clouse RE. Complications related to feeding tube placement. *Curr Opin Gastroenterol*. 2007;23:178–182.
117. Boullata JI, Carrera AL, Harvey L, et al. ASPEN safe practices for enteral nutrition therapy [formula: see text]. *JPEN J Parenter Enter Nutr*. 2017;41:15–103.
118. MacLeod JB, Lefton J, Houghton D, et al. Prospective randomized control trial of intermittent versus continuous gastric feeds for critically ill trauma patients. *J Trauma*. 2007;63:57–61.
119. van Nieuwenhoven CA, Vandenbroucke-Grauls C, van Tiel FH, et al. Feasibility and effects of the semirecumbent position to prevent ventilator-associated pneumonia: a randomized study. *Crit Care Med*. 2006;34:396–402.
120. Nguyen NQ, Chapman M, Fraser RJ, et al. Prokinetic therapy for feed intolerance in critical illness: one drug or two? *Crit Care Med*. 2007;35:2561–2567.
121. Ireton-Jones CS, Baxter CR. Nutrition for adult burn patients: a review. *Nutr Clin Pract*. 1991;6:3–7.
122. Casaer MP, Mesotten D, Hermans G, et al. Early versus late parenteral nutrition in critically ill adults. *N Engl J Med*. 2011;365: 506–517.
123. Yarandi SS, Zhao VM, Hebbar G, Ziegler TR. Amino acid composition in parenteral nutrition: what is the evidence? *Curr Opin Clin Nutr Metab Care*. 2011;14:75–82.
124. Mirtallo J, Canada T, Johnson D, et al. Safe practices for parenteral nutrition. *JPEN J Parenter Enter Nutr*. 2004;28:S39–S70.
125. McClave SA, Martindale RG, Vanek VW, et al. Guidelines for the provision and assessment of nutrition support therapy in the adult critically ill patient: society of critical care medicine (SCCM) and American society for parenteral and enteral nutrition (A.S.P.E.N.). *JPEN J Parenter Enter Nutr*. 2009;33:277–316.
126. Singer P, Berger MM, Van den Berghe G, et al. ESPEN guidelines on parenteral nutrition: intensive care. *Clin Nutr*. 2009;28:387–400.
127. Ziegler TR. Parenteral nutrition in the critically ill patient. *N Engl J Med*. 2009;361:1088–1097.
128. Fong YM, Marano MA, Barber A, et al. Total parenteral nutrition and bowel rest modify the metabolic response to endotoxin in humans. *Ann Surg*. 1989;210:449–456. discussion 456–457.
129. Barret JP, Jeschke MG, Herndon DN. Fatty infiltration of the liver in severely burned pediatric patients: autopsy findings and clinical implications. *J Trauma*. 2001;51:736–739.
130. Herndon DN, Stein MD, Rutan TC, et al. Failure of TPN supplementation to improve liver function, immunity, and mortality in thermally injured patients. *J Trauma*. 1987;27:195–204.
131. Kondrup J, Allison SP, Elia M, et al. ESPEN guidelines for nutrition screening 2002. *Clin Nutr*. 2003;22:415–421.
132. Graves C, Saffle J, Cochran A. Actual burn nutrition care practices: an update. *J Burn Care Res*. 2009;30:77–82.
133. Graves C, Saffle J, Morris S. Comparison of urine urea nitrogen collection times in critically ill patients. *Nutr Clin Pract*. 2005;20: 271–275.
134. Konstantinides FN, Radmer WJ, Becker WK, et al. Inaccuracy of nitrogen balance determinations in thermal injury with calculated total urinary nitrogen. *J Burn Care Rehabil*. 1992;13:254–260.
135. Rettmer RL, Williamson JC, Labbe RF, Heimbach DM. Laboratory monitoring of nutritional status in burn patients. *Clin Chem*. 1992; 38:334–337.
136. Cynober L, Prugnaud O, Lioret N, et al. Serum transthyretin levels in patients with burn injury. *Surgery*. 1991;109:640–644.
137. van den Berghe G, Wouters P, Weekers F, et al. Intensive insulin therapy in critically ill patients. *N Engl J Med*. 2001;345: 1359–1367.
138. Jeschke MG, Finnerty CC, Suman OE, et al. The effect of oxandrolone on the endocrinologic, inflammatory, and hypermetabolic responses during the acute phase postburn. *Ann Surg*. 2007;246: 351–360. discussion 360–362.
139. Porro LJ, Herndon DN, Rodriguez NA, et al. Five-year outcomes after oxandrolone administration in severely burned children: a randomized clinical trial of safety and efficacy. *J Am Coll Surg*. 2012;214:489–502. discussion 502–504.
140. Herndon DN, Rodriguez NA, Diaz EC, et al. Long-term propranolol use in severely burned pediatric patients: a randomized controlled study. *Ann Surg*. 2012;256:402–411.
141. Flores O, Stockton K, Roberts JA, et al. The efficacy and safety of adrenergic blockade after burn injury: a systematic review and meta-analysis. *J Trauma Acute Care Surg*. 2016;80:146–155.
142. Gibran NS, Wiechman S, Meyer W, et al. Summary of the 2012 ABA burn quality consensus conference. *J Burn Care Res*. 2013; 34:361–385.
143. Pierre EJ, Barrow RE, Hawkins HK, et al. Effects of insulin on wound healing. *J Trauma*. 1998;44:342–345.
144. Thomas SJ, Morimoto K, Herndon DN, et al. The effect of prolonged euglycemic hyperinsulinemia on lean body mass after severe burn. *Surgery*. 2002;132:341–347.
145. Hemmila MR, Taddonio MA, Arbabi S, et al. Intensive insulin therapy is associated with reduced infectious complications in burn patients. *Surgery*. 2008;144:629–635. discussion 635–637.
146. Gore DC, Wolf SE, Sanford A, et al. Influence of metformin on glucose intolerance and muscle catabolism following severe burn injury. *Ann Surg*. 2005;241:334–342.
147. Jeschke MG, Abdullahi A, Burnett M, et al. Glucose control in severely burned patients using metformin: an interim safety and efficacy analysis of a phase II randomized Controlled trial. *Ann Surg*. 2016;264:518–527.
148. Branski LK, Herndon DN, Barrow RE, et al. Randomized controlled trial to determine the efficacy of long-term growth hormone treatment in severely burned children. *Ann Surg*. 2009;250: 514–523.
149. Takala J, Ruokonen E, Webster NR, et al. Increased mortality associated with growth hormone treatment in critically ill adults. *N Engl J Med*. 1999;341:785–792.
150. Elijah IE, Branski LK, Finnerty CC, Herndon DN. The GH/IGF-1 system in critical illness. *Best Pract Res Clin Endocrinol Metab*. 2011; 25:759–767.
151. El-Ghazely MH, Mahmoud WH, Atia MA, Eldip EM. Effect of probiotic administration in the therapy of pediatric thermal burn. *Ann Burns Fire Disasters*. 2016;29:268–272.
152. Mayes T, Gottschlich MM, James LE, et al. Clinical safety and efficacy of probiotic administration following burn injury. *J Burn Care Res*. 2015;36:92–99.
153. Haberal M, Sakallioglu Abali AE, Karakayali H. Fluid management in major burn injuries. *Indian J Plast Surg*. 2010;43:S29–S36.
154. Pham TN, Cancio LC, Gibran NS. American Burn Association practice guidelines burn shock resuscitation. *J Burn Care Res*. 2008;29:257–266.
155. Dickerson RN, Gervasio JM, Riley ML, et al. Accuracy of predictive methods to estimate resting energy expenditure of thermally-injured patients. *JPEN J Parenter Enter Nutr*. 2002;26:17–29.

156. Cave MC, Hurt RT, Frazier TH, et al. Obesity, inflammation, and the potential application of pharmaconutrition. *Nutr Clin Pract.* 2008;23:16–34.
157. McClave SA, Frazier TH, Hurt RT, et al. Obesity, inflammation, and pharmaconutrition in critical illness. *Nutrition.* 2014;30: 492–494.
158. Renz EM, Cancio LC, Barillo DJ, et al. Long range transport of war-related burn casualties. *J Trauma.* 2008;64:S136–S144. discussion S144–145.
159. Ennis JL, Chung KK, Renz EM, et al. Joint theater trauma system implementation of burn resuscitation guidelines improves outcomes in severely burned military casualties. *J Trauma.* 2008;64: S146–S151. discussion S151–152.
160. Caldwell NW, Serio-Melvin ML, Chung KK, et al. Follow-up evaluation of the U.S. Army Institute of Surgical Research Burn flow sheet for en route care documentation of burned combat casualties. *Mil Med.* 2017;182:e2021–e2026.
161. Shields BA, Doty KA, Chung KK, et al. Determination of resting energy expenditure after severe burn. *J Burn Care Res.* 2013;34: e22–28.
162. White CE, Renz EM. Advances in surgical care: management of severe burn injury. *Crit Care Med.* 2008;36:S318–S324.
163. Wolf SE, Kauvar DS, Wade CE, et al. Comparison between civilian burns and combat burns from operation Iraqi freedom and operation enduring freedom. *Ann Surg.* 2006;243:786–792. discussion 792–795.

Index

'*Note*: Page numbers followed by "f" indicate figures, "t" indicates tables and "b" indicates boxes.'

D

N

R

S

Contents of Volume 1

Section D

Other Dietary Components

Section E

Cross Discipline Topics